MW01042476

Geometric, Physical, and Visual Optics

GEOMETRIC, PHYSICAL, AND VISUAL OPTICS

Second Edition

Michael P. Keating, Ph.D.

Professor, Michigan College of Optometry,
Ferris State University,
Big Rapids, Michigan

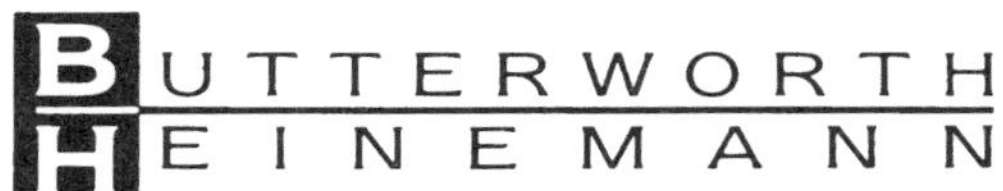

BOSTON OXFORD AUCKLAND JOHANNESBURG MELBOURNE NEW DELHI

A member of the Reed Elsevier group

Every effort has been made to ensure that the drug dosage schedules within this text are accurate and conform to standards accepted at time of publication. However, as treatment recommendations vary in the light of continuing research and clinical experience, the reader is advised to verify drug dosage schedules herein with information found on product information sheets. This is especially true in cases of new or infrequently used drugs.

Recognizing the importance of preserving what has been written, Butterworth-Heinemann prints its books on acid-free paper whenever possible.

Library of Congress Cataloging-in-Publication Data

Keating, Michael P.
Geometric, physical, and visual optics
1. Optics 2. Optometry
I. Title
617.7′5
ISBN: 0-7506-7262-5

British Library Cataloguing-in-Publication Data

The publisher offers special discounts on bulk orders of this book.
For information, please contact:

Manager of Special Sales
Butterworth-Heinemann
225 Wildwood Avenue
Woburn, MA 01801-2041
Tel: 781-904-2500
Fax: 781-904-2620

For information on all Butterworth-Heinemann publications available, contact our World Wide Web home page at: http://www.bh.com

10 9 8 7 6 5 4 3 2 1

Printed in the United States of America

For all who have been supportive—especially family, friends, colleagues, teachers, and my wife Mary Jean.

Contents

Preface to the Second Edition

While the basic philosophy of the first edition is retained in the second edition, there are two significant modifications. One is a change in the order of the chapters. The chapters on introductory astigmatism, prisms, and prism in lenses (which were Chapters 15, 17, and 18 in the first edition) are now Chapters 10, 11, and 12. This brings the core of the basic optics material for optometry students together in the first 12 chapters of the book.

The second significant modification follows a review of each chapter for the purpose of either updating the information, adding pertinent material, and/or improving (i.e., rewriting or condensing) the material. The review has resulted in minor changes in virtually all chapters, and extensive changes in four chapters (13, 16, 19, and 20). The review also resulted in over 70 figure revisions from the first edition to the second edition.

The first 9 chapters contain minor changes that are designed to improve the pedagogical value of the chapters. In addition Chapter 9 contains a new section on axial magnification. Chapter 10 (Astigmatism: On Axis) is not only moved forward (from Chapter 15) but has certain sections that have been rewritten, including a more coherent presentation on the Jackson Cross Cylinder Test for cylinder power refinement. The chapter on prisms in lenses (old Chapter 18) has been split into two parts. The first part of the chapter (with minor revisions) is now Chapter 12. Chapter 12 also contains an added section on retinoscopy reflex motion. The second part of the original Chapter 18 (which deals with the off-axis meridians of spherocylindrical lenses) is now part of Chapter 13.

On the whole, this book is not a matrix optics book. However matrices are used extensively in two chapters—13 and 16. Matrices are a simple, yet powerful tool in dealing both conceptually and quantitatively with optical systems (including the human eye) and in dealing with the off-axis aspects of astigmatism. The use of matrices has lead to significant increases in our knowledge of astigmatism and the statistics of refractive errors particularly over the last 10 years. Furthermore there are now inexpensive hand-held calculators that automatically perform matrix calculations (as well as personal computer software that does the same). So one just enters the numbers, presses the "calculate" button, and "presto" the answer appears.

Chapter 13 uses the dioptric power matrix, which is the most fundamental way of representing astigmatism in all contexts. Parts of Chapter 13 are rewritten from the old Chapters 16 and 18, while other parts are new. Chapter 16 (old 12) discusses system matrices. My experience over 20 years is that my optometry students consider this material easier than many other aspects of optics, and in particular easier than the principal plane system for understanding composite optical systems including the corrected or uncorrected human eye. The system matrix approach also has the advantage that it is easily extended to spherocylindrical (astigmatic) systems.

Chapters 14, 15, 17, and 18 all contain minor modifications. Also a section was added to Chapter 18 to connect prism effectivity and dynamic spectacle magnification considerations. Chapter 19 (Stops and Related Effects) was extensively rewritten. Sections of Chapter 20 on aberrations were rewritten (particularly the section on the optical origins of coma), and a section was added on oblique central refraction in spherocylindrical lenses with oblique principal meridians.

The physical optics Chapters 21 through 25 all have minor changes. In addition: Chapter 22 contains an added section on apodized apertures, an updated discussion of zone plates, a new discussion of diffractive lenses, and a proof of Snell's law. Chapter 23 contains an expanded introductory discussion on multiple incoherent scattering. Chapter 24 contains an added discussion of the Doppler shift, and an added discussion on the similarities and differences between the propagation of a Gaussian laser beam versus the propagation of waves from a point source. A new appendix reviewing basic trigonometry has been added. As in the first edition, there is also an appendix on basic matrix algebra.

There are certain sections of the text that I skip in the courses that I teach. In my proposal for the section edition, I had suggested eliminating those sections. However the anonymous content expert reviewers of the proposal liked those sections and wanted them left in the text. So they are still there. In a few cases, the reviewers suggested eliminating sections that I consider important, so those sections are also still there.

I believe that for many optometry students, there are concepts in optics that need "percolation" time before understanding occurs. This percolation time is built into the book in that certain concepts are introduced in one chapter, and then returned to in a later chapter.

I have received very positive compliments on the first edition from many students that have used it as a required text. I have also received (unsolicited) some very positive compliments on the first edition from optometrists who originally learned optics from other texts, and then for a variety of reasons needed to improve their optics knowledge in certain areas. In particular, most in this latter group have expressed that they wished this text had been the required text for their original optics courses. It is certainly the goal of the second edition to be equally as successful.

I need to thank all the people at the Michigan College of Optometry at Ferris State University for their support and encouragement. In addition, I need to thank my colleague and co-teacher Dr. Vince King for his feedback and advice. I also need to specially thank Michigan College of Optometry students Erin Miller and Jackie Scarbrough, who did considerable work on proofing and critiquing the first drafts of the second edition. My thanks also to Michigan College of Optometry students Darren Smarch and Kyle Schaub who proofread the later drafts, and to Karen Blanzy and Jacquie Beiser of the Ferris Media Production Department for their work on the figures that are new to the second edition. Finally, I wish to thank Mary Jean Keating, my wife and friend of 30 plus years, for her support and understanding during the extra hours that it took to produce both the first and the second editions of this book.

Preface to the First Edition

This basic textbook, written primarily for optometry students, contains an integrated approach to geometric, physical, and introductory visual optics. This book is nontraditional in the integration, sequencing, and conceptual development of the material. The nontraditional aspects include an early emphasis on image formation, the use of the vergence-dioptric power approach from the beginning, the relation of vergence to the geometric properties of wavefronts, and the interchangeability of the wavefront representation with the ray presentation. This approach has worked extremely well for me and for my students over a 15-year period. In particular, the integration of visual optics makes the optometry students feel that basic optics is highly relevant to their profession. I wrote the book so that others can share in the benefits.

The mathematical level of the book assumes a knowledge of algebra and trigonometry. While some introductory knowledge of calculus is helpful, it is not necessary for the level of this text. Since the advent of calculators and microcomputers, basic matrix algebra is being increasingly incorporated into high school and undergraduate algebra courses. After paraxial image formation by spherical systems is covered (Chapters 1 through 11), I do take advantage of matrices in some chapters (particularly 12, 16, and a little of 18). Appendix A covers the needed matrix algebra.

For optometry students, the sections on astigmatism are a very important part of this book. Chapter 15 gives an integrated treatment of the on-axis aspects, while Chapter 16 treats the more difficult off-axis aspects.

There is an emphasis in the book on developing intuition and conceptual understanding, so that the numbers means something to the reader. Chapters 2 through 4 emphasize concepts that are sometimes lost in the rush to get to the equations and calculations of Chapter 5 and beyond. I have included many worked examples, but I strongly encourage students to first work out their own solutions before checking mine. Due to the needs of optometry students, the physical optics chapters are more qualitative than the geometric optics chapters.

There are optical effects everywhere we look, and I have tried to incorporate them into this book so that the world becomes optically alive to the reader. This is, perhaps surprisingly, true of physical optics as well as geometric optics. Visual optics in particular is illustrated by the many characters that appear in the book.

In many cases, subsequent chapters in the book build on previous chapters. For example, Chapter 7 is a long chapter, but in fact most of the concepts have already been developed in previous chapters, and Chapter 7 goes fairly easily despite its length. Chapter 3 is very short, but the concepts are fundamental and often not dealt with very extensively in optics texts.

There is no doubt that parts of optics are conceptually difficult because many of the concepts require formal operational reasoning (as opposed to concrete operational). This is part of the fun and challenge of teaching it well.

While this book was written primarily for optometry students, I believe that it offers benefits for other students interested in the vergence approach to optics and vision. This might include physics undergraduates students as well as perceptual psychology students.

Geometric, Physical, and Visual Optics

CHAPTER 1

Optics, Light, and Vision

1.1 THE SEARCH FOR SOLUTIONS

"That's one small step for man. One giant leap for mankind." So stated Neil Armstrong, Jr., as he stepped down onto the moon's surface. The problem was how to send men to the moon and bring them back alive. The solution required commitment and financial resources, as well as scientific and technical knowledge.

How was the knowledge acquired? How do we proceed in developing new knowledge and solving new scientific problems? In *The Search for Solutions*, Horace Judson lists nine problem-solving techniques of the scientific method: investigation, evidence, trial and error, patterns, context, modeling, prediction, adaptation, and theory. Judson's capsulized summaries of these techniques are:

- *Investigation* Each of us discovers our world by investigation—tasting, watching, smelling, listening—so that eventually we turn bits and pieces of experience into generalizations and categories.
- *Evidence* We need information to solve problems. For the scientist, gathering evidence is just the first step. Each clue must then be tested and retested, verified and interpreted.
- *Trial and error* Trial and error is as basic as learning itself, and errors are essential to the process. Problem solvers must organize and direct a plan of attack, order priorities, determine the essential elements to combine, and then decide how a desired result is to be obtained.
- *Patterns* Science is the search for patterns, and patterns are not just pictures but predictions. Thus, the ability to discern patterns, to organize and reorganize the fruits of vision and evidence, is indispensable.
- *Context* To see an object within its framework means to see it in context. All problem solving requires trained powers of observation, an attitude of mind ready for the unexpected, and an eagerness to examine every clue that chance presents.
- *Modeling* Problem solving requires that models be used at every stage from definition to solution. As simple representations of complex forms, processes, and functions, they reduce risk, cost, and complexity to manageable size.
- *Prediction* Some of our oldest endeavors are to learn to avoid the destructive aspects of the environment, to capitalize on the positive factors, and to plan ahead. Prediction is the search for laws on which to base such forecasts.
- *Adaptation* Frequently, problems change as they are being solved. As a consequence, solutions have to adapt to complex new realities. Feedback is the systematic adaptive response to situations in which the problem and solution are in constant changing relationship.
- *Theory* The universal human need to tell stories and explain events forms the foundation of theory making. Theories enable both the scientist and the layperson to see significance in seemingly random events and objects.

These techniques are just as essential to optics as they are to the space program. The optics that this book addresses are a simplified model of the complex optical world. As stated by Judson, "the modeling step reduces complexity to a manageable size."

There have been many scientific advances that, like the lunar landing, were the result of the well-established developmental plan; however, the most revolutionary advances frequently occur unexpectedly. In those particular cases, the people involved in looking for the general patterns and context discover fundamental and important scientific phenomena for which they were not specifically looking. Patterns, context, adaptation, and prediction are all important in this process. This book is based on experimental investigations, evidence, and trial and errors of many people. Hopefully, the reader will also have the opportunity to recreate and experience firsthand some of these experimental investigations.

1.2 THE SCOPE OF OPTICS AND ITS SUBFIELDS

The main body of optics deals with light and its behavior. As such, optics is a branch of physics. The impact of optics on modern humans is enormous. Microscopes opened the ultrasmall world of bacteria, histology, and biological cells. Telescopes opened the ultralarge world of planets, stars, and galaxies, and enabled humans to study distant terrestrial objects, including enemy armies and wild animals. Cameras opened an incredible world of information capture and provided an aesthetic medium that produces beautiful results in the hands of an artistic photographer. Interferometers contribute to the ultraprecision world of modern manufacturing. Spectacle and contact lenses enable many of us to overcome the visual handicap of optical defects in our eyes.

As time passed, the borders of optics pushed out to include nonvisible parts of the electromagnetic spectrum, especially the infrared and ultraviolet regions. Optics combined with electronics to produce television, photocopiers, and night-vision scopes. Lasers, fiber optics, thin films, spatial filtering, computerized image analysis and enhancement, and robot vision are areas of current activity and development.

Theories involving the nature of light, its speed, and its interaction with matter have another impressive legacy. These theories were intimately involved with two of the greatest conceptual revolutions of modern man: Einstein's special theory of relativity and the quantum theory of matter. Relativity is a fascinating topic, but it lies outside the scope of this book. Some aspects of quantum theory are presented in later chapters.

Historically, optics has been divided into two subareas: geometric optics and physical optics. Geometric optics deals with the image-forming properties of lenses, mirrors, and prisms, and as such, is very important to visual optics. Physical optics deals with the physical character and behavior of light and its interaction with matter. Physical optics can be further subdivided into such areas as wave optics, quantum optics, and Fourier optics.

1.3 AN OVERVIEW OF THE HUMAN VISUAL PROCESS

Modern man is well aware of the optical images formed by slide and motion picture projectors as well as with camera television images. In developed countries, even elementary school children are aware that the human eye forms an optical image on the retina. Typically, modern man is less aware that his perceived image can differ significantly from his retinal image. This difference is due to the physiology and perceptual psychology of the human visual system. The study of vision is formally called physiological optics. It is interdisciplinary in that it includes the physiology and perceptual psychology of the visual system as well as visual optics.

Figure 1.1 shows a flow chart of the human visual process. The process begins with a primary light source that serves as the initial generator of the light. Some examples are the sun, fire, tungsten filament light bulbs, fluorescent lights, light emitting diodes (LEDs), and lasers. The light from the primary source illuminates an object. On a molecular scale, the object absorbs the incident light and then reradiates some of it. The reradiated light diverges away from the object and is incident on the eye. The object that absorbs and reradiates is called a secondary source of light. Some examples include sailboats illuminated by sunlight, actors and actresses illuminated by floodlights, a raccoon illuminated by a flashlight, as well as most of the other objects that we see. The cornea and the crystalline lens of each eye converge the incident light to form a small inverted image of the object on

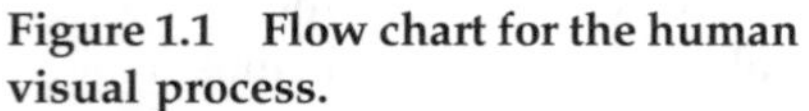
Figure 1.1 Flow chart for the human visual process.

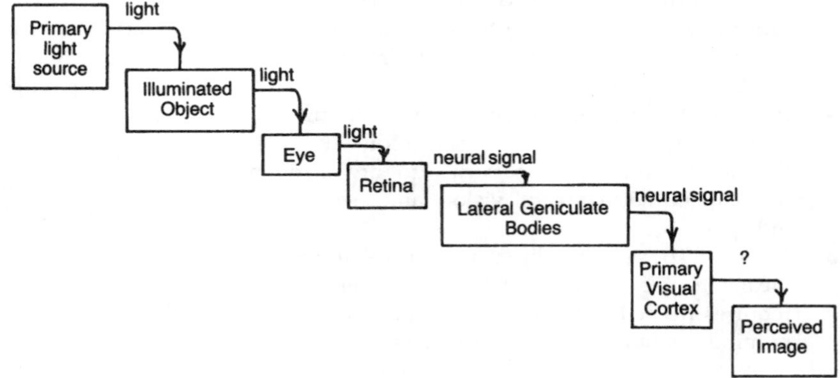

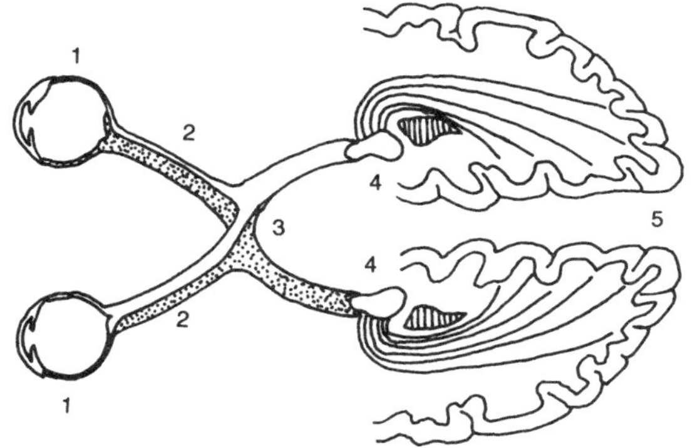

Figure 1.2 Schematic representation of the human visual system (top view).

the retina of each eye. Light is the carrier of information from the secondary source to the retina of the eye.

The retina is composed of ten layers. The rod and cone layer absorbs light, and the energy gained is used to generate neural signals. The neural signals are processed in some of the intermediate layers of the retina so that the signals leaving the retina as a whole are different from the signals that left the layer of rods and cones. The neural signals then proceed via the optic nerve fibers to the lateral geniculate bodies of the thalamus. There the fibers synapse, and the signals are processed further and sent to the primary visual cortex, which is adjacent to the back of the skull. The primary visual cortex has a mass of interconnections to and from other parts of the brain, and the resulting electrophysiological activity somehow results in the visually perceived image. The whole neural process is amazing in that the neural signals that travel the visual pathway are basically the same types of signals that travel the other neural pathways, such as the auditory pathway; yet, one results in a perceived image and the other results in perceived sound.

Figure 1.2 shows a schematic representation of the human visual system as viewed from above. The components represented are the two eyes with their respective optic nerves, the optic chiasm, the lateral geniculate bodies, and the primary visual cortex.

Humans can function quite well monocularly. However, in general, binocular visual performance is better than monocular visual performance. In particular, binocular depth perception is better than monocular depth perception.

1.4 PERCEPTUAL ASPECTS OF THE VISUAL PROCESS

Normal individuals perceive one three-dimensional image. The distal stimulus for this image is the illuminated world. The proximal stimuli are the two-dimensional retinal images of the right and left eyes. Our normal visual experience is coordinated with our motor experience. Not only do we see the coffee cup on the left side of the desk top, we can also reach out and pick it up. This coordination typically leads to a *seeing is believing* philosophy.

On the other hand, vision has many illusionary aspects to it. Two examples are given to illustrate some of the illusionary aspects of vision. The first example is a binocular example in that it depends on information from both eyes. The second example occurs when viewing with only one eye, so it is a monocular example.

The first example is the hole-in-the-hand illusion. People with normal binocular vision may perceive this illusion as follows. Take a sheet of paper and roll it into a small tube. Hold the tube close to your right eye and look through it at a distant object. Place your left hand, palm inward, against the left outer edge of the tube at a point near the far end of the tube. Your left eye is looking at the palm of your hand while your right eye is looking through the tube at the distant object. The perceived three-dimensional image is that of looking through a hole in your hand at the distant object. Here the visual system has taken two separate retinal images and processed them into one three-dimensional perceived image.

The second example is the moon illusion. Unlike the first example, the moon illusion can be observed monocularly as well as binocularly. When a full moon first rises above the horizon, it is frequently perceived as being much larger than when it is higher in the sky. This illusion occurs despite the fact that the retinal image size of the moon is the same regardless of its elevation in the sky. The difference in the perceived size is due to the difference in the visual information or cues between the two different situations. The horizon apparently provides the visual cues that fool the perceptual system.

These illusions, as well as many others, are discussed in a number of perceptual psychology books. This book discusses visual optics and characteristics of the retinal image. You should keep in mind that the retinal images are the stimuli for the perceived image and not the perceived image itself.

1.5 THE EYE

Insofar as image formation is concerned, the human eye can be compared to a camera. A camera has a dark interior chamber so that the desired image is not washed out by stray light. A camera also has a variable

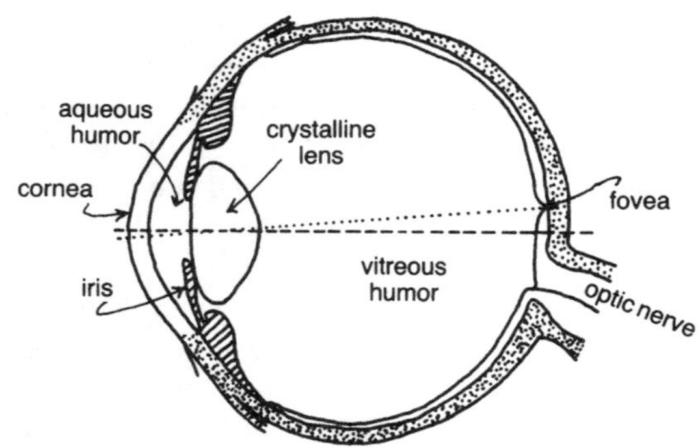

Figure 1.3 Simplified diagram of the human eye.

aperture to let in more or less light and an adjustable focus in order to image objects at different distances. The human eye has each of these three features.

Figure 1.3 is a simplified diagram of the eye. The cornea is the curved transparent front surface of the eye and is the major converging element of the eye. The tear film on the front of the cornea fills in the irregularities in the corneal surface and is thus important to the optical quality of the cornea.

A chamber filled with a transparent watery liquid called the aqueous humor follows the cornea. Near the rear of the aqueous humor chamber is the iris. The iris is opaque but has an opening at its center called the pupil. The iris contains involuntary muscles, which enable it to constrict or dilate, thus changing the size of the pupil.

Behind the iris and the aqueous humor lies the crystalline lens. The crystalline lens is a transparent high-protein material that is surrounded by fibers connecting it to the ciliary muscle. Contraction of the ciliary muscle results in changes in the focusing power of the eye. This process, referred to as accommodation, enables the eye to view near objects as well as distant objects. As the crystalline lens ages, it becomes less flexible, and consequently a person's ability to accommodate is slowly lost with time.

The crystalline lens is followed by a dark chamber, which is filled with a transparent gelatinous substance called the vitreous humor. The retina is the rear boundary of this chamber.

The rods and cones in the retina absorb some of the incident light and convert the energy into a neural signal. The rods and cones are not distributed uniformly. The region of the retina most sensitive to detail is the foveal area, which has many closely packed cones and only a few rods. Away from the fovea, the cones become progressively less dense and the number of rods increases. The peripheral region of the retina, dominated by the rods, is best at light and motion detection, while the foveal area, dominated by cones, is best at form detection, color detection, and resolution of fine detail. There are no rods or cones at the place where the optic nerve leaves the retina, so this area is blind.

1.6 ELECTROMAGNETIC RADIATION

Visible light is electromagnetic radiation that the retinal rods and cones are capable of absorbing, with the subsequent generation of a neural signal in the visual pathways. Visible light constitutes only a small part of the electromagnetic spectrum. From long to short wavelengths, the electromagnetic spectrum includes radio waves, television waves, radar waves, microwaves, infrared radiation, visible light, ultraviolet radiation, X-rays, and gamma rays.

The emitters and absorbers of electromagnetic radiation are the electrically charged particles of matter. The outer atomic electrons are the usual emitters and absorbers of visible light. The atomic and molecular structure of a material determines the intrinsic absorption properties of the electrons in the material.

All components of the electromagnetic spectrum propagate through a vacuum with a speed c of about 3×10^8 m/s (the actual value is 299,792,458 m/s). The speed of electromagnetic radiation in a vacuum is one of the fundamental constants of the world. The speed c is independent of both the speed of the source of the radiation and the speed of the detector of the radiation. These are two of the experimental foundations of the special theory of relativity.

The propagation of electromagnetic radiation through space can be described by wave equations. The vacuum wavelengths of electromagnetic radiation range from 10^{-13} m to 10^5 m. The interaction of electromagnetic radiation with matter is wavelength-dependent. Consequently, wavelengths are one of the ways used to classify the components of the spectrum. The vacuum wavelengths for visible light range from about 400–700 nm (one nanometer (nm) equals 10^{-9} m).

The ability of waves to propagate around corners is referred to as diffraction. (We are familiar with the diffraction of sound waves.) The ability of a wave to bend around a corner depends on its wavelength. The longer the wavelength, the more the wave bends. The shorter the wavelength, the less it bends. Thus, the diffraction of electromagnetic radiation is more apparent for the longer wavelength components of the spectrum. This is evident in the names of the longer wavelength components (radio waves, television waves, microwaves) versus the shorter wavelength components (X-rays, gamma rays).

The 400–700 nm wavelengths of visible light are relatively small; hence, diffraction of light is often negligible. In these situations we talk of straight line or rectilinear propagation of the light. Nevertheless, particularly when light propagates through a small opening, such as the spaces in a bird's feather, diffraction can become a dominant effect. For a small pupil size, diffraction introduces some blur into the retinal image of the human eye. Diffraction is discussed in later chapters of this book together with other wave effects, such as interference and polarization.

The quantum theory of matter attributes wave propagation properties to all particles including electrons, protons, and neutrons. The quantum theory also states that electromagnetic radiation is composed of zero rest mass particles called photons. Typical light levels consist of stupendous numbers of photons. A 60-watt light bulb puts out about 10^{19} photons/s. Millions of photons can be added to or removed from the 10^{19} level without any visible effect. Therefore, we are not aware of the particle nature of light. The wave nature of light is simply a manifestation of the wave propagation properties of the individual photons.

1.7 WAVELENGTHS AND COLOR

Human vision is wonderful in that we not only see objects, but we see them in color. Color vision depends on the fact that there are three different types of cones in the retina, each type of which absorbs maximally at a different wavelength of incident light. Each of the three sets of cones then generates neural signals that are then processed and ultimately produce the perceptual color response.

The optical stimulus for color is the wavelength distribution of the incident light. Light that has an equal mixture of all visible wavelengths is the stimulus for a white, gray, or black response depending on the amount of light coming from the object and its background. Light that consists of a single wavelength is the stimulus for a pure color response. Light of a single wavelength is thus called monochromatic light. The color response for monochromatic light ranging from long to short wavelengths is: red, orange, yellow, green, blue (indigo), violet. Indigo is actually a deep blue and not considered a separate color. (The name ROY G BIV, is often used to remember the wavelength ordering of the spectrum.) Table 1.1 gives the color responses as a function of incident vacuum wavelengths. Note that in the electromagnetic spectrum, infrared is next to visible red, and ultraviolet is next to visible violet. You should keep in mind that as the wavelength is changed, one color smoothly blends into another color. Hence, 590 nm light looks orangish-yellow, while 560 nm light looks greenish-yellow, etc.

Table 1.1 Color Response versus Vacuum Wavelength

Color Response	*Vacuum Wavelength (nm)*
Red	780–620
Orange	620–590
Yellow	590–560
Green	560–490
Blue	490–450
Indigo	450–430
Violet	430–380

Monochromatic light that consists of an incident wavelength of 530 nm typically generates a pure or saturated green response. Incident light that has equal amounts of all wavelengths together with an extra amount of 530 nm wavelength generates a desaturated green response. When the amount of 530 nm light is increased, the response moves toward the saturated green. When the amount of 530 nm light is decreased, the response further desaturates and moves toward white. However, a desaturated green response can also be generated by combinations of longer and shorter wavelengths that do not contain 530 nm and that by themselves do not generate a green response. In addition, light containing 530 nm together with longer wavelengths stimulates a color perception that tends toward yellow or orange. Thus, light of wavelength 530 nm is not intrinsically green, but instead is a stimulus to the green response.

Benham's top provides a neat example of the psychophysiological dependence of color perception. The top has a black and white pattern on it. When the top is rotated at the correct frequency, flashing colored spots appear on it. Somehow the varying light levels from the rotating black and white pattern are neurally processed to give the perceived color responses.

The psychophysiological dependence of color perception can also be noted by viewing the same central color against different surrounding backgrounds. The perceptual appearance of the central color changes slightly but definitely when the surrounding background color is changed. This perceptual change occurs even though the central color is physically unchanged.

While color is clearly recognized as a perceptual response, it is still convenient to tag or label monochromatic light by the color responses listed in Table 1.1. In other words, monochromatic light of vacuum wavelength 530 nm is referred to as green light, monochromatic light of vacuum wavelength 650 nm is referred to as red light, and monochromatic light of vacuum wavelength 460 nm is referred to as blue light.

1.8 ABSORPTION

Different materials have different absorption strengths for visible light. In many cases, the absorption strength of a material is also a function of the incident wavelength. A material may absorb the long (or red) wavelengths more than the short (or blue) wavelengths. Wavelength-dependent absorption is called selective absorption.

The total amount of light absorbed in a medium depends on the absorption strength and on the distance that the light travels in the medium. A strong absorber is usually opaque, but when made thin enough it can transmit a significant percentage of the incident light.

Gold, like other metals, is a strong absorber and is opaque for a typical thickness. However, a thin film of gold, deposited by vacuum evaporation techniques, transmits a significant percentage of light. The transmission of the thin gold film is actually a selective transmission. Gold absorbs more strongly in the red part of the spectrum. Thus, the transmitted light is greenish-blue.

At the other extreme are weak absorbers. Weak absorbers are usually transparent, but even a weak absorber can become opaque if the thickness is great enough. Water absorbs red light weakly. In typical quantities, such as in fishbowls, bathtubs, and swimming pools, water is transparent for all wavelengths including red. However, in oceans illuminated by sunlight, the red light fails to penetrate deeper than 30 m.

Clear glass is evenly transparent for a normal thickness. Tinted glass, as in stained glass windows, has a reduced transmission for the absorbed wavelengths.

1.9 REFLECTION

Transmission of light through a medium is decreased by any absorption that may be present. In addition to absorption, the amount of transmitted light can be reduced by surface reflection. The word reflection comes from the Latin word *reflectere*, which means *to bend back*. Reflection is a surface or boundary phenomenon. In general, whenever light is incident on a surface or a boundary between two different mediums, some of the incident light is reflected or bent back. The percent of the light reflected, and the wavelength dependence of that percentage, depends on the materials involved and the angle of incidence of the incident light.

On a molecular level, the reflection process involves an interaction of the incident light with the electrons in the atoms and molecules of the surface layers. There is a connection between a material's absorption properties and its reflection properties. Strong absorbers, such as metals, are strong reflectors. Weak absorbers, such as water and clear glass, are weak reflectors.

Reflection is classified as either specular or diffuse. The word specular means mirror-like. Specular reflection occurs when the surface is smooth and is the reflection involved in the formation of images by mirrors or other smooth surfaces such as a pond of water. Diffuse reflection occurs when the surface is rough.

Let us consider specular reflection first. Under rectilinear propagation conditions, the direction that light is traveling can be represented by straight lines called rays. Figure 1.4a shows a ray incident on a smooth surface. The line perpendicular to the surface is called the *normal* to the surface. The *angle of incidence* of the ray is defined as the angle θ_i that the ray makes with the normal. The *angle of reflection* is defined as the angle θ_s that the reflected ray makes with the normal. The law of reflection states that the angle of reflection θ_s is equal to the angle of the incidence θ_i, or mathematically,

$$\theta_i = \theta_s \tag{1.1}$$

The law of reflection is easy to determine and was known by the ancient Greeks. The law of reflection is independent of the wavelength of the incident light.

Figure 1.4b shows three parallel rays incident on the smooth surface. The law of reflection applies to each ray so the three reflected rays are still parallel. Figure 1.4c shows three rays diverging from a point source of light. Again, the law of reflection applies to each ray. A scaled drawing easily shows that the reflected rays appear to be diverging away from a point below the surface. This is the image point that an observer looking at the reflected light would see. Flat bathroom mirrors as well as smooth water surfaces form reflected images in this manner.

Now let us consider diffuse reflection. Figure 1.5 shows four parallel rays incident on a rough surface. Here the law of reflection still applies for each ray; however, the incident angles of each ray are different and, consequently, the reflected light is diffused in all directions. In diffuse reflection, the information carried by the incident light beam is lost and no reflected image of the original source can be seen. Instead, the diffusing surface itself becomes a secondary source.

Figure 1.4 Reflections from smooth surfaces: a, one ray; b, parallel rays; c, position of the reflected image.

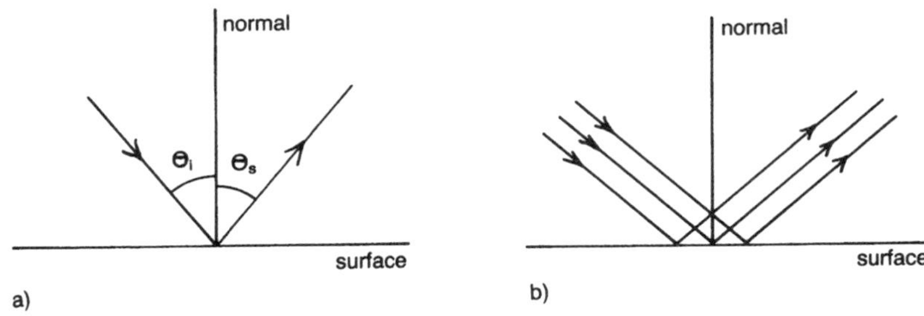

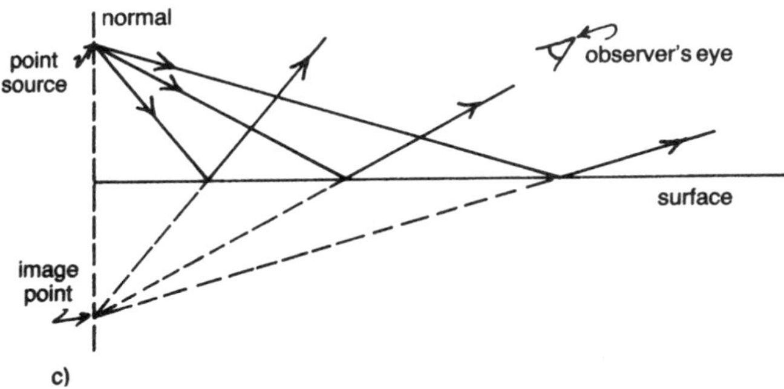

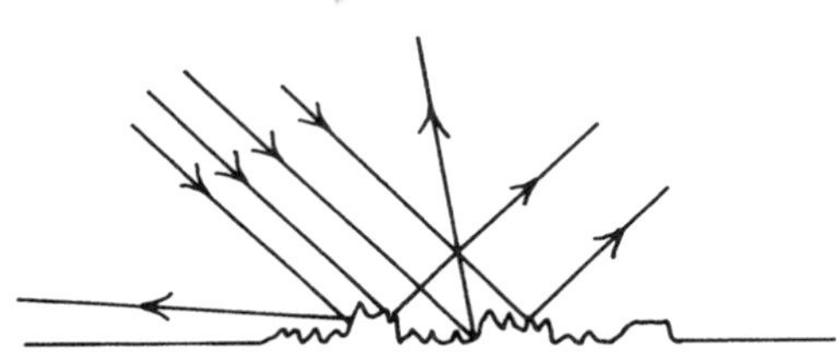

Figure 1.5 Reflection from a rough surface.

Suppose we take a rough metal surface that gives perfectly diffuse reflection and start polishing it smooth. At some stage, a reflected image starts to become visible. Initially, the image is a degraded or poor quality image, and as the polishing continues the images clears to that formed by specular reflection from a perfectly smooth surface. The reflection from the partially polished surface has a specular-like component that produces the image plus a diffuse-like component that degrades the image. Many naturally occurring surfaces give this type of mixed reflection.

The percent of light reflected can be selective. Gold absorbs reds more strongly than the blues and consequently reflects reds more strongly than blues. This can be observed by looking at the color of the image of either a white light bulb or of a blue sky formed by reflection off a smooth gold surface. In contrast to gold, silver absorbs and reflects uniformly across the visible spectrum, and so reflection from a silver surface does not modify the color appearance. Transparent materials also reflect uniformly across the visible spectrum.

1.10 SCATTERING

In an optically homogeneous material, a light beam is attenuated either by absorption in the medium or by reflection at the boundaries between the mediums. However, when the material is not optically homogeneous, scattering at each of the inhomogeneous particles can also attenuate the light beam. (As a model for homogeneous and inhomogeneous materials, you might think of vanilla ice cream as homogeneous and chocolate chip ice cream as inhomogeneous.)

The amount of scattering depends on the relative properties of the inhomogeneous material and on the number of inhomogeneous particles. Scattering occurs throughout the inhomogeneous material and, just as for absorption, the attenuation of a light beam is a function of the total thickness of the scattering medium.

Scattering can also be selective or nonselective. The blue sky is a familiar example of selective scattering. Air molecules are very weak light scatterers. They do, as does any object much smaller than visible light wavelengths, scatter blue light more than red light (i.e., shorter wavelengths more than longer wavelengths). Thus, when we look at the sky away from the sun, it appears blue because it is the scattered light that is reaching our eye. In Figure 1.6, the observer at *A* looking toward *C* sees the scattered light, which is predominately blue. The observer at *B* looking toward *C* sees the setting sun. The light reaching *B*'s eye has lost more blue light than red light due to scattering by

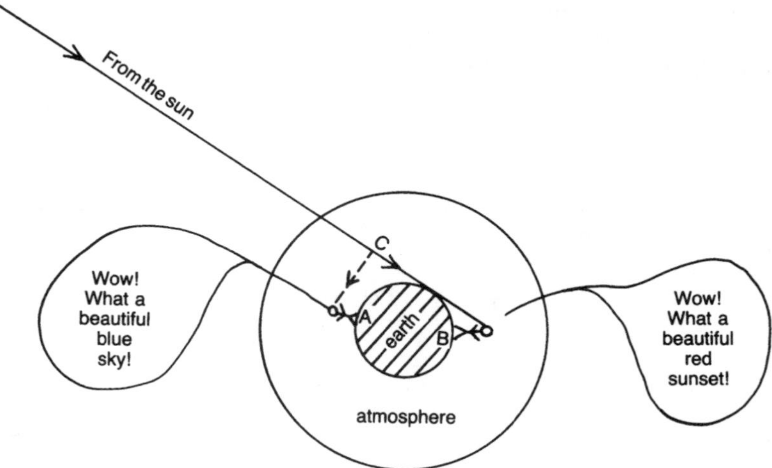

Figure 1.6 Some effects of atmospheric light scattering.

the air molecules as well as by suspended dust in the lower atmosphere, so the observer at *B* sees a reddish or orangish setting sun. The predominately bluish scattering characteristic of molecules or particles that are smaller than the wavelength of light is called Rayleigh scattering.

The moon has no atmosphere. Therefore, if one were to stand on the moon and look at the sky away from the sun, the sky would appear black because there is no scattering of light. Can you guess how a lunar sunset would appear?

Clouds contain either water droplets or ice crystals suspended in the air, while fogs contain suspended water droplets. The suspended water droplets are gigantic relative to the air molecules. Each water droplet scatters light predominately by surface reflections. The scattering from the water droplets is essentially wavelength-independent so the scattered light looks white. Since multiple scattering can occur in clouds and fogs, some of the scattered light emerges in the forward direction. A frequent effect of this type of scattering is that the forward-scattered light also enters the eye causing a contrast reduction in the retinal image of distant objects. The distant objects then seem to be in a haze or may even become invisible.

Materials that diffuse or scatter transmitted light are called *translucent* materials. They are sometimes beneficial as in supplying softer lighting, and sometimes detrimental as in dense fogs.

1.11 THE SPEED OF LIGHT IN A MEDIUM

When light enters a transparent medium from a vacuum, it slows down. The speed of the light in the medium is characteristic of that medium and of the wavelength of the incident light. The index of refraction n of the medium is a ratio of the speed c of the light in a vacuum to the speed v_m of the light in the medium, or

$$n = c/v_m \tag{1.2}$$

Equation 1.2 can be rearranged to give

$$v_m = c/n \tag{1.3}$$

For incident light of wavelength 588 nm, the indices of refraction of some common transparent materials are: water, 1.33; plastic, 1.44–1.71; crown glass, 1.523; other glasses, 1.50–1.90; diamond, 2.4. The index of refraction of air at 20 °C and 1 atmosphere of pressure is 1.0003. For a transparent material, the index of refraction is typically slightly higher for the short wavelengths (violets and blues) compared to the long wavelengths (reds). Since this dependence is slight, it is ignored until Chapter 20.

1.12 REFRACTION

When you stick a straight object such as a ballpoint pen into some water, the object appears to be bent at the water surface. Actually, the object remains straight, but the light traveling through the surface is bent. The bending of light at a surface is called refraction. The word refraction comes from the Latin word *refractus*, which means *to break back*.

Refraction occurs because of the speed change that light undergoes when it changes mediums. Consider light waves in air incident on a flat water surface. Assume that the index of refraction of the air is 1.00, and that the index of refraction of the water is 1.33. For a distant point source the incident wavefronts are flat,

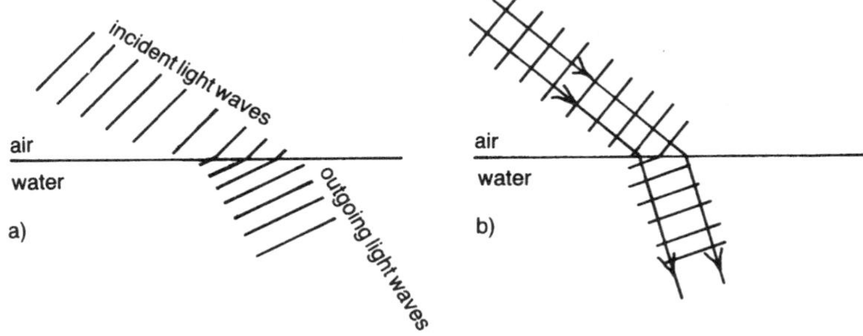

Figure 1.7 Refraction at a flat air–water interface: a, wavefronts; b, wavefronts and rays.

as shown in Figure 1.7a, and are perpendicular to the direction of travel, as shown by the rays in Figure 1.7b.

The lower edge of the incident wavefront enters the water first, and hence slows down first. Thus, in the same amount of elapsed time, that part of the wavefront in the water travels a smaller distance than that part of the wavefront in air. The net effect is that the wavefront becomes skewed so that its direction of travel in the water is different from that in the air. The rays indicating the direction of travel are perpendicular to the wavefront. In both air and water the rays are straight lines, but at the air–water boundary the rays are bent. The law of refraction states that the angle of incidence θ_i, made with the normal to the surface, is related to the angle of refraction θ_r, made with the normal to the surface, by the equation

$$n_1 \sin \theta_i = n_2 \sin \theta_r \quad (1.4)$$

where n_1 is the index of refraction of the medium in which the light is incident, and n_2 is the index of refraction of the medium in which the light leaves (Figure 1.8).

When the angles θ_i and θ_r are small, Eq. 1.4 can be simplified by its small angle approximation,

$$n_1 \theta_i = n_2 \theta_r \quad (1.5)$$

For light in air ($n = 1.00$) incident on a flat water ($n = 1.33$) surface at an incident angle of 6°, Eq. 1.5 gives the angle of refraction as:

$$(1.00)6^\circ = (1.33)\theta_r$$
$$\theta_r = 6^\circ/1.33 = 4.5^\circ$$

For light going from air into water the rays get bent toward the normal. In fact, Eq. 1.4 or 1.5 shows that bending toward the normal occurs whenever the light is entering the higher index medium. When light travels from the higher index medium to the lower index medium, then Eq. 1.4 or 1.5 shows that the rays get bent away from the normal.

The ancient Greeks studied the phenomenon of refraction. Ptolemy of Alexandria made accurate measurements on the refraction angles in A.D. 130 but failed to determine a describing equation. Later, about A.D. 1000, the Moslem scholar known as Alhazen extended the currently known knowledge of optics and studied refraction, but also failed to determine a describing equation. By A.D. 1611, Johannes Kepler had determined the equation (Eq. 1.5) that describes refraction for small angles, but it was not until A.D. 1621 that Willebrord Snell empirically discovered an equation that described refraction for large as well as small angles. Snell's equation, while correct, did not have the form shown in Eq. 1.4. In A.D. 1637, René Descartes was the first to publish the law of refraction in the form given in Eq. 1.4. There is a historical controversy about whether Descartes independently discovered the law of refraction or whether he was aware of Snell's previous but unpublished work. As a result of this controversy, the law of refraction is variously called Snell's Law or Descartes' Law, or sometimes the Snell–Descartes Law.

The determination of the long hidden law of refraction was a crucial and necessary step in the development of high quality optical instruments. However in

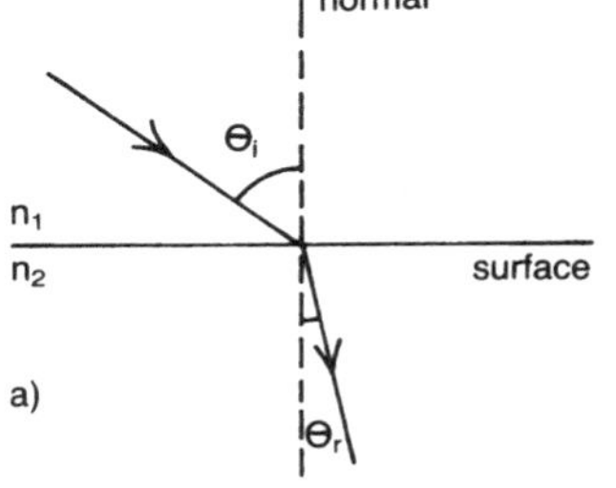

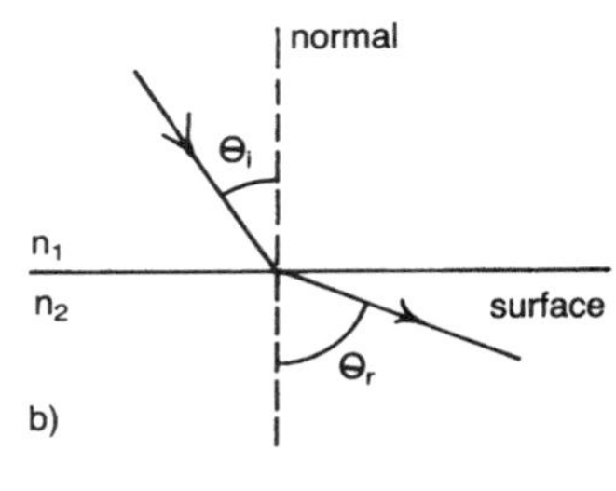

Figure 1.8 Refraction angles: a, $n_2 > n_1$; b, $n_2 < n_1$.

the 1600s there was still disagreement about the answer to the question "What is light?" The law of refraction (Eq. 1.4) derived by Descartes matches the experimental data, but Descartes derived the equation by using a particle model of light that incorrectly assumed that light speeds up when it goes from air to a higher index medium such as water.

In 1657, Pierre de Fermat took exception to Descartes' assumptions and rederived the law of refraction by using his *Principle of Least Time.* According to Fermat's principle, the actual ray path that light takes from a point A in a medium of index n_1 to a point B in a medium of index n_2 is the path that takes the least time. With the assumption that light slows down when it enters a higher index medium, Fermat used his Least Time Principle to derive Eq. 1.4.

Fermat's Principle refers to the behavior of light, but makes no assumptions on what light is. Still later in the 1600s, Christian Huygens rederived the law of refraction by using a wave model of light also with the assumption that light slows down when it goes from air to a higher index medium such as water. (Huygens' derivation is shown in Section 22.16.)

In 1873, James Clerk Maxwell combined the description of the electromagnetic phenomena known at that time into four equations. Maxwell then argued by symmetry that a term was missing in the equations. When Maxwell put in the missing term, he was able to derive (predict) that accelerating electrically charged particles should radiate energy, and that this energy (now called electromagnetic radiation) propagated through space as waves. Furthermore, when Maxwell used his equations to calculate the speed of these predicted electromagnetic waves, he got a value that matched the speed of light. This led Maxwell to propose that light was electromagnetic radiation. We can in fact start with Maxwell's electromagnetic equations and from them rederive the law of refraction. We can also show that the modern version of Fermat's Least Time Principle is a mathematical result of Maxwell's equations.

1.13 RECTILINEAR PROPAGATION, SHADOWS, AND MIRAGES

In most situations, light exhibits a definite straight line or rectilinear propagation. In nature, rectilinear propagation is observed when shafts of sunlight propagate in straight lines through holes between adjacent clouds. (Such shafts spreading across the sky are called crepuscular rays.)

Shadows are another manifestation of rectilinear propagation. You are no doubt familiar with your own shadow and well aware that you can count your fingers by looking at the shadow of your hand, or even use your hands to make shadows that resemble those of wolves, elephants, etc. You can also tell the direction of the primary light source by noting the relative locations of the shadow and the object that is blocking the light.

It is interesting to note that the ancient Greeks believed the Earth was round, not flat as was believed by the later Europeans. As one of the supports for this belief, the Greeks cited the shape of the Earth's shadow seen on the moon during a lunar eclipse. They contended that the shadow indicated a spherical Earth and not a flat Earth. To make a reasonable estimate of the radius of the Earth, the Greeks also used the slightly different angles that shadows made at high noon in deep holes that were located many miles apart from each other.

When more than one light source is present, then partial shadows can be formed as well as full shadows. A full shadow is called an umbra while a partial shadow is called a penumbra.

Shadows provide some relief on hot summer days, but they have an even more important use. Shadows provide information or cues about the three-dimensionality of solid objects, and these cues are used by our visual system as an aid in depth perception.

The law of rectilinear propagation breaks down in those situations in which diffraction of light waves becomes important. The law of rectilinear propagation also breaks down when a medium is not optically isotropic. (Isotropic means uniform in all directions.) The index of refraction of air is temperature dependent. On occasion, this temperature dependence can lead to observable effects. The air directly above a hot surface on a sunny summer day is warmer than the air at higher levels above the surface. Because of this, the index of refraction of the air smoothly changes as a function of altitude above the surface, so the air is not optically isotropic.

Light rays propagating through the hotter air near the surface bend upward while the rays at higher levels above the surface remain straight. The result is a mirage. The person can see both the object and a shimmering inverted image of it (Figure 1.9). This type of mirage is called an inferior mirage because the image appears below the object. Automobile drivers are familiar with the inferior mirage as the shimmering "water" on the road ahead. The shimmering water is actually an inferior mirage of the sky above. Next time you see this inferior mirage, check for the inverted image of an automobile or truck in front of you.

There are many other types of mirages depending on the index profile. These include the superior mirage and the fata-morgana mirage. To pursue mirages would unfortunately lead us away from the

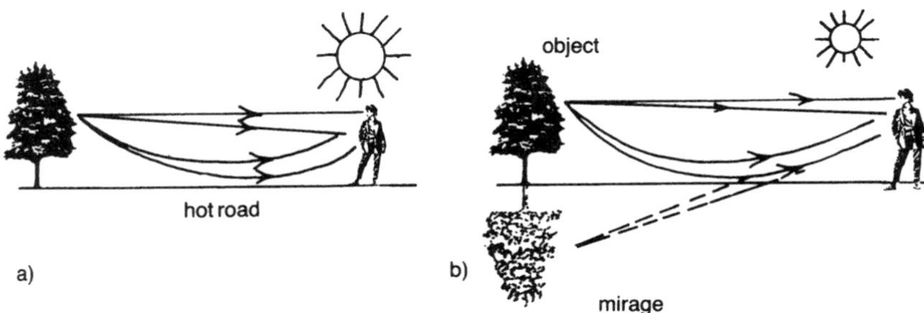

Figure 1.9 a, Curved rays; b, the inferior mirage.

goals of this book, just as desert mirages have allegedly misled thirsty travelers.

PROBLEMS

1. Light travels at a speed of 1.8×10^8 m/s in a transparent medium. What is the refractive index of the medium?
2. The refractive index of water is 1.33. What is the speed of light in water?
3. Light in air is incident on glass ($n = 1.523$). When the angle of incidence is 52°, what is the angle of refraction? Does the light bend toward or away from the normal?
4. Light in air is incident on plastic ($n = 1.66$) at an angle of 3.5°. Use the small angle approximation of Snell's Law to find the angle of refraction. Now use the exact version of Snell's Law to find the angle of refraction. How close are the answers from the two methods?
5. Light in water ($n = 1.33$) is incident on a water–air interface at a 4.0° incident angle. Use the small angle version of Snell's Law to find the angle of refraction. Does the ray bend toward or away from the normal?
6. Light in polycarbonate ($n = 1.586$) is incident on a polycarbonate–air interface. When the angle of incidence is 37°, what is the angle of refraction?
7. At the proper testing distance, a 20/20 (or 6/6) letter subtends an angle of 5′ at a patient's eye. (Recall that there are 60′ in a degree.) Can the small angle approximation of Snell's Law be used for incident angles of 5′? Provide a numerical example that supports either a yes or no answer.
8. What is an isotropic medium?
9. What is a homogeneous medium?
10. When a normal observer looks at a red leaf that is illuminated by white light, does the light that is diffusely reflected from the leaf and incident on the observer's eye contain an abundance of short wavelengths or an abundance of long wavelengths? What wavelengths were most absorbed by the leaf?
11. When a normal observer looks at a bright blue sports car that is illuminated by white light, does the light that is diffusely reflected from the sports car and incident on the observer's eye contain an abundance of short wavelengths or an abundance of long wavelengths? What wavelengths were most absorbed by the car?
12. When a full moon is high in the sky, it appears white. However, on a clear night, when the full moon first rises, it appears orangish. Why?
13. Specify the vacuum wavelengths that are in the middle of the following regions of the visible light spectrum: orange, yellow, green, and blue.

CHAPTER 2

The Geometric Behavior of Light

2.1 POINT SOURCES, WAVEFRONTS, AND RAYS

The geometric optics theory of image formation is built on the concept of point sources and point images. Consider an isolated point source in a uniform medium. The isolated point source emits light waves equally in all directions and the waves travel away from the source at the same speed. The light waves leaving the point source are represented by the wavefronts in Figure 2.1a. Since the wavefronts propagate away from the source at the same speed in all directions, they have a spherical shape. Each of the diverging spherical wavefronts is centered on the point source.

Figure 2.1b shows a point source embedded in the surface of a wall. The embedded point source emits light in the geometrically allowed directions. In the case of the embedded point source, the diverging wavefronts are again parts of concentric spheres centered on the point source.

If the medium is not uniform, then the wavefronts will not propagate away at equal speeds. Figure 2.2 shows a situation in which the lower half of the medium is uniform but the upper half is not. The index of refraction in the upper half of the medium decreases as a function of vertical distance above the point source. While the wavefronts in the lower half of the medium are spherical, the wavefronts in the upper half of the medium lose their sphericity because the waves propagating upward are moving faster than the waves propagating outward or downward.

A ray is defined as a trajectory orthogonal to the wavefronts. When given the wavefronts, one can draw the rays by having them pass perpendicular to each wavefront. Figure 2.3 presents the rays for the situation shown in Figure 2.2. Since the medium is not uniform in the upper half of Figure 2.3, the wavefronts there are not spherical. Since the wavefronts are not spherical, the rays are curved instead of straight even though they are drawn in perpendicular to each wavefront. These curved rays are the type that can occur in mirages, atmospheric refraction, or gradient index materials. (The acronym for *gr*adient *in*dex is *GRIN*.) In the lower half of Figure 2.3, the medium is uniform,

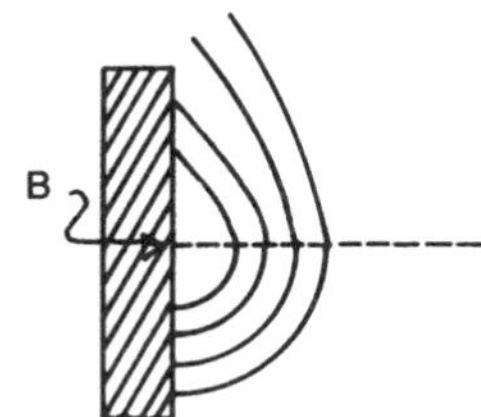

Figure 2.2 Wavefront propagation in a medium that is nonuniform above the dashed line and uniform below.

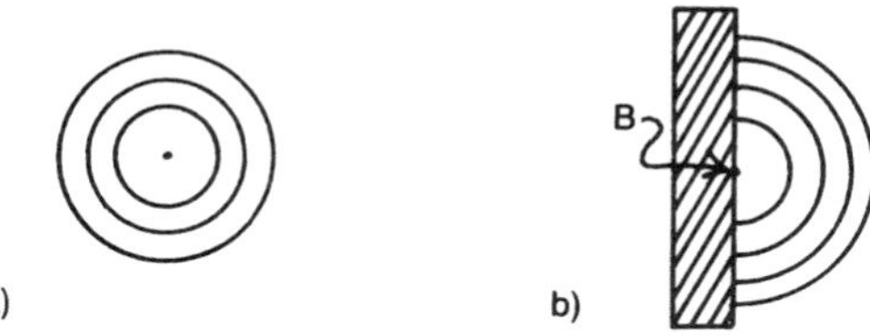

Figure 2.1 a, Diverging waves from an isolated point source; b, diverging waves from a point source embedded at B.

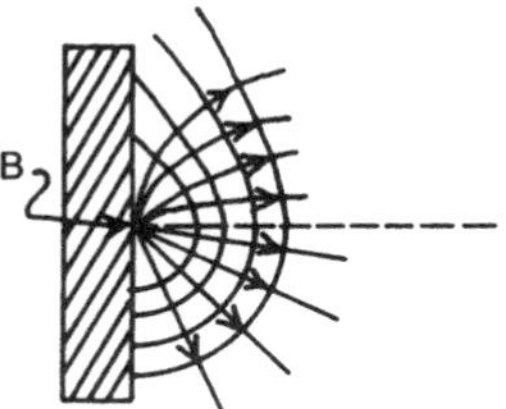

Figure 2.3 The rays for propagation in a nonuniform (top) region versus uniform (bottom).

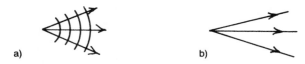

Figure 2.4 Uniform propagation from a point source: a, spherical diverging wavefronts and rays; b, rays only.

so the wavefronts there are spherical in shape. Consequently, the rays form straight lines pointing away from the point source.

Rays and wavefronts provide interchangeable information. When the positions of the wavefronts are known, then one can always draw the rays. Conversely, when the positions of the rays are known, then one can always draw the wavefronts. In discussing the optics of image formation, it is sometimes conceptually easier to use the rays, while at other times it is conceptually easier to use the wavefronts.

In most situations the rays represent the direction in which the electromagnetic energy propagated by the wave is traveling. The exception occurs in light propagation through certain anisotropic crystals. The crystal case is not of major concern in this book.

The situations of major interest in this book are the situations involving an isotropic homogeneous medium. Therefore, the wavefronts diverging from a point source are spherical in shape, and the corresponding rays are straight lines pointing away from the point source. The collection of rays or wavefronts coming from a single point source is called a homocentric (or monocentric) *bundle*. A cross section of a homocentric bundle and its point source is called a *pencil* (Figure 2.4).

2.2 CONVERGING WAVEFRONTS, POINT IMAGES, AND BLUR CIRCLES

The ideal imaging system takes incoming spherical diverging wavefronts and changes them into outgoing spherical converging wavefronts. The outgoing wavefronts then converge to a point as shown in Figure 2.5a. This point is called the image point. Figure 2.5a represents the imaging process in terms of the wavefronts, Figure 2.5b shows the rays as well as the wavefronts, and Figure 2.5c shows the rays only.

The outgoing converging wavefronts shown in Figure 2.5a are all parts of concentric spheres. Each of the wavefronts is centered on the same point. The converging light leaving the system forms the point image and then diverges away from it. Since the converging wavefronts are spherical, the rays leaving the system

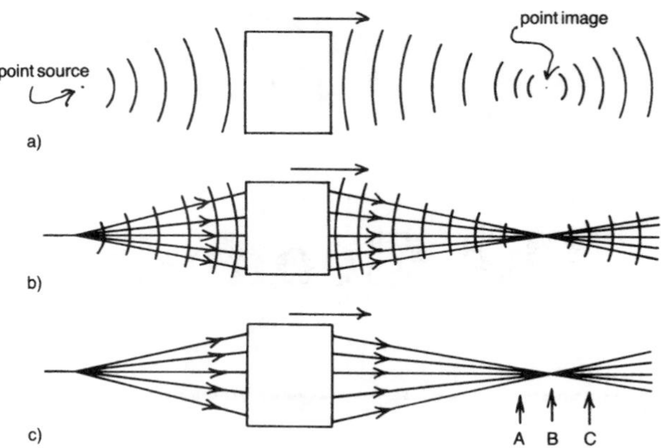

Figure 2.5 Ideal imaging process. The optical system is represented by the box: a, wavefronts; b, wavefronts and rays; c, rays only.

are straight lines that point toward the image point (as shown in Figures 2.5b and c). The rays remain straight and after passing through the image point diverge away from it.

When the apertures in the optical system are circular, then a screen placed in front of the image point would have a circular illumination patch on it (e.g., at position A in Figure 2.5c). The circular illumination patch is called a *blur circle*. The outer rays specify the diameter of the blur circle. As the screen is moved back to the image position (position B in Figure 2.5c), the blur circle decreases in size and becomes a point. When the screen is moved past the image position (e.g., toward position C in Figure 2.5c), the blur circle increases in size.

As discussed in Chapter 1, theories are actually models of the real world. The concept of a point image occurs in the model represented by the theory of geometric optics. In the real world only approximate point images occur. The optical system may not be perfect so that the converging wavefronts leaving are not perfectly spherical and a perfect point image is not formed. Such deviations from perfection are called *aberrations* and are discussed in Chapter 20.

Even more fundamentally, light propagates through space in a wavelike manner and waves exhibit diffraction effects. All optical systems have some apertures in them. Even a single lens has a finite size and therefore is not only a lens but also an aperture. The finite size apertures cause some diffraction of the light waves, which prevents the formation of a perfect point image. Nevertheless, in many cases the apertures are much larger than the wavelength of the light, and the diffraction effects are so small that the image can be considered a point image. Consequently, the theory of geometric optics is tremendously useful

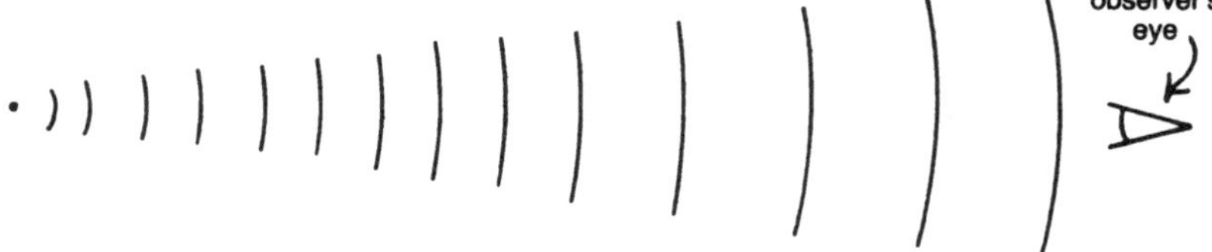

Figure 2.6 Diverging spherical wavefront. Each wavefront is centered on the point source.

in describing the image formation process even though it neglects diffraction. Note that the behavior of a system with smaller and smaller apertures eventually begins to deviate from the geometric optics description.

For the present, assume that diffraction is negligible and that the wavefronts leaving an optical system are spherical wavefronts. This assumption holds well for regions near the axis of the optical system, or more mathematically, for regions in which the *paraxial approximation* (literally "near the axis") is valid. To be classified as paraxial, a ray must be near the axis and make a small angle with the axis. When this condition is met, we can use the small angle version of the law of refraction for paraxial rays (Eq. 1.5).

2.3 DIVERGING WAVEFRONTS, PLANE WAVES, AND OPTICAL INFINITY

Everyone who has driven a car or ridden a bicycle is intuitively familiar with the concept of curvature. One must slow the car or bike down in order to negotiate a sharp or highly curved turn. On the other hand, one can speed through a gradual or relatively flat turn that has a small curvature.

Consider the diverging wavefronts shown in Figure 2.6. Each of the wavefronts is part of a sphere that is centered on the point source. The wavefronts nearest the point source have a high curvature while the wavefronts farthest from the point source have a smaller curvature. In fact, the wavefront farthest from the point source is part of an extremely large sphere and, in the localized region shown, is almost flat.

From Figure 2.6, it is clear that the spherical diverging wavefronts lose curvature as they move out away from the point source. In a localized region far away from the point source the wavefronts are very flat (as shown on the right in Figure 2.6). In the local regions where the wavefronts become very flat, they are referred to as *plane waves* (plane meaning flat). When the object point is far enough away so that the waves coming from it can be considered plane waves, the object point is said to be at *optical infinity*.

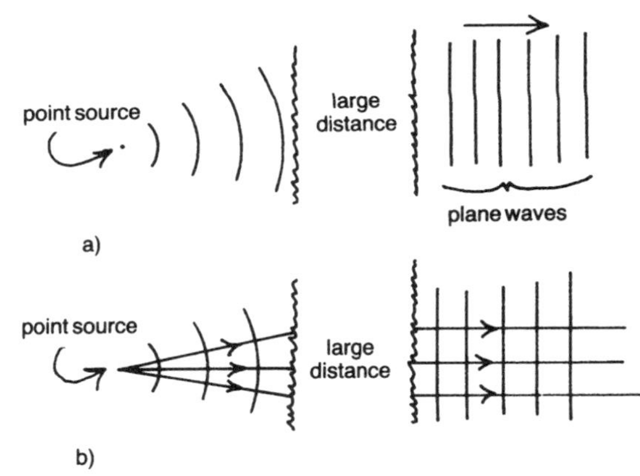

Figure 2.7 Plane waves that originated at the point source: a, wavefronts; b, wavefronts and rays.

Figure 2.7a shows another representation of the plane wave case. The wavefronts on the right are effectively flat because they have traveled a sufficiently large distance from the point source. Figure 2.7b shows the corresponding rays. When the wavefronts are flat, then the rays drawn in perpendicular to the wavefronts are parallel to each other. These parallel rays can be thought of as being very slightly divergent. However, in the plane wave region the degree of divergence is so slight that the rays are effectively parallel to each other. Even though these rays are then drawn as parallel, one should keep in mind that they originated at the point source at optical infinity.

Figure 2.8a shows converging spherical wavefronts leaving an optical system. Each of the converging wavefronts is spherical and centered on the image point. The converging wavefronts gain curvature as they travel away from the optical system toward the image point. In particular, the closer the wavefronts are to the image point, the greater the wavefront curvature.

Suppose the light leaving an optical system is only very slightly convergent. In this case, the convergent wavefronts leaving the system have only the minutest amount of curvature, and the image point, which is located at the center of curvature of the converging

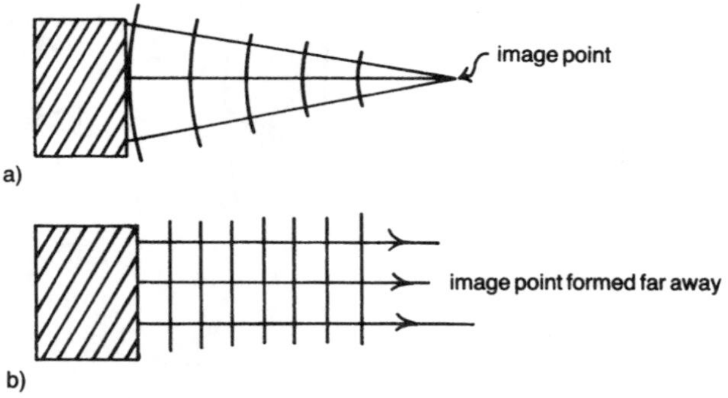

Figure 2.8 a, A converging bundle leaving a system; b, very slightly converging bundle leaving a system.

wavefront, is exceedingly far away. Then we say that the image point is at optical infinity, and it is convenient to approximate the very slightly converging wavefronts by plane waves. The rays representing the light are really very slightly convergent, but for all intents and purposes they can be considered parallel to each other, at least in the region immediately behind the optical system.

2.4 THE CONCEPT OF VERGENCE

The index of refraction of a vacuum is, by definition, exactly 1. The index of refraction of air is just slightly larger (typically 1.0003). For now, the small difference is neglected, and the index of air is assumed to equal 1.

As discussed in the previous sections, the wavefronts associated with point objects and point images are spherical. From calculus, the curvature of a sphere is equal to the reciprocal of the radius of the sphere. In air ($n = 1$), the curvature of the spherical wavefront is directly related to the degree of convergence or divergence of the light at the position of the wavefront.

The quantitative measure of the degree of convergence or divergence of light in air at a particular position is called the *vergence* of the light. For light in air, the vergence at a position is equal to the curvature of the wavefront at that position. The unit for vergence is the diopter (D), which is dimensionally equal to the reciprocal of a meter (m). Let V stand for the vergence of the light at a particular position, Q stand for the curvature of the wavefront at that position, and q stand for the radius of curvature of the wavefront. Mathematically,

$$V = Q \tag{2.1}$$

and for a sphere,

$$Q = \frac{1}{q} \tag{2.2}$$

Therefore,

$$V = \frac{1}{q} \quad q \text{ in meters} \tag{2.3}$$

In order to distinguish converging light from diverging light, a negative vergence value is used for diverging light and a positive vergence value is used for converging light. Equations 2.1 through 2.3 can be put in absolute values and then used to get the magnitude of the vergence. The appropriate plus or minus sign can then be inserted depending on whether the light is converging or diverging.

Alternatively, one can use q as a directed distance instead of just a magnitude and establish a plus-minus sign convention for q. The sign convention for q is as follows. Always measure q from the wavefront to the center of curvature of the wavefront. When the directed distance from the wavefront to the center of curvature of the wavefront is in the same direction that the light is traveling, then q is a positive value. If the directed distance from the wavefront to the center of curvature of the wavefront is opposite to the direction that the light is traveling, then q is a negative value. With these sign conventions, q is always negative for a diverging wave and positive for a converging wave.

In Figure 2.9a, a diverging wavefront is propagating to the right. The center of curvature of the diverging wavefront is at point A, which is to the left of the wavefront. The directed distance from the wavefront to its center of curvature is opposite to the direction that the wavefront is traveling; therefore, q is negative. In Figure 2.9b, a converging wavefront is propagating to the right. The center of curvature of the converging wavefront is at point B, which is to the right of the wavefront. The directed distance from the wavefront to point B is in the same direction that the light is propagating, so q is positive. The values q, Q, and V in Eqs. 2.1 through 2.3 are all negative for diverging light and all positive for converging light. Note, the fundamental assignment was that diverging light has

Figure 2.9 a, A diverging wavefront propagating to the right; b, a converging wavefront propagating to the right.

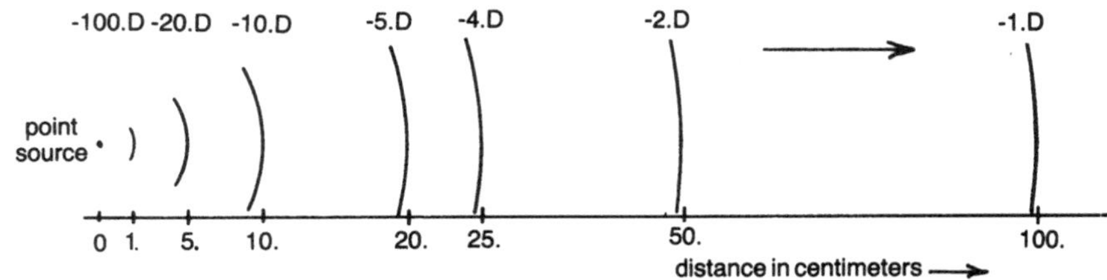

Figure 2.10 Vergence values for wavefronts diverging from a point source.

a negative vergence and that converging light has a positive vergence.

Consider the diverging waves shown in Figure 2.10. Since the wavefronts are diverging, the vergence of each wavefront is going to be negative. Consider the wavefront that is a distance of 5 cm or 0.05 m from the point source. The directed distance from this wavefront to the point source is opposite to the direction that the light is traveling, so the radius q is negative. Therefore, q equals -0.05 m. Then from Eq. 2.3,

$$V = \frac{1}{(-0.05\,\text{m})} = -20.00\,\text{D}$$

For the wavefront that is a distance of 25 cm or 0.25 m from the point source, q is -0.25 m. Then,

$$V = \frac{1}{(-0.25\,\text{m})} = -4.00\,\text{D}$$

In Figure 2.11, the center of curvature of each of the converging wavefronts is at the point image position. Since the light is converging, the vergence of each wavefront is positive. The wavefront on the left is 1 m from the point image. The directed distance from the wavefront to the point image is in the direction that the light is propagating; therefore, q equals $+1$ m. From Eq. 2.3,

$$V = \frac{1}{(+1\,\text{m})} = +1.00\,\text{D}$$

The next wavefront is 0.5 m from the point image, and from Eq. 2.3,

$$V = \frac{1}{(+0.5\,\text{m})} = +2.00\,\text{D}$$

2.5 VERGENCE: CONVERSION FACTORS

Frequently, the distances of optical interest are expressed in centimeters (cm) or in millimeters (mm), instead of in meters. The distances can be converted to meters and then Eq. 2.3 is used to calculate vergence. However, sometimes it is quicker and intuitively easier to use the conversion factor explicitly in the vergence equation.

Suppose the radius q is expressed in centimeters. Since there are 100 cm/m, Eq. 2.3 becomes

$$V = \frac{1}{q/(100\,\text{cm/m})} \tag{2.4}$$

When algebraically simplified, Eq. 2.4 results in

$$V = \frac{100\,\text{cm/m}}{q(\text{in cm})} \tag{2.5}$$

Equation 2.5 shows that the conversion factor can be written in the numerator.

Again consider a diverging wavefront at a distance of 0.05 m or 5 cm from a point source (see Figure 2.10). Here q equals -5 cm. Then, from Eq. 2.5,

$$V = \frac{100\,\text{cm/m}}{-5\,\text{cm}} = -20.00\,\text{D}$$

which is the same value as before.

Similarly, for the wavefront at a distance of 0.25 m in or 25 cm from the point source, q equals -25 cm. Then,

$$V = \frac{100\,\text{cm/m}}{-25\,\text{cm}} = -4.00\,\text{D}$$

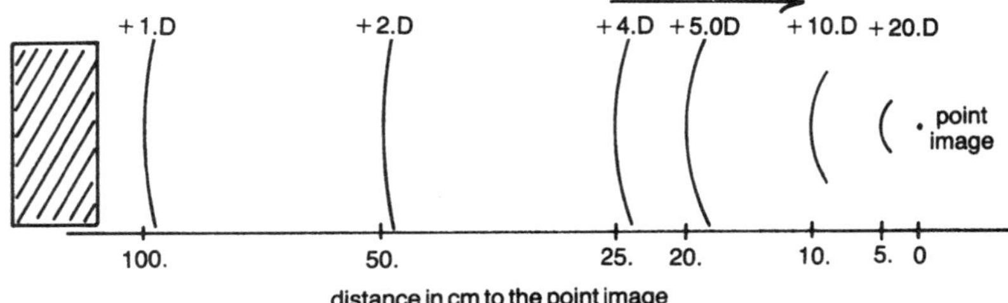

Figure 2.11 Vergence values for converging wavefronts.

Table 2.1 Vergence Values for Diverging Light

Distance from Point Source $|q|$ *(cm)*	*Vergence (V) (in air) (D)*
1	−100.00
5	−20.00
10	−10.00
20	−5.00
25	−4.00
50	−2.00
100	−1.00
200	−0.50
500	−0.20
1000	−0.10
∞	0

Table 2.1 shows the vergence values for diverging wavefronts as a function of the distance (absolute value) from the point source. Note in Table 2.1 that the vergence gets closer to zero as the wavefronts move further from the point source. This is a result of the flattening of the diverging waves as they move away from the point source (Figure 2.10). For large enough distances, the vergence is effectively zero and the waves are considered plane waves. The distance is then designated by the infinity symbol (∞).

In terms of Eq. 2.5, when the absolute value of q, labeled $|q|$, is a very large number, then V is a very small number. As $|q|$ gets larger and larger, V gets closer and closer to zero. In the limit of $|q|$ going to ∞, V goes to zero.

In Figure 2.11, the center of curvature of each of the converging wavefronts is at the point image position. Since the light is converging, the vergence of each wavefront is positive. The wavefront on the left is 100 cm from the point image. The directed distance from the wavefront to the point image is in the direction that the light is propagating. Therefore, q is +100 cm. From Eq. 2.5,

$$V = \frac{100\,\text{cm/m}}{+100\,\text{cm}} = +1.00\,\text{D}$$

Table 2.2 Vergence Values for Converging Light

Distance to Point Image (cm)	*Vergence (D)*
100	+1.00
50	+2.00
25	+4.00
20	+5.00
10	+10.00
5	+20.00

The next wavefront is 50 cm from the point image, and from Eq. 2.5,

$$V = \frac{100\,\text{cm/m}}{+50\,\text{cm}} = +2.00\,\text{D}$$

The vergence values for the other wavefronts are found similarly and are listed in Table 2.2. Note that the vergence of the converging light increases as the light moves closer to the point image position. This occurs because the curvature of the converging wavefronts is increasing as the light moves closer to the image position.

When the radius q is expressed in millimeters, then q can be converted to meters and the reciprocal taken to get the vergence (Eq. 2.3). Alternatively, the conversion factor can be put in algebraically, in which case it again ends up in the numerator, and

$$V = \frac{1000\,\text{mm/m}}{q(\text{in mm})} \tag{2.6}$$

As an example, consider a converging wavefront with a 20 mm radius of curvature. (Note, by the sign convention chosen the vergence must be positive since the light is converging.) From Eq. 2.6,

$$V = \frac{1000\,\text{mm/m}}{(+20\,\text{mm})} = +50.00\,\text{D}$$

For a diverging wavefront 2 mm away from the point source,

$$V = \frac{1000\,\text{mm/m}}{(-2\,\text{mm})} = -500.00\,\text{D}$$

The metric system conversion factors are multiples of 10 and are all extremely easy to use. If the radius of the wavefront is given in inches or feet, then the conversion factors are not convenient multiples of ten. There are 2.54 cm/in or (1/2.54) in/cm. The reciprocal of 2.54 is 0.394. In one meter there are 100 cm and, consequently, 39.4 in. The conversion factor of 39.4 in/m can be used to get the relationship,

$$V = \frac{39.4\,\text{in/m}}{q(\text{in in})} \tag{2.7}$$

As an example, consider the vergence of a diverging wavefront located 13 in from a point source.

$$V = \frac{39.4\,\text{in/m}}{-13\,\text{in}} = -3.03\,\text{D}$$

The conversion factor of 39.4 is not as easy to work with as the metric system units, particularly when a calculator is not available. For cases in which precision is not needed, the conversion factor of

39.4 in/m is approximated by 40 in/m. With this approximation,

$$V \approx \frac{40\,\text{in/m}}{q(\text{in in})} \tag{2.8}$$

Now reconsider the example immediately above. There, a diverging wavefront was 13 in away from the point source. From Eq. 2.8,

$$V \approx \frac{40\,\text{in/m}}{-13\,\text{in}} = -3.08\,\text{D}$$

The difference between the approximate value (−3.08 D) and the exact value (−3.03 D) is 0.05 D. In most visual optics cases this difference is negligible.

2.6 UPSTREAM AND DOWNSTREAM VERGENCE CHANGES

This section discusses examples of how to compute vergences either upstream or downstream from the location of a known vergence value. As mentioned in the last section, one can use the absolute values of the radius of curvature q of the wavefronts and get the correct sign for the vergence by checking whether the light is diverging or converging. The latter method has the advantage that one does not have to worry about the correct plus-minus sign for q. More importantly, it helps one to think in terms of whether the light is converging or diverging. All the examples in this section are worked using the absolute value of the radius of curvature.

EXAMPLE 2.1
Consider diverging light traveling to the right as shown in Figure 2.12. The vergence of the light at point A is −10.00 D. What is the vergence of the light at point B, which is 15 cm downstream from A?

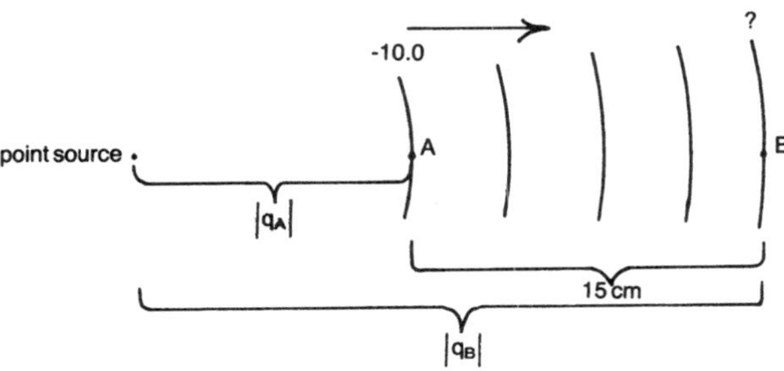

Figure 2.12 Downstream vergence example.

A good problem solver tries to anticipate or predict what characteristics the answer will have. From the sketch, the wavefronts at B are still diverging and are flatter than the wavefronts at A. Therefore, the expected vergence at B is minus and is a number smaller in magnitude than 10.00 D (i.e., we expect a number like −8 D or −4 D as opposed to a number like −12 D or −16 D). Now that we have our expectations, let's do the calculation.

The magnitude of the radius of curvature of the wavefront at A is

$$|q_A| = \left|\frac{100\,\text{cm/m}}{V_A}\right|$$

or

$$|q_A| = \left|\frac{100\,\text{cm/m}}{-10.00\,\text{D}}\right| = 10.00\,\text{cm}$$

From Figure 2.12, the radius of curvature of the wavefront at B is greater in magnitude than that at A, or

$$|q_B| = |q_A| + 15\,\text{cm}$$

and

$$|q_B| = 10\,\text{cm} + 15\,\text{cm} = 25\,\text{cm}$$

The magnitude of the vergence V_B of the wavefront at B is then

$$|V_B| = \left|\frac{100\,\text{cm/m}}{25\,\text{cm}}\right| = 4.00\,\text{D}$$

Since the light is diverging, V_B is minus, or

$$V_B = -4.00\,\text{D}$$

The answer qualitatively agrees with our anticipated results that the wavefront would be flatter.

EXAMPLE 2.2
In Figure 2.13, the vergence of light at position C is −2.00 D. What is the vergence at position D, which is 30 cm upstream from position C?

Since diverging wavefronts lose curvature as they propagate, the wavefront at D is more highly curved than the wavefront at C. The conventional terminology is that the wavefront at D is *steeper* than the wavefront at C. (Therefore, we expect that the vergence at D is more minus than the vergence at C (i.e., we expect numbers like −5 D or −10 D as opposed to −1 D or −0.5 D).

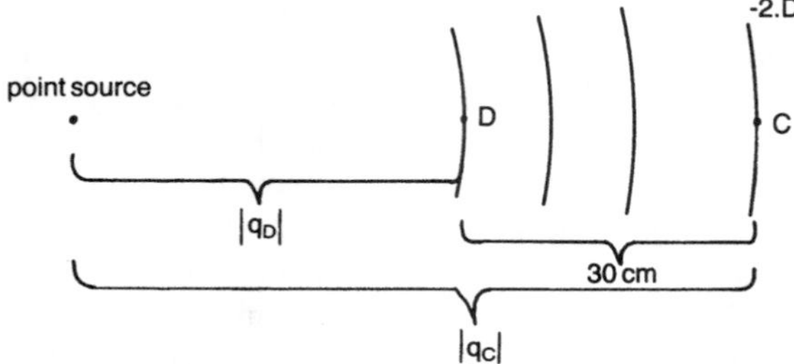

Figure 2.13 Upstream vergence example.

The magnitude of the radius of curvature of the wavefront at position C is

$$|q_C| = \left|\frac{100\,\text{cm/m}}{-2.00\,\text{D}}\right| = 50\,\text{cm}$$

From Figure 2.13, the radius of the wavefront at D is shorter than the radius of the wavefront at C, or

$$|q_D| = |q_C| - 30\,\text{cm}$$

and

$$|q_D| = 50\,\text{cm} - 30\,\text{cm} = 20\,\text{cm}$$

Then,

$$|V_D| = \left|\frac{100\,\text{cm/m}}{20\,\text{cm}}\right| = 5.00\,\text{D}$$

Since the light is diverging, the vergence is negative and

$$V_D = -5.00\,\text{D}$$

which agrees with our anticipated results.

EXAMPLE 2.3

The vergence of light at point C is +18.12 D. What is the vergence of the light at point B, which is 36.75 cm upstream? Try doing a quick sketch to convince yourself that V_B should be positive and less than +18.12 D. Then verify that the vergence at position B is +2.37 D.

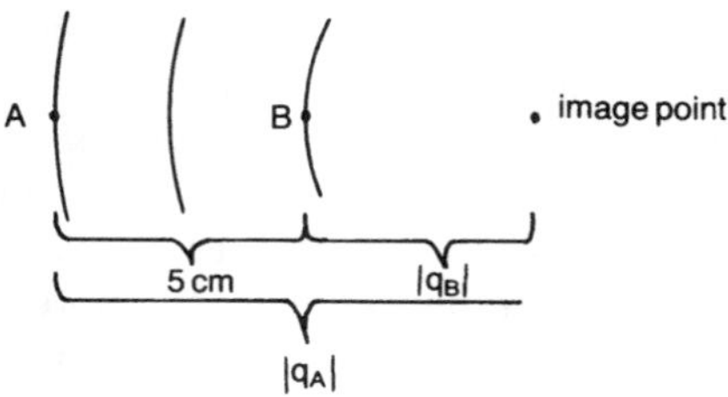

Figure 2.14 Downstream vergence example.

EXAMPLE 2.4

Consider converging light traveling to the right (Figure 2.14). The vergence of the light at point A is +8.00 D. What is the vergence at point B, which is 5 cm downstream from A? The magnitude of the radius of curvature of the wavefront at A is

$$|q_A| = \left|\frac{100\,\text{cm/m}}{8.00\,\text{D}}\right| = 12.50\,\text{cm}$$

The wavefronts are still converging at point B, so the wavefront there is steeper than at point A (see Figure 2.14). Therefore, we expect the vergence at B to be a number like +10 D, +15 D, or +20 D, as opposed to +6 D, +4 D, or +2 D.

From the sketch, the magnitude of the radius of curvature at B is

$$|q_B| = 12.5\,\text{cm} - 5\,\text{cm} = 7.5\,\text{cm}$$

Then,

$$|V_B| = \left|\frac{100\,\text{cm/m}}{7.5\,\text{cm}}\right| = 13.33\,\text{D}$$

Since the light is converging at point B, the vergence is positive and

$$V_B = +13.33\,\text{D}$$

EXAMPLE 2.5

As a final example in this section, consider light at position A with a vergence of +25.00 D (Figure 2.15). What is the vergence of the light at a position 15 cm downstream? (Try working it out before you read the solution and be sure to try to anticipate the results.)

The solution is as follows. The magnitude of the radius of curvature of the wavefront at A is

$$|q_A| = \left|\frac{100\,\text{cm/m}}{25.00\,\text{D}}\right| = 4.00\,\text{cm}$$

A quick sketch shows that the light converges to a point image 4 cm, downstream from A and then diverges away from that position. Therefore, the wavefront at position B will be diverging.

From the sketch, the magnitude of the radius of curvature of the diverging wavefront at B is

$$|q_B| = 15\,\text{cm} - 4\,\text{cm} = 11\,\text{cm}$$

The magnitude of the vergence at B is

$$|V_B| = \left|\frac{100\,\text{cm/m}}{11\,\text{cm}}\right| = 9.09\,\text{D}$$

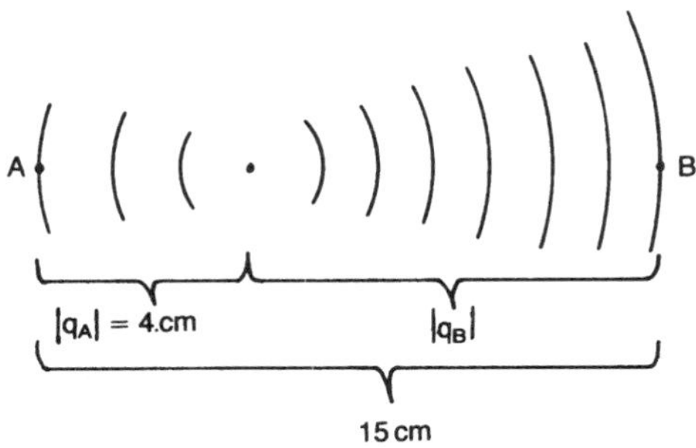

Figure 2.15 Downstream vergence example for point image between wavefronts.

Since the wavefront is diverging,

$$V_B = -9.09\,\text{D}$$

2.7 GENERALIZED OR REDUCED VERGENCE

For light propagating in a medium in which the index of refraction differs from one, we can generalize the definition of vergence as follows: The vergence of light at a position A in a medium of refractive index n is equal to n times the curvature of the wavefront at position A. Mathematically,

$$V = nQ \tag{2.9}$$

where Q is the curvature and V is the vergence. Then from Eq. 2.2 for spherical wavefronts

$$V = \frac{n}{q} \tag{2.10}$$

where q is the radius of curvature.

The index of refraction is a dimensionless number; thus, the units remain the same as before. The vergence V is in diopters when the radius q is in meters. Alternatively, conversion factors can be used in the numerator when q is expressed in units other than meters.

As an example, consider a point source in water ($n = 1.33$). What is the vergence of the light in the water at a distance of 28 cm from the point source? According to the sign convention,

$$q = -28\,\text{cm}$$

and from Eq. 2.10,

$$V = \frac{(1.33)(100\,\text{cm/m})}{(-28\,\text{cm})}$$

or

$$V = \frac{(133\,\text{cm/m})}{(-28\,\text{cm})} = -4.75\,\text{D}$$

Note that the vergence is negative as it should be for diverging light.

Historically, generalized vergence has been referred to by the name of *reduced vergence*. The rationale for this terminology and the generalized definition of vergence will be given in Chapter 8.

Note that if the light is in air, then n equals one and the equations in this section then become identical to the equations in the previous sections. Further, numerical examples of light in media other than air will be deferred to Chapter 7.

2.8 EXTENDED SOURCES AND BEAMS

Common objects such as trees, people, and books consist of many different point sources. (Conceptually, we might consider each atom in the object as a point source.) A primary or secondary source consisting of laterally separated point sources is called an *extended source*. Each point source on the extended source puts out its own bundle of light. The collection of all the bundles put out by the points on the source is called a *beam*.

The beam from typical primary and secondary extended sources is a diverging beam made up of a collection of diverging bundles. Consider the beam from a common flashlight. At night, the path of the flashlight beam is frequently visible due to light scattering off dust or suspended water droplets present in the air. The beam itself spreads out or diverges as it moves away from the flashlight. The diverging beam is made up of many individual diverging bundles, each of which originated from its own specific point on the tungsten filament of the flashlight's bulb (Figure 2.16).

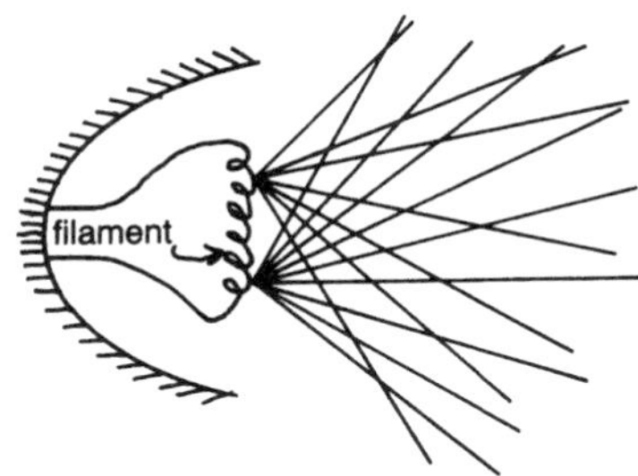

Figure 2.16 A diverging beam made up of diverging bundles.

Figure 2.17 The light leaving the lens consists of a diverging beam made up of converging bundles.

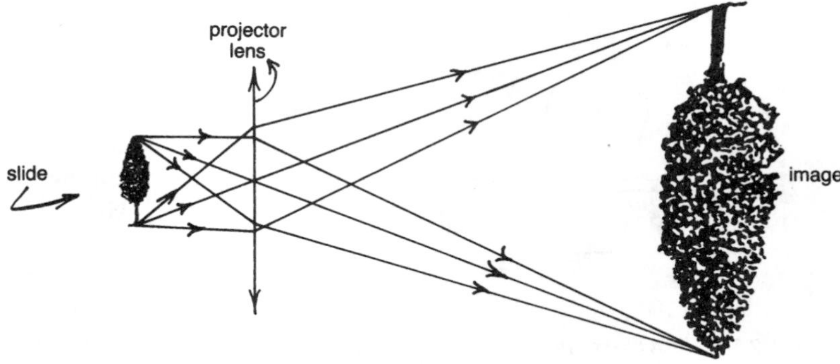

Let us now consider the beam coming from a slide or motion picture projector. The beam leaving the projector is also frequently visible due to light scattering off dust, smoke, or suspended water droplets in the air. The beam is diverging or spreading out as it moves away from the projector. However, the diverging beam leaving the projector is made up of converging bundles rather than diverging bundles. Figure 2.17 shows the image formation portion of the projector system. The bundle leaving the bottom point on the object is converged by the projector lens and eventually forms the top image point. The bundle leaving the top point on the object is converged by the lens and eventually forms the bottom image point. The extreme top and bottom rays are the beam boundaries. The beam is clearly spreading out or diverging even though each individual bundle is converging. A flashlight beam never forms an image on a screen because the individual bundles are diverging. A projector beam forms an image on a screen because the individual bundles are converging. The image on the screen is larger than the projector lens because the projector beam is diverging.

Figure 2.18 shows a converging lens that forms an extended image that is smaller than the size of the lens. The individual bundles leaving the lens are converging, which is why the image is formed. In this case, the beam leaving the lens is shrinking in size or converging as it moves away from the lens. The individual converging bundles form the image, but the converging beam is responsible for the image size being smaller than the lens size.

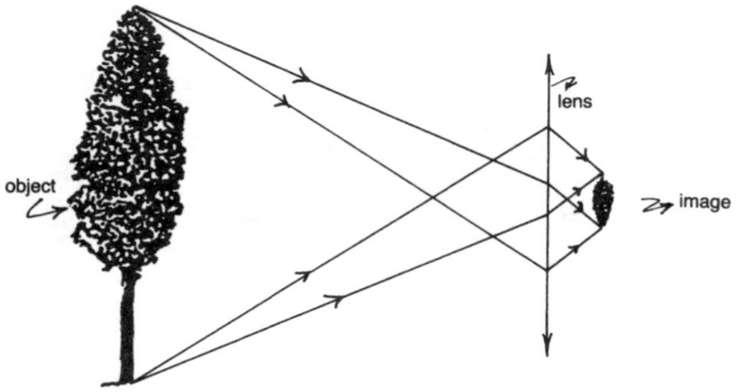

Figure 2.18 The light leaving the lens consists of a converging beam made up of converging bundles.

The above examples show that a diverging beam can be made with either diverging or converging bundles, and that a converging beam can be made with converging bundles. There is a fourth logical possibility—that of a converging beam made with diverging bundles. Is such a case physically possible? The answer is yes. This situation is treated later in connection with the discussion of the exit pupil of an optical system. (In the meantime, you might contemplate how such a system would be set up.)

Since both beams and bundles can have converging and diverging properties, what do we mean by converging light? The standard usage is that the term converging light means the individual bundles are converging. The beam may or may not be converging. The light coming out of the movie projector is then referred to as converging light because the bundles are converging. The term diverging light means that the individual bundles are diverging.

2.9 EXTENDED IMAGES AND BLUR

Figure 2.19 represents light from a tree being converged by a lens and forming a clear inverted image of the tree at position *A*. Two bundles of rays are shown, and each bundle forms its respective point image at position *A*.

When the object points all subtend a small enough angle directly in front of the lens, then the cross-sectional shape of each bundle is well approximated by a circle. If the screen is moved to position *B*, which is closer to the lens, each bundle forms a blur circle

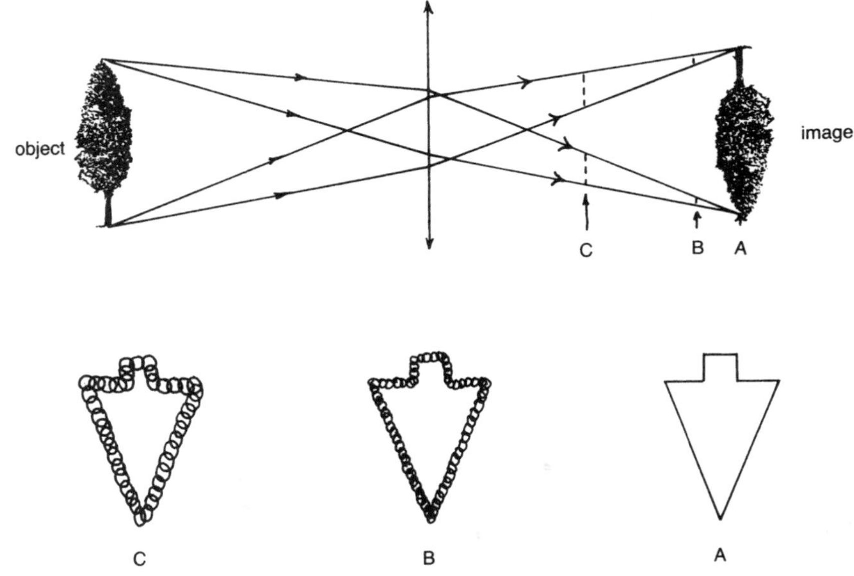

Figure 2.19 Effect of blur circle size on an extended image.

instead of a point image. The result is a blurred image on the screen. The blurred image can be simulated by drawing a small circle at each place that a point would occur in the clear image. The result is still a recognizable tree, but fine detail (such as a bird's nest) may be lost. If the screen is moved to position *C*, which is still closer to the lens, the blur circles get even larger and more information is lost. As the process continues, the blur circles eventually get large enough so that no information about the tree is present on the screen.

Each of these steps is simulated by drawing the blur circles larger and larger as in Figure 2.19. A similar sequence would occur if the screen were moved from the clear image position back away from the lens.

2.10 PINHOLES OR IMAGE FORMATION BY BLUR MINIMIZATION

If the screen is left at a blurred image position, placing an aperture next to the lens and making the aperture smaller reduces the amount of blur. This reduces the cross-sectional size of each bundle, and consequently each blur circle is smaller. This blur minimization is sometimes called the *pinhole effect*.

Figure 2.20a represents light coming from two points on an arrow object. Assume that the arrowhead is red and the bottom of the arrow is green. The light is incident on a screen, but because of the divergence of the incident bundles, no image is formed and no information about the arrow is present on the screen.

Figure 2.20b shows a circular aperture placed between the object and the screen. The aperture limits

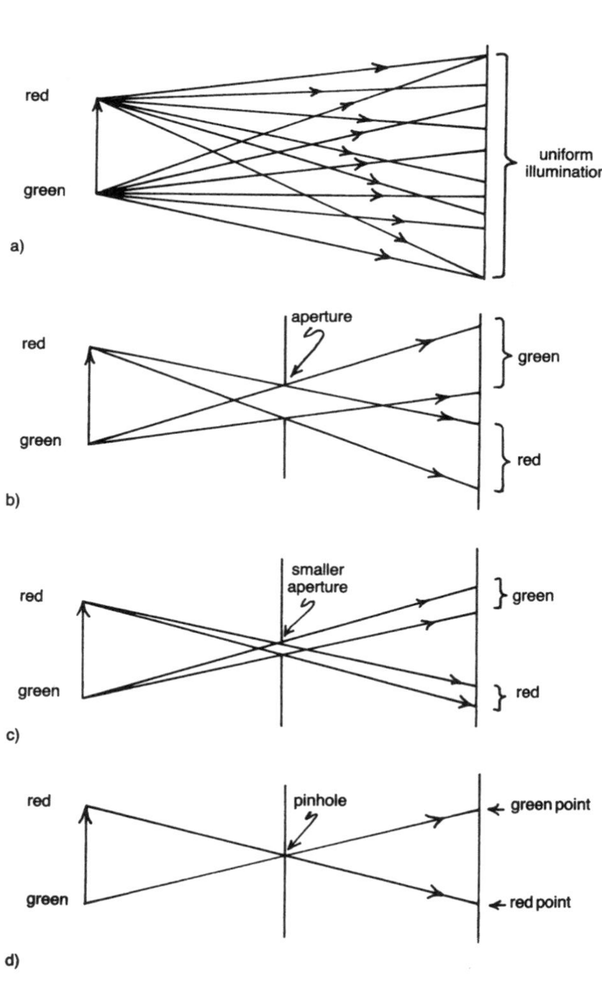

Figure 2.20 The pinhole effect.

the size of each bundle, and the illumination pattern on the screen now has a definite red illuminated region on the bottom and a definite green illuminated region on the top. These illumination patches act just like blur circles, and the illumination pattern on the screen resembles an inverted blurred image of the arrow object.

Figure 2.20c shows the aperture narrowed down further. The effective blur circles decrease further in size, and a less blurred inverted image appears on the screen.

If diffraction did not exist, one could make the aperture so small that only one ray from each object point would pass through. The illumination distribution on the screen would then have one-to-one correspondence with the object. In other words, a clear image would be formed. This is called the pinhole effect because a small aperture, such as a pinhole, is needed to form a clear image. In nature, pinhole images are sometimes accidentally formed by small holes in curtains or leaves.

The pinhole does not provide a perfect image because of diffraction. When the aperture is still large, diffraction is negligible. As the aperture is made smaller, the amount of diffraction steadily increases and the light waves start bending as they pass through the aperture, just as sound waves bend upon passing through a doorway. As the aperture size is decreased, the diffraction eventually overwhelms the reduction in blur gained by the pinhole effect. Even so, pinholes are optically useful.

The image formed by a pinhole is due to blur minimization and is not due to convergence of the light. Therefore, the position of the image screen behind the pinhole is not crucial. As the screen is moved, a clear image remains; however, the image will change in size.

Figure 2.21 shows an object of size O and an image of size I. The horizontal line is drawn through the center of the pinhole aperture normal to the aperture plane. The object stretches from the horizontal line to the point A. The aperture is a horizontal distance u from the object. An image screen is placed a horizontal distance v from the aperture.

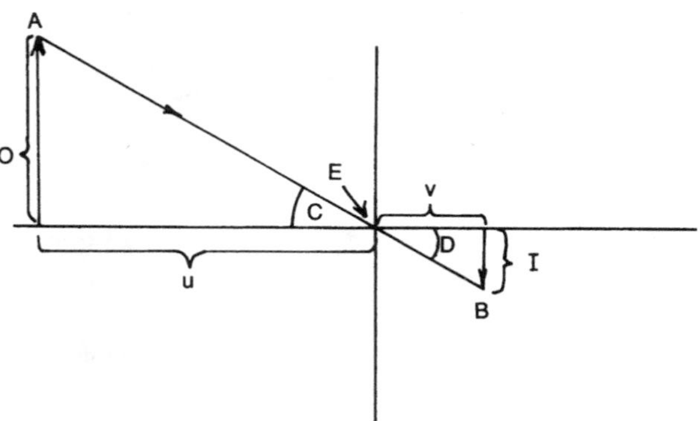

Figure 2.21 Pinhole imaging parameters.

The ray from the top of the object (point A) passes straight through the pinhole and goes to the image point B. The ray from the bottom of the object travels straight through the pinhole along the horizontal line. The angles C and D are formed by these two rays, and angle C equals angle D since angles on the opposite sides of intersecting lines are equal. From the triangles shown,

$$\tan C = \frac{|O|}{|u|}$$

and

$$\tan D = \frac{|I|}{|v|}$$

Since $C = D$, it follows that

$$\frac{|I|}{|v|} = \frac{|O|}{|u|} \tag{2.11}$$

(The absolute value signs are used in Eq. 2.11 so that we do not have to worry about plus and minus signs at this time.)

Equation 2.12 can be solved for any one of the four entities contained in it provided the other three are known. For example, what image size is produced on a screen 10 cm behind a pinhole that is placed 20 m from a 5 m tall elephant? From Eq. 2.11,

$$|I| = |O|\frac{|v|}{|u|}$$

or

$$\begin{aligned} |I| &= \frac{(5\,\text{m})(0.1\,\text{m})}{20\,\text{m}} \\ &= \frac{0.5\,\text{m}}{20} = \frac{50\,\text{cm}}{20} = 2.5\,\text{cm} \end{aligned}$$

If the screen is moved further back from the pinhole, the image remains clear but is larger. Objects that are closer to the pinhole than the elephant would also be imaged on the screen, but their size would be larger.

Historically, a device known as the camera obscura, which originally consisted of a hole in the wall of a darkroom, was used to form images by the pinhole effect. This principle was used by Aristotle, Alhazen, Leonardo da Vinci and Johannes Kepler, and by the late 1600s, small hand-held camera obscuras were popular in Europe.

The eye of the cuttlefish nautilus works on the camera obscura principle. The nautilus eye has no lens. It has an open pinhole that fills with seawater on immersion. A rattlesnake has a typical vertebrate eye. However, a rattlesnake also has infrared pits that work on the pinhole principle and supply enough information to enable the rattlesnake to strike a localized infrared target to within an angular accuracy of 5°.

The pinhole effect can be used to clear a blurred image behind a lens, again by minimizing the blur circle sizes. Blurred vision can be the result of an optical defect of the eye, but might also be the result of an ocular or neural pathology. A pinhole can sometimes be used to distinguish between these two cases. If one's vision is blurred and a pinhole clears it, this indicates an optical problem. If one's vision is blurred and a pinhole does not clear it, this indicates a pathological problem. Thus, the pinhole is a tool for optometrists and ophthalmologists. (With certain conditions, the pinhole test can give false positives and/or false negatives, so the eye doctor needs to understand more than the basic principles indicated here.)

2.11 REFRACTING STATES OF THE EYE

In the *emmetropic* eye, the cornea and unaccommodated crystalline lens converge the light from a distant object and form a clear image on the retina (Figure 2.22a). Remember that the ciliary muscle around the crystalline lens is relaxed when the eye is unaccommodated. The unaccommodated emmetrope can then see distant objects clearly.

When the object is moved closer to the eye, the divergence of the incident light increases. (For example, a point source 25 cm away from the eye produces a wavefront that when incident on the eye has a vergence of −4.00 D; whereas, a distant point source produces a wavefront that when incident on the eye has a vergence of zero.) The unaccommodated emmetropic eye will converge the light from the near object, but the converging light runs into the retina before the point images are formed. Consequently, blur circles occur on the retina instead of point images (Figure 2.22b). In this case, the near object appears blurred to the unaccommodated emmetrope. When the ciliary muscle contracts, converging power is added to the crystalline lens and the point image is pulled forward onto the retina. Thus, the accommodated emmetropic eye can clearly see the near object (Figure 2.22c).

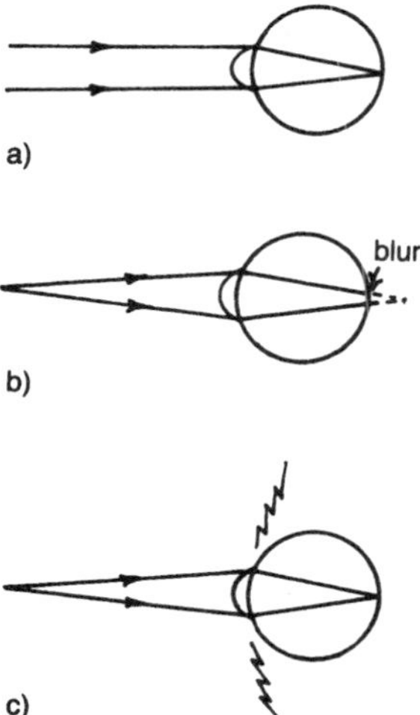

Figure 2.22 Emmetrope: a, unaccommodated and viewing a distant object; b, unaccommodated and viewing a near object; c, accommodated for the near object.

The emmetrope can clearly view a range of objects from far to near by changing the amount of accommodation. The nearer the object, the more accommodation is required. When the ciliary muscle contracts maximally, maximum accommodation occurs. As an object is brought closer and closer to the eye, the maximum amount of accommodation is eventually reached. If the object continues to be brought closer to the eye, it begins to blur. Just as a person cannot sprint at full speed for very long, so too a person cannot accommodate maximally for very long. If the object is held at a point requiring a considerable amount of accommodation, fatigue eventually occurs, accommodation decreases, and the near object appears blurred.

The maximum amount of accommodation available declines as a natural part of aging. This is apparently due to the fact that the crystalline lens grows in layers like an onion. The interior or core of the lens hardens with age and slowly ceases to change its shape when the ciliary muscle contracts. The symptom of the loss of accommodative ability is that the aging emmetrope has to hold things further away to see them clearly. When an older emmetrope can no longer see near objects clearly, the condition is called *presbyopia* or "old age" vision.

The *myopic* eye is an eye that is too long for the converging power of the eye (Figure 2.23a). The unaccommodated myopic eye forms the image of a distant object in front of the retina somewhere in the vitreous humor. The light then diverges from this point and blur circles are formed on the retina. If the myopic eye accommodates, the point image is formed even further in front of the retina and the retinal blur gets worse.

When the distant object is moved closer to the unaccommodated myopic eye, the divergence of the incident light wave is increased and the image moves back towards the retina. At some near object position, the object will be close enough so that the image point

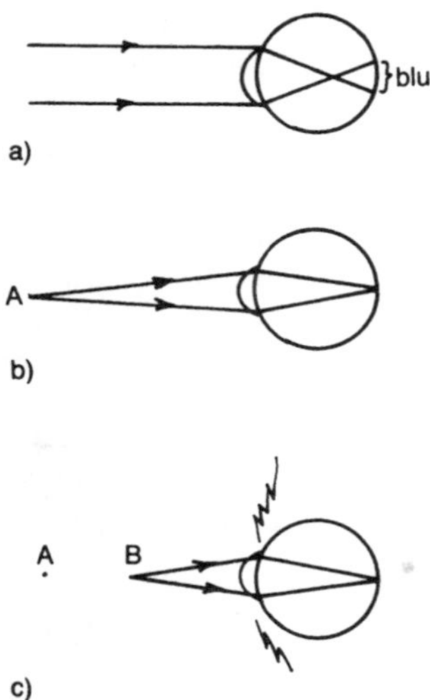

Figure 2.23 Myope: a, unaccommodated and viewing a distant object; b, unaccommodated and viewing a near object at *A*: c, accommodated and viewing a near object at *B*.

is formed on the retina. At this point the unaccommodated myopic eye can clearly see the near object (position *A* in Figure 2.23b). If the myope now accommodates, objects closer than *A* can be seen clearly (position *B* in Figure 2.23c). The condition of *myopia* is commonly called *nearsightedness* since an uncorrected myope cannot clearly see distant objects but is able to clearly see near objects.

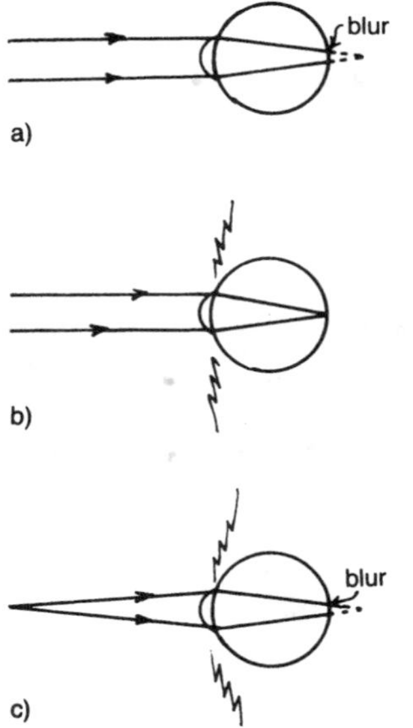

Figure 2.24 Hyperope: a, unaccommodated and viewing a distant object; b, accommodated and viewing a distant object; c, accommodated and viewing a near object.

The *hyperopic* eye is an eye that is too short for the converging power of the eye (Figure 2.24a). The unaccommodated hyperopic eye converges light from a distant object, but the image points are not yet formed when the light reaches the retina, so the retinal image is blurred.

When the hyperopic eye accommodates, the light inside the eye converges faster and the point images are pulled forward onto the retina. In this case, the accommodated hyperopic eye can clearly see a distant object (Figure 2.24b). The hyperopic eye uses up accommodation for a distant object and needs even more for a near object. Depending on the amount of hyperopia and the amount of accommodation, the hyperopic eye may not have enough accommodation left for a near object (Figure 2.24c). The result is that the uncorrected hyperope sees distant objects clearly (by accommodating), but near objects are blurred. Thus, the condition of *hyperopia* is commonly called *farsightedness.*

Unaccommodated hyperopic and myopic eyes viewing a distant object both produce spherical converging wavefronts inside the eye, and these spherical converging wavefronts can form point images. The optical defect is that the image points do not lie on the retina. Myopes and hyperopes are collectively called *spherical ametropes.* (Ametrope literally means not an emmetrope.) Another optical defect of the eye occurs when the converging wavefronts are not spherical, and, consequently, a point image is not formed anywhere. The resulting condition is called *astigmatism.* Stigmatus is the Latin word for point and astigmatism literally means no point. Astigmatism is discussed in Chapter 10.

Occasionally, cataracts develop and grow in the crystalline lens. The cataracts degrade vision by scattering light, which causes the retinal image to become washed out. One cure for cataracts is to surgically remove the crystalline lens. The resulting eye has no accommodative abilities but is correctable with spectacle lenses, contact lenses, or intraocular lens implants. An eye without a crystalline lens is called an *aphakic* eye (*a* = without; *phakic* = Latin for lens).

PROBLEMS

1. What is the vergence of the light at a distance of 8 cm from a point source? At 42 cm? At 123 cm? Draw a sketch of the wavefronts and indicate whether the wavefronts are gaining or losing curvature as they move away from the point source.
2. What is the vergence of converging light at 83 cm from the image point? At 32 cm? At 13 cm? At 4 mm? Draw a sketch of the wavefronts and indicate whether the wavefronts are gaining or losing curvature as they move towards the image point.

3. The light at position A has a vergence of +4.50 D. What is the vergence at position B, which is 14 cm downstream from position A? At a point C, which is 43 cm downstream from position A?
4. The light at position A has a vergence of −15.50 D. What is the vergence at position B, which is 21 cm downstream from position A?
5. The light at position A has a vergence of +13.50 D. What is the vergence at position B, which is 3 cm upstream from position A?
6. The light at position A has a vergence of −6.30 D. What is the vergence at position B, which is 9 cm upstream from position A? At position C, which is 37 cm upstream from A?
7. A point source is under water ($n = 1.33$). What is the vergence in the water at a distance of 11 cm from the source? At 21 cm from the source?
8. A point source is in air. What is the vergence of the light 6 in from the point source? At 17 in?
9. Given a −8.00 D diverging wavefront in air, how far (in cm) is the wave from its point source? For a −6.00 D wavefront?
10. Given a +7.00 D converging wavefront, how far (in cm) is the image point? For a +3.00 D wavefront?
11. An object is 6 m from a pinhole. A screen is placed 15 cm behind the pinhole. When the object is 2 m tall, what is the size of the image?
12. If the screen in no. 11 is moved closer to the pinhole, what happens to the image? If the screen is moved further from the pinhole, what happens to the image?
13. If the screen is fixed 15 cm from a pinhole, what happens to the image as the object is moved closer to the pinhole?
14. A piece of film 3 cm × 5 cm is placed 10 cm from a pinhole. What would be the linear field of view of this pinhole in object space at a distance of 25 m from the pinhole?

CHAPTER 3

Optical Objects and Images

3.1 OPTICALLY REAL VERSUS PHYSICALLY REAL OBJECTS

Figure 3.1 shows light waves from a specific source, a tree, incident on a specific optical system, a camera. The tree is a physically real entity. However, the optical stimulus for the camera is provided exclusively by the incident divergent light waves. These waves leave the tree, travel across the space between the tree and the camera, and are then incident on the camera.

Suppose that light waves identical to those coming from the tree can be artificially generated without the tree present. In that case, the optical stimulus for the camera would be unchanged and the camera would photograph a "tree" even though no tree is physically present.

A hologram can be used to artificially generate such light waves. Holograms are usually made optically, but some can also be computer generated. The hologram is a recording of a light wave interference pattern. When properly illuminated, the interference pattern artificially generates the light waves identical to those coming from the tree (Figure 3.2). Not only does the camera photograph the tree, but a human observer looking at the waves coming from the hologram sees the tree complete with three-dimensional depth and parallax effects.

In the aforementioned cases, the optical system responds identically regardless of whether the incident diverging light waves are coming from the physically real source or were artificially generated by the hologram. Since optical systems respond to the incident light, it is useful to separate the concept of an optically real object from that of a physically real object. We say that an optical system has an *optically real object* whenever the light incident on the system is diverging. The optically real object may or may not be physically real.

The location of an optically real object point can be specified in terms of the diverging spherical wavefront that is incident on the optical system (Figure 3.3). The location assigned to the optically real object point for the system is at the center of curvature of the

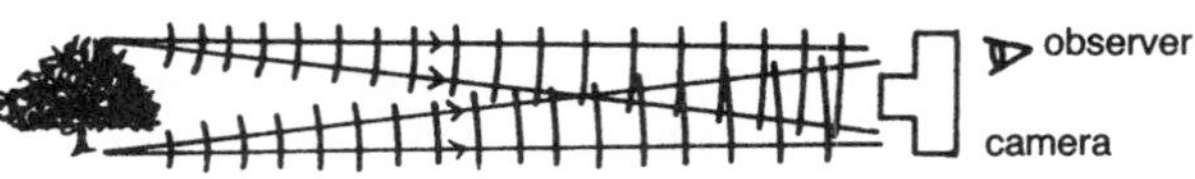

Figure 3.1 An observer photographing a tree.

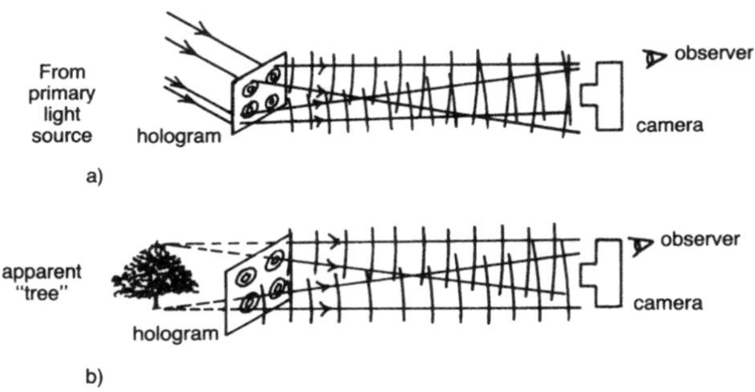

Figure 3.2 a, The hologram generates light waves identical to those coming from the tree; b, the apparent tree as seen by the camera and the observer.

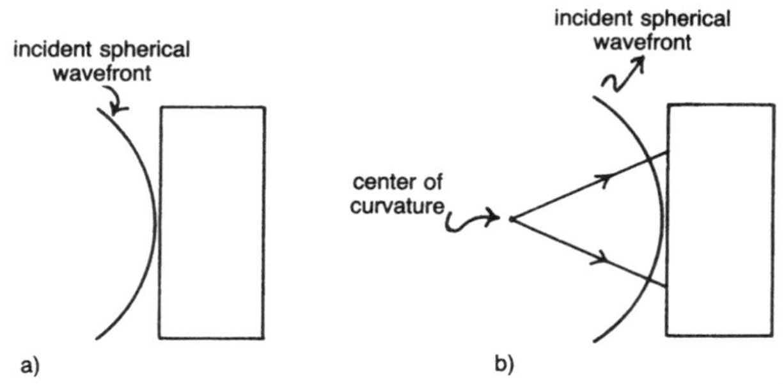

Figure 3.3 a, Incident spherical wavefront; b, locating the center of curvature of the incident wavefront.

incident spherical wavefront. If a physically real object point produced the incident diverging light wave, then the center of curvature of the wavefront is located at the physically real object point. However, if a hologram, lens, or mirror produced the diverging light wave, then there is no physically real object point at the location assigned to the optically real object point.

The rays associated with the incident diverging wavefront will, when extended back, intersect at the center of curvature of the wavefront. Since the center of curvature is the assigned object point, the incident rays appear to be diverging away from the assigned object position regardless of whether a physically real object is there or not. Figure 3.2b shows the location for a point on the tree produced by the hologram.

3.2 OPTICALLY REAL VERSUS PHYSICALLY REAL IMAGES

Figure 3.4a shows an optical system with diverging light incident on it and converging light leaving it. The relative distribution of visible electromagnetic radiation in the object plane is recreated in the image plane. The actual electromagnetic radiation at the image plane constitutes the *physically real image*.

In Figure 3.4b, a brick wall has been placed between the back of the system and the position of the physically real image. The wall stops the electromagnetic radiation from reaching the plane of the physically real image. However, the wavefronts leaving the back of the optical system are still converging and still have the same curvature that they had prior to the placement of the brick wall. Furthermore, the angles between the different converging bundles leaving the back of the system are still the same. In effect, the placement of the brick wall had no effect on the converging light waves that are immediately behind the system.

In analyzing the action of the system, it then becomes useful to say that the system has an *optically real image* whenever converging light leaves the system. The system has a physically real image only if the bundles in the converging light are actually allowed to form point images. In the brick wall case, we would say that the system has an optically real image, but not a physically real image.

The position assigned to an optically real image point is at the center of curvature of the converging spherical wavefront that is leaving the back of the system (Figure 3.5a). When the brick wall is not present, the bundle actually converges to form the physically real image point at the center of curvature of the exiting wavefront (Figures 3.5b and c). When the brick wall is present, the light is converging toward the center of curvature of the exiting wavefront but is stopped before reaching it (Figure 3.5d). In other words, the optically real image point is the point toward which the light is converging.

The center of curvature of the wavefront that is leaving the system can be located by drawing in the corresponding rays. These rays are of course converging and will pass through the center of curvature in those cases where the physically real image is formed.

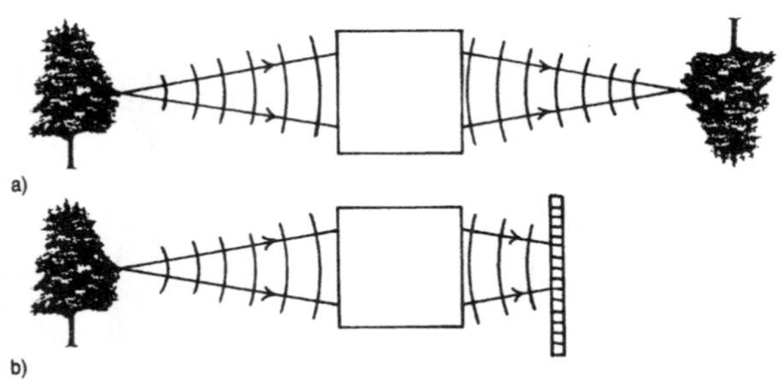

Figure 3.4 a, Converging light forms a physically real image; b, converging light is still leaving the system, but a brick wall stops formation of the physically real image.

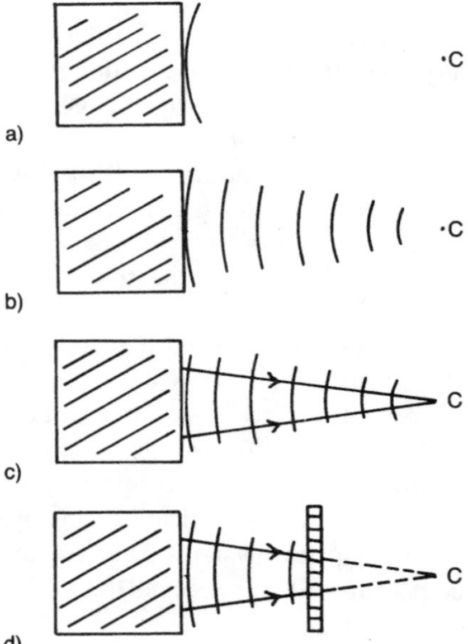

Figure 3.5 A converging wavefront leaving the system: a, exiting wavefront and its center of curvature *C*; b, wavefronts converging to *C*; c, wavefronts and rays; d, brick wall does not change location of *C* but blocks light from reaching *C*.

In the brick wall case, the rays are pointing toward the center of curvature when the wall stops them, but the rays can still be extended straight ahead to locate the center of curvature. The ray extensions are the dashed lines in Figure 3.5d.

Brick walls are not usually introduced as discussed above. However, in a multiple-component optical system, lenses or mirrors are frequently placed in the path of converging bundles and thus prevent the formation of the physically real image. The concept of the optically real image is then useful in analyzing the components that formed the converging bundles.

3.3 REAL IMAGES AS OBJECTS FOR THE EYE

In our everyday lives, we are familiar with the real images formed by movie and slide projectors. The light leaving the projector system is converging and a screen is placed at the position of the clear image. The light then diffusely reflects from the screen, and the now diverging bundles travel to the various observers' eyes (Figure 3.6a). The physically real image on the screen serves as the real object for the observers' eyes.

On the other hand, a real image can also be directly viewed without the use of a screen. When no screen is present, each bundle of the converging light leaving the lens system forms a point image and then diverges away from that point. To view the real image directly, the observer needs to move his eye into the path of the diverging light (Figure 3.6b). The physically real image for the lens directly serves as the real object for the observer's eye.

The real image for a single lens is inverted relative to the original object and, depending on the object distance, may be larger or smaller than the original object. In Figure 3.6c, the original object is a tree and the observer is looking at the small inverted real image of the tree. Since the real image is inverted, it is particularly easy for the observer to realize that he is looking at the real image and not at the original object.

The real image is, in effect, floating out in air with no solid objects around it and, as such, is called an *aerial image*. Consequently, the observer may have depth perception difficulties. The image may be perceived as being on the other side of the lens when in fact the image is between the lens and the observer. This misperception is due to the absence of the normal perceptual cues when viewing the aerial image.

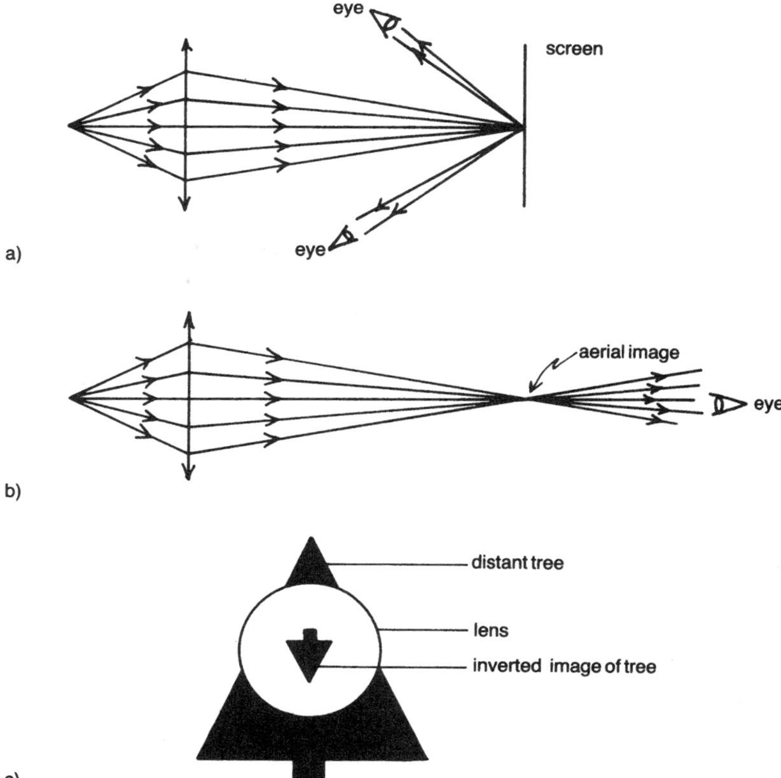

Figure 3.6 a, A screen makes an image visible to different observers; b, an aerial image viewed without a screen; c, appearance of a real aerial image to the observer.

Remember that the reason the observer sees the object, whether it is the real tree or the inverted real image of the tree, is that the refracting elements of the observer's eye form a real image on the retina. In Figure 3.6c, the inverted real image that the lens forms is serving as the real object for the eye and is thus the distal stimulus for the observer's visual perception. The proximal stimulus for the observer's visual perception is the retinal image formed by the refracting elements of the eye.

3.4 VIRTUAL IMAGES

Virtual, *adjective*: Being in essence or in effect though not formally recognized or admitted, for example, He was a virtual saint.

In our everyday lives, we are familiar with the images formed by mirrors. However, your image formed by a flat bathroom mirror is not a real image. The light leaving the bathroom mirror is diverging, not converging. Nevertheless, the mirror's image is clearly visible and has some of its own characteristics. For example, when you wave your left hand at your image in the mirror, it waves its right hand back at you.

Spherical diverging mirrors are now commonly used for security purposes as well as for giving an increased field of view in automobile and truck mirrors. Your image formed by a spherical diverging mirror is smaller than you, but it still waves its right hand when you wave your left hand. Again, the image is not a real image because the light leaving the mirror is diverging and not converging. While the images of these mirrors are not real, they are certainly visible and have the attributes of an image.

Images analogous to those of mirrors can also be formed by lenses (or even by holograms). In general, whenever diverging light is leaving an optical system, we say that the system has a *virtual image*. Virtual images cannot be formed on a screen because converging light is needed to form images on screens. However, virtual images can serve as optically real objects for our eyes or for other optical systems such as cameras. In fact it makes no optical difference to an eye or camera whether it is looking at a real or virtual image. In each case, the light incident on the eye or camera is diverging.

The position assigned to a virtual image point is at the center of curvature of the diverging spherical wavefront that is leaving the back of the system (Figure 3.7). The rays associated with the exiting diverging wavefront will, when extended back, intersect at the center of curvature point that is the assigned image position. The ray extensions are the dashed lines in Figure 3.7. In other words, the position assigned to the virtual image point is the point from which the light appears to be diverging.

For a flat mirror, the position assigned to the virtual image (i.e., at the center of curvature of the diverging wavefront that leaves the mirror) is where the image perceptually appears to be. When you stand 1 m in front of your bathroom mirror, your image appears to be 1 m behind it. Note that no light is physically present behind the mirror. You can build a brick wall against the back of your bathroom mirror and it won't affect your image in the mirror.

Figure 3.8a shows a tree in front of a diverging lens. For each point on the tree, the lens creates a virtual image point, and its position is assigned to be at the center of curvature of the wavefront leaving the back of the lens. An observer looking through the lens at the

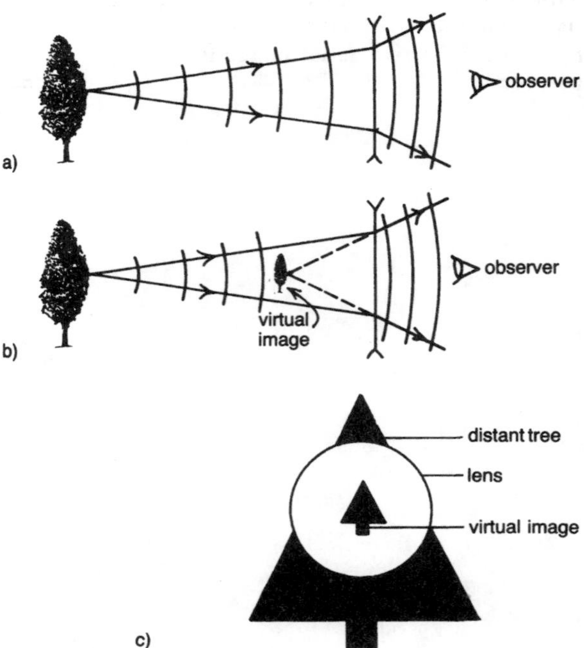

Figure 3.8 a, Wavefronts for light passing through a diverging lens; b, rays showing virtual image location; c, appearance of virtual image to the observer.

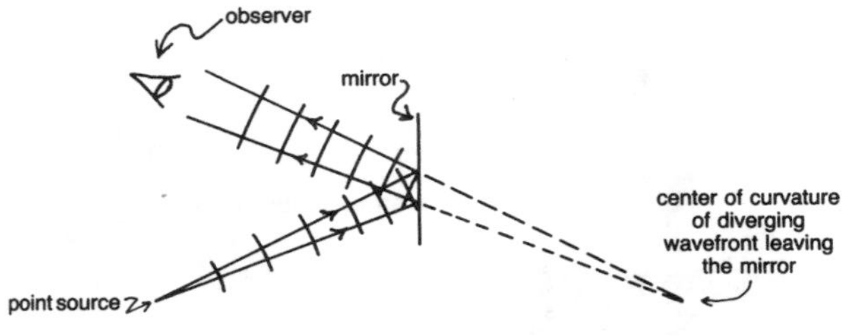

Figure 3.7 Observer viewing a mirror's image.

large tree sees the virtual image, which is the small, erect tree.

The virtual image is specified by the diverging wavefronts that leave the lens. These wavefronts then travel to the next optical system, which can be an observer's eye. The object for the observer's eye is then an optically real object that is specified by the diverging wavefronts incident on the eye. The physically real entities are the diverging light waves that leave the lens and are incident on the eye. The virtual image of the diverging lens is the optically real object for the observer's eye, and is the distal stimulus for the observer's visual perception. The retinal image that the eye forms is physically real and is the proximal stimulus for the observer's visual perception. Diverging corrective lenses are the spectacle or contact lens corrections for myopia.

3.5 VIRTUAL OBJECTS

When an optical system has diverging wavefronts incident on it, we say that the object is an optically real object and we assign its position at the center of curvature point of the incident diverging wavefront. As discussed in Section 3.1, there may or may not be a physically real object at that point. The geometric information carried by the incident waves is encoded in the curvature of the wavefronts and in the angles that the different bundles make with each other.

In general, it makes no difference to the optical system whether the incident light is diverging or converging. When diverging light is incident on a strong enough converging system, the exiting light is converging, and when converging light is incident on the same converging system, the system simply converges the light even more. When diverging light is incident on a diverging system, the system diverges the light even more, and when converging light is incident on the same diverging system, the system still has a divergent effect on the light. (The exiting light is either less convergent or may even be divergent depending on the diverging strength of the system.)

When the light incident on the system is converging, the object for the system is clearly not real. However, just as in the case of incident diverging waves, the incident converging waves carry geometric information encoded in the curvature of the wavefronts and in the angles that the individual bundles make with each other. Optically, objects for systems are defined in terms of this incoming information. Consequently, when the incident light is converging, we say that the system has a *virtual object*. The position assigned to a virtual object point is at the center of the curvature of the incident converging spherical wavefront.

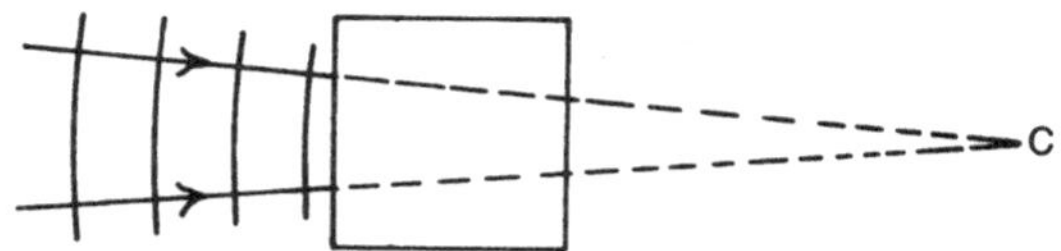

Figure 3.9 Converging light incident on a system. The center of curvature *C* of the incident wavefront serves as the location for the virtual object.

For a convergent wavefront incident on the front surface of a system, the center of curvature is located behind the front surface (Figure 3.9). The rays associated with the incident converging wavefront are pointing toward the center of curvature when they hit the front of the system. The ray extensions (the dashed lines in Figure 3.9) pass through the center of curvature point. Hence, the rays incident on the front surface of the system are converging toward the virtual object position.

Normally, the light leaving a source (either primary or secondary) is diverging. Therefore, to get converging light incident on an optical system, that light must leave the source and then be converged by some preceding optical system. The converging light leaving the first system is then incident on the second system. The second system, with the incident converging light, has a virtual object. The wavefronts leaving the first system and traveling to the second system specify both the real image for the first system and the virtual object for the second system. In effect, the real image for system one is the virtual object for system two (Figure 3.10).

Hyperopes are corrected by converging lenses. When a corrected hyperope views a distant object, the light leaving the correcting lens and incident on the hyperope's eye is converging. The optically real image of the correcting lens serves as the virtual object for the hyperope's eye. The optical position of this virtual object is at the center of curvature of the wavefront incident on the cornea. Since this wavefront is converging, the assigned position is behind the eye. However, while the optics of the hyperope's eye are

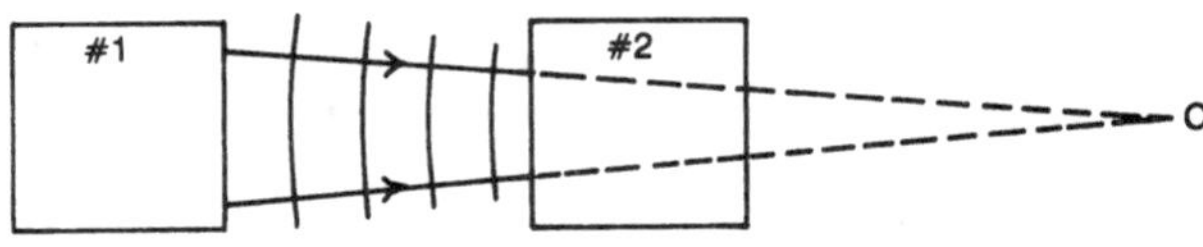

Figure 3.10 The converging light leaving system #1 is incident on system #2. The wavefronts are all centered on *C*.

analyzed with the virtual object position, remember that the proximal stimulus for the hyperope's visual perception is the physically real retinal image of the hyperope's eye. Just as with an emmetrope or a myope, the hyperope perceives the object to be in front of the eye.

3.6 OBJECT AND IMAGE SUMMARY

The aforementioned definitions for optical objects were in terms of the wavefront that is actually incident on the system. *When you encounter the word object, you should immediately think in terms of what the incident wavefront is doing.* The aforementioned definitions for optical images were in terms of the wavefront that is actually leaving the system. *When you encounter the word image, you should immediately think in terms of what the exiting wavefront is doing.*

The discussion given in the previous sections of this chapter is summarized below for quick reference.

Whenever diverging light is incident on an optical system, the system is said to have an *optically real object*. Note, the object may not be physically real. The position assigned to an optically real object point is at the center of curvature of the incident diverging wavefront. Consequently, the position assigned to the optically real object is at the place from which the incident light appears to be diverging.

Whenever converging light is incident on an optical system, the system is said to have a *virtual object*. This can happen only when some previous system has converged the light. The position assigned to a virtual object point is at the center of curvature of the incident converging wavefront. Consequently, the position assigned to the virtual object is at the place toward which the incident light is converging.

Whenever converging light leaves an optical system, the system is said to have an *optically real image*. (A physically real image exists only when the bundles are actually allowed to form their point images.) The position assigned to an optically real image point is at the center of curvature of the exiting converging wavefront. Consequently, the position assigned to the optically real image is at the place toward which the exiting light is converging.

Whenever diverging light leaves an optical system, the system is said to have a *virtual image*. The position assigned to a virtual image point is at the center of curvature of the exiting diverging wavefront. Consequently, the position assigned to the virtual image is at the place from which the light appears to be diverging.

3.7 THE IMAGE FOR SYSTEM 1 IS THE OBJECT FOR SYSTEM 2

Figure 3.11 shows four different two-lens systems. In each case, a physically real object point is located at position A in front of the first lens (L_1), and a physically real image point is located at position C behind the second lens (L_2). In each example, the image for the first lens and the object for the second lens are located at point B. Depending on the example, the image for the first lens is either real or virtual, and the object for the second lens is either real or virtual.

In Figure 3.11a, the light leaving the first lens is converging and a real image is actually formed at position B. The light waves that converge to form the image point at position B then diverge away from there and are incident on the second lens. Clearly, the real image for the first lens serves as the real object for the second lens. Note that the wavefront leaving the first lens is converging and has its center of curvature at B, while the wavefront incident on the second lens is diverging and also has its center of curvature at B.

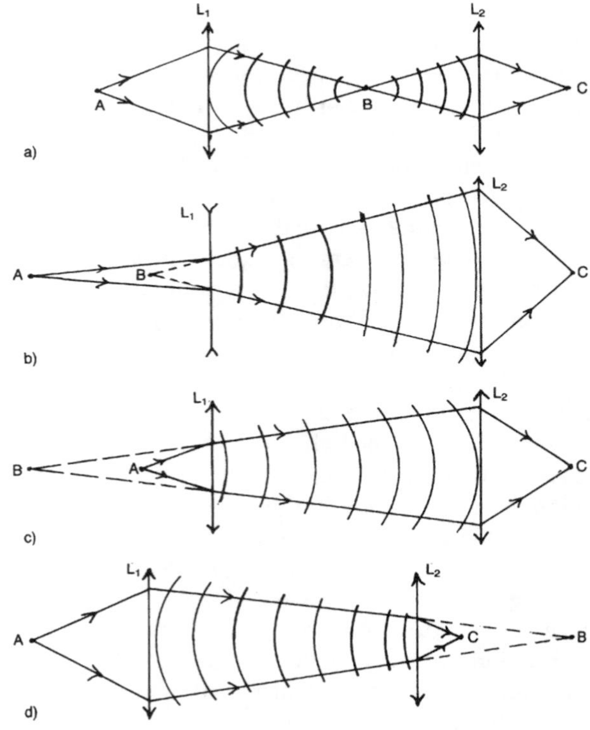

Figure 3.11 Object and image positions for four different two-lens systems. In each case A is the object for L_1, B is the image for L_1 and the object for L_2, C is the image for L_2.

In Figure 3.11b, the first lens is a diverging lens. The light incident on it is diverging, and the light leaving it is diverging even more. The center of curvature of the wavefront leaving the first lens is at B. We say that the first lens has a virtual image, and the location assigned to the image is at B. The diverging wavefronts that leave the first lens propagate across the space between the two lenses and are incident on the second lens. The second lens has an optically real object. The center of curvature of the diverging wavefront incident on the second lens is also at B, as are the centers of curvature of all the diverging wavefronts between the first and second lenses. The position assigned to the object for the second lens is at B. In effect, the virtual image for the first lens serves as the real object for the second lens.

In Figure 3.11c, the first lens is a converging lens. However, the light incident on the first lens has a high enough divergence so that the light emerging from it is still divergent. The first lens did have a converging effect since the divergence of the exiting light is less than the divergence of the incident light. All of the wavefronts traveling from the first lens to the second lens are diverging and have their centers of curvature located at B. Since the wavefront emerging from the first lens is divergent and has its center of curvature located at B, we say that the first lens has a virtual image located at B. Since the wavefront incident on the second lens is diverging and also has its center of curvature located at B, we say that the second lens has an optically real object located at B. In effect, the virtual image for the first lens serves as the real object for the second lens.

In Figure 3.11d, the light leaving the first lens is converging. The converging light is then incident on the second lens. All of the converging wavefronts traveling from the first lens to the second lens have a common center of curvature located at B. Since the wavefront emerging from the first lens is converging, we say that the first lens has an optically real image, and we assign the image position to be at B, which is the center of curvature of the wavefront leaving the first lens. Note that in this case, no physically real image point exists at B. The wavefront incident on the second lens is converging. We say that the second lens has a virtual object, and we assign the object position to be at the center of curvature of the wavefront incident on the second lens. The center of curvature of the wavefront incident on the second lens is also at B. In effect, the optically real image of the first lens serves as the virtual object for the second lens.

In each of these four cases, the light leaving the first lens propagates across the space between the two lenses and is incident on the second lens. The light that leaves the first lens carries information about the image of the first lens. The light incident on the second lens carries information about the object for the second lens, but the information carried by the light leaving the first lens is the same information that the light is carrying when it is incident on the second lens. Since the information transferred is the same, we say *that the image of the first lens is the object for the second lens.*

The preceding statement can be extended to other optical systems including mirrors. Consider your bathroom mirror. Use your face as the object for the mirror. The mirror forms a virtual image of your face. The mirror's virtual image serves as the (optically real) object for your eye. The object for system two (your eye) is the image for system one (the mirror).

3.8 CONJUGATE POINTS AND THE PRINCIPLE OF REVERSIBILITY

The *principle of reversibility* states that rays representing the path of light through a system would, upon reversal of their direction, retrace their original path back through the system. Reversibility at a reflecting or a refracting surface follows directly from the law of reflection (Eq. 1.1) or the law of refraction (Eq. 1.4).

Suppose in the situations shown in Figure 3.11 that the light is reversed and made to travel through the two lenses from right to left. According to the principle of reversibility, only the direction indicators on the rays need to be changed. The ray positions and angles remain unchanged.

In the reversed (i.e., right to left) situation, lens L_2 has a real object at C and either a real or a virtual image at B. In the reversed situation for the first three figures (Figures 3.11a, b and c), the image for L_2 is optically real, while in the fourth figure (Figure 3.11d), the image for L_2 is still at B but is now virtual.

In each of the two-lens examples, the two points B and C are coupled together. In the left to right situation, B was the object point and C the image point, while in the reversed situation, C was the object point and B the image point. Because of the coupling between B and C, they are labeled as *conjugate points* for lens L_2. For L_2, the statement "C is conjugate to B" means, that for light traveling to the right, B is the object and C is the image, while in the reversed case, C is the object and B is the image.

For lens L_1 the conjugate points in each case are A and B. For the left to right case, A is the object point and B is the image point, while for the reversed case, B is the object point and A is the image point.

In the left to right situation for the two-lens system (both L_1 and L_2), the original object in each case was at A and the final image was at C. In the reversed situation, the system object was at C and the system image was at A. Thus, the conjugate points for the two-lens system are A and C.

The ability to determine and use conjugate points is an important skill in analyzing optical systems. As illustrated by the above discussion, it is crucial to recognize which lens or lenses are involved. In particular, A is conjugate to B for the first lens. However, for both lenses together, A is conjugate to C. (You should take some time to think about this. In fact you might even try making up your own two- or three-lens example and analyzing it.)

3.9 OBJECT SPACE/IMAGE SPACE

The word space has several different definitions and uses. The word space in *object space* or *image space* is used in an abstract mathematical sense. A definition of the mathematical use of the word space is as follows: an aggregate or set of points or things that have a common property. Consider the original four cases in Figure 3.11 again. The light is traveling to the right and in each case, the assigned object point for lens L_2 was point B. In the first three cases, point B was the position of an optically real object for L_2 and was in front of (to the left of) L_2. In the last case, point B was the position of a virtual object for L_2 and was located behind (to the right of) L_2. Remember that in all the cases, the object position was taken to be at the center of curvature of the wavefront that is physically incident on L_2.

The set of all points, rays, or ray extensions associated with the light incident on an optical system constitutes the object space for the system. For L_2, all the points B are in this set, that is, are in the object space for L_2. Note, the object space for L_2 is a mathematical set that includes points both to the left and to the right of L_2. *The requirement for belonging to the object space set is not where the point is, but only that the point be associated with the incident light.*

For each of the original (left to right) cases shown in Figure 3.11, the image for lens L_1 is located at point B. In the first and last cases, the image for L_1 is real and point B is located to the right of L_1, while in the second and third cases, the image for L_1 is virtual and point B is located to the left of L_1. Remember that the image position was defined as the center of curvature of the wavefront that is physically leaving L_1.

The set of points, rays, or ray extensions associated with the light leaving an optical system constitutes the image space for the system. In the original cases of Figure 3.11, the points B are all in the image space for L_1. Note that the image space set for L_1 includes points that are both left and right of L_1. *The requirement for belonging to the image space set is not where the point is, but only that the point be associated with the light leaving the system.*

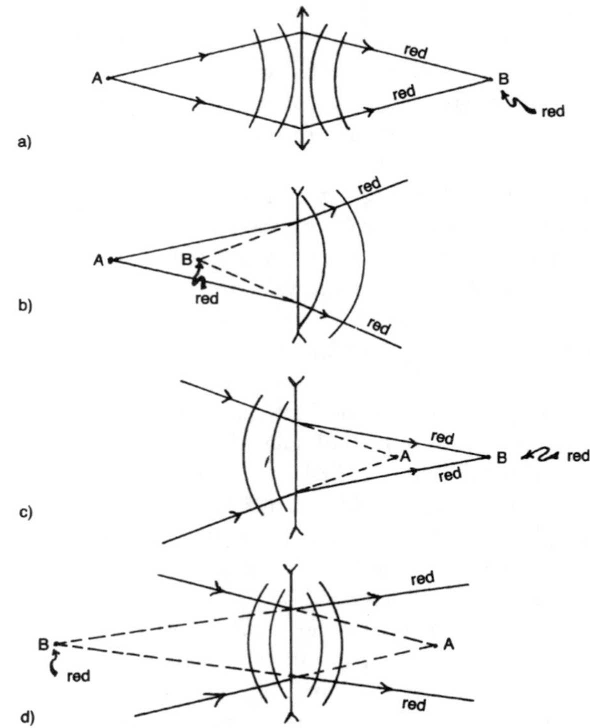

Figure 3.12 The lens in each case is a red tinted lens. The light leaving the lens is red, and the image *B* is red.

It may be helpful in initially learning the object space/image space concepts to think about imaging with a tinted lens (sunglasses are common examples of tinted lenses). Figure 3.12 shows four examples of imaging with a tinted lens. In each example, the light is traveling left to right.

In Figure 3.12a, a white point source is placed in front of a red tinted converging lens. The incident rays, drawn in black, represent the incident white light. The exiting rays, drawn in red, represent the transmitted red light. Point A is in object space and point B is in image space.

In Figure 3.12b, the white point source is placed in front of a red tinted diverging lens. The incident rays are black representing the incident diverging light. The outgoing rays are red and represent the exiting light, which is more divergent than the incident light. The image is virtual and the associated position is at the center of curvature of the exiting wavefront. This center of curvature is located by extending the outgoing red rays backward until they intersect at point B. Clearly, point A is in object space. Point B is associated with the red light leaving the lens. Therefore, it is in image space even though it is to the left of the lens.

In Figures 3.12c and d, a previous lens, which is not shown, has been used to generate white converging light incident on the red tinted diverging lens. In Figure 3.12c, the object for the diverging lens is virtual and is located at the center of curvature of the incident wavefront. The center of curvature is found by extending the incident black rays forward until they intersect at point A. Point A is shown in black since it is associated with the incident white light and not with the exiting red light. The light leaving the lens is still converging, but not as convergent as the incident light. A real image is formed at point B. In this case, point A is in the object space set (or simply, in object space), and point B is in the image space set (or simply, in image space), even though they are both to the right of the lens.

In Figure 3.12d, the incident white light is converging, but the degree of convergence is not as high as in part c. Consequently, the diverging lens has enough power to make the outgoing red light divergent. Both the image and the object points are virtual. The object point is at A, represented in black, and the image point is at B, represented in red. Point A is in object space even though it is to the right of the lens, and point B is in image space even though it is to the left of the lens.

In conclusion, when you see the term object space, you should think in terms of the convergence or divergence of the light incident on the system even if the object is virtual and located behind the system. When you see the term image space, you should think in terms of the convergence or divergence of the light leaving the system even if the image is virtual and located in front of the system. Once learned, the object space/image space concepts serve as a useful tool in dealing with multiple-component systems.

PROBLEMS

1. A flat bathroom mirror reflects light without changing the vergence. Suppose you stand in front of the bathroom mirror and look at your image in the mirror. Is the image formed by the mirror real or virtual? The mirror's image serves as the object for your eye. Does your eye have a physically real object, an optically real object, or a virtual object? When you hold your right hand up, does your image in the mirror hold its right or its left hand up?
2. Consider lens 2 in Figure 3.13. Which point (A, B, C, or D) is the object position for lens 2? Does lens 2 have a real or virtual object? Which point serves as the image for lens 2? Is the image for lens 2 real or virtual? Is lens 2 a converging or a diverging lens? What point is the center of curvature of the wavefront incident on lens 2?
3. Consider lens 1 in Figure 3.13. Which point (A, B, C, or D) is the image position for lens 1? Does lens 1 have a real or virtual image? Is lens 1 a converging or a diverging lens?
4. Consider lens 3 in Figure 3.13. Which point (A, B, C, or D) is the object position for lens 3? Does lens 3 have a real or a virtual object? Is lens 3 converging or diverging? What point serves as the center of curvature for the wavefront incident on lens 3?
5. Consider Figure 3.14. Point B is in the object space for which lens (1, 2, 3, 4, or 5)? What lens is point B in the image space for?
6. Consider Figure 3.14. Point D is in the object space for which lens (1, 2, 3, 4, or 5)? What lens is point D in the image space for?
7. Consider Figure 3.14. What lens (1, 2, 3, 4, or 5) is point E in the object space for? What lens is point E in the image space for?
8. Consider Figure 3.14. List the converging lenses. List the diverging lenses.
9. Consider Figure 3.14. For lens 2, what point is conjugate to point C? Now consider lens 2 and 3 as one system. For lens 2 and 3 as one system, what point is conjugate to C?
10. Consider Figure 3.14. There is light blue water between lens 1 and 2. There is light green jello between lens 2 and 3. There is light red water between lens 3 and 4. Draw the wavefronts that have point E as their center of curvature. We want to represent point E by the color of the medium that these wavefronts are in. What color should we use for E?

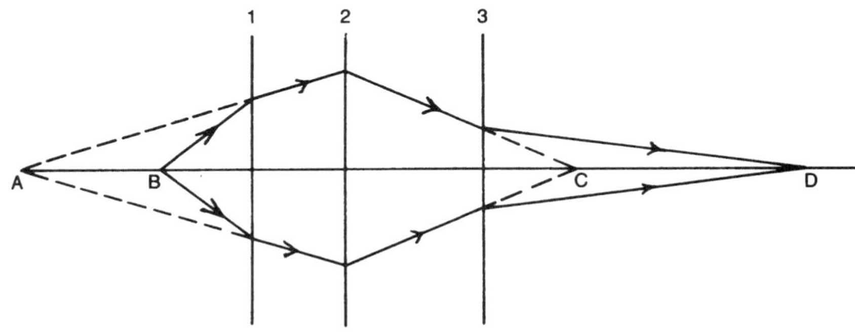

Figure 3.13 Three-lens system referred to in problem nos. 2 through 4.

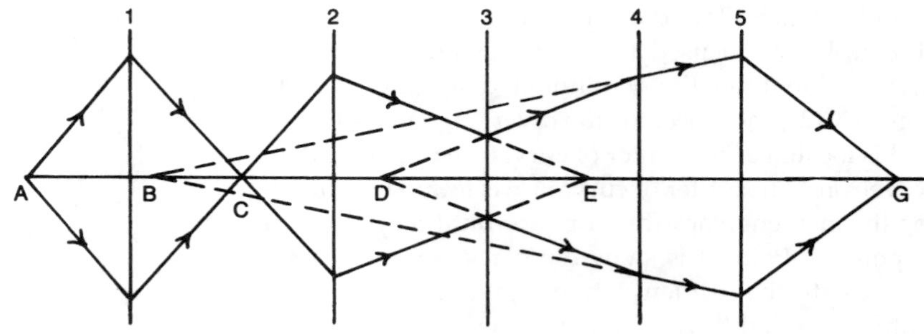

Figure 3.14 Five-lens system referred to in problem nos. 5 through 10.

11. A myope wears a diverging spectacle correction. When the myope looks through the spectacle lens at a distant tree, is the optical object for his eye the tree, or the image of the tree formed by the spectacle lens? Is the image of the spectacle lens real or virtual? Is the object for the myope's cornea real or virtual?
12. A hyperope wears converging spectacle lenses. When the hyperope looks through the spectacle lens at a distant tree, converging light leaves the spectacle lens and is incident on the hyperope's cornea. Does the hyperope's cornea have a real or virtual object? Where is the center of curvature of the wavefront that is incident on the hyperope's cornea? The spectacle corrected hyperope has a real image on the retina. For the spectacle lens eye system, what is the retinal image conjugate to?
13. Which is the better statement: "Seeing is believing" or "Sight is an illusion"? Why?

CHAPTER 4

Thin Lenses and Ray Diagrams

4.1 HOW SPHERICAL LENSES WORK

The long glass rod shown in Figure 4.1a has a spherical surface on the front. Plane waves from a distant point source are incident from the left. In Figure 4.1b, the first wavefront is entering the glass. The speed of the wavefront in the glass is slower than its speed in the air. Consequently, the center of the wavefront, which enters the glass first, slows down first and starts lagging behind the edges. The result is that the wavefronts in the glass become converging wavefronts. Within the accuracy of the paraxial approximation, the converging wavefronts are spherical and form a point image at position E in Figure 4.1c.

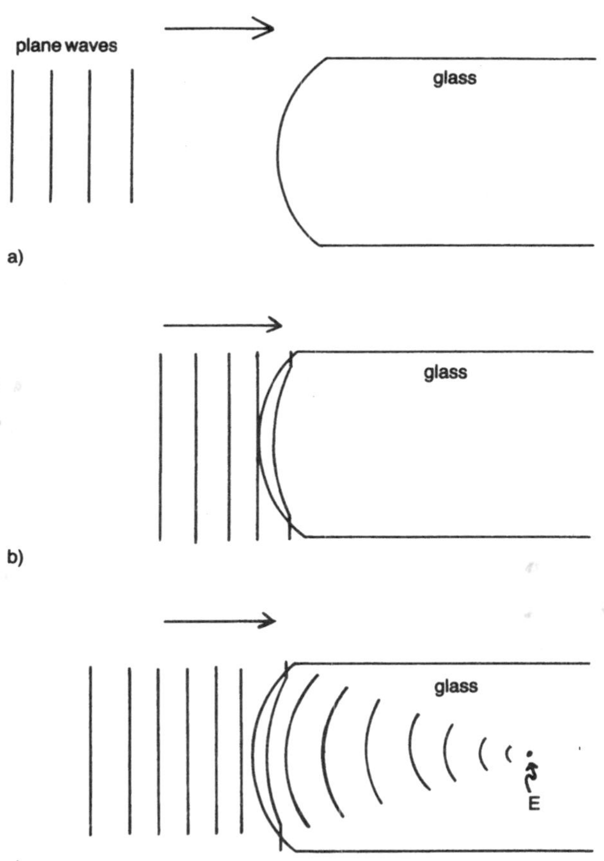

Figure 4.1 a, Plane waves in air incident on a glass rod with a convex spherical surface; b, in the glass, the middle of the wavefront lags behind the edges; c, the wavefronts in the glass converge to *E*.

Figure 4.2 shows plane waves in the glass incident from the opposite direction on the same spherical glass surface. As the first wavefront approaches the surface, the edges of the wavefront enter the air (before the center of the wavefront) and speed up. Consequently, the edges of the wavefront start leading the center of the wavefront that is still in the glass. Within the accuracy of the paraxial approximation, the exiting wavefronts in air are converging and spherical and form a point image at G.

The spherical glass surface in Figures 4.1 and 4.2 has the physical property of its center bulging out into the air. This surface converges plane waves no matter which way the waves travel through the surface, i.e.,

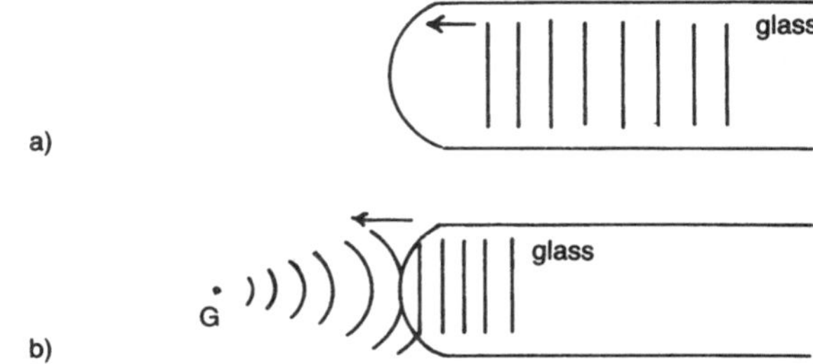

Figure 4.2 a, Plane waves in the glass incident on the convex surface of the previous figure; b, in the air, the wavefront edges lead the middle resulting in light converging to *G*.

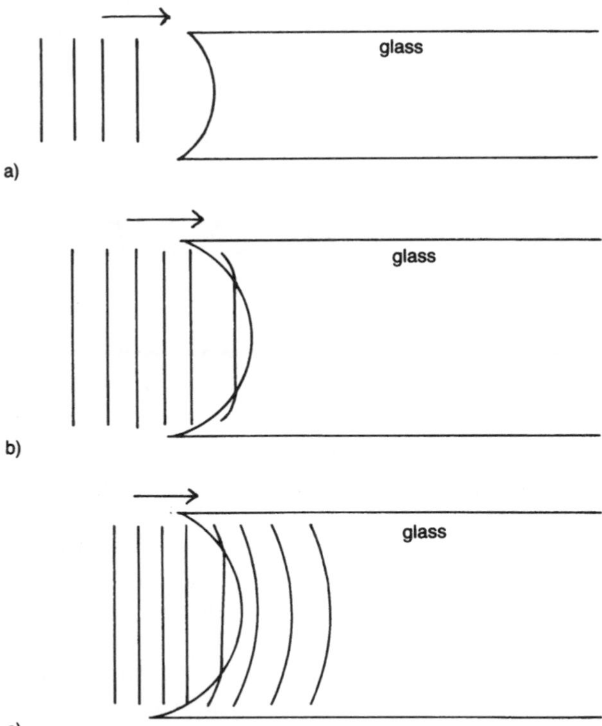

Figure 4.3 **a, Plane waves in air incident on a concave air–glass interface; b, in the glass, the edges of the wave lag behind the middle; c, the resulting diverging wavefronts in the glass.**

plane waves initially in the air are converged when passing into the glass (Figure 4.1), and plane waves initially in the glass are converged when passing into the air (Figure 4.2).

Figure 4.3 shows plane waves in air incident on a spherical glass surface in which the air bulges into the center of the glass surface. The edges of the plane waves enter the glass surface first and are consequently slowed down before the center section of the plane wave. Thus, when the entire wavefront has entered the glass, the edges are lagging behind the center. Within the accuracy of the paraxial approximation, the wavefronts in the glass are spherical diverging wavefronts.

Figure 4.4 shows plane waves in the glass incident from the opposite direction on the same spherical surface shown in Figure 4.3. Here, the middle of the wavefront enters the air first and thus speeds up first. Hence, the middle of the emerging wavefront leads the edges, so that the wavefront that emerges into the air is again diverging.

The glass surface shown in Figures 4.3 and 4.4 has the physical property such that, at its center, the air

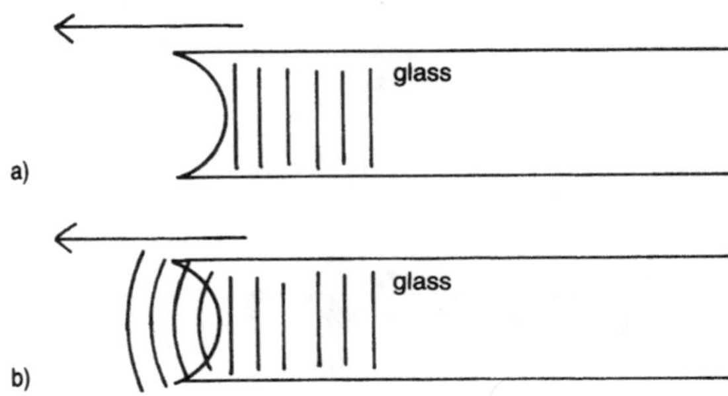

Figure 4.4 **a, Plane waves in the glass incident on the concave interface of the previous figure; b, in the air, the middle of the wavefronts leads the edges resulting in diverging waves.**

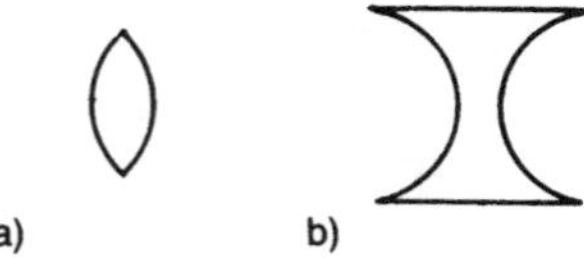

Figure 4.5 **a, A converging lens with two converging surfaces; b, a diverging lens with two diverging surfaces.**

bulges into the glass. Note that this surface diverges plane waves traveling in either direction, i.e., plane waves initially in the air are diverged when passing into the glass (see Figure 4.3), and plane waves initially in the glass are diverged when passing into the air (see Figure 4.4).

Figure 4.5a shows a converging glass lens made with two spherical surfaces. In the center, each glass surface bulges out into the air. Each of the surfaces contributes to the converging action of the lens. *A converging lens is thicker in the middle than it is at the edges.*

Figure 4.5b shows a diverging glass lens made with two spherical surfaces. In the center, each glass surface is indented so that the air bulges into the glass. Each glass surface contributes to the diverging action of the lens. *A diverging lens is thinner in the middle than it is at the edges.*

Figure 4.6 shows two more glass lenses made with spherical surfaces. In each case, the left surface of the

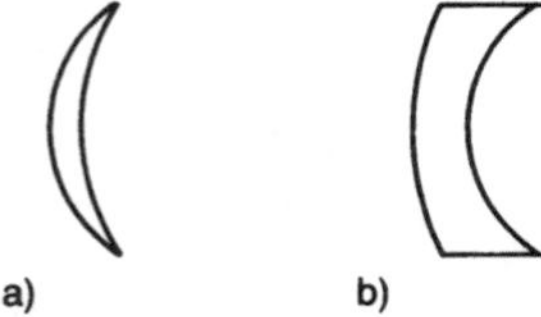

Figure 4.6 **a, A converging lens with one converging and one diverging surface; b, a diverging lens with one converging and one diverging surface.**

lens is convergent and the right surface of the lens is divergent. The net converging or diverging effect depends on the converging or diverging power of the individual surfaces. In Figure 4.6a, the converging surface (left) has more power than the diverging surface (right). Consequently, the net effect of the lens is to converge light. The tip-off that the lens in Figure 4.6a is a converging lens is that it is thicker in the middle than it is at the edges.

In Figure 4.6b, the diverging surface (right) has more power than the converging surface (left). The net effect of the lens is a diverging effect. The tip-off that the lens in Figure 4.6b is a diverging lens is that it is thinner in the middle than it is at the edges.

4.2 OPTICAL AXIS

Figure 4.7 shows a diverging lens. Each surface of the lens is spherical. The center of curvature of the left spherical surface is marked C_1, and the center of curvature of the right spherical surface is marked C_2. The dashed lines shown in Figure 4.7a complete the spheres for which C_1 and C_2 are the respective centers of curvature.

Figure 4.7b shows a straight line drawn through the centers of curvature of both spherical surfaces (i.e., through C_1 and C_2). This line is a symmetry axis for the lens. A clockwise or counter-clockwise rotation of the lens around this axis produces no change in the lens image. The line through the centers of curvature of the two spherical surfaces is called the optical axis of the lens. Figure 4.8 shows the respective centers of curvature, C_1 and C_2, for the left and right spherical surfaces of several other lenses together with the optical axis.

Whenever a line passes through the center of curvature of a sphere, it is normal to the sphere's surface. Since the optical axis passes through the center of curvature of each spherical surface of a lens, it is normal to each surface. For the diverging lenses shown in Figures 4.7 and 4.8, the optical axis passes through the thinnest portion of the lens, while for the converging lenses, the optical axis passes through the thickest portion of the lens.

The small angle approximation to Snell's law related the incident angle of a light ray to the angle of refraction of the light ray by the equation,

$$n_1\theta_i = n_2\theta_r \tag{4.1}$$

The angle of incidence θ_i and the angle of refraction θ_r are defined relative to the normal for a surface. When an incident ray is normal to a surface, the angle of incidence θ_i is zero. Therefore, from Eq. 4.1, the angle of refraction θ_r must also be zero. So a ray incident normal to a surface passes straight through the surface without bending.

Consider an incident ray lying on the optical axis of a spherical lens. The optical axis is normal to both of the surfaces, so the angles of incidence and refraction of the ray are equal to zero for both surfaces. Thus, a ray coming in along the optical axis does not bend while passing through the lens. The ray leaves the lens still traveling along the optical axis.

In order for two points to be conjugate points, any ray associated with the object point must, after passing through the lens, also be associated with the image point. Since a ray incident along the optical axis is not bent by the lens, any object point (real or virtual) lying on the optical axis has a conjugate image point that also lies on the optical axis.

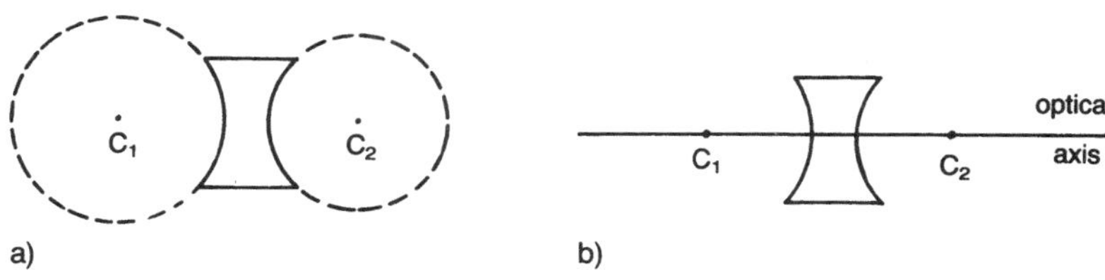

Figure 4.7 **C_1 and C_2 are the respective centers of curvature for the spherical surfaces of the lens. The optical axis is the line that passes through C_1 and C_2.**

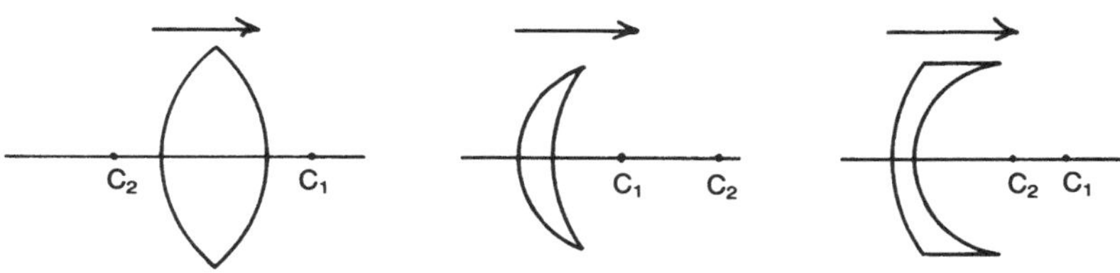

Figure 4.8 **C_1 and C_2 are the respective centers of curvature for the spherical surfaces of each lens, and the connecting line is the optical axis.**

4.3 THIN LENSES

The central thickness of the lenses discussed in the previous sections is the thickness of the lenses along the optical axis. When the central thickness of a lens is small enough, the converging and diverging properties of the lens in air are independent of the shape or form of the lens as well as the direction in which the light is traveling through the lens. In this case, the lens is called a *thin lens.* All converging thin lenses are represented by the symbol shown in Figure 4.9. Figure 4.10 shows the symbol for all diverging thin lenses.

The optical axis of a thin lens is drawn normal to the lens as shown in Figure 4.11. The point on the lens through which the optical axis passes is called the *optical center* of the lens.

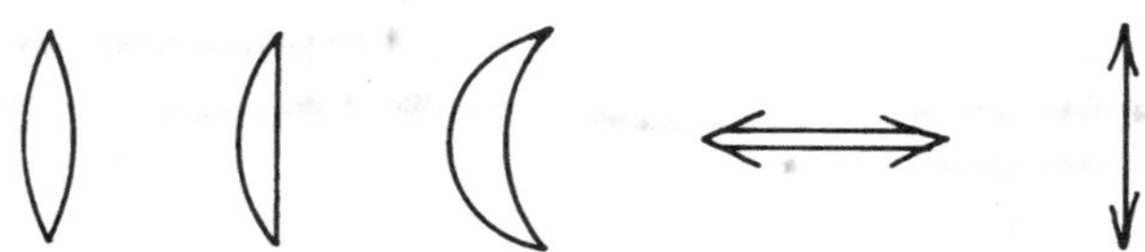

Figure 4.9 Thin converging lenses and the shape-independent representation.

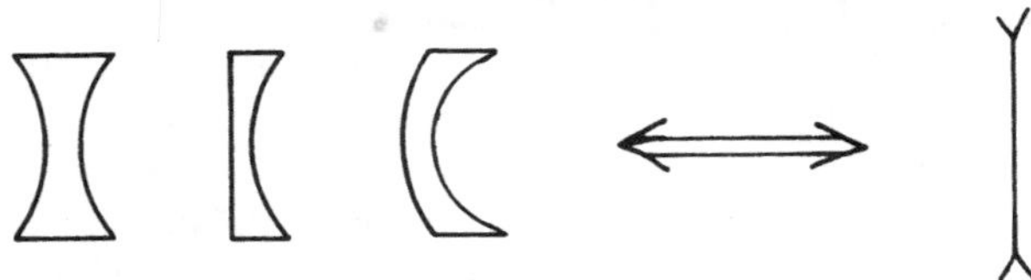

Figure 4.10 Thin diverging lenses and the shape-independent representation.

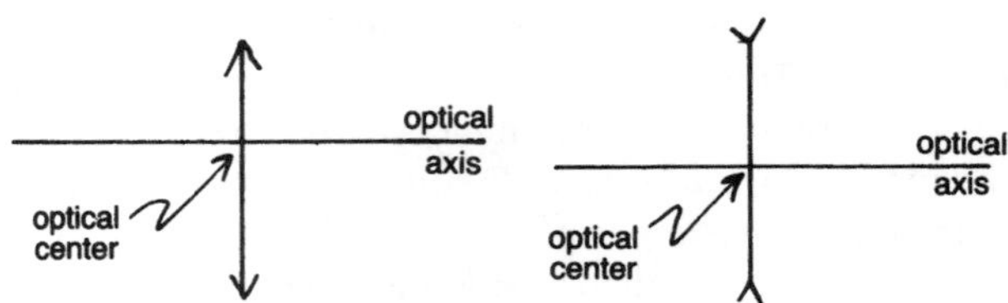

Figure 4.11 The optical center and optical axis for thin lenses.

4.4 SECONDARY FOCAL POINT (F_2)

The secondary focal point (F_2) for a thin lens is defined as the on-axis image point that results when a bundle of plane waves is incident normally on the lens. An alternative definition is that the secondary focal point F_2 for a thin lens is the on-axis image point conjugate to an on-axis object point at optical infinity. The two definitions are equivalent since the on-axis object point at optical infinity results in incident plane waves. Since an axial object point is always conjugate to an axial image point, F_2 is always located on the optical axis.

Figure 4.12 shows the situation for a thin converging lens. The wavefronts from the distant axial point source are effectively flat, or plane waves, when they reach the lens. The lens converges the light and a real image point is formed at F_2 on the axis behind the lens.

Figure 4.13 shows the situation for a thin diverging lens. The basic definition of the secondary focal point is still the same, i.e., the secondary focal point is the axial image point conjugate to an axial object point at optical infinity. Again, the waves incident on the lens from the distant axial object point are effectively flat or plane waves. The lens diverges the waves and the axial image point, F_2, is virtual and located at the

Figure 4.12 a, Plane waves incident on a converging lens resulting in waves that converge to the secondary focal point; b, wavefronts and rays; c, rays only.

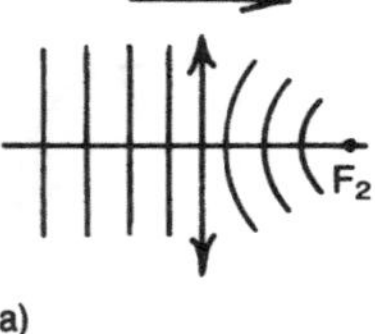

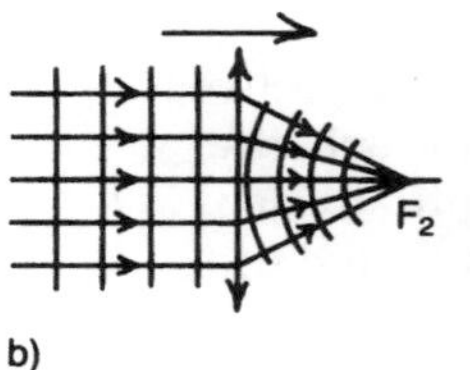

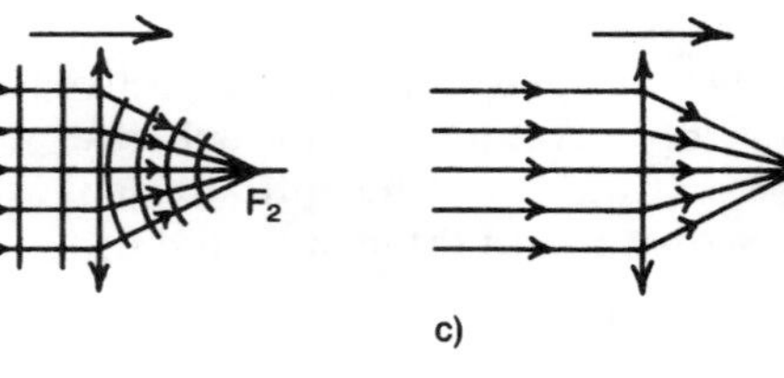

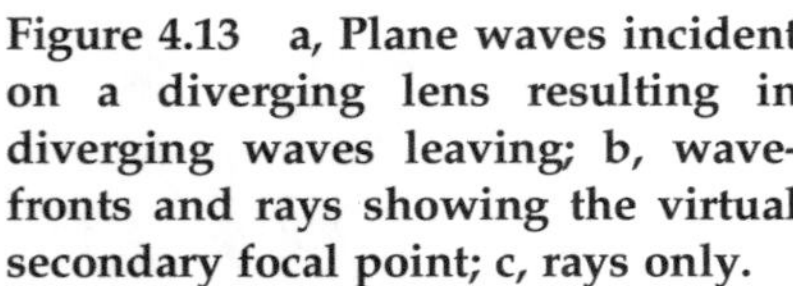

Figure 4.13 a, Plane waves incident on a diverging lens resulting in diverging waves leaving; b, wavefronts and rays showing the virtual secondary focal point; c, rays only.

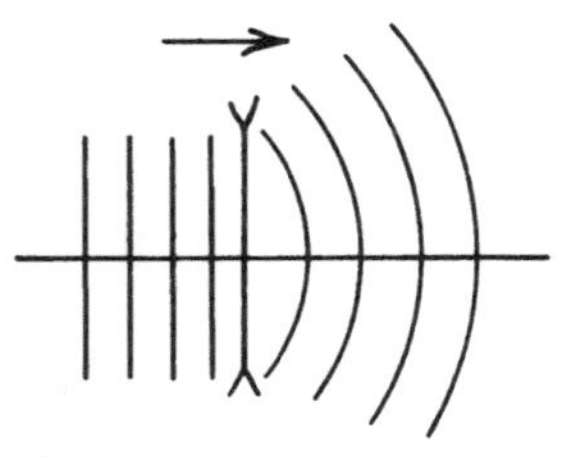

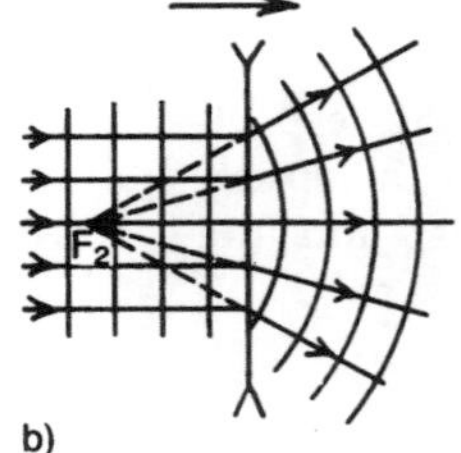

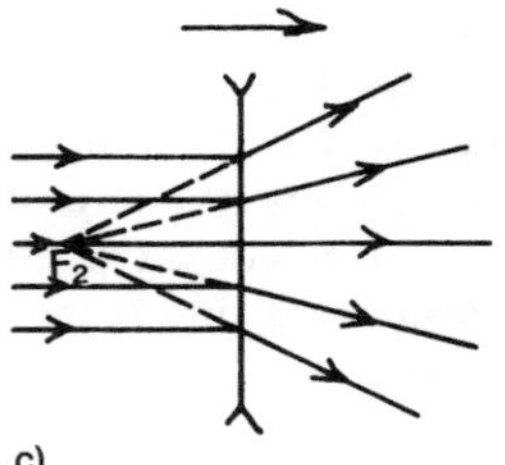

center of curvature of the exiting diverging wavefront. This position is found in Figures 4.13b and c by extending the outgoing rays back until they intersect. (The extensions are dashed.)

For incident light traveling to the right, F_2 lies to the right of a converging lens (see Figure 4.12) and to the left of a diverging lens (see Figure 4.13). However, for the diverging lens case, keep in mind that F_2 is a point in image space. F_2 is associated with the light leaving the lens (i.e., the light physically to the right of the lens) and not with the plane waves incident on the lens.

The location of F_2 relative to the lens is a measure of the converging or diverging power of the lens. A strong lens has F_2 located close to the lens, while a weak lens has F_2 located far away from the lens.

4.5 PRIMARY FOCAL POINT (F_1)

The primary focal point (F_1) is defined as the on-axis object point that results in plane waves leaving the lens. An alternative definition is that the primary focal point F_1 is the on-axis object point that is conjugate to an on-axis image point at optical infinity.

Figure 4.14 shows the situation for a thin converging lens. The wavefronts incident on the lens are diverging, while the wavefronts exiting the lens are plane waves. The rays leaving the lens are effectively parallel to each other and to the optical axis since one of the rays is traveling along the axis. Clearly, for a thin converging lens, F_1 is a real object point.

Figure 4.15 shows the situation for a thin diverging lens. In order to get plane waves to leave the diverging lens, the incident light must be converging. The object point is located at the center of curvature of the incident wavefront and is virtual. The virtual object point can be located by extending the incident rays forward until they intersect. Again, the rays representing the light leaving the lens are all parallel to each other and to the optical axis since one of the rays is traveling along the axis.

For incident light traveling to the right, F_1 lies to the left of a converging lens (see Figure 4.14) and to the right of a diverging lens (see Figure 4.15). However, for the diverging lens case, keep in mind that F_1 is a point in object space. F_1 is associated with the light incident on the lens, i.e., the light physically to the left of the lens, and not with the plane waves that are exiting the lens.

The location of F_1 relative to the lens is a measure of the converging or diverging power of the lens. A strong lens has F_1 located close to the lens, while a weak lens has F_1 located far away from the lens.

4.6 EQUIDISTANCE OF FOCAL POINTS FOR A THIN LENS IN AIR

When the central thickness of a lens in air is small enough, then the imaging properties of the lens are independent of the lens shape and of the direction the light travels through the lens. This was the thin lens assumption. Let us apply this assumption to a converging lens.

In Figure 4.16a, incident plane waves are traveling to the right and the secondary focal point, F_2, is located 10 cm to the right of the lens. In Figure 4.16b,

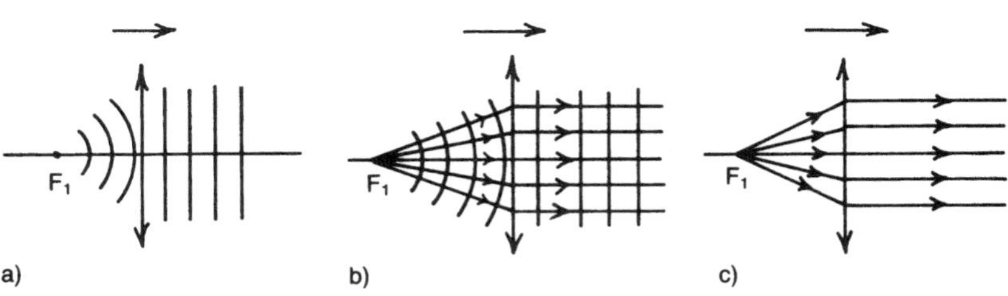

Figure 4.14 a, Wavefronts diverging from the primary focal point result in plane waves leaving; b, wavefronts and rays; c, rays only.

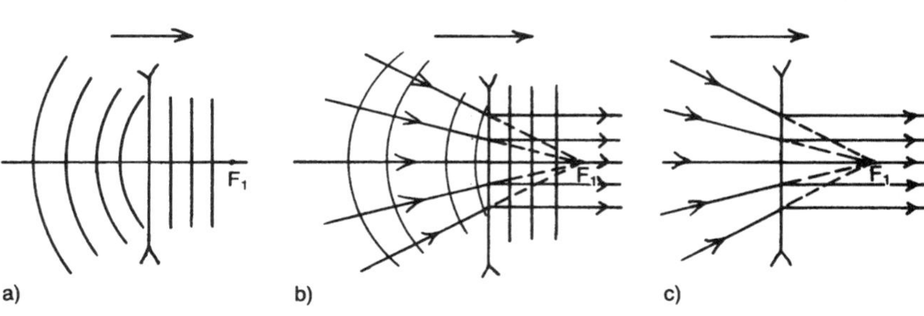

Figure 4.15 a, Converging wavefronts incident on a diverging lens resulting in plane waves leaving. The center of curvature of the incident wavefront is the primary focal point; b, wavefronts and rays; c, rays only.

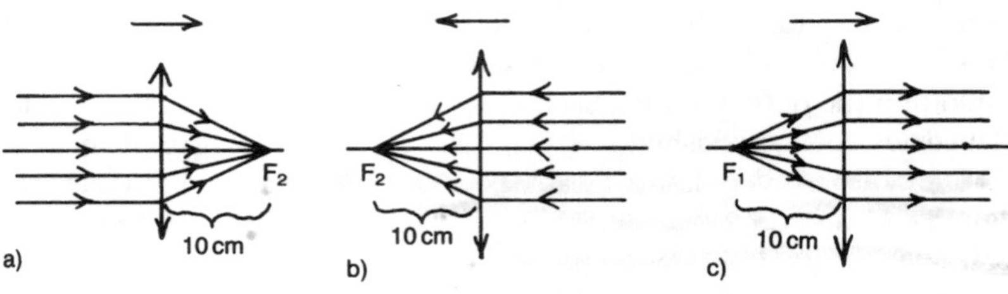

Figure 4.16 a, Plane waves incident from the left give a secondary focal point 10 cm right of the lens; b, plane waves incident from the right give a secondary focal point 10 cm to the left of the lens; c, the principle of reversibility shows that the primary focal point is also 10 cm from the lens.

plane waves incident on the same lens are traveling to the left. In this case, since the imaging properties of the thin lens in air are independent of the direction in which the light is traveling, F_2 is now located 10 cm to the left of the lens.

According to the principle of reversibility, rays travel the same path backward through a system; thus, only the direction indicators on the rays need to be changed. Figure 4.16c shows the principle of reversibility applied to Figure 4.16b. However, in the reversed situation (Figure 4.16c), the light is diverging away from the point 10 cm to the left of the lens and plane waves are leaving the lens. Consequently, the point labeled F_2 in Figure 4.16b becomes the primary focal point, F_1, for the same lens in Figure 4.16c.

Since the imaging properties of the thin lens in air are independent of the direction in which the light is traveling, then by comparing Figures 4.16a and c, one can see that the primary and secondary focal points are both 10 cm from the lens. This argument can be repeated for any focal length. Therefore, the primary and secondary focal points for any thin lens in air are always equidistant from the lens. Note the argument also shows that the primary and secondary focal points simply change places when light travels in the opposite direction through a lens.

4.7 PREDICTABLE RAYS/ CONVERGING LENSES/ OFF-AXIS OBJECT POINTS

Figure 4.17 shows the rays used in defining the primary and secondary focal points for a thin converging lens in air. The secondary focal point, F_2, is an on-axis image point conjugate to optical infinity, while the primary focal point, F_1, is an on-axis object point conjugate to optical infinity.

Figure 4.18 shows an extended object located a finite distance in front of a thin converging lens. Our initial interest is in the off-axis point at the top of the object. The figure shows some of the incident diverging rays from the top object point.

We cannot predict how most of the rays in Figure 4.18 will leave the lens. However, we can use Figure 4.17 to predict how two of the rays will leave the lens. In Figure 4.17a, the incident rays are all parallel to the axis and the exiting rays all point toward F_2. Consequently, any incident ray that is parallel to the axis will point toward F_2 when it leaves the lens. One of the incident rays in Figure 4.18 is parallel to the axis; therefore, it must point toward F_2 when it leaves the lens. Figure 4.19a shows this ray by itself, and Figure 4.19b shows this ray together with the other incident rays.

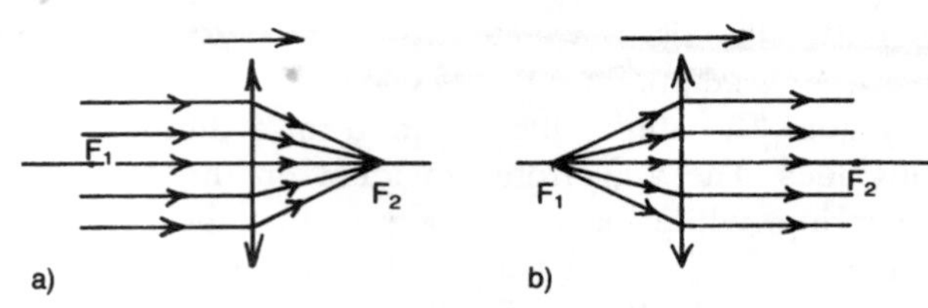

Figure 4.17 Diagrams used to predict the respective behavior of rays associated with the focal points of a converging lens.

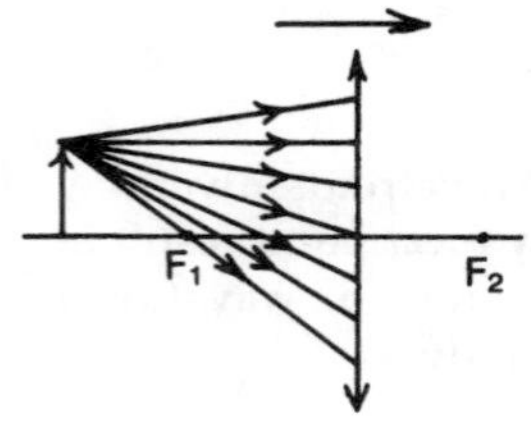

Figure 4.18 Diverging rays incident on a lens.

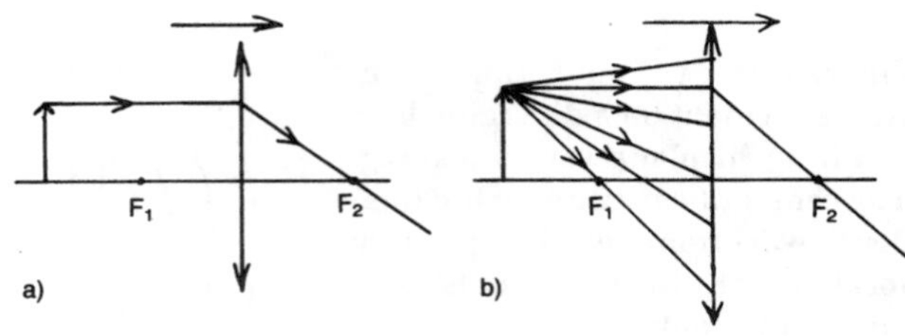

Figure 4.19 a, Isolation of the predictable ray incident parallel to the axis; b, path of predictable ray.

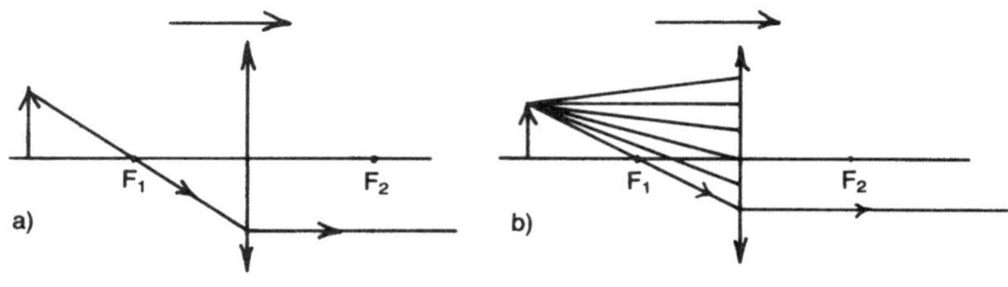

Figure 4.20 a, Isolation of the predictable ray through the primary focal point; b, path of the predictable ray.

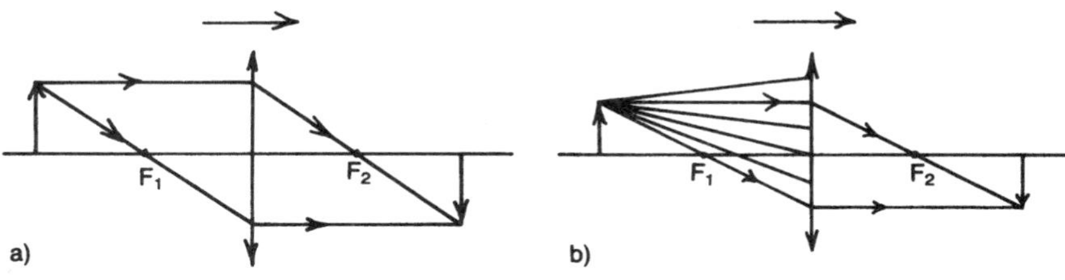

Figure 4.21 a, Isolation of the two predictable rays and resultant image location; b, predictable rays among the others.

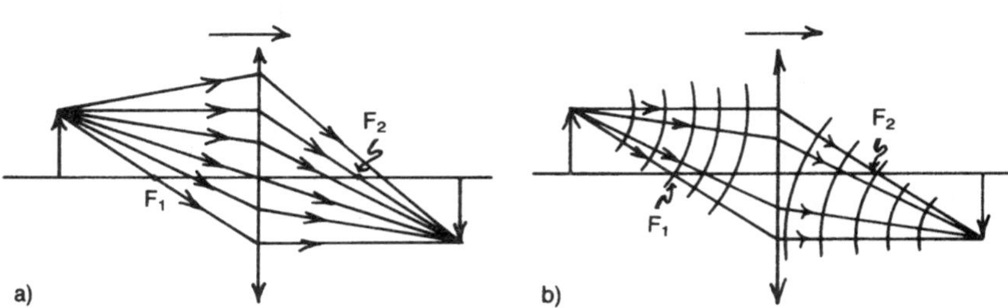

Figure 4.22 a, Once the image point is known, all exiting rays must go there; b, wavefronts and rays.

In Figure 4.17b, the incident rays all originate at F_1 and the exiting rays are all parallel to the axis. Based on Figure 4.17b, we can predict that any incident ray that, as far as the lens is concerned, appears to be coming from F_1 will leave the lens parallel to the axis. For the off-axis object point in Figure 4.18, one of the incident rays leaves the object point and passes through F_1 before hitting the lens. Hence, this ray will leave the lens parallel to the axis. Figure 4.20a isolates this ray and Figure 4.20b shows this ray together with the other incident rays.

Taken together, the two predictable rays shown in Figures 4.19 and 4.20 are sufficient to indicate whether the light leaving the lens is converging or diverging. Figure 4.21a shows an isolation of the two rays and Figure 4.21b shows the two rays along with the other incident rays.

The two exiting rays indicate that the light leaving the lens is converging. The conjugate image point is real and is located at the place where the two rays intersect. Now that the conjugate off-axis image point is located, all the other incident rays can be traced through the lens. These rays must also pass through the image point (Figure 4.22a). (Figure 4.22b also shows the incident diverging wavefronts and the exiting converging wavefronts.)

The object under discussion lies in a plane that is perpendicular to the optical axis of the lens. Under paraxial conditions, the image also lies in a plane perpendicular to the axis. Since an axial object point must be conjugate to an axial image point, we can locate the axial image point by simply drawing a perpendicular line from the off-axis image point to the axis (Figures 4.21 and 4.22).

Consider a second ray trace example for the same thin converging lens. The object is now placed between F_1 and the lens. Figure 4.23 shows some

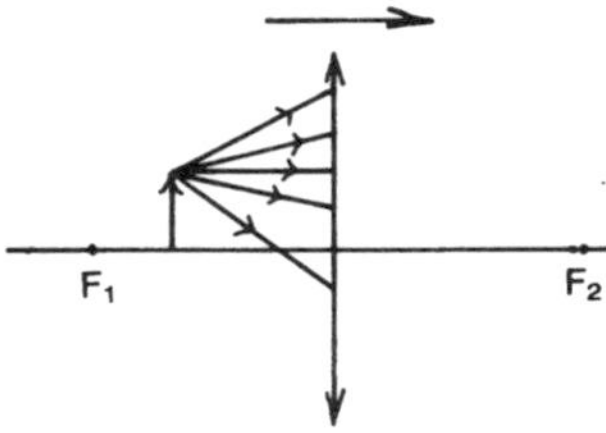

Figure 4.23 Incident rays for object inside the primary focal point.

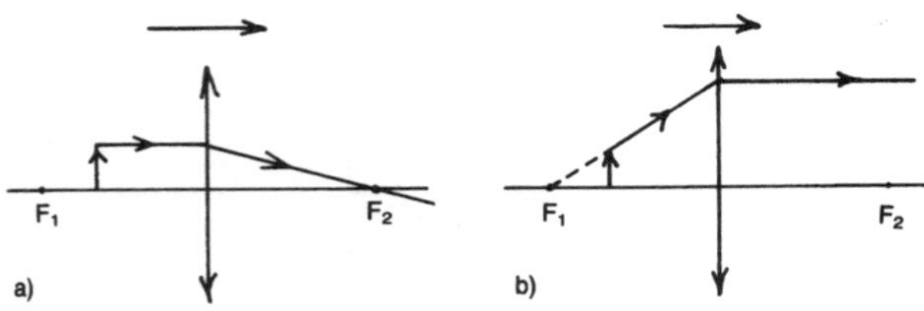

Figure 4.24 Predictable rays associated with the focal points.

incident diverging rays. Again, most of these diverging rays are not predictable. However, one of the incident rays is parallel to the axis; therefore, we can use Figure 4.17a as a guide to see that this ray must exit the lens pointing toward F_2. Figure 4.24a isolates this ray. Another of the incident rays in Figure 4.23 hits the lens and, as far as the lens is concerned, appears to be coming from F_1. We can use Figure 4.17b as a guide to see that this ray must exit the lens parallel to the axis. Figure 4.24b isolates this ray.

Figure 4.25a shows both of the predictable rays. The exiting rays indicate that the outgoing light is diverging. Consequently, the image is virtual and can be located by extending the rays backward until they intersect (Figure 4.25b). The virtual image is erect relative to the object and larger than the object. (This is an example of a simple magnifying lens.)

All of the outgoing rays must appear to be coming from the same virtual image point. So, the remaining rays can now be traced as shown in Figure 4.26a. Figure 4.26b also shows the incident diverging wavefronts and the exiting diverging wavefronts. In Figure 4.26b, the exiting wavefronts have less divergence than the incident wavefronts.

4.7.1 Instructional Comment

Ray diagrams of the type discussed can greatly aid an individual in developing optics intuition. These diagrams can be drawn to scale on graph paper, and that is sometimes necessary. However, in developing optics intuition, I believe that the main utility of ray diagrams is gained from being able to do a *quick and dirty* freehand sketch that provides the needed information. Therefore, I urge beginners to practice such sketches.

A common pitfall of some beginners is to try to memorize all the possible types of ray diagrams. Let that be anathema. I believe that one should learn to quickly draw the predictable rays and then trust the ray diagram. In this way, much less memory is required and the skill gained will tend to remain long after one's memorized results have been forgotten.

> If I give you some fish, you eat for a day.
> If I teach you to fish, you eat for a lifetime.
> —Old Chinese Proverb

4.8 NODAL RAYS

Figure 4.27 is a repeat of Figure 4.22a in which the object was located outside the primary focal point, F_1, and a conjugate real image was formed. Some of the incident rays are bent down upon passing through the lens and some of the incident rays are bent up upon passing through the lens. Between the bent-up rays

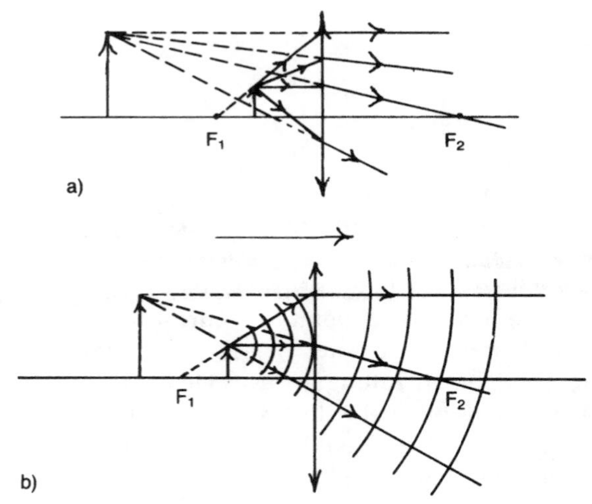

Figure 4.26 a, Ray behavior for virtual image; b, rays and wavefronts.

Figure 4.25 Virtual image location from the predictable rays: a, actual rays; b, backward extensions to locate the image.

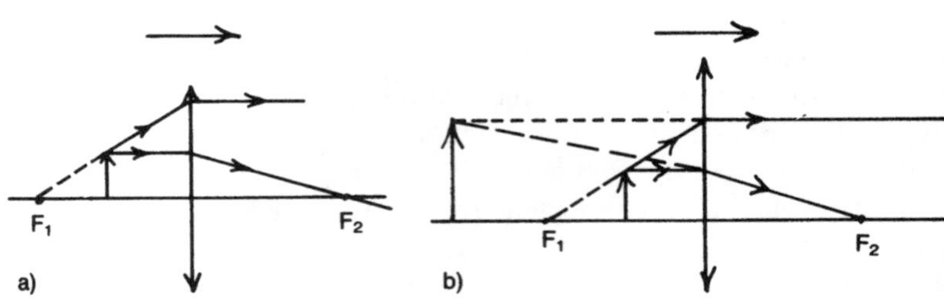

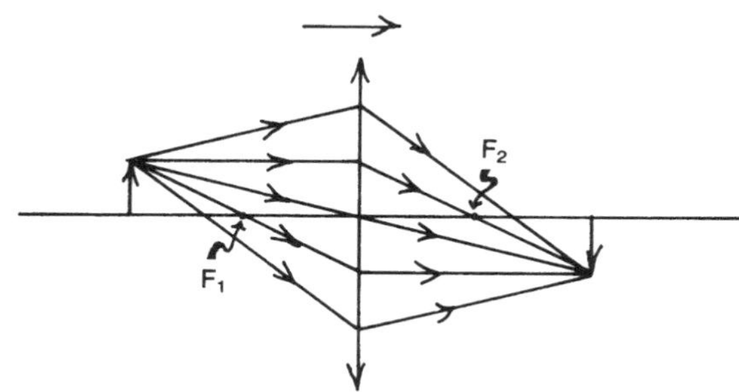

Figure 4.27 Ray diagram showing some rays bend down and other bend up, while the nodal ray passes through the optical center.

and the bent-down rays, there must be a ray that passes straight through the lens without being bent. Inspection of Figure 4.27 shows that the unbent ray passes through the lens at the same point that the optical axis passes through the lens. This point was previously named the optical center of the lens.

The latter property is a general property for thin lenses and gives us a third predictable ray to use. Namely, any ray passing through the optical center of a thin lens passes straight through without bending. The ray that does not bend is called the nodal ray, and the optical center of the thin lens is the nodal point for the thin lens.

4.9 FURTHER EXAMPLES: CONVERGING LENSES

In order to let the ray diagram convey the information intended, the following convention is used. *A ray that is actually representing light physically present at that point in space is drawn as a solid line. Extensions of the ray either forwards or backwards into regions of space where the light associated with the ray is not physically present is shown as a dashed line.*

Consider the dashed line in Figure 4.24b. There, the ray of interest left the object and was incident on the lens as if it had come from the primary focal point, F_1. The ray was drawn in solid from the object to the lens, but the extension of the ray from the object to F_1, was drawn in dashed.

In Figure 4.25a, the two exiting rays, drawn solid, are diverging. Figure 4.25b shows the backward extensions of the exiting rays in order to locate the virtual image. These extensions are dashed. The extensions are associated with the exiting light and not with the light that is physically incident on the lens.

Figure 4.28a shows a real object placed outside F_1 of the lens. The incident ray parallel to the axis is shown in Figure 4.28b, and it exits the lens pointing toward

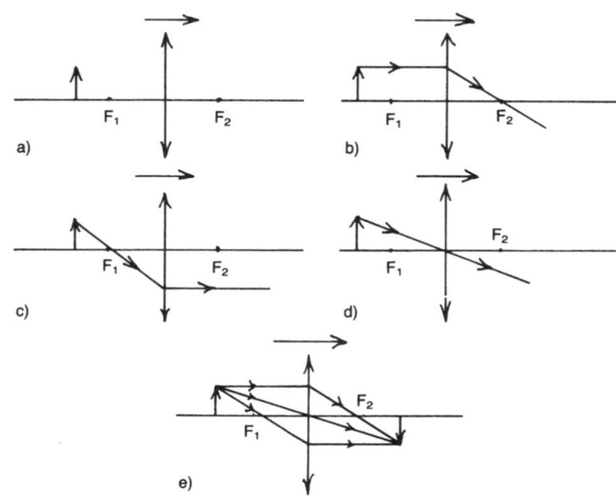

Figure 4.28 a, Object outside the primary focal point; b, predictable incident ray parallel to the axis; c, predictable ray through the primary focal point; d, predictable ray through the optical center; e, image location by the three predictable rays.

point F_2. The ray incident on the lens that passes through F_1 exits parallel to the axis as shown in Figure 4.28c. The nodal ray is shown in Figure 4.28d. Finally, all the rays are shown in Figure 4.28e.

Figure 4.29a shows converging light incident on the lens. The light has been converged by a preceding optical system, which is not shown. Since the incident light is converging, the object for the lens is virtual and the location assigned to the virtual object is at the center of curvature of the wavefront incident on the lens. The location of the virtual object is found by extending the converging rays forward until they intersect. These extensions are shown as the dashed lines.

Out of all the incident converging rays, three are predictable as discussed previously. Figure 4.29b isolates the nodal ray. Since the nodal ray passes straight through the lens without bending, it is drawn entirely as a solid line.

Figure 4.29c shows the incident ray that is parallel to the axis. This ray exits the lens pointing toward F_2. (Recall Figure 4.17a for the general behavior of incident rays that are parallel to the axis.)

Figure 4.29d shows the incident ray that passes through F_1 and exits parallel to the axis. (Recall Figure 4.17b for the general behavior of rays incident through F_1.)

Figure 4.29e shows all three of the incident predictable rays. The exiting rays, drawn solid and to the right of the lens, show that the light leaving the lens is converging and forms a real image, which is erect and smaller relative to the virtual object.

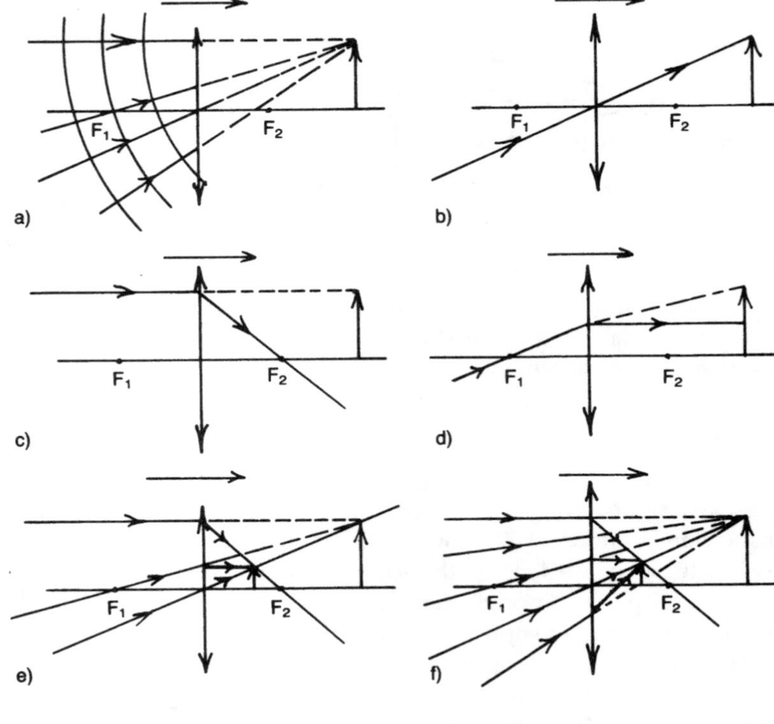

Figure 4.29 a, Converging wavefronts and rays incident on a converging lens; b, the nodal ray; c, the ray incident parallel to the axis; d, the ray incident through the primary focal point; e, image location by the three predictable rays; f, other rays.

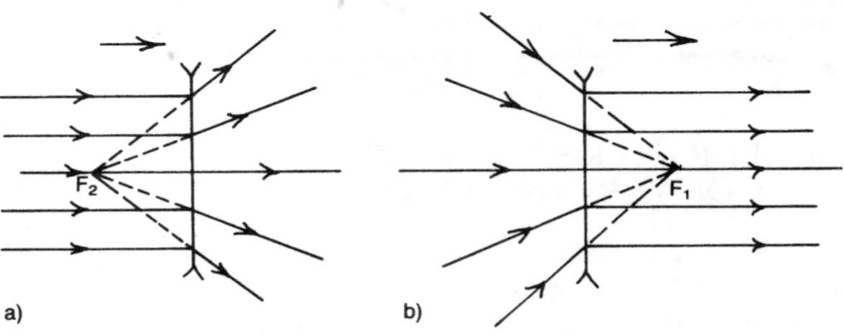

Figure 4.30 Rays associated with the primary and secondary focal points of a diverging lens.

Note that in this case, the lens took the incident converging light and converged it even more, which is what one might expect a converging lens to do. Once the conjugate image point is located, all the other incident rays can then be traced through the system. Some of these other rays are shown in Figure 4.29f.

4.10 PREDICTABLE RAYS/ DIVERGING LENSES/ OFF-AXIS OBJECT POINTS

The secondary focal point, F_2, is the axial image point that is conjugate to an axial object point at optical infinity. In other words, F_2 is the on-axis image point that results when plane waves are incident on the lens. For a thin diverging lens, F_2 is a virtual image point. Figure 4.30a shows the rays associated with F_2 for a thin diverging lens. Each incident ray parallel to the axis is bent by the lens and appears to be coming from F_2 when it exits the lens. Figure 4.30a shows that for a thin diverging lens any incident ray parallel to the axis must appear to be coming from F_2 when it leaves the lens.

The primary focal point, F_1, is the on-axis object point that results in plane waves leaving the lens. Clearly, to get plane waves leaving a diverging lens, the incident light must be converging. Thus, F_1 must be a virtual object point. Figure 4.30b shows the rays associated with F_1 for a thin diverging lens. Based on Figure 4.30b, any incident ray pointing toward F_1 of a thin diverging lens leaves the lens parallel to the axis. Remember that F_1 and F_2 are equidistant from the lens.

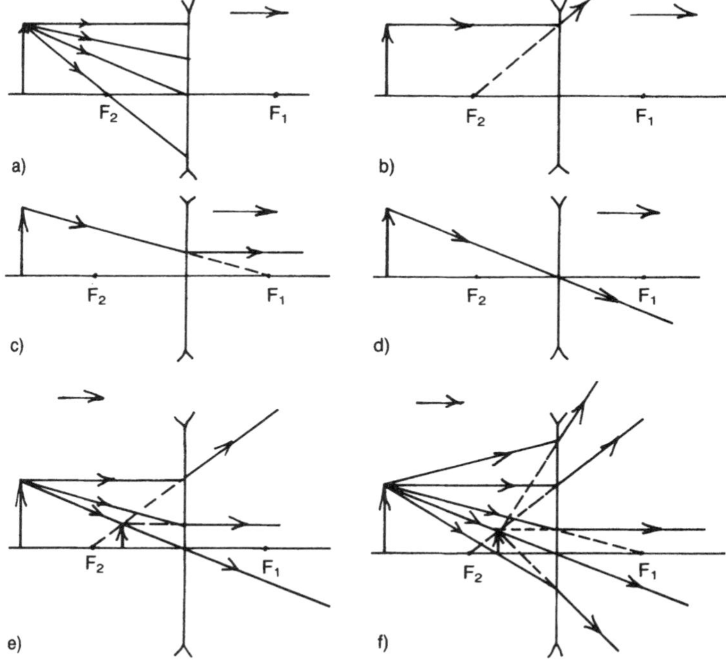

Figure 4.31 a, Diverging rays incident on a diverging lens; b, the predictable ray parallel to the axis; c, the predictable ray pointing toward the primary focal point; d, the nodal ray; e, image location by the three predictable rays; f, other rays.

Figure 4.31a shows the rays from a near extended object located in front of a thin diverging lens. Three of these rays are predictable. Figure 4.31b isolates the incident ray parallel to the axis. In accordance with Figure 4.30a, this ray appears to be coming from F_2 when it leaves the lens. Figure 4.31c isolates the incident ray that is pointing toward F_1. In accordance with Figure 4.30b, this ray leaves the lens parallel to the axis. Figure 4.31d shows the nodal ray. Figure 4.31e shows all three of the predictable rays. The exiting rays indicate that the light leaving the lens is diverging. Figure 4.31f shows that the virtual image position is located by extending the exiting rays backward until they intersect. The virtual image is erect and smaller relative to the object.

Figure 4.32 shows a case of converging light incident on a diverging thin lens. The incident light was converged by a preceding optical system, which is not shown. The location of the virtual object is at the center of curvature of the incident wavefront. The location is found by extending the incident converging rays forward until they intersect (Figure 4.32a).

Out of all the incident rays in Figure 4.32a, three are predictable. Figure 4.32b isolates the incident ray parallel to the axis. In accordance with Figure 4.30a, this ray appears to be coming from F_2 when it exits the lens. Figure 4.32c isolates the incident ray that is pointing toward F_1. In accordance with Figure 4.30b, this ray exits the lens parallel to the axis. Figure 4.32d shows the nodal ray. Figure 4.32e shows all three of the incident predictable rays with their corresponding exiting rays. The exiting rays are converging to form

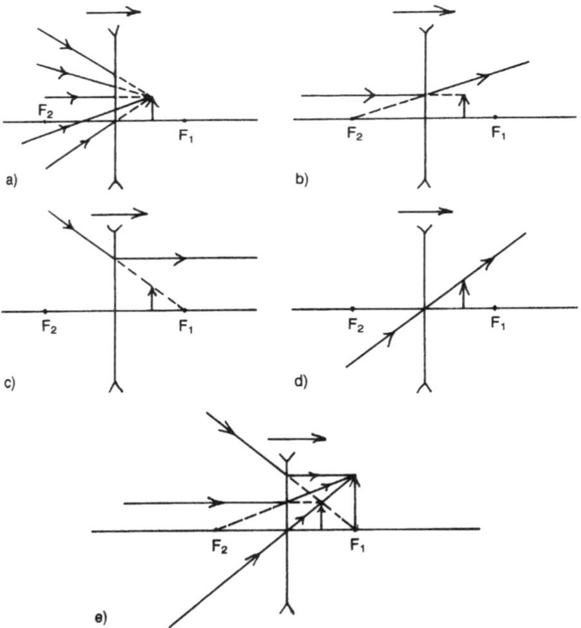

Figure 4.32 a, Converging rays incident such that the virtual object is inside the primary focal point; b, the predictable ray parallel to the axis; c, the predictable ray pointing toward the primary focal point; d, the nodal ray; e, real image location by the three predictable rays.

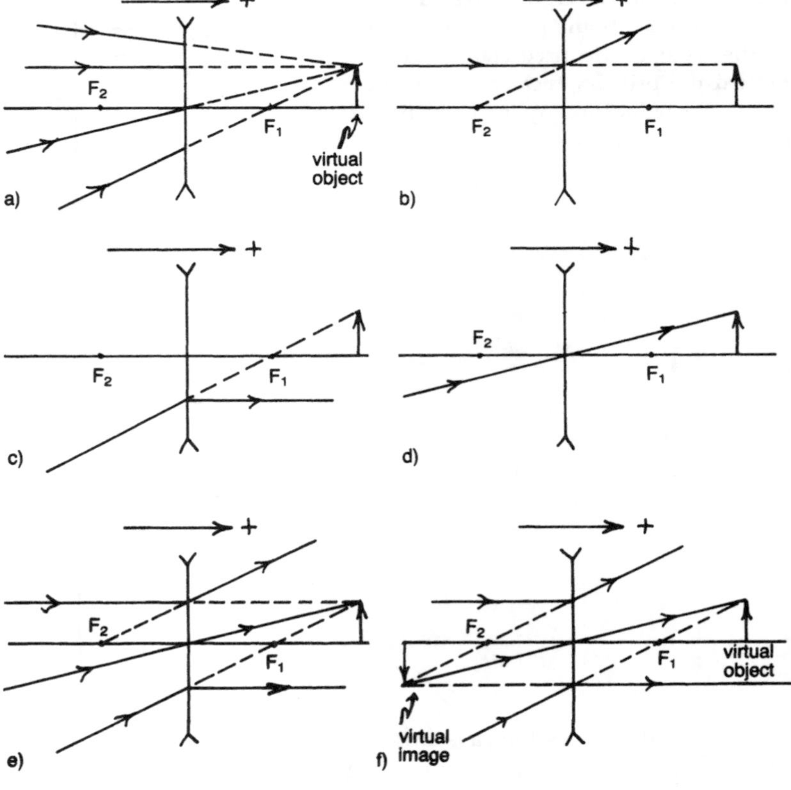

Figure 4.33 a, Converging rays incident such that the virtual object is outside the primary focal point; b, the predictable ray incident parallel to the axis; c, the predictable ray pointing toward the primary focal point; d, the nodal ray; e, the three predictable rays; f, ray extensions locating the virtual image.

a real image that is erect and larger relative to the virtual object. Note in this case that the light leaving the lens is not as convergent as the light incident on the lens.

Figure 4.33a again considers converging light incident on a diverging lens. As compared to the previous example, the incident light is less convergent. The virtual object is located by extending the incident rays forward until they intersect. Figure 4.33b isolates the incident ray parallel to the axis. This ray appears to be coming from F_2 when it leaves the lens. Figure 4.33c isolates the incident ray that is pointing toward F_1 and is parallel to the axis when it leaves. Figure 4.33d isolates the nodal ray.

Figure 4.33e shows all three of the predictable rays. The exiting rays are diverging and the image is virtual. The position of the virtual image is located by extending the exiting rays backward until they intersect as shown in Figure 4.33f. In this case, the virtual image is inverted and the same size as the virtual object. Keep in mind that the virtual image is associated only with the light physically leaving the lens (i.e., on the right in Figure 4.33f), and that the virtual object is associated only with the light physically incident on the lens (i.e., on the left in Figure 4.33f). (You might want to consider a tinted lens and color code the rays for this situation.)

4.10.1 Instructional Comment

Again, these types of ray diagrams can be done on graph paper, and that is sometimes necessary. However, I believe the greatest benefit is gained by learning to quickly draw a freehand sketch that is accurate enough to supply the needed information. The beginner should avoid memorizing these ray diagrams. Instead, by remembering the three predictable rays, one should be able to draw a ray diagram and trust the results.

4.11 COMMON FEATURES

The predictable rays involve the nodal point and the focal points. The nodal point is at the optical center of a lens for both converging and diverging lenses. When plane waves along the axis are incident on the front of a lens, the resulting image point is the secondary focal point, F_2, which is located at the center of curvature of the exiting wavefront. For light incident on the front of

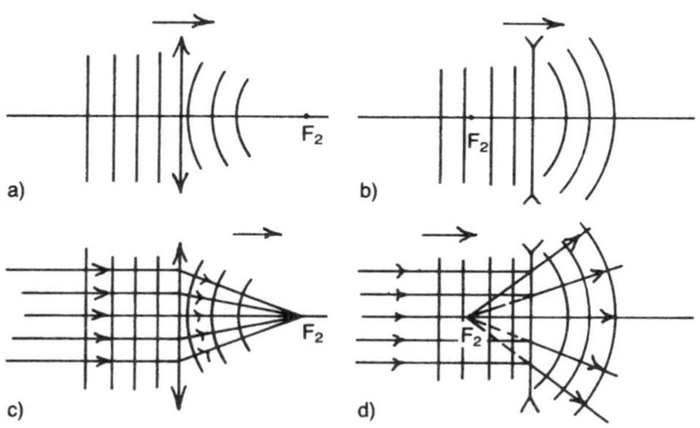

Figure 4.34 Common features of wavefronts and rays associated with the secondary focal point.

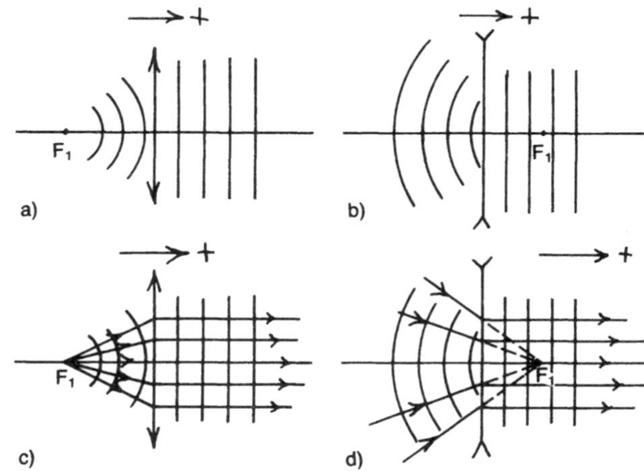

Figure 4.35 Common features of wavefronts and rays associated with the primary focal point.

a lens, the center of curvature of the exiting wavefront is behind a converging lens and in front of a diverging lens (Figures 4.34a and b, respectively). For both converging and diverging lenses, the parallel rays associated with the incident plane waves are always associated with F_2 when exiting the lens. The exiting rays point toward F_2 for a converging lens and point away from F_2 for a diverging lens (Figures 4.34c and d, respectively). In both cases, the rays are easily drawn in from the wavefront diagrams.

When plane waves leave the back of a lens, the original object point is the primary focal point, F_1. To get plane waves leaving a converging lens, the incident light waves must be diverging. To get plane waves leaving a diverging lens, the incident light must be converging. The location of the primary focal point is at the center of curvature of the incident wavefront. The center of curvature of the incident wavefront is in front of a converging lens and behind a diverging lens (Figures 4.35a and b, respectively). For both converging and diverging lenses, the parallel rays associated with the exiting plane waves are always associated with F_1 when entering the lens. The incident rays point away from F_1 for a converging lens and point toward F_1 for a diverging lens (Figures 4.35c and d, respectively). In both cases, the rays are easily drawn in from the wavefront diagrams.

4.12 SCALING OF RAY DIAGRAMS

The vertical scale on a ray diagram is frequently different than the horizontal scale. Figure 4.36 shows a case where the vertical scale spacing is 1 cm per mark and the horizontal scale spacing is 10 cm per mark. Scale differences are used so that ray diagrams are large enough to see. If the 10 cm per mark were used for both vertical and horizontal scales, the ray diagram would be squashed along the horizontal axis and the details would be hard to see. If the 1 cm per mark scale were used, the ray diagram would be too large for convenient use. The different scales enable the ray diagram to be compact with the details still visible. Note, with different scales the angles are distorted and can look large even though they are, in reality, small angles made by paraxial rays.

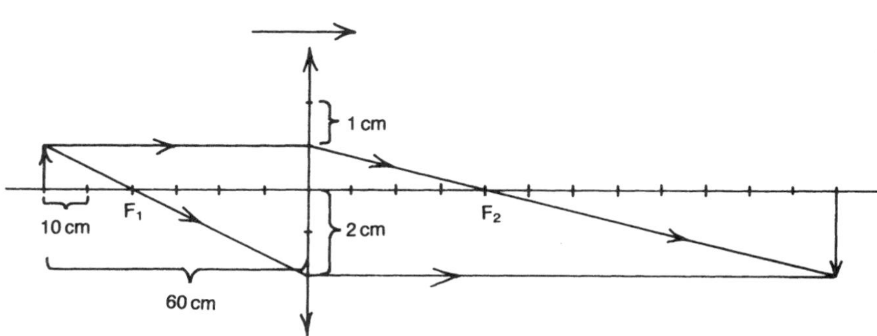

Figure 4.36 Horizontal and vertical scaling differences.

PROBLEMS

1. An extended object is midway between a converging lens and its primary focal point. Draw a ray diagram to locate the image. Is the image real or virtual, erect or inverted, larger or smaller?
2. An extended object is midway between F_1 and $2F_1$ for a converging lens. Draw a ray diagram to locate the image. Is the image real or virtual, erect or inverted, larger or smaller?
3. An extended object is at $4F_1$ for a converging lens. Draw a ray diagram to locate the image. Is the image real or virtual, erect or inverted, larger or smaller?
4. A converging lens with a secondary focal length of g has a virtual extended object located a distance g from the lens. Draw a ray diagram to locate the image. Indicate approximately the location of the image. Is it real or virtual, erect or inverted, larger or smaller?
5. For a diverging lens and a real near object, locate the image by drawing a ray diagram. Is the image real or virtual, larger or smaller, erect or inverted?
6. A diverging lens has a virtual primary focal point. Draw a ray diagram to locate the image for a virtual object located midway between the primary focal point and the lens. Is the image real or virtual, larger or smaller, erect or inverted?
7. A diverging lens has a virtual primary focal point. A virtual object is located twice as far from the lens as the primary focal point. Find the image by drawing a ray diagram. Is the image real or virtual, erect or inverted? Is the image larger, smaller, or the same size?

CHAPTER 5

Thin Lens Equations

5.1 THIN LENS VERGENCE EQUATION

The thin lens in air in Figure 5.1a has a diverging wavefront incident on it and a converging wavefront leaving it. The degree of divergence or convergence of these wavefronts at the lens is specified quantitatively by their vergence. The action of the thin lens on paraxial wavefronts can be described by a simple vergence equation:

$$V = P + U \tag{5.1}$$

where U is the vergence of the wavefront incident on the lens, V is the vergence of the wavefront exiting the lens, and P is called the *dioptric power* of the lens (Equation 5.1 is derived in Chapter 7). The dioptric power P is a characteristic of the lens and is a measure of the lens' converging or diverging power. The units of the vergence U and V are diopters, so from Eq. 5.1 the units of P must also be in diopters. P is positive for converging lenses and negative for diverging lenses.

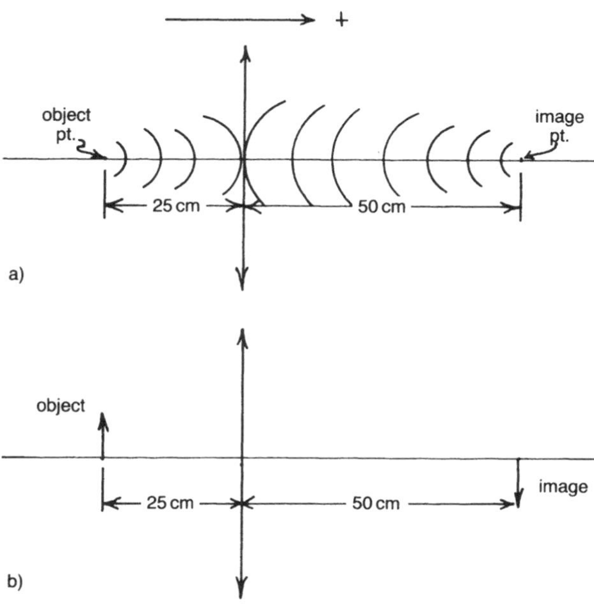

Figure 5.1 a, Wavefronts converged by a lens; b, extended real object and conjugate real image.

If the vergence U of the wavefront incident on the lens is $-4.00\,\text{D}$ and the vergence V of the wavefront exiting the lens is $+2.00\,\text{D}$, then from Eq. 5.1 the dioptric power P of the lens is

$$P = V - U$$
$$P = +2.00\,\text{D} - (-4.00\,\text{D})$$

or

$$P = +6.00\,\text{D}$$

The dioptric power of a lens does not change when the incident vergence changes. Suppose the vergence U incident on the $+6.00\,\text{D}$ lens is changed to $-9.00\,\text{D}$. Then the exiting vergence V is

$$V = P + U$$
$$P = +6.00\,\text{D} + (-9.00\,\text{D})$$

or

$$V = -3.00\,\text{D}$$

When plane waves are incident on the $+6.00\,\text{D}$ lens, U equals zero and the exiting vergence V numerically equals the dioptric power P of the lens:

$$V = P + U$$
$$V = P + 0\,\text{D}$$

or

$$V = P = +6.00\,\text{D}$$

Note that the exiting vergence depends on both the dioptric power of the lens and the incident vergence.

The exiting vergence, therefore, equals the dioptric power of the lens only when plane waves are incident on the lens.

5.2 OBJECT AND IMAGE DISTANCES

An object for a thin lens in air is labeled real or virtual depending on whether the incident light is diverging or converging. The position assigned to the object point is at the center of curvature of the incident wavefront that hits the lens. An image for a lens is labeled real or virtual depending on whether the exiting light is converging or diverging. The position assigned to the image point is at the center of curvature of the wavefront that is just leaving the lens.

Both the object point and image point can be on either side of a lens. For example, for light traveling to the right, a real object point might be 15 cm in front of the lens (to the left) while a virtual object point might be 15 cm behind the lens (to the right). A sign convention is used to distinguish between these cases.

The object distance u and image distance v are directed distances along the optical axis measured from the lens to the object and from the lens to the image respectively. The positive direction is the direction along the optical axis that the light is traveling when it leaves the lens.

In Figure 5.1a, light leaves the lens traveling to the right, which thus becomes the positive direction (indicated by the symbol, $\rightarrow +$). The image distance v, measured from the lens to the image position, is in the same direction that the exiting light is traveling and is therefore positive ($v = +50.0\,\text{cm}$). The object distance u, measured from the lens to the object position, is opposite to the direction that the exiting light is traveling and is therefore negative ($u = -25.0\,\text{cm}$).

Note that the object distance u is the radius of curvature of the wavefront incident on the lens. The vergence U of this wavefront (in diopters) equals the reciprocal of the object distance (in meters), or

$$U = \frac{1}{u} \tag{5.2}$$

The image distance v is the radius of curvature of the wavefront that is just leaving the lens. The vergence V of this wavefront (in diopters) equals the reciprocal of the image distance (in meters), or

$$V = \frac{1}{v} \tag{5.3}$$

When the distances are not expressed in meters, then conversion factors can be used in the numerator, as discussed in Section 2.5. In Figure 5.1, $u = -25.0\,\text{cm}$ and from Eq. 5.2,

$$U = \frac{100\,\text{cm/m}}{-25.0\,\text{cm}} = -4.00\,\text{D}$$

while $v = +50.0\,\text{cm}$ and from Eq. 5.3,

$$V = \frac{100\,\text{cm/m}}{+50.0\,\text{cm}} = +2.00\,\text{D}$$

These vergence values correspond to the +6.00 D lens discussed in the previous section.

In Figure 5.2, the light leaving the lens is again traveling to the right. The incident light is converging and the center of curvature of the incident wavefront is 20.0 cm to the right of the lens. The light leaving the

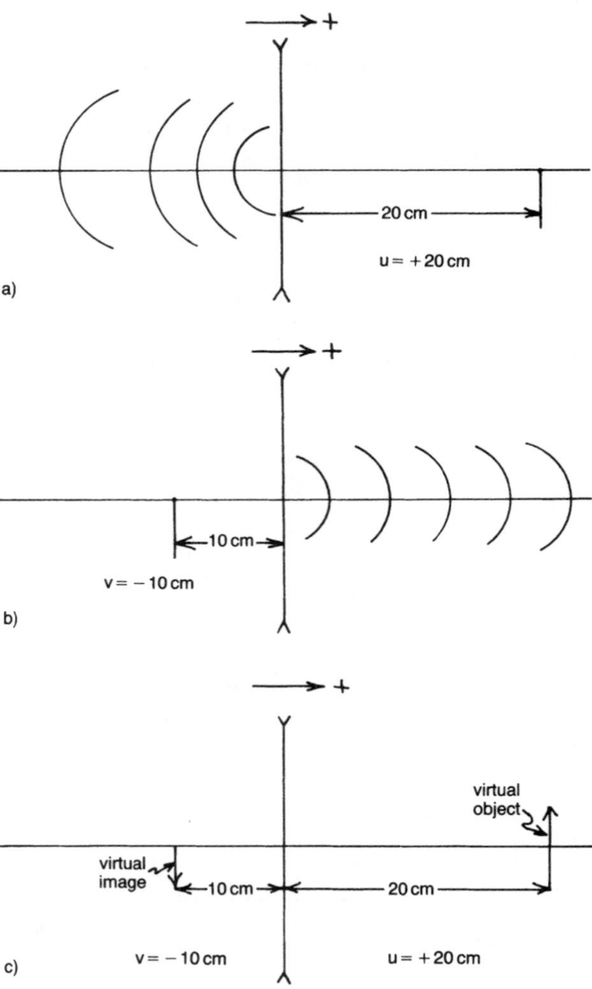

Figure 5.2 **a, Converging wavefronts incident on a diverging lens; b, diverging wavefronts leaving the lens; c, extended virtual object and conjugate virtual image.**

lens is diverging and the center of curvature of the exiting wavefront is 10.0 cm to the left of the lens. Here,

$$u = +20.0\,\text{cm}$$
$$U = \frac{1}{u} = \frac{100\,\text{cm/m}}{+20.0\,\text{cm}} = +5.00\,\text{D}$$

and

$$v = -10.0\,\text{cm}$$
$$V = \frac{1}{v} = \frac{100\,\text{cm/m}}{-10.0\,\text{cm}} = -10.00\,\text{D}$$

We can start with Eq. 5.1 and use it to find the dioptric power for this lens.

$$V = P + U$$

or

$$P = V - U$$
$$= -10.00\,\text{D} - (+5.00\,\text{D}) = -15.00\,\text{D}$$

5.3 DIOPTRIC POWER: FOCAL LENGTH RELATIONSHIPS

The secondary focal length, f_2, is a directed distance along the optical axis of a lens and is measured from the lens to the secondary focal point F_2. For plane waves incident on the lens, the image point occurs at the secondary focal point, or

$$v = f_2$$

When plane waves are incident on the lens, the incident vergence U equals zero and the exiting vergence V is equal to the dioptric power P of the lens, or

$$V = P + U = P$$

From Eq. 5.3,

$$V = \frac{1}{v}$$

By combining the above three equations

$$P = \frac{1}{f_2} \tag{5.4}$$

Equation 5.4 relates the secondary focal length (in meters) of the lens to the dioptric power (in diopters). (Some authors use Eq. 5.4 as the defining equation for dioptric power of a thin lens in air instead of the more general vergence equation, 5.1.) When the secondary focal length is expressed in units other than meters, the appropriate conversion factor can be used in the numerator.

The primary focal length, f_1, is a directed distance along the optical axis of a lens and is measured from the lens to the primary focal point F_1. When plane waves are leaving the lens, the object is at the primary focal point, or

$$u = f_1$$

For plane waves leaving the lens, $V = 0$ and from Eq. 5.1,

$$V = 0 = P + U$$

or

$$P = -U$$

From Eq. 5.2,

$$U = \frac{1}{u}$$

Then, by combining the above equations,

$$P = -\frac{1}{f_1} \tag{5.5}$$

Equation 5.5 relates the primary focal length (in meters) of the lens to the dioptric power (in diopters). When the primary focal length is expressed in units other than meters, the appropriate conversion factor can be used in the numerator.

Note, from Eqs. 5.4 and 5.5,

$$f_2 = -f_1$$

which confirms that for a thin lens in air the focal points are equidistant from and on opposite sides of the lens.

The focal lengths for the +4.00 D lens in Figure 5.3 are:

$$f_2 = \frac{1}{P} = \frac{100\,\text{cm/m}}{+4.00\,\text{D}} = +25.00\,\text{cm}$$
$$f_1 = -\frac{1}{P} = -\frac{100\,\text{cm/m}}{+4.00\,\text{D}} = -25.00\,\text{cm}$$

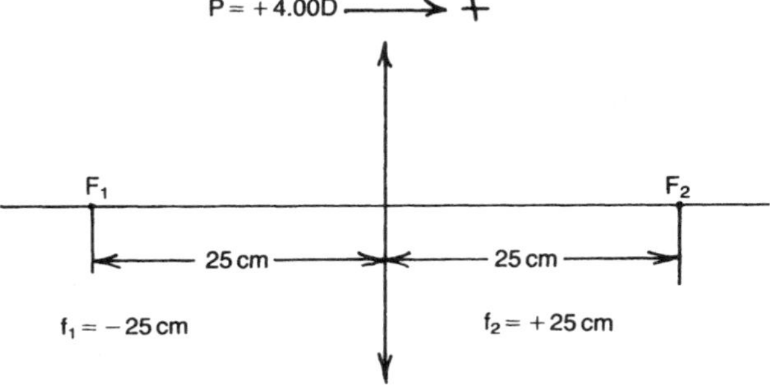

Figure 5.3 Primary and secondary focal lengths for a +4.00 D thin lens.

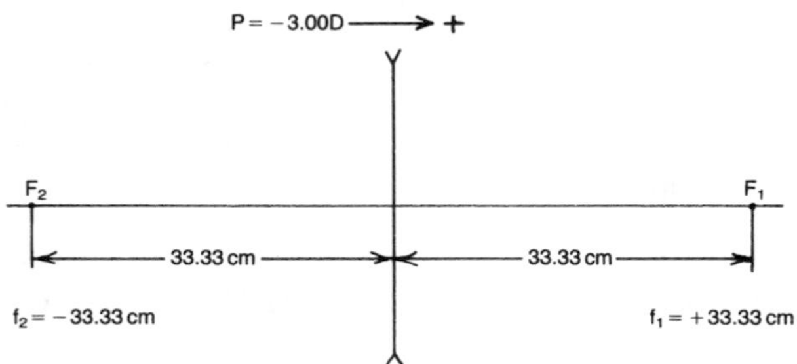

Figure 5.4 Primary and secondary focal lengths for a −3.00 D thin lens.

In this case, the focal points are both real.

The focal lengths for the −3.00 D lens in Figure 5.4 are:

$$f_2 = \frac{1}{P} = \frac{100}{-3.00\,\text{D}} = -33.33\,\text{cm}$$
$$f_1 = -\frac{1}{P} = \frac{-100}{-3.00\,\text{D}} = +33.33\,\text{cm}$$

In this case, the focal points are both virtual.

5.4 LATERAL MAGNIFICATION

The images of extended objects are typically larger or smaller than the object. The ratio of the image size to the object size is called the *lateral magnification* (m). Let O be the object size and I be the image size. Assume O is positive if the object point is above the optical axis and negative if the object point is below the axis. Similarly, assume I is positive if the image point is above the axis and negative if the image point is below the axis. Then,

$$m = \frac{I}{O} \tag{5.6}$$

A positive lateral magnification (m) indicates that the image is erect relative to the object and a negative m indicates the image is inverted relative to the object. A lateral magnification m greater than 1 indicates the image is larger than the object and an m less than 1 indicates the image is smaller than the object. Assume that the object size O is +4.0 cm and the image size I is −2.0 cm. Then from Eq. 5.6, the lateral magnification m is

$$m = \frac{-2.0\,\text{cm}}{+4.0\,\text{cm}} = -0.5$$

Figure 5.5 shows the nodal ray for a lens that has a real object and a real image. Since the nodal ray is a straight line, the angle w subtended by the object at

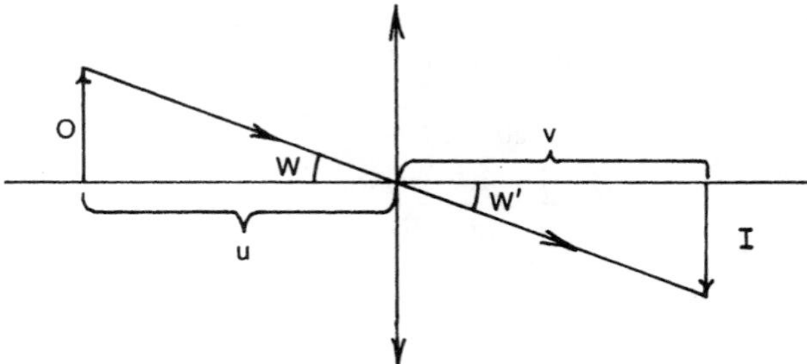

Figure 5.5 Geometry relating object and image size.

the nodal point is equal in magnitude to the angle w' subtended by the image at the nodal point. Then,

$$\tan w' = \frac{I}{v}$$

and

$$\tan w = \frac{O}{u}$$

Since $w = w'$, the above equations give

$$\frac{I}{v} = \frac{O}{u}$$

or

$$\frac{I}{O} = \frac{v}{u}$$

Therefore, from Eq. 5.6,

$$m = \frac{v}{u} \tag{5.7}$$

Equation 5.7 shows that the lateral magnification is equal to the linear ratio of the image distance to the object distance. For this reason, lateral magnification is sometimes called *linear magnification*.

Since the object and image distances are reciprocally related to the vergences U and V, we can combine Eqs. 5.7, 5.2, and 5.3 to obtain

$$m = \frac{U}{V} \tag{5.8}$$

Equation 5.8 shows that a knowledge of U and V is sufficient to compute the lateral magnification.

5.5 EXAMPLES

It is a good problem solving technique to predict what characteristics an answer should have before doing any calculations. In working these examples, I suggest that a quick ray diagram sketch initially be made. This

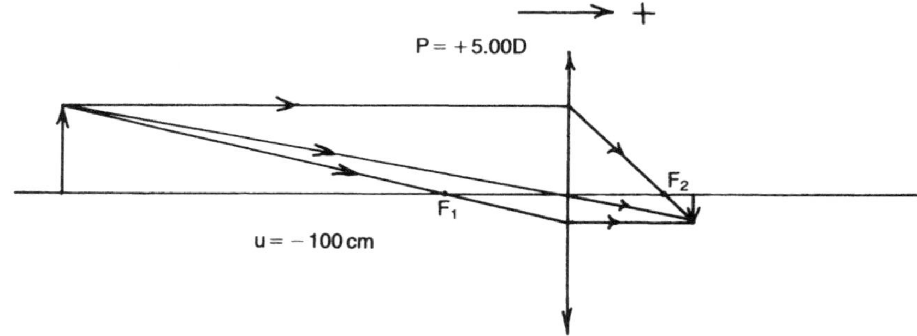

Figure 5.6 Ray diagram for a real object 100 cm in front of a +5.00 D lens.

sketch provides the predictions for what the numerical answer should be. If the answers do not correlate with the predictions, that is a tip-off that something is wrong. If this does occur, then double-check the ray diagram (might have to be more accurate this time) and the numerical calculations.

EXAMPLE 5.1

A real object is located 100 cm in front of a +5.00 D lens. Where is the conjugate image? Is it real or virtual, erect or inverted, larger or smaller?

The primary and secondary focal lengths for a +5.00 D lens are, from Eqs. 5.4 and 5.5,

$$f_2 = \frac{1}{P} = \frac{100\,\text{cm/m}}{+5.00\,\text{D}} = +20.00\,\text{cm}$$

$$f_1 = -\frac{1}{P} = -\frac{100\,\text{cm/m}}{+5.00\,\text{D}} = -20.00\,\text{cm}$$

From a ray diagram sketch (Figure 5.6), the predictions are: the image is real, inverted, smaller, and located at about 25 cm. Now, let us calculate the numbers.

$$u = -100.0\,\text{cm}$$

$$U = \frac{1}{u} = \frac{100\,\text{cm/m}}{-100\,\text{cm}} = -1.00\,\text{D}$$

The negative U value agrees with the fact that the light incident on the lens is diverging. From Eq. 5.1,

$$V = P + U$$
$$= +5.00\,\text{D} + (-1.00\,\text{D}) = +4.00\,\text{D}$$

The positive V value indicates that the light leaving the lens is converging, which agrees with the ray diagram.

$$v = \frac{1}{V} = \frac{100\,\text{cm/m}}{+4.00\,\text{D}} = +25.0\,\text{cm}$$

The image distance of +25 cm agrees well with the prediction.

$$m = \frac{U}{V} = \frac{-1.00\,\text{D}}{+4.00\,\text{D}} = -0.25$$

The lateral magnification of −0.25 indicates that the image is inverted and 0.25 times as large as the object. Both items agree with the ray diagram.

EXAMPLE 5.2

A real object is placed 30 cm from a +5.00 D lens. Is the conjugate image real or virtual, erect or inverted, larger or smaller? What is the image distance? (You might try this example yourself before looking at the solution.)

The focal points for the +5.00 D lens are 20.0 cm away as found in Example 5.1. From a ray diagram sketch (Figure 5.7), the predictions are that the image is real, inverted, larger, and about 60 cm from the lens. The calculations follow:

$$u = -30.0\,\text{cm}$$

$$U = \frac{1}{u} = \frac{100}{-30\,\text{cm}} = -3.33\,\text{D}$$

The negative U value agrees with the fact that the light incident on the lens is diverging.

$$V = P + U$$
$$= +5.00\,\text{D} + (-3.33\,\text{D}) = +1.67\,\text{D}$$

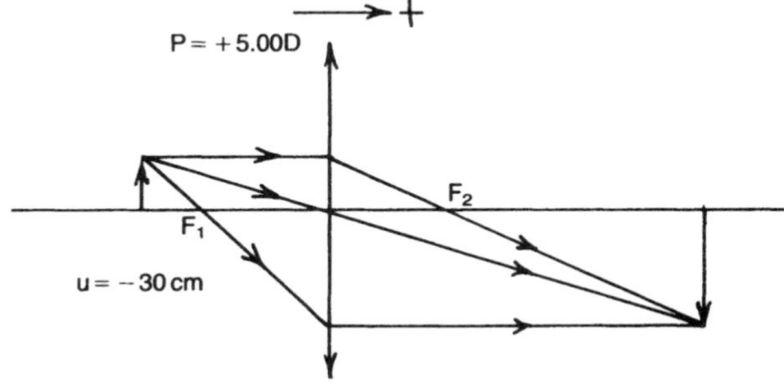

Figure 5.7 Ray diagram for a real object 30 cm in front of +5.00 D lens.

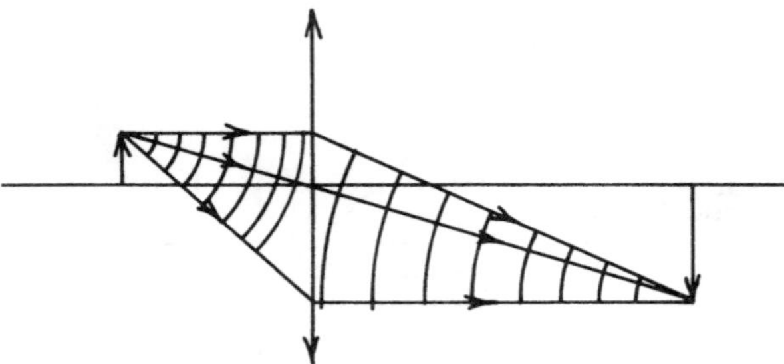

Figure 5.8 Wavefronts for Figure 5.7. Vergence values can be calculated for any of the wavefronts.

The positive V value indicates that the light leaving the lens is converging, which agrees with the ray diagram.

$$v = \frac{1}{V} = \frac{100}{+1.67\,\text{D}} = +60.0\,\text{cm}$$

The image distance also agrees with the ray diagram.

$$m = \frac{U}{V} = \frac{-3.33\,\text{D}}{+1.67\,\text{D}} = -2.0$$

The lateral magnification indicates that the image is inverted and twice as large as the object. Note that the lateral magnification can also be calculated from Eq. 5.7:

$$m = \frac{v}{u} = \frac{+60\,\text{cm}}{-30\,\text{cm}} = -2.0$$

The vergence U incident on the lens is −3.33 D. The vergence V leaving the lens is +1.67 D. The wavefronts are shown in Figure 5.8. It is instructive to calculate the vergence of the light at places other than the lens. For example, what is the vergence of the light at a point 40 cm behind the lens?

All of the wavefronts leaving the lens are spherical and have their centers of curvature at the image point. The image point is 60 cm behind the lens, so the wavefront 40 cm behind the lens is 20 cm from the image point and so has a radius of curvature of 20 cm. Therefore, the vergence of the wavefront 40 cm behind the lens is +5.00 D (i.e., 100/20 cm).

What is the vergence of the light at a point 5 cm in front of the lens? All of the wavefronts incident on the lens are diverging and have their centers of curvature located at the object point. The object point is 30 cm in front of the lens. Therefore, the wavefront 5 cm in front of the lens is 25 cm from the object point and has a vergence of −4.00 D.

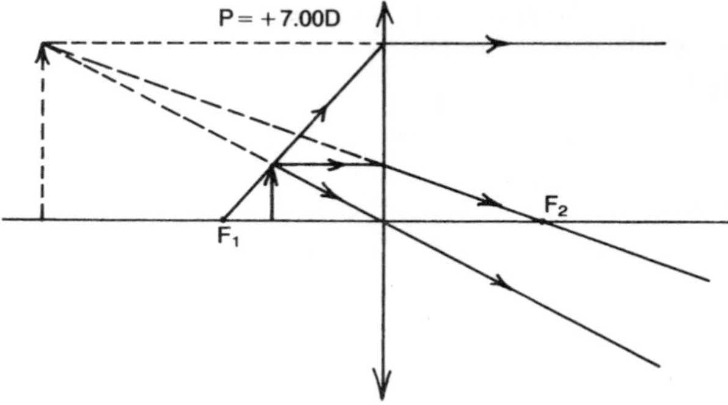

Figure 5.9 Ray diagram for real object 10 cm in front of a +7.00 D lens.

EXAMPLE 5.3

A real object is placed 10 cm in front of a +7.00 D lens. Is the image real or virtual, larger or smaller, erect or inverted? What is the image distance? (Again, try this example yourself before looking at the solution.)

The focal lengths for a +7.00 D lens are:

$$f_2 = \frac{1}{P} = \frac{100}{+7.00\,\text{D}} = +14.3\,\text{cm}$$

$$f_1 = -\frac{1}{P} = -\frac{100}{+7.00\,\text{D}} = -14.3\,\text{cm}$$

From a ray diagram sketch (Figure 5.9), the predictions are that the image is virtual, erect, larger, and the image distance is about 30 cm in magnitude. The calculations follow:

$$u = -10\,\text{cm}$$

$$U = \frac{1}{u} = \frac{100}{-10.0\,\text{cm}} = -10.00\,\text{D}$$

The negative U value agrees with the fact that the light incident on the lens is diverging.

$$V = P + U$$
$$= +7.00\,\text{D} + (-10.00\,\text{D}) = -3.00\,\text{D}$$

The negative V value indicates that the light leaving the lens is diverging, which agrees with the ray diagram. Then,

$$v = \frac{1}{V} = \frac{100}{-3.00\,\text{D}} = -33.33\,\text{cm}$$

$$\text{m} = \frac{U}{V} = \frac{-10\,\text{D}}{-3\,\text{D}} = +3.33$$

The lateral magnification indicates that the image is erect relative to the object and 3.33 times larger than the object. Note that in this case the light leaving the converging lens is

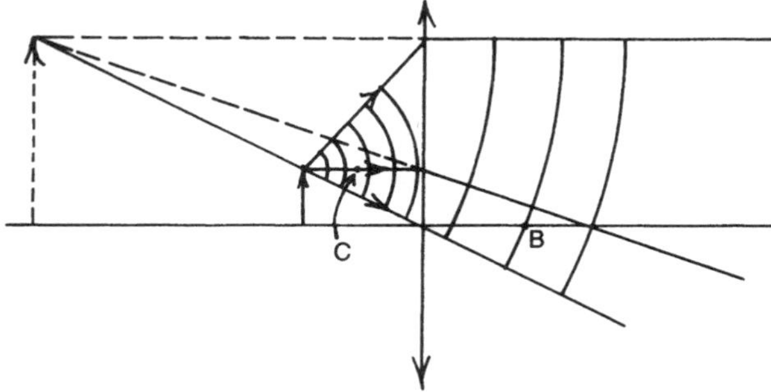

Figure 5.10 Wavefronts for Figure 5.9. *C* and *B* show positions for vergence values in front of and behind the lens, respectively.

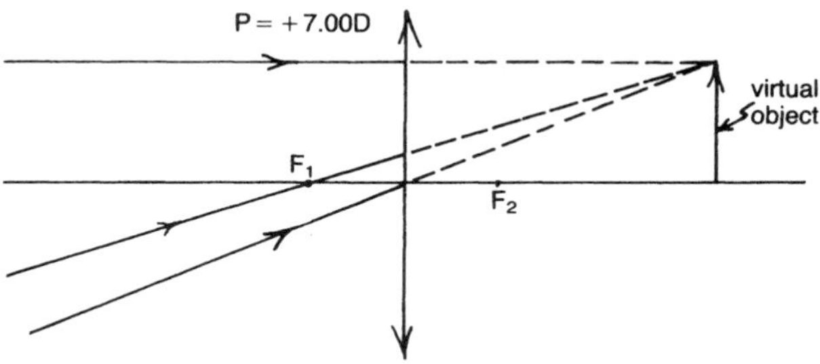

Figure 5.11 Incident rays for a virtual object located 50 cm from a +7.00 D lens.

diverging (−3.00 D) but not as divergent as the incident light ($U = -10.00$ D). A plus lens used as a magnifying lens works like this.

Let us consider the vergence of light at a point *B* that is 10 cm behind the lens. The diverging wavefront just leaving the lens has a radius of 33.3 cm (Figure 5.10). All the other diverging wavefronts behind the lens are further from the virtual image, so their radii will be greater than 33.3 cm. Therefore, the radius of the wavefront at point B is 43.3 cm and the vergence of the wavefront is:

$$V_B = \frac{100}{-43.3\,\text{cm}} = -2.31\,\text{D}$$

Note that the vergence of the wavefront leaving the lens was −3.00 D and that the vergence 10 cm behind the lens is −2.31 D.

What is the vergence of light at a point *C* that is 6 cm in front of the lens? The center of curvature of all the diverging wavefronts incident on the lens is at the real object that is 10 cm in front of the lens. Since point *C* is 6 cm in front of the lens, then point *C* is 4 cm from the object. Therefore, the wavefront at *C* has a vergence of −25.00 D. Note that the vergence of the wavefront incident on the lens was −10.00 D and that the vergence 6 cm in front of the lens is −25.00 D.

EXAMPLE 5.4

A virtual object is located 50 cm from a +7.00 D lens. Is the conjugate image real or virtual, larger or smaller, erect or inverted? What is the image distance?

The virtual object means that the incident light is converging and the center of curvature of the incident converging wavefront is located 50 cm behind the lens (Figure 5.11). The focal points are located 14.3 cm from the +7.00 D lens (Example 5.3). From a ray diagram sketch (Figure 5.12), the predictions are that the image is real, erect, smaller, and located at about 10 cm. The calculations follow:

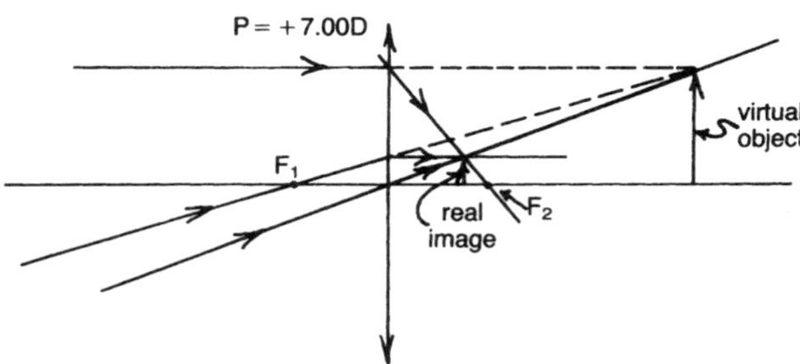

Figure 5.12 Real image location for the Figure 5.11.

$$u = +50\,\text{cm}$$

Light leaves the lens going to the right. The positive object distance agrees with this since the positive direction is the direction in which the light is traveling when it leaves the lens.

$$U = \frac{100}{+50\,\text{cm}} = +2.00\,\text{D}$$

Here is the best place to check for signs. Since the incident light is converging, *U* must be positive, otherwise something is wrong.

$$\begin{aligned} V &= P + U \\ &= +7.00\,\text{D} + (+2.00\,\text{D}) = +9.00\,\text{D} \end{aligned}$$

The positive *V* value indicates that the light leaving the lens is converging, which agrees with the ray diagram.

$$v = \frac{1}{V} = \frac{100}{+9.00\,\text{D}} = +11.1\,\text{cm}$$

$$m = \frac{U}{V} = \frac{+2\,\text{D}}{+9\,\text{D}} = +0.22$$

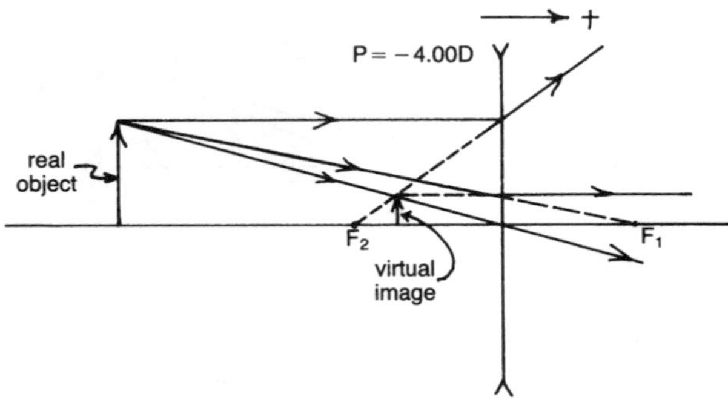

Figure 5.13 Ray diagram for a real object 50 cm in front of a −4.00-D lens.

The lateral magnification indicates that the image is erect and only 0.22 times as large as the object. This agrees with our ray diagram. In this example, the incident light is already converging ($U = +2.00$ D), and the lens converges it even more ($V = +9.00$ D).

EXAMPLE 5.5

A real object is located 50 cm in front of a −4.00 D lens. Is the conjugate image real or virtual, larger or smaller, erect or inverted? What is the image distance?

The primary and secondary focal lengths for the −4.00 D lens are:

$$f_2 = \frac{1}{P} = \frac{100}{-4.00\,\text{D}} = -25.0\,\text{cm}$$
$$f_1 = -\frac{1}{P} = \frac{-100}{-4.00\,\text{D}} = +25.0\,\text{cm}$$

Remember that for a minus lens, the focal points are both virtual and F_2 is located in front of the lens. From a ray diagram sketch (Figure 5.13), the predictions are that the image is virtual, erect, smaller, and located at about 15 cm. The calculations follow:

$$u = -50\,\text{cm}$$

Light leaves the lens going to the right. The negative object distance agrees with this since the positive direction is the direction in which the light is traveling when it leaves the lens.

$$U = \frac{100}{-50\,\text{cm}} = -2.00\,\text{D}$$

The negative U value agrees with the fact that the light incident on the lens is diverging.

$$V = P + U$$
$$= -4.00\,\text{D} + (-2.00\,\text{D}) = -6.00\,\text{D}$$

The negative V value indicates that the light leaving the lens is diverging, which agrees with the ray diagram.

$$v = \frac{1}{V} = \frac{100}{-6.00\,\text{D}} = -16.7\,\text{cm}$$
$$m = \frac{U}{V} = \frac{-2\,\text{D}}{-6\,\text{D}} = +0.33$$

The lateral magnification indicates that the image is erect and 0.33 times smaller than the object. In this case, the lens took the incident light ($U = -2.00$ D) and diverged it even more ($V = -6.00$ D).

EXAMPLE 5.6

A virtual object is located 8 cm from a −4.00 D lens. Where is the conjugate image? What is the lateral magnification? Is the image real or virtual? (Remember, you should try this first yourself.)

The focal points are virtual and 25 cm from the lens (Example 5.5). The virtual object means that the incident light is converging and the center of curvature of the incident converging wavefront is located 8 cm behind the lens. From a ray diagram sketch (Figure 5.14), the predictions are that the image is real, erect, larger, and located at about 12 cm. The calculations follow:

$$u = +8\,\text{cm}$$
$$U = \frac{100}{+8\,\text{cm}} = +12.50\,\text{D}$$

The positive U value agrees with the fact that the light incident on the lens is converging.

$$V = P + U$$
$$V = -4.00\,\text{D} + (+12.50\,\text{D}) = +8.50\,\text{D}$$

The positive V value indicates that the light leaving the lens is converging, which agrees with the ray diagram.

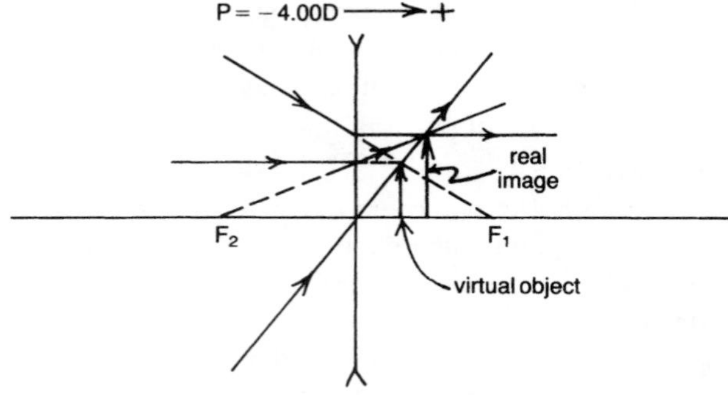

Figure 5.14 Ray diagram for a virtual object located 8 cm from a −4.00 D lens.

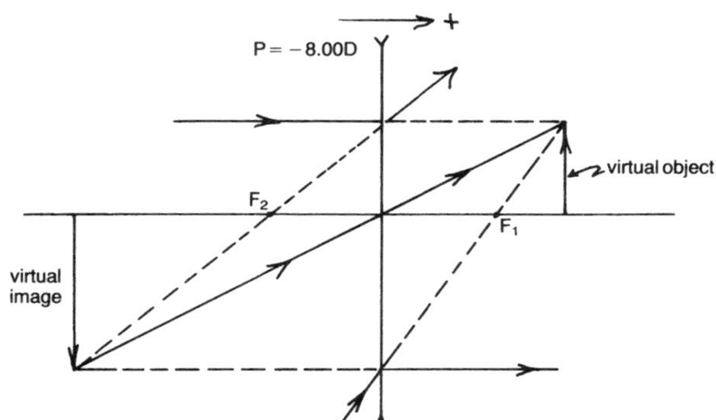

Figure 5.15 Ray diagram for a virtual object located 20 cm from a −8.00 D lens.

$$v = \frac{1}{V} = \frac{100}{+8.50\,\text{D}} = +11.8\,\text{cm}$$
$$m = \frac{U}{V} = \frac{+12.50\,\text{D}}{+8.50\,\text{D}} = +1.47$$

The lateral magnification indicates that the image is erect and 1.47 times larger than the object.

EXAMPLE 5.7

A virtual object is located 20 cm from a −8.00 D lens. Is the conjugate image real or virtual, erect or inverted, larger or smaller? What is the image distance?

The primary and secondary focal lengths for the −8.00 D lens are:

$$f_2 = \frac{1}{P} = \frac{100}{-8.00\,\text{D}} = -12.5\,\text{cm}$$
$$f_1 = -\frac{1}{P} = \frac{-100}{-8.00\,\text{D}} = +12.5\,\text{cm}$$

Again, the virtual object means that the incident light is converging and the center of curvature of the incident converging wavefront is located 20 cm behind the lens (see Figure 5.11).

From the ray diagram sketch (Figure 5.15), the predictions are that the image is virtual, inverted, larger, and the image distance is about 30 cm. The calculations follow:

$$u = +20\,\text{cm}$$
$$U = \frac{100}{+20\,\text{cm}} = +5.00\,\text{D}$$

The positive U value agrees with the fact that the light incident on the lens is converging.

$$V = P + U$$
$$= -8.00\,\text{D} + (+5.00\,\text{D}) = -3.00\,\text{D}$$

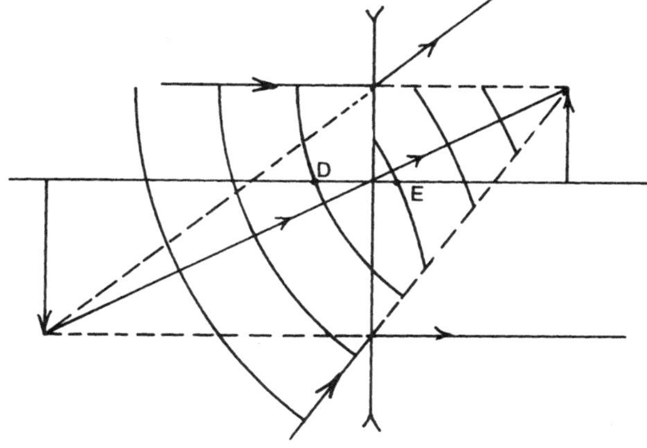

Figure 5.16 Wavefronts for vergence calculations at positions in front of or behind the lens (*D* and *E* respectively).

The negative V value indicates that the light leaving the lens is diverging, which agrees with the ray diagram.

$$v = \frac{1}{V} = \frac{100}{-3.00\,\text{D}} = -33.3\,\text{cm}$$
$$m = \frac{U}{V} = \frac{+5\,\text{D}}{-3\,\text{D}} = -1.67$$

The lateral magnification indicates that the image is inverted and 1.67 times larger than the object.

What is the vergence at a point D that is 5 cm in front of the lens and at a point E that is 5 cm behind the lens (Figure 5.16)? The light in front of the lens is converging. Each incident wavefront has its center of curvature at the virtual object position 20 cm behind the lens. So, the wavefront at point D has a radius of curvature of 25 cm. Its vergence is

$$U_D = \frac{100}{+25\,\text{cm}} = +4.00\,\text{D}$$

Note that this wavefront with a vergence of +4.00 D at a point 5 cm in front of the lens has a vergence of +5.00 D when it hits the lens. Also note that the dashed rays associated with the virtual image do not have anything to do with the incident light. These dashed rays are in image space because they are associated only with the light leaving the lens.

The light behind the lens is diverging, and each wavefront has its center of curvature located at the virtual image position 33.3 cm in front of the lens. So, the radius of curvature of the wavefront at point E is 38.3 cm (i.e., 33.3 cm + 5 cm). The vergence is

$$V_E = \frac{100}{-38.3\,\text{cm}} = -2.61\,\text{D}$$

Note that the diverging wavefront leaving the lens has a vergence of −3.00 D and at a point 5 cm downstream it has a vergence of −2.61 D.

5.6 BOUNDARY ROLE OF THE FOCAL POINTS

Besides the conjugate relationship of the focal points with optical infinity and the use of the focal points in drawing predictable rays, the focal points also serve as boundaries in the imaging process. Consider a real object located in front of a converging lens of dioptric power P. When the object is between optical infinity and the primary focal point F_1, then the negative vergence U of the incident diverging wavefront is not enough to overcome the positive dioptric power P. The vergence V of the wavefront leaving the lens is positive, the light leaving is converging, and the resulting real image is a finite distance behind the lens. When the real object is at F_1, then plane waves leave the lens, V is zero, and the image is at optical infinity. When the real object is between F_1 and the lens, the negative incident vergence U is great enough to overcome the positive dioptric power P. The exiting vergence V is negative, the light leaving is diverging, and the resulting virtual image is located a finite distance in front of the lens. (I suggest that you make some quick ray diagrams to check the above assertions.)

In the case of a virtual object for the converging lens, the incident light is converging and U is positive. Then, from $V = P + U$, V is always greater than P; and from the reciprocal relations $v = 1/V$ and $f_2 = 1/P$, the image distance v is less than the secondary focal length f_2. As a result, the real image is trapped between the lens and the secondary focal point F_2.

A real object in front of a diverging lens always results in diverging light leaving the lens. In the equation $V = P + U$, P and U are both negative, so V is more negative than P. Again, from the reciprocal relations $v = 1/V$ and $f_2 = 1/P$, the image distance v is negative and smaller in magnitude than f_2. Thus, the virtual image is trapped between F_2 and the lens.

In the case of a virtual object for the diverging lens, the converging incident light gives a positive value for the incident vergence U. When the virtual object is located between the lens and the (virtual) primary focal point F_1, the positive vergence U is great enough to overcome the negative dioptric power P. Consequently, V is positive, the exiting light is converging, and the resulting real image is located a finite distance behind the lens. When the virtual object is at F_1, then plane waves leave the lens and the image is at optical infinity. When the virtual object is located between F_1 and optical infinity, then the positive U is not great enough to overcome the negative P. Thus, the exiting vergence V is negative, the exiting light is diverging, and the resulting virtual image is located a finite distance in front of the lens. (Again, I suggest that you make some quick ray diagrams to check the above assertions.)

5.7 THE SYMMETRY POINTS

In developing intuition about the optics of lenses, it is helpful to consider the special case where the lateral magnification equals −1. In this case, the image is the same size as the object but is inverted relative to the object. Let us start by finding the object distance that results in $m = -1$. From Eq. 5.8,

$$m = \frac{U}{V} = -1$$

or

$$V = -U$$

From Eq. 5.1,

$$V = P + U$$

When we combine the above two equations, we get

$$-2U = P$$

Since $U = 1/u$ and $P = -1/f_1$, it follows that

$$-\frac{2}{u} = -\frac{1}{f_1}$$

or

$$u = 2f_1$$

Thus, when the object distance is twice the primary focal length, the resulting lateral magnification is equal to −1. It is easily shown that the image distance in this case is twice the secondary focal length, or

$$v = 2f_2$$

The axial points at $2f_1$ and $2f_2$ are conjugate points and are labeled $2F_1$ and $2F_2$, respectively. These conjugate points are called the *symmetry points* of the lens. The *symmetry planes* contain the symmetry points and are perpendicular to the optical axis of the lens.

EXAMPLE 5.8

Find the symmetry points of a +5.00 D lens.

From Example 5.1, the primary focal length f_1 of the lens is −20.0 cm and the secondary focal length f_2 is +20.0 cm. From the above discussion, the symmetry points are located at

$$u = 2f_1 = 2(-20.0\,\text{cm}) = -40.0\,\text{cm}$$

and

$$v = 2f_2 = 2(+20.0\,\text{cm}) = +40.0\,\text{cm}$$

We can use Eq. 5.7 to check the lateral magnification:

$$m = \frac{v}{u} = \frac{+40.0\,\text{cm}}{-40.0\,\text{cm}} = -1$$

As an alternate check, we can take the object distance of −40 cm and compute the resulting image distance and lateral magnification.

$$U = \frac{1}{u} = \frac{100}{-40.0\,\text{cm}} = -2.50\,\text{D}$$

The negative U value agrees with the fact that the light incident on the lens is diverging.

$$\begin{aligned} V &= P + U \\ &= +5.00\,\text{D} + (-2.50\,\text{D}) = +2.50\,\text{D} \\ v &= \frac{100}{+2.50\,\text{D}} = +40.0\,\text{cm} \end{aligned}$$

and

$$m = \frac{U}{V} = \frac{-2.50\,\text{D}}{+2.50\,\text{D}} = -1$$

The ray diagram is shown in Figure 5.17.

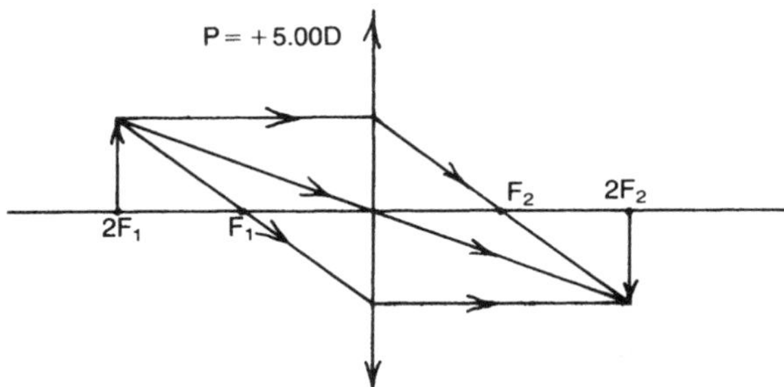

Figure 5.17 The symmetry points for a converging (plus) lens.

EXAMPLE 5.9

Find the symmetry points for a −20.00 D lens.

The primary and secondary focal lengths are:

$$f_2 = \frac{1}{P} = \frac{100}{-20.00\,\text{D}} = -5.0\,\text{cm}$$

$$f_1 = -\frac{1}{P} = -\frac{100}{-20.00\,\text{D}} = +5.0\,\text{cm}$$

Again,

$$u = 2f_1 = 2(+5.0\,\text{cm}) = +10.0\,\text{cm}$$

and

$$v = 2f_2 = 2(-5.0\,\text{cm}) = -10.0\,\text{cm}$$

Here the object and image points are both virtual. One check on the lateral magnification is

$$m = \frac{v}{u} = \frac{-10.0\,\text{cm}}{+10.0\,\text{cm}} = -1$$

As an alternate check, we can find the vergences and use Eq. 5.8. Here,

$$U = \frac{1}{u} = \frac{100}{+10.0\,\text{cm}} = +10.00\,\text{D}$$

The positive U value agrees with the fact that the object is virtual and that the light incident on the lens is converging.

$$\begin{aligned} V &= P + U \\ &= -20.00\,\text{D} + (+10.00\,\text{D}) = -10.00\,\text{D} \\ v &= \frac{100}{-10.00\,\text{D}} = -10.0\,\text{cm} \end{aligned}$$

and

$$m = \frac{U}{V} = \frac{+10.00\,\text{D}}{-10.00\,\text{D}} = -1$$

Note that the light leaving the lens is diverging and the image is virtual. The ray diagram is shown in Figure 5.18.

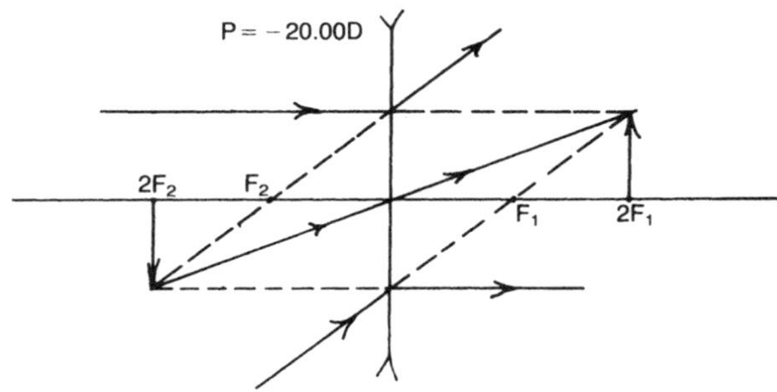

Figure 5.18 The symmetry points for a diverging (minus) lens.

Table 5.1 Lateral Magnification as Object Distance Goes to Zero

u (cm)	*v (cm)*	*m*
−2.000	−2.500	+1.250
−1.000	−1.111	+1.111
−0.500	−0.526	+1.053
−0.250	−0.256	+1.026
−0.125	−0.127	+1.013
−0.0625	−0.0629	+1.0063

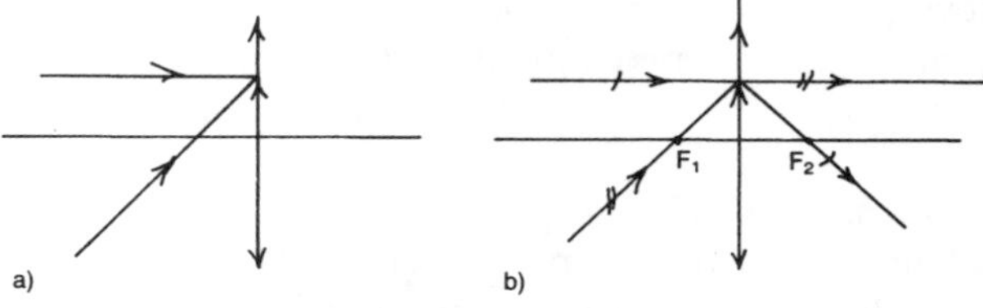

Figure 5.19 a, Converging rays forming an image at a thin lens; b, single notched ray is bent down at the lens, and double notched ray comes out parallel to the axis.

5.8 UNIT LATERAL MAGNIFICATION

What happens to the lateral magnification as an object is moved closer and closer to a lens? Let's consider a specific case with a +10.00 D lens. First, set the object at 2 cm in front of the lens.

$$u = -2\,\text{cm}$$

$$U = \frac{1}{u} = \frac{100}{-2.0\,\text{cm}} = -50.0\,\text{D}$$

$$V = P + U$$

$$= +10.00\,\text{D} + (-50.0\,\text{D}) = -40.0\,\text{D}$$

$$v = \frac{100}{-40.0\,\text{D}} = -2.5\,\text{cm}$$

$$m = \frac{U}{V} = \frac{-50.00\,\text{D}}{-40.0\,\text{D}} = +1.25$$

The image distance is −2.5 cm and the lateral magnification is +1.25. Now set the object at 1 cm, in front of the lens and repeat the calculations. The image distance v becomes −1.111 cm and the lateral magnification m becomes +1.111. The calculations can be repeated as the object is moved closer and closer to the lens. The results are shown in Table 5.1.

Note from the table that the smaller the object distance becomes, the closer the image distance gets to the object distance and the closer the lateral magnification gets to +1. In the limit of the object distance going to zero, the image distance goes to zero and the lateral magnification goes to +1.

The physical meaning of the +1 limit is that a *thin* lens has no optical effect when the object distance is zero. One way to observe this is to lay a thin lens directly on some letters in a book. The letters appear the same size with or without the lens over them.

Another way to have an object at the lens is to use a previous lens to converge light and form an image at the second lens. The image for the first lens is the object for the second lens, and the second lens object distance u_2 is zero. Figure 5.19 is a ray diagram for this case.

Figure 5.19a shows two rays representing the incident converging light. As usual, the incident ray parallel to the axis passes through F_2 when it leaves the lens, and the incident ray passing through F_1 leaves the lens parallel to the axis. The two outgoing rays are diverging away from the same point on the lens toward which the incoming rays converged. The object distance is zero, the image distance is zero, and the lateral magnification is +1.

5.9 OBJECT MOVEMENT/IMAGE MOVEMENT

Let us consider what happens to the image as an object for a converging lens is moved smoothly through space. Figure 5.20 helps to visualize the situation. The light incident on the lens is traveling to the right. The object positions are represented as points on a distorted circle. *The points on the left half of the circle represent real object points, while the points on the right half of the circle represent virtual object points.*

The circle depicts the fact that there are two ways to reach optical infinity. A real object can be moved left from the lens until it reaches optical infinity, or a virtual object can be moved right from the lens until it reaches optical infinity. As a real object is moved left, the incident light is initially diverging but loses negative vergence until all the waves incident on the lens effectively become plane waves. As a virtual object is moved right, the incident light is initially converging but loses positive vergence until all the waves incident on the lens again effectively become plane waves.

In Figure 5.21, an object is moved counter-clockwise around the circle starting from optical infinity, passing through the lens, and ending back at optical infinity. The points marked on the circle include the primary (F_1) and secondary (F_2) focal points as well as the symmetry points $2F_1$ and $2F_2$. The A on the outside of the circle marks the starting position for the real object at optical infinity. Its real conjugate image point is at F_2 and is marked on the inside of

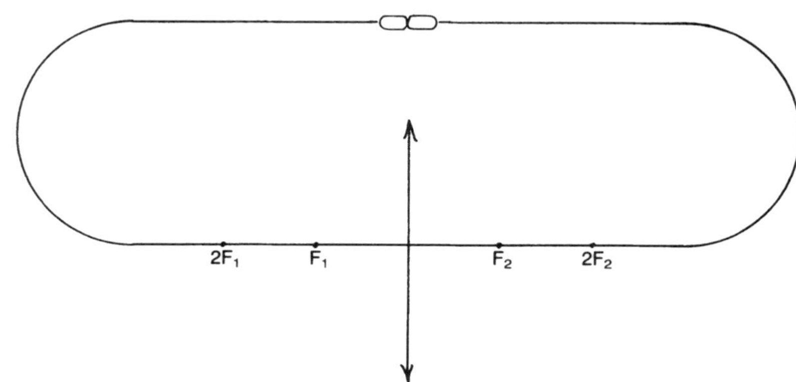

Figure 5.20 Distorted circle to help visualize object movement/image movement relations.

the circle by A′. As the real object is moved counter-clockwise from optical infinity to $2F_1$, its image moves counter-clockwise from F_2 to $2F_2$. The object position at $2F_1$ is marked on the inside by B, and its conjugate image position at $2F_2$ is now marked on the inside by B'. As the object is moved from $2F_1$ to F_1, its image moves from $2F_2$ to optical infinity. At F_1, the object position is represented on the inside by C, and its image position at optical infinity is represented on the inside by C'. As the real object continues its counter-clockwise movement, this time from F_1 to the lens, its conjugate image also continues its counter-clockwise movement, starting from optical infinity (becoming virtual at this stage) and traveling all the way from optical infinity until it finally catches up with the object at the lens. The conjugate object and image positions at the lens are marked D and D'. Next, as the object becomes virtual and moves counter-clockwise from the lens to optical infinity (object position D to A), its conjugate image becomes real once again, moving from the lens to F_2, (image position D' to A'). Both the object and its conjugate image have completed a full counter-clockwise trip around the circle.

A similar circle can be constructed for a minus lens (see the problems).

5.10 ERECT AND INVERTED RELATIONSHIPS: SINGLE LENSES

For a single thin lens, a real image is always inverted relative to a conjugate real object. One can easily prove this statement from the lateral magnification equation, $m = U/V$. For a real object, the incident light is diverging and U is negative. For a real image, the exiting light is converging and V is positive. A negative U value divided by a positive V value gives a negative m value, which indicates inversion.

For a single thin lens, a virtual image is always erect relative to a conjugate real object. Here, U is again negative, but now V is also negative since the exiting light is diverging. A negative U value divided by a negative V value results in a positive m value, which indicates the image is erect relative to the object.

Similarly, one can show that for a single thin lens a real image is always erect relative to a conjugate

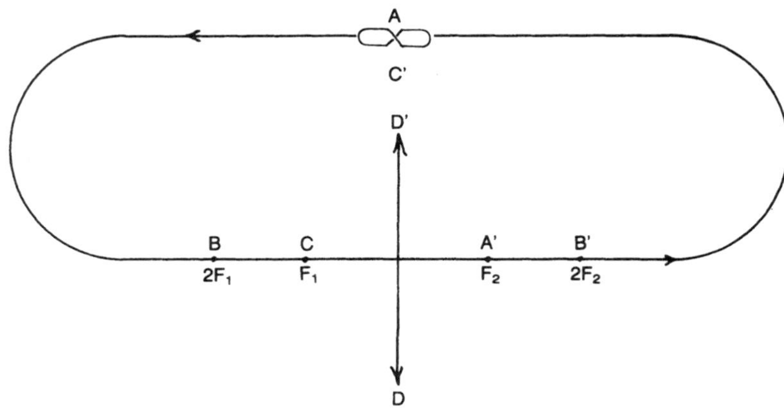

Figure 5.21 ***A′*, *B′*, *C′*, and *D′*** **are the respective image positions conjugate to the object positions *A*, *B*, *C*, and *D*.**

virtual object, and a virtual image is always inverted relative to a conjugate virtual object.

5.11 TWO-LENS SYSTEMS

Consider a lens of dioptric power P_1 placed at distance d in front of a second lens of dioptric power P_2. The light that leaves the first lens is incident on the second lens, so the image for the first lens is the object for the second lens. The final image position can be found by successively applying $V = P + U$ to each lens.

A special equation can be derived for the total lateral magnification m_t in the two-lens system. Let O_1 and I_1 be the respective object and conjugate image sizes for the first lens, and let O_2 and I_2 be the respective object and conjugate image sizes for the second lens. The total lateral magnification m_t is defined as the ratio of the final image size I_2 to the original object size O_1, or

$$m_t = \frac{I_2}{O_1}$$

The above equation can be multiplied and divided by O_2.

$$m_t = \frac{I_2}{O_1}\frac{O_2}{O_2}$$

or

$$m_t = \frac{I_2}{O_2}\frac{O_2}{O_1}$$

Since the image for lens one is the object for lens two, $I_1 = O_2$. We can then substitute I_1 for O_2:

$$m_t = \frac{I_2}{O_2}\frac{I_1}{O_1}$$

The lateral magnifications m_1 and m_2 for lenses one and two are, respectively,

$$m_1 = \frac{I_1}{O_1}$$
$$m_2 = \frac{I_2}{O_2}$$

By combining the above three equations, one finds that

$$m_t = m_2 m_1 \tag{5.9}$$

The total lateral magnification is the product of the lateral magnifications for each individual lens. This statement is easily extended to multiple lens systems containing more than two lenses. In particular, for a system of n thin lenses,

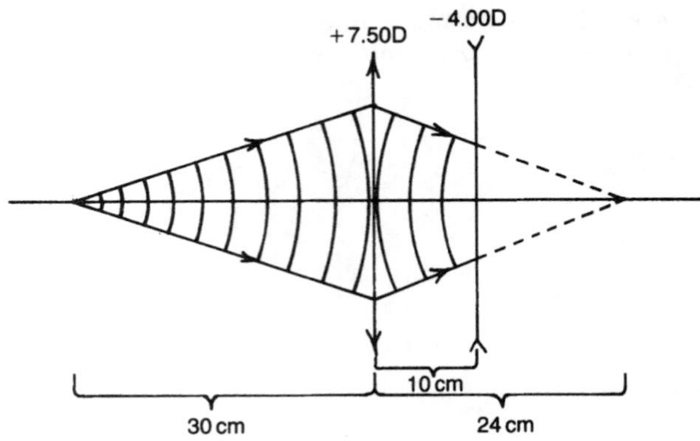

Figure 5.22 Rays and wavefronts in a two-lens system. There are downstream vergence changes between the two lenses.

$$m_t = \mathrm{m}_n \mathrm{m}_{n-1} \ldots \mathrm{m}_2 \mathrm{m}_1 \tag{5.10}$$

EXAMPLE 5.10

A +7.50 D lens is placed 10 cm in front of a −4.00 D lens. A real object is placed 30 cm in front of the +7.50 D lens. Find the final image position and the total lateral magnification, and state whether the final image is real or virtual.

For lens 1:

$$u_1 = -30\,\text{cm}$$
$$U_1 = \frac{1}{u_1} = \frac{100}{-30.0\,\text{cm}} = -3.33\,\text{D}$$
$$V_1 = P_1 + U_1$$
$$= +7.50\,\text{D} + (-3.33\,\text{D}) = +4.17\,\text{D}$$

$$v_1 = \frac{100}{+4.17\,\text{D}} = +24.0\,\text{cm}$$
$$m_1 = \frac{U_1}{V_1} = \frac{-3.33\,\text{D}}{+4.17\,\text{D}} = -0.80$$

Figure 5.22 schematically shows the diverging light incident on lens 1 and the converging light leaving it. The light incident on the second lens is converging so the object for the second lens is virtual. Note from Figure 5.22 that the image for lens 1 is located a distance of 14 cm (i.e., 24 cm – 10 cm) past lens 2.

For lens 2:

$$u_2 = 24\,\text{cm} - 10\,\text{cm} = +14\,\text{cm}$$
$$U_2 = \frac{1}{u_2} = \frac{100}{+14.0\,\text{cm}} = +7.14\,\text{D}$$

The converging wavefront leaving the first lens has a vergence of +4.17 D. From the figure, the

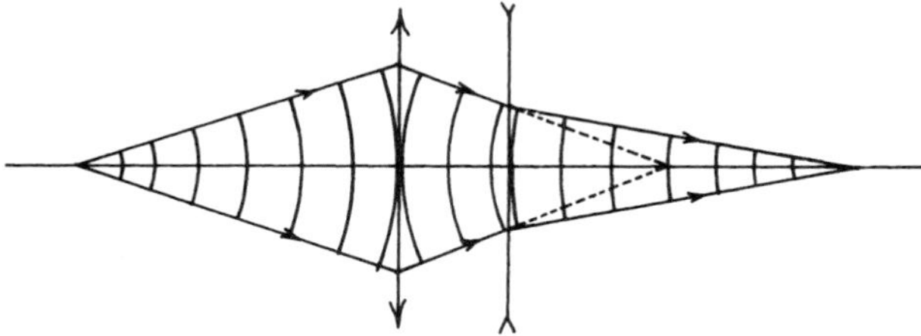

Figure 5.23 Rays and wavefronts leaving the second lens of the previous figure.

converging wavefronts gain curvature as they cross the gap between the two lenses so that the vergence of the converging wavefront incident on the second lens is +7.14 D.

$$V_2 = P_2 + U_2$$
$$= -4.00\,\text{D} + (+7.14\,\text{D}) = +3.14\,\text{D}$$
$$v_2 = \frac{100}{+3.14\,\text{D}} = +31.8\,\text{cm}$$
$$m_2 = \frac{U_2}{V_2} = \frac{+7.14\,\text{D}}{+3.14\,\text{D}} = +2.27$$

All the axial wavefronts are schematically represented in Figure 5.23.

The total lateral magnification is

$$m_t = m_2 m_1 = (+2.27)(-0.80) = -1.82$$

The final image is real, inverted, and 1.82 times larger than the original object.

An off-axis ray diagram can be used to confirm the above results. The secondary focal lengths for the two lenses are, respectively,

$$(f_2)_1 = \frac{1}{P_1} = \frac{100}{+7.50\,\text{D}} = +13.3\,\text{cm}$$
$$(f_2)_2 = \frac{1}{P_2} = \frac{100}{-4.00\,\text{D}} = -25.0\,\text{cm}$$

The first part of the ray diagram is shown in Figure 5.24a. Once the image I_1 is located, all the rays for the first lens can be drawn. In particular, we want to pick those rays that will also turn out to be the predictable rays for the second lens. Figure 5.24b shows the completion of the ray diagram. Figure 5.24c shows just the actual ray paths.

EXAMPLE 5.11

A +12.00 D lens is located 5 cm in front of a +8.00 D lens. An object is located 5 cm in front of the +12.00 D lens. Where is the final image? Is it real or virtual? What is the total lateral magnification?

$$u_1 = -5\,\text{cm}$$
$$U_1 = \frac{1}{u_1} = \frac{100}{-5\,\text{cm}} = -20.00\,\text{D}$$
$$V_1 = P_1 + U_1$$
$$V_1 = +12.00\,\text{D} + (-20.00\,\text{D}) = -8.00\,\text{D}$$
$$v_1 = \frac{100}{-8\,\text{D}} = -12.5\,\text{cm}$$
$$m_1 = \frac{U_1}{V_1} = \frac{-20.00\,\text{D}}{-8.00\,\text{D}} = +2.50$$

Figure 5.25 schematically shows the diverging light incident on lens 1 and the diverging light leaving it. The light incident on the second lens is diverging so the object for the second lens is real. From Figure 5.25, it is easy to see that the total distance from the virtual image to lens 2 is 17.5 cm.

Then,

$$u_2 = -(12.5\,\text{cm} + 5\,\text{cm}) = -17.5\,\text{cm}$$
$$U_2 = \frac{1}{u_2} = \frac{100}{-17.5\,\text{cm}} = -5.71\,\text{D}$$

Note that the vergence of the diverging wavefront leaving the first lens is −8.00 D. The diverging wavefronts lose curvature as they cross the gap between the two lenses so that the vergence of the light incident on the second lens is −5.71 D.

$$V_2 = P_2 + U_2$$
$$V_2 = +8.00\,\text{D} + (-5.71\,\text{D}) = +2.29\,\text{D}$$
$$v_2 = \frac{100}{+2.29\,\text{D}} = +43.7\,\text{cm}$$
$$m_2 = \frac{U_2}{V_2} = \frac{-5.71\,\text{D}}{+2.29\,\text{D}} = -2.49$$

The total lateral magnification is

$$m_t = m_2 m_1 = (-2.49)(+2.50) = -6.22$$

The final image is real, inverted relative to the object, and 6.22 times larger than the original object (Figure 5.26).

5.12 TWO THIN LENSES IN CONTACT

An important aspect of separated two-lens systems is the vergence change of the light as it propagates from lens 1 to lens 2. Therefore, the vergence of the light incident on lens 2 is, in general, not equal to the vergence of the light leaving lens 1.

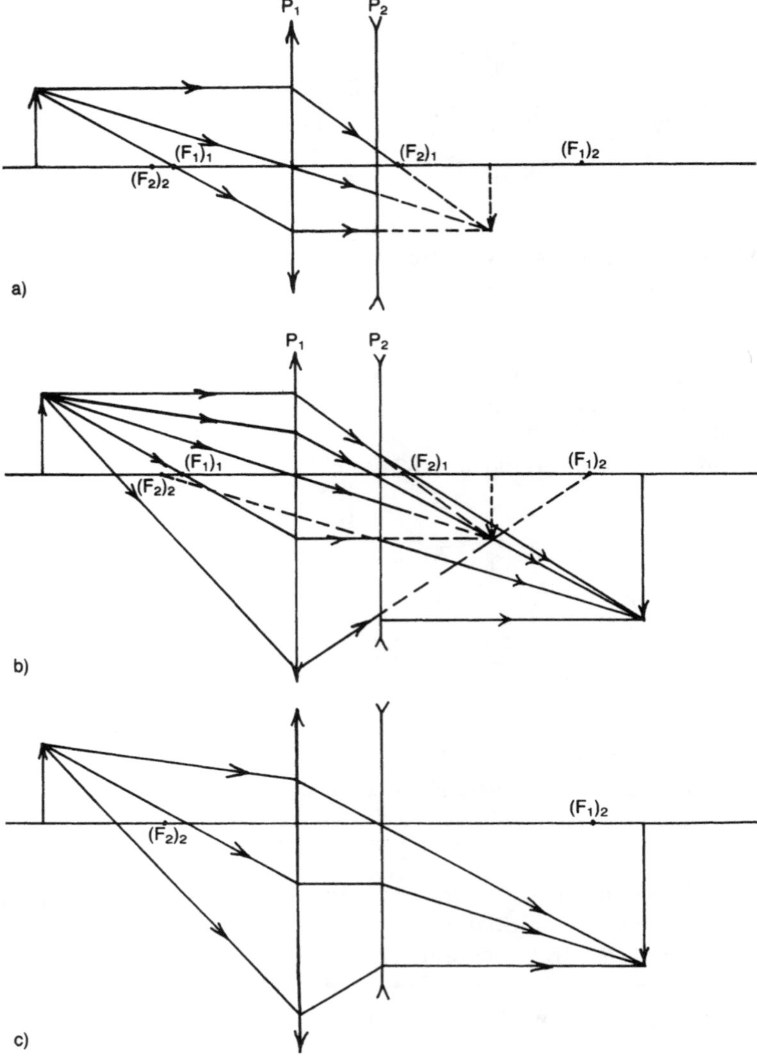

Figure 5.24 **a, The image of the first lens is the object for the second lens; b, image location for the second lens; c, actual ray paths without extensions.**

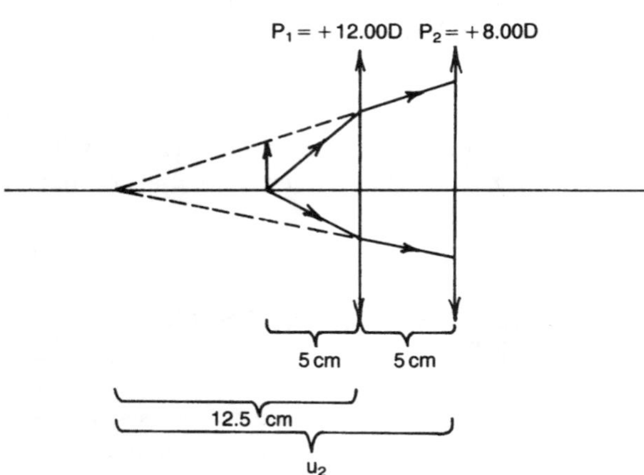

Figure 5.25 **Axial rays showing that the virtual image for the first lens is the real object for the second lens.**

Let us now consider the case in which two lenses are placed in contact with each other. The separation is zero, and the light leaving lens 1 is immediately incident on lens 2. Consequently, for the two thin lenses in contact with each other, the vergence of the light incident on lens 2 is always equal to the vergence of the light leaving lens 1, or

$$U_2 = V_1$$

In this case, we can simplify the two-lens problem considerably. For lens 1,

$$V_1 = P_1 + U_1$$

and for lens 2,

$$V_2 = P_2 + U_2$$

Figure 5.26 Extended ray diagram for Figure 5.25.

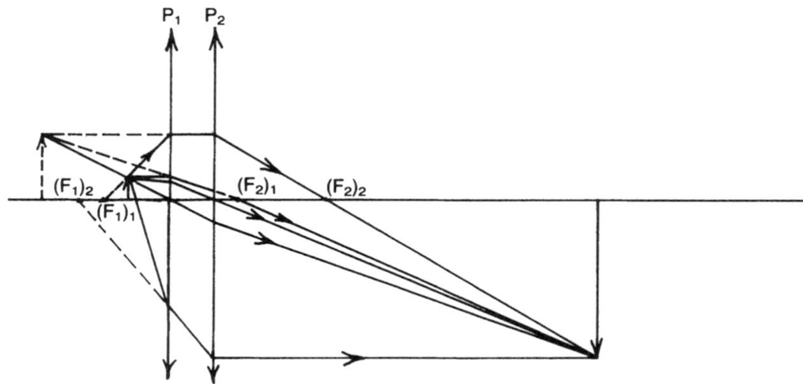

V_1 can be substituted into the above equation for U_2 to give

$$V_2 = P_2 + V_1$$

The substitution for V_1 then results in

$$V_2 = P_2 + P_1 + U_1$$

or

$$V_2 = (P_2 + P_1) + U_1$$

The above equation relates the incident vergence U_1 to the exiting vergence V_2. Furthermore, the above equation shows that the relationship is of the form

$$V_2 = P_t + U_1 \tag{5.11}$$

where,

$$P_t = P_2 + P_1 \tag{5.12}$$

Equation 5.11 shows that the two thin lenses in contact with each other simply act like one thin lens with a dioptric power of P_t. Equation 5.12 states that dioptric powers are additive for thin lenses in contact with each other.

EXAMPLE 5.12

A +4.00 D thin lens is placed in contact with a +7.00 D thin lens. A real object is located 40.0 cm in front of the combination. Where is the final image? Is it real or virtual? What is the lateral magnification?

From Eq. 5.12, the two thin lenses in contact act like a single thin lens with a power of

$$P_t = (+4.00\,\text{D}) + (+7.00\,\text{D}) = +11.00\,\text{D}$$

Then,

$$u_1 = -40\,\text{cm}$$

and

$$U_1 = \frac{100}{-40.0\,\text{cm}} = -2.50\,\text{D}$$

From Eq. 5.11,

$$V_2 = +11.00\,\text{D} + (-2.50\,\text{D}) = +8.50\,\text{D}$$

The light leaving the combination is converging and the image is real. The image distance is

$$v_2 = \frac{100}{+8.50\,\text{D}} = +11.8\,\text{cm}$$

The lateral magnification is

$$m_t = \frac{U_1}{V_2} = \frac{-2.50\,\text{D}}{+8.50\,\text{D}} = -0.29$$

EXAMPLE 5.13

What single lens acts like a +3.00 D thin lens and a −8.00 D thin lens held together?

From Eq. 5.12,

$$P_t = (+3.00\,\text{D}) + (-8.00\,\text{D}) = -5.00\,\text{D}$$

A −5.00 D thin lens acts exactly like the combination.

EXAMPLE 5.14

A thin lens with a secondary focal length of +50.00 cm is held in contact with a second thin lens. The secondary focal length of the combination is +16.67 cm. What is the secondary focal length of the unknown lens?

You might need to be careful here. Equation 5.12 says that the dioptric powers are additive. This does not mean that the secondary focal lengths are additive.

The dioptric power of lens 1 is

$$P_1 = \frac{1}{f_2} = \frac{100}{+50.0\,\text{cm}} = +2.00\,\text{D}$$

Figure 5.27 Projector lens ray diagram showing that the image size depends on the geometric relationship between two different bundles.

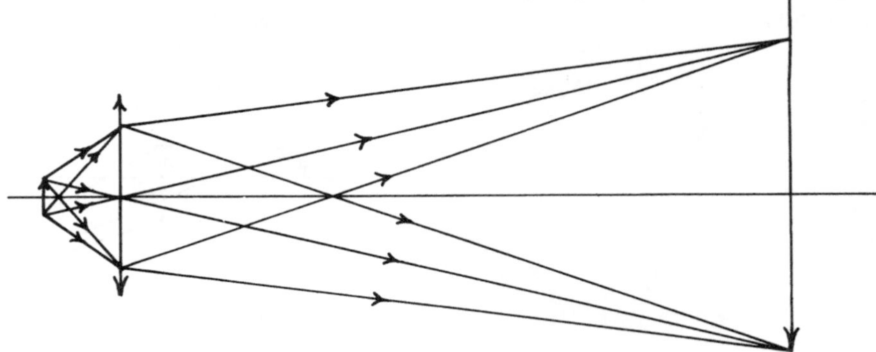

The dioptric power of the combination is

$$P_t = \frac{1}{f_2} = \frac{100}{+16.67\,\text{cm}} = +6.00\,\text{D}$$

Then from Eq. 5.12, the dioptric power of the unknown (second) lens is

$$P_2 = P_t - P_1$$
$$P_2 = (+6.00\,\text{D}) - (+2.00\,\text{D}) = +4.00\,\text{D}$$

The secondary focal length of the originally unknown lens is

$$f_2 = 100/(+4.00\,\text{D}) = +25.0\,\text{cm}$$

The secondary focal lengths of the two thin lenses are, respectively, +50 cm and +25 cm, while the secondary focal point of the combination is +16.67 cm. Clearly the focal lengths are not additive.

The dioptric power additivity for thin lenses in contact results from the fact that there is no vergence change between the two lenses. For two separated thin lenses, there will generally be a vergence change between the two lenses, and the dioptric powers are not additive.

The additivity of the dioptric powers is easily extended to include n thin lenses in contact with each other, or

$$P_t = P_n + P_{n-1} + \cdots + P_2 + P_1 \qquad (5.13)$$

5.13 BUNDLES, BEAMS, AND LATERAL MAGNIFICATION

A movie (or slide) projector forms a large image on a distant screen. Figure 5.27 represents the image formation by a single thin lens projector. The light beam leaving such a projector is a diverging beam. (This beam is frequently visible in movie theaters due to light scattering off dust particles in the air.) The diverging beam is composed of individual converging bundles. The fact that the real image is formed is due to these individual converging bundles. The fact that the image size is larger than the lens size is due to the diverging beam.

The image size is determined not by an individual bundle, but rather by the geometric relationship between at least two different bundles. (Note that an axial bundle could also be drawn in Figure 5.27.) The lateral magnification, defined as the image size divided by the object size, depends on the relationship between at least two different bundles, i.e., it is not considered a property of one, individual, solitary bundle. This two-bundle dependence has important implications in the next section and in the optics of spherocylindrical lenses.

5.14 IMAGE SIZES FOR DISTANT OBJECTS

When an object is far away from a thin lens, the vergence U of the wavefront incident on the lens is very close to zero. In this case, we frequently use the plane wave approximation and set the vergence U equal to zero. Use of the plane wave approximation does not significantly affect the calculation of the image distance v since the image distance is a property of a single bundle. The lateral magnification, however, is a property of at least two bundles (Section 5.13). Consequently, use of the plane wave approximation can significantly affect image size calculations.

The lateral magnification equation, $m = U/V$, shows that if U is very close to zero, then m is very small. From Eq. 5.6, the image size I in terms of m is

$$I = mO$$

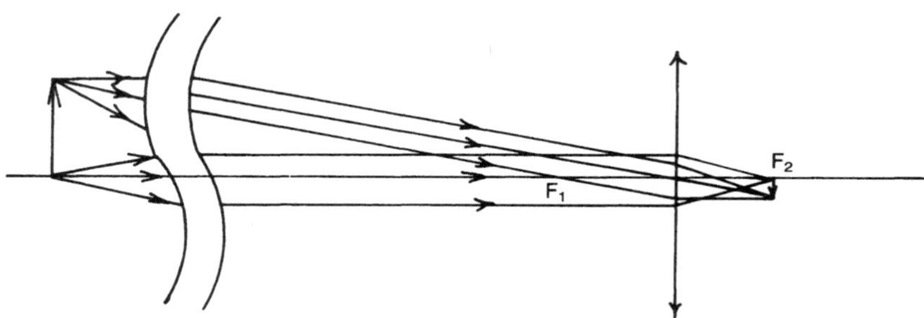

Figure 5.28 Rays showing two different incident bundles from a distant object. The image is inverted and at the secondary focal point.

where O is the object size. A very small m can be offset by a large object size O, so that I is not necessarily a small value. However, the plane wave approximation ($U = 0$) leads to $m = 0$ and, consequently, $I = 0$, which is clearly wrong for large enough objects. Either the small U value must be kept and not set equal to zero, or an alternate method is needed to calculate image sizes for distant objects.

Let us consider an alternate method. Figure 5.28 represents a real object located far away from a thin converging lens. Two bundles are shown: one from the top of the object and one from the axial object point.

The object is far enough away so that the plane wave approximation can be used and each bundle by itself can be represented by parallel rays. The rays from the axial point are parallel to the axis since one of the rays coincides with the axis. The rays from the off-axis point are parallel with each other but not with the axis. Note that there are two predictable rays in the off-axis bundle: one through the nodal point of the lens (the optical center), and the other through the primary focal point F_1. The extended image is formed in the secondary focal plane of the lens.

Figure 5.29 shows only the nodal ray from the off-axis point. The nodal ray forms a straight line between the conjugate object and image points. The angle w is the angle that the object subtends at the nodal point of the lens, and the angle w' is the angle that the image subtends at the nodal point. Since the nodal ray is a straight line between the conjugate object and image points then the angles w and w', are equal. From the figure,

$$\tan w' = |I|/f_2$$

It follows that

$$|I| = f_2 \tan w \tag{5.14}$$

where w has been substituted for w'.

Equation 5.14 is the alternate equation for the image size when the object is distant. It avoids the lateral magnification difficulties with the ultrasmall lateral magnification values.

EXAMPLE 5.15

A full moon subtends an angle of 0.5° at the earth's surface. A real image of the full moon is formed by a +1.00-D thin lens. What is the size of the image?

The secondary focal length of a +1.00 D lens is +100 cm. From Eq. 5.14,

$$\begin{aligned}|I| &= (+100\,\text{cm})\tan(0.5°)\\ &= (+100\,\text{cm})(0.0087)\\ &= 0.87\,\text{cm} = 8.7\,\text{mm}\end{aligned}$$

Often even a large distant object, such as the moon, subtends a small angle at the lens. When this occurs, the small angle approximation for the tangent can be used so that Eq. 5.14 results in

$$|I| = f_2 w \tag{5.15}$$

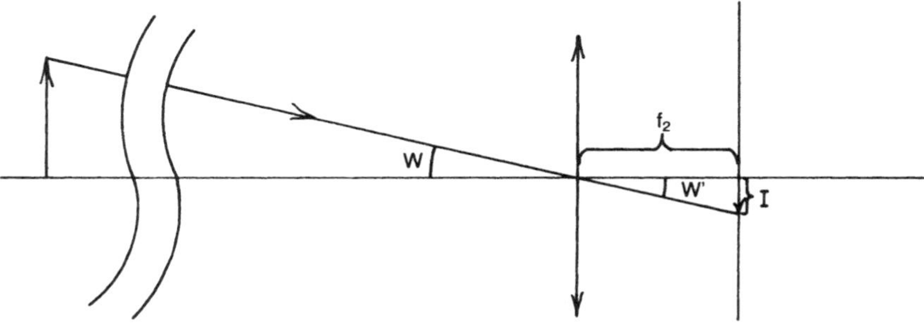

Figure 5.29 Nodal ray to determine the image size for distant object.

where w is expressed in radians. When the small angle approximation is used for the full moon example, the result is again 8.7 mm. In fact, the percent difference between the small angle method and the tangent method is less than 0.01% in this case.

Can a large object ever be imaged with zero size? A typical star is larger than the planet Earth, but so far away that its subtended angle at the planet Earth is very, very small. Consequently, the subtended angle w is effectively zero, and from Eq. 5.15 the image size I is then zero. As a result, when a person looks at a star on a clear night, the person's retinal image of the star is effectively a point image. (If you are driving, be sure to park before checking the stars.) You might also note some radial streaks of light around the point image of the star. These radial streaks are due to diffraction from the structure of the crystalline lens sutures. The twinkling of the stars is due to atmospheric turbulence. If you get a ride on the space shuttle, you can observe the stars without having to look through the atmosphere.

5.15 REVERSIBILITY AND FINDING THE OBJECT

Many of the previous examples in this chapter deal with finding the image once the object is given. Suppose instead that the image is given and we are asked to find the object. One approach is to use the thin lens vergence equation, solve for the incident vergence U, and then find the object distance u.

Another approach is to use the principle of reversibility. Section 3.8 discussed the fact that two conjugate points, A and B, are conjugate no matter which way the light is passing through the system. When A is the object point, then B is the image point. When the light direction is reversed, then B becomes the object point and A becomes the image point. If the image point B is known and the conjugate object point A is needed, then the direction of the light can be reversed, B considered as the object point, and A found as the conjugate image. The following example uses the reversibility method.

EXAMPLE 5.16

A +9.00 D thin lens in air has a real image located 20 cm behind it. Where is the conjugate object and is it real or virtual?

Figure 5.30a shows an on-axis sketch of the given situation and Figure 5.30b shows the reversed situation. Remember that the dioptric power P remains +9.00 D no matter which way the light travels through the lens.

For the reversed situation, the positive direction is to the left and a real object is located 20 cm from the lens. Then,

$$u_{rev} = -20\,\text{cm}$$

$$U_{rev} = \frac{1}{u_{rev}} = \frac{100}{-20\,\text{cm}} = -5.00\,\text{D}$$

$$V_{rev} = P_{rev} + U_{rev}$$

$$= +9.00\,\text{D} + (-5.00\,\text{D}) = +4.00\,\text{D}$$

and

$$v_{rev} = \frac{100}{+4.00\,\text{D}} = +25.0\,\text{cm}$$

Note that for the reversed case in Figure 5.30b the positive direction is to the left, so the real image at +25 cm is to the left of the lens. Consequently, for light traveling in the original direction (to the right), the object is real and located 25 cm to the left of the lens (Figure 5.30a).

From the above discussion, there are at least two approaches that one can use in finding the object once the image is known. For visual optics purposes, there are some conceptual advantages to using the reversibility method as given in Example 5.16. In particular, the reversibility method facilitates the understanding of the optics of retinoscopy and ophthalmoscopy.

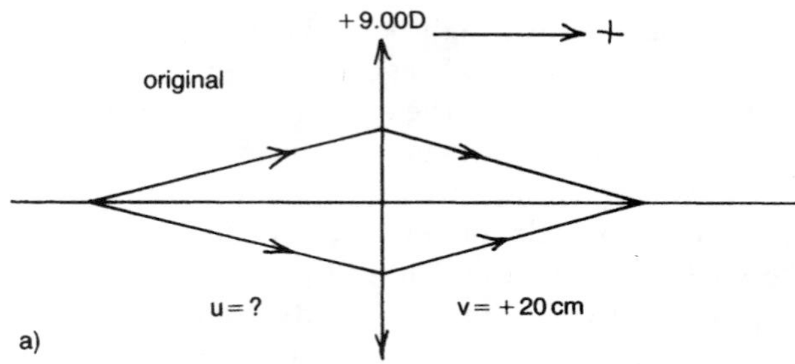

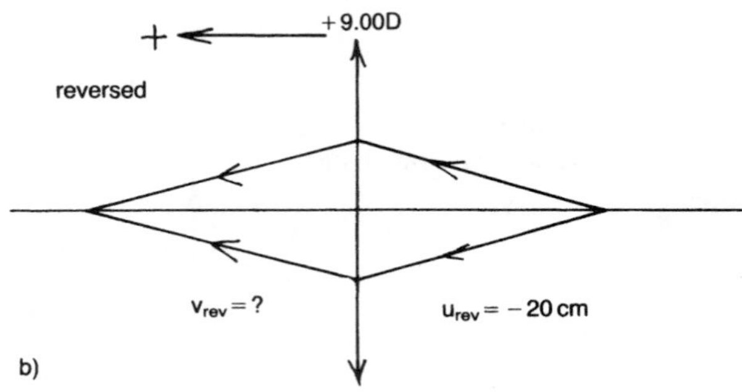

Figure 5.30 Principle of reversibility: a, original light traveling right; b, reversed light traveling left.

PROBLEMS

For problems 1 through 10, find the image, specify whether it is real or virtual, and give the lateral magnification. Draw an extended ray diagram to confirm your calculations. Also, calculate the vergence of the wavefront 5 cm in front of the lens and the vergence of the wavefront 5 cm behind the lens.

1. +6.00 D lens, real object 50 cm from the lens.
2. +6.00 D lens, real object 25 cm from the lens.
3. +6.00 D lens, real object 10 cm from the lens.
4. +6.00 D lens, virtual object 10 cm from the lens.
5. +6.00 D lens, virtual object 30 cm from the lens.
6. −7.00 D lens, real object 40 cm from the lens.
7. −7.00 D lens, real object 10 cm from the lens.
8. −7.00 D lens, virtual object 10 cm from the lens.
9. −7.00 D lens, virtual object 20 cm from the lens.
10. −7.00 D lens, virtual object 50 cm from the lens.
11. What is the secondary focal length of a +14.00 D lens? Of a −8.00 D lens?
12. The primary focal length of a lens is −15.0 cm. What is the dioptric power of the lens?
13. A 20 mm tall real object is located 28.0 cm from a +5.50 D thin lens. What is the image size?
14. Give the object distance that results in a lateral magnification of −1.0 for a +6.50 D lens and for a −4.50 D lens.
15. Give the object distance that results in a lateral magnification of +1.0 for a +2.50 D lens and for a −8.00 D lens.
16. A +5.50 D lens has a real image located 35 cm from the lens. Is the conjugate object real or virtual? What is the object distance?
17. A +5.00 D lens has a real image located 12 cm from the lens. Is the conjugate object real or virtual? What is the object distance?
18. A −7.50 D lens has a virtual image located 9 cm from the lens. Is the conjugate object real or virtual? What is the object distance?
19. A +8.20 D lens forms a real image that is inverted and 4 times the size of the object. What is the image distance? What is the object distance?
20. A real object is 20 cm from a thin lens. The conjugate image is erect and 3 times larger than the object. What is the lens power?
21. A real object is located 40 cm in front of a +6.50 D thin lens. The +6.50 D thin lens is located 20 cm in front of a −10.00 D thin lens. What is the vergence of light that exits the −10.00 D lens? What is the total lateral magnification?
22. A real object is located 34.0 cm in front of a lens of unknown power. A +7.00 D thin lens is located 10.0 cm behind the first lens. The second lens has a real image located 29.0 cm from it. What is the dioptric power of the first lens?
23. A real object is located 13 cm in front of a lens of dioptric power P. A real image is located on a screen placed a distance x behind the lens. A −7.00 D lens is placed between the object and the lens at a distance of 5 cm from the lens. Relative to the minus lens, where must the object be placed in order to again have an image on the screen? Remember that neither P nor x changes.
24. A thin lens of dioptric power P has a distant object and a real image located on a screen that is at distance x behind the lens. A +5.00 D thin lens is then placed against the lens of power P. What thin lens located 14.0 cm in front of the +5.00 D lens will again result in a clear image on the screen? Remember that neither P nor x changes.
25. What single lens is equivalent to a +9.00 D thin lens combined with a −6.00 D thin lens?
26. For a distant tree, a thin lens held 19.0 cm in front of a wall results in an inverted image on the wall. When a second thin lens of unknown power is combined with the first, the real image is on the wall only when the combination is held 69.0 cm from the wall. What is the dioptric power of the second lens?
27. A distant building subtends an angle of 90 min at a +2.00 D thin lens. What is the size of the image (in mm)?
28. A person stands 3.6 m from the camera in which the lens is a single thin lens. The person is 250 cm tall and her image is 35.2 mm tall. What is the dioptric power of the camera lens? What is the secondary focal length of the lens?
29. Section 5.9 contains a distorted circle representation of the object movement/image movement relation for a plus thin lens. Construct the object movement/image movement circle for a minus thin lens.

CHAPTER 6

Thin Lens Eye Models

6.1 EMMETROPES

The simplest optical model of the eye is a thin lens and screen model. The thin lens represents the cornea and the crystalline lens while the screen represents the retina. Air is assumed to be between the lens and the screen. A typical dioptric power for the lens representing the unaccommodated human eye is +60.00 D.

An emmetrope is a person who can clearly see a distant object without accommodating. The light that reaches the eye from the distant object consists of plane waves. The unaccommodated emmetropic eye converges the plane waves and forms a clear image on the retina. In the thin lens and screen model of the unaccommodated emmetropic eye, the screen, which represents the retina, is placed at the image point conjugate to optical infinity.

Consider Amy who is an emmetrope and has an unaccommodated eye with +60.00 D power. What should the lens–screen separation be in a model simulating Amy's eye? One method for answering this question is to find the image position for incoming plane waves. From Eq. 5.1,

$$V = P + U$$
$$= +60.00\,\text{D} + (0\,\text{D}) = +60.00\,\text{D}$$

and

$$v = \frac{1000\,\text{mm/m}}{+60.00\,\text{D}} = +16.67\,\text{mm}$$

The image distance is 16.67 mm and the screen should be placed that distance behind the +60.00 D lens in order to simulate Amy's eye (Figure 6.1a).

A distant object is conjugate to the secondary focal point of a lens. An alternate solution for the emmetropic lens–screen distance is to recognize that the secondary focal point of the unaccommodated emmetropic eye coincides with the retina. Thus, the lens–screen distance is just equal to the secondary focal length of the lens. From Eq. 5.4, the secondary focal length is

$$f_2 = \frac{1}{P}$$

or

$$f_2 = \frac{1000\,\text{mm/m}}{+60.00\,\text{D}} = +16.67\,\text{mm}$$

Brian is an emmetrope whose eye is simulated with a lens–screen separation of 18.00 mm. What is the power of the lens in the model for Brian's unaccommodated eye? In this example, the image distance for a distant

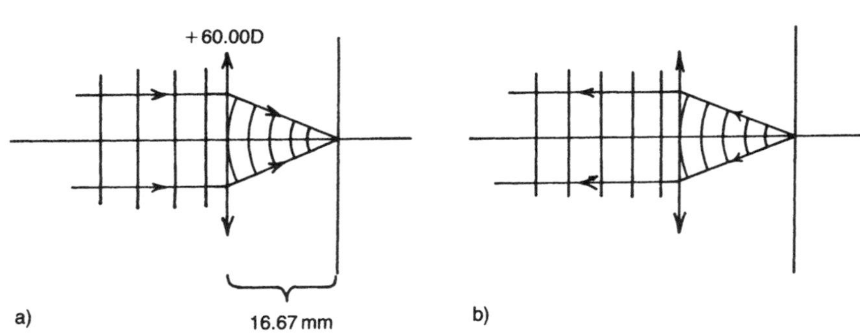

Figure 6.1 a, Plane waves from a distant object incident on a thin lens and screen model of an emmetropic eye; b, the reversed situation when the retina is the object, plane waves emerge from the emmetropic eye.

object is 18.00 mm which is thus the secondary focal length for the eye. Therefore,

$$P = \frac{1}{f_2}$$
$$= \frac{1000\,\text{mm/m}}{18\,\text{mm}} = +55.56\,\text{D}$$

Brian's unaccommodated eye has a dioptric power less than the typical value of +60.00 D but is still emmetropic because the eye is longer than the 16.67 mm lens–screen separation corresponding to the +60.00-D emmetropic eye.

We usually think in terms of light entering the eye. However, consider the situation when an examiner uses an ophthalmoscope or a retinoscope to examine the eye. The light is initially directed into the eye to illuminate the retina (just as you turn on the room lights to illuminate a wall). The retina then acts as a secondary source with the diffusely reflected light diverging away from it and emerging from the eye.

Figure 6.1a shows plane waves from a distant object point entering an unaccommodated emmetropic eye model. The image point is on the retina. According to the principle of reversibility, light diverging from a point on the retina retraces the same path back out of the eye. (In Figure 6.1a, simply reverse the arrow direction on each ray.) Therefore, the light emerging from the unaccommodated emmetropic eye consists of plane waves with the image point at optical infinity (Figure 6.1b).

The far point of an eye is the point conjugate to the axial retinal point for the unaccommodated eye. For the unaccommodated eye, an object point at the far point results in an image point on the retina (light is incident on the eye), and an object point on the retina results in an image point at the far point (light is emerging from the eye). The far point is also known by its Latin name, *punctum remotum.*

The far point of an emmetrope is at optical infinity. In the following sections, two types of ametropes, myopes and hyperopes, are discussed. The far point for ametropes is not at optical infinity.

6.2 MYOPES

Myopes are nearsighted. When a myope views a distant object, the eye converges the light to form a clear image in front of the retina (i.e., in the vitreous humor) resulting in a blurred image on the retina. When the object is brought closer to the myopic eye, the divergence of the incident light increases and the image moves back towards the retina. Eventually, the image is formed on the retina and the near object appears clear to the unaccommodated myope. In this case the near object is located at the far point of the myope's eye. It is a characteristic of a myopic eye that its far point is a real point located a finite distance in front of the eye.

Cindy is a myope whose unaccommodated eye is simulated by a +58.00 D lens and a 20 mm lens–screen distance. One way to check that the model is simulating a myopic eye is to determine if the light from a distant object point is imaged in front of the retina.

For incident plane waves, the image is at the secondary focal plane. Then,

$$f_2 = \frac{1}{P}$$
$$= \frac{1000}{+58\,\text{D}} = +17.24\,\text{mm}$$

The lens–screen distance is 20 mm. Consequently, the clear image is formed in front of the screen representing the retina (Figure 6.2a). While this calculation shows that Cindy's eye is myopic, it does not determine the amount of myopia.

One way to determine the amount of myopia is to take the retina as the object and consider the light that emerges from the eye, as occurs in ophthalmoscopy and retinoscopy. In the reversed case, the object distance u for the retina is -20 mm (Figure 6.2b). Then,

$$u = -20\,\text{mm}$$
$$U = \frac{1000}{-20\,\text{mm}} = -50.00\,\text{D}$$

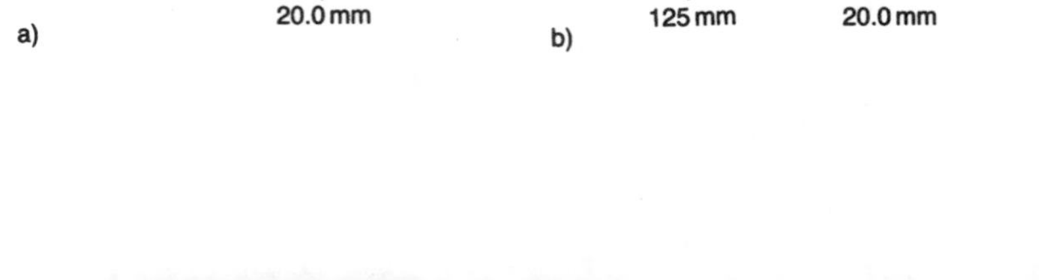

Figure 6.2 a, Rays from a distant point incident on a myopic eye; b, when the retina is the object, the waves emerging from a myopic eye are converging.

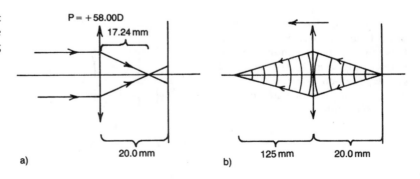

Since

$$V = P + U$$
$$= +58.00\,\text{D} + (-50.00\,\text{D}) = +8.00\,\text{D}$$

and

$$v = \frac{100}{+8.00\,\text{D}} = +12.5\,\text{cm}$$

The light emerging from Cindy's eye has a convergence of +8.00 D. Note that plane waves emerge from an emmetropic eye. Cindy's myopic eye needs 8.00 D less converging power in order to be emmetropic. The 8.00 D is a measure of Cindy's refractive error.

The converging light coming out of Cindy's eye forms a real image at 12.5 cm in front of the eye (Figure 6.2b). The real image point at 12.5 cm is conjugate to the retina and, consequently, is the far point of Cindy's eye. By reversibility, an object placed at the far point results in a clear image on the retina. (In Figure 6.2b, the position of the rays would be unchanged, but the arrows on the rays would be reversed and point to the right.) For an object point at 12.5 cm in front of the eye, the light incident on the eye would have a divergence of −8.00 D. This −8.00 D, in effect, offsets or neutralizes the 8.00 D of excess converging power in the eye, resulting in a clear image on the retina.

A contact lens correction is a correcting lens that sits on the cornea. In the thin lens and screen model, the contact correction is simulated by a thin lens placed against the front of the thin lens representing the eye. What contact lens would correct Cindy for distant vision?

To get a clear image on the retina of her unaccommodated eye, Cindy must have a vergence of −8.00 D incident on the cornea. Plane waves come from a distant object, so the contact lens must be a lens that produces a vergence of −8.00 D from the incident plane waves. From the thin lens vergence equation, the contact lens must have a power of −8.00 D.

In the above example, the dioptric power of a distance vision contact lens was equal to the vergence of the light incident on the cornea when the object was at the far point of the eye. This is true in general, and is shown algebraically as follows. Let U_{fp} be the vergence of the light incident on the cornea when the object is at the far point of the eye, P_c be the dioptric power of the contact lens, U_c the vergence of the light incident on the contact lens, and V_c the vergence of the light exiting the contact lens.

From Eq. 5.1,

$$P_c = V_c - U_c$$

Then since $U_c = 0$, it follow that

$$P_c = V_c$$

Since the light leaving the contact lens is immediately incident on the cornea, there is no downstream vergence change. Furthermore, the vergence of the light entering the cornea must equal U_{fp} in order to get a clear image on the retina. Therefore,

$$V_c = U_{fp}$$

From the above two equations,

$$P_c = U_{fp} \qquad (6.1)$$

In the case of the myope Cindy, Eq. 6.1 gives the −8.00 D contact lens power. Remember that Eq. 6.1 is general and applies to hyperopes as well as to myopes.

Dan is a myope whose unaccommodated eye has a power of +62.00 D. The far point of Dan's eye is located 50 cm in front of the eye. In the thin lens and screen model, what is the lens–screen distance? What contact lens correction does Dan require?

When an object is placed at Dan's far point, a clear image will be formed on the retina. In this case,

$$u_{fp} = -50\,\text{cm}$$

and

$$U_{fp} = \frac{100}{-50\,\text{cm}} = -2.00\,\text{D}$$

Since

$$V = P + U_{fp}$$
$$= +62.00\,\text{D} + (-2.00\,\text{D}) = +60.00\,\text{D}$$

and

$$v = \frac{100}{+60.00\,\text{D}} = +16.67\,\text{mm}$$

The lens–screen separation for Dan's eye is 16.67 mm. This happens to be the same lens–screen separation of a typical emmetrope. Dan's +62.00-D power is 2.00 D more than the typical emmetrope, and the U_{fp} of −2.00 D simply neutralizes the +2.00 D error.

Dan's distance vision contact correction must take incoming plane waves and convert them into light of −2.00 D vergence. Hence, Dan's contact lens power P_c is −2.00 D, which is the same result that Eq. 6.1 gives.

The amount of myopia is directly quantified by the absolute value of U_{fp}, which was 8.00 D and 2.00 D respectively for Cindy and Dan. An alternative conceptual quantification of the amount of myopia is in

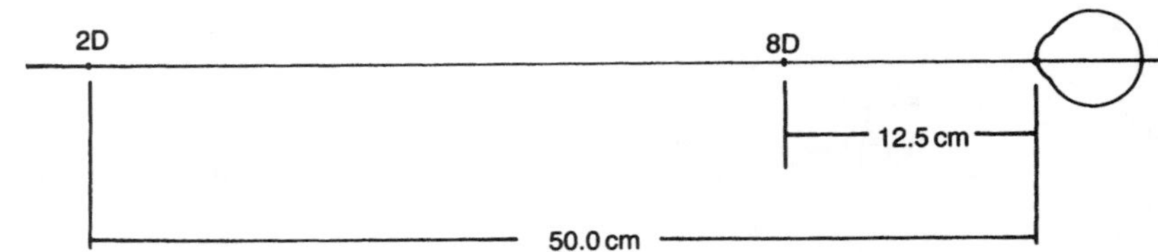

Figure 6.3 Far point location for a 2 D and an 8 D myope.

terms of the far point location. The closer the far point is to optical infinity, the less the degree of myopia and the closer the eye is to being emmetropic. The closer the far point is to the eye, the greater the degree of myopia. Dan, the 2.00 D myope, had a far point 50 cm in front of the eye, while Cindy, the 8.00 D myope, had a far point 12.5 cm in front of the eye. Note that in all cases the far point for a myope is a real point as opposed to a virtual point (Figure 6.3).

The concept of the far point, and hence U_{fp}, is particularly useful. Once the far point is known, then the correcting lens for the eye can be determined even if the internal dimensions of the eye are not known.

6.3 HYPEROPES

An unaccommodated hyperopic eye is too short to clearly image a distant object on the retina (Figure 6.4a). When an unaccommodated hyperope looks at a distant object, the eye converges the light, but the converging light runs into the retina before the image is formed. Hence, the retinal image is blurred. To get a clear image on the retina of an unaccommodated hyperope, the light incident on the eye must be converging. This means that the far point of a hyperope's eye is virtual and located a finite distance behind the eye (Figure 6.4b).

Fay has an unaccommodated eye that is simulated by a +60.00 D thin lens and a screen located 16 mm behind the lens. Since the typical +60.00 D eye has a length of 16.67 mm, Fay's eye is clearly too short and is therefore hyperopic. What is the degree of hyperopia and where is the far point for Fay's eye?

Again, as in retinoscopy, we will consider the light emerging from the eye when the retina serves as the object (Figure 6.4c). Then,

$$u = -16\,\text{mm}$$

and

$$U = \frac{1000}{-16\,\text{mm}} = -62.50\,\text{D}$$

From $V = P + U$,

$$V = +60.00\,\text{D} + (-62.50\,\text{D}) = -2.50\,\text{D}$$

and

$$v = \frac{100}{-2.50\,\text{D}} = -40.0\,\text{cm}$$

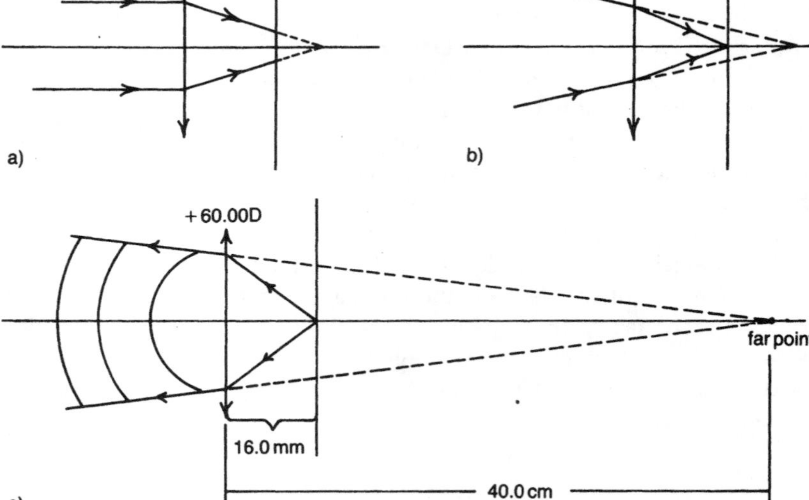

Figure 6.4 a, Rays from a distant point incident on an unaccommodated hyperopic eye; b, converging incident light (virtual far point) is needed to get an image on the hyperope's retina; c, when the retina is the object, diverging light leaves the hyperopic eye resulting in a virtual image at the far point.

The light emerging from Fay's eye is diverging and has a vergence of −2.50 D. The image point is virtual, located 40 cm behind the +60.00 D lens, and is the far point for Fay's eye.

Plane waves emerge from an emmetropic eye. Fay has diverging light of −2.50 D emerging from her eye. Fay's eye is lacking 2.50 D of converging power. This 2.50 D is the degree of hyperopia.

Since Fay's eye is lacking +2.50 D, light entering her eye must be converging and have a vergence of +2.50 D in order to produce a clear retinal image. In other words, to obtain a clear retinal image, the object for the eye must be virtual and located 40 cm behind the eye at the far point. Then $u_{fp} = +40\,\text{cm}$ and $U_{fp} = +2.50\,\text{D}$. (In Figure 6.4c, the rays would be unchanged except that the arrows would be reversed and point to the right.)

A contact lens correction that enables Fay to see a distant object without accommodating must take incident plane waves and produce exiting light of vergence +2.50 D. A +2.50 D contact lens does this. We can also find the power of the contact lens from Eq. 6.1, which gives

$$P_c = U_{fp} = +2.50\,\text{D}$$

George is a hyperope whose unaccommodated eye is simulated by a +54.00 D thin lens and a typical lens–screen distance of 16.67 mm. Where is George's far point? What distance vision contact lens correction does George require?

A typical emmetropic model eye has a dioptric power of +60.00 D and a lens–screen distance of 16.67 mm. George's lens–screen distance is 16.67 mm, but George only has +54.00 D of power. Hence, George is lacking +6.00 D of converging power. In other words, George has 6.00 D of hyperopia.

Alternatively, we can determine the amount of hyperopia by taking the retina as the object and considering the light emerging from the eye. Thus,

$$u = -16.67\,\text{mm}$$

and

$$U = \frac{1000}{-16.67\,\text{mm}} = -60.00\,\text{D}$$

From $V = P + U$,

$$V = +54.00\,\text{D} + (-60.00\,\text{D}) = -6.00\,\text{D}$$

and

$$v = \frac{100}{-6.00\,\text{D}} = -16.67\,\text{cm}$$

The light leaving George's eye is diverging and has a vergence of −6.00 D. Plane waves emerge from an emmetropic eye, so the −6.00 D vergence confirms that George is lacking 6.00 D of power (i.e., George has 6.00 D of hyperopia). The image conjugate to the retina is virtual and located 16.67 cm behind the +54.00 D lens. This is the far point for George's eye.

To get a clear retinal image, the light incident on George's eye must have a vergence U_{fp} equal to +6.00 D. Consequently, the contact lens correction necessary for George to clearly see a distant object without accommodating is +6.00 D.

Fay was a 2.50 D hyperope and had a virtual far point located 40 cm behind her eye, while George was a 6.00 D hyperope and had a virtual far point located 16.67 cm behind his eye. Note that the closer the far point is to optical infinity, the lesser the degree of hyperopia and the closer the eye is to being emmetropic. The closer the far point is to the eye, the greater the degree of hyperopia (Figure 6.5).

6.4 SPECTACLE LENS CORRECTIONS

While contact lens corrections sit on the cornea, spectacle lens corrections are mounted in a frame and sit a certain distance in front of the cornea. The distance from the back of the spectacle lens to the cornea is called the *vertex distance*. Because of the vertex distance, the dioptric power of a spectacle correction can differ from the dioptric power of the contact lens correction. The reason for this difference is that the wavefronts that leave the back of the spectacle lens gain or lose curvature as they cross the gap to the cornea.

Helen has a far point that is real and located 10 cm in front of her cornea. What contact lens correction and

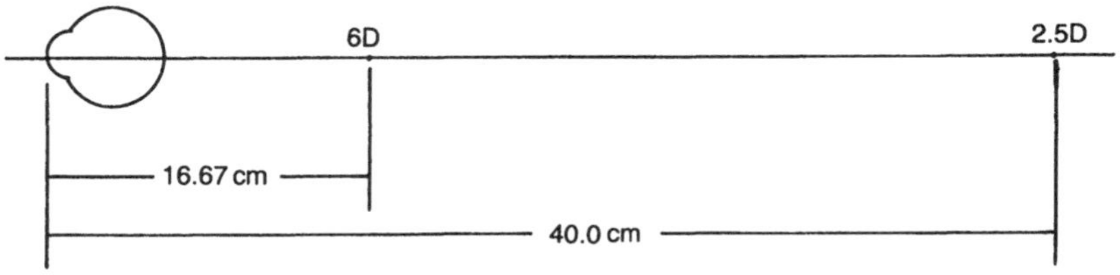

Figure 6.5 Far point location for a 2.5 D and a 6.0 D hyperope.

6D
2.5D
16.67 cm
40.0 cm

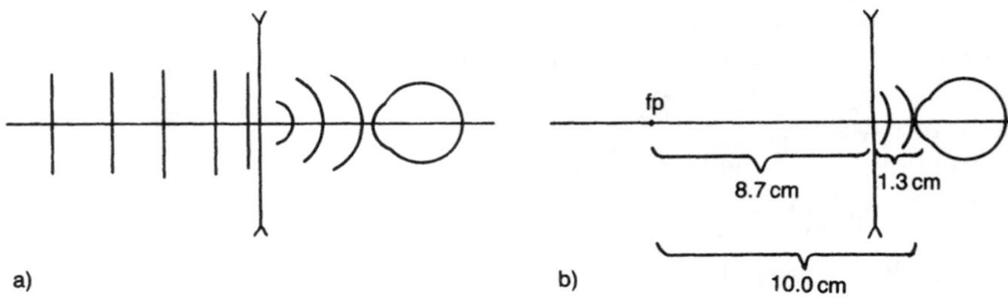

Figure 6.6 a, Plane waves incident on a spectacle correction for a myopic eye. The vergence of the wavefront incident on the cornea must be −10.00 D; b, geometry to get vergence of the wavefront leaving the spectacle lens.

what spectacle lens correction does Helen need for distance vision? Assume a vertex distance of 13 mm.

First of all, since Helen's far point is in front of her eye, Helen is a myope and needs diverging light incident on her cornea. Secondly, Helen's far point is relatively close to her eye, so Helen is a fairly high myope. When an object is placed at Helen's far point,

$$u_{fp} = -10.0\,\text{cm} \quad \text{and} \quad U_{fp} = -10.00\,\text{D}$$

Helen needs a vergence of −10.00 D incident on her cornea. From Eq. 6.1, Helen's distance vision contact lens correction is then −10.00 D.

The distance vision spectacle lens correction must take incoming plane waves and diverge them in such a manner that the vergence of the light reaching the cornea is −10.00 D (Figure 6.6a). Since the diverging wavefronts lose curvature as they travel across the gap from the spectacle lens to the cornea, the vergence leaving the spectacle lens must be more minus than −10.00 D.

For the proper correction, the wavefront incident on the cornea must be spherical and centered on the far point of the eye that is 10 cm in front of the cornea. In fact, all of the wavefronts in the bundle leaving the lens and traveling to the cornea must be spherical and centered on the far point. In other words, for incident plane waves the spectacle lens's image is at the eye's far point (i.e., the image for lens 1, the spectacle, is the object for lens 2, the eye). The wavefront leaving the spectacle lens is 13 mm or 1.3 cm closer to the far point than the wavefront incident on the cornea. Therefore, the radius of curvature of the wavefront leaving the spectacle lens is 10 cm minus 1.3 cm, or 8.7 cm (Figure 6.6b). The radius is negative since the wavefront is diverging, and the vergence leaving the spectacle lens is

$$V = \frac{100}{-8.7\,\text{cm}} = -11.50\,\text{D}$$

Since plane waves are incident on the spectacle lens for distance vision ($U = 0$), the dioptric power of the lens is

$$P = V - U = -11.50\,\text{D}$$

Helen's distance vision spectacle correction worn at a vertex distance of 13 mm is −11.50 D, while Helen's contact lens correction is −10.00 D. Note that the spectacle correction and contact correction were determined by knowing the far point location of Helen's eye and without knowing the dioptric power or length of the eye.

Ian wears a +5.00 D distance vision contact lens correction. What is Ian's distance vision spectacle lens correction worn at a vertex distance of 15 mm?

Ian is hyperopic, and from Eq. 6.1,

$$U_{fp} = P_c = +5.00\,\text{D}$$

resulting in

$$u_{fp} = \frac{100}{+5.00\,\text{D}} = +20.0\,\text{cm}$$

Ian's far point is virtual and located 20 cm behind the cornea.

The spectacle lens correction must be a converging lens. However, the converging wavefronts leaving the back of the spectacle lens gain curvature as they cross the gap between the lens and the cornea. Therefore, the vergence leaving the spectacle lens must be less positive than the incident vergence of +5.00 D that is required on the cornea (Figure 6.7a).

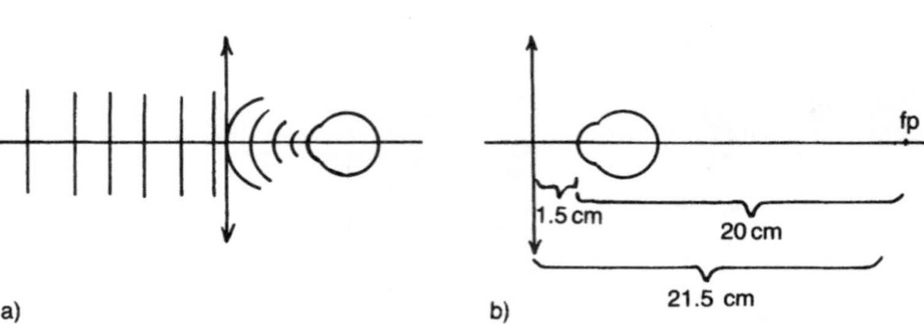

Figure 6.7 a, Plane waves incident on a spectacle correction for a hyperopic eye. The vergence of the wavefront incident on the cornea must be +5.00 D; b, geometry to get vergence of the wavefront leaving the spectacle lens.

All the converging wavefronts in the bundle between the spectacle lens and the cornea are centered on the far point. (In other words, the image of the spectacle lens, which is lens 1, must be at the far point of the eye, which is lens 2.) The radius of curvature of the wavefront incident on the cornea is 20 cm. The radius of curvature of the wavefront leaving the spectacle lens is 1.5 cm longer, or 21.5 cm (Figure 6.7b). Then the vergence of the wavefront leaving the lens is

$$V = \frac{100}{+21.5\,\text{cm}} = +4.65\,\text{D}$$

Since the incident waves from a distant object are plane waves, the dioptric power of the spectacle lens must then be +4.65 D. (Note that as expected the +4.65 D is positive and less than +5.00 D.)

It is important to keep in mind whether the wavefronts traveling across the gap between a spectacle lens and the cornea are gaining or losing curvature. Simple sketches like Figures 6.6a and 6.7a quickly supply this information.

The amount of vergence change across the gap depends on the power of the lens involved. High powered lenses, either plus or minus, produce large vergence changes, while low powered lenses produce small vergence changes. Changes smaller than 0.25 D are usually considered clinically insignificant. Changes of 0.25 D or greater are considered clinically significant.

Jeremy has a distance vision spectacle correction of −6.25 D. The vertex distance is 12 mm. What is Jeremy's distance vision contact lens power?

In Jeremy's case, the diverging wavefronts leaving the spectacle lens become flatter as they travel to the cornea (Figure 6.6a). Therefore, the contact lens power will be less minus than −6.25 D.

The center of curvature of the wavefront leaving the spectacle lens is

$$v = \frac{100}{-6.25\,\text{D}} = -16.0\,\text{cm}$$

The point 16 cm in front of the spectacle lens is the far point of Jeremy's eye. Each of the wavefronts crossing the gap is spherical and centered on the far point. The cornea is 1.2 cm further away, so the wavefront incident on the cornea has a radius of magnitude 17.2 cm. The radius is negative, and the vergence of the wavefront incident on the cornea is

$$U_{fp} = \frac{100}{-17.2\,\text{cm}} = -5.81\,\text{D} = \rho_c$$

An aphakic eye has no crystalline lens and is thus lacking plus power. The far point of an aphake is similar to that of a high hyperope: virtual and a finite distance behind the eye. Consider Karen, an aphake, who needs a distance vision spectacle lens correction of +14.25 D at a vertex distance of 15 mm. Karen chooses a frame that gives a vertex distance of 12 mm. What lens power does Karen need for the new frame?

For incident plane waves, light of vergence +14.25 D would leave the spectacle lens, which is 15 mm from the cornea. Since the wavefronts gain curvature as they move toward the cornea, the vergence at a distance of 12 mm from the cornea will be greater than +14.25 D (Figure 6.8a).

The center of curvature of the wavefront leaving the spectacle lens is at the far point of Karen's eye. The radius of curvature, which is also the image distance for the lens, is

$$v = \frac{100}{+14.25\,\text{D}} = +7.02\,\text{cm}$$

The vergence at 12 mm from the cornea (i.e., 3 mm behind the spectacle lens, Figure 6.8b) is

$$V = \frac{100}{(7.02 - 0.3)\,\text{cm}} = \frac{100}{6.72\,\text{cm}} = +14.88\,\text{D}$$

For distance vision, a spectacle lens placed 12 mm from Karen's eye must take incoming plane waves and change them into converging waves with a vergence of +14.88 D. From $P = V - U$, the power of the spectacle lens is then +14.88 D. Note that the +14.88 D lens at a vertex distance of 12 mm is a change of

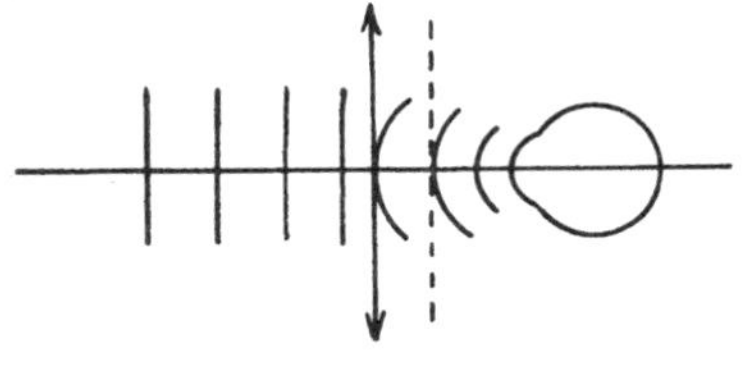

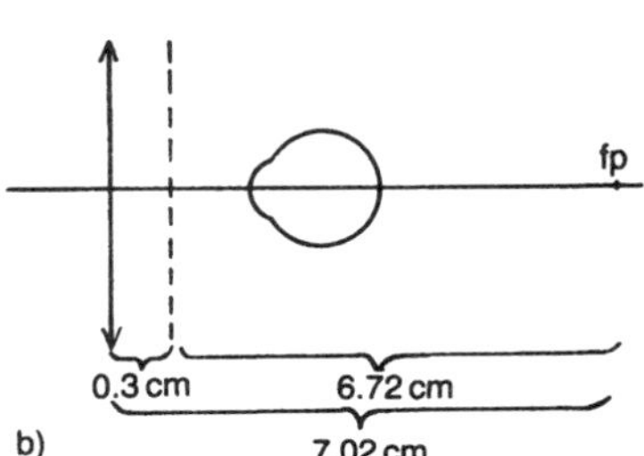

Figure 6.8 a, Downstream vergence changes involved in a vertex distance change for an aphakic correction; b, geometry to calculate resulting differences in spectacle correction power.

+0.63 D from the +14.25 D lens at a vertex distance of 15 mm, and this difference is clinically significant.

6.5 LENS EFFECTIVITY TERMINOLOGY

In the previous sections we saw that the power of a distance spectacle correction can differ from that of a contact correction because of the change in vergence of the wavefronts as they move from the spectacle plane to the eye. Historically, this phenomenon has been described under the name of lens effectivity. Instead of directly mentioning the change in vergence, people would refer to the effect of the spectacle lens at the cornea.

Consider a vertex distance of 12 mm. Then, the effect of a +10.00 D spectacle lens at the eye is +11.36 D. This statement means that for plane waves incident on the +10.00 D lens, the vergence of the light leaving the lens is +10.00 D, but the vergence of the light at the eye is +11.36 D.

Plus lenses are said to gain plus effectivity as they move away from the eye. This statement assumes that plane waves are incident on the lens, so this is simply another way of stating that converging wavefronts gain curvature as they travel from the spectacle lens to the eye.

Minus lenses are said to lose minus effectivity, or to gain plus effectivity, as they move away from the eye. Again, this statement assumes that plane waves are incident on the lens, so this also is simply another way of stating that diverging wavefronts lose curvature as they travel from the spectacle lens to the eye.

The gain in plus effectivity or loss in minus effectivity statements may not accurately describe what happens when diverging or converging light is incident on a spectacle lens because there the vergence incident on the lens may be changing in the opposite manner as the effectivity changes.

What is actually changing in the effectivity cases is the vergence of the wavefronts as they travel from one position to the other. Therefore, the name vergence effectivity is more appropriate than lens effectivity. However, the lens effectivity terminology is useful for those who are not familiar with vergence.

6.6 OCULAR ACCOMMODATIVE DEMAND

In dealing with distance vision corrections, we consider only unaccommodated eyes. Let us now take accommodation into account.

The crystalline lens in the eye adds converging power when the eye accommodates. In our thin lens and screen model, we can simulate this change by adding power to the thin lens. In the model, let P_u be the power of the unaccommodated eye, and P_a be the power of the accommodated eye. The amount of ocular accommodation A_o is the difference in the two values, or

$$A_o = P_a - P_u \tag{6.2}$$

Let v_e be the distance between the thin lens and the screen. Since the eye does not change length when it accommodates, v_e is a constant. In order to have a clear retinal image, the vergence V_e of the light leaving the thin lens representing the eye must equal the reciprocal of v_e, or

$$V_e = \frac{1}{v_e} \tag{6.3}$$

When the object is at the far point of the eye and the eye is unaccommodated, then the retinal image is clear and

$$V_e = P_u + U_{fp} \tag{6.4}$$

When the object is moved inside the far point to a point x, i.e., closer to the eye, then the eye accommodates to maintain a clear retinal image, and

$$V_e = P_a + U_x \tag{6.5}$$

where U_x is the vergence incident on the cornea when the object is at point x. Figure 6.9 shows the case for a myope.

We can subtract Eq. 6.5 from Eq. 6.4 to get

$$0 = P_u + U_{fp} - P_a - U_x$$

or

$$P_a - P_u = U_{fp} - U_x \tag{6.6}$$

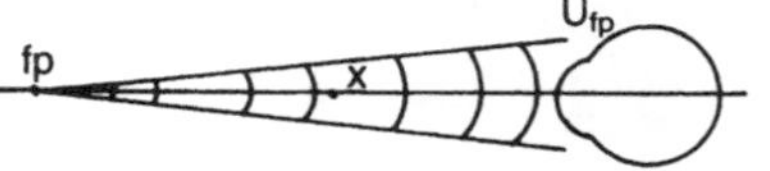

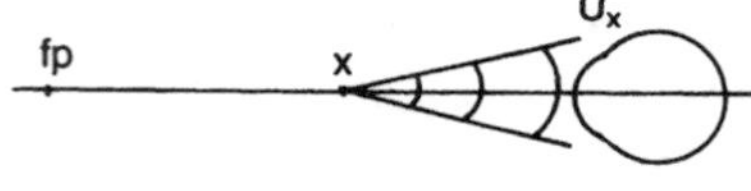

Figure 6.9 a, Wavefronts from the far point incident on a myopic eye; b, wavefronts from a point x inside the far point.

Then from Eq. 6.2,

$$A_o = U_{fp} - U_x \tag{6.7}$$

Equation 6.7 states that the amount A_o of ocular accommodation needed to maintain a clear retinal image must just offset (or neutralize) the increase in vergence incident on the eye when the object is moved in from the far point to the point x. In real eyes, the amount of accommodation that actually occurs (the accommodative response) may not match the accommodation needed. To distinguish the two, the amount of accommodation needed is called the *ocular accommodative demand*. Equation 6.7 is the fundamental working equation for computing the ocular accommodative demand.

Larry is an uncorrected myope with a far point 40 cm in front of his eye. So,

$$U_{fp} = \frac{100}{-40\,\text{cm}} = -2.50\,\text{D}$$

Suppose Larry looks at a book 25 cm in front of his eye. How much accommodation is needed for Larry to have a clear retinal image?

When the book is 25 cm in front of Larry's eye, the vergence incident on Larry's eye when he looks at the book is

$$U_x = \frac{100}{-25\,\text{cm}} = -4.00\,\text{D}$$

From Eq. 6.7, the ocular accommodative demand is

$$\begin{aligned} A_o &= U_{fp} - U_x \\ &= -2.50\,\text{D} - (-4.00\,\text{D}) \\ &= +1.50\,\text{D} \end{aligned}$$

When uncorrected, Larry has an ocular accommodative demand of +1.50 D when viewing the book at 25 cm.

Suppose Larry holds the book only 10 cm in front of his cornea. How much accommodation is needed then? In this case,

$$U_x = \frac{100}{-10\,\text{cm}} = -10.00\,\text{D}$$

From Eq. 6.7,

$$\begin{aligned} A_o &= U_{fp} - U_x \\ &= -2.50\,\text{D} - (-10.00\,\text{D}) \\ &= +7.50\,\text{D} \end{aligned}$$

Larry's ocular accommodative demand for the object at 10 cm is +7.50 D.

Suppose Larry looks at an object 1 m from his eye. In this case, the image inside Larry's eye would be formed in front of his retina resulting in a blurred retinal image. If Larry accommodates, the image is pulled even further in front of the retina, thus increasing the amount of retinal blur. We say that the object appears blurred because it is outside Larry's far point. Suppose we blindly went ahead and calculated the ocular accommodative demand anyway. For an object at 1 m, $U_x = -1.00$ D. Then,

$$\begin{aligned} A_o &= U_{fp} - U_x \\ &= -2.50\,\text{D} - (-1.00\,\text{D}) \\ &= -1.50\,\text{D} \end{aligned}$$

The negative value indicates a need for less plus power (in this case, 1.50 D less plus). Since we assumed that an unaccommodated eye has the least plus power and that accommodation adds plus power, then a negative value for A_o indicates that the object is outside the far point. (There is physiological evidence for a positive resting level of accommodation, but that does not change the basic considerations here.)

6.7 NEAR POINT AND RANGE OF CLEAR VISION: MYOPE

As a person moves an object closer and closer to his eye, more and more accommodation is needed to maintain a clear retinal image. Eventually, the maximum amount is reached. The maximum amount of accommodation is called the *amplitude of accommodation* (A_m).

The near point of an eye is the point conjugate to the axial retinal point of the maximally accommodated eye. The near point is also known by its Latin name, *punctum proximum*. The near point can be found as a special case of Eq. 6.7 by setting A_o equal to the amplitude of accommodation A_m. The points that successively become conjugate to the retina as a person increases his or her accommodation constitute the person's range of clear vision.

Suppose Larry, the myope in the preceding section, has an amplitude of accommodation of 9.00 D. Where is Larry's near point?

We can solve Eq. 6.7 for U_x to get

$$U_x = U_{fp} - A_o$$

Larry's far point was 40 cm, and

$$U_{fp} = -2.50\,\text{D}$$

When A_o is set equal to the 9.00 D amplitude of accommodation, the point x is the near point.

$$U_x = -2.50\,\text{D} - (9.00\,\text{D}) = -11.50\,\text{D}$$

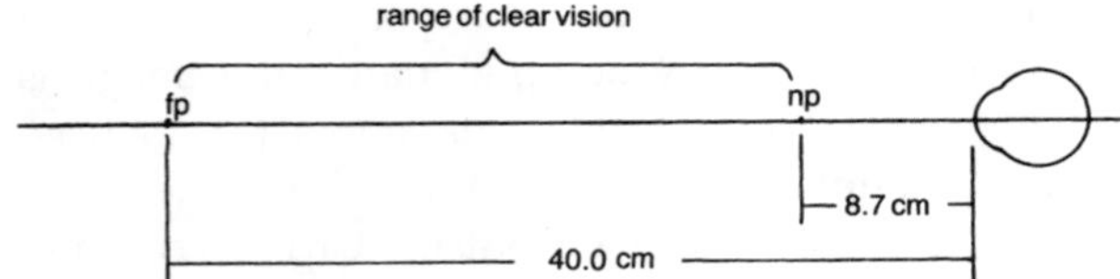

Figure 6.10 Range of clear vision for a myope.

Then,

$$u_x = \frac{1}{U_x}$$

or

$$u_{np} = u_x = \frac{100}{-11.50\,\text{D}} = -8.70\,\text{cm}$$

Larry's range of clear vision extends from his far point at 40 cm to his near point at 8.7 cm (Figure 6.10).

Now consider Marcie who wears a −5.00 D distance vision contact correction and has a 3.00 D amplitude of accommodation. What is Marcie's uncorrected range of clear vision?

From Eq. 6.1,

$$U_{fp} = -5.00\,\text{D} \quad \text{and} \quad u_{fp} = -20.0\,\text{cm}$$

From Eq. 6.7,

$$U_x = U_{fp} - A_o$$

or

$$U_x = -5.00\,\text{D} - 3.00\,\text{D} = -8.00\,\text{D}$$

Finally,

$$u_{np} = u_x = \frac{100}{-8.00\,\text{D}} = -12.5\,\text{cm}$$

Marcie's uncorrected range of clear vision extends from her far point at 20 cm to her near point at 12.5 cm.

The amplitude of accommodation gradually diminishes with age. At the age of 8 years, the amplitude of accommodation is approximately 14.00 D, at 20 years it has fallen to 11.00 D, at 30 years it is approximately 9.00 D, and at the age of 50 years it is less than 2.00 D. Because of the decline of the amplitude of accommodation with age, a person's near point steadily recedes from the eye and approaches the far point.

6.8 RANGE OF CLEAR VISION: EMMETROPE

Accommodation is particularly easy to calculate for the emmetrope. The general equation is again Eq. 6.7:

$$A_o = U_{fp} - U_x$$

However, for an emmetrope, U_{fp} is zero.

Norman is an emmetrope who looks at a poster 50 cm from his eye. What is Norman's ocular accommodative demand?

Here,

$$U_x = \frac{100}{-50\,\text{cm}} = -2.00\,\text{D}$$

and from Eq. 6.7,

$$A_o = 0 - (-2.00\,\text{D}) = +2.00\,\text{D}$$

If Norman moves the poster in to a point 25 cm in front of his eye, then

$$U_x = \frac{100}{-25\,\text{cm}} = -4.00\,\text{D}$$

and

$$A_o = 0 - (-4.00\,\text{D}) = +4.00\,\text{D}$$

For an object 20 cm in front of his eye, Norman has an ocular accommodative demand of +5.00 D, and for an object 10 cm in front of his eye he has an ocular accommodative demand of +10.00 D.

Octavia is an emmetrope with a 7.00 D amplitude of accommodation. What is Octavia's range of clear vision?

To find Octavia's near point: use Eq. 6.7, set A_o equal to the amplitude of accommodation, and solve for U_x.

$$U_x = U_{fp} - A_o$$

But U_{fp} is zero, therefore,

$$U_x = 0 - (+7.00\,\text{D}) = -7.00\,\text{D}$$

and

$$u_{np} = u_x = \frac{100}{-7.00\,\text{D}} = -14.3\,\text{cm}$$

Octavia's near point is 14.3 cm, in front of her eye. Since Octavia is an emmetrope, her far point is at optical infinity. Octavia's range of clear vision extends from optical infinity to 14.3 cm in front of her eye.

As Octavia ages, her near point will move out away from her eye toward her far point at optical infinity. Eventually, she will have difficulty seeing near objects, a signal that presbyopia has arrived.

6.9 RANGE OF CLEAR VISION: HYPEROPE

A hyperope does not have enough converging power in the unaccommodated eye. Since accommodation adds plus converging power, it can be used to over-

Figure 6.11 Point x is conjugate to the retina for an 8.00 D hyperope who is accommodating 3.00 D.

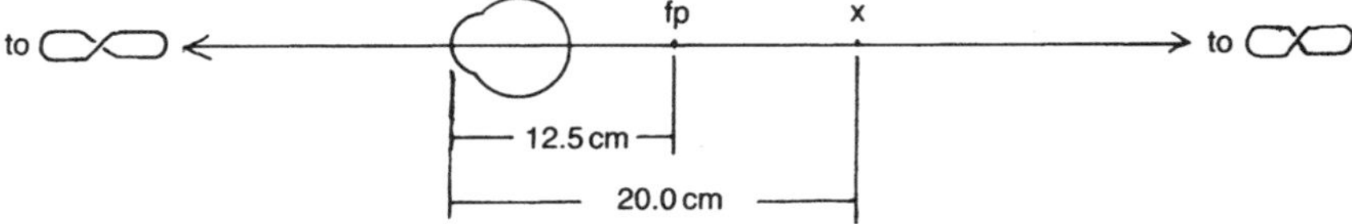

come some or all of the hyperopia. Since the uncorrected hyperope uses accommodation to see distant objects, he or she may not have enough left for near objects. Furthermore, the ciliary muscle, like any muscle in the body, is subject to fatigue under conditions of exertion for long periods of time. Therefore, while a high hyperope may be able to see a distant object clearly by accommodating, he may not be able to sustain the accommodation.

An uncorrected hyperope has a virtual far point. As the hyperope accommodates, the virtual point conjugate to the retina moves away from the eye and toward optical infinity. If a hyperope has enough accommodation, an object at optical infinity can be imaged clearly on the retina. Whatever accommodation is left can then be used to see real objects that are closer than optical infinity.

Consider Paul, a hyperope who needs a +8.00 D contact lens. From Eq. 6.1,

$$U_{fp} = P_c = +8.00\,\text{D}$$

and

$$u_{fp} = \frac{100}{+8.00\,\text{D}} = +12.5\,\text{cm}$$

Paul's far point is virtual and located 12.5 cm behind his cornea. (Here the virtual object means that the light incident on Paul's cornea must be converging in order to get a clear image on the retina.)

When Paul accommodates 3.00 D, what point is conjugate to his retina? From Eq. 6.7,

$$A_o = U_{fp} - U_x$$
$$+3.00\,\text{D} = +8.00\,\text{D} - U_x$$

or

$$U_x = +8.00\,\text{D} - (+3.00\,\text{D}) = +5.00\,\text{D}$$

Then,

$$u_x = \frac{100}{+5.00\,\text{D}} = +20.0\,\text{cm}$$

When Paul accommodates 3.00 D, the point conjugate to his retina remains virtual, but moves from 12.5 cm to 20.0 cm. An uncorrected 5.00 D hyperope has a far point at 20.0 cm, so in a sense, by using 3.00 D of accommodation Paul can now function as a 5.00 D hyperope instead of an 8.00 D hyperope (Figure 6.11).

What is Paul's ocular accommodative demand to see an object at optical infinity? From Eq. 6.7,

$$A_o = U_{fp} - U_x$$

For the object at optical infinity $U_x = 0$, and since

$$U_{fp} = +8.00\,\text{D}$$

it follows that

$$A_o = +8\,\text{D} - 0\,\text{D} = +8.00\,\text{D}$$

When uncorrected, Paul needs to accommodate +8.00 D to clearly see an object at optical infinity. In effect, Paul neutralizes the 8.00 D of hyperopia by accommodating 8.00 D.

What is Paul's ocular accommodative demand to read a book held 25 cm in front of his eye? Now,

$$U_x = \frac{100}{-25\,\text{cm}} = -4.00\,\text{D}$$

From Eq. 6.7,

$$A_o = U_{fp} - U_x$$

or

$$A_o = +8.00\,\text{D} - (-4.00\,\text{D}) = +12.00\,\text{D}$$

Paul's ocular accommodative demand to read the book 25 cm in front of his eye is +12.00 D.

Note that Paul needed 8.00 D to see an object at optical infinity. In order to get from optical infinity to a book that is 25 cm in front of his eye, Paul requires an additional 4.00 D of accommodation. The 8.00 D plus 4.00 D provides the total ocular accommodative demand of 12.00 D that Paul needs to read the book. Figure 6.12 provides a circular representation of Paul's accommodation.

6.10 RANGE OF CLEAR VISION: SUMMARY

The circular representation can be used to represent the range of clear vision for the myope and emmetrope as well as for the hyperope. Figure 6.13 shows

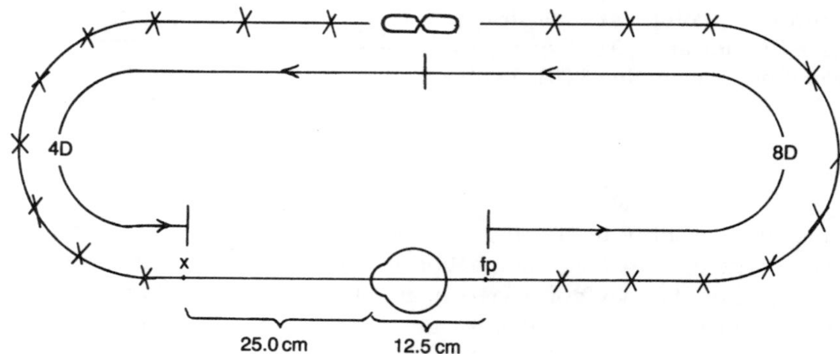

Figure 6.12 Range of clear vision as an 8.00 D hyperope accommodates 12.00 D.

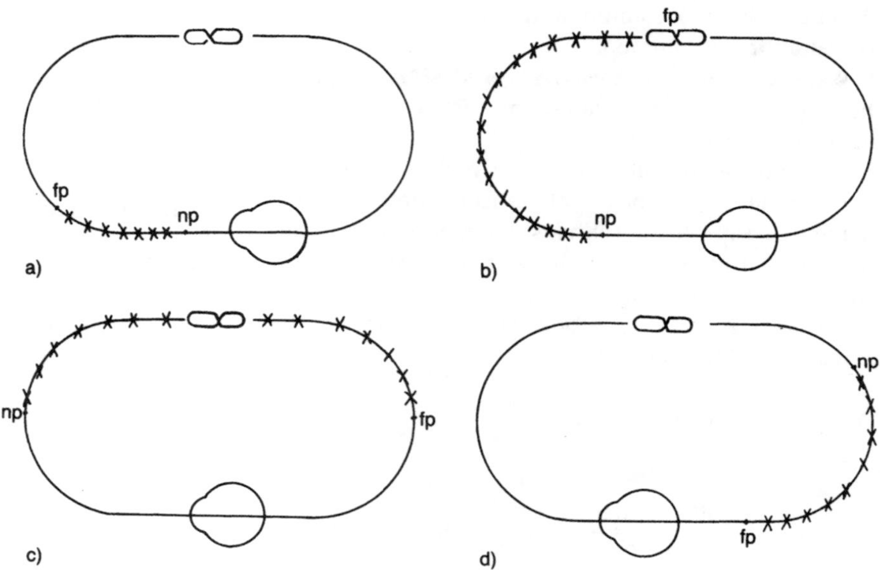

Figure 6.13 Ranges of clear vision: a, myope; b, emmetrope; c, low hyperope; d, high hyperope.

four cases. In each case, the eye is looking left. The points on the left half of the circle represent optically real points, while the points on the right half of the circle represent virtual points. The far point of a myope is a real point located a finite distance in front of the eye, while the far point of a hyperope is a virtual point located a finite distance behind the eye. The far point of an emmetrope is at optical infinity.

The first case is that of a myope. The far point is real and a finite distance in front of the eye. The near point is also real and closer to the eye than the far point. Distance objects are not included in the range of clear vision.

The second case is that of an emmetrope. The far point is at optical infinity, and the near point is real and closer to the eye than the far point.

The third case is that of a hyperope with enough accommodation to overcome the hyperopia and see some near real objects. The far point is virtual and a finite distance behind the eye, while the near point is real and a finite distance in front of the eye. The range of clear vision includes optical infinity.

The fourth case is that of a hyperope who does not have enough accommodation to overcome the hyperopia. The far point is virtual and located a finite distance behind the eye, and the near point is also virtual and located a finite distance behind the eye. The near point is closer to optical infinity than the far point. No real object points are imaged on the retina.

In each of the cases, the range of clear vision extends counter-clockwise from the far point to the near point. The region inside, or counter-clockwise from, the near point is the region where objects are not clearly imaged on the retina because the person does not have enough accommodation available. The region outside, or clockwise from, the far point is the region where objects are not clearly imaged on the retina because the unaccommodated eye already has too much converging power, and the clear image is formed in the vitreous humor in front of the retina.

Suppose each of the eyes represented in Figure 6.13 has a 4.00 D amplitude of accommodation and the respective refractive states are: 3.00 D myopia, emmetropia, 3.00 D hyperopia, and 6.00 D hyperopia. The respective far points are then: real and 33.3 cm in front of the eye; at optical infinity; virtual and 33.3 cm behind the eye; and virtual and 16.67 cm behind the eye. You should now be able to show that the respective near points are: real and 14.3 cm in front of the eye; real and 25.0 cm in front of the eye; real and 100.0 cm in front of the eye; and virtual and 50.0 cm behind the eye. Note the near point variation even though each has a 4.00 D amplitude of accommodation.

6.11 SPECTACLE ACCOMMODATIVE DEMAND

Consider an unaccommodated emmetrope with a 10.00 D amplitude of accommodation. When this emmetrope puts on a −8.00 D contact lens and looks at a distant object, the object will appear blurred (and maybe not even visible). However, if the emmetrope accommodates 8.00 D, the distant object will appear clear. In other words, in the thin lens eye model the 8.00 D of accommodation neutralizes the −8.00 D contact lens.

Suppose the emmetrope looks through a −8.00 D spectacle lens at the distant object. Again the emmetrope can accommodate to neutralize the spectacle lens and see the distant object clearly. In this case, we tend to say the −8.00 D spectacle lens causes 8.00 D of accommodation, but, in fact, the actual ocular accommodative demand is not 8.00 D. For the distant object, the vergence of the light leaving the spectacle lens is −8.00 D, but 14 mm downstream the vergence incident on the eye is −7.19 D. The vergence U_{fp} is zero for the emmetrope, so the emmetrope's ocular accommodative demand is +7.19 D.

In the above case, we label the 8.00 D as the spectacle accommodative demand. The spectacle accommodative demand is related (but not equal) to the ocular accommodative demand. Clinically, it is expedient to think in terms of the spectacle accommodative demand even though it can differ from the ocular accommodative demand.

Another example of spectacle accommodative demand is that of a spectacle corrected ametrope looking through the spectacle lenses at a near object. Assume that the spectacle corrected ametrope can see a distant object clearly without accommodating. For the distant object, the vergence incident on the spectacle lens is zero. When the object is 25 cm from the spectacle lens, the vergence incident on the spectacle lens is −4.00 D. To see this object clearly, the person has to accommodate enough to neutralize the 4.00 D change. The 4.00 D is the spectacle accommodative demand. We can find the actual amount of accommodation needed by the eye (the ocular accommodative demand) by calculating U_{fp} and U_x (the vergence incident on the eye) and using Eq. 6.7. This is shown in the next section.

We can formalize the above argument by defining the spectacle accommodative demand A_s as the difference in the vergences incident on the spectacle lens. For the distance object (no accommodation) the incident vergence is zero. For the near object, the vergence incident on the spectacle lens is U_s. The spectacle accommodative demand is the difference between the two vergences incident on the spectacle lens, or

$$A_s = 0 - U_s$$

Then,

$$A_s = -U_s \tag{6.8}$$

EXAMPLE 6.1

Bobby Brickbat is wearing a distance vision spectacle correction. What is the spectacle accommodative demand when Bobby holds his bat 20 cm from his spectacle lens and examines it for a suspected crack?

For the bat at 20 cm (the proximal object),

$$U_s = -5.00\,\text{D}$$

and

$$A_s = -(-5.00\,\text{D}) = +5.00\,\text{D}$$

Note that the power of the spectacle lens does not matter for the spectacle accommodative demand. However, the spectacle lens power does matter for the ocular accommodative demand.

6.12 OCULAR ACCOMMODATIVE DEMAND THROUGH SPECTACLES

Figure 6.14 shows a spectacle corrected hyperope looking first at a distant object (Figure 6.14a), and then at a near object (Figure 6.14b). For the distant object, plane waves are incident on the spectacle lens, and the vergence leaving the spectacle lens is equal to the power P_s of the spectacle lens. Converging light leaves

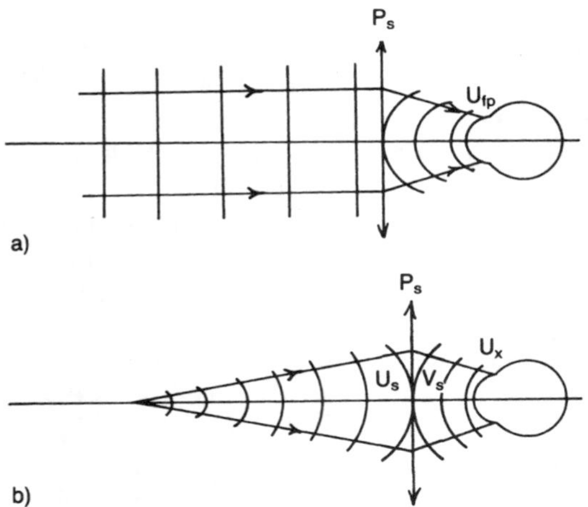

Figure 6.14 a, A spectacle-corrected hyperope viewing a distant object; b, the spectacle-corrected hyperope viewing a near object.

the spectacle lens, and the vergence U_{fp} incident on the cornea is greater than P_s. For the near (proximal) object, the vergence V_s leaving the spectacle lens is less than P_s, and again a vergence change occurs across the gap between the lens and the eye. The vergence incident on the eye is U_x. From Eq. 6.7, the ocular accommodative demand is

$$A_o = U_{fp} - U_x$$

Because of the vergence changes across the gap between the lens and the eye, the ocular accommodative demand and the spectacle accommodative demand may differ.

EXAMPLE 6.2a

Hilda is hyperope with a +12.00 D spectacle correction at a 14 mm vertex distance. What is Hilda's spectacle and ocular accommodative demands when looking at a tapestry located 25 cm in front of her spectacle lens?

For the tapestry (the proximal object), the vergence incident on the spectacle lens is

$$U_s = -4.00\,\text{D}$$

From Eq. 6.8, Hilda's spectacle accommodative demand is

$$A_s = -(-4.00\,\text{D}) = +4.00\,\text{D}$$

For the tapestry, the light leaving the spectacle lens has a vergence

$$\begin{aligned} V_s &= P_s + U_s \\ &= +12.00\,\text{D} + (-4.00\,\text{D}) = +8.00\,\text{D} \end{aligned}$$

For a +8.00 D vergence, the vergence U_x at a distance 14 mm downstream is +9.01 D. When plane waves are incident on the +12.00 D lens, the vergence leaving is +12.00 D, and the vergence U_{fp} 14 mm downstream is +14.42 D. From Eq. 6.7, the ocular accommodative demand is

$$\begin{aligned} A_o &= U_{fp} - U_x \\ &= +14.42\,\text{D} - (+9.01\,\text{D}) = +5.41\,\text{D} \end{aligned}$$

So while Hilda's spectacle accommodative demand is +4.00 D, her ocular accommodative demand is +5.41 D.

EXAMPLE 6.2b

Myra is myope with a −12.00 D spectacle correction at a 14 mm vertex distance. What is Myra's spectacle and ocular accommodative demands when looking at the tapestry located 25 cm in front of her spectacle lens?

As in Example 6.1a, the spectacle accommodative demand is

$$A_s = +4.00\,\text{D}$$

For the tapestry, the light leaving the spectacle lens has a vergence

$$\begin{aligned} V_s &= P_s + U_s \\ &= -12.00\,\text{D} + (-4.00\,\text{D}) = -16.00\,\text{D} \end{aligned}$$

For a −16.00 D vergence, the vergence U_x at a distance 14 mm downstream is −13.07 D.

When plane waves are incident on the −12.00 D lens, the vergence leaving is −2.00 D, and the vergence U_{fp} 14 mm downstream is −10.27 D. From Eq. 6.7, the ocular accommodative demand is

$$\begin{aligned} A_o &= U_{fp} - U_x \\ &= -10.27\,\text{D} - (-13.07\,\text{D}) = +2.80\,\text{D} \end{aligned}$$

So while Myra's spectacle accommodative demand is +4.00 D, her ocular accommodative demand is only +2.80 D.

Note that while the spectacle accommodative demand was the same for Hilda and Myra, the ocular accommodative demands are very different. Hilda, the hyperope, has an ocular accommodative demand that is higher than the spectacle accommodative demand; while Myra, the myope, has an ocular accommodative demand that is lower than the spectacle accommodative demand. This difference is due to the vergence effectivity changes between the spectacle lens and the eye. In effect, for an object at the same distance, spectacle corrected hyperopes have to accommodate more than spectacle corrected myopes.

While the previous examples clearly show this ocular accommodation effect, they do not provide an intuitive feeling for the result. We can derive an algebraic approximation that helps supply intuition. First, we need to consider an algebraic equation for downstream vergence.

6.13 THE DOWNSTREAM VERGENCE EQUATION

We have been numerically solving downstream vergence problems since Chapter 2. Here we use the same technique to derive an algebraic equation for the downstream vergence problem.

Figure 6.15a shows converging wavefronts in the same bundle. The wavefront at position 2 is a distance d downstream from position 1. The wavefront at position 1 has a radius of curvature q_1 and the wavefront at position 2 has a radius of curvature of q_2. From the figure, it is clear that

$$q_2 = q_1 - d$$

The vergence of the wavefront at position 2 is given by

$$V_2 = \frac{1}{q_2}$$

where q_2 is in meters. Then,

$$V_2 = \frac{1}{q_1 - d}$$

provided q_1 and d are in meters. The numerator and the denominator of the above equation can each be divided by q_1 with the result that

$$V_2 = \frac{1/q_1}{1 - d/q_1}$$

Since the vergence at position 1 is given by

$$V_1 = \frac{1}{q_1}$$

the expression for V_2 becomes

$$V_2 = \frac{V_1}{1 - dV_1}, \quad d \text{ in meters} \qquad (6.9)$$

Equation 6.9 relates the vergence at position 1 to the vergence at position 2 that is a distance d downstream. For this reason, I like to call Eq. 6.9 the downstream vergence equation. However, one can also say that Eq. 6.9 gives the effect at a distance d downstream of the vergence at position 1. Therefore, it can also be referred to as a vergence effectivity equation.

Equation 6.9 is a general equation, and can be derived from diverging wavefronts as well as from converging wavefronts (Figure 6.15b). Note the diopter is the reciprocal of a meter, and the distance d in Eq. 6.9 must be in meters so that the product dV_1 is dimensionless.

EXAMPLE 6.3

For converging wavefronts (Figure 6.15a), when the vergence at position 1 is +4.00 D, what is the vergence at position 2, which is 15 cm downstream?

Note that you should also be able to work this particular problem numerically in your head by using the techniques of Chapter 2. From Eq. 6.9,

$$V_2 = \frac{+4.00\,\text{D}}{1 - (0.15\,\text{m})(+4.00\,\text{D})}$$

$$= \frac{+4.00\,\text{D}}{1 - 0.60} = +10.00\,\text{D}$$

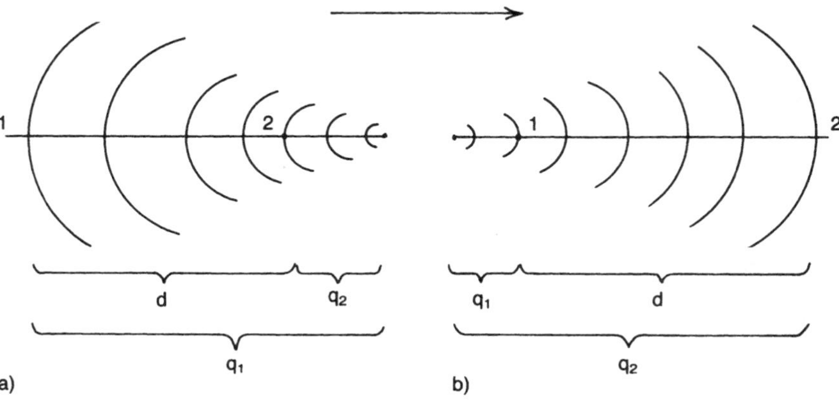

Figure 6.15 Downstream vergence geometry: a, converging wavefronts; b, diverging wavefronts.

EXAMPLE 6.4

For diverging wavefronts (Figure 6.15b), when the vergence at position 1 is $-20.00\,\mathrm{D}$, what is the vergence at position 2, which is a distance of 45 cm downstream?

Again from Chapter 2, you should be able to work this problem numerically in your head without using Eq. 6.9. From Eq. 6.9,

$$V_2 = \frac{-20.00\,\mathrm{D}}{1-(0.45\,\mathrm{m})(-20.00\,\mathrm{D})} = \frac{-20.00\,\mathrm{D}}{1-(-9.00)} = -2.00\,\mathrm{D}$$

We can also solve Eq. 6.9 for V_1 in terms of V_2, in which case the result is the upstream vergence equation

$$V_1 = \frac{V_2}{1+dV_2}, \quad d \text{ in meters} \tag{6.10}$$

6.14 APPROXIMATION FOR ACCOMMODATION THROUGH SPECTACLE LENSES

Figure 6.14 shows the situation for the ocular accommodative demand through spectacle lenses. For vergence incident on the eye, the fundamental equation is

$$A_o = U_{fp} - U_x$$

When the person is looking at the distant object, plane waves are incident on the spectacle lens and, consequently, the vergence of the light leaving the spectacle lens is equal to the dioptric power of the lens. Then from the downstream vergence Eq. 6.9, the vergence U_{fp} incident on the eye is

$$U_{fp} = \frac{P_s}{1-dP_s}$$

When the person looks at the near (proximal) object the vergence incident on the spectacle lens is U_s and the vergence leaving the spectacle lens is V_s. Then the vergence U_x incident on the eye is

$$U_x = \frac{V_s}{1-dV_s}$$

When the expressions for U_{fp} and U_s are substituted into the accommodation equation, the result is

$$A_o = \frac{P_s}{1-dP_s} - \frac{V_s}{1-dV_s} \tag{6.11}$$

Equation 6.11 gives the ocular accommodative demand in terms of the dioptric power of the spectacle lens, the vergence V_s of the light leaving the spectacle lens, and the vertex distance d. It is clear from Eq. 6.11 that the vertex distance has an effect, but it is not clear what the pattern of that effect is. We can make the pattern emerge by considering some approximations to Eq. 6.11.

Consider an equation of the form

$$y = \frac{1}{1-x} \tag{6.12}$$

When x is small relative to 1, the equation can be approximated by

$$y \approx 1 + x \tag{6.13}$$

For example,

$$y = \frac{1}{1-0.10} = 1.11$$

while the approximation gives

$$y \approx 1 + 0.10 = 1.10$$

The approximation gets better for smaller x values and worse for larger x values.

The vergence effectivity terms in Eq. 6.11 have the form of Eq. 6.12 with x equal to either dP_s or dV_s with d in meters. When these terms are small relative to 1, we can use the approximation, Eq. 6.13, in Eq. 6.11 to obtain

$$A_o \approx P_s(1+dP_s) - V_s(1+dV_s)$$

or

$$A_o \approx P_s - V_s + d(P_s^2 - V_s^2)$$

Now,

$$P_s^2 - V_s^2 = (P_s - V_s)(P_s + V_s)$$

Since

$$V_s = P_s + U_s$$

$$-U_s = P_s - V_s$$

We can combine the above four equations to obtain

$$A_o \approx -U_s + d(-U_s)(P_s + V_s) \approx -U_s[1 + d(P_s + V_s)]$$

and

$$A_o \approx -U_s[1 + d(2P_s + U_s)]$$

In our approximation, we want a simple expression that gets us close to the exact value. In situations where U_s is smaller than $2P_s$, we can further simplify the approximate expression to

$$A_o \approx -U_s[1 + 2dP_s] \tag{6.14}$$

From Eq. 6.8, the spectacle accommodative demand A_s is equal to $-U_s$, so

$$A_o \approx A_s[1 + 2dP_s] \tag{6.15}$$

Equation 6.15 is an approximation to Eq. 6.11. According to Eq. 6.15, the difference between the ocular accommodative demand and the spectacle accommodative demand is due to the $2dP_s$ term. However, this term has opposite effects for myopes and hyperopes. For hyperopes, the spectacle lens power P_s is positive and the term adds so that A_o is greater than A_s. For myopes, P_s is negative and the term subtracts so that A_o is less than A_s.

Consider Myra, the myope in Example 6.2b. Myra has a −12.00 D spectacle lens at a 14 mm vertex distance. In Example 6.2b, Myra looks at an object that is 25 cm from her spectacle lens, and her spectacle accommodative demand is +4.00 D. Then from Eq. 6.15, the ocular accommodative demand is

$$\begin{aligned} A_o &\approx +4.00\,\text{D}[1 + 2(0.014\,\text{m})(-12.00\,\text{D})] \\ &\approx +4.00\,\text{D}[1 - 0.34] = +2.66\,\text{D} \end{aligned}$$

Here the approximation confirms that for the Myra, the myope, A_o is less than A_s. In Example 6.2b, the exact ocular accommodative demand for Myra was +2.80 D, which was the result of several downstream vergence calculations. Here the simple approximation gets us within 0.16 D of the exact result. The approximation would be better for objects that are farther away than 25 cm, and worse for objects that are closer than 25 cm.

Consider Hilda, the hyperope in Example 6.2a. Hilda has a +12.00 D spectacle lens at a 14 mm vertex distance. In the example, Hilda views an object 25 cm from her spectacle lens, and her spectacle accommodative demand is +4.00 D. Then from Eq. 6.15, the ocular accommodative demand is

$$\begin{aligned} A_o &\approx +4.00\,\text{D}[1 + 2(0.014\,\text{m})(+12.00\,\text{D})] \\ &\approx +4.00\,\text{D}[1 + 0.34] = +5.36\,\text{D} \end{aligned}$$

The numbers for Hilda the hyperope confirm that A_o is greater than A_s. In Example 6.2a, the exact ocular accommodative demand for Hilda was +5.41 D, which was the result of several downstream vergence calculations. The simple approximation gets us within 0.05 D of the exact result. The approximation would be better for objects that are farther away than 25 cm, and worse for objects that are closer than 25 cm.

We can also use the approximation to estimate corrected near points for Myra and Hilda. Suppose that each has a 6.00 D ocular amplitude of accommodation. What are their respective near points while wearing their spectacle corrections?

Here we can set A_o equal to 6.00 D, solve for A_s, and then find the corresponding object point for the spectacle lens. First consider Hilda, the hyperope. From Eq. 6.15,

$$\begin{aligned} A_s &\approx \frac{A_o}{1 + 2dP_s} \\ &\approx \frac{6.00\,\text{D}}{1 + [2 \cdot 0.014\,\text{m}\ (+12.00\,\text{D})]} \\ &\approx \frac{6.00\,\text{D}}{1 + 0.34} \approx +4.49\,\text{D} \end{aligned}$$

From Eq. 6.8,

$$U_s = -A_s \approx -4.49\,\text{D}$$

So,

$$u_s = \frac{100}{-4.49\,\text{D}} = -22.3\,\text{cm}$$

According to these numbers, when Hilda uses all of her accommodation, the object that is conjugate to the retina is located approximately 22.3 cm from her spectacle lens. This is her corrected near point.

Now consider Myra, the myope.

$$\begin{aligned} A_s &\approx \frac{A_o}{1 + 2dP_s} \\ &\approx \frac{6.00\,\text{D}}{1 + [2 \cdot 0.014\,\text{m}\ (-12.00\,\text{D})]} \\ &\approx \frac{6.00\,\text{D}}{1 - 0.34} \approx +9.04\,\text{D} \end{aligned}$$

From Eq. 6.8,

$$U_s = -A_s \approx -9.04\,\text{D}$$

So,

$$u_s = \frac{100}{-9.04\,\text{D}} = -11.1\,\text{cm}$$

According to these numbers, Myra's corrected near point is approximately 11.1 cm in front of her spectacle lens.

Note that Myra and Hilda each had the same ocular amplitude of accommodation, but they have different corrected near points through their spectacle lens because of the different accommodative demands. Both Myra and Hilda have very strong corrections.

When the calculations are done for a myope and a hyperope with *low* dioptric power corrections, there is very little difference in their corrected near points.

These results show that moderate to high spectacle corrected hyperopes have a larger accommodative demand than moderate to high spectacle corrected myopes. Based on these results, we would expect that moderate to high spectacle corrected hyperopes would start experiencing presbyopia symptoms at an earlier age than spectacle corrected moderate to high myopes.

6.15 ACCOMMODATION THROUGH CONTACT LENSES

The differences in accommodative demand in the spectacle corrected cases were due to the different vergence changes that occurred between the spectacle lens and the eye. However, contact lens corrections sit on the eye; therefore, no vergence changes occur between the contact lens and the eye.

We can consider a contact lens as a spectacle lens with a zero vertex distance. In this case, Eq. 6.15 becomes exact, and shows that

$$A_o = A_s$$

So, for a contact corrected ametrope, the ocular accommodative demand equals the spectacle accommodative demand (spectacle at zero vertex distance). In turn, Eq. 6.8 gives

$$A_o = -U_c \tag{6.16}$$

where the subscript s (for spectacle) has been changed to c (for contact).

We can also derive Eq. 6.16 from first principles. Let P_c be the power of the contact lens, U_c be the vergence incident on the contact lens, and V_c be the vergence of the light exiting the contact lens. Then,

$$V_c = P_c + U_c$$

The light leaving the contact lens is immediately incident on the eye with no vergence change. Therefore,

$$U_x = V_c$$

From Eq. 6.7, the ocular accommodative demand is given by

$$A_o = U_{fp} - U_x$$

where the vergences U_{fp} and U_x are incident on the cornea. From Eq. 6.1,

$$U_{fp} = P_c$$

By combining the above three equations, we get

$$A_o = P_c - V_c$$

From the basic $V = P + U$ equation,

$$-U_c = P_c - V_c$$

and the ocular accommodative demand equation simplifies to

$$A_o = -U_c \tag{6.16}$$

For the contact corrected ametropes, the vergence of the light incident on the contact lens is equal to the vergence of the light incident on the cornea of an emmetrope who is standing at the same distance from the object. Thus, in the thin lens and screen model, all contact corrected ametropes have the same ocular accommodative demand as an emmetrope.

For example, a myope wearing a −4.00 D contact lens correction and viewing an object 50 cm in front of the lens has a U_c of −2.00 D, and from Eq. 6.16 an ocular accommodative demand of +2.00 D. Similarly, a hyperope wearing a +4.00 D contact correction and viewing an object 50 cm in front of the lens has an ocular accommodative demand of +2.00 D. An emmetrope viewing the same object 50 cm in front of his or her eye also has an ocular accommodative demand of +2.00 D.

For Myra and Hilda in the previous section, the contact corrections are −10.27 D and +14.43 D, respectively. The ocular accommodative demand for the contact corrected girls to see the tapestry 25 cm from the spectacle plane, or 26.4 cm from the eye is found as follows:

$$U_c = \frac{100}{-26.4\,\text{cm}} = -3.79\,\text{D}$$

and

$$A_o = -U_c = +3.79\,\text{D}$$

The accommodative demand of 3.79 D is the same as that of an emmetrope viewing the tapestry held 26.4 cm in front of the cornea.

Myra, the myope, needs 2.80 D of accommodation to see the tapestry when spectacle corrected and 3.79 D when contact corrected. Hilda, the hyperope, requires 5.41 D of accommodation to see the tapestry when spectacle corrected but only 3.79 D when contact corrected. In general, when a hyperope changes from a contact correction to a spectacle correction, more ocular accommodation is needed. When a myope changes from a contact correction to a spectacle correction, less ocular accommodation is required. Keep in mind that

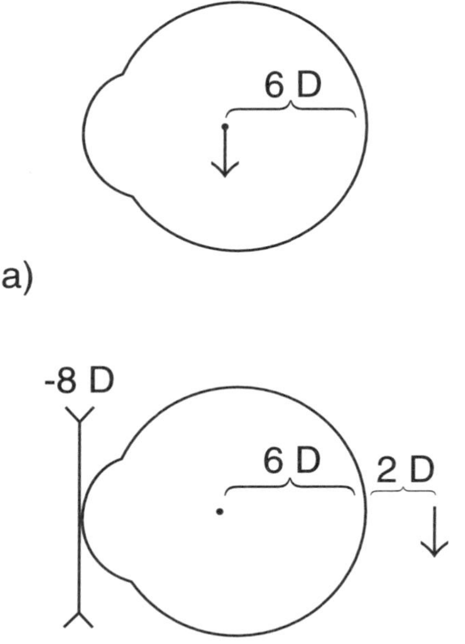

Figure 6.16 a, For a distant object, uncorrected clear image location for Quinn, a 6.00 D ocular myope; b, clear image location for Quinn wearing a –8.00 D lens. The –8.00 D lens pushes the clear image 8.00 D back, so that it is 2.00 D behind the retina.

any difference has to be 0.25 D or greater to be clinically significant and that low hyperopes and myopes may not show any clinically significant differences.

6.16 OVER/UNDER MINUS OR PLUS

Suppose that a lens in front of an eye is not the proper correcting lens. Then the "corrected far point" is not at optical infinity and the person will not function like an emmetrope. There are several ways to analyze this situation. A particularly simple way is to consider the clear image locations relative to the retina.

Quinn is a myope who needs a −6.00 D distance vision contact lens but instead is given a −8.00 D contact lens. What ametrope does Quinn function like while wearing the −8.00 D lens?

When Quinn is uncorrected and viewing a distant object, the clear image formed by his eye is in the vitreous humor and his retinal image is blurred. We can describe this situation by saying that Quinn's clear image is 6.00 D in front of the retina (Figure 6.16a). Then a −6.00 D contact lens moves the clear image back onto the retina and corrects Quinn for distance vision. However when Quinn wears the −8.00 D lens, the clear image is moved back from 6.00 D in front of the retina to 2.00 D behind the retina (Figure 6.16b). Here Quinn is over-minused by 2.00 D, and functions like a 2.00 D hyperope.

The dioptric locations used in the previous paragraph are relative to the retina, and not to the lens representing Quinn's eye. For example, when the thin lens–screen eye model for Quinn's eye is a +64.00 D lens located 17.24 mm in front of the retina, the clear image of a distant object is at

$$v = \frac{1000}{+64.00\,\text{D}} = 15.63\,\text{mm}$$

This is the image position that is "6.00 D in front of the retina." Note that the 6.00 D was not used in this calculation. Fundamentally, the 6.00 D of myopia by itself tells us that U_{fp} is −6.00 D, and the far point location for Quinn's uncorrected eye is 16.67 cm in front of the cornea. With the −8.00 D lens on, Quinn functions like a 2.00 D hyperope, and his "corrected" far point is virtual and 50 cm behind the cornea (i.e., in this case, $U_{\text{fp}} = +2.00\,\text{D}$, in order to overcome the 2.00 D of over-minus).

Now consider Rita, a presbyopic hyperope, who needs a +5.00 D spectacle lens but is given a +3.00 D spectacle lens. When uncorrected and viewing a distant object, the optically real image for Rita's eye is located 5.00 D behind the retina (Figure 6.17a). The +3.00 D lens pulls the image 3.00 D forward (i.e., closer to the retina), so that now it is only 2.00 D behind the retina (Figure 6.17b). Rita is underplussed by 2.00 D, and functions like a 2.00 D spectacle hyperope while wearing the +3.00 D lens.

When uncorrected, Rita's far point is virtual and 20 cm (i.e., 100/5.00 D) behind the spectacle plane. While wearing the +3.00 D lens, Rita still needs an incident vergence of +2.00 D on the spectacle lens in order to get a clear image on her retina, so her "corrected far point" is virtual and 50 cm behind the spectacle lens. (Rita was presbyopic and so has no accommodation left. If Rita was younger, so that she had an amplitude of accommodation greater than 2.00 D, she could overcome the 2.00 D deficit with accommodation.)

Sam is a hyperope who requires a +3.00 D contact lens but is given a +4.00 D contact lens. When uncorrected, Sam's eye has an optically real image 3.00 D behind the retina. When the +4.00 D contact lens is placed on Sam's eye, it pulls the image 4.00 D forward, so it is now 1.00 D in front of the retina. With the +4.00 D lens on, Sam is overplussed by 1.00 D, and functions like a 1.00 D myope.

Tina is a myope who needs a −8.50 D spectacle lens but instead is given a −7.00 D spectacle lens. In Tina's

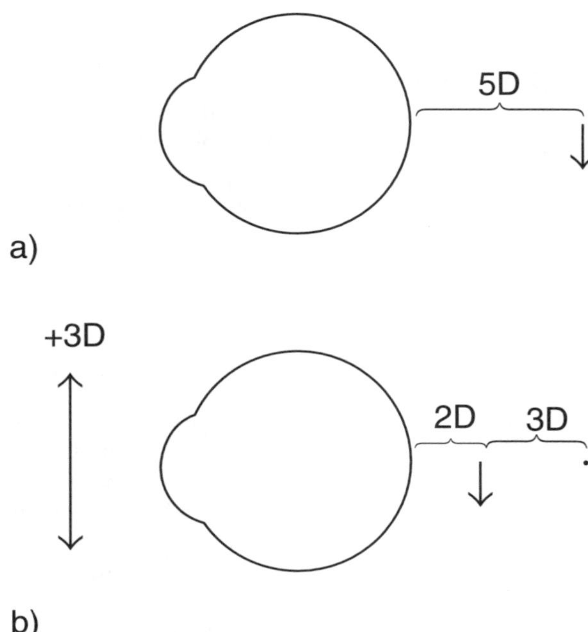

Figure 6.17 a, For a distant object, uncorrected clear image location for Rita, a 5.00 D spectacle hyperope; b, clear image location for Rita wearing a +3.00 D lens. The 3.00 D lens pulls the clear image 3.00 D forward, which leaves it 2.00 D behind the retina.

uncorrected eye, the clear image is 8.50 D in front of her retina (as measured at the spectacle plane). When Tina puts on the −7.00 D spectacle lens, it moves the image 7.00 D back towards the retina, which leaves the image 1.50 D in front of the retina. Tina is underminused by 1.50 D, and functions as a 1.50 D spectacle myope with the −7.00 D lens on.

Any person who is overplussed or underminused functions like a myope. When these people view a distant object without accommodating, their eye forms the clear image in the vitreous humor and the retinal image is blurred. When they accommodate, the clear image is pulled even further away from the retina and the blur of the retinal image increases. These people are sometimes said to be *fogged* because their distance vision is blurred and accommodation blurs it even more.

Any person who is underplussed or overminused functions like a hyperope. Accommodation can be used to compensate for the underplussed or overminused amount.

Ursula is wearing a +3.50 D spectacle lens. While wearing these spectacles, she has a "far point" that is real and 40 cm in front of her spectacle plane. What is Ursula's proper correction?

When the object is at the real far point 40 cm in front of the spectacle plane, the vergence incident on the spectacle plane is −2.50 D. This indicates that Ursula needs an additional −2.50 D in her spectacle correction (or +3.50 D − 2.50 D = +1.00 D). More formally,

$$\begin{aligned} V_s &= P_s + U_s \\ &= +3.50\,\text{D} + (-2.50\,\text{D}) = +1.00\,\text{D} \end{aligned}$$

So when unaccommodated, Ursula needs +1.00 D leaving the spectacle plane. This light propagates to the eye, is converged by the eye, and forms a clear retinal image. For a distance correction, $U_s = 0$, and since V_s needs to be +1.00 D, the lens power P_s is +1.00 D.

6.17 RANGE OF CLEAR VISION THROUGH VARIOUS LENSES

Suppose that Randy (an ametrope) while looking through a +4.00 D lens in the spectacle plane, can clearly see real objects ranging from 100 cm to 20 cm in front of the lens. What is Randy's range of clear vision when the +4.00 D lens is replaced by a +6.00 D lens?

One way to proceed is to figure the range of clear vision bounds needed for the vergence leaving the spectacle plane. For the object at 100 cm in front of the +4.00 D lens (the unaccommodated situation), the vergence leaving the lens is +3.00 D. For the object at 20 cm in front of the +4.00 D lens (maximal accommodation), the vergence leaving the lens is −1.00 D. Randy can handle vergences leaving the spectacle plane ranging from +3.00 D down to −1.00 D. Then for the +6.00 D lens (unaccommodated case),

$$\begin{aligned} U_s &= V_s - P_s \\ &= +3.00\,\text{D} - 6.00\,\text{D} = -3.00\,\text{D} \end{aligned}$$

For the +6.00 D lens (accommodated case),

$$\begin{aligned} U_s &= V_s - P_s \\ &= -1.00\,\text{D} - 6.00\,\text{D} = -7.00\,\text{D} \end{aligned}$$

Here the range of incident vergences is from −3.00 D to −7.00 D, or Randy's range of clear vision through the +6.00 D lens is 33.3 cm in to 14.3 cm.

In the above analysis, we figured out that Randy needed +3.00 D of vergence leaving the spectacle plane in the unaccommodated case ($V_s = +3.00$ D). When Randy looks at a distant object, the light incident on the spectacle plane consists of plane waves ($U_s = 0$). So if we want Randy corrected to see at distance without an ocular accommodative demand, we need a spectacle correction that changes plane waves into a converging light with a +3.00 D vergence, or

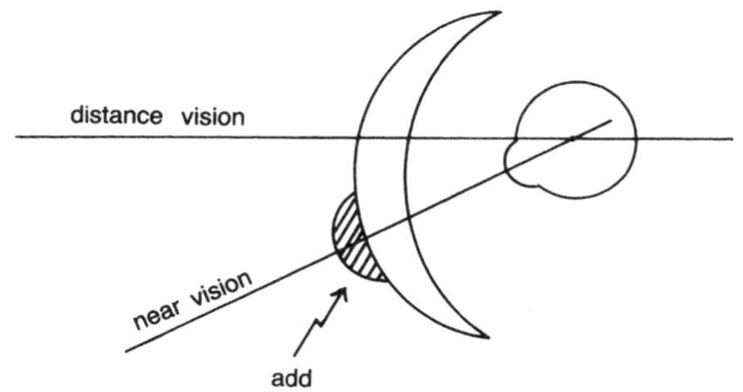

Figure 6.18 A bifocal lens.

$$P_s = V_s - U_s = +3.00\,\text{D}$$

So Randy's distance correction is +3.00 D.

In the maximally accommodated case, Randy needed a vergence of −1.00 D leaving the spectacle lens. So Randy's amplitude of accommodation in terms of the spectacle accommodative demand is +3.00 D − (−1.00 D) = +4.00 D. Through the +3.00 D lens, Randy's range of clear vision consists of real object points from optical infinity to 25 cm in front of the eye.

A bifocal lens is a lens with a distance vision area of one power and a near vision area of a higher plus (or less minus) power. The difference between the near vision power and the distance vision power is called the add. An unsophisticated bifocal can be achieved by simply gluing a small plus lens to the distance vision lens (Figure 6.18).

We could consider the +4.00 D lens of the above example as the near vision region of a +3.00 D distance vision lens with a +1.00 D add. Similarly, the +6.00-D lens can be considered as a +3.00 D distance vision lens with a +3.00 D add for near vision. Note that increasing the add makes the range of clear vision closer and smaller. This is an important feature in the clinical selection of an add.

6.18 RETINAL IMAGE SIZES

Retinal images are small and inverted relative to the real world object. Consider a 2 m tall basketball player standing 10 m from a typical emmetrope. In the thin lens and screen model, the typical lens–screen distance was 16.67 mm. From the nodal ray,

$$\tan w = \frac{|O|}{10\,\text{m}}$$

and

$$\tan w = \frac{|I|}{16.67\,\text{mm}}$$

Therefore,

$$\frac{|I|}{16.67\,\text{mm}} = \frac{|O|}{10\,\text{m}}$$

Then for $|O| = 2$ m, we can solve for $|I|$ to get 3.33 mm. So the retinal image of the 2 m tall basketball player is only 3.33 mm in size.

The letters on a 20/20 visual acuity line subtend an angle of 5′ with the fine detail subtending an angle of 1′. The retinal image size of such a letter is,

$$\frac{|I|}{16.67\,\text{mm}} = \tan(5')$$

Since there are 60′ per degree, then 5′ equates to 0.083°. Therefore,

$$|I| = 16.67\,\text{mm}\ \tan(0.083°) = 0.0241\,\text{mm}$$

or

$$|I| = 24.1\,\mu\text{m}$$

where μm stands for micrometer. (Note 1 μm = 10^{-6} m. That's small!)

An alternate method for dealing with the tangents of small angles is to use the small angle approximation in which the tangent is replaced by the angle itself expressed in radians. For the above case, 5′ equals 0.083°. Let us convert the angle to radians:

$$\theta = 0.083°/(57.3°/\text{radian}) = 1.45 \times 10^{-3}\ \text{radians}$$

Then,

$$\begin{aligned}|I| &= 1.67\,\text{mm}\ \tan\theta\\ &\approx 1.67\,\text{mm}\,\theta\\ &\approx 1.67\,\text{mm}(1.45 \times 10^{-3})\\ &\approx 24.1 \times 10^{-3}\,\text{mm} = 24.1\,\mu\text{m}\end{aligned}$$

6.19 RETINAL IMAGE SIZES: SPECTACLE VERSUS CONTACT LENSES

Retinal image sizes of corrected ametropes differ depending on whether a contact correction or a spectacle correction is used. Figure 6.19a shows the nodal ray for a contact corrected myope viewing a distant off-axis object point. The nodal ray specifies the retinal image size I_c. When the myope is corrected with a spectacle lens, the same incident ray is bent up by the spectacle lens and is no longer the nodal ray of the eye (Figure 6.19b). Figure 6.19c shows a ray (solid lines), which after being bent by the spectacle lens

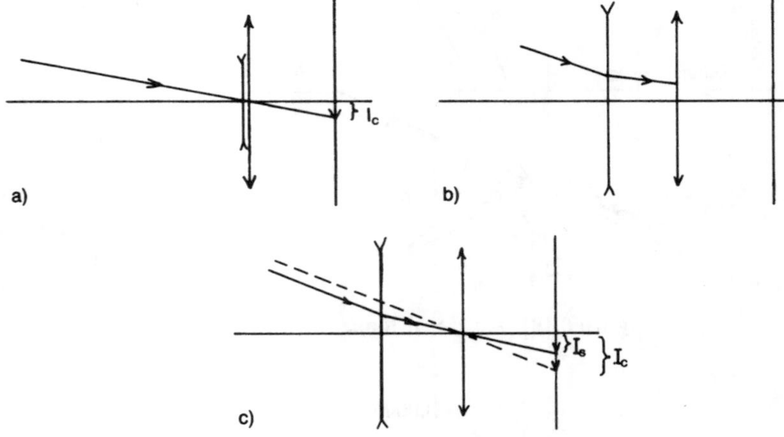

Figure 6.19 a, Image size for a contact-corrected myope; b, deviation of ray by the spectacle correction; c, superposition to compare spectacle and contact-corrected retinal image sizes.

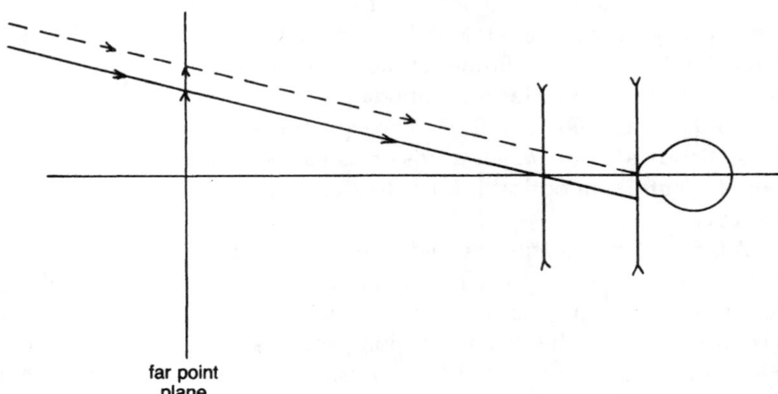

Figure 6.20 Spectacle versus contact lens image sizes in a myope's far point plane.

becomes the nodal ray for the eye and specifies the retinal image size I_s. For comparison purposes, the nodal ray (dashed line) for the contact lens is superimposed on Figure 6.19c. The two rays, solid and dashed, are parallel in object space because they come from the same distant object point. For the myope, the path of the ray traveling through the spectacle lens shows that the spectacle corrected retinal image is smaller than the contact corrected retinal image. Many myopes prefer contact lenses to spectacle lenses because of the larger retinal image size they get with the contact lenses.

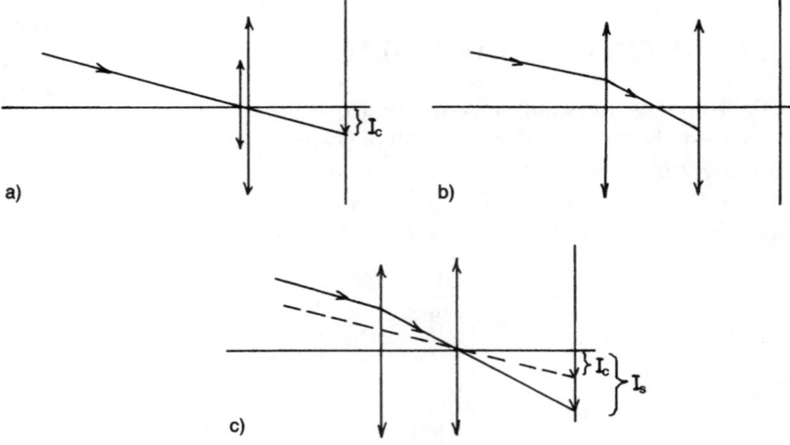

Figure 6.21 a, Image size for a contact corrected hyperope; b, deviation of ray by the spectacle lens; c, superposition to compare spectacle and contact corrected retinal image sizes.

Figure 6.22 Spectacle versus contact corrected image sizes in a hyperope's far point plane.

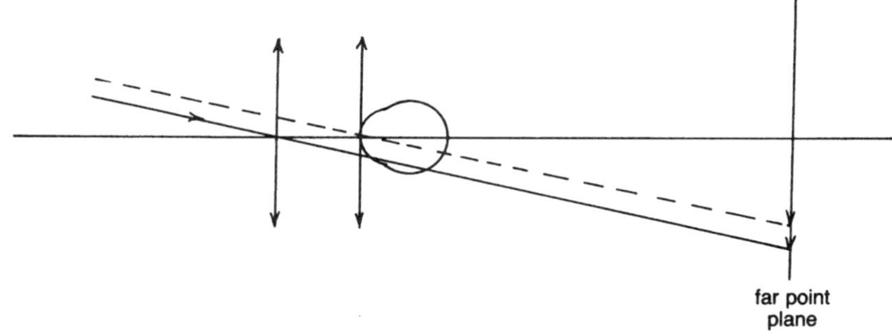

Another way to reach the same conclusion is to consider the image size of the two different correcting lenses. The image of these correcting lenses is the object for the eye, and this image is formed in the far point plane of the eye. The image size in the far point plane is easily determined by considering the nodal ray for the correcting lens. Figure 6.20 shows a superposition of the spectacle lens case (solid line) and the contact lens case (dashed line). The two incident nodal rays are parallel to each other because they come from the same distant object point. Clearly, the contact lens image in the far point plane is larger than the spectacle lens image in the far point plane. Since the correcting lens images are both formed in the far point plane and both serve as the object for the eye, then the contact corrected retinal image will be larger than the spectacle corrected retinal image. For high myopes who switch back and forth between contacts and spectacles, this effect is clearly noticeable.

Similar diagrams for a hyperope are shown in Figures 6.2la,b and c. Figure 6.21a shows the nodal ray for the contact corrected eye. Figure 6.21b shows that this ray is not the nodal ray for the eye when a spectacle correction is worn. Figure 6.21c shows the nodal ray (solid) for the eye when a spectacle lens is worn together with a superposition of the nodal ray (dashed) for the contact corrected eye. The hyperope's retinal image is larger when spectacle corrected. This is exactly opposite to that of the myope.

Figure 6.22 shows the correcting lens image sizes in the hyperope's far point plane. The dashed ray is the nodal ray for the contact lens, while the solid ray is the nodal ray for the spectacle lens. Note that in the far point plane the spectacle lens image is larger than the contact lens image. Consequently, since these images serve as the object for the eye, then the spectacle corrected retinal image for the hyperope will be larger than the contact corrected retinal image.

Table 6.1 Retinal Image Size Comparison: Same Ametrope

Ametrope	*Contact Corrected*	*Spectacle Corrected*
Myope	Larger	Smaller
Hyperope	Smaller	Larger

Table 6.1 summarizes the qualitative findings of this section. Note that we are talking about the retinal image size of the same ametrope when corrected by spectacle lenses versus contact lenses. We are not comparing different ametropes. A quantitative treatment is given in Chapter 18.

PROBLEMS

For each of the next four problems, represent the unaccommodated eye by a +60.00 D thin lens and a screen (retina) located a distance x behind the lens. The amplitude of accommodation is listed as A. For the uncorrected eye, find the far point and near point, sketch the range of clear vision, classify the refractive error (myopia, hyperopia, emmetropia), and give the distance vision correction at the cornea and the distance vision correction at a spectacle plane located 15 mm from the cornea.

1. Sally Jones, age 30, $x = 19.9$ mm, $A = 7.00$ D.
2. Richard Nixit, age 55, $x = 13.9$ mm, $A = 1.25$ D.
3. Roger Stub, age 25, $x = 16.0$ mm, $A = 8.50$ D.
4. Thelma Elf, age 43, $x = 17.2$ mm, $A = 2.50$ D.
5. Molly Finnigan is a 4.50 D ocular myope with a 6.00 D amplitude of accommodation. When uncorrected, can Molly clearly see the fine print in a book held 40 cm from her cornea? If not, why not? If so, what is the ocular accommodative demand?
6. Mike Finnigan is a 3.50 D ocular hyperope with a 5.00 D amplitude of accommodation. When uncorrected, can Mike clearly see the fine print in a book held 40 cm from his cornea? If not, why not? If so, what is the ocular accommodative demand?
7. Jim Finnigan is a 1.50 D ocular myope with a 2.00 D amplitude of accommodation. When uncorrected, can Jim clearly see the fine print in a book held

40 cm from his cornea? If not, why not? If so, what is the ocular accommodative demand?

8. Katie Finnigan is a 2.00 D ocular hyperope with a 5.50 D amplitude of accommodation. When uncorrected, can Katie clearly see the fine print in a book held 40 cm from her cornea. If not, why not? If so, what is the ocular accommodative demand?
9. Rose Opal has a +13.50 D distance vision spectacle correction at a 12 mm vertex distance. Rose looks through her spectacles at a statue located 19 cm in front of the spectacles. What is the spectacle accommodative demand? What is Rose's ocular accommodative demand? (Compare the exact and the approximate answers.)
10. Zeke Feldstein has a −9.50 D distance vision spectacle correction at a 13 mm vertex distance. Zeke looks through his spectacles at a small automotive part that he holds 14 cm in front of his spectacles. What is the spectacle accommodative demand? What is Zeke's ocular accommodative demand? (Compare the exact and the approximate answers.)
11. Wilhelmina Roads puts on a +5.00 D spectacle lens that has an 11 mm vertex distance. With the +5.00 D lens, Wilhelmina can clearly see real objects at a distance of 37–75 cm from the lens. When the +5.00 D lens is replaced by a +4.00 D lens (same vertex distance), what is Wilhelmina's range of clear vision? What is Wilhelmina's distance vision correction (same vertex distance)? What is Wilhelmina's range of clear vision through her spectacle correction?
12. Elroy Frost puts on a −1.50 D spectacle lens at a 13 mm vertex distance. With the −1.50 D lens, Elroy can clearly see real objects from 26 cm to 50 cm from the lens. What is Elroy's range of clear vision through a +1.00 D spectacle lens (same vertex distance)? What is Elroy's distance vision spectacle correction? What is his range of clear vision through his correction?
13. Jill Harkins is an emmetrope with an unaccommodated eye represented by a +64.00 D thin lens and screen (retina). What retinal image size (in microns) does Jill have when viewing a distant object that subtends an angle of 16′?

CHAPTER 7

Single Spherical Refracting Interfaces

7.1 CONVEX/CONCAVE TERMINOLOGY

Consider the spherical glass ($n = 1.50$) surface shown in Figure 7.1. In the middle, the glass bulges out into the air. In Section 4.1, we saw qualitatively that such a surface converges plane waves no matter which way the waves propagate through the surface. Consequently, a spherical glass surface with the glass in the middle bulging into the air is always a converging surface.

The surface is actually an interface between two different optical media, air and glass. Some other examples of optical interfaces are water and glass, plastic and water, oil and glass, air and the cornea of the eye, the aqueous humor and the front surface of the crystalline lens, and the back surface of the crystalline lens and the vitreous humor. In general, when the interface is spherical and the middle of the higher index media bulges out into the lower index media, then the interface is converging no matter which way the light propagates through the interface. Figure 7.2 shows examples of converging interfaces. Conversely, when the middle of a lower index media bulges into a higher index media, then a spherical interface diverges incident light no matter which way the waves propagate through the interface. Figure 7.3 shows some diverging spherical interfaces.

Historically, people have sought to identify surfaces by their geometric characteristics rather than their optical characteristics. The word *convex* is defined as being curved outward like the exterior of a sphere. The word *concave* is defined as being curved inward like the interior of a bowl or the interior of a cave.

Figure 7.4a shows a glass lens with two converging surfaces. The lens itself is thus a converging lens. As

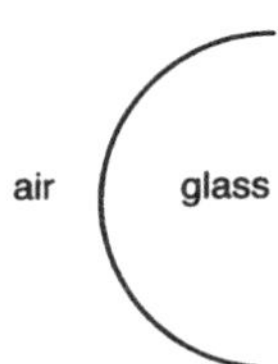

Figure 7.1 A spherical interface.

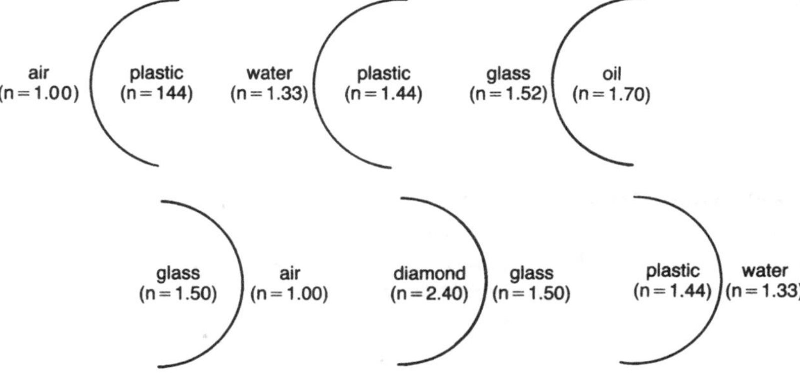

Figure 7.2 Converging interfaces, all convex to the lower index medium.

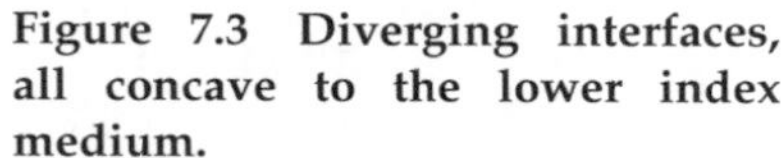

Figure 7.3 Diverging interfaces, all concave to the lower index medium.

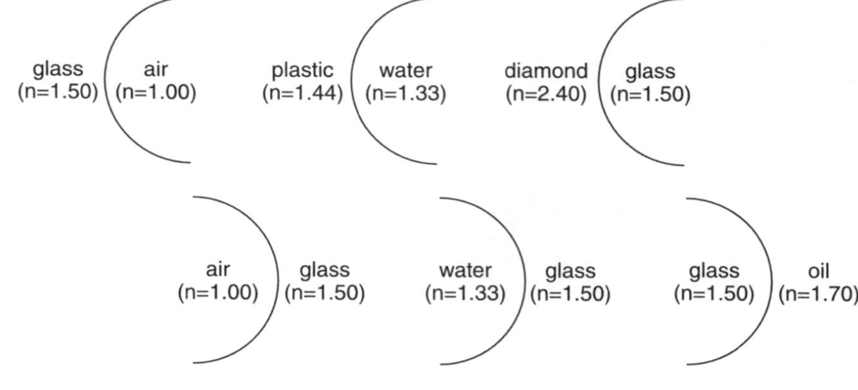

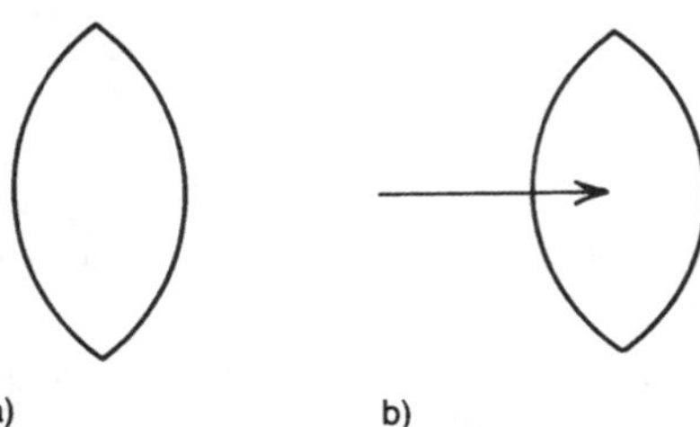

Figure 7.4 Biconvex lens.

viewed from the outside, which is where a human observer would be, each surface is convex. This lens is conventionally called a biconvex lens.

However, a discrepancy in terminology has developed in the description of each surface. Consider Figure 7.4b, which shows light incident from the left on the biconvex lens. Initially the light in air approaches the left surface of the lens, and this surface viewed from the left is convex. Then the light enters the glass and approaches the right surface of the lens. But the right surface of the lens, as viewed from inside the glass, is curved inward like the inside of a bowl. Consequently, some authors call the right surface concave, but according to such terminology, the biconvex lens, in which biconvex literally implies two convex sides, has a convex left side and a concave right side.

In order to avoid the above illogical terminology, let us label a surface or interface as being convex or concave from the perspective of the lower index medium, regardless of which way the light is traveling. Thus, let us call the right surface of the lens in Figure 7.4b convex. With this convention, a biconvex lens has a convex left side and a convex right side, as one might expect.

With the assignment of convex and concave being made from the perspective of the lower index medium, then a convex refracting interface always turns out to be a converging interface (see Figures 7.1 and 7.2), and a concave refracting interface always turns out to be a diverging interface (see Figure 7.3). (When referring to other books, be sure to check what terminology they are using.)

7.2 SAGITTAS AND THE SAGITTAL APPROXIMATION

The next two sections deal with the derivation of the vergence equation for a single spherical refracting interface. If you wish to study the equation and related examples before going through the derivation, then skip to Section 7.4.

The sagittal approximation is frequently used in geometric optics to quantitatively treat the relationship between the curvature of a spherical surface and the dioptric power of that surface, as well as the relationship between the curvature of a wavefront and the vergence of that wavefront. Before treating the sagittal approximation, we derive and discuss an exact equation for the sagitta.

Figure 7.5a shows a cross-section of a long horizontal glass rod with a spherical front surface. The center of curvature of the surface is labeled C. The horizontal line

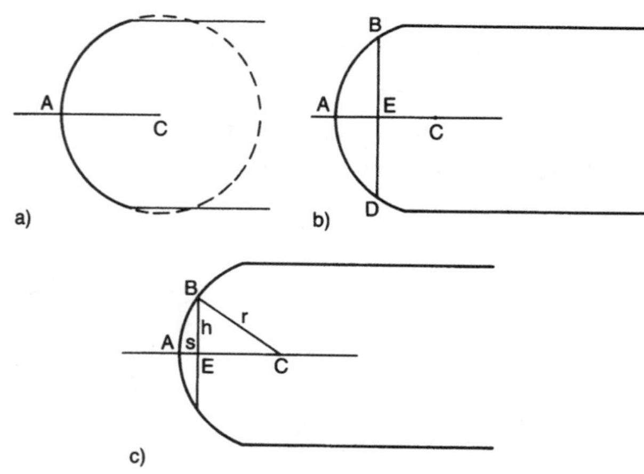

Figure 7.5 Spherical interface and sagitta.

through C is normal (i.e., perpendicular to) the spherical surface at point A. In Figure 7.5b, a line called a chord is perpendicular to the normal line. The chord intersects the surface of the sphere at points B and D, and intersects the normal at point E. The line segment AE, which is normal to the surface, is called the sagitta. The point A is called the vertex or pole of the sphere.

Let r equal the radius of curvature of the sphere, and s equal the length of the sagitta. In Figure 7.5c, r equals both the length AC and the length BC. Let h equal half the chord length, which is the length BE. Let g equal the length EC. Then from the Pythagorean theorem applied to the triangle BEC,

$$r^2 = g^2 + h^2$$

or

$$g = \sqrt{r^2 - h^2} \tag{7.1}$$

From Figure 7.5c,

$$AC = AE + EC$$

or

$$r = s + g$$

and

$$s = r - g \tag{7.2}$$

By substituting Eq. 7.1 into Eq. 7.2, we obtain

$$s = r - \sqrt{r^2 - h^2} \tag{7.3}$$

Equation 7.3 is an exact relationship between the sagittal length s, the half chord length h, and the radius of curvature of the spherical interface or wavefront.

EXAMPLE 7.1a

A spherical convex glass surface, as in Figure 7.5, has a radius of curvature of 20.0 cm. What is the sagittal length for a chord length of 36.0 cm?

The half cord length is 18.0 cm. Then,

$$\begin{aligned} s &= 20.0\,\text{cm} - \sqrt{(20.0\,\text{cm})^2 - (18.0\,\text{cm})^2} \\ &= 20.0\,\text{cm} - \sqrt{(400 - 324)\,\text{cm}} \\ &= 20.0\,\text{cm} - 8.72\,\text{cm} = 11.28\,\text{cm} \end{aligned}$$

EXAMPLE 7.1b

A spherical convex glass surface, as in Figure 7.5, has a radius of curvature of 10.00 cm. What is the sagittal length for a chord length of 1.80 cm?

The half chord length h is 0.9 cm. Then,

$$\begin{aligned} s &= 10\,\text{cm} - \sqrt{(10\,\text{cm})^2 - (0.9\,\text{cm})^2} \\ &= 10\,\text{cm} - \sqrt{(100 - 0.81)\text{cm}} \\ &= 10\,\text{cm} - 9.96\,\text{cm} = 0.04\,\text{cm} = 0.40\,\text{mm} \end{aligned}$$

In Example 7.1b, h^2 is much smaller than r^2. In this case, we can accurately approximate Eq. 7.3 by a simpler equation. First, rewrite Eq. 7.3 as

$$s = r - r\sqrt{1 - (h^2/r^2)} \tag{7.4}$$

From calculus, the square root can be approximated by a Taylor series expansion:

$$\sqrt{1 - (h^2/r^2)} = 1 - \frac{h^2}{2r^2} - \frac{h^4}{8r^4} - \frac{h^6}{16r^6} - \cdots \tag{7.5}$$

When h^2 is much smaller than r^2, only the first two terms of the expression are significant, or

$$\sqrt{1 - (h^2/r^2)} \approx 1 - \frac{h^2}{2r^2} \quad \text{when } h^2 \ll r^2$$

The square root is equivalent to an exponential of 1/2, which is the source of the 2 in the denominator of the second term.

When we substitute the above equation into Eq. 7.4, we obtain

$$s \approx r - r\left(1 - \frac{h^2}{2r^2}\right)$$

or

$$s \approx r - r + \frac{h^2}{2r}$$

Finally,

$$s \approx \frac{h^2}{2r} \quad \text{provided } h^2 \ll r^2 \tag{7.6}$$

Equation 7.6 is called the *sagittal approximation*. It provides a very simple relationship between s, h, and r. Furthermore, since the curvature R of a sphere is equal to the reciprocal of the radius r, it follows from the sagittal approximation that

$$s = \frac{h^2}{2}R \quad \text{provided } h^2 \ll r^2 \tag{7.7}$$

Equation 7.7 shows that the sagittal length s is directly proportional to the curvature R of the sphere for those situations is which the approximation is accurate.

EXAMPLE 7.2

Use the sagittal approximation to calculate s for the surface used in Example 7.1b.

There, the radius r was 10 cm and the half chord length h was 0.9 cm. From Eq. 7.6,

$$s = \frac{(0.9\,\text{cm})^2}{2(10\,\text{cm})} = \frac{0.81\,\text{cm}^2}{20\,\text{cm}} = 0.04\,\text{cm}$$

or

$$s = 0.4\,\text{mm}$$

which is the same value obtained with the exact equation.

For those who are not familiar with the Taylor series expansion, there is a more intuitive way to obtain the sagittal approximation. First, we need to take the exact sagittal equation, Eq. 7.3, and solve for r. From Eq. 7.3,

$$s - r = -\sqrt{r^2 - h^2}$$

Square both sides to obtain

$$(s - r)^2 = r^2 - h^2$$

Then,

$$s^2 - 2rs + r^2 = r^2 - h^2$$

or

$$s^2 - 2rs = -h^2$$

We can solve for r to obtain

$$r = \frac{s^2 + h^2}{2s} \tag{7.8}$$

Equation 7.8 is still an exact relationship between s, h, and r. However, when h^2 is much less than r^2, then s^2 is also much less than h^2. For example, in the Example 7.1b,

$$s^2 = (0.04\,\text{cm})^2 = 0.0016\,\text{cm}^2$$

while

$$h^2 = (0.9\,\text{cm})^2 = 0.81\,\text{cm}^2$$

When s^2 is much less than h^2, s^2 can be neglected in the numerator of Eq. 7.8, and then

$$r = \frac{h^2}{2s}$$

or

$$s = \frac{h^2}{2r}$$

which is the sagittal approximation.

As shown in the next section, the sagittal approximation is immensely useful. However when h^2 is not small relative to r^2, we need to use the exact relationship, Eq. 7.3, instead of the sagittal approximation. (Specifically, for the values in Example 7.1a, the sagittal approximation gives 8.10 cm, which is considerably different from the 11.28 cm exact value.)

7.3 DERIVATION OF THE VERGENCE EQUATION

Figure 7.6 shows a long glass rod with a convex spherical surface. The spherical surface is optically a single spherical refracting interface (SSRI) between air and glass.

The medium that the light is initially in has a refractive index n_1. The medium that the light is in when leaving the interface has a refractive index n_2. The incident wavefront (in medium n_1) is diverging, while the exiting wavefront (in medium n_2) is converging. The incident wavefront is just touching the interface at point B, which is the vertex of the interface. The exiting wavefront has moved to point C on the normal to the interface.

The time t for the wavefront to move from B to C, in terms of the directed distance BC and the velocity w_2 of the wavefront in the second medium, is

$$t = \frac{BC}{w_2}$$

During this time, the part of the incident wavefront at point E has moved from E to H. In the paraxial approximation, the path of the wavefront in going from E to H is well approximated by the horizontal line defined by the points E, F, G, and H. In other words, any vertical movement is negligible relative to the horizontal movement. In moving from E to H, the wavefront enters the second medium at G. The time t that it takes for the wavefront to get from E to

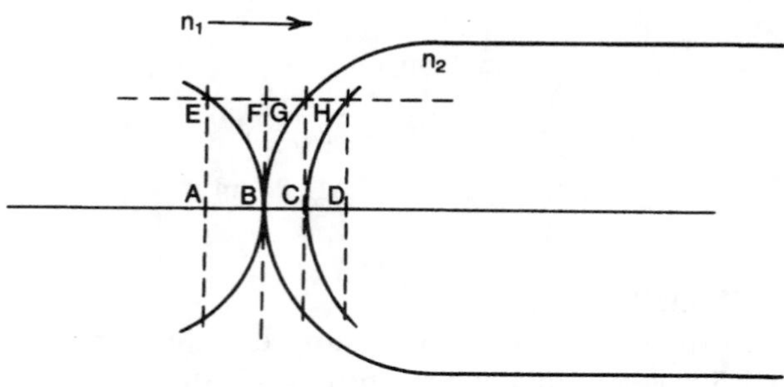

Figure 7.6 Wavefronts passing through the spherical interface.

F to G to H, in terms of the directed distances EF, FG, and GH, and the velocities w_1 and w_2 of the wavefront in the first and second mediums, respectively, is

$$t = \frac{EF}{w_1} + \frac{FG}{w_1} + \frac{GH}{w_2}$$

Since the two previous equations are for the same period of time, they can be set equal to each other resulting in

$$\frac{EF}{w_1} + \frac{FG}{w_1} + \frac{GH}{w_2} = \frac{BC}{w_2} \tag{7.9}$$

The respective velocities w_1 and w_2 of the light in the first and second media are related to the speed of light c in a vacuum, and the respective indices of refraction n_1 and n_2 by the equations

$$w_1 = \frac{c}{n_1} \quad \text{and} \quad w_2 = \frac{c}{n_2}$$

When the velocity relationships are substituted into Eq. 7.9 and the common factor c is cancelled on both sides of the equation, the result is

$$n_1EF + n_1FG + n_2GH = n_2BC \tag{7.10}$$

In general, the index of refraction n times a distance along a wavefront direction (or ray) is called the *optical path length*. Equation 7.10 is an example of a general principle that states: When a wavefront propagates from one place to another, the optical path lengths for different parts of the wavefront are equal. Note that it is the optical path lengths that are equal, as opposed to the actual path lengths.

From Figure 7.6, the following distance equalities hold:

$$EF = AB$$
$$FG = BC$$
$$GH = CD$$

Furthermore, the directed distance AB is opposite in sign to the directed distance BA, or

$$AB = -BA$$

By using the preceding distance equalities in Eq. 7.10, we obtain

$$-n_1BA + n_1BC + n_2CD = n_2BC$$

or

$$n_2CD = (n_2 - n_1)BC + n_1BA \tag{7.11}$$

The distances CD, BC, and BA are the respective sagittas of the exiting wavefront, the single spherical refracting interface, and the incident wavefront. Under paraxial conditions, the sagittal approximation is accurate. Then,

$$BC = \frac{h^2}{2r}$$

where r is the radius of curvature of the interface and h is the half-chord length,

$$BA = \frac{h^2}{2u}$$

where u is the radius of curvature of the incident wavefront (u is then, by definition, the object distance), and

$$CD = \frac{h^2}{2v}$$

where v is the radius of curvature of the exiting wavefront (v is then, by definition, the image distance).

By substituting the sagitta relationships into Eq. 7.11 and canceling the common factor $h^2/2$ on both sides, we obtain

$$\frac{n_2}{v} = \frac{(n_2 - n_1)}{r} + \frac{n_1}{u} \tag{7.12}$$

But n_2/v is the vergence V of the exiting wavefront, and n_1/u is the vergence U of the incident wavefront. So,

$$V = \frac{n_2 - n_1}{r} + U \tag{7.13}$$

Equation 7.13 is a vergence equation for the single spherical refracting interface. Evidently, the dioptric power P is given by

$$P = \frac{n_2 - n_1}{r} \tag{7.14}$$

in which case, Eq. 7.13 can be written as

$$V = P + U \tag{7.15}$$

7.4 DIOPTRIC POWER

The derivation in the preceding section shows that the vergence equation

$$V = P + U \tag{7.16}$$

describes the paraxial imaging, by a single spherical refracting interface. The (generalized) vergence U of the incident wavefront is given by

$$U = n_1/u \tag{7.17}$$

where n_1 is the index of the medium that the light is initially in and u is the radius of curvature of the incident wavefront. The radius of curvature u of the incident wavefront is, by definition, the object distance for the interface. The (generalized) vergence V of the wavefront exiting the interface is given by

$$V = n_2/v \tag{7.18}$$

where n_2 is the index of the medium that the light is in after it passes through the interface and v is the radius of curvature of the wavefront leaving the interface. The radius of curvature v of the wavefront leaving the interface is, by definition, the image distance. The sign convention is the same as for thin lenses. In fact, the only difference between the basic SSRI equations and the thin lens in air equations is the appearance of the refractive indices.

The derivation of Eq. 7.16 also provided the relationship between the dioptric power P of the spherical interface, the radius of curvature r, and the indices of refraction n_1 and n_2:

$$P = \frac{n_2 - n_1}{r} \tag{7.19}$$

The same sign convention is used for u, v, and r. The directed distance r is the distance from the interface to its center of curvature C. The directed distance r is positive when it is in the same direction that the light is traveling when it leaves the interface and negative when it is opposite to the direction that the light is traveling when it leaves the interface.

Since the radius r is reciprocally related to the curvature R of the interface, then Eq. 7.19 can be written as

$$P = (n_2 - n_1)R \tag{7.20}$$

Equation 7.20 says that the dioptric power of the interface increases when the curvature of the interface increases (i.e., the surface gets steeper), and decreases when the curvature of the interface decreases (i.e., the surface gets flatter). The equation also says that the dioptric power of the interface increases when the difference in the refractive indices increases, and decreases when the difference in the refractive indices decreases.

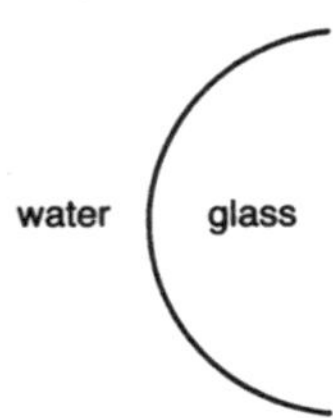

Figure 7.7 Convex interface.

The dioptric power P is expressed in diopters with 1 D being dimensionally equal to the reciprocal of 1 m. In Eq. 7.19, either r must be expressed in meters, or a conversion factor must be used. Just as with vergence, the conversion factor can be explicitly written in the numerator.

EXAMPLE 7.3a

A spherical convex interface between water of index 1.33 and glass of index 1.53 has a radius of curvature of 10 cm (Figure 7.7). What is the dioptric power of the interface when light is incident from the water side?

Before calculating, you should be able to tell whether the interface is converging or diverging. Here the interface is convex, so it must be converging and P must be positive.

The parameters for the calculations are:

$$n_1 = 1.33 \quad n_2 = 1.53 \quad \text{and } r = +10\,\text{cm}$$

Then from Eq. 7.19,

$$P = \frac{n_2 - n_1}{r} = \frac{(1.53 - 1.33)100\,\text{cm/m}}{+10\,\text{cm}} = \frac{+20\,\text{cm/m}}{+10\,\text{cm}} = +2.00\,\text{D}$$

EXAMPLE 7.3b

What is the dioptric power of the above interface when light is incident from the glass side?

We already know that the interface is a converging interface for light going either way. Therefore, P must be positive for light going either way.

For the reversed direction,

$$n_1 = 1.53 \quad n_2 = 1.33 \quad \text{and} \quad r = -10\,\text{cm}$$

Then,

$$P = \frac{n_2 - n_1}{r} = \frac{(1.33 - 1.53)100\,\text{cm/m}}{-10\,\text{cm}} = \frac{-20\,\text{cm/m}}{-10\,\text{cm}} = +2.00\,\text{D}$$

Note that the dioptric power of the interface is +2.00 D no matter which way the light is propagating through the interface. The sign of the radius of curvature r does change since it depends on the sign convention for directed

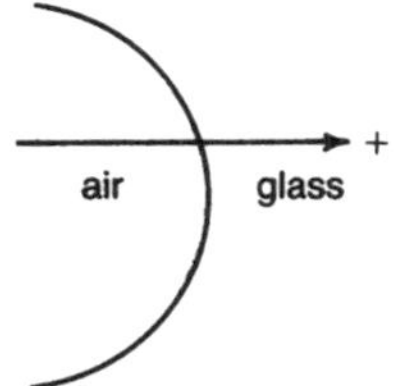

Figure 7.8 **Concave interface.**

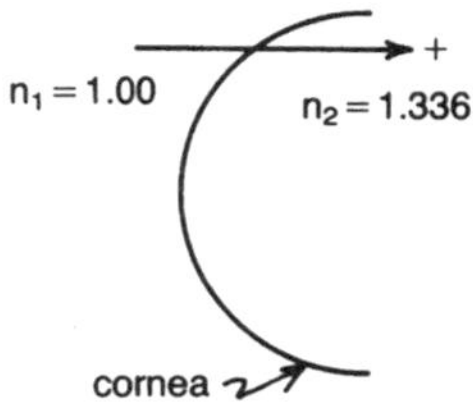

Figure 7.9 **Cornea modeled as an SSRI.**

distances. However, the sign of the difference in indices also changes with the result that the sign of the dioptric power P is invariant with respect to the direction that the light is propagating.

EXAMPLE 7.4

A spherical concave interface between air ($n = 1.00$) and glass ($n = 1.50$) has a radius of curvature of magnitude 5 cm. What is the dioptric power of the interface when light is incident from the air side?

Note before calculating: Since the interface is concave, it is diverging and the dioptric power should be negative. From Figure 7.8,

$$n_1 = 1.00 \quad n_2 = 1.50 \quad \text{and} \quad r = -5\,\text{cm}$$

Then,

$$P = \frac{n_2 - n_1}{r} = \frac{(1.50 - 1.00)100\,\text{cm/m}}{-5\,\text{cm}} = \frac{50\,\text{cm/m}}{-5\,\text{cm}} = -10.00\,\text{D}$$

What is the dioptric power of the above interface when the light is incident from the glass side?

The interface is still divergent, so P must be negative. Here,

$$n_1 = 1.50 \quad n_2 = 1.00 \quad \text{and} \quad r = +5\,\text{cm}$$

Since

$$P = \frac{n_2 - n_1}{r} = \frac{(1.00 - 1.50)100\,\text{cm/m}}{+5\,\text{cm}} = \frac{-50\,\text{cm/m}}{+5\,\text{cm}} = -10.00\,\text{D}$$

Again note that the dioptric power of the interface is -10.00 D, irrespective of which way the light travels through the interface.

EXAMPLE 7.5

As shown in Figure 7.9, the cornea and aqueous humor of the eye can be approximated as an SSRI between air and the ocular contents ($n = 1.336$). A typical radius of curvature of the cornea is 7.5 mm. What is the dioptric power of the cornea?

The cornea is convex, so P must be positive. For light going into the eye,

$$n_1 = 1.00 \quad n_2 = 1.336 \quad \text{and} \quad r = +7.5\,\text{mm}$$

Then,

$$P = \frac{n_2 - n_1}{r} = \frac{(1.336 - 1.000)1000\,\text{mm/m}}{+7.5\,\text{mm}} = \frac{336\,\text{mm/m}}{+7.5\,\text{mm}} = +44.80\,\text{D}$$

A typical cornea has a dioptric power of almost +45 D, while a typical human eye has a dioptric power of +60 D. Clearly, the cornea is the strongest converging element of the eye.

7.5 FOCAL POINTS

The secondary focal point (F_2) is the axial image point that results when plane waves are incident on the interface. Alternatively, the secondary focal point is the axial image point conjugate to optical infinity. The paraxial rays associated with the secondary focal point are shown in Figure 7.10a.

Frequently, we use a larger scale vertically so that we can easily see the rays (Section 4.12). The larger vertical scale stretches out the spherical surface so that it appears flat on the ray diagram (Figure 7.10b). This is equivalent to saying that the paraxial rays are refracted at or near the vertex point of the interface. As an aid in remembering which way the spherical surface is actually curving, little curves at the top and bottom of the vertical line represent the interface. The center of curvature C provides the same information, but not as quickly.

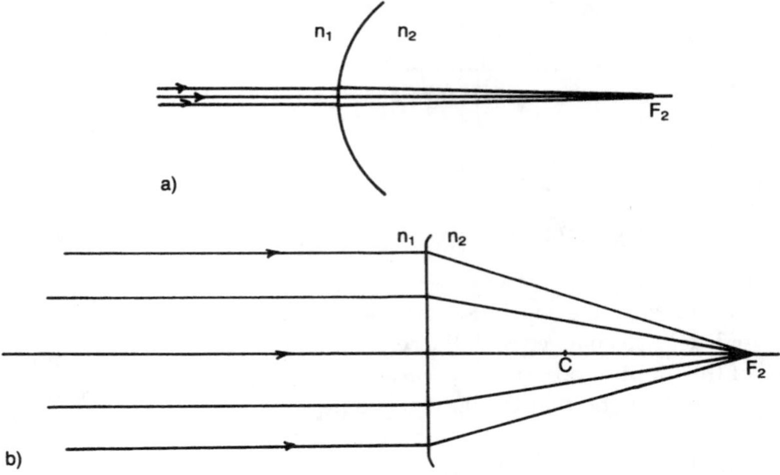

Figure 7.10 Paraxial rays: a, actual; b, scaled.

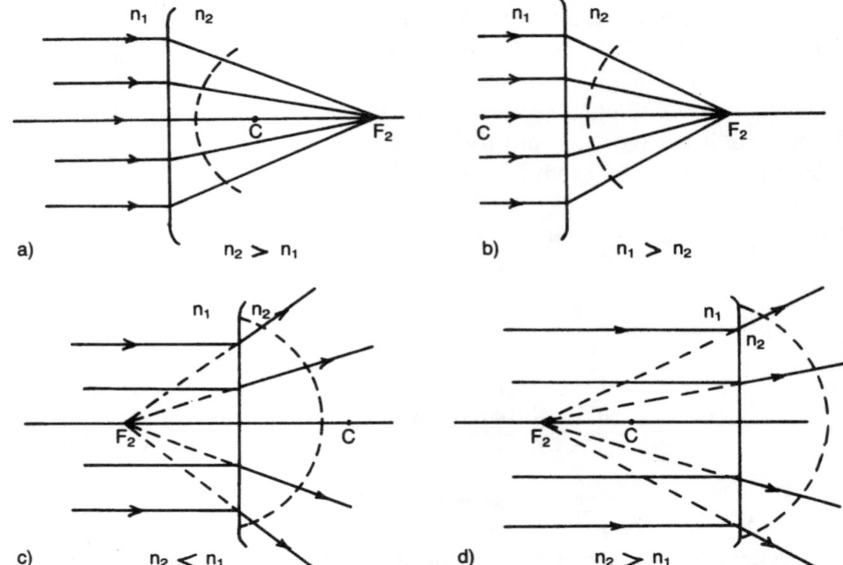

Figure 7.11 Predictable rays associated with the secondary focal point.

The secondary focal point is a real image point for a converging SSRI and a virtual image point for a diverging SSRI (Figure 7.11). Once the location of the secondary focal point is known, the incident parallel rays become predictable, and can be used in a ray diagram.

The secondary focal length f_2 is the image distance when the object is at optical infinity, or alternatively it is the directed distance from the interface to the secondary focal point F_2. To find the secondary focal length, we use

$$V = P + U$$

and set U equal to zero (incident plane waves). Then,

$$V = P$$

Since

$$V = \frac{n_2}{v}$$

and for this case

$$f_2 = v$$

one can combine the above three equations to obtain

$$P = \frac{n_2}{f_2} \tag{7.21}$$

The primary focal point (F_1) is the axial object point that results in plane waves leaving the interface. Alternatively, the primary focal point is the axial object point conjugate to optical infinity. The primary focal

Figure 7.12 Predictable rays associated with the primary focal point.

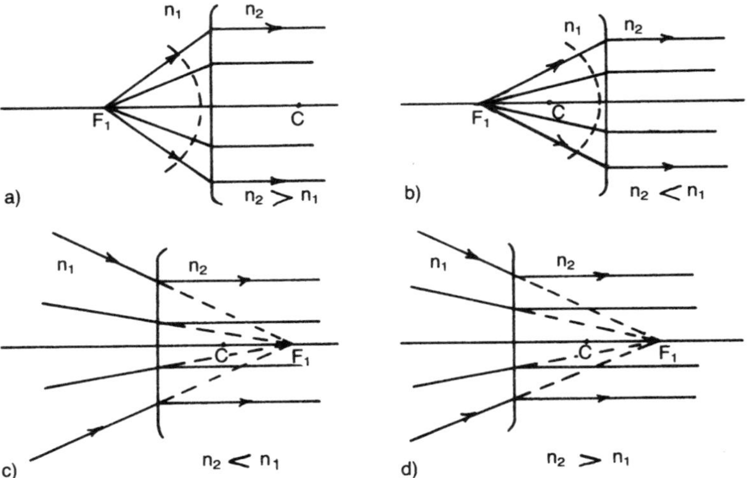

point is a real object point for a converging interface and a virtual object point for a diverging interface (Figure 7.12).

The rays that originate at the primary focal point all leave the interface parallel to the axis. Once the location of F_1 is known, any incident ray associated with F_1 becomes predictable, and can be used in a ray diagram.

The primary focal length f_1 is the object distance for which the conjugate image point is at optical infinity, or alternatively it is the directed distance from the interface to F_1.

To find the primary focal length, use

$$V = P + U$$

and set V equal to zero (exiting plane waves). Then,

$$P = -U$$

Since

$$U = \frac{n_1}{u}$$

and for this case

$$f_1 = u$$

we can combine the above three equations to obtain

$$P = -\frac{n_1}{f_1} \tag{7.22}$$

Equations 7.21 and 7.22 are similar to Eqs. 5.4 and 5.5 for the focal lengths of a thin lens in air except that now the indices of the different media appear. The primary and secondary focal points are not equidistant from the interface since n_1 and n_2 are not equal. By equating 7.21 and 7.22, we obtain

$$\frac{f_2}{n_2} = -\frac{f_1}{n_1} \tag{7.23}$$

or

$$\frac{f_2}{f_1} = -\frac{n_2}{n_1} \tag{7.24}$$

Equation 7.24 shows that in magnitude, the ratio of the focal lengths equals the ratio of the indices of refraction. The larger the difference in the indices of refraction, the larger the difference in the focal lengths. It also follows that the longer focal length is always associated with the higher index medium and vice versa.

The secondary focal length is the image distance for incident plane waves. As such, the secondary focal length is really the radius of curvature of the wavefront that leaves the interface when plane waves are incident. *The exiting wavefront is physically in the medium of index n_2, and the secondary focal length is then associated with n_2 as is indicated mathematically in Eq. 7.21.* This is true even when the secondary focal point is virtual, in which case the exiting wavefront is diverging (see Figures 7.11c and d).

Similarly, the primary focal point is the object point conjugate to optical infinity. As such, the primary focal length is really the radius of curvature of the incident wavefront that results in plane waves leaving the interface. *The incident wavefront is physically in the medium of index n_1, and the primary focal length is then associated with n_1, as is evident mathematically in Eq. 7.22.* This is true even when the primary focal point is virtual, in which case the incident wavefront is converging (see Figures 7.12c and d).

Besides Eq. 7.23 and 7.24, another relationship exists between the focal lengths. By adding Eq. 7.21 and 7.22 together, we obtain

$$f_2 + f_1 = \frac{n_2}{P} - \frac{n_1}{P}$$

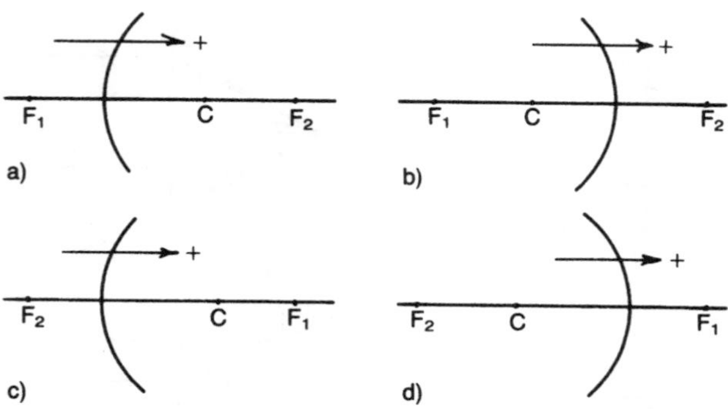

Figure 7.13 Center of curvature and focal points.

or

$$f_2 + f_1 = \frac{n_2 - n_1}{P}$$

But from Eq. 7.19,

$$r = \frac{n_2 - n_1}{P}$$

so

$$f_2 + f_1 = r \tag{7.25}$$

Equation 7.25 says that the radius of curvature of the interface is equal to the sum of the primary and secondary focal lengths of the interface. This relationship is a useful self-consistency check when doing SSRI calculations. It is also useful in setting up "quick and dirty" ray diagrams.

In Figure 7.13a, F_2 and C are both on the right side of the interface. From Eq. 7.25,

$$f_1 = r - f_2$$

or in absolute values

$$|f_1| = |r - f_2| = |CF_2|$$

where CF_2 is the distance from the center of curvature C to F_2. Consequently, when making a quick ray diagram for this case, one can select the horizontal scale, plot C and F_2, and then simply insert F_1 on the opposite side at a distance equal to CF_2.

A similar relationship exists for Figures 7.13b and c in which C and F_1 are on the same side. From Eq. 7.25,

$$f_2 = r - f_1$$

or in absolute values

$$|f_2| = |r - f_1| = |CF_1|$$

where CF_1 is the distance from C to F_1. Consequently, for the cases where C and F_1 are on the same side, the distance f_2 is equal to the distance CF_1.

EXAMPLE 7.6

In Example 7.3, there was a +2.00 D SSRI between water ($n = 1.33$) and glass ($n = 1.53$). What are the focal lengths for the +2.00 D interface?

For light incident from the water side,

$$n_1 = 1.33 \quad \text{and} \quad n_2 = 1.53$$

From Eq. 7.21,

$$f_2 = \frac{n_2}{P} = \frac{(1.53)100\,\text{cm/m}}{+2.00\,\text{D}}$$

or

$$f_2 = \frac{153\,\text{cm/m}}{+2.00\,\text{D}} = +76.5\,\text{cm}$$

The secondary focal point is 76.5 cm behind the interface (Figure 7.14).

From Eq. 7.22,

$$f_1 = -\frac{n_1}{P}$$

or

$$f_1 = -\frac{133\,\text{cm/m}}{+2.00\,\text{D}} = -66.5\,\text{cm}$$

The primary focal point is 66.5 cm in front of the interface.

Let us use Eq. 7.25 as a self-consistency check. From Example 7.3, the radius of curvature of this interface is +10 cm. From Eq. 7.25,

$$\begin{aligned} r &= f_1 + f_2 \\ &= -66.5\,\text{cm} + 76.5\,\text{cm} = +10.0\,\text{cm} \end{aligned}$$

which checks.

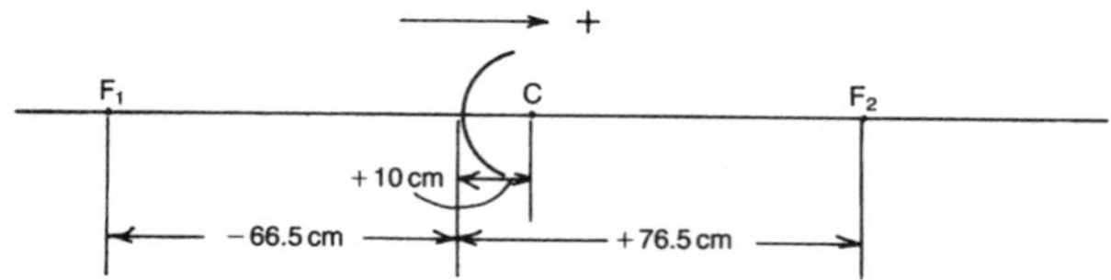

Figure 7.14 A +2.00-D SSRI.

EXAMPLE 7.7

In Example 7.4, a −10.00 D SSRI between air and glass ($n = 1.50$) had a radius of curvature of

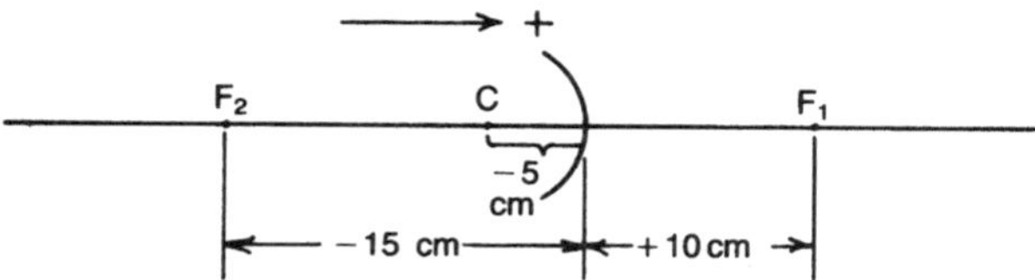

Figure 7.15 An SSRI with a −15 cm secondary focal length.

−5 cm for light incident from the air side. What are the focal lengths?

Here, $n_1 = 1.00$ and $n_2 = 1.50$. From Eq. 7.21,

$$f_2 = \frac{n_2}{P} = \frac{(1.50)100\,\text{cm/m}}{-10.00\,\text{D}} = \frac{150\,\text{cm/m}}{-10.00\,\text{D}} = -15.0\,\text{cm}$$

The secondary focal point is virtual and 15 cm in front of the interface (Figure 7.15). From Eq. 7.22,

$$f_1 = -\frac{n_1}{P} = \frac{-(1.00)100\,\text{cm/m}}{-10.00\,\text{D}} = +10.00\,\text{cm}$$

The primary focal point is virtual and located 10 cm behind the interface.

The self-consistency check is:

$$r = f_1 + f_2 = (10.0\,\text{cm}) + (-15.0\,\text{cm}) = -5.0\,\text{cm}$$

which checks.

EXAMPLE 7.8

A single spherical refracting interface between plastic ($n = 1.40$) and diamond ($n = 2.40$) has a primary focal length of +40.00 cm and a secondary focal length of −23.33 cm. What is the dioptric power of the interface?

The secondary focal length is negative so the interface is a diverging interface and P must be negative.

Since the longer focal length is associated with the higher index medium, the primary focal length (+40.00 cm) is associated with the diamond ($n = 2.40$). Thus, the incident light is in the diamond, and

$$n_1 = 2.40 \quad \text{while} \quad n_2 = 1.40$$

Then either Eq. 7.21 or Eq. 7.22 can be used to calculate P. From Eq. 7.22,

$$P = -\frac{n_1}{f_1} = \frac{-(2.40)100\,\text{cm/m}}{+40.00\,\text{cm}} = \frac{-240\,\text{cm/m}}{+40.00\,\text{cm}} = -6.00\,\text{D}$$

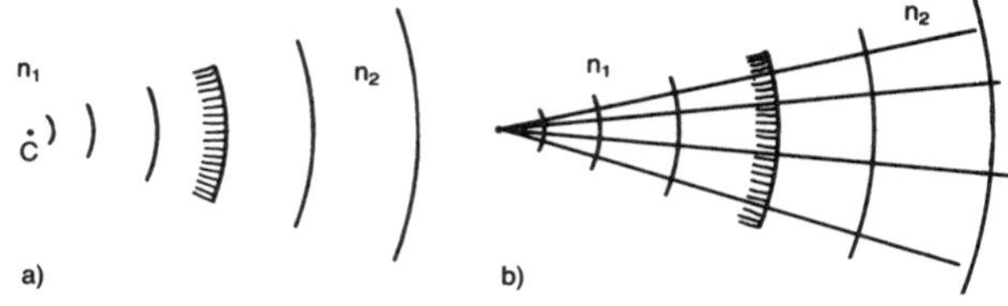

Figure 7.16 Point source at the center of curvature: a, wavefronts; b, wavefronts and rays.

You should check that Eq. 7.21 gives the same value for P.

7.6 THE NODAL POINT

Consider a point source located at the center of curvature of an SSRI (Figure 7.16). The wavefronts leaving the point source are spherical and centered on the point source. Since the point source is located at the center of curvature of the interface, the wavefront reaching the interface has the same curvature as the interface, and all parts of the wavefront enter the second medium at the same time. Consequently, the whole wavefront changes speed at the same instant, and no curvature change occurs as the wavefront passes through the interface. The wavefronts leaving the interface are spherical and still centered on the center of curvature of the interface.

Since there is no wavefront curvature change, the rays associated with the wavefronts are straight lines that pass through the interface without bending (Figure 7.16b). This is consistent with Snell's Law,

$$n_1 \sin\theta_i = n_2 \sin\theta_r$$

since a ray from the center of curvature is normal to the interface. Here the incident angle θ_i is equal to zero, and thus the angle of refraction θ_r, is also zero.

The rays that pass straight through an interface are the nodal rays, and hence the nodal point of an SSRI is at the center of curvature of the interface (Figure 7.17). For a thin

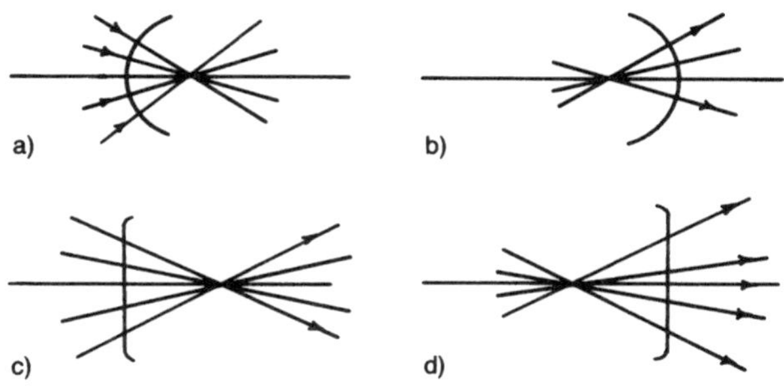

Figure 7.17 Nodal rays: a, b, actual; c, d, scaled.

lens in air, the nodal point is at the lens itself, but for an SSRI the nodal point is at C and not at the vertex of the SSRI.

The displacement of the nodal point away from the interface is a result of the asymmetry of the SSRI. A thin lens in air is symmetric in the sense that the same media is on both sides of the lens. An SSRI has a different medium on each side, and thus is asymmetric.

In general, any ray associated with the nodal point (either passing through it or pointing toward or away from it) is a predictable ray, and passes straight through the interface without bending. The paraxial ray diagrams with the expanded vertical scale are shown in Figures 7.17c and d.

7.7 LATERAL MAGNIFICATION

Figure 7.18 shows a real object, its conjugate real image, and the nodal ray connecting the object and image. The image size is I and the object size is O. As before, the sizes are considered positive for objects or images above the axis and negative for objects and images below the axis. The lateral magnification m is defined as the ratio of the image size I to the object size O, or

$$m = I/O \tag{7.26}$$

The image subtends the angle w' at the nodal point C, and from Figure 7.18,

$$\tan w' = \frac{-I}{v - r}$$

The object subtends the angle w at the nodal point C and from Figure 7.18,

$$\tan w = \frac{O}{-u + r}$$

Note that u is a negative quantity in Figure 7.18, so that $-u$ is a positive quantity.

Since the nodal ray is a straight line, the angles w and w' are equal and from the above two equations

$$\frac{-I}{v - r} = \frac{O}{-u + r}$$

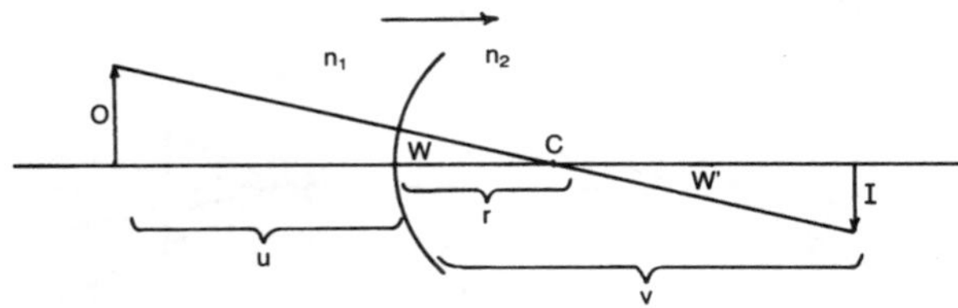

Figure 7.18 Nodal ray and image size.

or

$$m = \frac{I}{O} = \frac{r - v}{r - u} \tag{7.27}$$

Equation 7.27 can be used to calculate the lateral magnification; however, an easier expression can be derived as follows

From Eq. 7.16,

$$V = P + U$$

which can be written as

$$\frac{n_2}{v} = \frac{n_2 - n_1}{r} + \frac{n_1}{u}$$

We can then find a common denominator:

$$\frac{n_2 ru}{vru} = \frac{n_2 vu}{vru} - \frac{n_1 vu}{vru} + \frac{n_1 rv}{vru}$$

We can eliminate the common denominator to obtain

$$n_2 ru = n_2 vu - n_1 vu + n_1 rv$$

or

$$n_2 ru - n_2 vu = -n_1 vu + n_1 rv$$

Then,

$$n_2 u(r - v) = n_1 v(r - u)$$

or

$$\frac{n_1 v}{n_2 u} = \frac{r - v}{r - u} \tag{7.28}$$

Equations 7.27 and 7.28 can be combined to give

$$m = \frac{n_1 v}{n_2 u} \tag{7.29}$$

Equation 7.29 is an equation for the lateral magnification m in terms of the image distance v, the object distance u, and the indices of refraction n_1 and n_2. Equation 7.29 differs from the corresponding Eq. 5.7 for a thin lens in air by the presence of the indices of refraction.

For an SSRI,

$$V = \frac{n_2}{v} \quad \text{and} \quad U = \frac{n_1}{u}$$

When the vergence equations are substituted into Eq. 7.29, the result is

$$m = \frac{U}{V} \tag{7.30}$$

Equation 7.30 is a straightforward relationship between the lateral magnification and the vergences

U and V. Furthermore, Eq. 7.30 is identical in form to Eq. 5.8 for thin lenses in air. This identity occurs because the vergences U and V implicitly contain the indices or refraction. Equation 7.30 makes lateral magnification calculations extremely easy.

7.8 IMAGING EXAMPLES

EXAMPLE 7.9

A goldfish in water ($n = 1.33$) is 60 cm from a +5.00 D water-high index glass ($n = 1.83$) interface (Figure 7.19). First, use a ray diagram to find the image, and determine whether it is virtual or real, erect or inverted, larger or smaller. Then answer the same questions by calculation.

In order to draw the ray diagram, we first need to find the focal points and the radius of curvature of the interface. Here $n_1 = 1.33$, $n_2 = 1.83$, $u = -40$ cm.

From Eq. 7.19,

$$r = \frac{n_2 - n_1}{P} = \frac{(1.83 - 1.33)100\,\text{cm/m}}{+5.00\,\text{D}} = \frac{50\,\text{cm/m}}{+5.00\,\text{D}} = +10.0\,\text{cm}$$

From Eq. 7.21,

$$f_2 = \frac{n_2}{P} = \frac{(1.83)100\,\text{cm/m}}{+5.00\,\text{D}} = \frac{183\,\text{cm/m}}{+5.00\,\text{D}} = +36.6\,\text{cm}$$

From Eq. 7.22,

$$f_1 = -\frac{n_1}{P} = \frac{-133\,\text{cm/m}}{+5.00\,\text{D}} = -26.6\,\text{cm}$$

Equation 7.25 can be used as a self-consistency check:

$$r = f_1 + f_2 = (-26.6\,\text{cm}) + (+36.6\,\text{cm}) = +10.0\,\text{cm}$$

Figure 7.20 shows F_1, F_2, C, and the predictable rays. From the ray diagram, the image is real,

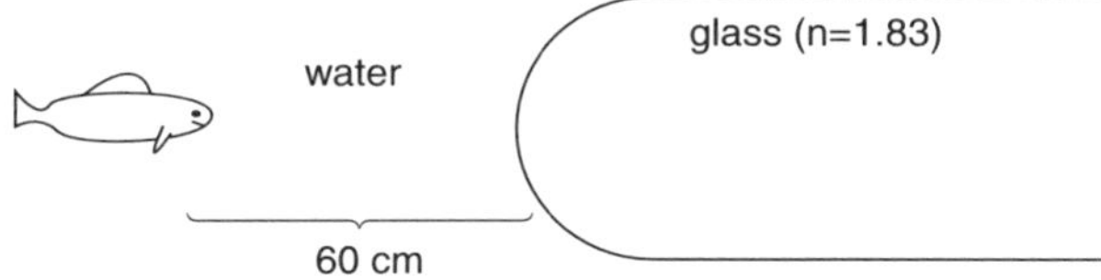

Figure 7.19 Goldfish example.

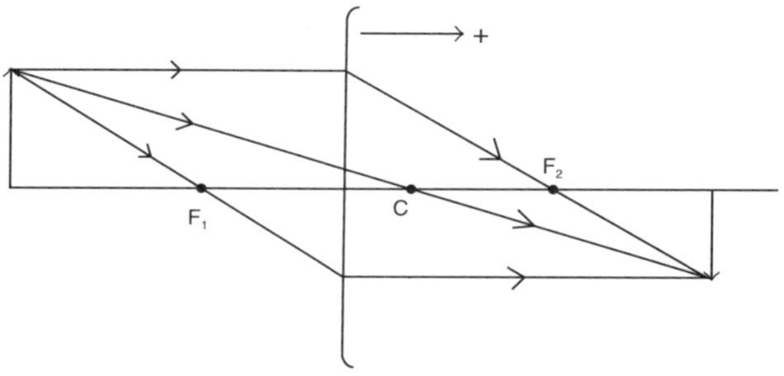

Figure 7.20 Ray diagram for Figure 7.19.

inverted, larger, and approximately 60 cm from the interface. Note that the nodal ray goes through C and not through the pole of the interface.

The calculations are:

$$U = \frac{n_1}{u} = \frac{(1.33)100\,\text{cm/m}}{-60\,\text{cm}} = \frac{133\,\text{cm/m}}{-60\,\text{cm}} = -2.22\,\text{D}$$

Then,

$$V = P + U = +5.00\,\text{D} + (-2.22\,\text{D}) = +2.78\,\text{D}$$

The light in the glass leaving the interface is converging, which agrees with the ray diagram.

$$v = \frac{n_2}{V} = \frac{183\,\text{cm/m}}{+2.78\,\text{D}} = +65.75\,\text{cm}$$

The image distance of +65.75 cm agrees with the ray diagram. The lateral magnification is

$$m = \frac{U}{V} = \frac{-2.22\,\text{D}}{+2.78\,\text{D}} = -0.80$$

The image is inverted and smaller than the object by a factor of 0.80, and that agrees with the ray diagram.

For instructional purposes, let us also use Eq. 7.29 to calculate m:

$$m = \frac{n_1 v}{n_2 u} = \frac{(1.33)(+65.75\,\text{cm})}{(1.83)(-60\,\text{cm})} = -0.80$$

Note that the indices are needed in the above equation, and that we cannot obtain m by merely taking the image distance over the object distance.

EXAMPLE 7.10

The goldfish in the previous example swims in to a distance of 14 cm in front of the interface.

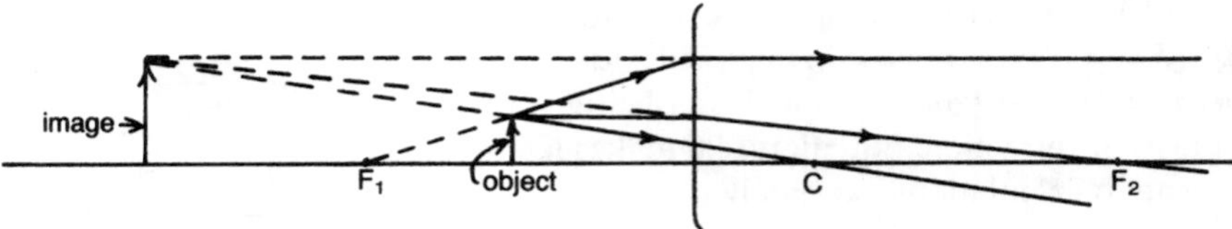

Figure 7.21 Goldfish inside the primary focal point.

Now where is the conjugate image? Is it real or virtual, erect or inverted, larger or smaller?

The focal points and nodal points are unchanged. The primary focal length is −26.6 cm, so the fish is inside F_1. Therefore, we would expect a virtual image that is erect and larger. A quick ray diagram (Figure 7.21) confirms these expectations.

The calculations are:

$$U = \frac{n_1}{u} = \frac{133\,\text{cm/m}}{-14\,\text{cm}} = -9.50\,\text{D}$$

Then,

$$V = P + U$$
$$= +5.00\,\text{D} + (-9.50\,\text{D}) = -4.50\,\text{D}$$

The light leaving the interface is in glass, and is diverging. The image distance is

$$v = \frac{n_2}{V} = \frac{183\,\text{cm/m}}{-4.50\,\text{D}} = -40.67\,\text{cm}$$

which agrees with the ray diagram. Note that the image position is at the center of curvature of the wavefronts leaving the interface and these wavefronts are physically in the glass.

The lateral magnification is

$$m = \frac{U}{V} = \frac{-9.50\,\text{D}}{-4.50\,\text{D}} = +2.11$$

So the image is erect and 2.11 times as large as the object, which also agrees with the ray diagram.

EXAMPLE 7.11

For the previous example compute the vergence of the light at 5 cm in front of the interface (point A in Figure 7.22), and at 5 cm behind the interface (point B in Figure 7.22).

The light incident on the interface had a vergence of −9.50 D. At 5 cm in front of the interface, the light is in water and is diverging. The wavefront there is curved more than the wavefront hitting the interface so that we expect the vergence to be more minus than −9.50 D. Position A is 5 cm closer to the object so the radius of curvature of a wavefront at A is 9 cm (i.e., 14 cm – 5 cm). The magnitude of the vergence is

$$|U_A| = \frac{(1.33)100\,\text{cm/m}}{9\,\text{cm}}$$

or

$$|U_A| = \frac{133\,\text{cm/m}}{9\,\text{cm}} = 14.78\,\text{D}$$

Since the wavefront is diverging,

$$U_A = -14.78\,\text{D}$$

The light leaving the interface has a vergence of −4.50 D. At 5 cm behind the interface, the light is in the glass and is diverging. The center of curvature of the diverging wavefront at B is at the image position that is 45.67 cm away from B (i.e, 40.67 cm + 5 cm). The magnitude of the vergence at B is

$$|V_B| = \frac{(1.83)(100\,\text{cm/m})}{45.67\,\text{cm}}$$
$$= \frac{183}{45.67} = 4.01\,\text{D}$$

Since the light is diverging at B, the vergence is negative and

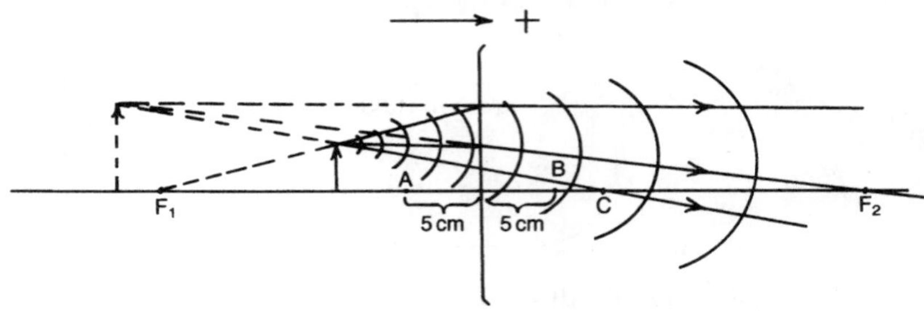

Figure 7.22 Wavefronts for vergence values.

$$V_B = -4.01\,\text{D}$$

Thus, the light lost about a half diopter of minus vergence in traveling from the interface to B.

EXAMPLE 7.12

A concave interface between air and plastic ($n = 1.44$) has a butterfly imbedded in the plastic at a distance of 10.0 cm from the interface. The conjugate image is virtual and located at a distance of −6.02 cm from the interface. What is the dioptric power of the interface? Also compute the lateral magnification and draw a ray diagram.

The interface is concave from the perspective of the lower index medium. Figure 7.23 shows a sketch of the given information. The light incident on the interface is in the plastic and is diverging. Here $n_1 = 1.44$, $n_2 = 1.00$, and $u = -10$ cm. Then,

$$U = \frac{n_1}{u} = \frac{144\,\text{cm/m}}{-10\,\text{cm}} = -14.4\,\text{D}$$

The light leaving the interface is in air and is diverging away from the virtual image position. In other words, a wavefront leaving the interface is in air and is centered on the virtual image. Here,

$$v = -6.02\,\text{cm}$$

Then,

$$V = \frac{n_2}{v} = \frac{100\,\text{cm/m}}{-6.02\,\text{cm}} = -16.6\,\text{D}$$

From the vergence equation,

$$P = V - U$$
$$= -16.6\,\text{D} - (-14.4\,\text{D}) = -2.2\,\text{D}$$

The lateral magnification is

$$m = \frac{U}{V} = \frac{-14.4\,\text{D}}{-16.6\,\text{D}} = +0.87$$

Alternatively,

$$m = \frac{n_1 v}{n_2 u}$$
$$= \frac{(1.44)(-6.02\,\text{cm})}{(1.00)(-10.0\,\text{cm})} = +0.87$$

We need to find the center of curvature and the focal points of the interface in order to draw the ray diagram. The radius of curvature is

$$r = \frac{n_2 - n_1}{P}$$
$$= \frac{(1.00 - 1.44)100\,\text{cm/m}}{-2.2\,\text{D}}$$
$$= \frac{-44\,\text{cm/m}}{-2.2\,\text{D}} = +20.0\,\text{cm}$$

The focal lengths are:

$$f_2 = \frac{n_2}{P} = \frac{100\,\text{cm/m}}{-2.2\,\text{D}} = -45.5\,\text{cm}$$

$$f_1 = -\frac{n_1}{P} = \frac{-144\,\text{cm/m}}{-2.2\,\text{D}} = +65.5\,\text{cm}$$

The self-consistency check is

$$r = f_1 + f_2$$
$$= +65.5\,\text{cm} + (-45.5\,\text{cm}) = +20.0\,\text{cm}$$

Figure 7.24 shows two of the three predictable rays. You should draw in the predictable ray associated with F_1.

EXAMPLE 7.13

For the situation in the preceding example, calculate the vergence of the light at a position 4 cm, in front of the interface (A in Figure 7.24), and at a position 5 cm behind the interface (B in Figure 7.24).

The wavefront that is physically at A is diverging, in the plastic, and centered on the object. The object is 10 cm from the interface, so position A is 6 cm from the object, and the radius of curvature of the diverging wavefront is then 6 cm in magnitude.

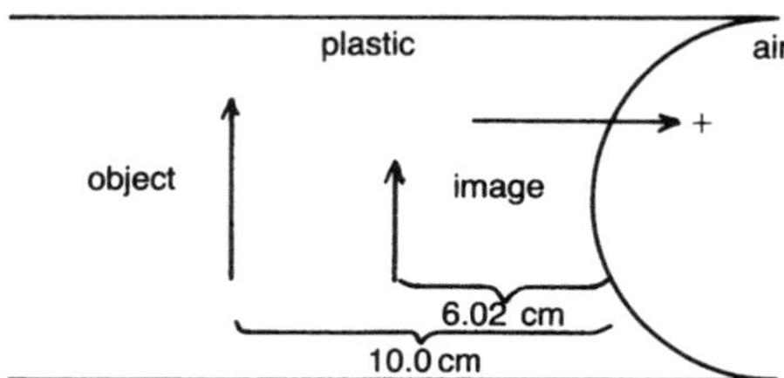

Figure 7.23 Butterfly example.

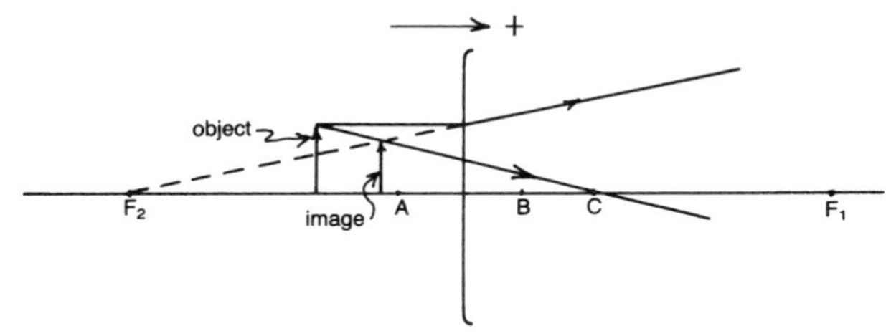

Figure 7.24 Ray diagram for Figure 7.23.

The magnitude of the vergence is

$$|U_A| = \frac{(1.44)(100\,\text{cm/m})}{6\,\text{cm}}$$
$$= \frac{144}{6} = 24.00\,\text{D}$$

or

$$U_A = -24.00\,\text{D}$$

The vergence of the wavefront incident on the interface was −14.4 D, which is consistent with the fact that the diverging wavefronts lose curvature as they propagate from A to the interface.

At B, the wavefront is diverging, in air, and is centered on the virtual image. The image is 6.02 cm from the interface. The radius of curvature of the wavefront at B has a magnitude of 11.02 cm (i.e., 6.02 cm + 5 cm). The magnitude of the vergence at B is

$$|V_B| = \frac{(1.00)100\,\text{cm/m}}{11.02\,\text{cm}} = 9.07\,\text{D}$$

or since the wavefront is diverging

$$V_B = -9.07\,\text{D}$$

The wavefront leaving the interface has a vergence of −16.6 D, and 5 cm downstream (at B) its vergence is −9.07 D.

EXAMPLE 7.14

Converging light in plastic is incident on the same plastic–air interface discussed in the previous two examples. The resulting virtual object is located 30.0 cm from the interface. Find the conjugate image, and specify whether it is real or virtual, larger or smaller, erect or inverted.

From Example 7.12,

$$r = +20\,\text{cm} \quad f_2 = -45.5\,\text{cm} \quad f_1 = +65.5\,\text{cm}$$
$$\text{and} \quad P = -2.2\,\text{D}$$

Figure 7.25 shows two predictable rays. The exiting rays show that the image is real, erect, and larger. You should draw in the predictable ray associated with F_2.

The calculations are:

$$u = +30\,\text{cm}$$
$$U = \frac{n_1}{u} = \frac{144}{+30} = +4.80\,\text{D}$$

Note that the incident converging wavefront is in the plastic. Then,

$$V = P + U$$
$$= -2.2\,\text{D} + (+4.80\,\text{D}) = +2.60\,\text{D}$$

The light leaving the interface is in air and converging in agreement with the ray diagram. The image distance is:

$$v = \frac{n_2}{V} = \frac{100}{2.60\,\text{D}} = +38.5\,\text{cm}$$

The lateral magnification is:

$$m = \frac{U}{V} = \frac{+4.80\,\text{D}}{+2.60\,\text{D}} = +1.85$$

So the image is erect and 1.85 times larger than the object.

For instructional purposes, calculate the vergence of the wavefront at C, the center of curvature of the interface. The wavefront at C is converging, in air, and centered on the real image that is 18.5 cm away from C (i.e., 38.5 cm − 20.0 cm). The vergence at C is:

$$V_C = \frac{100}{+18.5\,\text{cm}} = +5.40\,\text{D}$$

Note that the wavefront leaving the interface has a vergence of +2.60 D, and its vergence has increased to +5.40 D at C.

7.9 THE SYMMETRY POINTS

For thin lenses in air, the plane $2F_1$ was conjugate to the plane $2F_2$, and the lateral magnification was −1. Let us now consider what conjugate plane gives a lateral magnification of −1 for an SSRI. Since

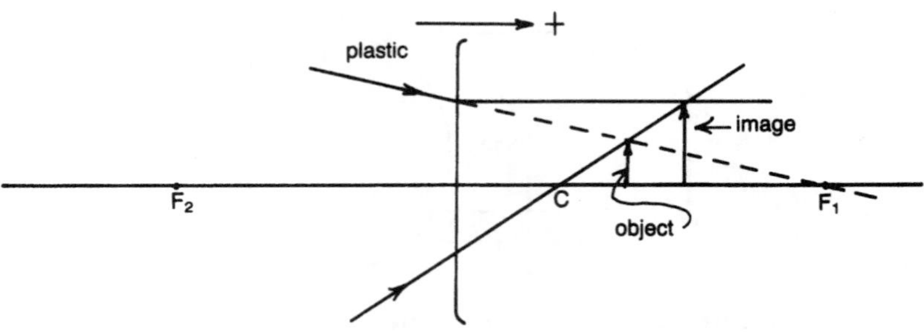

Figure 7.25 Incident converging light in the plastic.

$$m = \frac{U}{V} = -1$$
$$U = -V$$

Then,

$$V = P + U$$

becomes

$$V = P - V$$

or

$$2V = P$$

and

$$V = \frac{P}{2}$$

Then the expressions for V and P in Eqs. 7.18 and 7.21 can be inserted to obtain

$$\frac{n_2}{v} = \frac{n_2}{2f_2}$$

or

$$v = 2f_2$$

The image plane is again at $2F_2$.

Similarly, it is easy to show that

$$u = -2f_1$$

so that the object plane is again at $2F_1$.

Therefore, just as for a thin lens in air, $2F_1$ is conjugate to $2F_2$ and the lateral magnification is -1. The axial points $2F_1$ and $2F_2$ are called the symmetry points, and the planes containing the symmetry points are called the symmetry planes. Since the primary and secondary focal points of an SSRI are not equidistant from the interface, the symmetry points are also not equidistant. When the interface is a converging interface, the symmetry points are both real, and when the interface is a diverging interface the symmetry points are both virtual.

EXAMPLE 7.15

Find the symmetry points for a $-8.00\,\text{D}$ single spherical refracting interface between glass ($n = 1.50$) and diamond ($n = 2.4$) with the light incident from the glass side.

Here $n_1 = 1.50$, and $n_2 = 2.40$. Then,

$$f_2 = \frac{n_2}{P} = \frac{240}{-8.00} = -30.0\,\text{cm}$$

and

$$f_1 = -\frac{n_1}{P} = \frac{-150}{-8.00} = +18.75\,\text{cm}$$

For the symmetry points:

$$u = 2f_1 = 2(+18.75\,\text{cm}) = +37.5\,\text{cm}$$
$$v = 2f_2 = 2(-30.0\,\text{cm}) = -60.0\,\text{cm}$$

The lateral magnification is:

$$m = \frac{n_1 v}{n_2 u} = \frac{(1.50)(-60.0\,\text{cm})}{(2.40)(+37.5\,\text{cm})} = -1.0$$

The radius of curvature of the interface is

$$r = f_1 + f_2 = +18.75\,\text{cm} + (-30.0\,\text{cm}) = -11.25\,\text{cm}$$

Figure 7.26 gives the ray diagram. You could also draw in the nodal ray. For instructional purposes, let us also consider the vergences U and V.

$$U = \frac{n_1}{u} = \frac{150}{+37.5\,\text{cm}} = +4.0\,\text{D}$$
$$V = \frac{n_2}{v} = \frac{240}{-60.0\,\text{cm}} = -4.0\,\text{D}$$

and then

$$m = \frac{U}{V} = \frac{+4.0\,\text{D}}{-4.0\,\text{D}} = -1.0$$

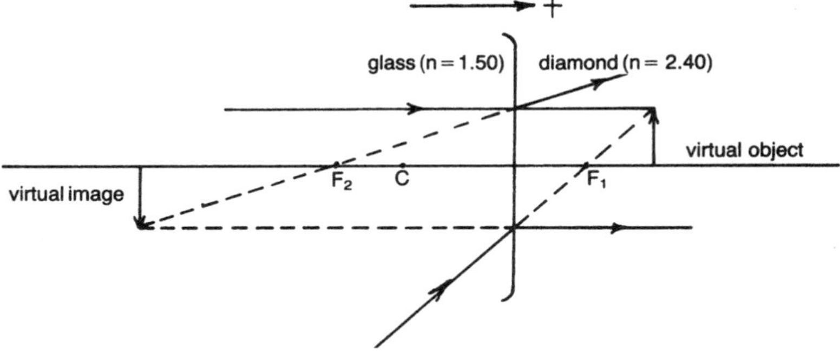

Figure 7.26 Symmetry points for a diverging interface.

7.10 UNIT MAGNIFICATION

For thin lenses in air, an object distance of zero resulted in an image distance of zero and a lateral magnification of +1. Let us check if this also holds for an SSRI.

From $V = P + U$,

$$\frac{n_2}{v} = P + \frac{n_1}{u}$$

Then,

$$\frac{n_2}{v} = \frac{uP + n_1}{u}$$

or

$$\frac{v}{n_2} = \frac{u}{uP + n_1}$$

As the object is moved closer and closer to the interface, u gets closer and closer to zero, and the uP term in the denominator becomes negligible compared to n_1. So in the limit of u going to zero.

$$\frac{v}{n_2} = \frac{u}{n_1}$$

Since

$$m = \frac{n_1 v}{n_2 u}$$

we can combine the above two equations to obtain

$$m = +1$$

Therefore, for an SSRI, an object distance of zero gives an image distance of zero and a lateral magnification of +1.

EXAMPLE 7.16

Consider a +6.00 D convex air–glass ($n = 1.50$) interface. Find the image distance and lateral magnification for a piece of paper in air at distances of 1 cm, 0.1 cm, and 0.01 cm. Does the lateral magnification go to +1 as u goes to zero?

Here $n_1 = 1.00$ and $n_2 = 1.50$. The calculations for 1 cm are:

$$u = -1\,\text{cm}$$

$$U = \frac{n_1}{u} = \frac{100}{-1} = -100\,\text{D}$$

$$V = P + U$$

$$= +6.00\,\text{D} + (-\,100\,\text{D}) = -94\,\text{D}$$

$$v = \frac{n_2}{V} = \frac{150}{-94\,\text{D}} = -1.60\,\text{cm}$$

$$m = \frac{U}{V} = \frac{-100\,\text{D}}{-94\,\text{D}} = +1.06$$

Table 7.1 Lateral Magnification as Object Distance Goes to Zero

u (cm)	*v (cm)*	*m*
−1.00	−1.60	+1.06
−0.10	−0.15	+1.006
−0.01	−0.015	+1.0006

The results for the other object distances are computed similarly, and shown in Table 7.1.

From the numerical results presented in Table 7.1, it is clear that as the object distance goes to zero, the image distance goes to zero and the lateral magnification goes to +1. This means that when an object is placed directly in contact with the SSRI, the interface essentially has no imaging effect.

7.11 THE NODAL PLANE

In addition to a zero object distance, there is another case in which the object and image are both the same distance away from the SSRI. This case involves the nodal point that is at the center of curvature C of the SSRI. Figure 7.27 shows an object in the nodal plane of a converging SSRI. Note that the focal points in Figure 7.27 are placed so as to satisfy Eq. 7.25. The two predictable rays show that the image is virtual, located in the same plane as the object, and larger than the object.

The ray diagram can be confirmed analytically as follows:

$$V = P + U$$

$$\frac{n_2}{v} = \frac{n_2 - n_1}{r} + \frac{n_1}{u}$$

Let $u = r$. Then,

$$\frac{n_2}{v} = \frac{n_2 - n_1}{r} + \frac{n_1}{r}$$

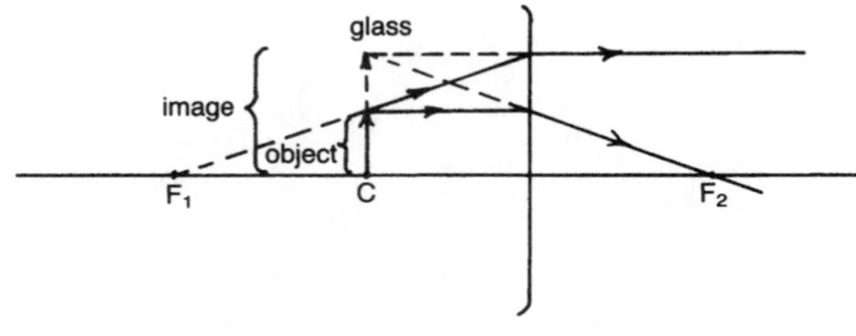

Figure 7.27 Object in the center of curvature plane.

or

$$\frac{n_2}{v} = \frac{n_2}{r}$$

and

$$v = r$$

The lateral magnification is

$$m = \frac{n_1 v}{n_2 u} = \frac{n_1 r}{n_2 r} = \frac{n_1}{n_2} \qquad (7.31)$$

The SSRI shown in Figure 7.27 is converging, and the higher index medium must be on the left. Therefore, for this case, n_1 must be greater than n_2. Consequently, m is greater than $+1$, and the image must be erect and larger than the object, which agrees with the ray diagram.

EXAMPLE 7.17

A glass ($n = 1.50$) hemisphere of radius 5 cm is used as a paperweight. A 2-mm tall letter is centered under the hemisphere (Figure 7.28). The light diverging away from the letter is in the glass so the letter effectively acts like an object in the glass. Since the letter is centered, it is at the center of curvature of the interface. Where is the conjugate image? What is its size? Here $n_1 = 1.50$ and $n_2 = 1.00$. Then,

$$u = r = -5\,\text{cm}$$

and the ray diagram in Figure 7.27 describes the situation. The dioptric power is given by

$$P = \frac{n_2 - n_1}{r} = \frac{(1.00 - 1.50)100\,\text{cm/m}}{-5\,\text{cm}} = \frac{-50}{-5} = +10.0\,\text{D}$$

The incident vergence is given by

$$U = \frac{n_1}{u} = \frac{150}{-5\,\text{cm}} = -30.0\,\text{D}$$

Then,

$$V = P + U = +10.0\,\text{D} + (-\,30.0\,\text{D}) = -20.0\,\text{D}$$

The light leaving the interface is in air and diverging. The image is virtual, and the image distance is

$$v = \frac{n_2}{V} = \frac{100}{-20.0\,\text{D}} = -5\,\text{cm}$$

which is equal to r.

The lateral magnification is

$$m = \frac{U}{V} = \frac{-30.0\,\text{D}}{-20.0\,\text{D}} = +1.50$$

The image size is

$$I = mO = (= 1.50)(2\,\text{mm}) = 3\,\text{mm}$$

An observer looking at the letter through the paperweight would see a virtual image at the same position as the letter but 1.5 times larger than the letter.

The adjective *apparent* is used to describe various aspects of the image formed by an optical system placed between the object and an observer's eye. In the previous example, the apparent position of the letter is 5 cm from the interface and its apparent size is 3 mm. Note that the word apparent refers to the characteristics of the interface's image (virtual in this case), and not necessarily to the visually perceived image of the observer.

In the preceding discussion, the image is larger than the object by the ratio of the indices of refraction. In general, an image at the center of curvature of the interface can be either larger or smaller than its conjugate image by the ratio of the indices of refraction. Figure 7.29 shows a ray diagram for a converging interface with a virtual object and a smaller real image at the center of curvature.

7.12 STRANGE CASES

Chapters 4, 5, and 6 developed optics intuition by considering thin lenses in air. Much of this intuition has

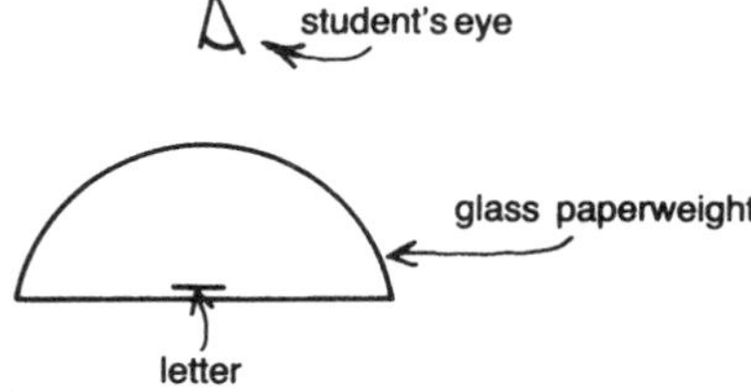

Figure 7.28 Paperweight example.

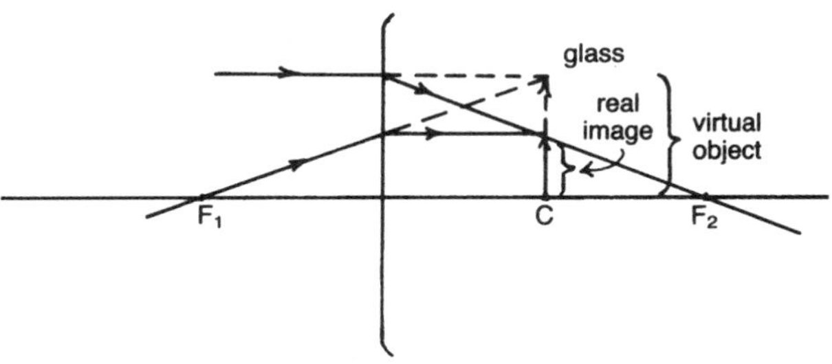

Figure 7.29 Virtual object at the center of curvature.

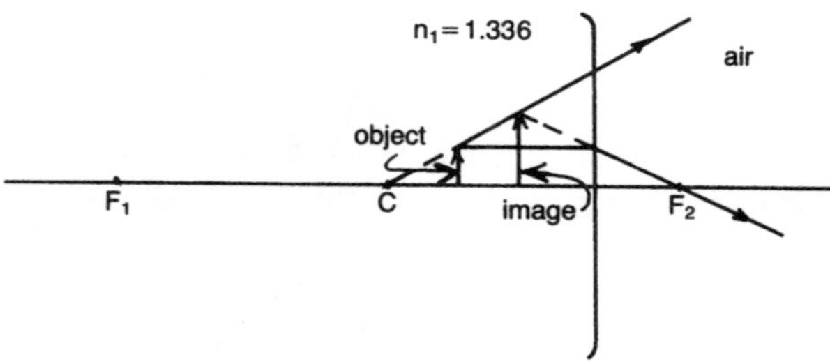

Figure 7.30 Real object inside the center of curvature for a converging interface.

carried over to the discussion of SSRIs. In particular, the role of the focal points F_1 and F_2 is the same, the symmetry points are again at $2F_1$ and $2F_2$, and an object distance of zero gives an image distance of zero with a lateral magnification of +1.

However, there is no thin lens in air analog for an object at the center of curvature of an SSRI. In that sense, an object at the center of curvature of an SSRI constitutes a strange case. Actually, all SSRI cases for which an object or an image falls between the interface and the center of curvature are strange in that they have no thin lens in air analog, and thus our thin lens in air intuition breaks down.

Consider the ray diagram in Figure 7.30. The interface is converging. The object is inside F_1 and inside C. Our thin lens in air intuition would tell us to expect the image to be virtual, larger, and further from the interface than the object. In the ray diagram, however, the two predictable rays show that while the image is indeed virtual and larger, it is closer instead of being further away.

EXAMPLE 7.18

Consider a simplified model of the anterior chamber of the eye (Figure 7.31). Assume that the cornea and the anterior chamber both have an index of 1.336, and that the cornea is spherical with a radius of curvature of 7.5 mm. The iris of the eye sits in the aqueous humor about 3.6 mm from the cornea. When you look at the iris you do not see the iris itself, but rather an image of the iris formed by the cornea. Find the image position and the lateral magnification.

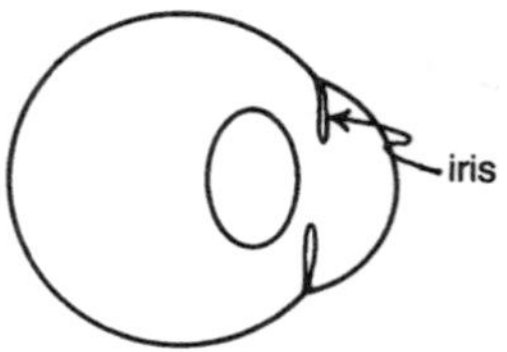

Figure 7.31 Iris as object for the cornea.

The light leaving the iris is initially in the aqueous humor. Therefore, $n_1 = 1.336$, $n_2 = 1.000$, and $r = -7.5$ mm. Then,

$$P = \frac{n_2 - n_1}{r} = \frac{(1.000 - 1.336)1000\,\text{mm/m}}{-7.5\,\text{mm}} = \frac{-336}{-7.5} = +44.8\,\text{D}$$

and

$$U = \frac{n_1}{u} = \frac{(1.336)1000\,\text{mm/m}}{-3.6\,\text{mm}} = \frac{1336}{-3.6} = -371.1\,\text{D}$$

From $V = P + U$,

$$V = +44.8\,\text{D} + (-371.1\,\text{D}) = -326.3\,\text{D}$$

The light leaving the cornea is in air and the image is virtual. The image distance is

$$v = \frac{n_2}{V} = \frac{1000\,\text{mm/m}}{-326.3\,\text{D}} = -3.06\,\text{mm}$$

So the virtual image is at 3.06 mm which is closer to the cornea than the iris is.
The lateral magnification is

$$m = \frac{U}{V} = \frac{-371.1\,\text{D}}{-326.3\,\text{D}} = +1.14$$

so the virtual image is larger than the iris. Thus, the apparent iris that you see is both closer and larger than the actual iris. You might keep this in mind the next time you are gazing into someone's beautiful eyes.

The pupil is the opening in the center of the iris, and if the virtual image of the iris is larger than the actual iris, then so too is the virtual image of the pupil larger than the actual pupil. In later chapters, we will come to call the virtual image of the pupil the eye's *entrance pupil*.

EXAMPLE 7.19

An object in air is located 12.5 cm from a −2.00 D air–glass ($n = 1.50$) interface. Find the conjugate image and specify whether it is real or virtual, erect or inverted, larger or smaller.

Here $n_1 = 1.00$ and $n_2 = 1.50$. The focal lengths and the radius of curvature can be determined from the usual equations. The results are as follows: $r = -25.0$ cm, $f_1 = +50.0$ cm, and $f_2 = -75.0$ cm.

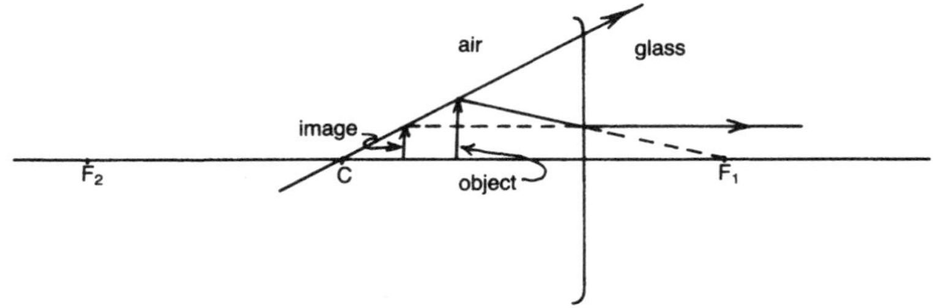

Figure 7.32 Real object inside the center of curvature for a diverging interface.

Figure 7.32 shows two of the predictable rays. (You should supply the third predictable ray.) According to our thin lens in air intuition, an object in front of a minus system would result in a virtual image that is erect, smaller, and closer. The ray diagram shows that this is a strange case because the virtual image is erect, smaller, and further from the interface than the object is. The calculations are as follows:

$$u = -12.5\,\text{cm}$$
$$U = -8.00\,\text{D}$$
$$V = P + U = -2.00\,\text{D} + (-8.00\,\text{D}) = -10.00\,\text{D}$$
$$v = \frac{n_2}{V} = \frac{150}{-10} = -15\,\text{cm}$$
$$m = \frac{U}{V} = \frac{-8.00\,\text{D}}{-10.00\,\text{D}} = +0.8$$

EXAMPLE 7.20

An ophthalmic crown glass ($n = 1.523$) lens has a front surface power of +14.00 D, a back surface power of −3.00 D, and a central thickness of 8 mm. What is the apparent thickness of this lens as viewed from the front?

The question is essentially asking for the image position of the back surface of the lens as seen through the front. The object distance is

$$u = -8\,\text{mm}$$

and $n_1 = 1.523$ while $n_2 = 1.000$. Then,

$$U = \frac{n_1}{u} = \frac{1523\,\text{mm/m}}{-8\,\text{mm}} = -190.4\,\text{D}$$
$$V = P + U$$
$$V = +14.00\,\text{D} + (-190.4\,\text{D}) = -176.4\,\text{D}$$
$$v = \frac{n_2}{V} = \frac{1000}{-176.4\,\text{D}} = -5.7\,\text{mm}$$

The image of the back surface is virtual and located 5.7 mm from the front surface. Thus, the apparent thickness, as seen from the front, is 5.7 mm.

7.13 OBJECT SPACE/IMAGE SPACE

The concepts of object space and image space were introduced in Section 3.9. The set of all points, rays, or ray extensions associated with the light incident on an SSRI constitutes the object space for the interface. All object space entities are associated with the index n_1. The set of all points, rays, or ray extensions associated with the light leaving the interface constitutes image space. All image space entities are associated with the index n_2.

Remember that object space and image space are mathematical sets. An object space point might be in front of the interface (as for a real object) or behind the interface (as for a virtual object). Similarly, an image space point might be behind the interface (as for a real image) or in front of the interface (as for a virtual image).

Consider a glass–air interface (Figure 7.33). *A "real image in air" immediately indicates that the light leaving the interface is in air and is converging. Similarly, a "virtual image in air" indicates that the light leaving the interface is in air and diverging.* Pay special attention to the fact that the virtual image in Figure 7.33b has no association with the incident light that is physically in the glass. Based on the information given so far, we do not know whether the incident light is converging or diverging. Remember that the virtual image point is the center of curvature of the exiting diverging wavefront that is physically in the air.

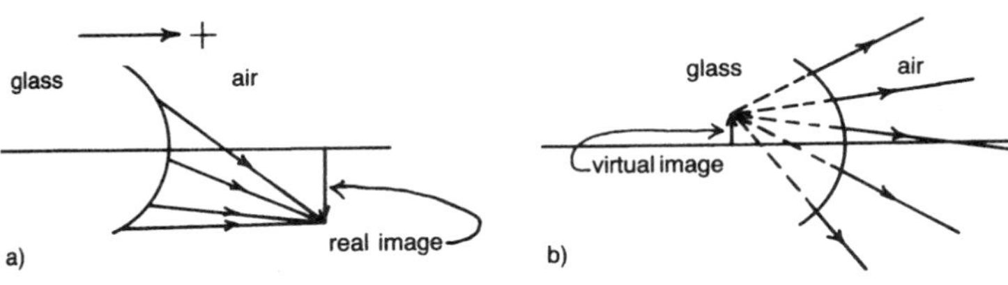

Figure 7.33 a, Real image in air; b, virtual image in air.

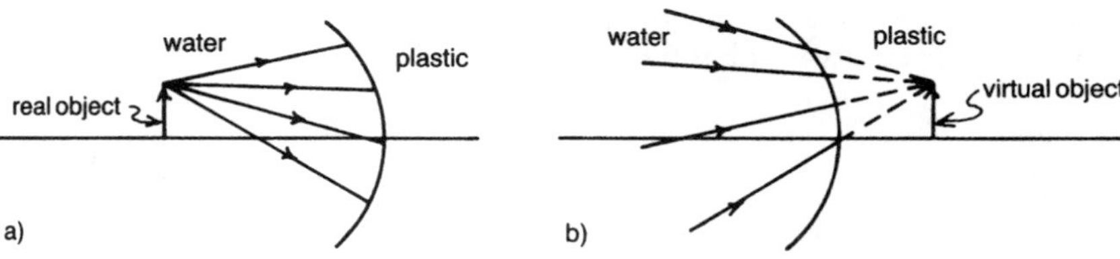

Figure 7.34 a, Real object in water; b, virtual object in water.

Figure 7.34 shows a water–plastic interface. *A "real object in water" indicates immediately that the light incident on the interface is in the water and is diverging. Similarly, a "virtual object in water" indicates that the light incident on the interface is in the water and is converging.* Pay special attention to the fact that the virtual object in Figure 7.34b has no association with the exiting light that is physically in the plastic. Based on the information given so far, we do not know whether the exiting light is converging or diverging. Remember that the virtual object point in Figure 7.34b is simply the center of curvature of the incident converging wavefront that is physically in the water.

Imagine an interface between glass and plastic with a virtual object in plastic. What does this mean in terms of the incident light? The "virtual object" indicates that the incident light is converging. "In plastic" indicates that the incident light is physically in the plastic. So converging light in the plastic is incident on the interface. The virtual object location is at the center of curvature of the incident converging wavefront. You should draw a sketch similar to Figure 7.34b for this situation.

Imagine an interface between beer and glass with a virtual image in the beer. What does this mean in terms of the exiting light? The "virtual image" indicates that the exiting light is diverging. "In beer" indicates that the exiting light is physically in the beer. So diverging light in the beer is leaving the interface. The virtual image location is at the center of curvature of the diverging wavefront that is leaving the interface. You should draw a sketch similar to Figure 7.33b for this situation.

As suggested in Section 3.9, it sometimes helps to color code the incident light and everything associated with it (i.e., everything in object space), and use a different color for the exiting light and everything associated with it (i.e., everything in image space).

7.14 IMAGING A DISTANT OBJECT

The calculation of the image size for a distant object in front of a thin lens in air was discussed in Section 5.14. There, the angle subtended at the nodal point of the thin lens in air was used to calculate the image size. The same technique can be used for a distant object in front of an SSRI, but now the nodal point is at the center of curvature of the interface and not at the interface itself.

Figure 7.35a shows a converging interface and the nodal ray for a distant object that subtends an angle w at the nodal point. The image is in the secondary focal plane, which is a distance of f_2 minus r from the nodal point. The angle w' that the image subtends at the nodal point is equal to w. From the triangle involving C, the optical axis, and the image:

$$|I| = (f_2 - r)\tan w. \tag{7.32}$$

Note that Eq. 7.32 has a different form than the analogous Eq. 5.14 for a thin lens in air.

EXAMPLE 7.21

A distant object in air is in front of a long glass ($n = 1.50$) rod with a +1.00 D front surface. The object subtends an angle of 2° at the interface. Where is the conjugate image? What is its size? Here,

$$f_2 = \frac{n_2}{P} = \frac{150}{+1} = +150\,\text{cm}$$

$$r_2 = \frac{n_2 - n_1}{P} = \frac{50}{+1} = +50\,\text{cm}$$

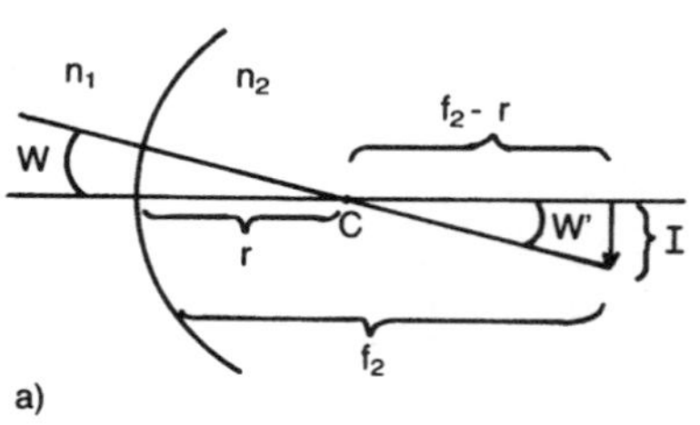

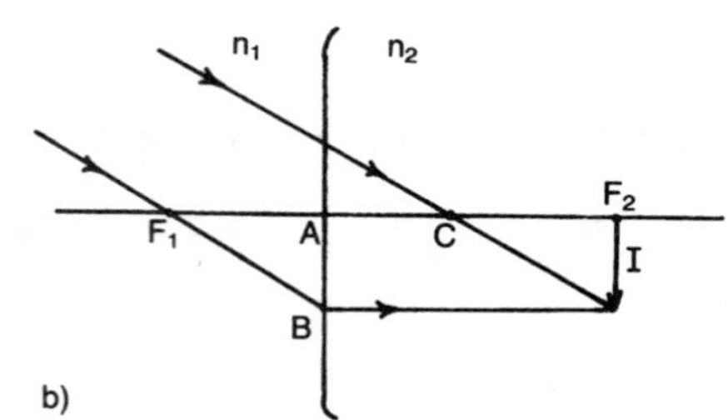

Figure 7.35 Image size for a distant object: a, nodal ray; b, ray associated with the primary focal point.

Then from Eq. 7.32,

$$\begin{aligned}|I| &= (150\,\text{cm} - 50\,\text{cm})\tan 2^\circ \\ &= (100\,\text{cm})(0.0349) = 3.49\,\text{cm}\end{aligned}$$

It is interesting to note that from Eq. 7.25,

$$-f_1 = f_2 - r$$

so that Eq. 7.32 can be written as

$$|I| = |f_1| \tan w \qquad (7.33)$$

Figure 7.35b shows the geometry involved. The parallel ray in image space shows that the distance AB is equal to the image size I, and then the above equation follows directly from the triangle ABF_1.

7.15 CHANGING MEDIA WITHOUT CHANGING CURVATURE

It is instructive to consider the dioptric power changes that occur for an SSRI when a media change occurs without a change in curvature.

EXAMPLE 7.22

Suppose we have a +2.00 D SSRI between water ($n = 1.33$) and glass ($n = 1.53$), and the water is drained off. What is the dioptric power of the resulting air–glass interface?

Let us assume that the light is initially incident in the water, although this assumption is not crucial since the dioptric power is invariant relative to the direction that the light is traveling. Here $n_1 = 1.33$ and $n_2 = 1.53$.
From Eq. 7.19,

$$\begin{aligned}r &= \frac{n_2 - n_1}{P} \\ &= \frac{(1.53 - 1.33)100\,\text{cm/m}}{+2.00\,\text{D}} \\ &= \frac{20}{2} = +10\,\text{cm}\end{aligned}$$

For the air–glass interface,

$$\begin{aligned}P &= \frac{n_2 - n_1}{r} \\ &= \frac{(1.53 - 1.00)100\,\text{cm/m}}{10\,\text{cm}} \\ &= \frac{53}{10} = +5.30\,\text{D}\end{aligned}$$

The dioptric power of the air–glass interface is +5.30 D, which is considerably higher than the +2.00 D of the water–glass interface. Since the curvature is unchanged, the increase is due to the change in the index difference.

Actually, in the case of changing media while the curvature is unchanged, the radius can be algebraically eliminated and an equation derived that relates the old dioptric power to the new dioptric power.

In the original situation, we first found the radius of curvature from

$$r = \frac{(n_2 - n_1)_{\text{old}}}{P_{\text{old}}}$$

Then we used r to get the new dioptric power from

$$P_{\text{new}} = \frac{(n_2 - n_1)_{\text{new}}}{r}$$

We can then combine the above two equations to obtain

$$P_{\text{new}} = \frac{(n_2 - n_1)_{\text{new}}}{(n_2 - n_1)_{\text{old}}} P_{\text{old}} \qquad (7.34)$$

Equation 7.34 says that to get the new dioptric power, one can take the old dioptric power, divide out the old difference in indices (which we do not want anymore), and multiply in the new difference in indices. When the new difference in indices is greater than the old difference in indices, the new dioptric power will be greater in magnitude than the old dioptric power. When the new difference in indices is less than the old difference in indices, then the new dioptric power will be less in magnitude than the old dioptric power.

EXAMPLE 7.23

Let us reconsider the case in Example 7.22. There, a +2.00 D water ($n = 1.33$) glass ($n = 1.53$) interface had the water drained off. Since the index difference increases, the new dioptric power is greater than the old dioptric power.

The old indices are:

$$n_2 = 1.53 \quad \text{and} \quad n_1 = 1.33$$

The new indices are:

$$n_2 = 1.53 \quad \text{and} \quad n_1 = 1.00$$

Then from Eq. 7.34,

$$\begin{aligned}P_{\text{new}} &= \frac{(1.53 - 1.00)}{(1.53 - 1.33)}(+2.00\,\text{D}) \\ &= \frac{0.53}{0.20}(+2.00\,\text{D}) \\ &= (2.65)(+2.00\,\text{D}) = +5.30\,\text{D}\end{aligned}$$

The +5.3 D is the same result as that obtained in the previous example, and the increase in dioptric power agrees with our expectations. Note that with a little practice, the next to the last step (the one containing 53/20) can be written down immediately.

EXAMPLE 7.24
Consider a −13.00 D air–polycarbonate ($n = 1.586$) interface. The room is suddenly flooded with water ($n = 1.333$). What is the dioptric power of the resulting water–plastic interface?

Stop! Before calculating, do you expect a dioptric power that is larger or smaller in magnitude?

The difference in indices decreases, so the dioptric power should decrease in magnitude. For the calculations, let us assume that the light is initially in air, although the assumption is not crucial. The old indices are:

$$n_1 = 1.00 \quad \text{and} \quad n_2 = 1.586$$

The new indices are:

$$n_1 = 1.333 \quad \text{and} \quad n_2 = 1.586$$

Then from Eq. 7.34,

$$P_{\text{new}} = \frac{(1.586 - 1.333)}{(1.586 - 1.000)}(-13.00\,\text{D}) = \frac{0.253}{0.586}(-13.00\,\text{D}) = -5.61\,\text{D}$$

The −5.61 D agrees with the expectations of a dioptric power smaller in magnitude.

7.16 LENS CLOCK READINGS

A lens clock (also known as a lens measure) is a three-legged device that actually measures the sagitta of a spherical surface (Figure 7.36). However, the sagitta is directly related to the curvature, and for a given set of indices the curvature is directly related to the dioptric power. Therefore, the lens clock can be calibrated directly in terms of the dioptric power of an assumed index of refraction.

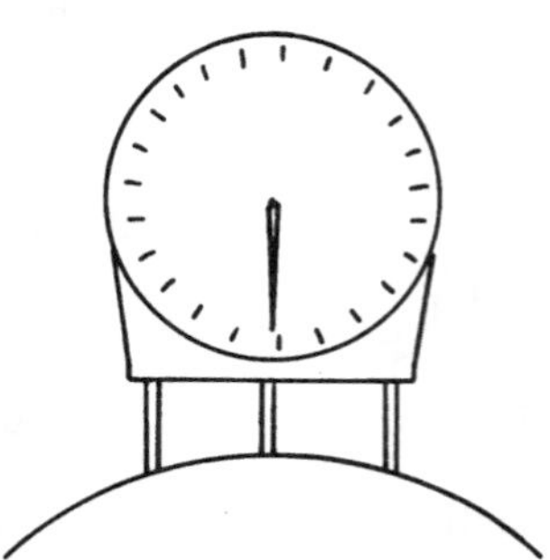

Figure 7.36 Lens clock.

The tools for making spectacle lenses are usually calibrated for a 1.53 index of refraction. A lens clock, calibrated for index 1.53, reads the true dioptric power on an air–glass SSRI provided 1.53 is the index of the glass or plastic spectacle lens material.

When the lens clock is used on an SSRI with an index different from the calibrated index, then it gives an incorrect reading. The true power may be calculated directly from the lens clock reading and the differences in indices.

The calculation is based on the fact that the lens clock is actually measuring a sagitta, and the sagitta is directly related to the curvature. When two SSRIs have the same curvature, the lens clock reading is the same on both surfaces. In effect, when going from one surface to the other, the media is being changed without changing the curvature. Hence, Eq. 7.34 can be used with the old dioptric power as the lens clock reading, and the new dioptric power as the true dioptric power of the surface, i.e.,

$$P_{\text{true}} = \frac{(n_2 - n_1)_{\text{true}}}{(n_2 - n_1)_{\text{clock}}} P_{\text{clock}} \tag{7.35}$$

The true dioptric power is larger in magnitude than the lens clock reading when the true index difference is larger than the assumed index difference, and vice versa.

EXAMPLE 7.25
A lens clock calibrated for an index of 1.53 reads −6.50 D on a spherical plastic interface with a 1.66 index. What is the true dioptric power to the nearest quarter diopter?

Stop! Before calculating, do you expect the true dioptric power to be larger or smaller in magnitude than the lens clock reading? From Eq. 7.35,

$$P_{\text{true}} = \frac{(1.66 - 1.00)}{(1.53 - 1.00)}(-6.50\,\text{D}) = \frac{66}{53}(-6.50\,\text{D}) = -8.09\,\text{D}$$

As expected, the true dioptric power is larger in magnitude than the lens clock reading since the 66 was multiplied in and the 53 was divided out. Note that with a little practice, the line containing 66/53 can be written down immediately.

EXAMPLE 7.26
A lens clock, calibrated for a 1.53 index, reads +14.00 D on a CR-39 hard resin plastic ($n = 1.50$) spherical surface. To the nearest quarter diopter, what is the true dioptric power of the interface? (Before calculating, do you expect the true dioptric power to be larger or smaller?)

The difference in indices is smaller than the difference assumed for the lens clock, so the true dioptric power is also smaller. From Eq. 7.35,

$$P_{true} = \frac{(1.50 - 1.00)}{(1.53 - 1.00)}(+\,14.00\,\text{D})$$
$$= \frac{50}{53}(+\,14.00\,\text{D}) = +13.21\,\text{D} \approx +13.25\,\text{D}$$

When properly used, lens clocks supply the needed information very quickly. However, lens clocks are not smart. The people who use the lens clocks must supply the intelligence. One can put a lens clock on a rock, and it might read +4.00 D. This does not mean the rock has dioptric power. The material, the index assumptions, and the fact that a lens clock is actually measuring a sagitta need to be kept in mind.

PROBLEMS

1. Given a convex air–glass ($n = 1.56$) SSRI with a 14 cm radius of curvature, calculate conjugate image positions and magnifications for the following object points. Include a ray diagram for each part. Also, calculate the vergence of the light 5 cm in front of the interface and 5 cm behind the interface.

   a. a real object in air 1 m from the interface.
   b. a real object in air 50 cm from the interface.
   c. a real object in air 35 cm from the interface.
   d. a real object in air 20 cm from the interface.
   e. a virtual object in air 14 cm from the interface.
   f. a virtual object in air 40 cm from the interface.
   g. a real object in glass 150 cm from the interface.
   h. a real object in glass 40 cm from the interface.
   i. a real object in glass 15 cm from the interface.
   j. a virtual object in glass 48 cm from the interface.

2. Given a concave air–glass ($n = 1.52$) SSRI with a 13 cm radius of curvature, calculate conjugate image positions and magnifications for the following object points. Include a ray diagram for each part, and calculate the vergence of the light 5 cm in front of and 5 cm behind the interface.

   a. a real object in air 50 cm from the interface.
   b. a real object in air 10 cm from the interface.
   c. a virtual object in air 20 cm from the interface.
   d. a virtual object in air 50 cm from the interface.
   e. a real object in glass 25 cm from the interface.
   f. a virtual object in glass 10 cm from the interface.
   g. a virtual object in glass 45 cm from the interface.

3. An air bubble is 5 cm from the center of a glass ($n = 1.61$) sphere of radius 12 cm. Where does the bubble appear to be to an observer, (a) when looking in at the side nearest the bubble? (b) when looking in at the side farthest from the bubble?
4. Given a plastic ($n = 1.49$) sphere of radius 10 cm, calculate where paraxial parallel incident rays come to a focus after passing through the center of the sphere.
5. A glass paperweight is hemispheric in shape. The glass refractive index is 1.60, and the radius of curvature of the spherical surface is 8.0 cm (convex). A centered printed letter is under the paperweight, flush against its flat face. The letter is 6 mm in length. Locate the position and size of the conjugate paraxial image.
6. A thick lens is made of CR-39 plastic, index 1.50. The convex front surface has a 5.0 cm radius of curvature. The concave back surface has a 10.0 cm radius of curvature. The lens is 9.0 cm thick. Considering the lens as two separated single spherical refracting surfaces find the primary and secondary focal points of the lens.
7. A real object in water ($n = 1.33$) is located 25 cm from a water–glass ($n = 1.63$) SSRI. The conjugate image is real and located in the glass 60.82 cm from the interface. What is the lateral magnification? What is the dioptric power of the interface?
8. A 10 cm long glass ($n = 1.53$) rod has a +6.00 D spherical front surface and a −2.00 D spherical back surface. For plane waves incident on the front, what is the vergence of the wavefront leaving the back surface?
9. Represent an aphakic eye with a +44.00 D cornea. If the cornea to retina length is 22.27 mm and the ocular index is 1.336, what is the aphake's spectacle correction at a 10 mm vertex distance?
10. Represent an eye by a +63.00 D SSRI between air and the ocular media ($n = 1.336$). If the length of the eye is 19.0 mm, what contact correction (if any) is needed?
11. A long plastic rod ($n = 1.44$) has a +3.80 D spherical front surface. What is the image size in the plastic for a distant object that subtends an angle of 3°?
12. Represent an emmetropic eye by a +56.00 D SSRI between air and the ocular media ($n = 1.336$). What is the retinal image size (in microns) for a distant letter that subtends an angle of 5′?
13. The anterior surface of the crystalline lens is an SSRI between the aqueous humor ($n = 1.336$) and the crystalline lens cortex ($n = 1.386$). If the radius of curvature is 10.0 mm, what is the dioptric power of this surface in the eye? If the crystalline lens is removed from the eye, and the anterior surface remains spherical with the same radius, what is the dioptric power of the air–crystalline lens interface?
14. An air–glass ($n = 1.53$) interface has a power of −10.00 D. If the room is filled with water ($n = 1.33$), what is the power of the water–glass interface? If the room is filled with oil ($n = 1.73$), what is the power of the oil–glass interface?
15. A lens clock calibrated for $n = 1.53$ reads +6.00 D on a spherical plastic ($n = 1.71$) surface. What is the true dioptric power of the interface?

CHAPTER 8

Plane Refracting Interfaces and Reduced Systems

8.1 PLANE INTERFACES AS A SPECIAL CASE OF SPHERICAL INTERFACES

Consider a series of single spherical refracting interfaces (SSRIs) where each successive interface is flatter than the preceding one. The SSRI equations in Chapter 7 hold for each of these interfaces. The limiting case of this series is a flat or plane interface, and hence, in the limit, the SSRI equations also hold for the flat interface.

As shown in Eq. 7.20, the dioptric power P of an SSRI is directly proportional to the curvature R of the interface. As spherical interfaces are made flatter, their curvature decreases and their dioptric power gets closer to zero. A flat or plane interface has zero curvature and zero dioptric power. Note that the radius r is reciprocally related to the curvature R, and hence r goes to infinity for a plane interface.

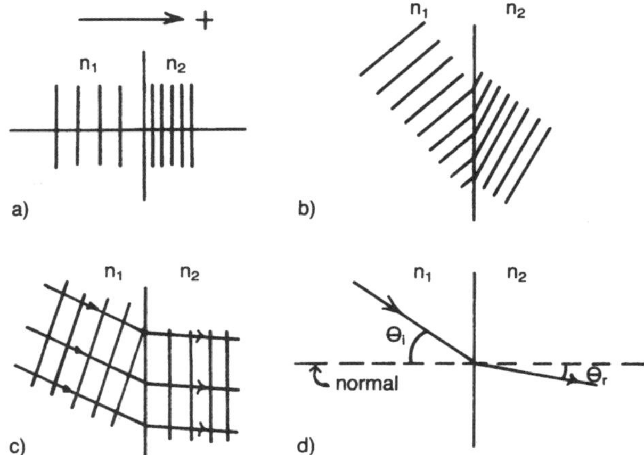

Figure 8.1 Plane waves incident on a flat interface: a, incident normal; b, incident at an angle to the normal; c, wavefronts and rays; d, one ray.

Consider plane waves in a medium of index n_1, incident on a plane refracting interface between media n_1 and n_2. When the incident plane waves are incident normal to the interface, all parts of the wavefront reach the interface at the same time and all parts change speed at the same time. The wavefronts leaving the interface are still plane waves and still normal to the interface (Figure 8.1a).

When the plane waves are incident on a plane interface at an angle to the normal, they are neither converged nor diverged so that the waves leaving the interface are still plane waves, as expected for a zero dioptric power interface. However, the direction of travel of the plane waves is deviated (Figure 8.1b). As discussed in Section 1.12, the direction of travel of the plane waves leaving the interface is related to the direction of travel of the incident plane waves by Snell's Law (Figures 8.1c and d),

$$n_1 \sin \theta_i = n_2 \sin \theta_r \tag{8.1}$$

When paraxial angles are involved, the small angle approximation to Snell's law is valid, i.e.,

$$n_1 \theta_i = n_2 \theta_r \tag{8.2}$$

When n_2 is greater than n_1, the rays bend toward the normal (Figure 8.1d). For example, the ray bends towards the normal when light in air is incident on a plane air–water interface. When n_1 is greater than n_2, the rays bend away from the normal (Figure 8.2). For example, the ray bends away from the normal when light in glass is incident on a plane glass–air interface.

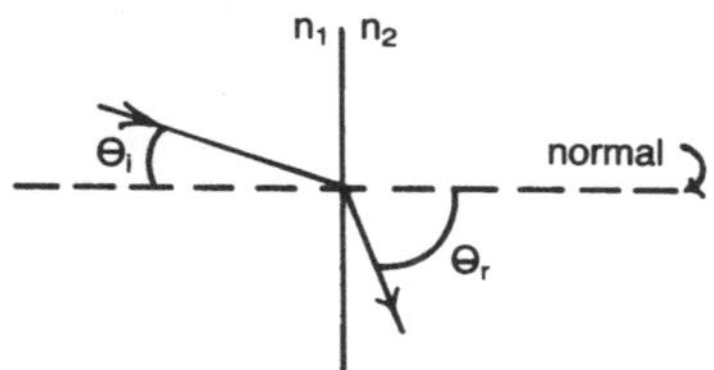

Figure 8.2 Ray incident in the higher index medium.

8.2 DIVERGING AND CONVERGING WAVEFRONTS

When diverging or converging wavefronts are incident on a plane interface, part of the wavefront reaches the interface first, and this part changes speed before the remaining parts. The result is that diverging or converging wavefronts change their curvature as they pass through plane interfaces. Figure 8.3a shows the wavefronts for a case in which n_1 is greater than n_2. Figure 8.3b shows the rays associated with the wavefronts.

Since n_1 is greater than n_2 each ray in Figure 8.3 bends away from the normal. The object point at A is real, and the image point at B is virtual and closer than the object to the interface. The image location can be determined from the vergence Eqs. 7.16 through 7.18. Since P is zero,

$$V = P + U$$

results in

$$V = U$$

where,

$$V = \frac{n_2}{v}$$

and

$$U = \frac{n_1}{u}$$

One can combine the above three equations to directly obtain

$$\frac{v}{n_2} = \frac{u}{n_1} \tag{8.3}$$

Equation 8.3 relates the object and image distance for the plane interface. (It is also possible to derive Eq. 8.3 directly from the small angle version of Snell's law without using the SSRI equations.)

EXAMPLE 8.1

A small fish is swimming in water ($n = 1.33$) 100 cm below the (plane) surface. To an observer in air, what is the apparent depth of the fish?

An observer in air looking at the fish underwater sees the virtual image of the fish. In Figure 8.3, A represents the position of the fish and B represents the position of the virtual image. The apparent depth of the fish is just the location of the virtual image. The fact that the rays bend away from the normal indicates that the virtual image of the fish is closer than 100 cm. In this case, $n_1 = 1.33, n_2 = 1.00$, and $u = -100$ cm. Then,

$$U = \frac{n_1}{u} = \frac{133}{-100\,\text{cm}} = -1.33\,\text{D}$$

Then

$$V = U = -1.33\,\text{D}$$

and from,

$$V = \frac{n_2}{v}$$

$$v = \frac{100}{-1.33\,\text{D}} = -75.2\,\text{cm}$$

Alternatively, we can use Eq. 8.3 directly.

$$\frac{v}{n_2} = \frac{u}{n_1}$$

$$\frac{v}{1.00} = \frac{-100\,\text{cm}}{1.33}$$

$$v = -75.2\,\text{cm}$$

The apparent depth of the fish is 75.2 cm below the water's surface.

EXAMPLE 8.2

A mayfly is flying 50 cm above a pond. A hungry trout swimming in the water below the pond's surface sees the mayfly. To the trout, what is the apparent height of the mayfly?

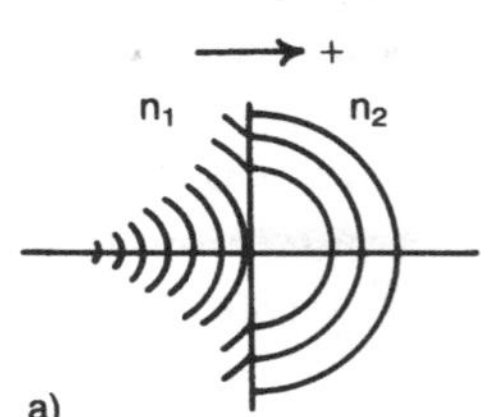

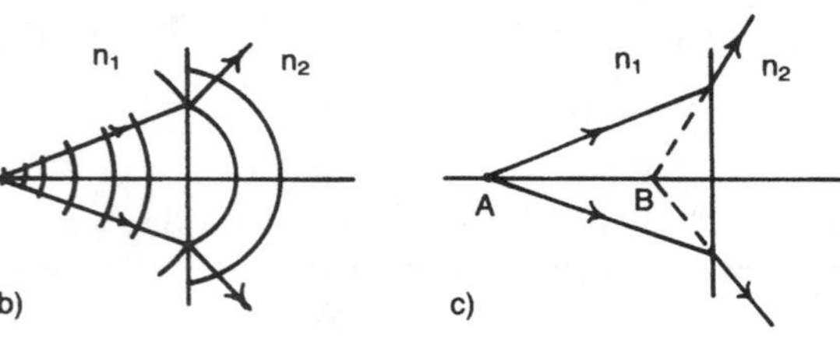

Figure 8.3 a, Diverging wavefronts incident on a flat interface; b, wavefronts and rays; c, rays only.

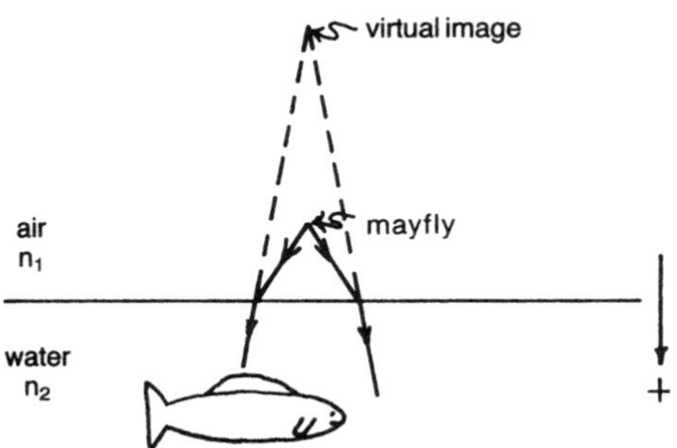

Figure 8.4 The virtual image of the mayfly serves as the object for the trout's eye.

Figure 8.4 shows the situation for the trout. The light leaving the mayfly is initially in air ($n_1 = 1.00$), and then enters the water ($n_2 = 1.33$). In this case, n_2 is greater than n_1, and the rays bend toward the normal. The trout sees a virtual image of the mayfly, and the virtual image is farther than the mayfly from the surface. From Eq. 8.3,

$$\frac{v}{1.33} = \frac{-50\,\text{cm}}{1.00}$$

or

$$v = -66.5\,\text{cm}$$

The apparent height of the mayfly is 66.5 cm above the surface.

EXAMPLE 8.3

What is the apparent thickness of a 9 cm thick flat glass ($n = 1.5$) slab?

An observer in air looking through the slab does not see the actual backside of the slab but instead sees the virtual image of the backside. By drawing a figure, such as Figure 8.3c, it is easy to predict that the apparent thickness will be less than the actual thickness.

The object distance u is -9 cm and from Eq. 8.3,

$$\frac{v}{1} = \frac{-9\,\text{cm}}{1.50}$$

or

$$v = -6\,\text{cm}$$

The apparent thickness is 6 cm as compared to the actual thickness of 9 cm. (Note the same principle applies to aquariums, which is why they look narrower than they actually are.)

The (reduced) vergence of a wavefront is equal to the index of the medium that the wavefront is in times the curvature of the wavefront. Even though the curvature of a converging or diverging wavefront changes at a plane interface, the (reduced) vergence of the wavefront does not change. This means that the curvature change is exactly offset by the index change.

8.3 LATERAL MAGNIFICATION

The lateral magnification m of an SSRI is equal to U/V. Since the vergences U and V are equal for a plane interface, m is $+1$. This is easily confirmed by using rays incident along the normal.

Figure 8.5 shows such a case for the fish underwater. The two rays incident normally are the vertical lines from the front and back of the fish. The respective virtual image points also lie along these two vertical lines, so the virtual image of the fish is the same size as the fish itself.

Whenever any object is brought closer to an observer, the observer's retinal image of the object gets larger even though the object's size is unchanged. This same principle holds when viewing virtual images.

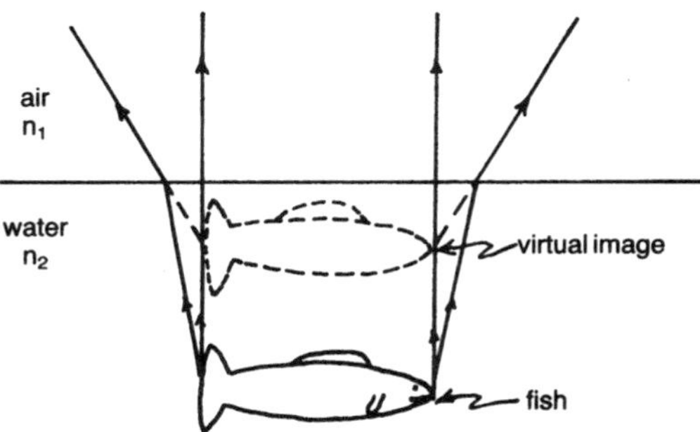

Figure 8.5 The virtual image is the same size as the object (the fish), so the lateral magnification is +1.

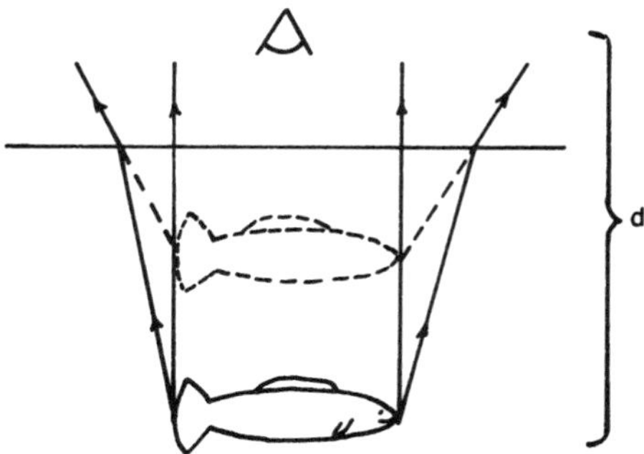

Figure 8.6 Comparison for the observer viewing a fish that is an actual distance *d* away. When the water is drained, the observer views the actual fish at the distance *d*. When the water is present, the observer views the virtual image at a distance less than *d*.

Figure 8.6 shows an observer looking at the submerged fish and then looking at the fish in air. The actual distance between the fish and the observer's eye is the same in each case. The observer looking at the submerged fish does not see the actual fish, but rather sees the virtual image of the fish at the apparent depth. Since the apparent depth is less than the actual depth, the observer's retinal image of the submerged fish is larger than when she looks at the fish in air. The lateral magnification of the plane interface is +1, so it does not cause the increase. Instead, the shortened object distance for the observer when viewing the virtual image causes the increase.

EXAMPLE 8.4a

An arrowhead, 3 cm in size, is imbedded 20 cm deep in a block of ice ($n = 1.33$) with flat sides. An emmetrope stands with his eye 5 cm from the block of ice (i.e., 25 cm from the arrowhead). Use the typical +60.00 D thin lens and screen model for the unaccommodated emmetrope's eye to calculate the accommodative demand and the retinal image size that the emmetrope has when observing the arrowhead.

Since n_1 is greater than n_2 Figure 8.3 applies to the situation. The emmetropic observer sees the virtual image of the arrowhead. The virtual image of the arrowhead is still 3 cm in size but is at an apparent depth given by Eq. 8.3.

$$\frac{v}{1} = \frac{-20\,\text{cm}}{1.33}$$

or

$$v = -15\,\text{cm}$$

The object distance for the emmetrope's eye is

$$u_x = -(15 + 5)\,\text{cm} = -20\,\text{cm}$$

For the emmetrope, U_{fp} is zero and the accommodative demand is

$$A_o = U_{fp} - U_x$$

or

$$A_o = -\left(\frac{100}{-20\,\text{cm}}\right) = +5\,\text{D}$$

In the thin lens and screen model for the emmetrope's eye, the screen is 16.67 mm from the lens. So the image distance for the emmetrope's eye is 16.67 mm, and the lateral magnification is

$$m = \frac{+16.67\,\text{mm}}{-200\,\text{mm}} = -0.0834$$

The retinal image size I is

$$I = mO$$
$$= (-0.0834)(30\,\text{mm}) = -2.50\,\text{mm}$$

EXAMPLE 8.4b

The ice in Example 8.4a melts, and the emmetrope can now hold the arrowhead in air 25 cm from his eye and look directly at it. Calculate the accommodative demand and the retinal image size of the emmetrope, and compare it with the results in Example 8.4a. Now,

$$u_x = -25\,\text{cm} \quad \text{and} \quad U_x = -4\,\text{D}$$

Then,

$$A_o = U_{fp} - U_x = +4\,\text{D}$$

The accommodative demand is less when the emmetrope is viewing the arrowhead in air as compared to viewing it in ice.

The image distance remains at 16.67 mm, so

$$m = \frac{v}{u} = \frac{+16.67\,\text{mm}}{-250.0\,\text{mm}} = -0.0667$$

and the retinal image size is

$$I = mO$$
$$= (-0.0667)(30\,\text{mm}) = -2.00\,\text{mm}$$

The emmetrope's retinal image size when the arrowhead is imbedded in the ice is 25% larger than when the ice is melted.

8.4 RAY TRACING THROUGH A FLAT SLAB IN EQUI-INDEX MEDIA

Figure 8.7 shows a ray passing through a flat slab of index n_2. The indices of the media in front of and behind the slab are n_1 and n_3, respectively. Assume that n_1 equals n_3.

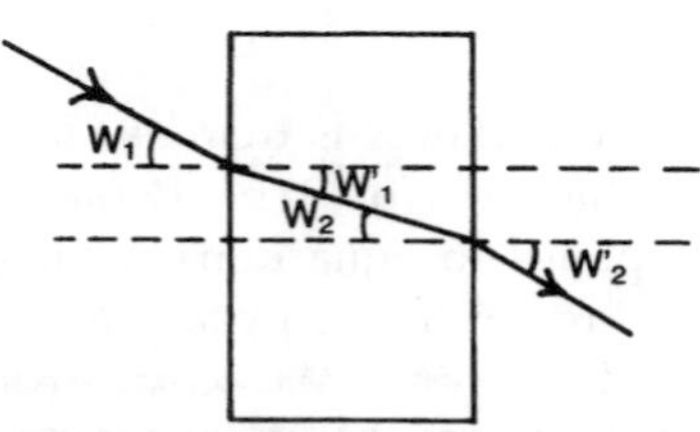

Figure 8.7 Ray through a flat slab.

The angles of incidence and refraction at the first surface are w_1 and w'_1, respectively. The angles of incidence and refraction at the rear surface are w_2 and w'_2 respectively. From Snell's law,

$$n_1 \sin w_1 = n_2 \sin w'_1$$
$$n_2 \sin w_2 = n_3 \sin w'_2$$

The two normals (at the front and back surfaces of the slab) are parallel. From geometry, the alternate interior angles to parallel lines are equal, and so w'_1 and w_2 are equal. Then from the above two equations,

$$\frac{n_3}{n_2} \sin w'_2 = \frac{n_1}{n_2} \sin w_1$$

or

$$n_3 \sin w'_2 = n_1 \sin w_1$$

But since n_3 equals n_1, it follows that

$$\sin w'_2 = \sin w_1$$

or

$$w'_2 = w_1$$

The equality of w'_2 and w_1 means that the outgoing ray in n_3 is parallel to the incident ray in n_1.

The fact that the outgoing ray is parallel to the incident ray makes it easy to quickly draw qualitative ray sketches for flat slabs in equi-index media. However, when n_1 is not equal to n_3, the outgoing ray is not parallel to the incident ray.

8.5 FLAT SLABS

Figure 8.8 shows a point source in air at a distance d_1 from the front surface of a glass slab. The slab itself has a thickness d_2, and an index n_g. A thin lens in air is located a distance d_3, behind the back surface of the slab. The object for the lens is the image formed by the back surface of the slab.

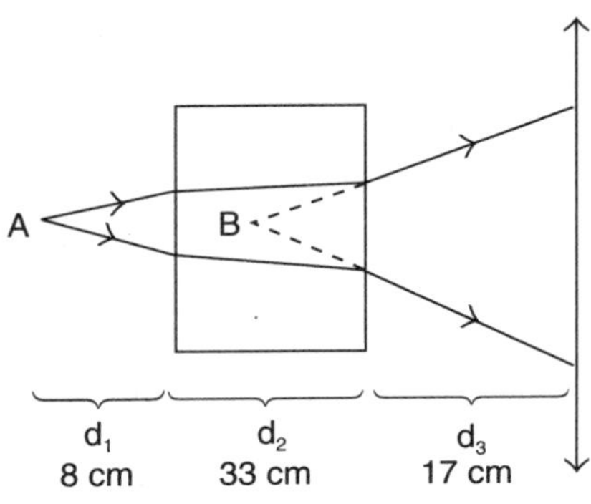

Figure 8.8 Flat slab in front of a lens.

Each of the diverging rays leaving the point source bends toward the normal on entering the slab and away from the normal on leaving the slab. The outgoing rays are parallel to the incident rays but displaced in such a manner that the virtual image for the back surface of the slab is closer than the actual point source to the lens.

Assume that the distances d_1, d_2, and d_3 are all positive. The object distance for the lens can be found by stepping through the slab. From Eq. 8.3, the image distance for the first surface is

$$\frac{v_1}{n_g} = \frac{-d_1}{1}$$

or

$$v_1 = -n_g d_1$$

In this case, v_1 is negative, and

$$u_2 = v_1 - d_2$$

Equation 8.3 applied to the second surface is

$$\frac{v_2}{1} = \frac{u_2}{n_g}$$

or

$$v_2 = -d_1 - \frac{d_2}{n_g}$$

The object distance for the lens is

$$u_3 = v_2 - d_3$$

or

$$u_3 = -\left[d_1 + \frac{d_2}{n_g} + d_3\right] \tag{8.4}$$

In Eq. 8.4, d_1 and d_3 are actual distances in air, while d_2 is a thickness of glass and is divided by the index n_g. Evidently, the thickness d_2 in glass of index n_g is equivalent to an air thickness of d_2/n_g.

By the same reasoning, it is easy to show that any thickness d of a material of index n is equivalent to an air thickness of d/n. Let's label the *equivalent air thickness* as $\bar{d}$, or

$$\bar{d} = \frac{d}{n} \tag{8.5}$$

Then we can write Eq. 8.4 as

$$u_3 = -[d_1 + \bar{d}_2 + d_3] \tag{8.6}$$

EXAMPLE 8.5

A 4 mm tall object in air is located 8 cm from the front surface of a 33 cm thick glass ($n = 1.50$) slab. A thin lens in air is located 17 cm behind the glass slab. What is the object distance for the lens? What is the size of the (apparent) object for the lens?

The object for the lens is the virtual image formed by the back surface of the slab, and Figure 8.8 shows the situation.

Equation 8.6 gives the object distance for the lens:

$$u_3 = -\left[8\,\text{cm} + \frac{33\,\text{cm}}{1.5} + 17\,\text{cm}\right]$$
$$= -[8 + 22 + 17]\,\text{cm} = -47\,\text{cm}$$

Note that the 33 cm of glass of index 1.5 is equivalent to 22 cm worth of air.

The lateral magnification for each plane surface is +1, so the size of the object for the lens is still 4 mm.

Equation 8.6 is easily extended to systems with multiple plane interfaces. Figure 8.9a shows three flat slabs in front of a thin lens in air. The object distance for the lens can be found by stepping through the plane interfaces, a somewhat slow process, or by setting up the equivalent air distances as shown in Figure 8.9b and writing directly that

$$u_{\text{lens}} = -[\bar{d}_1 + \bar{d}_2 + \bar{d}_3 + d_4] \tag{8.7}$$

EXAMPLE 8.6

A butterfly is imbedded 7 cm deep in a plastic ($n = 1.44$) slab. The plastic is covered by 16 cm of water ($n = 1.33$), and a 5 cm layer of oil ($n = 1.72$) is floating on the water. A camera is held in the air so that its lens is 10 cm above the top surface of the oil (see Figure 8.9). What distance must the camera be focused for?

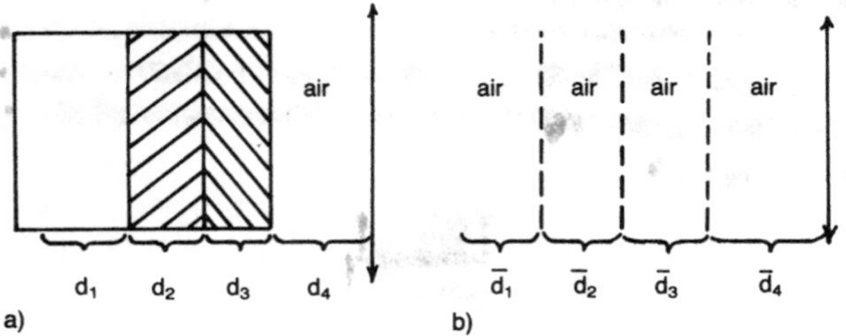

Figure 8.9 a, A series of plane interfaces in front of a lens; b, the equivalent air (or reduced) system.

The object for the camera is the virtual image that the top oil surface forms. From the equivalent air system, the object distance for the camera lens is

$$u_{\text{lens}} = -\left[\frac{7}{1.44} + \frac{16}{1.33} + \frac{5}{1.72} + 10\right]\text{cm}$$
$$= -[4.86 + 12.03 + 2.91 + 10]\,\text{cm}$$
$$= -29.80\,\text{cm}$$

Note that the 7 cm of plastic is equivalent to 4.86 cm of air, the 16 cm of water is equivalent to 12.03 cm of air, and the 5 cm of oil is equivalent to 2.91 cm of air. Note also that the apparent depth of the butterfly is 19.80 cm from the top oil surface, and finally the virtual image of the butterfly at the apparent depth is the same size as the imbedded butterfly.

Whenever the refractive index n is greater than 1, the equivalent air distance $\bar{d}$ is less than the actual distance d. For this reason, the equivalent air distance is usually called the *reduced distance*. In the preceding example, the reduced distance for the 7 cm of plastic was 4.86 cm, the reduced distance for the 16 cm of water was 12.03 cm, and the reduced distance for the 5 cm of oil was 2.91 cm. In this context, *reduced* is a synonym for *equivalent air*.

EXAMPLE 8.7

A 3 cm thick oil layer ($n = 1.72$) floats on top of 26.6 cm of water ($n = 1.33$), which in turn is on a 27 cm thick flat glass slab ($n = 1.50$). A camera is held so that its lens is 4 cm above the oil's top surface. A beetle is clearly imaged in the camera when it is focused for an object distance of 21.53 cm. Where is the actual beetle?

One method of solving this problem is to step back through the surfaces, again a slow process. An alternate method is to use the equivalent air (or reduced) system to determine the apparent location of the beetle relative to the apparent boundaries of the different media.

Figure 8.10 shows the reduced system. The reduced thicknesses are:

$$\bar{d}_{\text{oil}} = \frac{3\,\text{cm}}{1.72} = 1.74\,\text{cm}$$
$$\bar{d}_{\text{water}} = \frac{26.6\,\text{cm}}{1.33} = 20.0\,\text{cm}$$
$$\bar{d}_{\text{glass}} = \frac{27\,\text{cm}}{1.50} = 18.0\,\text{cm}$$

The dashed lines in the figure mark the positions corresponding to the media boundaries.

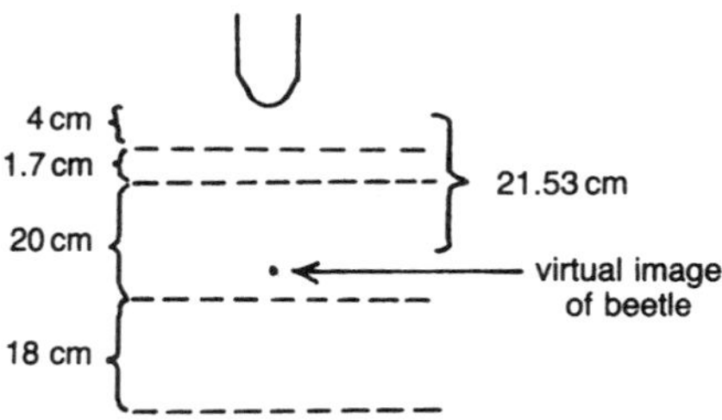

Figure 8.10 Reduced (equivalent air) system for beetle example.

The object distance for the camera is 21.53 cm. In the reduced (or equivalent air) system, the beetle is at distance x below the marker corresponding to the oil–water interface, and

$$x = 21.53\,\text{cm} - 4\,\text{cm} - 1.74\,\text{cm} = 15.79\,\text{cm}$$

The 15.79 cm is the reduced (or equivalent air) distance corresponding to an actual distance in the water. We can then find the actual water distance by unreducing, or

$$\begin{aligned} d_{\text{water}} &= n_{\text{water}}\bar{d}_{\text{water}} \\ &= (1.33)(15.79\,\text{cm}) = 21.0\,\text{cm} \end{aligned}$$

The actual beetle is located in the water 21 cm below the oil–water interface.

8.6 CONVERGING LIGHT AND REDUCED SYSTEMS

The techniques for plane interfaces work for converging light as well as for diverging light. The problems may be solved either by stepping through the interfaces or by using a reduced system.

EXAMPLE 8.8

Converging light in air is incident on an air–water ($n = 1.33$) interface. When the vergence of the incident wavefront is +4.00 D, where is the image for the interface located?

Before calculating, you should draw a ray sketch to see what characteristics you expect the answer to have. The incident light is converging, so the interface has a virtual object (shown at A in Figure 8.11). Since the rays are initially in the lower index medium, they bend towards the normal. The result is that the image, shown at B, is real and farther than the (virtual) object from the interface.

For this situation, $n_1 = 1.00$ and $n_2 = 1.33$. $P = 0$ for the plane interface, so

$$V = U = +4.00\,\text{D}$$

Then,

$$v = \frac{n_2}{V} = \frac{133}{+4\,\text{D}} = +33.25\,\text{cm}$$

which confirms that the image is real and farther from the interface than the virtual object. The image would be visible on a screen placed in the water 33.25 cm from the interface.

Alternatively, Eq. 8.3 can be used. Here,

$$u = \frac{100}{+4\,\text{D}} = +25\,\text{cm}$$

Then,

$$\frac{v}{n_2} = \frac{u}{n_1}$$

gives

$$\frac{v}{1.33} = \frac{+25\,\text{cm}}{1.00}$$

or

$$v = (1.33)(+25\,\text{cm}) = +33.25\,\text{cm}$$

The lateral magnification for the interface is still +1, so the real image is the same size as the virtual object.

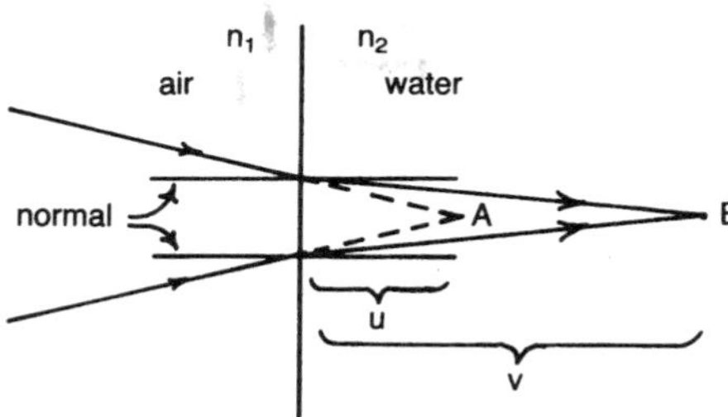

Figure 8.11 Converging light incident on a flat interface.

EXAMPLE 8.9

An 8 mm spider is suspended on a web 40 cm in front of a +8.50 D lens. The lens has 4 cm of air behind it followed by a 12 cm thick glass ($n = 1.5$) slab, a 13.3 cm thickness of water, and a 25 cm thick plastic ($n = 1.44$) slab. Where is the physically real image of the spider? What is the image size?

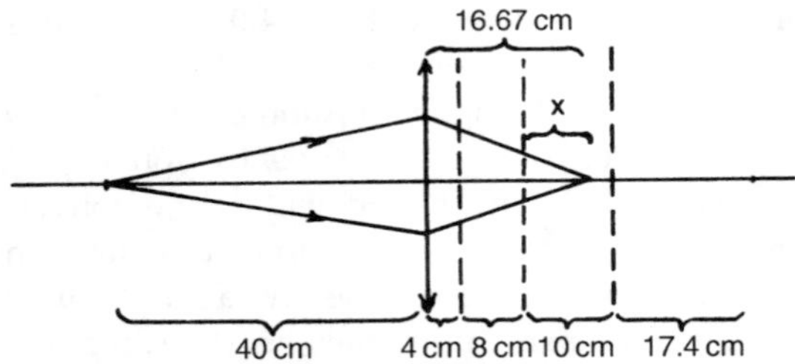

Figure 8.12 Reduced system for spider example.

Figure 8.12 shows the reduced system. The reduced distances are:

$$\bar{d}_{\text{glass}} = \frac{12\,\text{cm}}{1.50} = 8\,\text{cm}$$
$$\bar{d}_{\text{water}} = \frac{13.3\,\text{cm}}{1.33} = 10\,\text{cm}$$
$$\bar{d}_{\text{plastic}} = \frac{25\,\text{cm}}{1.44} = 17.4\,\text{cm}$$

For the lens,

$$u = -40\,\text{cm}$$
$$U = \frac{100}{-40\,\text{cm}} = -2.5\,\text{D}$$
$$V = P + U$$
$$= +8.50\,\text{D} + (-2.50\,\text{D}) = +6.00\,\text{D}$$
$$\bar{v} = \frac{100}{+6.00\,\text{D}} = +16.67\,\text{cm}$$

and

$$m = \frac{U}{V} = \frac{-2.50\,\text{D}}{+6.00\,\text{D}} = -0.42$$

In the actual system, the lens' image is optically real but not physically real. In the reduced system, the image is 16.67 cm from the lens. As shown in Figure 8.12, the image is located in the region corresponding to the water at a distance of x past the marker corresponding to the glass–water boundary, and

$$x = 16.67 - 4 - 8 = 4.67\,\text{cm}$$

The 4.67 cm is the equivalent air or reduced distance corresponding to the actual distance in the water. Therefore, in the actual system, the physically real image is in the water at a distance of

$$(1.33)(4.67\,\text{cm}) = 6.21\,\text{cm}$$

from the glass–water interface. The image would be visible on a screen placed in the water at this position.

The lateral magnification for each plane interface is +1, so the total lateral magnification is +1 times the lateral magnification m of the lens. The image size is

$$I = mO = (-0.42)(8\,\text{mm}) = 3.33\,\text{mm}$$

8.7 SINGLE SPHERICAL REFRACTING INTERFACES AND REDUCED SYSTEMS

A reduced (equivalent air) system can also be set up for a single spherical refracting interface (SSRI). In the reduced system, a thin lens in air supplies the convergence or divergence that the SSRI supplies in the actual system. As shown below, all corresponding vergences in the reduced and the actual systems are equal, and consequently *the dioptric power of the thin lens in the reduced system must be equal to the dioptric power of the actual SSRI.*

Consider an object in a medium of refractive index n_1 at a distance u in front of an SSRI of dioptric power P. The image is in a medium of index n_2 at a distance v away from the interface. Figure 8.13 shows an example of such a system. In the actual SSRI system, the vergence equations are:

$$U_a = \frac{n_1}{u} \quad \text{and} \quad V_a = \frac{n_2}{v}$$

The dioptric power of the SSRI is P_a and

$$V_a = P_a + U_a$$

The reduced (equivalent air) object distance $\bar{u}$ is given by

$$\bar{u} = \frac{u}{n_1}$$

The reduced (equivalent air) image distance $\bar{v}$ is given by

$$\bar{v} = \frac{v}{n_2}$$

In the reduced (equivalent air) system corresponding to the SSRI, the incident vergence is given by

$$U_r = \frac{1}{\bar{u}}$$

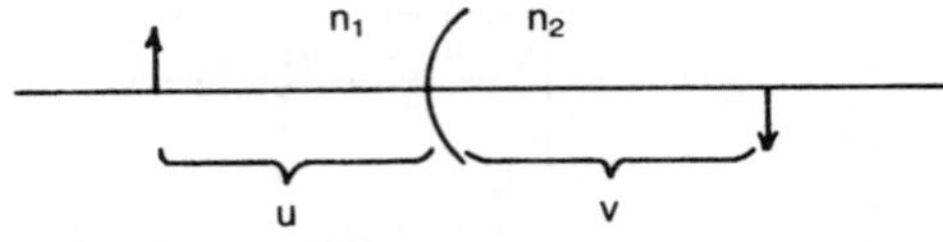

Figure 8.13 Actual system.

and the exiting vergence is given by

$$V_r = \frac{1}{\bar{v}}$$

The dioptric power of the thin lens in the reduced system is P_r, and

$$V_r = P_r + U_r$$

By substituting the equation for the reduced distance $\bar{u}$ into the above equation for U_r, we see that

$$U_r = \frac{1}{(u/n_1)} = \frac{n_1}{u} = U_a$$

where U_a is the vergence in the actual system. By substituting the expression for the reduced distance $\bar{v}$, we find that

$$V_r = \frac{1}{(v/n_2)} = \frac{n_2}{v} = V_a$$

where V_a is the exiting vergence in the actual system. Since the corresponding vergences are equal, the subscripts can be dropped:

$$U = U_a = U_r$$

and

$$V = V_a = V_r$$

It then follows that the dioptric power of the thin lens in the reduced system must be equal to the dioptric power of the actual SSRI, or

$$P = P_a = P_r$$

The lateral magnification of an SSRI is equal to the vergence ratio U/V. Since the respective vergences are the same in the actual system and in the reduced system, the lateral magnification is the same in the two systems. Thus for a given object size O, the image size I is the same in the actual and in the reduced system.

EXAMPLE 8.10

A real object in water ($n = 1.33$) is 66.5 cm in front of a +6.00 D water–glass ($n = 1.50$) interface. The conjugate image is real and located in the glass 37.5 cm from the interface (see Figure 8.13). Set up the equivalent air system and verify that the vergences and the lateral magnification are equal in the two systems.

The reduced object distance is

$$\bar{u} = \frac{-66.5\,\text{cm}}{1.33} = -50.0\,\text{cm}$$

and the reduced image distance is

$$\bar{v} = \frac{+37.5\,\text{cm}}{1.50} = +25.0\,\text{cm}$$

Thus, the reduced system consists of a +6.00 D thin lens in air with the (real) object located 50 cm in front of the lens and the (real) image located 25 cm behind the lens.

In the reduced system:

$$U = \frac{100}{-50.0\,\text{cm}} = -2.00\,\text{D}$$

and

$$V = \frac{100}{+25.00\,\text{cm}} = +4.00\,\text{D}$$

From U and V, it is clear that the dioptric power of the thin lens in the reduced system must be +6.00 D.

In the actual system:

$$U = \frac{133}{-66.5\,\text{cm}} = -2.00\,\text{D}$$

and

$$V = \frac{150}{+37.5\,\text{cm}} = +4.00\,\text{D}$$

The respective vergences are equal, and in both systems the lateral magnification is U/V or -0.5.

EXAMPLE 8.11

A real object in plastic ($n = 1.44$) is located 18 cm in front of a +3.00 D plastic–water ($n = 1.33$) interface. The conjugate image is virtual and located -26.6 cm from the interface. Set up the

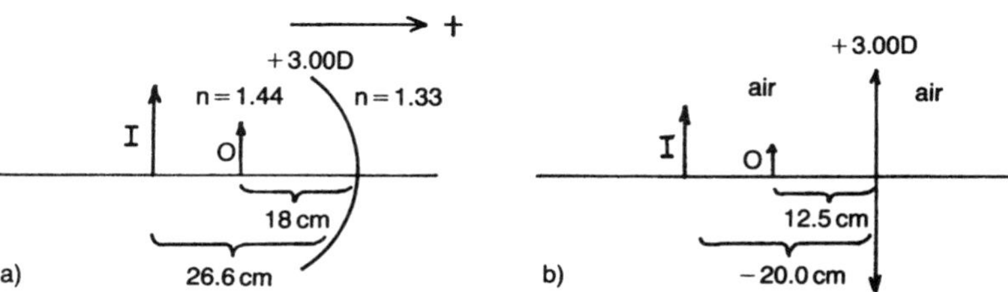

Figure 8.14 a, Actual system; b, reduced system.

reduced system, and verify that the vergences are equal.

Figure 8.14a shows the actual system and Figure 8.14b shows the reduced system. The thin lens in the reduced system has a power of +3.00 D. The reduced object distance is given by

$$\bar{u} = \frac{u}{n_1} = \frac{-18\,\text{cm}}{1.44} = -12.5\,\text{cm}$$

Now look at Figure 8.14a again. What index should we use to reduce the image distance? The correct answer is the index of water. Remember that a virtual image is defined by an exiting diverging wavefront, and in this case the *exiting diverging wavefront is physically in the water*. The image point itself is simply the center of curvature of the diverging wavefront that leaves the interface. The equation for the reduced image distance indicates the index automatically (and hopefully it now makes sense).

$$\bar{v} = \frac{v}{n_2} = \frac{26.6\,\text{cm}}{1.33} = -20.0\,\text{cm}$$

The vergences in the reduced system are:

$$U = \frac{100}{-12.5\,\text{cm}} = -8.00\,\text{D}$$

and

$$V = \frac{100}{-20.0\,\text{cm}} = -5.00\,\text{D}$$

In the actual system:

$$U = \frac{144}{-18.0\,\text{cm}} = -8.00\,\text{D}$$

and

$$V = \frac{133}{-26.6\,\text{cm}} = -5.00\,\text{D}$$

The vergences in the two systems are indeed equal.

EXAMPLE 8.12

A real object is in air 68 cm from a +7.00 D air–glass ($n = 1.50$) interface. Suddenly, the room floods with oil ($n = 1.70$). Now the object is in oil 68 cm from an oil–glass interface. Set up the reduced system, and use it to find the image and the lateral magnification.

Be careful when setting the dioptric power for the interface in the reduced system. The power of the thin lens must be equal to the power of the interface in the actual system. The actual interface is now an oil–glass interface. From Eq. 7.34, the new dioptric power is

$$\begin{aligned} P_{\text{new}} &= \frac{(n_2 - n_1)_{\text{new}}}{(n_2 - n_1)_{\text{old}}} P_{\text{old}} \\ &= \frac{(1.50 - 1.70)}{(1.50 - 1.00)}(+7.00\,\text{D}) \\ &= \frac{-20}{+50}(+7.00\,\text{D}) = -2.80\,\text{D} \end{aligned}$$

Note that with the flood of high index oil, the interface changes from converging to diverging. The dioptric power of the thin lens in the reduced system is −2.80 D.

The reduced object distance is

$$\bar{u} = \frac{u}{n_1} = \frac{-68\,\text{cm}}{1.70} = -40\,\text{cm}$$

Then,

$$U = \frac{100}{-40\,\text{cm}} = -2.50\,\text{D}$$

and

$$V = P + U$$

gives

$$V = -2.80\,\text{D} + (-2.50\,\text{D}) = -5.30\,\text{D}$$

The reduced image distance is

$$\bar{v} = \frac{100}{-5.30\,\text{D}} = -18.9\,\text{cm}$$

The light leaving the actual interface is diverging and in the glass. Therefore, the actual image distance is found by unreducing.

$$v = n_2\bar{v} = (1.50)(-18.9\,\text{cm}) = -28.3\,\text{cm}$$

Again, pay special attention to the fact that the image space index is n_2 (or 1.50 in this case) regardless of whether the image is real or virtual. In the actual system, the exiting wavefront is physically in the glass. Virtual simply means the wavefront is diverging instead of converging.

The lateral magnification is

$$m = \frac{U}{V} = +0.47$$

8.8 SYSTEMS WITH MULTIPLE SPHERICAL SURFACES

Reduced systems greatly simplify the calculations of a system of multiple plane interfaces. Reduced systems

Figure 8.15 a, Actual; b, reduced.

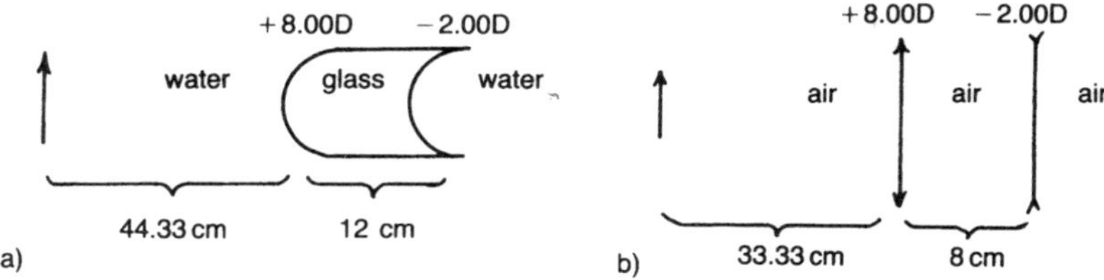

also simplify the calculations for systems of multiple spherical surfaces. In the reduced system, the multiple spherical interface system is equivalent to a series of thin lenses in air. In the reduced system calculations, the refractive indices are used only at the beginning and at the end. This eliminates the possibility of using the wrong refractive index midway in the calculations. In addition, a bonus occurs if the image space happens to consist of air ($n = 1$). Then the reduced image space answers are automatically equal to the actual image space answers.

Another advantage is that several different actual systems can have the same reduced system. In such cases, the reduced system analysis provides information about each of the different actual systems. (In effect, the different actual systems with the same reduced system are all optically equivalent.)

In the next series of examples, both the actual system calculations and the reduced system calculations are done. You should compare the two systems.

EXAMPLE 8.13a

As shown in Figure 8.15a, a real object is in water 44.33 cm from a +8.00 D water–glass interface. The glass is 12 cm thick and has a −2.00 D back interface with water. The refractive indices of the water and glass are 1.33 and 1.50 respectively. Where is the final image? What is the total lateral magnification?

The calculations for the actual system are:

$$u_1 = -44.33\text{ cm}$$

$$U_1 = \frac{133}{-44.33\text{ cm}} = -3.00\text{ D}$$

$$V_1 = P_1 + U_1$$

$$= +8.00\text{ D} + (-3.00\text{ D}) = +5.00\text{ D}$$

The light leaving the interface is in the glass, and

$$v_1 = \frac{150}{+5.00\text{ D}} = +30.00\text{ cm}$$

The object distance for the −2.00 D interface is then

$$u_2 = +30.00\text{ cm} - 12\text{ cm} = +18\text{ cm}$$

The light incident on the interface is still in the glass so

$$U_2 = \frac{150}{+18\text{ cm}} = +8.33\text{ D}$$

$$V_2 = P_2 + U_2$$

$$= -2.00\text{ D} + 8.33\text{ D} = +6.33\text{ D}$$

The light leaving the interface is in water so

$$v_2 = \frac{133}{+6.33\text{ D}} = +21\text{ cm}$$

The final image is real and located 21 cm behind the glass–water interface.

The total lateral magnification is

$$m_{tot} = m_1 m_2$$

$$= \frac{U_1}{V_1}\frac{U_2}{V_2}$$

$$= (-0.60)(+1.32) = -0.79$$

EXAMPLE 8.13b

Use the reduced system and rework Example 8.13a.

The reduced system consists of a +8.00 D thin lens in air separated by a distance $\bar{d}$ from a −2.00 D thin lens in air. Here,

$$\bar{d} = \frac{12\text{ cm}}{1.50} = 8\text{ cm}$$

The reduced object distance for the first lens (see Figure 8.15b) is

$$\bar{u}_1 = \frac{-44.33\text{ cm}}{1.33} = -33.33\text{ cm}$$

Then,

$$U_1 = \frac{100}{-33.33\text{ cm}} = -3.00\text{ D}$$

$$V_1 = P_1 + U_1$$

$$= +8.00\text{ D} + (-3.00\text{ D}) = +5.00\text{ D}$$

$$\bar{v}_1 = \frac{100}{+5.00\text{ D}} = +20\text{ cm}$$

Figure 8.16 a, Actual; b, reduced.

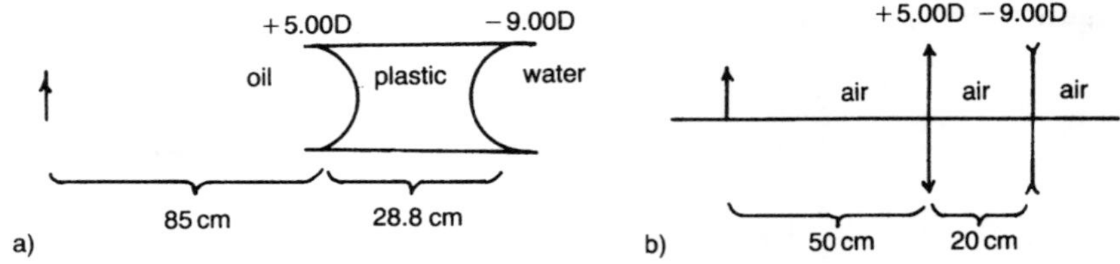

The reduced object distance for the −2.00 D interface is then,

$$\bar{u}_2 = +20\,\text{cm} - 8\,\text{cm} = +12\,\text{cm}$$

$$U_2 = \frac{100}{+12\,\text{cm}} = +8.33\,\text{D}$$

$$V_2 = P_2 + U_2$$

$$= -2.00\,\text{D} + 8.33\,\text{D} = +6.33\,\text{D}$$

$$\bar{v}_2 = \frac{100}{+6.33\,\text{D}} = +15.8\,\text{cm}$$

In the actual system, the light leaving the −2.00 D interface is in water, and so the actual image distance is

$$v_2 = 1.33\bar{v}_2$$

$$= (1.33)(+15.8\,\text{cm}) = +21.0\,\text{cm}$$

which agrees with the results in Example 8.13a. Since the vergences in the reduced system are identical to the corresponding vergences in the actual system, the computations for the total lateral magnification are exactly the same as in Example 8.13a.

EXAMPLE 8.14a

Figure 8.16a shows a system consisting of a +5.00 D oil–plastic interface followed by a −9.00 D plastic–water interface. The plastic is 28.8 cm thick, and the refractive indices of the oil, plastic, and water are 1.70, 1.44, and 1.33 respectively. A real object is in the oil 85 cm in front of the +5.00 D interface. Where is the final image? What is the total lateral magnification?

The calculations for the actual system are:

$$u_1 = -85\,\text{cm}$$

$$U_1 = \frac{170}{-85\,\text{cm}} = -2.00\,\text{D}$$

$$V_1 = P_1 + U_1$$

$$= +5.00\,\text{D} + (-2.00\,\text{D}) = +3.00\,\text{D}$$

The light leaving the interface is in the plastic, and

$$v_1 = \frac{144}{+3.00\,\text{D}} = +48.00\,\text{cm}$$

The object distance for the −9.00 D interface is then,

$$u_2 = +48.00\,\text{cm} - 28.8\,\text{cm} = +19.20\,\text{cm}$$

The light incident on the interface is still in the plastic so

$$U_2 = \frac{144}{+19.20\,\text{cm}} = +7.50\,\text{D}$$

$$V_2 = P_2 + U_2$$

$$= -9.00\,\text{D} + 7.50\,\text{D} = -1.50\,\text{D}$$

The light leaving the interface is in the water so

$$v_2 = \frac{133}{-1.50\,\text{D}} = -88.67\,\text{cm}$$

The final image is virtual and located 88.67 cm to the left of the plastic–water interface.

The total lateral magnification is

$$m_{tot} = m_1 m_2$$

$$= \frac{V_1}{V_1}\frac{U_2}{v_2}$$

$$= (-0.67)(-5.00) = +3.33$$

The final image is erect and 3.33 times larger than the object.

EXAMPLE 8.14b

Solve Example 8.14a by using the reduced system.

Figure 8.16b shows the reduced system. The dioptric powers in the reduced system are the same as those in the actual system, namely, +5.00 D and −9.00 D. The lenses are separated by the reduced distance d where

$$\bar{d} = \frac{28.8\,\text{cm}}{1.44} = 20.0\,\text{cm}$$

The calculations for the reduced system are:

$$\bar{u}_1 = \frac{-85\,\text{cm}}{1.70} = -50\,\text{cm}$$

$$U_1 = \frac{100}{-50\,\text{cm}} = -2.00\,\text{D}$$

$$V_1 = P_1 + U_1$$

$$= +5.00\,\text{D} + (-2.00\,\text{D}) = +3.00\,\text{D}$$

Figure 8.17 a, Actual; b, reduced; c, focal points in actual system.

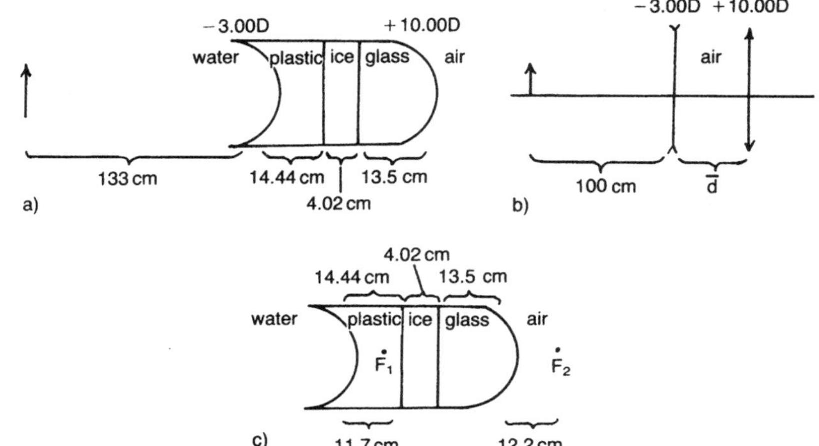

$$\bar{v}_1 = \frac{100}{+3.00\,\text{D}} = +33.33\,\text{cm}$$

$$\bar{u}_2 = +33.33\,\text{cm} - 20.0\,\text{cm} = +13.33\,\text{cm}$$

$$U_2 = \frac{100}{+13.33\,\text{cm}} = +7.50\,\text{D}$$

$$V_2 = P_2 + U_2$$

$$= -9.00\,\text{D} + 7.50\,\text{D} = -1.50\,\text{D}$$

$$\bar{v}_2 = \frac{100}{-1.50\,\text{D}} = -66.67\,\text{cm}$$

In the reduced system, the final image is virtual and located 66.67 cm to the left of the −9.00 D lens. In the actual system, the light leaving the −9.00 D interface is in the water. So the actual image distance is

$$v_2 = 1.33\bar{v}_2$$

$$= (1.33)(-66.67\,\text{cm}) = -86.67\,\text{cm}$$

Note that the vergences at each step in Examples 8.14a and b are identical. Therefore, the total lateral magnification is the same in both the reduced and in the actual system. Consequently, the image size I is the same in both the reduced and in the actual system.

The above examples show the equivalency of the actual system and the reduced system. However, in general, the numerical round-off errors are different in the actual system versus the reduced system. So when comparing the two systems, one needs to keep in mind the number of significant figures.

EXAMPLE 8.15

A real object is in water 133 cm from −3.00 D water–plastic interface. The refractive indices of the water and plastic are 1.33 and 1.44, respectively. The plastic is 14.44 cm thick and followed by a 4.02 cm thick slab of ice ($n = 1.34$). The ice is followed by 13.5 cm of glass ($n = 1.50$). The back surface of the glass is a +10.00 D glass–air interface. The plastic–ice and ice–glass interfaces are plane interfaces (Figure 8.17a). Where is the final image? What is the lateral magnification?

Since the system has some plane interfaces, it is easier to work this problem with the reduced system. The reduced system consists of a −3.00 D thin lens in air at a distance of $\bar{d}$ in front of a +10.00 D thin lens in air (Figure 8.17b). The reduced distance $\bar{d}$ is given by

$$\bar{d} = \frac{14.44\,\text{cm}}{1.44} + \frac{4.02\,\text{cm}}{1.34} + \frac{13.5\,\text{cm}}{1.50} = 22.0\,\text{cm}$$

The reduced object distance for the −3.00 D lens is

$$\bar{u}_1 = \frac{-133\,\text{cm}}{1.33} = -100\,\text{cm}$$

Then,

$$U_1 = \frac{100}{-100\,\text{cm}} = -1.00\,\text{D}$$

$$V_1 = P_1 + U_1$$

$$= -3.00\,\text{D} + (-1.00\,\text{D}) = -4.00\,\text{D}$$

$$\bar{v}_1 = \frac{100}{-4.00\,\text{D}} = -25\,\text{cm}$$

$$\bar{u}_2 = -(25\,\text{cm} + 22\,\text{cm}) = -47\,\text{cm}$$

$$U_2 = \frac{100}{-47\,\text{cm}} = -2.13\,\text{D}$$

$$V_2 = P_2 + U_2$$

$$= +10.00\,\text{D} + (-2.13\,\text{D}) = +7.87\,\text{D}$$

$$\bar{v}_2 = \frac{100}{7.87\,\text{D}} = +12.7\,\text{cm}$$

In the actual system, the final medium is air ($n = 1.00$), so it is trivial to find the actual distance.

$$v_2 = 1.00\bar{v}_2 = (1.00)(+12.7\,\text{cm}) = +12.7\,\text{cm}$$

The lateral magnification is the same in both the reduced and the actual system. From the reduced system,

$$\begin{aligned} m_{\text{tot}} &= m_1 m_2 \\ &= \frac{U_1}{V_1}\frac{U_2}{V_2} \\ &= \left(\frac{-1\,\text{D}}{-4\,\text{D}}\right)\left(\frac{-2.13\,\text{D}}{+7.87\,\text{D}}\right) \\ &= (+0.25)(-0.27) = -0.068 \end{aligned}$$

8.9 FRONT AND BACK VERTEX POWERS

Consider a centered multiple refracting interface system with an image space index of n_i (the refractive index of the medium behind the system), and an object space index of n_o (the refractive index of the medium in front of the system) (Figure 8.18a). Three dioptric values are used to characterize the paraxial imaging properties of such refractive systems. These values are the equivalent dioptric power, the back vertex dioptric power, and the front vertex or neutralizing dioptric power.

In the basic vergence equation, $V = P + U$, the dioptric power P is operative for any incident vergence U. Of the three dioptric values for refractive systems, only the equivalent dioptric power is operative for any incident vergence. The front and back vertex powers are operative only for situations involving plane waves, and thus are not real dioptric powers in the $V = P + U$ sense. Here only the back vertex and neutralizing powers are discussed. The equivalent dioptric power is discussed in Chapters 15 and 16.

The *back vertex power* of a system is the vergence V_b of the light leaving the back of the system when plane waves are incident on the front ($U_1 = 0$); i.e., for $U_1 = 0$, $P_v = V_b$. For plane waves incident along the optical axis, the final image point is the system's secondary focal point F_2. The back focal length f_b is the distance from the back vertex of the system to F_2 and as such is just the radius of curvature of the wavefront leaving the back of the system. Figure 8.18b shows a converging wavefront leaving the back resulting in a real F_2. Figure 8.18c shows a diverging wavefront leaving the back resulting in a virtual F_2. Since P_v is equal to the vergence V_b, which in turn equals the image space index divided by the radius of curvature of the wavefront, it follows that

$$P_v = \frac{n_i}{f_b} \tag{8.8}$$

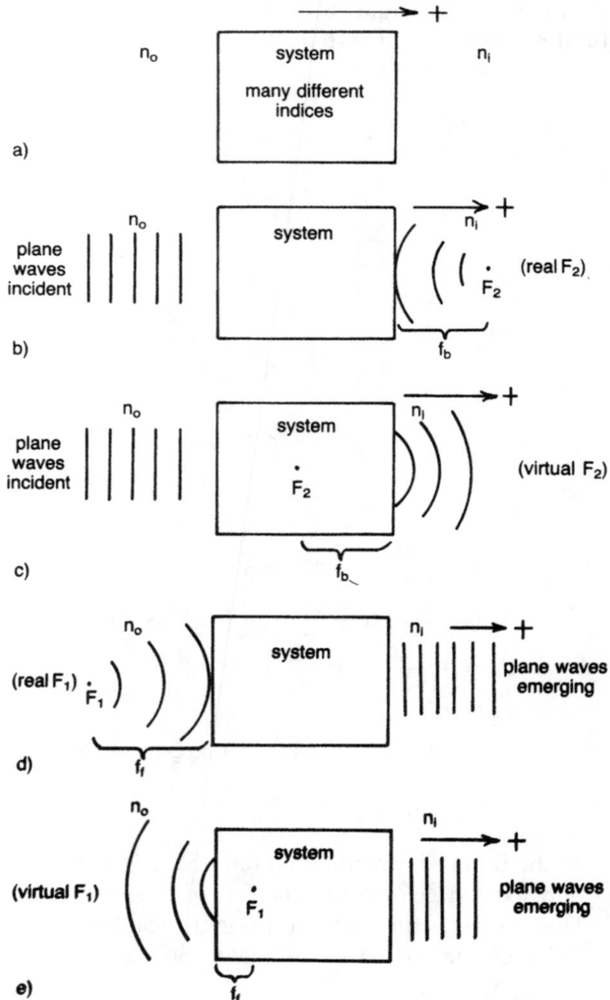

Figure 8.18 a, Paraxial representation of multi-interface system; b, positive back vertex power; c, negative back vertex power; d, positive (or plus) neutralizing power; e, negative (or minus) neutralizing power.

Before considering the neutralizing power of a thick system, let's first consider a +3.00 D thin lens in air. In order to get plane waves leaving the lens, what must the incident vergence U be? From $V = P + U$, $U = V - P$. For plane waves leaving, $V = 0$, and so $U = -3.00\,\text{D}$. Note that here the dioptric power P is opposite in sign to the incident vergence U.

Now consider the thick system. Let U_1 be the vergence of the light incident on the front of the system.

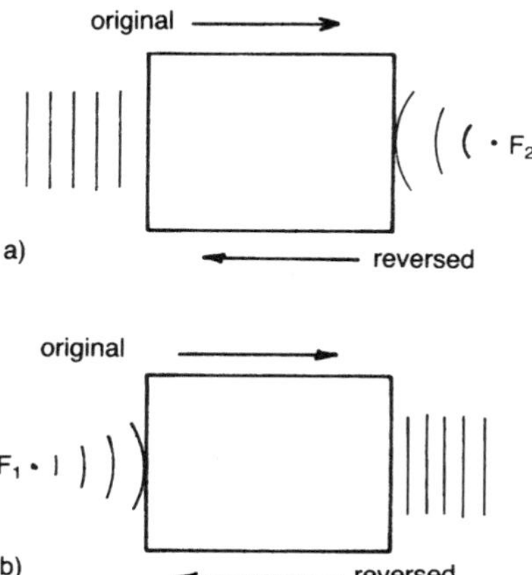

Figure 8.19 Principle of reversibility and vertex powers.

When plane waves leave the back of the system ($V_b = 0$), we say the system neutralizes the vergence U_1 or that the system has a *neutralizing dioptric power* P_n of $-U_1$ i.e., for $V_b = 0$, $P_n = -U_1$. (The minus sign is present for the same reason that it was present in the thin lens example of the previous paragraph.) For example, when light of vergence −3.00 D is incident on a system with a neutralizing power of +3.00 D, then plane waves leave the back of the system. The neutralizing power P_n is also called the *front vertex power*.

When plane waves leave a system along the optical axis, the initial object point is the system's primary focal point F_1. The front focal length f_f is the distance from the front vertex of the system to F_1, and thus is the radius of curvature of the incident wavefront. In this case,

$$U_1 = \frac{n_o}{f_f}$$

and

$$P_n = -\frac{n_o}{f_f} \tag{8.9}$$

Figure 8.18d shows a system with a positive P_n. For emerging plane waves, the incident light is diverging and F_1 is real. Figure 8.18e shows a system with a negative P_n. For emerging plane waves, the incident light is converging and F_1 is virtual.

Consider a system with a back vertex power of +7.00 D. When plane waves are incident on the system, the vergence of the converging light leaving the back vertex is +7.00 D. Now reverse the light. When the light is reversed, diverging light of vergence −7.00 D is incident on the back surface of the system, and according to the principle of reversibility, plane waves leave the front vertex (Figure 8.19a). For the reversed situation, the system has a neutralizing dioptric power of +7.00 D; i.e., it neutralizes light of vergence −7.00 D. In general, when the light through a system is reversed, the original back vertex power becomes the new neutralizing power. (Another way of saying this is that the original back vertex power becomes the new front vertex power.)

Similarly, consider light of vergence −5.00 D incident on a system with a neutralizing power of +5.00 D. Then plane waves leave the back of the system. Now reverse the light so that the plane waves are incident on the back of the system. From the principle of reversibility, the light emerging from the front vertex of the system now has a vergence of +5.00 D (Figure 8.19b). Thus, in the reversed situation, the original neutralizing power of +5.00 D plays the role of back vertex power. In general, when the light through a system is reversed, the original neutralizing power becomes the new back vertex power. (Another way of saying this is that the original front vertex power becomes the new back vertex power.)

EXAMPLE 8.16

Find the neutralizing and back vertex powers of the system in Example 8.15 (see Figure 8.17a).

Since the vergences are the same in the actual and in the reduced system, we can use the reduced system. The reduced system consists of a −3.00 D thin lens 22 cm in front of a +10.00 D thin lens (Figure 8.17b). To find the back vertex power, consider plane waves incident on the system front (the −3.00 D lens). Then,

$$U_1 = 0$$
$$V_1 = -3.00\,\text{D}$$
$$v_1 = -33.33\,\text{cm}$$
$$u_2 = -(33.33\,\text{cm} + 22.00\,\text{cm}) = -55.3\,\text{cm}$$
$$U_2 = -1.81\,\text{D}$$
$$V_2 = +10.00\,\text{D} + (-1.81\,\text{D}) = +8.19\,\text{D}$$

So

$$P_v = +8.19\,\text{D}$$

The easiest way to find the neutralizing power (or front vertex power) is to reverse the light and let plane waves be incident on the back lens. For the reversed system, relabel the lens as

$$P_1 = +10.00\,\text{D} \quad \text{and} \quad P_2 = -3.00\,\text{D}$$

Then,

$$U_1 = 0$$
$$V_1 = +10.00\,\text{D}$$
$$\bar{v}_1 = +10.00\,\text{cm}$$
$$\bar{u}_2 = +10.00\,\text{cm} - 22.00\,\text{cm} = -12.00\,\text{cm}$$
$$U_2 = -8.33\,\text{D}$$
$$V_2 = -3.00\,\text{D} + (-8.33\,\text{D}) = -11.33\,\text{D}$$

So in the reversed system

$$(P_v)_{rev} = -11.33\,\text{D}$$

or in the original system

$$P_n = -11.33\,\text{D}$$

EXAMPLE 8.17

Find F_1 and F_2 for the system in the previous two examples.

In the actual system, the image space index n_i is 1.00 and the object space index n_o is 1.33. From Eq. 8.8,

$$f_b = \frac{n_i}{P_v} = \frac{100}{+8.19\,\text{D}} = +12.2\,\text{cm}$$

F_2 is real and located +12.2 cm behind the back vertex of the system.

From Eq. 8.9,

$$f_f = -\frac{n_o}{P_n} = -\frac{133}{-11.33\,\text{D}} = +11.7\,\text{cm}$$

F_1 is virtual and located 11.7 cm behind the front vertex of the system (Figure 8.17c).

Note that the back vertex power provides information only when plane waves are incident on a system, and the neutralizing power provides information only when plane waves are leaving a system. For the system in Example 8.15, the back vertex power is +8.19 D, and the neutralizing or front vertex power is −11.33 D. Clearly, the two vertex powers can be very different, but this is not always the case.

Consider a thin lens of dioptric power P. When plane waves are incident on the lens:

$$V = P + U = P$$

so the back vertex power of the thin lens is equal to P. When plane waves leave the lens:

$$V = 0 = P + U$$

or

$$P = -U$$

so the neutralizing power of the thin lens is equal to P. Thus, for a thin lens of power P, the back vertex power and the neutralizing power are both equal to P. As shown in Chapter 15, the equivalent dioptric power also equals P.

8.10 VERTEX NEUTRALIZATION

Consider two optical systems A and B that are in contact with each other, with A in front of B. Assume that whenever plane waves are incident on A, plane waves leave B. Then we say that the systems have neutralized each other. What condition is needed for this to happen?

Since plane waves are incident on A, the vergence leaving it is equal to its back vertex power $(P_v)_A$. Since the systems are in contact, this vergence is incident on B without change. For plane waves to leave B, the vergence incident on it must equal $-(P_n)_B$, where $(P_n)_B$ is the neutralizing power of system B. Therefore, the condition is that the back vertex power of system A is equal in magnitude but opposite in sign to the neutralizing power of system B, or

$$(P_v)_A = -(P_n)_B \tag{8.10}$$

EXAMPLE 8.18

System B has a neutralizing power of +4.00 D and a back vertex power of +7.00 D. System B is placed in contact with the back of system A. What parameters must A have to neutralize B?

To get plane waves out of B, the vergence incident on it must equal −4.00 D. Therefore, the vergence leaving A must be −4.00 D, and A must have a back vertex power of −4.00 D. Equation 8.10 gives the same result. Note that the information given does not specify the neutralizing power of A. Also, the back vertex power of B is not useful here since plane waves are not incident on B.

EXAMPLE 8.19a

A system has a neutralizing power of −3.75 D and a back vertex power of −6.25 D. What thin lens placed against the back of the system will neutralize it?

When plane waves are incident on the front of the system, the vergence of the light leaving the back is −6.25 D. Therefore, a +6.25 D thin lens is needed to give plane waves leaving.

EXAMPLE 8.19b

For the same system, what thin lens placed against the front of the system will neutralize it?

To get plane waves leaving the back of the system, the vergence of the light incident on the front must be +3.75 D. The thin lens in front of the system must take incident plane waves and convert them to the needed vergence. A +3.75 D thin lens will do the job.

8.11 REDUCED ANGLES

Figure 8.20a shows a paraxial ray incident on a spherical surface. The object space index is n. The axial point is a distance d from the surface. The ray makes an angle ϕ with the axis and hits the surface at a distance y above the axis. Therefore,

$$\tan\phi \approx \phi = \frac{y}{d}$$

Figure 8.20b shows the same ray in a reduced system. Now the axial point is a (reduced) distance $\bar{d}$ from the surface, where

$$\bar{d} = \frac{d}{n}$$

Since image sizes are the same in an actual system and in a reduced system, it follows that the lateral distance

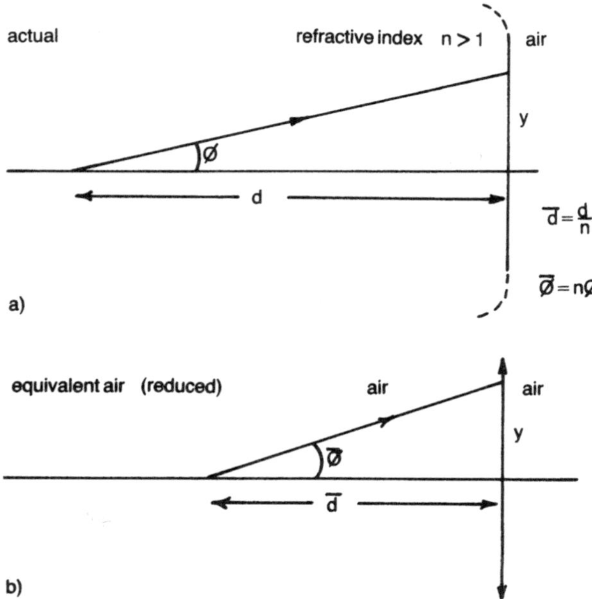

Figure 8.20 a, Actual ray angle; b, reduced ray angle.

y is the same in the two systems. The (reduced) angle $\bar{\phi}$ that the ray makes with the axis is given by

$$\bar{\phi} \approx \tan\bar{\phi} = y/\bar{d}$$

We can then substitute for the reduced distance to obtain

$$\bar{\phi} = y/\bar{d} = \frac{y}{d/n} = n\frac{y}{d}$$

or

$$\bar{\phi} = n\phi \tag{8.11}$$

Equation 8.11 relates the reduced angle $\bar{\phi}$ to the angle ϕ in the actual system. Remember that reduced is a synonym for equivalent air. While a reduced distance $\bar{d}$ is smaller than the actual distance d, the reduced angle $\bar{\phi}$ is the larger than the actual angle ϕ.

PROBLEMS

1. A butterfly is 18.5 cm above the surface on a pond ($n = 1.33$). What is the apparent height of the butterfly as seen by a fish under water in the pond? If the fish is 250 cm below the pond's surface, what is the apparent depth of the fish as seen by the butterfly?
2. While tubing down the Muskegon River ($n = 1.33$), a student notices a rock that appears to be 80 cm vertically below the surface. What is the actual depth of the rock?
3. A real object is located 12.5 cm in front of a 15 cm thick glass ($n = 1.50$) slab. A lens is located 7 cm from the back surface of the slab. What is the vergence of the wavefront incident on the lens? What is the equivalent air thickness (reduced thickness) of the slab?
4. A submarine has a 12 cm thick polycarbonate ($n = 1.58$) window with flat sides. A 3.25 D uncorrected hyperope in the submarine views a tropical fish in the water ($n = 1.33$) outside the window. What is the ocular accommodative demand when the fish is 21 cm from the outside of the submarine's window and when the lens representing the hyperope's eye is 15 cm from the inside of the window?
5. A lens in air has exiting light of vergence +3.50 D. Seven centimeters behind the lens is a flat air–glass ($n = 1.53$) interface. The glass is 11 cm thick followed by a flat glass–water ($n = 1.33$) interface. The water is 9 cm thick followed by a flat water–plastic ($n = 1.44$) interface. The plastic is 5 cm thick followed by a flat plastic–air interface. Where and in what medium is the physically real image formed?
6. Find the reduced (equivalent air) system for a 7 cm thick plastic ($n = 1.61$) lens with a +7.00 D front surface and a −3.00 D back surface. Specify a lower index plastic ($n = 1.44$) lens (surface powers and central thickness) that has the same reduced system.

7. A system consists of an ophthalmic crown (n = 1.523) glass component in front of a barium crown (n = 1.617) glass component. The ophthalmic crown glass is 4 cm thick and has a +10.00 D front surface. The barium crown component is 3 cm thick and has a −4.00 D back surface. The interface between the two glass types is flat. Find the reduced system, the back vertex power, and the neutralizing power.
8. A +2.00 D thin lens is located 6 cm in front of a −6.00 D thin lens, which in turn is 3 cm in front of a +7.00 D thin lens. What is the back vertex power? What is the neutralizing power?
9. A +8.00 D thin lens is located 15 cm in front of a −10.00 D thin lens. Find the back vertex power and the neutralizing power of the system.
10. A three lens system has a +3.00 D neutralizing power, and a +7.00 D back vertex power. Relative to the front surface of the system, where can an object be placed in order for plane waves to leave the back of the system?
11. A system has a distant object, a +4.00 D neutralizing power, and a +6.50 D back vertex power. What thin lens placed against the front of the system results in plane waves leaving the back of the system?
12. A system has a distant object, a −5.00 D neutralizing power, and a +8.00 D back vertex power. What thin lens placed against the back of the system results in plane waves leaving the thin lens?
13. What is the neutralizing power of a +4.50 D thin glass (n = 1.53) lens?
14. A system has a distant object, a +5.00 D back vertex power, and a +12.00 D neutralizing power. Which of the following systems placed against the back of the first system will result in plane waves leaving the back of the second system.

a. neutralizing power −5.00 D, back vertex power anything.
b. neutralizing power −12.00 D, back vertex power anything.
c. neutralizing power −7.00 D, back vertex power anything.
d. neutralizing power −17.00 D, back vertex power anything.
e. back vertex power −5.00 D, neutralizing power anything.
f. back vertex power −12.00 D, neutralizing power anything.
g. back vertex power −7.00 D, neutralizing power anything.
h. back vertex power −17.00 D, neutralizing power anything.

CHAPTER 9

Lenses Revisited

9.1 LENS SHAPES

A lens consists of two refractive surfaces separated by a certain thickness. The words convex and concave are frequently used to classify lenses as well as to classify the individual surfaces. A convex lens is a converging lens, and a concave lens is a diverging lens.

Converging lenses in air tend to be thicker in the middle than at the edge. A converging lens with two converging surfaces is called a biconvex lens (Figure 9.1a). When the two converging surfaces have the same curvature, the lens is called equiconvex (Figure 9.1b). When a converging lens has one plane surface and one converging surface, the lens is called planoconvex (Figure 9.1c). When a converging lens has a converging surface and a diverging surface, the lens is called meniscus-convex (Figure 9.1d). (The word meniscus comes from the Greek word *meniskos*, which means moon. A meniscus convex lens is crescent-shaped like a new moon.)

Diverging lenses in air tend to be thinner in the middle than at the edge. A diverging lens with two diverging surfaces is called a biconcave lens (Figure 9.2a). When the two diverging surfaces have the same curvature, the lens is called equiconcave (Figure 9.2b). When a diverging lens has one plane surface and one diverging surface, the lens is called planoconcave (Figure 9.2c). When a diverging lens has a converging surface and a diverging surface, the lens is called meniscus-concave (Figure 9.2d).

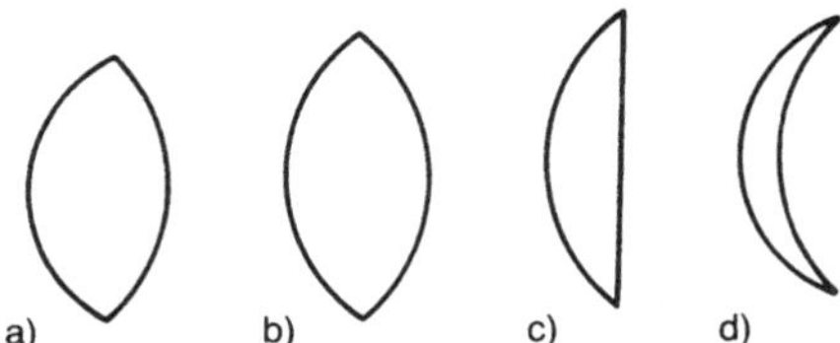

Figure 9.1 Converging lenses: a, biconvex; b, equiconvex; c, planoconvex; d, meniscus-convex.

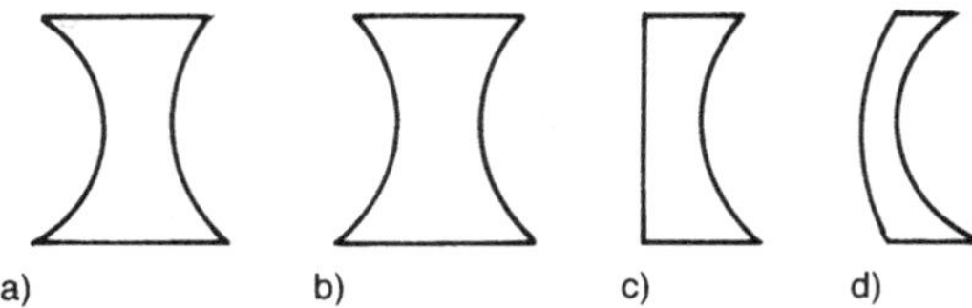

Figure 9.2 Diverging lenses: a, biconcave; b, equiconcave; c, planoconcave; d, meniscus-concave.

While the shape of a *thin* lens is not optically important, the shape of a *thick* lens is. Ophthalmic lenses used to correct the eye typically have a meniscus shape with the convex surface away from the eye and the concave surface toward the eye (Figures 9.1d and 9.2d).

9.2 THIN LENS POWER

In general, the optics of a lens depends on the dioptric powers of the front and back surface of the lens, and on the reduced thickness of the lens. Figure 9.3 shows light incident on the convex surface of a meniscus-convex lens. P_1 and P_2 are the dioptric powers of the front and back surfaces, respectively. The surface powers are related to the refractive indices and radii of curvature by

$$P_1 = \frac{n_2 - n_1}{r_1} \quad \text{and} \quad P_2 = \frac{n_3 - n_2}{r_2} \tag{9.1}$$

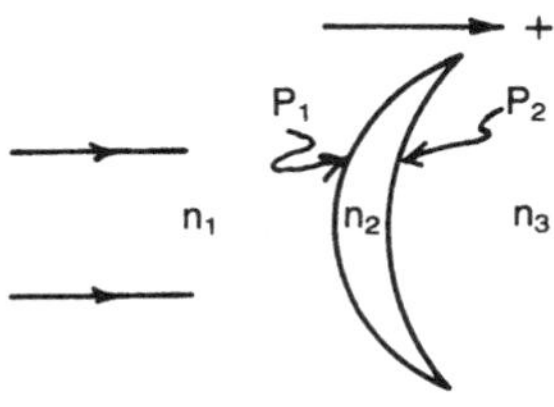

Figure 9.3 Lens surface powers.

where r_1 and r_2 are the respective radii of curvature of the surfaces, n_2 is the refractive index of the lens material, and where n_1 and n_3 are the respective refractive indices for the mediums in front of and behind the lens.

Let U_1 and V_1 be the respective incident and exiting vergence of the light at the first surface. Let U_2 and V_2 be the respective incident and exiting vergence of the light at the second surface. The vergence equations at each surface are:

$$V_1 = P_1 + U_1 \quad \text{and} \quad V_2 = P_2 + U_2$$

When the central thickness of the lens is small enough, no significant vergence changes occur as the light travels across the lens, and

$$U_2 = V_1$$

Then,

$$V_2 = P_2 + V_1$$

and we can substitute for V_1 to obtain

$$V_2 = P_2 + P_1 + U_1$$

which can be written as

$$V_2 = P_t + U_1 \tag{9.2}$$

with

$$P_t = P_2 + P_1 \tag{9.3}$$

Equation 9.2 directly relates any vergence U_1 incident on the thin lens to the vergence V_2 leaving it. P_t is the dioptric power of the thin lens. According to Eq. 9.3, P_t is the sum of the surface powers P_1 and P_2. The refractive index and the surface curvature information is hidden in P_t and does not explicitly occur in Eq. 9.2.

Since addition is commutative, we can interchange P_1 and P_2 in Eq. 9.3. Thus, within the accuracy of the paraxial approximation, the shape of a thin lens is not important. It follows that the front and back vertex power of a thin lens (Section 8.9) are both equal to P_t.

EXAMPLE 9.1

A thin MR6 plastic ($n = 1.60$) biconvex lens has surface radii of magnitude 12 cm and 20 cm, respectively (Figure 9.1a). What is the dioptric power of the lens?

Unless specified otherwise, we assume the lens is in air. Since the lens is biconvex, the surface powers are both positive. From Eq. 9.1,

$$P_1 = \frac{(1.60 - 1.00)100\,\text{cm/m}}{+12\,\text{cm}}$$

or

$$P_1 = \frac{60}{12} = +5.00\,\text{D}$$

Similarly,

$$P_2 = \frac{-60}{-20} = +3.00\,\text{D}$$

From Eq. 9.3,

$$P_t = (+5.00\,\text{D}) + (+3.00\,\text{D}) = +8.00\,\text{D}$$

EXAMPLE 9.2

A thin CR-39 plastic ($n = 1.50$) meniscus-convex lens has a side with a 25 cm radius of curvature and a side with a 5 cm radius of curvature. What is the dioptric power of the lens?

First, we need to decide which side is the convex side and which side is the concave side. Since the lens is meniscus-convex (Figure 9.1d), the convex side is steeper and the concave side is flatter, and the resulting lens power should be positive. The side with the 5 cm radius of curvature is steeper than the side with the 25 cm radius of curvature, so the convex side has the 5 cm radius of curvature.

Assume the light is incident on the convex side. Then for the convex side, Eq. 9.1 gives

$$P_1 = \frac{50}{+5} = +10.00\,\text{D}$$

For the concave side:

$$P_2 = \frac{-50}{+25} = -2.00\,\text{D}$$

Then,

$$P_t = (+10.00\,\text{D}) + (-2.00\,\text{D}) = +8.00\,\text{D}$$

The lenses in the above two examples are made out of different materials and have different shapes, but both are +8.00 D thin lenses.

EXAMPLE 9.3

A −4.50 D thin meniscus-concave glass lens has one side with a 10 cm radius of curvature and the other side with a 25 cm radius of curvature. What is the refractive index of the lens material?

Again we first need to decide which side is the convex side and which side is the concave side. Since the lens is meniscus-concave (Figure 9.2d), the convex side is flatter and the concave side is steeper. So the convex side has the 25 cm radius of curvature.

Assume the light is incident on the convex side. Then from Eqs. 9.1 and 9.3,

$$P_t = -4.50\,\text{D} = P_1 + P_2$$

$$-4.50\,\text{D} = \frac{(n_2 - 1)100\,\text{cm/m}}{25\,\text{cm}} + \frac{(1 - n_2)100\,\text{cm/m}}{10\,\text{cm}}$$

$$= [(n_2 - 1)4] + [(1 - n_2)10]$$

and it follows that

$$n_2 = 1 + \left(\frac{-4.50}{-6}\right) = 1.75$$

9.3 THICK LENSES: FRONT AND BACK VERTEX POWERS

When a lens is thick enough there is a significant vergence change across the interior of the lens, so the vergence U_2 incident on the back surface of the lens is not equal to the vergence V_1 leaving the front surface, i.e.,

$$U_2 \neq V_1$$

As a result, Eqs. 9.2 and 9.3 do not hold for thick lenses.

When plane waves are incident on the front of a lens, the vergence of the light leaving the back surface is called the back vertex power P_v (Section 8.9). In other words, when $U_1 = 0$, $P_v = V_2$. The back vertex power is a characteristic of a lens. *The back vertex power is the parameter specified in a prescription for a distance vision ophthalmic correction.*

When a thick lens neutralizes incident vergence of $-U_1$ (i.e., gives plane waves leaving), the lens' neutralizing dioptric power P_n is equal to minus U_1, i.e., when $V_2 = 0$, $P_n = -U_1$. The neutralizing power is a characteristic of the lens, and in general is not equal to the back vertex power. The neutralizing power is also called the front vertex power. Remember that both the front and back vertex powers are not real dioptric powers in the $V = P + U$ sense, because both are operative only in their respective plane wave situations.

EXAMPLE 9.4a

What is the back vertex power of an ophthalmic crown glass ($n = 1.523$) lens with a central thickness of 2 cm and with front and back surface powers of +12.00 D and −4.00 D, respectively?

Before calculating, one should first think about the characteristics expected for the answer. What is the expected answer if the lens was thin? The expected answer for a thin lens is the sum of the surface powers or +8.00 D in this case. A thin lens has no significant vergence change across the interior of the lens. A 2 cm thickness is large for a lens. For plane waves incident on the +12.00 D front surface, the converging light that crosses the interior of the lens gains vergence (i.e., the converging wavefronts gain curvature). Thus we expect the back vertex power will be greater than +8.00 D.

This example can be worked either with the reduced system or with the actual system. Let us use the reduced system since that minimizes the use of the refractive index. The reduced central thickness $\bar{d}$ is

$$\bar{d} = \frac{2\,\text{cm}}{1.523} = 1.31\,\text{cm}$$

The reduced system consists of a $P_1 = +12.00$ D thin lens in air 1.31 cm in front of a $P_2 = -4.00$ D thin lens in air. The calculations are:

$$U_1 = 0$$

$$V_1 = P_1 + U_1 = +12.00\,\text{D}$$

$$\bar{v}_1 = \frac{100}{+12.00\,\text{D}} = +8.33\,\text{cm}$$

$$\bar{u}_2 = +8.33\,\text{cm} - 1.31\,\text{cm} = +7.02\,\text{cm}$$

$$U_2 = \frac{100}{+7.02\,\text{cm}} = +14.25\,\text{D}$$

(Note the light waves gain +2.25 D of vergence while crossing the interior of the lens—i.e., the difference between 14.25 D and 12.00 D). Then,

$$V_2 = P_2 + U_2 = -4.00\,\text{D} + (+14.25\,\text{D})$$

and

$$P_v = V_2 = +10.25\,\text{D}$$

The answer agrees with our expectations and is greater than the thin lens value by the +2.25 D of vergence gained by the converging light as it crossed the interior of the lens.

EXAMPLE 9.4b

What is the neutralizing power of the lens in Example 9.4a?

The easiest way to find the neutralizing power is to use the reduced system, reverse the light, and consider plane waves incident on the back of the lens. (Before calculating be sure to make your own estimates for what the answer should be.) In the reversed system, we relabel the lenses as

$$P_1 = -4.00\,\text{D} \quad \text{and} \quad P_2 = +12.00\,\text{D}$$

The calculations are:

$$U_1 = 0$$
$$V_1 = P_1 + U_1 = -4.00\,\text{D}$$
$$\bar{v}_1 = \frac{100}{-4.00\,\text{D}} = -25.0\,\text{cm}$$
$$\bar{u}_2 = -(25.0\,\text{cm} + 1.31\,\text{cm}) = -26.31\,\text{cm}$$
$$U_2 = \frac{100}{-26.31\,\text{cm}} = -3.80\,\text{D}$$
$$V_2 = P_2 + U_2 = +12.00 + (-3.80\,\text{D})$$
$$P_n = V_2 = +8.20\,\text{D}$$

So in the forward system, when light of vergence $U_1 = -8.20\,\text{D}$ is incident on the front surface, plane waves leave the back surface. The neutralizing dioptric power of the lens is then $P_n = -U_1 = +8.20\,\text{D}$.

The lens in this example has a back vertex power of +10.25 D and a neutralizing (or front vertex) power of +8.20 D. The difference of the values from each other and from the thin lens value of +8.00 D comes from the different vergence changes across the interior of the lens.

EXAMPLE 9.5

A high index glass ($n = 1.70$) lens has a central thickness of 4 cm, a front surface power of +6.00 D, and a back surface power of −15.00 D. What are the front and back vertex powers of the lens?

What are the expectations? The thin lens results would be −9.00 D. For the back vertex power, the converging light across the interior adds plus vergence to the −9.00 D (or reduces the minus), so we expect a minus power with less magnitude than 9.00 D. For the neutralizing power (in the reversed system), the diverging light loses minus vergence across the interior, so again we expect a minus power with less magnitude than 9.00 D.

In the reduced system:

$$\bar{d} = \frac{4\,\text{cm}}{1.70} = 2.35\,\text{cm}$$

The calculations for the back vertex power are:

$$P_1 = +6.00\,\text{D} \quad \text{and} \quad P_2 = -15.00\,\text{D}$$

For

$$U_1 = 0$$
$$V_1 = P_1 + U_1 = +6.00\,\text{D}$$
$$\bar{v}_1 = \frac{100}{+6.00\,\text{D}} = +16.67\,\text{cm}$$
$$\bar{u}_2 = +16.67\,\text{cm} - 2.35\,\text{cm} = +14.31\,\text{cm}$$
$$U_2 = \frac{100}{+14.31\,\text{cm}} = +6.98\,\text{D}$$
$$V_2 = P_2 + U_2 = -15.00\,\text{D} + 6.98\,\text{D}$$
$$P_v = V_2 = -8.02\,\text{D}$$

which agrees with our expectations that the result would be less minus than the thin lens value of −9.00 D.

In the reversed system, the calculations for the neutralizing power are:

$$P_1 = -15.00\,\text{D} \quad \text{and} \quad P_2 = +6.00\,\text{D}$$
$$U_1 = 0$$
$$V_1 = P_1 + U_1 = -15.00\,\text{D}$$
$$\bar{v}_1 = \frac{100}{-15.00\,\text{D}} = -6.67\,\text{cm}$$
$$\bar{u}_2 = -(6.67\,\text{cm} + 2.35\,\text{cm}) = -9.02\,\text{cm}$$
$$U_2 = \frac{100}{-9.02\,\text{cm}} = -11.09\,\text{D}$$
$$V_2 = P_2 + U_2 = +6.00\,\text{D} + (-11.09\,\text{D})$$
$$P_n = V_2 = -5.09\,\text{D}$$

which also agrees with our expectations that the result would be less minus than the thin lens value of −9.00 D.

This lens has a back vertex power of −8.02 D and a front vertex (or neutralizing) power of −5.09 D. Again, the difference is due to the different vergence changes across the interior of the lens.

Consider a polycarbonate ($n = 1.586$) spectacle correction with a central thickness of 3 mm, a +4.00 D front surface, and a −2.00 D back surface. The back vertex power is +2.03 D, and the neutralizing power is +2.01 D. The sum of the surface powers is +2.00 D. Variations much smaller than 0.25 D are negligible in ophthalmic correcting lenses, so this polycarbonate lens can be treated as a thin lens.

Consider a meniscus-convex Fluoroperm 60 ($n = 1.473$) rigid contact lens correction with a 0.36 mm central thickness, a 6.30 mm front surface radius, and a 7.80 mm back surface radius. The front and back surface powers are +75.08 D and −60.64 D, respectively. The sum of the surface powers is +14.44 D. The back vertex power is +15.84 D, and the neutralizing power is +15.33 D. The contact lens has a small central thickness, but the surface powers are high. Therefore, *a clinically significant vergence change occurs across the interior of the contact lens, and this contact lens must be treated as a thick lens instead of a thin lens.* Clearly, the surface powers as well as the central thickness must be taken into account in deciding whether or not a lens can be treated as thin!

9.4 THIN LENSES IN DIFFERENT MEDIA

Typically, lenses are used in air and so the thin lens power P_t is the power of the lens in air. Suppose the medium in front of or behind the lens is changed. What happens to the dioptric power? To answer this question, we need to know the refractive index n_2 of the lens material.

Let n_1 be the refractive index of the medium in front of the lens (the object space index), n_2 be the refractive index of the lens material, and n_3 be the refractive index of the medium behind the lens (the image space index). When the object space index n_1 is changed, the front interface power P_1 changes according to Eq. 7.34:

$$(P_1)_{new} = \frac{(n_2 - n_1)_{new}}{(n_2 - n_1)_{old}}(P_1)_{old} \tag{9.4}$$

When the image space index n_3 is changed, the back interface power P_2 changes according to

$$(P_2)_{new} = \frac{(n_3 - n_2)_{new}}{(n_3 - n_2)_{old}}(P_2)_{old}$$

or

$$(P_2)_{new} = \frac{(n_2 - n_3)_{new}}{(n_2 - n_3)_{old}}(P_2)_{old} \tag{9.5}$$

In general, the new thin lens dioptric power can be calculated by adding the new interface powers together.

A simplification occurs when the object and image space indices remain equal during the change. Then, since n_1 is equal to n_3, Eqs. 9.4 and 9.5 can be added to give

$$P_{new} = \frac{(n_2 - n_1)_{new}}{(n_2 - n_1)_{old}} P_{old} \tag{9.6}$$

where P_{new} is the new thin lens power and P_{old} is the old thin lens power, i.e.,

$$P_{new} = (P_1)_{new} + (P_2)_{new}$$

and

$$P_{old} = (P_1)_{old} + (P_2)_{old}$$

Note that in Eq. 9.6 the interface powers have dropped out and only the total thin lens powers remain.

EXAMPLE 9.6

A +13.00 D thin Spectralite lens (mid-index plastic, $n = 1.537$) is dropped into water ($n = 1.333$). What is the power of the lens while under water?

From Eq. 9.6,

$$P_{new} = \frac{(1.537 - 1.333)}{(1.537 - 1.000)}(+13.00\text{ D})$$
$$= \frac{204}{537}(+13.00\text{ D}) = +4.94\text{ D}$$

EXAMPLE 9.7

Assume the crystalline lens of the human eye is thin and has a refractive index of 1.400. The power of the lens in the eye is about +19 D. What is the power of the crystalline lens in air?

In the eye, the crystalline lens is bounded on the front by the aqueous humor, and on the back by the vitreous humor, both of which have a refractive index of 1.336. From Eq. 9.6,

$$P_{new} = \frac{(1.400 - 1.000)}{(1.400 - 1.336)}(+19\text{ D}) = +119\text{ D}$$

Actually, the crystalline lens powers are very high, so it should be treated as a thick lens.

9.5 ANOTHER EYE MODEL

Previously, we dealt with thin lenses in air and single spherical refracting interface eye models. Now consider a slightly more sophisticated eye model. The cornea is represented as a +47.00 D SSRI between air and the aqueous humor ($n = 1.336$), while the crystalline lens is represented as a +19.00 D thin lens with the aqueous humor in front of it and the vitreous humor ($n = 1.336$) behind it. The distance from the cornea to the crystalline lens is 3.6 mm, and the distance from the crystalline lens to the retina is 21 mm. What is the ocular refractive status of this eye?

The easiest way to answer this question is to reduce the system and reverse the light. The reduced system consists of a +47.00 D lens located 2.70 mm (i.e., 3.6/1.336) in front of a +19.00 D lens, which in turn is located 15.72 mm (i.e., 21/1.336) in front of the retina. Then in the reversed system:

$$U_1 = \frac{1000\text{ mm/m}}{-15.72\text{ mm}} = -63.61\text{ D}$$
$$V_1 = P_1 + U_1 = +19.00\text{ D} + (-63.61\text{ D})$$
$$= -44.61\text{ D}$$
$$\bar{v}_1 = \frac{1000}{-44.61\text{ D}} = -22.42\text{ mm}$$
$$\bar{u}_2 = -(22.42\text{ mm} + 2.70\text{ mm}) = -25.12\text{ mm}$$
$$U_2 = \frac{1000}{-25.12} = -39.81\text{ D}$$
$$V_2 = P_2 + U_2 = +47.00\text{ D} + (-39.81\text{ D})$$
$$= +7.19\text{ D}$$

and

$$\bar{v}_2 = \frac{100\text{ cm/m}}{+7.19\text{ D}} = +13.91\text{ cm}$$

The light coming out of the eye is converging and has a vergence of magnitude 7.19 D. This eye is a 7.19 D ocular myope. The far point is real and located a distance of 13.91 cm in front of the eye.

What (thick) spectacle lenses worn at a vertex distance of 12 mm corrects this eye for distance vision? For this model, assume the vertex distance is from the back vertex of the lens to the cornea.

To get a clear image on the retina, the vergence incident on the cornea must be −7.19 D. The far point is 13.91 cm minus 1.2 cm or 12.71 cm from the spectacle plane. The vergence V_b leaving the back of the spectacle lens must be

$$V_b = -\frac{100}{12.71\ \text{cm}} = -7.87\ \text{D}$$

At this vertex distance, any spectacle lens with a back vertex power of −7.87 D corrects the eye for distance vision.

9.6 EXPLODING A SINGLE SPHERICAL REFRACTING INTERFACE

Figure 9.4a shows a system with water ($n = 1.33$) in front, air ($n = 1.00$) in the middle, and glass ($n = 1.53$) behind. Both the concave water–air interface and the convex air–glass interface have a radius of curvature of 4 cm. From

$$P = \frac{n_2 - n_1}{r}$$

the dioptric powers of the two interfaces are, respectively,

$$P_1 = \frac{-33}{+4} = -8.25\ \text{D}$$

and

$$P_2 = \frac{+53}{+4} = +13.25\ \text{D}$$

Let U_1 be the vergence of the light in water incident on the first interface and V_1 be the vergence of the light in air leaving the first interface. Let U_2 be the vergence of the light in air incident on the second interface and V_2 be the vergence of the light in glass leaving the second interface. The vergence equations at the two interfaces are:

$$V_1 = P_1 + U_1 \quad \text{and} \quad V_2 = P_2 + U_2$$

In general, there is a vergence change across the air gap so that U_2 is not equal to V_1.

Suppose the air gap is so thin that no significant vergence change occurs across it. Then,

$$V_1 = U_2$$

and similar to the thin lens situation, the above three equations can be combined to give

$$V_2 = P_s + U_1$$

where

$$P_s = P_1 + P_2$$

Then,

$$P_s = +13.25\ \text{D} + (-8.25\ \text{D}) = +5.00\ \text{D}$$

Consider a single spherical water–glass interface with a radius of curvature of 4 cm (Figure 9.4b). The dioptric power of the water–glass interface is

$$P = \frac{(1.53 - 1.33)100}{+4\ \text{cm}} = \frac{20}{+4} = +5.00\ \text{D}$$

Essentially, the +5.00 D water–glass interface acts paraxially just like the system consisting of the −8.25 D water–air interface separated by a thin air gap from the +13.25 D air–glass interface. This means that, for analysis purposes, we can conceptually split the water and glass apart, and consider a thin air layer in between them.

The above argument can be repeated for any SSRI between media of refractive index n_o and n_i. Thus, the interface can be split in two with a thin air gap in between. (Conceptually, you might think of one molecular layer of air.) The curvature of each interface remains the same as the original interface. A system with each interface split in this manner is sometimes called an *exploded system*. Exploded systems are useful in the analysis of contact lens corrections.

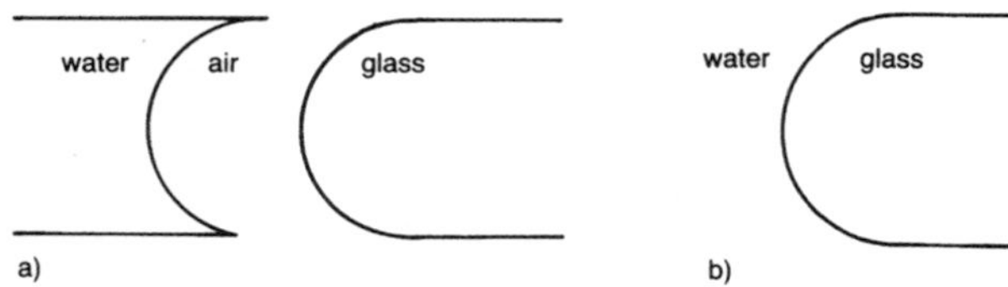

Figure 9.4 a, Two interfaces each with a 4-cm radius of curvature; b, single interface with 4 cm of curvature.

EXAMPLE 9.8

Find the exploded system for a −2.00 D spherical refracting interface between plastic ($n = 1.44$) and high index glass ($n = 1.74$).

Figures 9.5a and b show the actual and the exploded system, respectively. One way to proceed is to find the radius of curvature r, and then

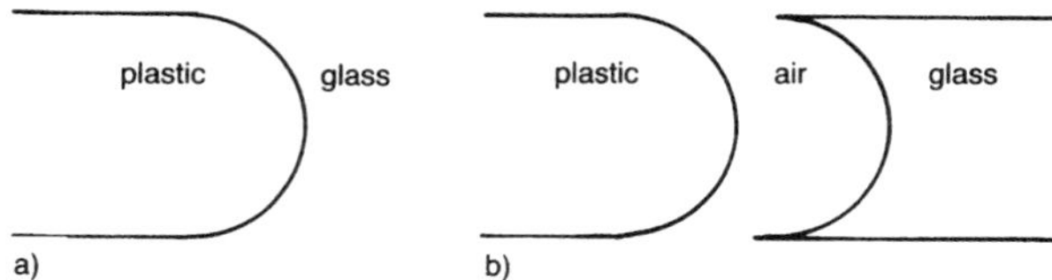

Figure 9.5 a, Plastic–glass spherical interface; b, exploded system.

calculate the powers in the exploded system. However, since the curvature is unchanged, we can also use Eqs. 9.4 and 9.5.

The old interface is between plastic and the high index glass. In the exploded system, the first new interface is between plastic and air, so

$$P_1 = P_{\text{new}} = \frac{1.00 - 1.44}{1.74 - 1.44}(-2.00\,\text{D})$$
$$= \frac{-44}{+30}(-2.00\,\text{D}) = +2.93\,\text{D}$$

In the exploded system, the second new interface is between air and high index glass. So,

$$P_2 = P_{\text{new}} = \frac{1.74 - 1.00}{1.74 - 1.44}(-2.00\,\text{D})$$
$$= \frac{+74}{+30}(-2.00\,\text{D}) = -4.93\,\text{D}$$

The exploded system consists of a +2.93 D plastic–air interface separated by a thin air layer from a −4.93 D air–glass interface. As a check, the sum should equal the original dioptric power:

$$P_s = P_1 + P_2 = +2.93\,\text{D} + (-4.93\,\text{D}) = -2.00\,\text{D}$$

which agrees.

9.7 CONTACT LENSES

Knowledge of the eye's far point enables us to calculate the vergence U_{fp} of light in air incident on the cornea that results in a clear retinal image. A spectacle lens correction sits in the air in front of the eye and has a back vertex power that gives the proper U_{fp} value. However, a contact lens correction sits on the cornea and wipes out the air–corneal interface. Nevertheless, we can use the exploded system concept and consider a thin layer of air (perhaps one molecular layer thick) between the contact lens and the cornea. This enables us to continue to use the U_{fp} information in the same manner as it is used for spectacle lenses.

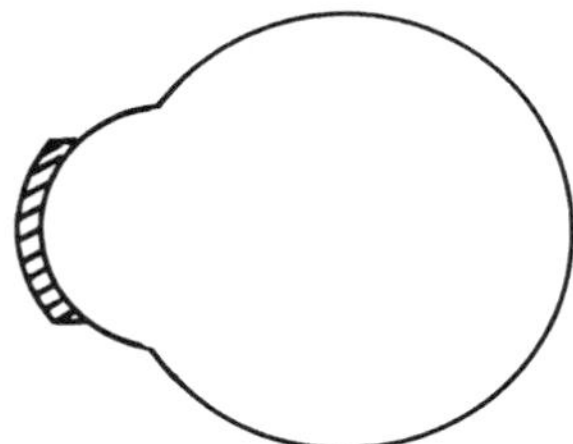

Figure 9.6 Contact lens correction.

EXAMPLE 9.9

The eye considered in Section 9.5 was a 7.19 D ocular myope, so U_{fp} equals −7.19 D. The cornea was a +47.00 D spherical refracting interface between air and the aqueous humor (n = 1.336). Consider a TransAir (n = 1.475) Rigid Gas Permeable (RGP) contact lens that has the same back surface radius of curvature as the cornea and a central thickness of 0.2 mm (Figure 9.6). What must the front surface power of the contact lens be?

The radius of curvature of the cornea is

$$r = \frac{n_2 - n_1}{P}$$
$$= \frac{(1.336 - 1.000)1000\,\text{mm/m}}{+47.00\,\text{D}}$$
$$= \frac{336}{+47.00\,\text{D}} = +7.15\,\text{mm}$$

Thus, the back surface of the contact lens has a radius of curvature of +7.15 mm. The back surface of the contact lens is a diverging surface in air. In the exploded system, the contact lens has a back surface power of

$$P = \frac{(1.00 - 1.475)1000\,\text{mm/m}}{+7.15\,\text{mm}}$$
$$= \frac{-475}{+7.15} = -66.43\,\text{D}$$

Contact lenses have large surface powers, so we expect a significant vergence change across the interior of the contact lens. For plane waves incident on the front of the contact lens, we want light of vergence −7.19 D coming out the back (in the exploded system). If we reverse the light, we then have light of vergence +7.19 D incident on the back surface of the contact lens and

$$V_1 = P_1 + U_1$$
$$= -66.43\,\text{D} + (+7.19\,\text{D}) = -59.24\,\text{D}$$
$$\bar{v}_1 = \frac{1000\,\text{mm/m}}{-59.24\,\text{D}} = -16.88\,\text{mm}$$

The reduced central thickness of the contact lens is

$$\bar{d} = \frac{0.20\,\text{mm}}{1.475} = 0.14\,\text{mm}$$

Then,

$$\bar{u}_2 = -(16.88 + 0.14)\,\text{mm} = -17.02\,\text{mm}$$

$$U_2 = \frac{1000}{-17.02\,\text{mm}} = -58.75\,\text{D}$$

Note that the vergence changed by 0.49 D (i.e., the difference between 59.24 D and 58.75 D) across the interior of the contact lens. Light of vergence −58.75 D is incident on the front surface of the contact lens, and plane waves must leave. Therefore, the front surface power must be +58.75 D. The radius of curvature of the front surface of the contact lens is

$$r = \frac{(1.475 - 1.00)1000}{+58.75\,\text{D}} = \frac{475}{+58.75\,\text{D}} = +8.09\,\text{mm}$$

EXAMPLE 9.10

A +9.25 D ocular hyperope has a cornea with a radius of curvature of 7.8 mm. A Boston 7 ($n = 1.429$) RGP contact lens has the same back surface radius of curvature as the cornea and a central thickness of 0.4 mm. What is the front surface radius of the distance vision contact correction?

First, explode the system. The back surface (diverging) power in the exploded system is

$$P = \frac{(1.000 - 1.429)1000}{+7.8\,\text{mm}} = \frac{-429}{+7.8\,\text{mm}} = -55.00\,\text{D}$$

The light emerging from the back surface in the exploded system should have a vergence of +9.25 D. (In other words the back vertex power P_v of the contact lens in air is +9.25 D). Now reverse the light. Then,

$$V_1 = P_1 + U_1$$
$$= -55.00\,\text{D} + (-9.25\,\text{D}) = -64.25\,\text{D}$$
$$\bar{v} = \frac{1000}{-64.25\,\text{D}} = -15.56\,\text{mm}$$

The reduced central thickness of the contact lens is

$$\bar{d} = \frac{0.40\,\text{mm}}{1.429} = 0.28\,\text{mm}$$

Then,

$$\bar{u}_2 = -(15.56 + 0.28)\,\text{mm} = -15.84\,\text{mm}$$

$$U_2 = \frac{1000}{-15.84\,\text{mm}} = -63.13\,\text{D}$$

Note that the vergence changed by 1.12 D across the interior of the contact lens, which is a clinically significant amount. Light of vergence −63.13 D is incident on the front surface of the contact lens, and plane waves must leave. Therefore, the front surface power must be +63.13 D. The radius of curvature of the front surface of the contact lens is then

$$r = \frac{(1.429 - 1.00)1000}{+63.13\,\text{D}} = \frac{429}{+63.13\,\text{D}} = +6.80\,\text{mm}$$

9.8 THE TEAR LENS EFFECT

Figure 9.7a shows a Rigid Gas Permeable (RGP) contact lens that has a back surface steeper (curved more) than the cornea. This fit creates a gap between the back of the contact lens and the cornea, and the gap fills up with tear fluid. The tears must now be taken into account in determining the correction. In an exploded system, the tears act like a converging lens (Figure 9.7b). In particular, the back vertex power P_v of the contact lens plus the tear lens power P_{tears} equals U_{fp}, which is the patient's Rx at the cornea:

$$\text{Rx} = P_v + P_{tears} \tag{9.7}$$

When a RGP contact lens has a back surface that is flatter than the cornea, the tears act like a minus lens in the exploded system (Figures 9.7c and d). For a contact lens fit with the same curvature as the cornea, the tears act like a thin plano lens (which is why we did not consider the tears in Section 9.7).

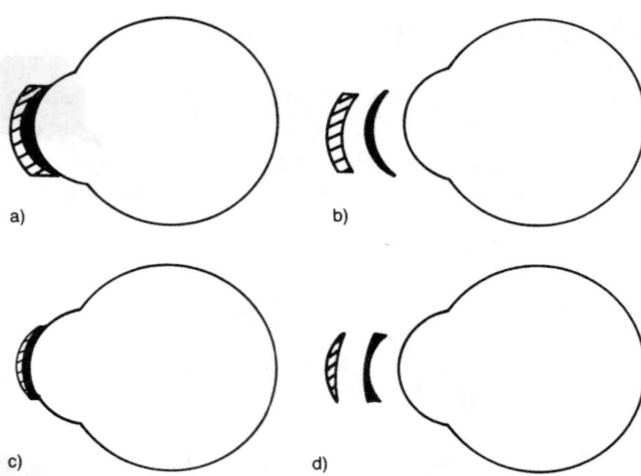

Figure 9.7 a, Tears (black) for minus contact lens that is fit steep; b, exploded system; c, tears (black) for a plus contact lens fit flat; d, exploded system.

EXAMPLE 9. 11

The patient in Example 9.10 was a 9.25 D ocular hyperope and had a cornea with a radius of curvature of 7.80 mm. When a RGP contact lens was fit with a back surface curvature that matched that of the cornea, the back vertex power of the contact lens was +9.25 D. Now suppose that a Boston ES ($n = 1.443$) RGP contact lens is fit with a back surface radius of 7.40 mm (Figure 9.8a). What back vertex power should be ordered for the contact lens? (That is, what should the back vertex power of the contact lens be in air?)

Since the back surface of the contact lens does not have the same curvature as the cornea, we need to take the tear layer into account. Assume the tears have a refractive index of 1.337. From Figure 9.8b, the tears act like a converging lens in the exploded system. The tear's front surface radius of curvature is 7.40 mm and the back surface radius is 7.80 mm. The surface powers of the tear lens in the exploded system are:

$$P_A = \frac{(1.337 - 1.000)1000}{+7.40\,\text{mm}} = \frac{337}{+7.40} = +45.54\,\text{D}$$

$$P_B = \frac{(1.000 - 1.337)1000}{+7.80\,\text{mm}} = \frac{-337}{+7.8} = -43.21\,\text{D}$$

The thin lens power of the tears is

$$P_t = +45.54\,\text{D}(-43.21\,\text{D}) = +2.34\,\text{D}$$

The patient's Rx is +9.25 D, so from Eq. 9.7,

$$P_v = +9.25\,\text{D} - (+2.34\,\text{D}) = +6.91\,\text{D}$$

The effect of the tear layer is to change the needed back vertex power of the contact lens in air. The patient is a 9.25 D ocular hyperope, but the tear lens corrects 2.34 D of the hyperopia. So the back vertex power of the contact lens in air needs only to be +6.91 D. (Clinically this would be rounded to the nearest quarter-diopter).

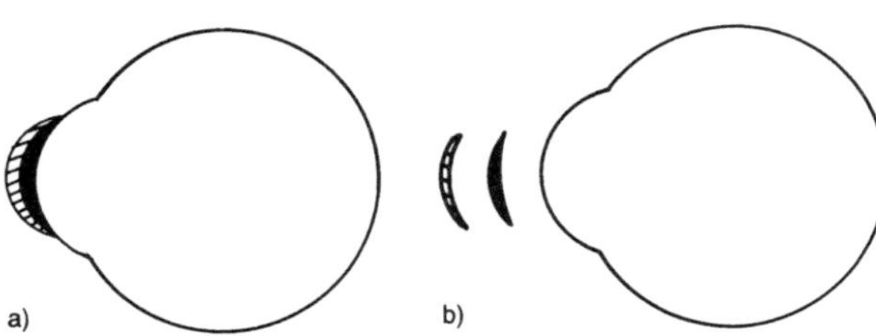

Figure 9.8 a, Tears (black) for a plus contact lens fit steep; b, exploded system.

EXAMPLE 9.12

Suppose the same 9.25 D ocular hyperope is fit with a Boston ES ($n = 1.443$) RGP contact lens that has a back surface radius of 8.00 mm. Now the back surface is flatter than the cornea (radius 7.8 mm), so in the exploded system, the tear lens acts like a diverging lens (Figure 9.7d). What back vertex power should be ordered for the contact lens? (That is, what should the back vertex power of the contact lens be in air?)

In the exploded system, the front surface power of the tear lens is

$$P_A = \frac{(1.337 - 1.000)1000}{+8.0\,\text{mm}} = \frac{337}{+8.0} = +42.13\,\text{D}$$

The cornea did not change, so the back surface power of the tear lens is the same as the previous example, or −43.21 D. The thin lens power of the tears is

$$P_t = +42.13\,\text{D} + (-43.21\,\text{D}) = -1.09\,\text{D}$$

The patient's Rx is +9.25 D, so from Eq. 9.7,

$$P_v = +9.25\,\text{D} - (-1.09\,\text{D}) = +10.34\,\text{D}$$

The effect of the tear layer is to change the needed back vertex power of the contact lens in air. The patient is a 9.25 D ocular hyperope, but the tears act like a −1.09 D lens. The contact lens must have additional plus power to overcome the tears as well as to correct the hyperopia.

9.9 NEWTON'S EQUATIONS

The single spherical refracting interface is the fundamental building block for the paraxial analysis of spherical refracting systems. The (reduced) vergence equation for a spherical system was heavily used by Allvar Gullstrand (1862–1930). The corresponding image distance–object distance equation was first introduced by Karl Gauss (1777–1855). There is an alternate formulation of the optics of an SSRI that is due to Issac Newton (1642–1727). The alternate analysis is as follows.

Figure 9.9 shows a paraxial ray parallel to the optical axis incident on a spherical interface. At the interface, the ray is bent down and passes through the secondary focal point and then on to the image position. The directed distance from the secondary focal

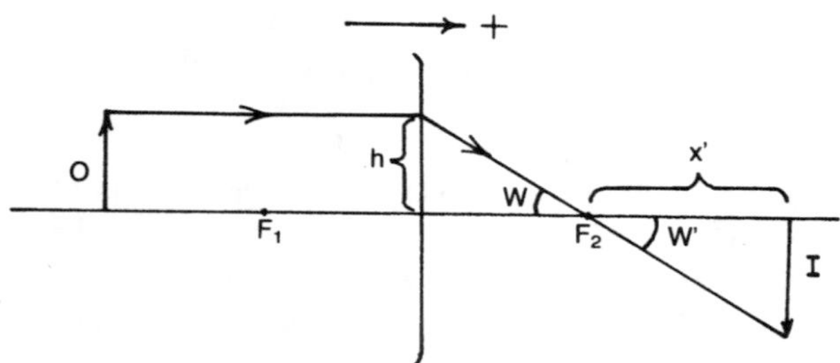

Figure 9.9 Ray giving x' dependence.

point to the image is called the *extra-focal image length* and is labeled x′. The incident ray hits the surface at a distance h from the axis, but since the incident ray is parallel to the axis, h equals the object size O. Since the angles labeled w and w' are equal, it is easily shown from the tangents of the angles that

$$\frac{-I}{x'} = \frac{O}{f_2}$$

Since the lateral magnification $m = I/O$, it follows that

$$m = -\frac{x'}{f_2} \tag{9.8}$$

Figure 9.10 shows a similar drawing for the object space ray that passes through the primary focal point. The directed distance from the primary focal point to the object is called the *extra-focal object length* and is labeled x. The ray leaves the surface a distance h from the axis, but since this ray is parallel to the axis, h is equal to the image size I. Since the ray angles w and w' at the primary focal point are equal, it follows from the tangents that

$$\frac{-I}{-f_1} = \frac{O}{-x}$$

and then

$$m = -\frac{f_1}{x} \tag{9.9}$$

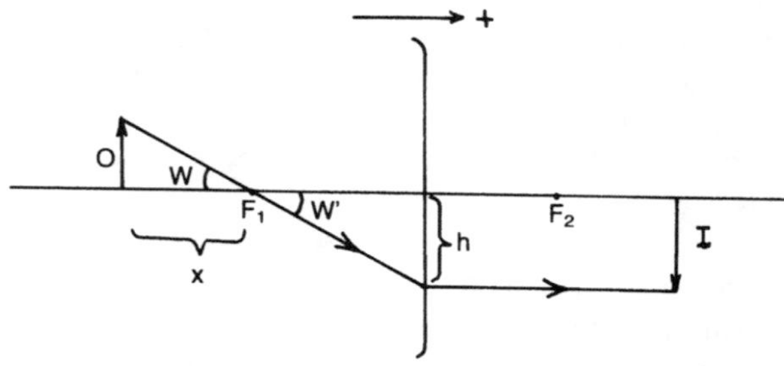

Figure 9.10 Ray giving x dependence.

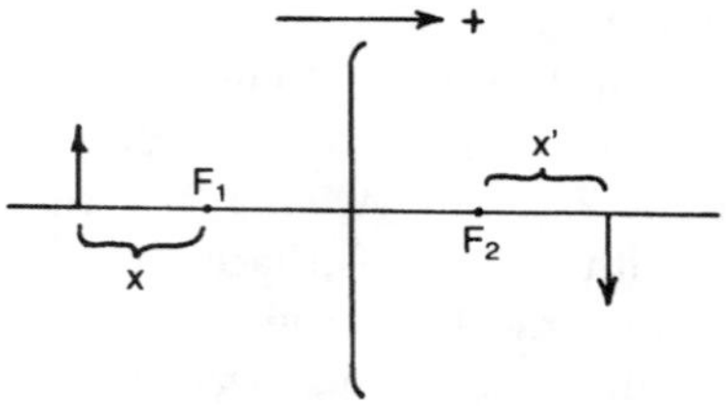

Figure 9.11 Newton's parameters. The real object is a distance x left of F_1, and the conjugate real image is a distance x' right of F_2.

We can set the right hand sides of Eqs. 9.8 and 9.9 equal to each other and obtain

$$xx' = f_1 f_2 \tag{9.10}$$

Equation 9.10 is called Newton's equation.

EXAMPLE 9.13

A real object in air is 45 cm in front of an air–glass ($n = 1.50$) interface. The primary focal length of the system is −20 cm, and the secondary focal length is +30 cm (Figure 9.11). Use Newton's equation to find the image, and then find the lateral magnification m.

The object is 25 cm in front of F_1, so the extra-focal distance x is −25 cm. Then from Eq. 9.10,

$$(-25\,\text{cm})x' = (-20\,\text{cm})(+30\,\text{cm})$$
$$x' = +24\,\text{cm}$$

The image is 24 cm past F_2. (An image at that position must be real.)

From Eq. 9.8,

$$m = -\frac{x'}{f_2} = -\left(\frac{+24\,\text{cm}}{+30\,\text{cm}}\right) = -0.8$$

Equation 9.9 could also be used for m. You should check the above results with the $V = P + U$ equations.

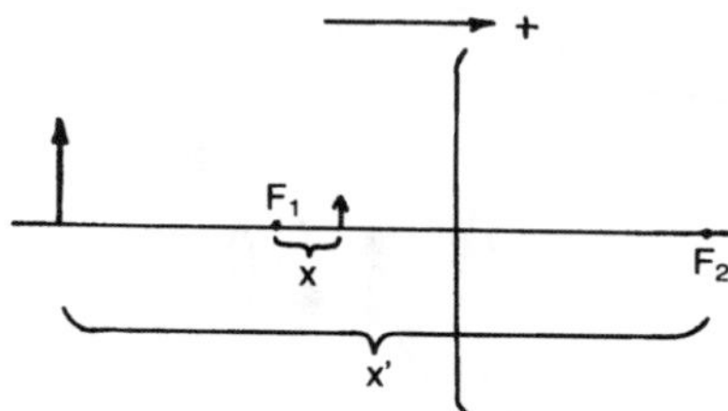

Figure 9.12 Newton's parameters. The real object is a distance x right of F_1, and the conjugate virtual image is a distance x' left of F_2.

EXAMPLE 9.14

The real object in the previous example is moved in to 15 cm in front of the interface. Figure 9.12 shows the situation for light traveling to the right. Use Newton's equation to find the image, and then find the lateral magnification.

The object is now 5 cm past F_1, so the extra focal distance x is +5 cm. Then from Eq. 9.10,

$$(+5\text{ cm})x' = (-20\text{ cm})(+30\text{ cm})$$
$$x' = -120\text{ cm}$$

The image is 120 cm to the left of F_2, or 90 cm to the left of the interface. (An image at that position must be virtual.)

From Eq. 9.9,

$$m = -\frac{f_1}{x} = -\left(\frac{-20\text{ cm}}{+5\text{ cm}}\right) = +4.0$$

Equation 9.8 could also be used for m. Again, you should check the above results with the $V = P + U$ equations.

The primary focal length can be eliminated from Newton's equation. From Eq. 7.23,

$$f_1 = -\frac{n_1 f_2}{n_2}$$

We can substitute the above result into Eq. 9.10 to obtain

$$\left(\frac{x}{n_1}\right)\left(\frac{x'}{n_2}\right) = -\left(\frac{f_2}{n_2}\right)^2 \qquad (9.11)$$

Newton's equation can also be derived for a thin lens in air. There, n_1 and n_2 are both equal to 1.00, and Newton's equation simplifies to

$$xx' = -(f_2)^2 \qquad (9.12)$$

EXAMPLE 9.15

A real object in air is located 18 cm in front of a diverging thin lens with a secondary focal length of −12 cm. Use Newton's equation to find the image, and then find the lateral magnification.

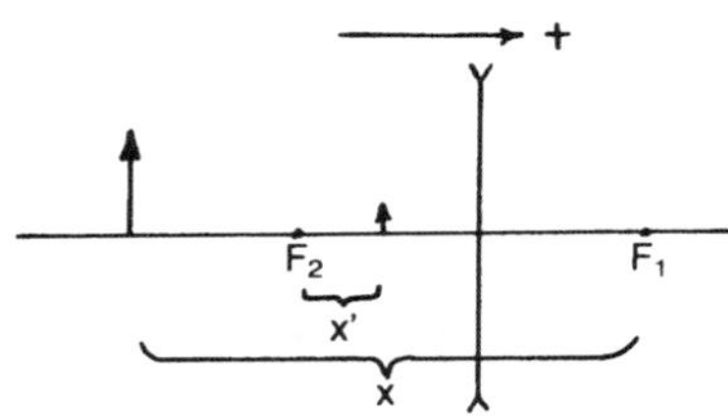

Figure 9.13 Newton's parameter for a diverging lens. The real object is a distance x left of F_1, and the conjugate virtual image is a distance x' right of F_2.

Figure 9.13 shows the diagram for light traveling to the right. The object is 30 cm to the left of F_1, so x is −30 cm. From Eq. 9.12,

$$(-30\text{ cm})\,x' = -(-12\text{ cm})^2$$
$$x' = +4.8\text{ cm}$$

The image is located 4.8 cm to the right of F_2, or 7.2 cm to the left of the lens. (An image at this location must be virtual.) From Eq. 9.8,

$$m = -\frac{x'}{f_2} = -\frac{+4.8\text{ cm}}{-12\text{ cm}} = +0.40$$

Newton's equation can also be written in terms of (reduced) vergences. For an SSRI, the vergence X of the incident wavefront at F_1, is given by

$$X = \frac{n_1}{x} \qquad (9.13)$$

while the vergence X' of the outgoing wavefront at F_2 is given by

$$X' = \frac{n_2}{x'} \qquad (9.14)$$

Then from Eqs. 9.10, 7.21, and 7.22,

$$XX' = -P^2 \qquad (9.15)$$

EXAMPLE 9.16

Rework Example 9.13 using Eq. 9.15.

In Example 9.13, $n_1 = 1.00$ and $n_2 = 1.50$. The secondary focal length of the interface is +30 cm, and the dioptric power of the interface is

$$P = \frac{n_2}{f_2} = \frac{150}{+30\text{ cm}} = +5.00\text{ D}$$

From Example 9.13, x is −25 cm. The object is then 25 cm in front of F_1, and the vergence X of the wavefront at F_1 is

$$X = \frac{(1.00)100\text{ cm/m}}{-25\text{ cm}} = -4.00\text{ D}$$

From Eq. 9.15,

$$X' = \frac{-P^2}{X} = \frac{-(+5.00\text{ D})^2}{-4.00\text{ D}}$$
$$= \frac{-25.00}{-4.00} = +6.25\text{ D}$$

The wavefront at F_2 is converging, and a real image is located a distance x' from F_2, where

$$x' = \frac{n_2}{X'} = \frac{(1.50)100\text{ cm/m}}{+6.25\text{ D}}$$
$$= \frac{150}{+6.25} = +24\text{ cm}$$

9.10 AXIAL MAGNIFICATION

Consider a convex SSRI with a real object at A and its conjugate real image at A', and a second real object at B with its conjugate real image at B'. The axial distance between the images at B' and A' is different than the axial distance between the objects at B and A. The axial magnification Ω is a measure of the axial image separation compared to the axial object separation. The concept of axial magnification applies only when both images are of the same type (i.e., either both real or both virtual) and when both objects are of the same type (i.e., either both real or both virtual). For real objects, the images can be either real or virtual, and similarly for virtual objects. Mathematically,

$$\Omega \equiv \frac{v_B - v_A}{u_B - u_A} \tag{9.16}$$

It is easy to show that the above equation is a simplified version of

$$\Omega = \left(\frac{v_B n_1}{u_B n_2}\right)\left(\frac{v_A n_1}{u_A n_2}\right)\left(\frac{n_2}{n_1}\right)\frac{\left(\frac{n_2}{v_A} - \frac{n_2}{v_B}\right)}{\left(\frac{n_1}{u_A} - \frac{n_1}{u_B}\right)}$$

From Eq. 7.29, the first bracket on the left side is the lateral magnification m_A for the object at A and the second bracket is the lateral magnification m_B for the object at B. Then from the vergence equations 7.17 and 7.18,

$$\Omega = m_B m_A \left(\frac{n_2}{n_1}\right)\frac{(V_A - V_B)}{(U_A - U_B)}$$

From $V = P + U$, the end bracket on the right side equals +1, so

$$\Omega = m_B m_A \left(\frac{n_2}{n_1}\right) \tag{9.17}$$

Equation 9.17 shows that the axial magnification for a SSRI is equal to the product of the respective lateral magnifications times the ratio of the image space index n_2 to the object space index n_1.

EXAMPLE 9.17

Consider a +10.00 D SSRI between air and glass of index 1.80. One real object (A) is 15 cm from the interface, while a second real object (B) is 12.5 cm from the interface. What is the axial magnification?

To check for consistency, we will calculate the axial magnification Ω both from the derived equation (9.17) and from the definition (Eq. 9.16). For this situation: $n_1 = 1.00$ and $n_2 = 1.80$. From $V = P + U$ and $m = U/V$, the respective image distances and magnifications are:

$$v_A = +54.0\,\text{cm} \quad \text{and} \quad m_A = -2$$
$$v_B = +90.0\,\text{cm} \quad \text{and} \quad m_B = -4$$

From Eq. 9.17,

$$\Omega = (-2)(-4)(1.80) = 14.40$$

From the definition (Eq. 9.16),

$$\Omega \equiv \frac{90\,\text{cm} - 54\,\text{cm}}{-12.5\,\text{cm} - (-15\,\text{cm})} = 14.40$$

and the two results agree.

In those situations where the objects are very close together (i.e., B is very close to A), Eq. 9.17 effectively simplifies to

$$\Omega = m^2\left(\frac{n_2}{n_1}\right) \tag{9.18}$$

where m is the lateral magnification for the object distance A. (Technically Eq. 9.18 is accurate in the limit of B going to A).

A similar derivation shows that that for a thin lens in air, Eqs. 9.17 and 9.18 give the axial magnification Ω provided both n_1 and n_2 are set equal to 1. Thus for a thin lens in air, the axial magnification Ω for objects at A and B equals the product of the lateral magnifications m_B and m_A. If the objects are very close together, then the axial magnification Ω for a thin lens in air effectively equals the square of the lateral magnification. As an example, for a real object 25.0 cm from a +12.00 D thin lens in air, the conjugate image is real, 12.5 cm from the lens, and the lateral magnification m is −0.50. For a second object very close to the first one, the axial magnification Ω is effectively $(-0.50)^2$, which is 0.25. In other words, the images are only 1/4 as far apart as the objects are.

PROBLEMS

1. A thin meniscus-convex polycarbonate ($n = 1.58$) lens has surfaces with radii of curvature of 9.0 cm and 6.0 cm, respectively. What is the dioptric power of the lens?
2. A thin meniscus-concave highlite glass ($n = 1.71$) lens has surfaces with 12.0 cm, and 8.0 cm, respective radii of curvature. What is the dioptric power of the lens?
3. A thin biconvex ophthalmic crown ($n = 1.523$) lens has radii of curvature of 16 cm and 25 cm, respectively. What is the dioptric power of the lens?

4. A thick ophthalmic crown ($n = 1.523$) lens has a front surface power of +12.00 D and a back surface power of −4.00 D. The central thickness is 5.0 cm. Find the back vertex power and the neutralizing power of the lens.
5. A thick plastic ($n = 1.49$) lens has a +5.00 D front surface and a −12.00 D back surface. The central thickness is 6.0 cm. Find the back vertex power and the neutralizing power.
6. A thick lens has a +4.00 D back surface power and a +7.00 D back vertex power. Find the back focal length for the lens.
7. A thick lens has a +5.00 D front surface power and a −3.00 D neutralizing power. What vergence must the incident wavefront have in order to get plane waves leaving the back of the lens? Find the primary focal point of the lens.
8. A thick lens has a +8.00 D neutralizing power and a +10.00 D back vertex power. What thin lens held against the back of the thick lens will neutralize it? (Plane waves out for plane waves in.)
9. Dr Fred Pepper is a 7.00 D ocular myope with a spherical cornea of radius of curvature 8.20 mm. Dr Pepper is fit with a contact lens that has a back surface radius of 8.20 mm. What is the front surface power and radius if the contact lens central thickness is 0.30 mm and it has a 1.49 index?
10. Maribell Maple is a 4.50 D ocular myope. Maribell's cornea has a 7.00 mm radius of curvature. Maribell is fit with a contact lens ($n = 1.49$) of back surface radius 7.20 mm. What back vertex power must the contact lens have in air? (Assume 1.333 is the refractive index of Maribell's tears.)
11. Baron Smith is a 3.50 D ocular hyperope. The baron's cornea has a 7.60 mm radius of curvature and the baron is fit with a contact lens ($n = 1.49$) of back surface radius of 7.90 mm. What back vertex power must the contact lens have in air? (Assume 1.333 is the refractive index of the baron's tears.)
12. Sugar Brains is a 4.25 D ocular hyperope. Sugar's cornea has a 7.50 mm radius of curvature. Sugar is fit with a contact lens ($n = 1.49$) with a back surface radius of 7.35 mm. What back vertex power must the contact lens have in air? (Assume 1.333 is the refractive index of Sugar's tears.)
13. Represent the cornea of an eye by a +45.00 D SSRI between air and the ocular media ($n = 1.336$). Represent the crystalline lens as a +20.00 D thin lens between the aqueous and vitreous humor ($n = 1.336$ each). The distance from the cornea to the crystalline lens is 4.0 mm, and the distance from the cornea to the retina is 20.0 mm. Where is the far point for this eye? Is it real or virtual? What correction is needed at the cornea?
14. A +14.00 D thin glass ($n = 1.523$) trial lens is placed underwater ($n = 1.33$). What is the power of the lens while underwater?
15. An SSRI between water ($n = 1.33$) and glass ($n = 1.73$) has a real object in water and a real image in glass at a distance of 20.0 cm from the secondary focal point. If the image is two times larger than the object, what is the dioptric power of the interface?
16. An SSRI between glass ($n = 1.61$) and air has a real object in glass at a distance of 13 cm from the primary focal point and a real image in air at a distance of 35 cm from the secondary focal point. What is the dioptric power of the interface?
17. A spherical concave ophthalmic crown ($n = 1.523$) surface is held against a convex spherical barium crown ($n = 1.617$) surface. The dioptric power of the barium crown–ophthalmic crown interface is +2.00 D. If the surfaces are slightly separated so that a thin air gap exists between them, what is the dioptric power of the air–ophthalmic crown interface, and what is the dioptric power of the air–barium crown interface? What is the sum of these two powers?
18. Given: Neil Deluded's eye has a +46.00 D cornea (represented as an SSRI between air and the cornea). For simplicity, let 1.336 be the refractive index of the cornea, aqueous humor, and vitreous humor. Deluded's crystalline lens (represented as a thin lens) is located 4 mm behind the cornea, and the retina is 17.48 mm behind the crystalline lens. Deluded is a 3.00 D ocular hyperope. Problem: Deluded's crystalline lens has developed cataracts and needs to be removed. In this case, it is desirable for the ophthalmologist to implant a new Intra-Ocular Lens (IOL) lens that is clear and also makes Deluded emmetropic. Treat the IOL as a thin lens of index 1.475. What is the dioptric power in the eye of the desired IOL? What is the dioptric power in air of this IOL?

CHAPTER 10

Astigmatism: On Axis

10.1 INTRODUCTION

The paraxial optics of spherical systems is built on the concept of point objects and conjugate point images. The latin word *stigmatus* means point, and systems that form point images are sometimes called *stigmatic* systems. An *astigmatic* system (''a''= not, ''*stigmatus*'' = point) forms line images instead of point images.

Astigmatism is quite common in the human eye. In some groups, over 80% of the people have some astigmatism. Astigmatism is optically corrected by cylindrical or spherocylindrical lenses.

This chapter deals with the on-axis or principal meridians of astigmatism. Chapter 13 deals with the off-axis or non-principal meridians.

10.2 CYLINDRICAL LENSES

Figure 10.1 shows a cylinder. Geometrically, we can generate a cylinder by taking two parallel lines, and rotating one around the other while maintaining the parallelism. The line that serves as the center of the rotation is called the *axis* of the cylinder. Each point on the cylinder's surface is equidistant from the axis.

A point on the line that is rotating traces out a circle around the axis. The radius of this circle is the distance from the point to the axis. A cylinder is flat along any meridian parallel to the axis, and has a circular cross section along any meridian perpendicular to the axis. For a cylindrical refracting or reflecting surface, the flat meridian is referred to as the *axis meridian*, and the perpendicular meridian with the circular cross section is referred to as the *power meridian*. The axis meridian and the power meridian are the *principal meridians* of the cylindrical surface.

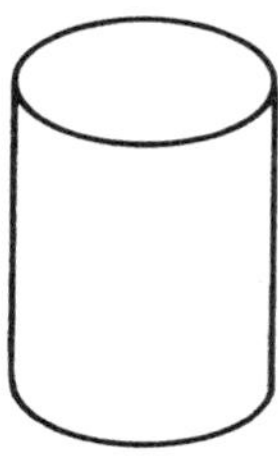

Figure 10.1 A cylinder with a vertical axis.

Figure 10.2 shows a series of lenses made with cylindrical and/or flat surfaces. The cylindrical lenses each have an axis meridian and a perpendicular power meridian. We can identify the axis meridian by the flat meridian on the cylindrical surfaces. The power meridian is the meridian in which the cylindrical surfaces have circular cross sections.

A real cylinder (such as a soft drink can, a roll of toilet paper, a sheet of paper rolled up to form a cylinder, etc.) helps in visualizing the three dimensional aspects of cylindrical lens optics. Imagine plane waves from a distant point source incident normally on a soft drink can with a vertical axis (as in Figure 10.1). If the can was a cylindrical lens, the plano vertical axis meridian would not provide any dioptric power to refract (bend) the wave vertically (up or down). However, the horizontal power meridian would refract (bend) the wave horizontally (left or right). In the paraxial region, this would result in a cylindrical wavefront leaving the lens (Figure 10.3). The cylindrical wavefronts, converging in the horizontal meridian, form a real vertical *line image* that coincides with the axis of the cylindrical wavefronts.

Figure 10.4a shows a planoconvex cylindrical lens with a vertical axis meridian and a horizontal power meridian. In order to analyze the ray behavior, we divide the lens into a series of thin horizontal segments (Figure 10.4b). The front surface of each horizontal segment is a cross section of the power meridian and has a circular shape. Each segment's back surface is flat.

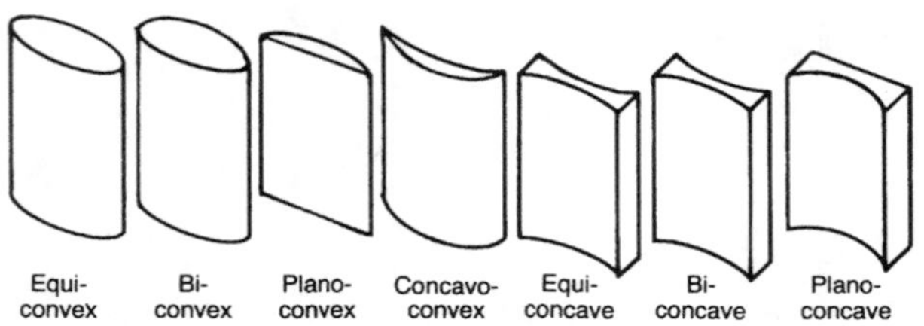

Figure 10.2 Cylindrical lenses.

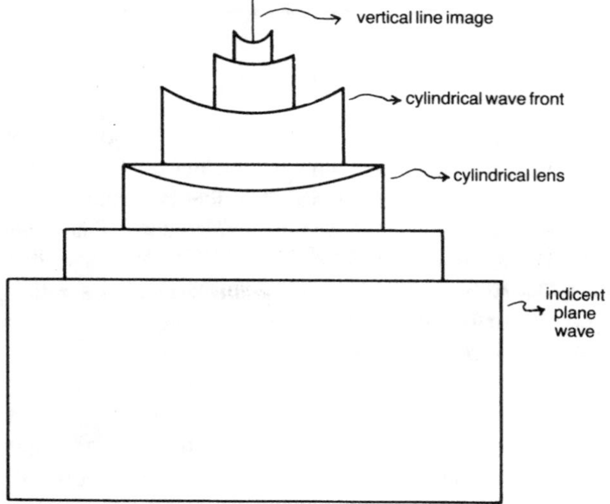

Figure 10.3 Wavefronts passing through a cylindrical lens.

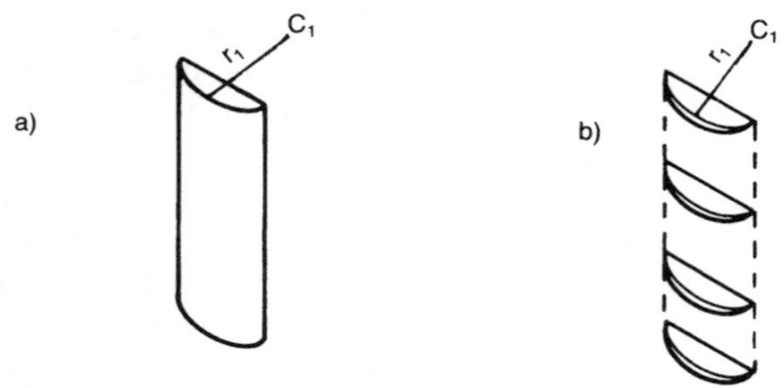

Figure 10.4 a, Power meridian curvature; b, sections of a cylindrical lens.

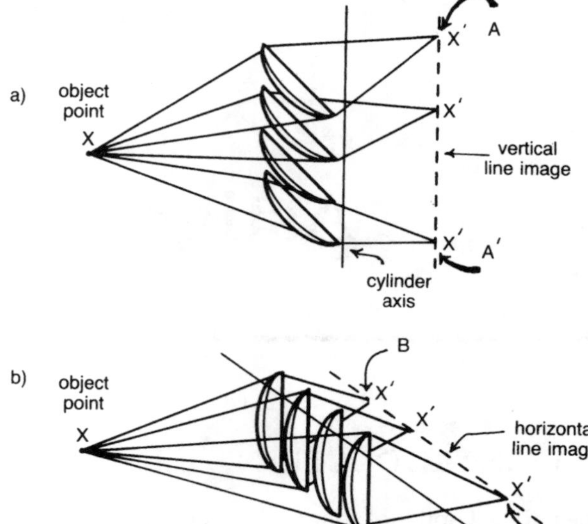

Figure 10.5 a, Line Image formation by section-vertical axis meridian; b, line image formation by section-horizontal axis meridian.

Figure 10.5a shows incident rays coming from a near object point. The thin top segment does not change the vertical angle that the rays make with the optical axis, but it does converge the rays horizontally (left or right) and forms a point image at A. The thin bottom segment also does not change the vertical angle that the rays are traveling, but it does converge the rays horizontally and forms a point image at A'. Each thin segment converges the rays only horizontally and forms its own point image (at the respective X' positions). Collectively, all the individual point images make a vertical line image. *Even though the real vertical line image is parallel to the axis meridian, it is the horizontal power meridian that is responsible for the convergence that forms the line.*

Figure 10.5b shows a planoconvex cylindrical lens with a horizontal axis meridian and a vertical power meridian. The lens is segmented vertically along the power meridian. The left thin segment does not change the horizontal angle of the rays, but does converge the rays vertically (up or down) and forms a point image at B. The right thin segment also does not change the horizontal angle of the rays, but converges the rays vertically and forms a point image at B'. Again, each thin segment forms its own point image. Collectively, all the point images form a real horizontal line image. *Note that the vertical power meridian is responsible for the convergence that forms the horizontal line image.*

When the plus cylindrical lens with a vertical axis is rotated clockwise toward a horizontal axis, the real vertical line image rotates clockwise with the lens. In particular, *the real line image is always parallel to the axis meridian and perpendicular to the power meridian that forms it.*

In Figure 10.4a, the axis meridian has flat surfaces of zero dioptric power. Since the power meridian of the cylindrical front surface has a circular cross section, its power is given by

$$P_1 = \frac{n_2 - n_1}{r_1} \tag{10.1}$$

where r_1 is the radius of curvature of the power meridian, n_1 is the refractive index of the medium in front of the surface, and n_2 is the refractive index of the lens. Since the back surface is plano, its power P_2 is zero. For a thin cylindrical lens, the total power in the power meridian is

$$P = P_1 + P_2 \tag{10.2}$$

From the power meridian, the location of the line image can be found from

$$V = P + U \tag{10.3}$$

EXAMPLE 10.1

A real point source is located 50 cm in front of a planoconvex cylindrical lens with a horizontal axis meridian and a vertical power meridian. The refractive index of the lens is 1.5, and the cylindrical power meridian's radius of curvature is 10 cm. Where is the real line image? What is its orientation?

For the vertical front surface cylindrical power meridian, Eq. 10.1 gives

$$P_1 = \frac{(1.50 - 1.00)100\,\text{cm/m}}{+10\,\text{cm}} = +5.00\,\text{D}$$

The back surface is plano, so $P_2 = 0$. The incident wavefront is spherical with $U = -2.00$ D. In the power meridian, Eqs. 10.2 and 10.3 give

$$V = +5.00\,\text{D} + (-2.00\,\text{D}) = +3.00\,\text{D}$$

The (real) line image position is

$$v = \frac{100\,\text{cm/m}}{+3.00\,\text{D}} = +33.3\,\text{cm}$$

As discussed in the previous paragraphs, power in the vertical principal meridian forms horizontal lines. One can observe the horizontal line image on a screen 33.3 cm behind the lens.

For a thin cylindrical lens with an object point at the (near) distance u, Figure 10.6a shows the ray behavior in the axis meridian and Figure 10.6b shows the ray behavior in the power meridian. There is no convergence in the axis meridian, and the rays go straight through without bending. The segment shown by the power meridian converges the rays and forms one point (A) on the line image at the distant v from the lens. The line image is perpendicular to the power meridian and lies in (or is parallel to) the axis meridian. Thus the line image itself can be drawn at the distance v in the axis meridian. Figure 10.6a shows that while the axis meridian does not form the line image, it does determine its length. Once the line image position v is determined from the power meridian calculations, the line image length can be determined from the similar triangles in the axis meridian.

EXAMPLE 10.2

A point image is located 25 cm in front of a thin +10.00 D cylindrical lens with a vertical axis meridian. The lens has a round aperture 40 mm in diameter placed against it. What is the location, length, and orientation of the real line image?

The line image is parallel to the axis meridian, or vertical in this case. The incident vergence U is −4.00 D. In the power meridian,

$$V = P + U$$
$$= +10.00\,\text{D} + (-4.00\,\text{D}) = +6.00\,\text{D}$$

and

$$v = +16.67\,\text{cm}$$

which is the location of the vertical line image.

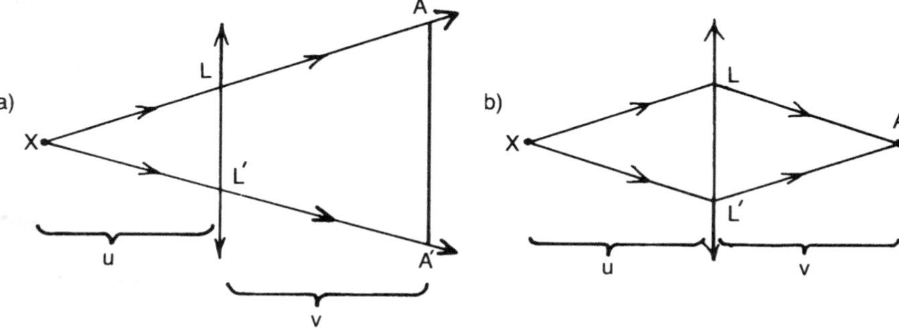

Figure 10.6 Cross-sectional ray diagrams: a, axis meridian; b, power meridian.

The axis meridian (vertical) has a ray diagram just like Figure 10.6a. In Figure 10.6a, the triangle XLL' is similar to the triangle XAA'. Then the line image length AA' is given by the equal base to height ratios:

$$\frac{AA'}{|u| + v} = \frac{LL'}{|u|}$$

The effective lens diameter is 40 mm or 4 cm. So,

$$\frac{AA'}{25\,\text{cm} + 16.67\,\text{cm}} = \frac{4\,\text{cm}}{25\,\text{cm}}$$

and

$$AA' = 6.67\,\text{cm}$$

The line image is 6.67 cm in length.

We can watch the formation of the line image by placing a screen directly behind the lens and then moving the screen toward the line image position. Figure 10.7 shows the cross-sectional illumination patterns that appear on the screen for the lens in the previous example. Initially, the illumination pattern is circular and the same size as the aperture. As the screen is moved back, the illumination pattern gets longer in the vertical meridian (since the vertical meridian is the axis meridian and supplies no convergence), and shorter in the horizontal meridian (since the horizontal meridian is the power meridian that supplies the convergence). The result on the screen is a vertically oriented elliptical blur pattern (paraxial approximation). As the screen is moved farther back, the ellipse continues to grow vertically and to shrink horizontally. The vertical line image occurs at the position where the ellipse has shrunk to a zero horizontal width. As the screen is moved past the line image position, the light starts to diverge in the horizontal meridian, and a vertically oriented blur ellipse again appears. At any position, one can determine the lengths of the major and minor axes of the blur ellipse from the similar triangles in Figures 10.6a and b.

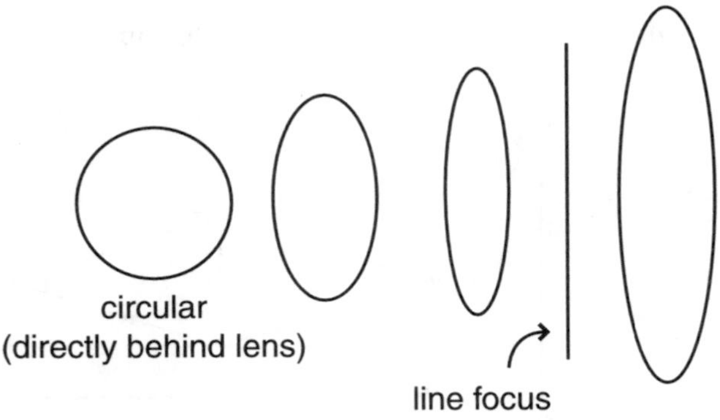

Figure 10.7 Image space illumination patterns for a point source.

It is helpful to analyze the optics of a cylindrical lens in terms of a *power cross*. The power cross shows the dioptric powers of the lens in the two principal meridians. The power cross for the +10.00 D cylinder with a vertical axis meridian has zero power vertically and +10.00 D horizontally:

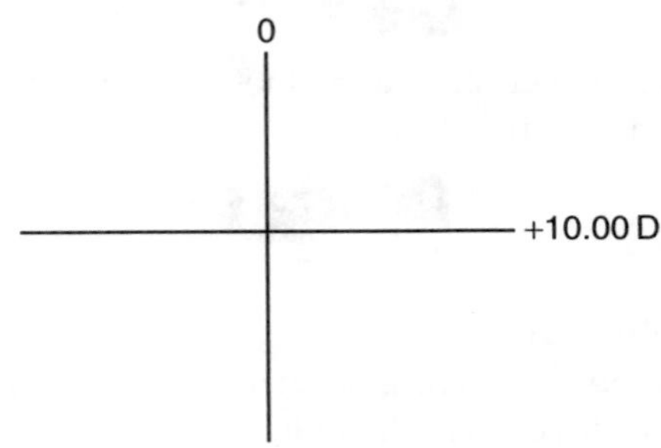

The power cross for a +7.00 D cylindrical lens with a horizontal axis meridian has zero power horizontally and +7.00 D vertically:

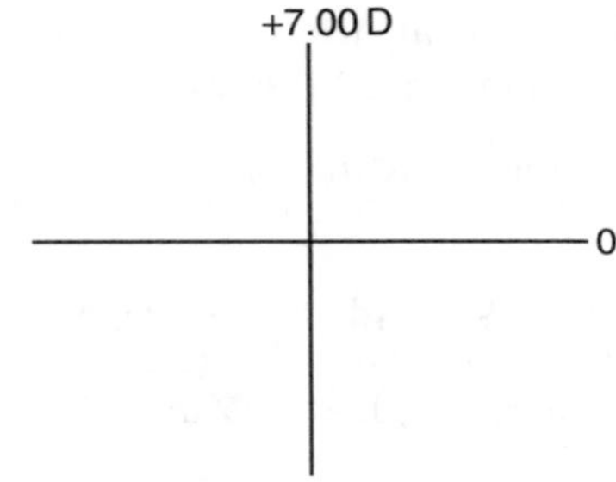

10.3 STANDARD AXIS NOTATION

A spherical lens has rotational symmetry around the optical axis of the lens. In other words, the spherical lens can be rotated clockwise or counter-clockwise around the optical axis with no optical effects. A cylindrical lens does not have rotational symmetry. When the cylindrical lens is rotated clockwise or counter-clockwise, the resulting line image rotates with it. Consequently, when a cylindrical lens is used to correct astigmatism, the orientation of the lens must be specified together with the power.

The coordinate system used to specify the orientation is set up in terms of the examiner's view when looking at the patient (Figure 10.8). This view is the so-called *contra-ocular view* (i.e., against the view of the

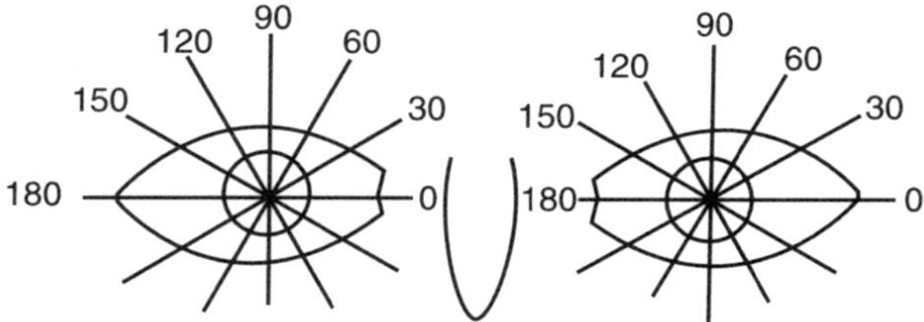

Figure 10.8 Coordinate system for cylinder orientation.

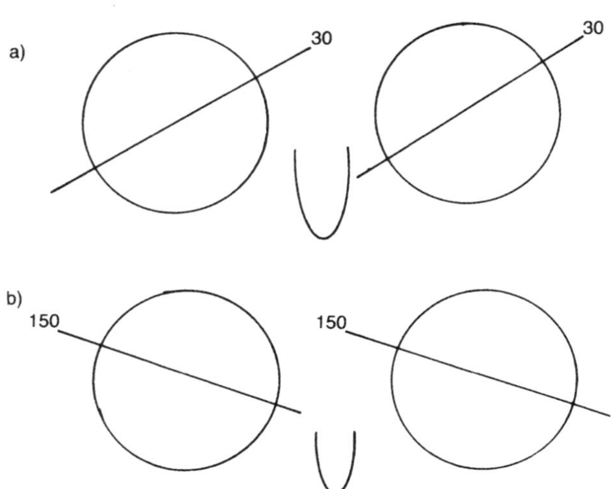

Figure 10.9 a, 30° meridians; b, 150° meridians.

patient's eye). Each meridian could be identified by two different angles. For example, the vertical meridian could be labeled 90 or 270. The degree sign is assumed and not usually written. We use the smaller of the two angles except in the case of the horizontal meridian. The horizontal meridian is labeled as the 180 meridian instead of the 0 meridian. (Zero is not used in order to avoid confusion between a cylindrical lens with a horizontal axis meridian and a spherical lens that does not have an axis meridian.)

As seen by the examiner, the first quadrant angles label the meridians clockwise from the top, and the second quadrant angles label the meridians counterclockwise from the top. Figure 10.9a shows the 30° meridians, while Figure 10.9b shows the 150° meridians.

The conventional way of specifying the orientation of a cylindrical lens is in terms of the axis meridian, although it would have been more logical to do in terms of the power meridian. A +3.00 D cylindrical lens with a vertical axis is labeled:

$$+3.00 \times 90$$

Diopters are assumed for the power and degrees are assumed for the meridian specification. Usually the D and the degree sign are not written. The × stands for the axis meridian, so the above mathematical expression literally stands for a +3.00-D cylindrical lens with an axis meridian of 90°. The expression is typically read: +3 axis 90. The corresponding power cross is

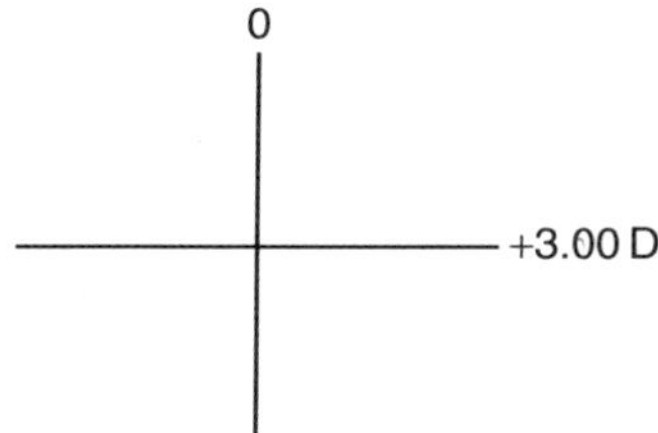

Consider a patient with a +2.00 × 30 lens in front of each eye. In Figure 10.10, the drawing for the patient's left eye shows how the lens would look if made with cylindrical surfaces, and the drawing for the patient's right eye shows the power cross. Figure 10.11 shows a similar case for a +4.50 × 150 lens in front of each eye.

Besides the symbol ×, which represents the axis meridian, the symbol @ is used to specify the power in a principal meridian. For the +3.00 × 90, there is +3.00 D @ 180 and 0 D @ 90. The power cross is a symbolic representation of the same information.

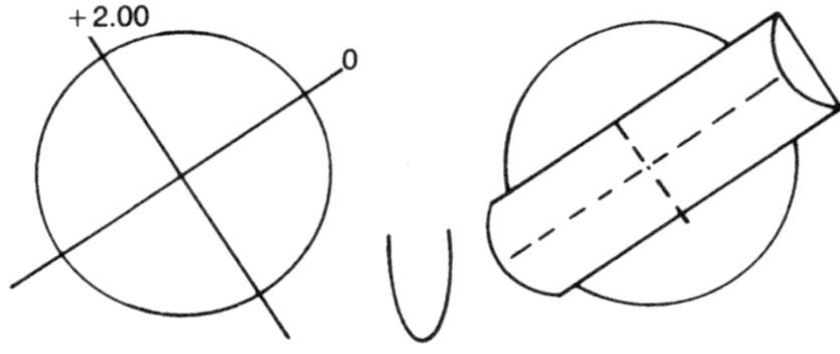

Figure 10.10 +2.00×30 lens in front of patient's left eye. Power cross in front of the right eye.

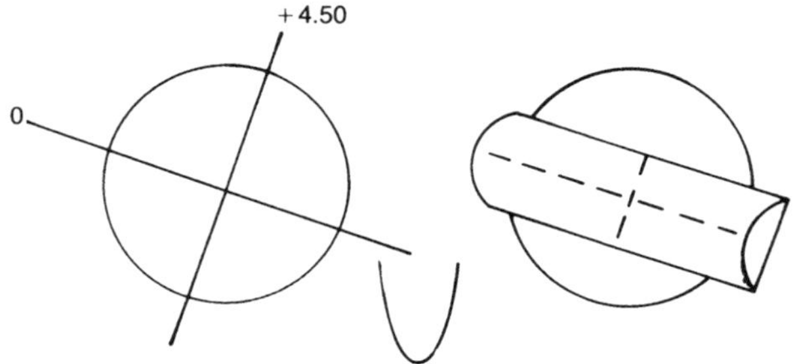

Figure 10.11 Same as previous figure for a +4.50×150.

10.4 PERPENDICULARLY CROSSED CYLINDRICAL LENSES

First consider two thin cylindrical lenses with axis meridians that are aligned. The power meridians are also aligned, and when these lenses are placed in contact with each other, the cylinder power adds. For example, a +3.00 × 60 combined with a +2.00 × 60 is equivalent to a +5.00 × 60. Similarly, a +7.00 × 135 combined with a −3.00 × 135 is equivalent to a +4.00 × 135.

Now consider a case of combining cylindrical lenses with perpendicular axis meridians. Example 10.2 considered a +10.00 D cylindrical lens with a vertical axis meridian (i.e., +10.00 × 90) together with a point source 25 cm in front of the lens. Suppose a +7.00 D cylindrical lens with a horizontal axis meridian (i.e., +7.00 × 180) is placed in contact with the +10.00 D cylindrical lens. The +7.00 × 180 has zero dioptric power in the horizontal meridian. Thus, the total power in the horizontal meridian is provided by the +10.00 × 90. Similarly, the +10.00 × 90 provides zero power in the vertical meridian, and the total power there is provided by the +7.00 × 180.

In terms of the power crosses for the individual lenses, we can add the vertical power of one with the vertical power of the other, and then the horizontal power of one with the horizontal power of the other.

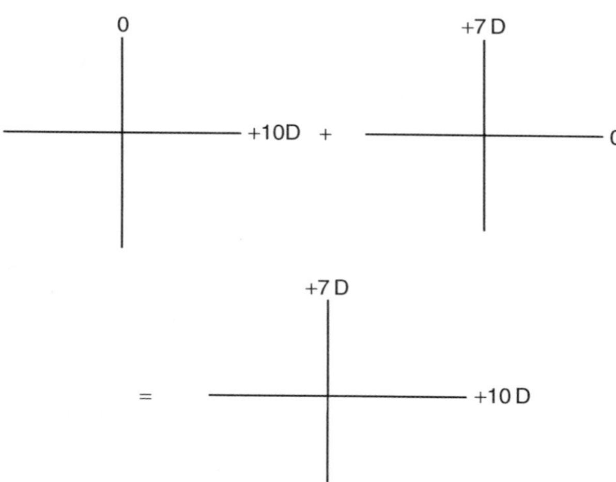

The power cross for the combination has +10.00 D power in the horizontal meridian and +7.00 D power in the vertical meridian.

For a point source 25 cm in front of a +10.00 × 90 lens by itself, a real vertical line image is formed 16.67 cm behind the lens (Example 10.2). When the +7.00 × 180 is combined with the +10.00 × 90, the horizontal power remains +10.00 D and the vertical line image is still formed 16.67 cm behind the lenses.

For a point source 25 cm in front of a +7.00 × 180 lens by itself, the vertical power meridian gives

$$V = P + U = +7.00\,\text{D} + (-4.00\,\text{D}) = +3.00\,\text{D}$$

and a real horizontal line image is formed 33.3 cm, behind the lens. When combined with the +10.00 ×90, the power in the vertical meridian is still +7.00 D, and a horizontal line image is still formed 33.3 cm behind the lens. We can track the vergences in each principal meridian with vergence crosses. Then $V = P + U$ in each meridian gives

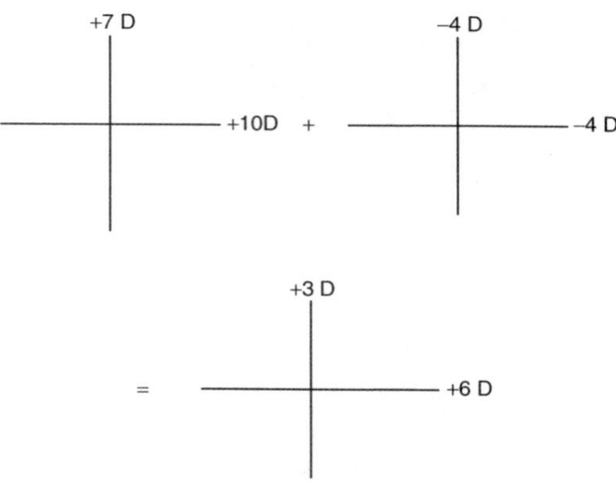

The +6.00 D vergence in the horizontal meridian is responsible for the formation of the vertical line image at 16.67 cm, while the +3.00 D vergence in the vertical meridian is responsible for the formation of the horizontal line image at 33.33 cm.

Figures 10.12a and b shows the corresponding cross-sectional ray diagrams. Figure 10.12a shows the horizontal meridian in which the rays converge to a point at 16.67 cm, and then diverge. (This point is actually on the vertical line image that would be perpendicular to the plane of the paper.) Figure 10.12b shows the vertical meridian in which the rays converge to a point at 33.33 cm. (This point is actually a point on the horizontal line image.) We can determine the length of the vertical line image from the similar triangles in Figure 10.12b, the cross-sectional view of the vertical meridian. Similarly, we can determine the length of the horizontal line image from Figure 10.12a, the cross-sectional view of the horizontal meridian. Note that the line image length is determined by the meridian perpendicular to the power meridian that forms the line.

Again, consider a circular aperture of diameter 40 mm placed against the two perpendicularly crossed cylindrical lenses. When a screen is placed directly behind the lenses, the illumination pattern on the

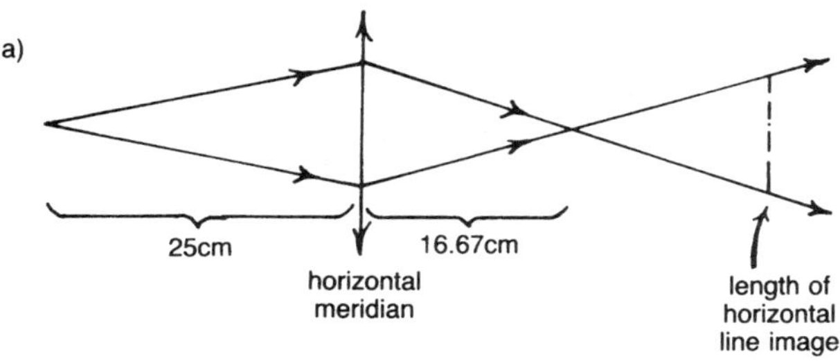

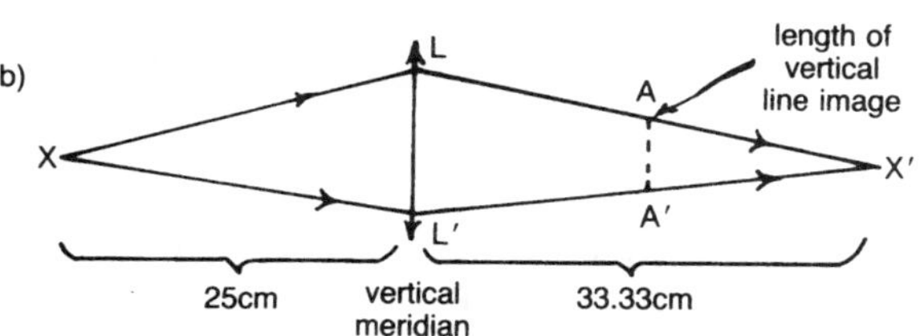

Figure 10.12 Cross-sectional ray diagrams for perpendicularly crossed lenses.

screen is circular. As the screen is moved back away from the lenses, convergence occurs in both meridians. Since convergence in the horizontal meridian occurs faster than the convergence in the vertical meridian, the resulting illumination pattern is a vertically oriented blur ellipse in which both the major and minor axes are less than 40 mm in length (Figure 10.13). As the screen is moved back to the 16.67 cm position, the convergence continues in both meridians, but since the horizontal meridian is converging faster, its length shrinks to zero first, and the vertically oriented blur ellipse turns into the vertical line image. Once the screen is moved past the vertical line image position, the light starts diverging in the horizontal meridian, while at the same time it is still converging in the vertical meridian. The result is again a vertically oriented blur ellipse. However, as the screen is moved farther back, the growing horizontal length becomes equal to the shrinking vertical length and the result is a blur circle called the *circle of least confusion*. Once the screen is moved past the circle of least confusion, the growing horizontal length becomes greater than the shrinking vertical length and the result is a horizontally oriented blur ellipse. As the screen moves toward the 33.33 cm position, the vertical meridian shrinks to zero length resulting in the horizontal line image. Once the screen is past the 33.33 cm position, the light in the vertical meridian starts to diverge, and again a horizontally oriented blur ellipse appears.

We have been considering only one point source in front of the lenses, so only one bundle is incident on the lens. In the single astigmatic bundle leaving the lens, the two line images are perpendicular to each other and are aligned with the principal meridians of the perpendicularly crossed lenses. Note that *all the light in the single astigmatic bundle passes through the first line image and then through the second line image.* At the second line image position in the single bundle, there is no blur from the first line image.

The entire three-dimensional astigmatic bundle is called the *conoid of Sturm* after J.F.C. Sturm who made the first systematic investigation of astigmatic bundles (1838). The linear distance between the two line images is called the *interval of Sturm.*

The position of least confusion lies between the two line images, and is characterized by equal lengths of the illumination patch in the principal meridians. When the aperture is circular, a blur circle occupies the position of least confusion. However, when the aperture has a different shape, the blur pattern at the position of least confusion is no longer a circle.

Consider a square aperture with horizontal and vertical sides placed against the two perpendicularly crossed cylindrical lenses. The line image orientations and positions remain the same. A screen placed directly behind the lenses has a square illumination pattern on it (Figure 10.14). As the screen is moved back, the convergence is faster in the horizontal meridian than in the vertical meridian, so the illumination pattern becomes a vertically oriented blur rectangle. The horizontal width shrinks to zero at the vertical line image position and then starts growing. The light in the vertical meridian is still converging, and a vertically oriented blur rectangle results. At the position of least confusion, the shrinking vertical length is equal to the growing horizontal length, and a square illumination pattern is formed. Past the least confusion position, the horizontal length is longer, and the

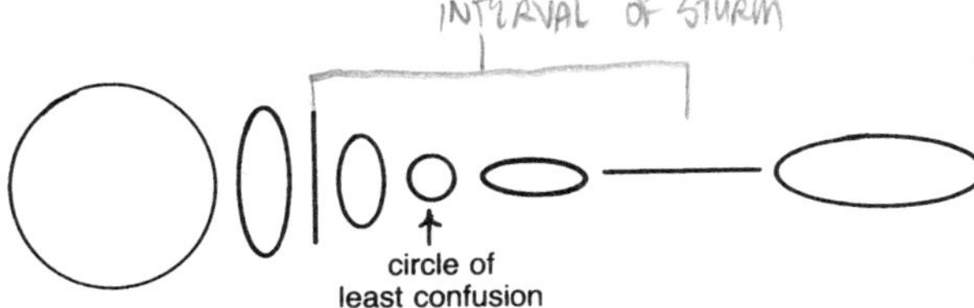

Figure 10.13 Cross-sectional illumination patterns for a circular aperture.

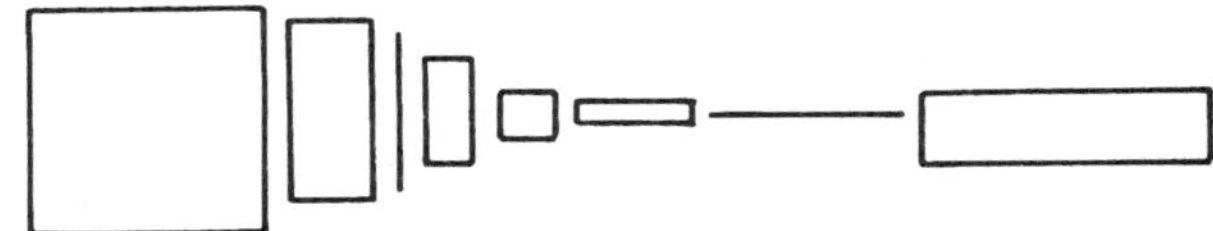

Figure 10.14 Cross-sectional illumination patterns for a square aperture.

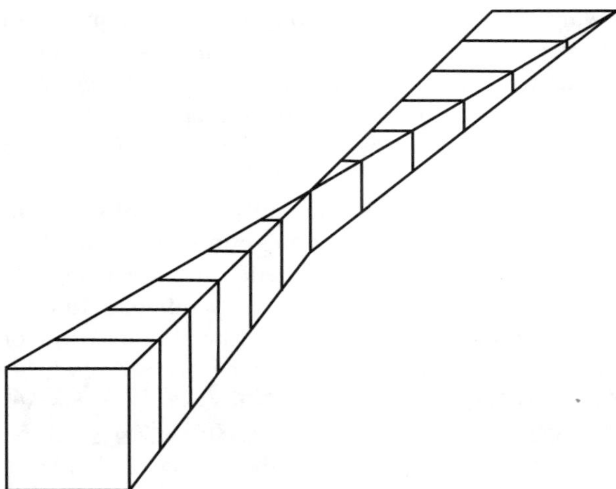

Figure 10.15 Solid figure of the conoid of Sturm for a square aperture.

illumination pattern becomes a horizontal rectangle that shrinks to zero vertically at the horizontal line image position. Once past the last line image position, both principal meridians are diverging and a horizontal rectangle again results.

Figure 10.15 shows the solid conoid that results for the square aperture with a single point source in front. Again note that all the light in the single bundle passes through the first line image, and then proceeds to the second line image.

The horizontal and vertical lengths of the blur ellipses, the blur rectangles, or the line images can be calculated from the similar triangles shown in Figure 10.12. In particular, the following example compares the line image lengths in the perpendicularly crossed cylinder case to the line image length in the case of the single plus cylinder in Example 10.2.

EXAMPLE 10.3

In Example 10.2, the point source was 25 cm in front of the $+10.00 \times 90$. The circular aperture had a diameter of 40 mm. The real line image was vertical, occurred at 16.67 cm, and had a length of 6.67 cm. What happens to this line image when the $+7.00 \times 180$ cylindrical lens is placed against the $+10.00 \times 90$?

From the previous discussion, the vertical line image is still formed at 16.67 cm. However, its length is now different, which can be observed by comparing Figures 10.6a and 10.12b. In Figure 10.12b, the triangle LL′X′ is similar to the triangle AA′X′. The length LL′ is equal to the diameter of the aperture, which is 40 mm or 4 cm. The length AA′ is equal to the length of the vertical line image. From the similar triangles,

$$\frac{33.3\,\text{cm}}{4\,\text{cm}} = \frac{16.67\,\text{cm}}{\text{AA}'}$$

and

$$\text{AA}' = 2\,\text{cm}$$

So while the vertical line image remains in the same position, it does get shorter when the +7.00 D cylindrical lens is added

EXAMPLE 10.4

Plane waves from a distant point source are incident on two perpendicularly crossed cylindrical lenses. A real horizontal line image is found 20 cm behind the lenses, and a real vertical line image is found 40 cm behind the lenses (Figure 10.16a). Draw the resultant power cross for the perpendicularly crossed cylindrical lenses, and specify their power and orientation.

The horizontal line image is formed by the convergence in the vertical meridian, and the vertical line image is formed by the convergence in the horizontal meridian. Since plane waves are incident, $U = 0$, and $P = V = 1/v$. Thus, the power cross for the lenses is

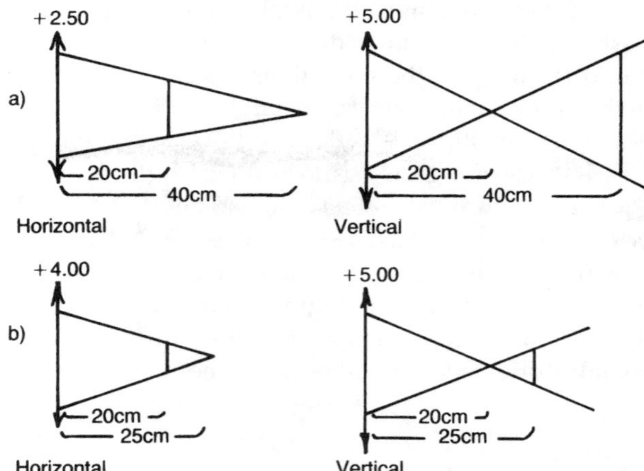

Figure 10.16 a, Cross sections of the conoid for a +2.50×90 combined with a +5.00×180; b, Cross sections when the +2.50×90 is changed to +4.00×90. The vertical line image moves closer to the horizontal line image and gets shorter. The horizontal line image stays in the same place and gets shorter.

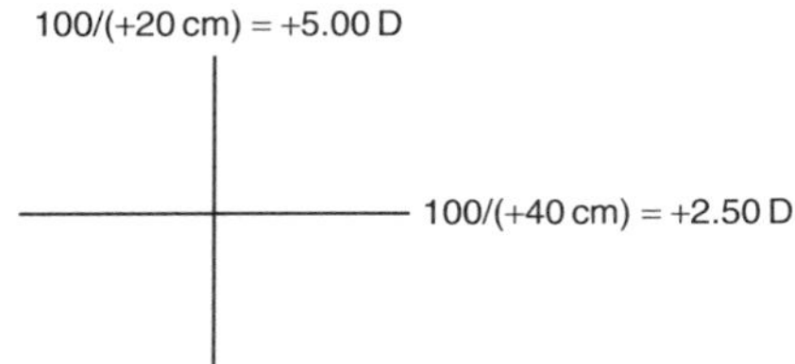

The two individual cylindrical lenses have respective power crosses of

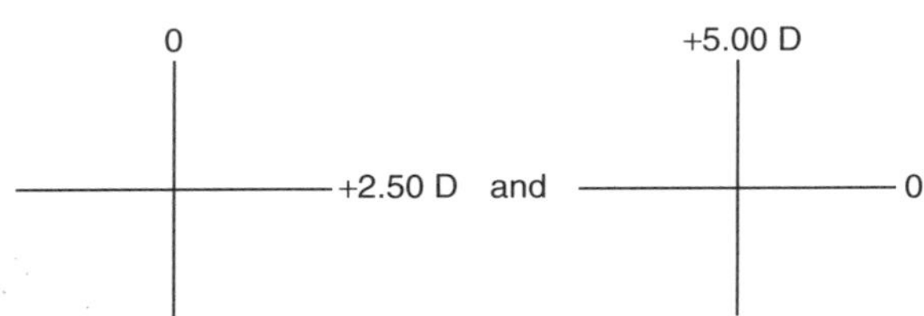

The individual cylindrical lenses are +2.50 × 90 and +5.00 × 180, respectively.

10.5 COLLAPSING THE CONOID BY EQUALIZING THE CROSS CYLINDERS

Figure 10.16a shows the ray diagrams for the image space rays of the previous example. Suppose the +2.50 × 90 is replaced with a +4.00 × 90. For incident plane waves, what happens to the line images?

The new power in horizontal meridian is +4.00 D, and since the power in the horizontal meridian forms the vertical line image, it now occurs at +25 cm and is shorter. The power in the vertical meridian is still +5.00 D, so the horizontal line image remains at +20 cm. However, since the line images are now closer together, the horizontal line image is also shorter (compare Figures 10.16a and b).

If the +4.00 × 90 is now changed to a +4.50 × 90, the vertical line now moves to +22.2 cm and gets shorter. Even though the horizontal line image remains at +20 cm, it also gets shorter. In general: *the closer the line images are to each other, the shorter both get.*

If the +4.50 × 90 is changed to a +5.00 × 90, we then have a +5.00 × 180 combined with a +5.00 × 90. Both the vertical and the horizontal meridians form their line images at 20 cm, but now both lines have zero length. In effect, the conoid has collapsed and a point image has formed at 20 cm. Furthermore, since the convergence is equal in the horizontal and vertical meridians, blur circles are formed instead of blur ellipses. The two +5.00 D perpendicularly crossed cylindrical lenses converge the light exactly as a +5.00 D spherical lens converges it.

We can repeat the above argument for any two perpendicularly crossed cylindrical lenses of equal power (e.g., +5.00 × 45 combined with +5.00 × 135). Hence, we have a general principle: *In the paraxial approximation, two thin perpendicularly crossed cylindrical lenses each of power P are equivalent to a single spherical lens of power P, and vice versa.*

The power cross

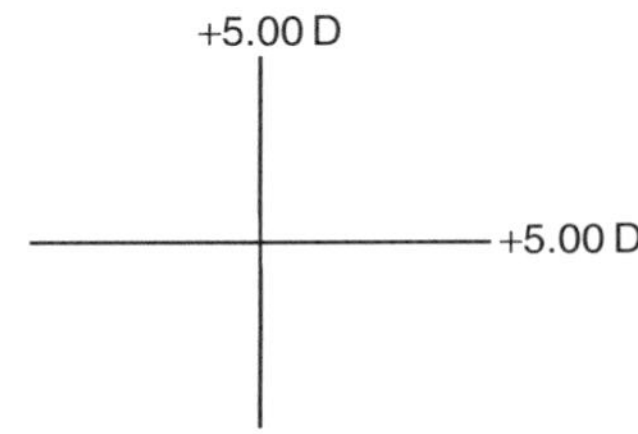

represents a +5.00 D spherical lens. Since the equivalence is good for any two perpendicularly crossed spherical lenses, the power cross

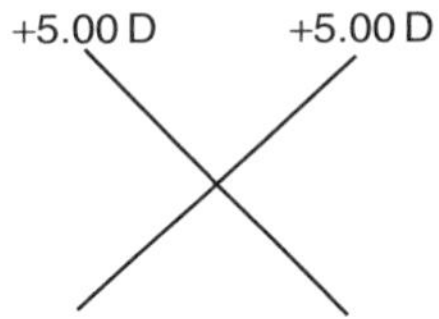

also represents the +5.00 D spherical lens. Similarly, any other orientation of the perpendicularly crossed lenses is equivalent to a sphere. The different possible orientations manifest the fact that a spherical lens is rotationally symmetric around its optical axis.

10.6 EQUIVALENT COMBINATIONS AND TRANSPOSITION

Consider plane waves from a distant point source incident on a +5.00 D spherical lens placed in contact with a +2.00 × 180 cylindrical lens. The expression for this combination is conventionally written +5.00 ⊂ +2.00 × 180. We can use power crosses to analyze the effects of the lenses. The power cross for the cylindrical lens is

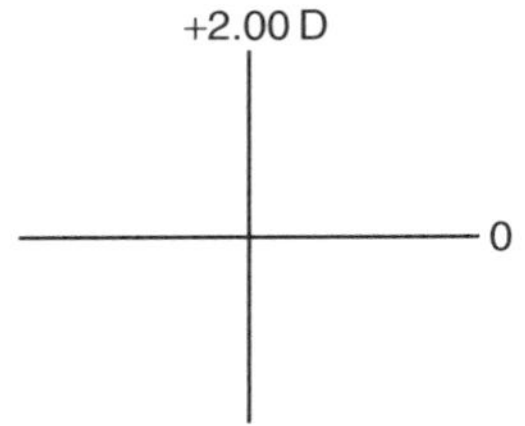

As discussed in the previous section, a possible power cross for the spherical lens is

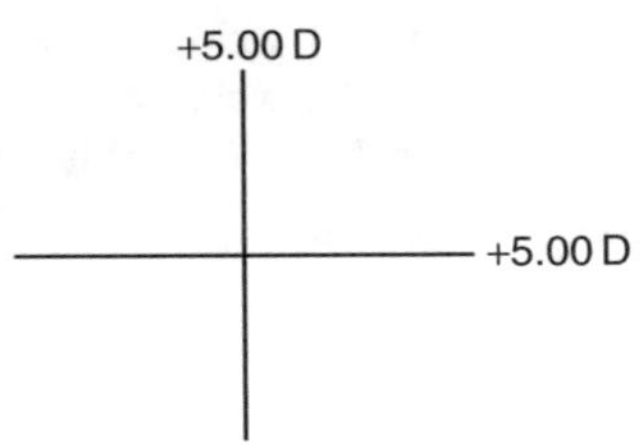

Then we can add the powers in the respective meridians to obtain the resultant power cross.

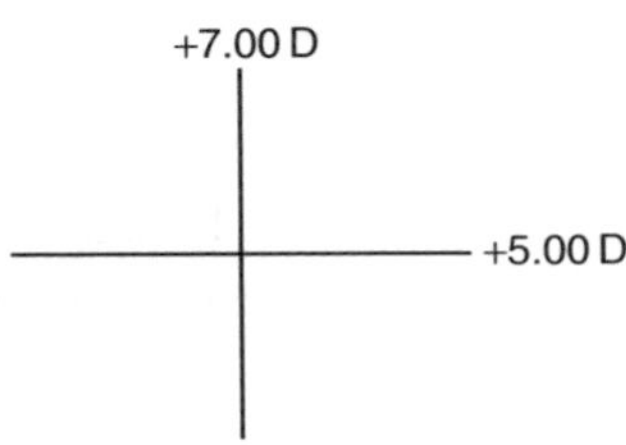

For the incident plane waves, the +7.00 D of power in the vertical meridian forms a real horizontal line image at +14.3 cm, and the +5.00 D of power in the horizontal meridian forms a real vertical line image at +20 cm.

This sphere–cylinder combination gives a typical conoid of Sturm. The same conoid can be generated with perpendicularly crossed cylindrical lenses. We can determine the lenses by noting that the above power cross is equal to

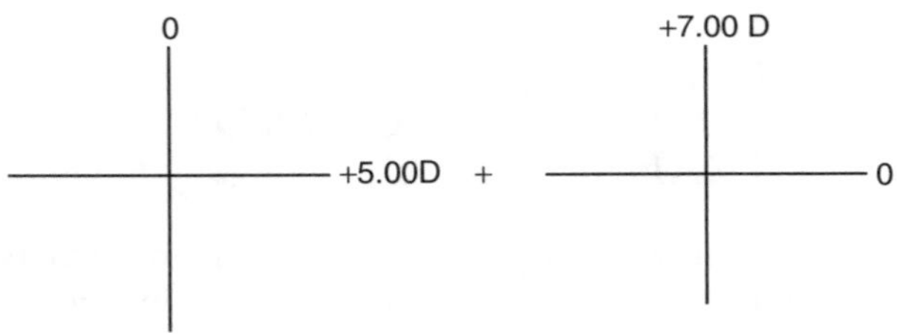

The left power cross is for a +5.00 × 90 and the right power cross is for a +7.00 × 180.

The sphere–cylinder combination above consists of a spherical lens combined with a plus cylindrical lens. There is a second sphere–cylinder combination that also gives the same conoid of Sturm. The second sphere–cylinder combination consists of a spherical lens together with a minus cylindrical lens. To find the second combination, note that the powers in the resultant power cross are +7.00 D and +5.00 D, and the spherical lens in the first combination is +5.00 D. The spherical lens in the second combination has the other power, namely, +7.00 D. The above power cross is then equal to the sum of the power cross for the +7.00-D sphere and the power cross for the unknown cylindrical lens.

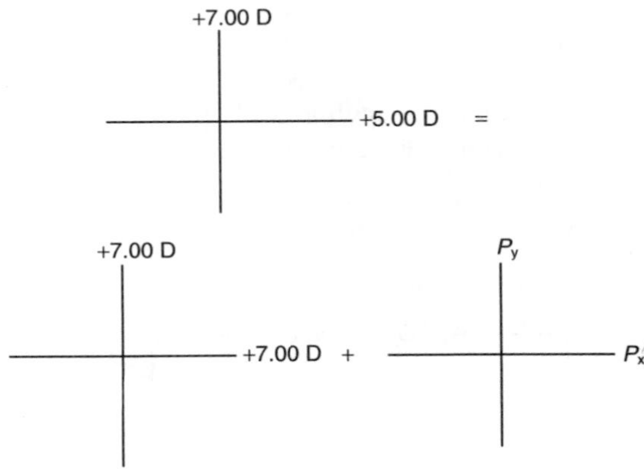

Subtraction in each principal meridian gives

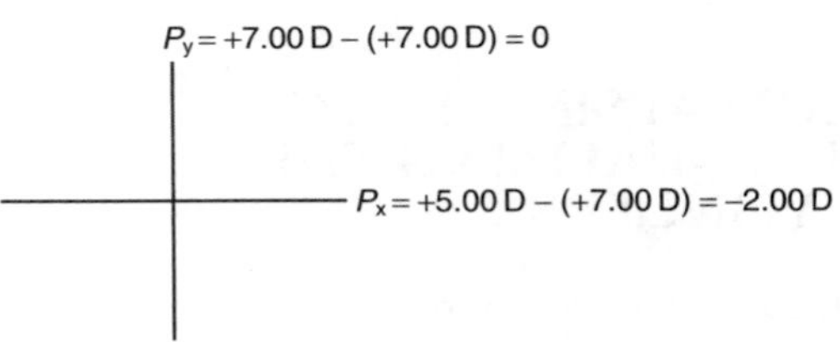

which is the power cross for a −2.00 × 90 cylindrical lens. So a +7.00 ◯ −2.00 × 90 combination gives the same power cross as a +5.00 ◯ +2.00 × 180.

In summary, the following three lens combinations are equivalent in the sense that they all give the same power cross and the same conoid of Sturm:

+ 5.00 × 90 combined with + 7.00 × 180
+ 5.00 ◯ +2.00 × 180
+ 7.00 ◯ −2.00 × 90

When comparing the perpendicularly crossed cylinder combination to the equivalent sphere–cylinder combinations, note that the respective powers (+5.00 D and +7.00 D) each serve as the spherical power in one of the sphere–cylinder combinations, and that the difference between the +7.00 D and the +5.00 D gives the magnitude (2.00 D) of the cylindrical lens power. Note also that the cylinder axis meridians are 90° different in the different sphere–cylinder combinations.

In general for any astigmatic power cross, there are three different lens combinations that will give the power cross. In visual optics, people usually mathematically write the astigmatic power cross information as one or the other of the sphere–cylinder combinations. (Optometrists usually write the sphere-minus cylinder combination while ophthalmologists usually write the sphere-plus cylinder combination.) An algebraic representation for the sphere-cylinder combination is $S \bigcirc C \times \theta$; where S represents the spherical dioptric power, C represents the cylindrical dioptric power, and θ represents the cylindrical axis meridian.

Given an astigmatic power cross, we can always work out the power cross solutions to find the equivalent sphere–cylinder combination. For those who perform refractions to find the astigmatism correction for humans, it is helpful to be able to write down the equivalent sphere–cylinder combination directly from a power cross. This can be done as follows.

To obtain the sphere-minus cylinder combination from the power cross: Pick the most plus power (or the least minus power) as the sphere power S. Then the minus cylinder power C is the difference between this least plus (or most minus) meridian and the most plus meridian. The minus cylinder axis meridian θ is the meridian picked for the sphere power (i.e., the meridian of most plus power).

For example, consider the power cross

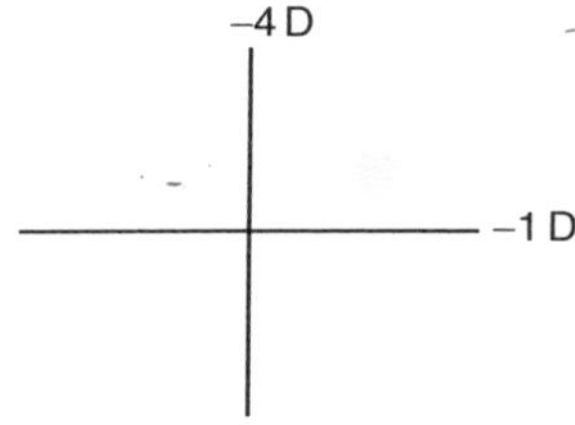

The equivalent sphere-minus cylinder combination is then $-1.00 \bigcirc -3.00 \times 180$. (You should check that the power cross solution also gives this.)

To obtain the sphere-plus cylinder combination from the power cross: Pick the least plus power (or the most minus power) as the sphere power. Then the plus cylinder power is the difference between this most plus (or least minus) meridian and the least plus meridian. The plus cylinder axis meridian is the meridian picked for the sphere power (i.e., the meridian of least plus power). For example, from the above power cross $-4.00 \bigcirc +3.00 \times 90$. (Again you should check that the power cross solution also gives this.)

Given the sphere–cylinder combination $S \bigcirc C \times \theta$, we can make separate power crosses for the sphere and the cylinder, and perform the respective additions to obtain the resultant power cross. However, it is also helpful to be able to write the power cross directly from the sphere–cylinder expression. We can do this as follows: In the meridian θ, the power is S (since the cylinder contributes zero power in the axis meridian). In the meridian perpendicular to θ, the power is equal to the sum $S + C$ (since the sphere contributes in all meridians and this is also the cylinder power meridian).

The process of going from the sphere-plus cylinder combination to the equivalent sphere-minus cylinder combination or vice versa is called *transposition*. The following power crosses reiterate the algebra of transposition. When θ is a first quadrant angle, the power cross for the combination is

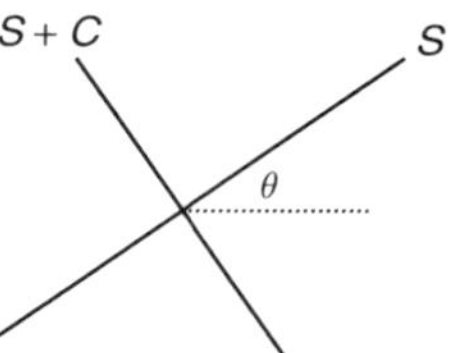

The other equivalent sphere–cylinder combination has a spherical power equal to the sum $S + C$. Thus the left power cross below for a sphere (power equal to $S + C$) plus the power cross on the right (with unknown powers P_1 and P_2) must equal the above power cross.

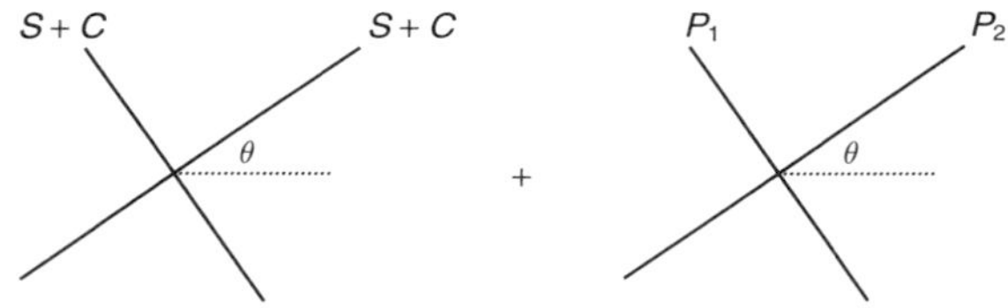

When we algebraically subtract in each principal meridian, we obtain the powers P_1 and P_2:

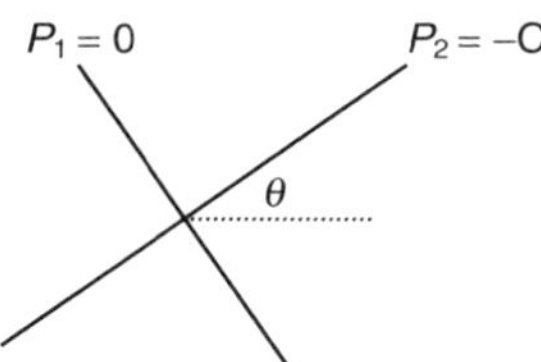

This is the power cross for a $-C \times (\theta + 90)$ cylindrical lens.

θ is a first quadrant angle in the above power crosses. When θ is a second quadrant angle, the cylinder axis meridian of the equivalent sphere–cylinder combination is $\theta - 90$. Thus a *synopsis of transposition* is:

Given a sphere–cylinder combination

$$S \bigcirc C \times \theta$$

the transposed combination is

$$(S + C) \bigcirc -C \times (\theta \pm 90)$$

EXAMPLE 10.5

For a +4.00 ○ −3.00 × 42 find the equivalent sphere–cylinder and perpendicularly crossed cylinder combinations. Also, write down the resultant power cross, and for incident plane waves specify the orientation and location of the line images.

The combination given is a sphere-minus cylinder. The equivalent combination is a sphere-plus cylinder. From the transposition rule, the equivalent sphere-plus cylinder is

[+4.00 + (−3.00)] ○ +3.00 × (42 + 90)

or

+1.00 ○ +3.00 × 132

The resultant power cross for the original combination can be obtained by adding the power crosses. Alternatively, one can proceed directly from the +4.00 ○ −3.00 × 42 lens, and note that only the sphere power (+4.00 D) contributes in the 42 meridian, while both the sphere and cylinder power contribute in the 132 meridian (i.e., +4.00 D + (−3.00 D) = +1.00 D). The resultant power cross is

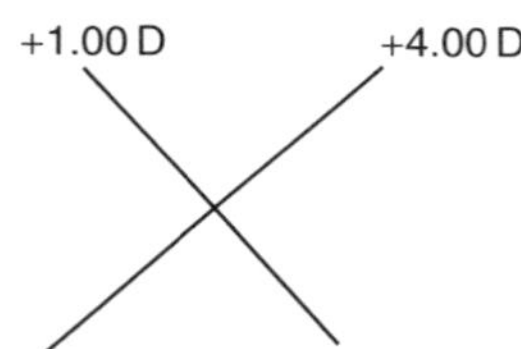

The resultant power cross is equal to

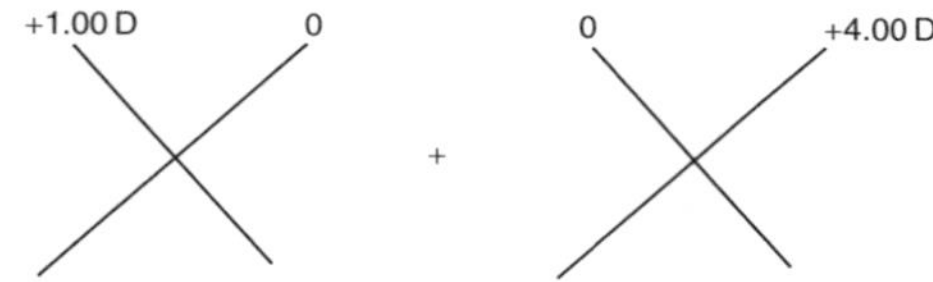

so the equivalent perpendicularly crossed cylinder combination is

+4.00 × 132 combined with +1.00 × 42

For incident plane waves, the +4.00 D of power in the 42 meridian gives a 132° line at 25 cm, and the +1.00 D of power in the 132 meridian gives a 42° line image at 100 cm.

EXAMPLE 10.6

Find the sphere-plus cylinder combination that is equivalent to +9.50 × 35 combined with +5.50 ×125.

The +9.50 × 35 lens has a 125 power meridian, while the +5.50 × 125 has a 35 meridian. The resultant power cross is

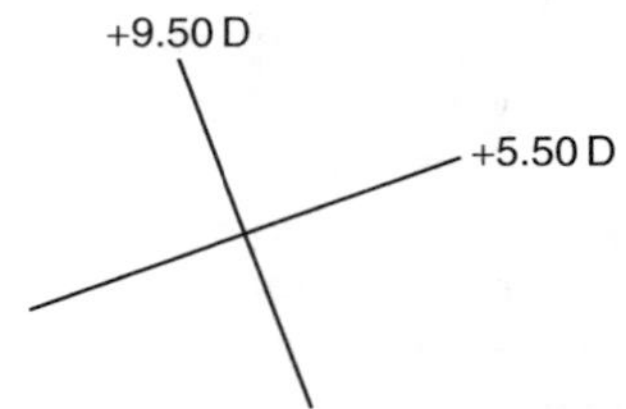

In the sphere-plus cylinder combination, the sphere has the least plus power, which is +5.50 D, and that meridian (35) is the cylinder axis meridian. The cylinder power is the difference or +4.00 D. The result is +5.50 ○ +4.00 × 35.

(Suppose you "incorrectly" picked +9.50 D for the sphere power. If you work the rest correctly, you would obtain +9.50 ○ −4.00 × 125. Then you can simply transpose to obtain +5.50 ○ +4.00 × 35.)

10.7 TORIC SURFACES

A conoid of Sturm can be generated by a single *toric* surface. Figure 10.17a shows a torus. An inflated inner tube (used for tires or for floating down rivers) is a common example of a torus. A perfect doughnut or bagel would be another example. The line in Figure 10.17b is the symmetry axis of the torus. The small circle has a radius r_1 and its center is a distance g from the symmetry axis. A rotation of the circle about the symmetry axis forms the torus.

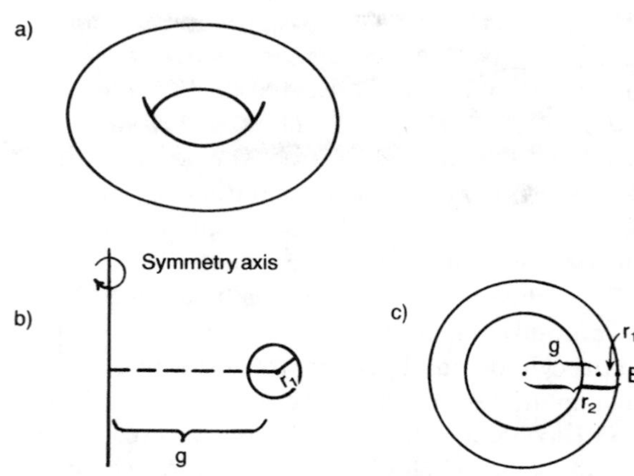

Figure 10.17 a, A torus; b, symmetry parameters; c, radii of curvature. (View is perpendicular to the symmetry axis.)

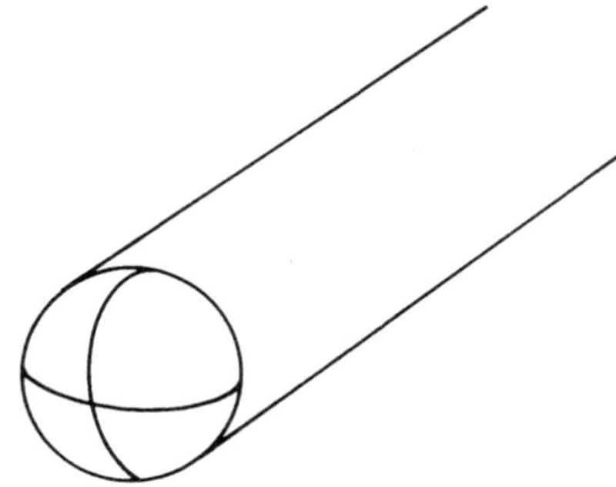

Figure 10.18 Toric interface on a long rod.

Consider cross sections that contain the point B on the outer surface of the torus. Two of the cross sections are circular in shape, and these two are perpendicular to each other. One is the small circle of radius r_1. The other is the circle of radius r_2 (where $r_2 = g + r_1$) formed by the rotation of point B around the symmetry axis of the torus (Figure 10.17c). The two circular cross sections are the principal meridians through point B.

Just as a spherical surface is part of a sphere, a toric surface is part of a torus. A refracting or reflecting surface can be toric in shape. The characteristics of the toric surface are the symmetry, as defined above, and the two perpendicular principal meridians with circular cross sections. Toric surfaces can have two convex principal meridians, two concave principal meridians, or one concave and one convex principal meridian.

Consider a long glass ($n = 1.5$) rod with a toric front surface. The principal meridians are both convex, and aligned with the vertical and horizontal meridians (Figure 10.18). The vertical meridian has a 20 cm radius of curvature, and the horizontal meridian has a 25 cm radius of curvature. We can represent the toric surface by a power cross aligned with the principal meridians, and calculate the refracting power in each principal meridian from

$$P = \frac{n_2 - n_1}{r}$$

Then,

$P_2 = 50/20 = +2.50$ D

$P_1 = 50/20 = +2.00$ D

The toric surface forms a conoid of Sturm in the glass rod. For a distant point source, $U = 0$ and the vergence V in the vertical meridian equals +2.50 D. The vertical principal meridian forms a horizontal line image, which from $v = n_2/V$ is a distance of 150/+2.50 D or +60 cm from the surface. The horizontal principal meridian forms the vertical line image, which is a distance of 150/+2.00 D or +75 cm from the surface.

The power cross for a toric surface has the same form as the power cross for a sphere–cylinder combination. As a result, the equations describing the toric dioptric parameters have the same form as those for sphere–cylinder combinations. For example, the toric surface with the above power cross can be described a +2.00 ◯ +0.50 × 180 surface. Alternatively, the same toric surface might be described as +2.50 ◯ −0.50 × 90.

The wavefronts leaving the toric surface are themselves toric in shape. In general, *toric wavefronts form a conoid of Sturm*. A cylindrical surface is a special case of a toric surface in which one of the radii goes to infinity and the corresponding meridian is flat. A spherical surface is a special case of a toric surface in which the two radii in the principal meridians are equal.

A lens made with a toric surface, or surfaces, generates a conoid of Sturm just like a sphere–cylinder combination or the equivalent perpendicularly crossed cylinder combination. A lens with one or more toric surfaces is called a *spherocylindrical* lens. A typical spherocylindrical spectacle lens has a spherical front surface and a toric back surface.

EXAMPLE 10.7

A point source is 100 cm in front of a thin spherocylindrical lens that has a +8.00 spherical front surface and a −3.00 ◯ −2.00 × 45 toric back surface. What are the line image positions and orientations? What is the sphere-minus cylinder equation that describes the lens?

First find the power cross for the lens. The toric back surface has 45 and 135 principal meridians. The spherical front surface can be represented by a power cross with +8.00 D of power in both the 45 and 135 meridians. We can write down the power cross for each surface, and then add the surface powers in the respective principal meridians to obtain the power cross for the thin lens.

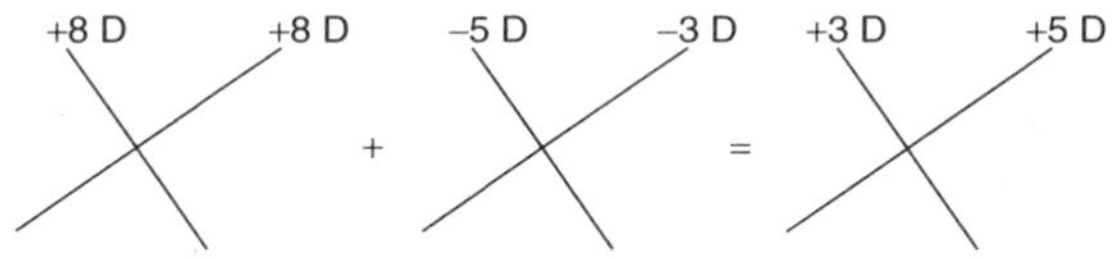

The power cross for the lens has +3.00 D of power in the 135 meridian and +5.00 D of power in the 45 meridian. The incident wavefront is spherical with $U = -1.00\,\text{D}$. We can apply $V = P + U$ in both principal meridians to obtain the vergence cross for the exiting toric wavefront:

+3 D +5 D + −1 D −1 D = +2 D +4 D

The exiting wavefront has +2.00 D vergence in the 135 meridian, and that meridian forms a 45° line image at +50 cm. The exiting wavefront has +4.00 D vergence in the 45 meridian forms a 135° line image at +25 cm.

To write a sphere-minus cylinder equation for the lens, consider the resultant power cross for the lens. The highest plus power was +5.00 D in the 45 meridian. The sphere-minus cylinder equation is then +5.00 ○ −2.00 × 45. (You can also verify this with power crosses.) Note that since the lens is thin, we could just add the spherical front surface power, +8.00 D, to the spherical power in the toric back surface equation, −3.00 ○ −2.00 × 45, to obtain the equation for the total lens +5.00 ○ −2.00 × 45.

10.8 EXTENDED OBJECTS AND MULTIPLE CONOIDS

The above discussion of astigmatism dealt only with a single point source and a single astigmatic bundle (i.e., a single conoid of Sturm). Extended objects consist of many point sources. Consider a target consisting of the five paraxial point sources shown in Figure 10.19a. One point source is centrally located. The others are above, below, left, and right of the center respectively. The object plane is 50 cm in front of a thin +7.00 ○ −3.00 × 180 spherocylindrical lens. What does the image of the points look like at various positions behind the lens?

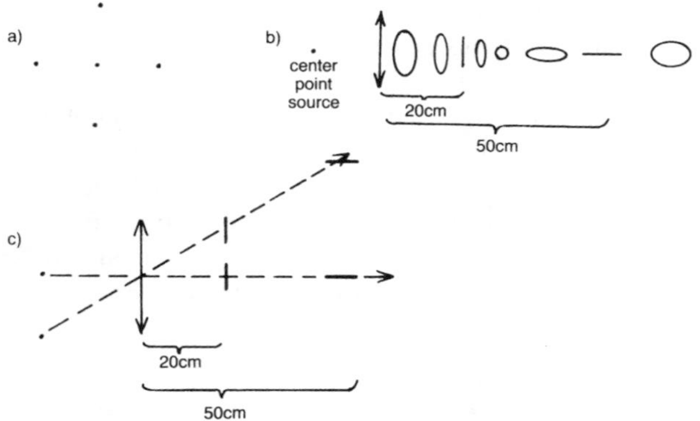

Figure 10.19 a, Array of point sources; b, a conoid for one point source; c, line images in the respective conoids from two different point sources.

We start by asking how the central point is imaged in the conoid. The power cross for the lens is

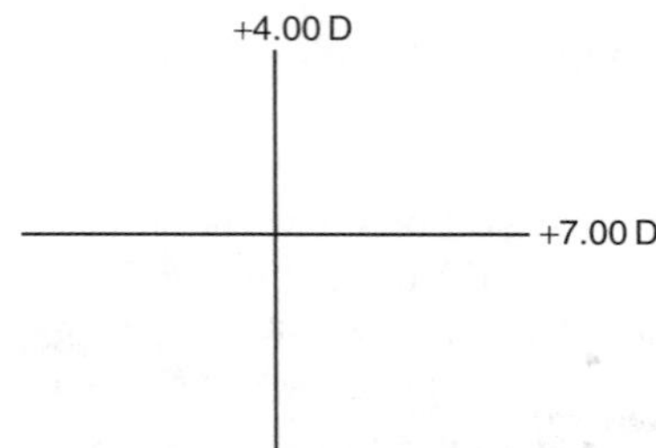

U is −2 D (spherical), so from $V = P + U$ the vergence cross for the toric wavefront leaving the lens is

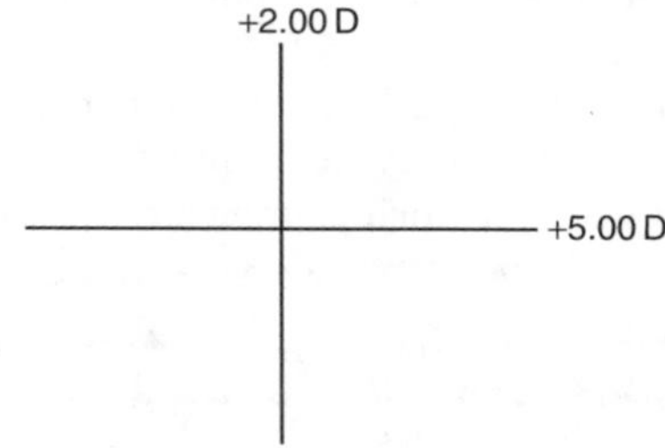

The +2.00 D vergence in the vertical meridian forms a horizontal line image +50 cm behind the lens, and the +5.00 D vergence in the horizontal meridian forms a vertical line image +20.0 cm behind the lens. Figure 10.19b shows the line images and the corresponding blur ellipses.

For the central point source, the chief ray in the astigmatic bundle lies on the optical axis. For the point source below the center, a different astigmatic bundle is formed, and its chief ray travels upward relative to the axis (Figure 10.19c). In the paraxial approximation, the vertical line image in the latter conoid is still in the +20 cm plane and the horizontal line image is still in the +50 cm plane. For the point source above the center, still another astigmatic bundle is formed and its chief ray travels downward relative to the axis. In fact, an astigmatic bundle is formed for each of the paraxial point sources, and the vertical line image in each astigmatic bundle is in the +20 cm plane and the horizontal line image is in the +50 cm plane.

Once we know how a single point is imaged, we can simulate how the collection of points constituting

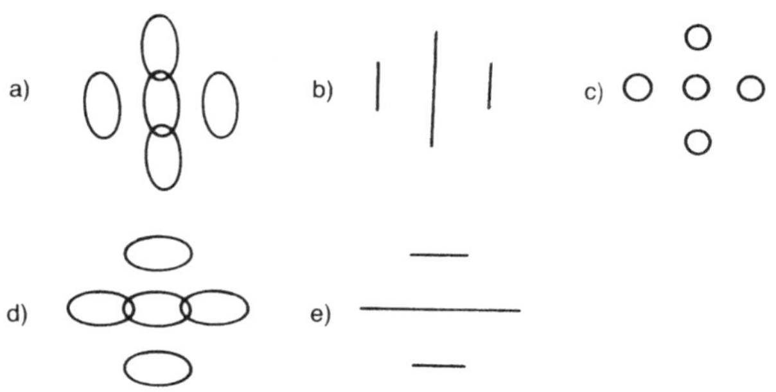

Figure 10.20 Illumination patterns at various locations for the object points of Figure 10.19a.

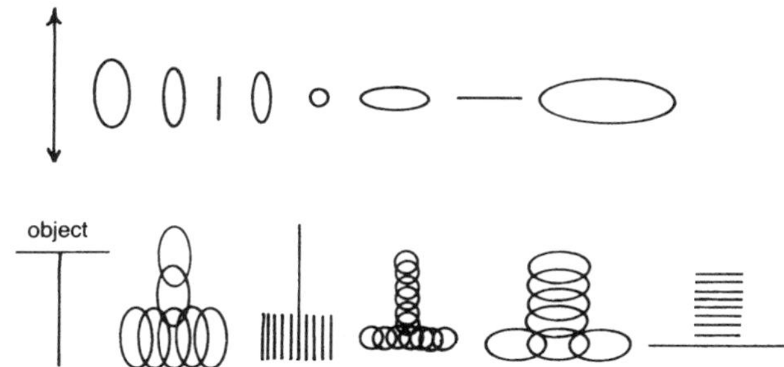

Figure 10.21 Illumination patterns at various locations for a single point object and simulation of illumination patterns for an extended object.

the extended target is imaged. In Figure 10.19b, the blur ellipse nearest the lens is vertically oriented. To simulate the illumination pattern for the five-point extended target, we center a vertically oriented blur ellipse on each of the five chief ray positions. As shown in Figure 10.20a, some or all of these blur ellipses may overlap.

For each astigmatic bundle, the vertical line image occurs at +20 cm. The illumination pattern at 20 cm for the five points is simulated by drawing a vertical line centered on the chief ray of each bundle (Figure 10.20b). The overlapping of the individual vertical line images gives the image the appearance of having a solid vertical line in the middle.

At the position of the circle of least confusion, the five-point image is simulated by drawing the blur circle centered at each chief ray (Figure 10.20c). At the position of the horizontally oriented blur ellipse, the five-point image is simulated by drawing a horizontally oriented blur ellipse at the position of each chief ray (note some overlapping in Figure 10.20d). At +50 cm, the position of the horizontal line image, the five-point image is simulated by drawing a horizontal line image centered on each chief ray position. As shown in Figure 10.20e, the resulting extended image appears to have a solid horizontal line.

Assume the five point sources are replaced by the letter T. Figure 10.21 shows the results of the simulation process for astigmatically imaging the letter T. In Figure 10.21, the top row shows the cross-sectional illumination patterns in the conoid of Sturm for a single astigmatic bundle. The second row shows the simulated illumination patterns for the letter T. To construct the simulations, first remember that the chief rays cross over the axis, so the image of the letter T is inverted.

At the position in the single conoid of the vertically oriented blur ellipse, a vertically oriented blur ellipse is drawn for each chief ray (i.e., at each point in the inverted T). The result shows that the horizontal bar in the T image is blurred more than the vertical bar. At the vertical line image position (+20 cm), a vertical line image is drawn for each chief ray or each point in the inverted T, i.e., the image of the horizontal bar in the inverted T consists of a series of vertical line images that results in a blurred horizontal bar. (Whether the blurred horizontal bar is visible or not depends on the amount of blur.) The image of the vertical bar in the inverted T consists of a series of overlapping vertical lines. The result is a clear vertical bar. At the circle of least confusion position, a blur circle is drawn for each point in the inverted T, and in this case the horizontal and vertical bars are equally blurred. The procedure is the same at the position of a horizontally oriented blur ellipse, in which case the vertical bar is blurred more than the horizontal bar. At the horizontal line image position, the horizontal line images at each chief ray position give a blurred vertical bar in the inverted T, while the overlapping horizontal line images give a clear horizontal bar.

Figure 10.22 shows a similar simulation in which the letter A is the object. The astigmatic images correspond to an inverted A. For the inverted A, the horizontal bar is clear at +50 cm, which is the horizontal line image position in a single astigmatic bundle. The

Figure 10.22 Simulated illumination patterns for the letter A as an object.

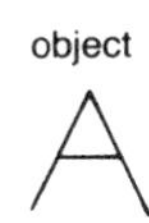

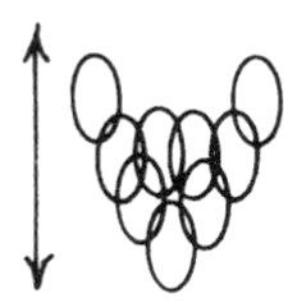

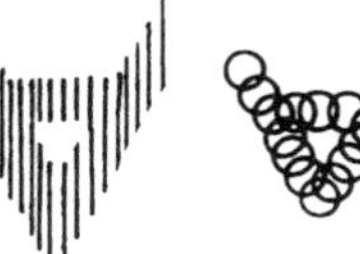

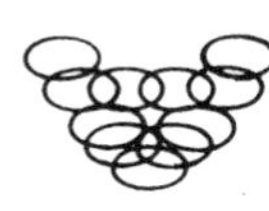

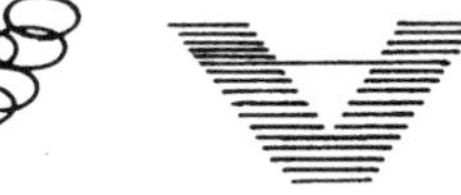

diagonal lines in the inverted A are not aligned with a principal meridian of the spherocylindrical lens, and as a result are not clear anywhere. (Note how the blur boundaries for the diagonal lines in the A differ at the vertical line image position compared to the horizontal line image position. In particular the bottom of the inverted A's blur patch is peaked or pointed at the vertical line image position, whereas it is flat at the horizontal line image position.)

For most image positions, there are differing amounts of blur for the different bars depending on the bar orientation. The only position where the amount of blur is equal for all orientations is at the circle of least confusion. For a complex target, the circle of least confusion then supplies equal information, regardless of orientation. In this case, the circle of least confusion is regarded as the best image position for a complex target. However, the amount of information supplied by the circle of least confusion is less than a clear image supplies.

Remember that for a single astigmatic bundle, all of the light first passes through one line image and then proceeds to the second line image. At one line image position, there is no information in the illumination pattern about the other line image (the top row in Figure 10.21). However, for an extended object, such as the letter T, there are multiple astigmatic bundles. The resulting illumination patterns at the position of one line image do give information about different bars or lines in the target. The amount of information depends on the amount of blur, which depends on the orientation of the bar. The only bars that have a clear image somewhere in the conoid are those that are aligned with the principal meridians of the conoid. (Incidentally, the process of simulating the illumination patterns on a point by point basis can be formalized mathematically and is called a *convolution*.)

10.9 THE CIRCLE OF LEAST CONFUSION AND THE SPHERICAL EQUIVALENT

Since the circle of least confusion has some special significance, let us figure out its exact position in the conoid. Consider a lens with a circular aperture of diameter h. Assume the exiting wavefront is converging and toric with a vergence V_1 in one principal meridian and a vergence V_2 in the other principal meridian. Figure 10.23 gives the corresponding ray diagrams. The first line image occurs at v_1 (which equals $1/V_1$), and the second line image occurs at v_2 (which equals $1/V_2$).

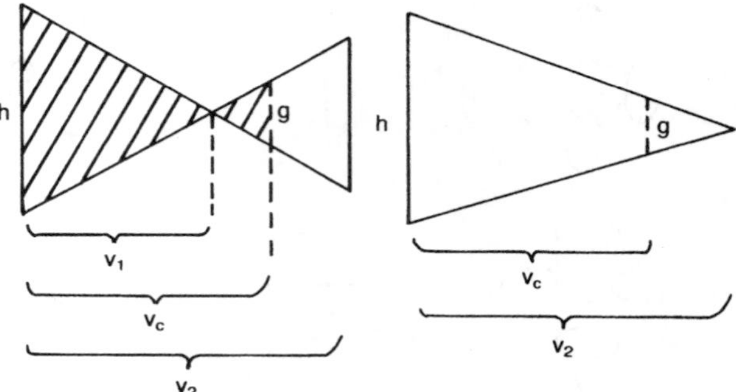

Figure 10.23 Geometry to find circle of least confusion location.

The circle of least confusion occurs between the two line images at the position v_c in which the cross sectional length g is the same for each principal meridian (dashed line in Figure 10.23). From the similar triangles in the left diagram,

$$\frac{h}{v_1} = \frac{g}{v_c - v_1}$$

From the similar triangles in the right diagram,

$$\frac{h}{v_2} = \frac{g}{v_2 - v_c}$$

We can solve each of the above two equations for g/h and set the results equal to each other to obtain

$$\frac{v_c - v_1}{v_1} = \frac{v_2 - v_c}{v_2}$$

or

$$\frac{v_c}{v_1} - 1 = 1 - \frac{v_c}{v_2}$$

It follows that

$$\frac{2}{v_c} = \frac{1}{v_1} + \frac{1}{v_2}$$

Let V_c be the dioptric location of the circle of least confusion:

$$V_c = \frac{1}{v_c}$$

where v_c is in meters.
Then,

$$2V_c = V_1 + V_2 \tag{10.4}$$

and finally

$$V_c = \frac{V_1 + V_2}{2} \tag{10.5}$$

Equation 10.5 says that *the circle of least confusion is located dioptrically halfway between the line images.* This does not mean that the circle of least confusion is located linearly halfway between the line images.

EXAMPLE 10.8

A point source is located 40 cm from a thin $+7.50 \bigcirc -4.00 \times 125$ spherocylindrical lens. Find the circle of least confusion position, and the line image positions and orientations.

The left power cross below is the power cross for the lens. The incident vergence U is -2.50 D (spherical). Then from $V = P + U$ is each principal meridian,

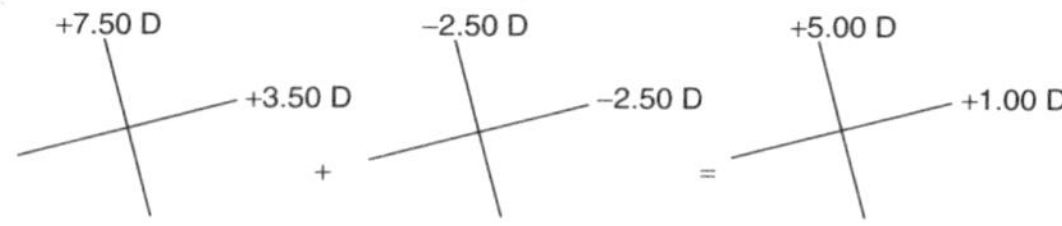

From Eq. 10.5,

$$V_c = \frac{+5.00\,\text{D} + 1.00\,\text{D}}{2} = +3.00\,\text{D}$$

(Note that 3 is halfway between 1 and 5.) The linear location of the circle of least confusion is

$$v_c = \frac{100}{+3.00\,\text{D}} = +33.3\,\text{cm}$$

The first line image is oriented at 35° and is located at

$$v_1 = \frac{100}{+5.00\,\text{D}} = +20.0\,\text{cm}$$

The second line image is oriented at 125° and is located at

$$v_2 = \frac{100}{+1.00\,\text{D}} = +100.0\,\text{cm}$$

Figure 10.24 summarizes the results. The linear halfway point between the two line images is the +60 cm position. Note that while the circle of least confusion is dioptrically halfway between the two line images, it is definitely not linearly halfway between. Instead, it is much closer to the first line image.

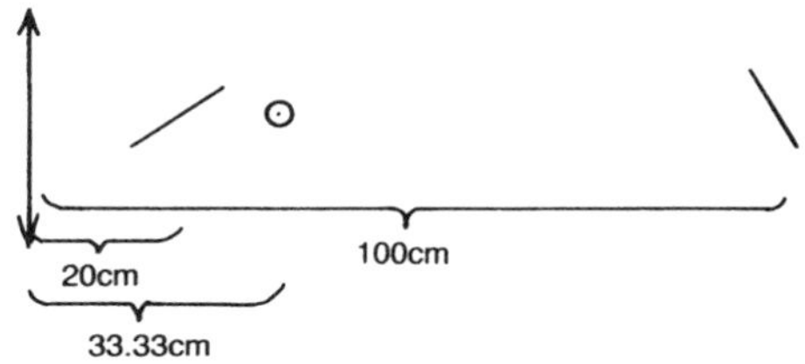

Figure 10.24 Circle of least confusion location.

When plane waves $U = 0$ are incident on a spherocylindrical lens of parameters $S \bigcirc C \times \theta$, the vergence V in each principal meridian is equal to the dioptric power P in that meridian:

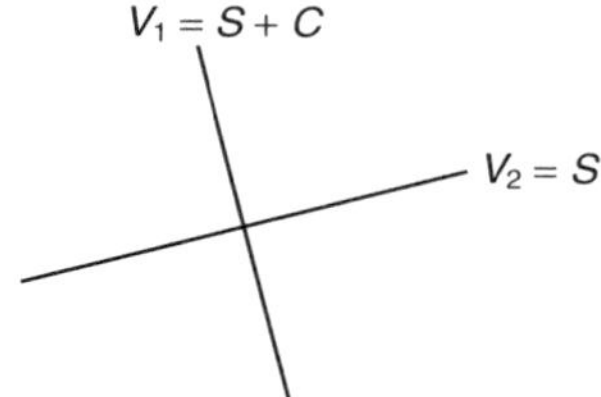

Equation 10.5 gives the dioptric location for the circle of least confusion:

$$V_c = \frac{(S + C) + S}{2} = S + \frac{C}{2}$$

For a complex target, the circle of least confusion is the best image position for the spherocylindrical lens. The spherical lens, which gives a point image at the same position as the circle of least confusion, is called the *spherical equivalent* (Sp Eq) of the spherocylindrical lens. The dioptric power of the Sp Eq is halfway between the principal meridian dioptric powers of the spherocylindrical lens. Alternatively, from the above equation,

$$\text{Sp Eq} = S + \frac{C}{2} \tag{10.6}$$

Note that the Sp Eq is independent of the cylinder axis θ. For a cylindrical lens, S is zero and the Sp Eq is equal to $C/2$. For a spherical lens, C is zero and the Sp Eq is just the sphere power S.

EXAMPLE 10.9

A point source is located 15 cm in front of a thin $+10.00 \bigcirc -6.00 \times 155$ spherocylindrical lens. What is the Sp Eq?

The Sp Eq is defined in terms of the dioptric parameters of the lens, so the point source location is irrelevant. From Eq. 10.6,

$$\text{Sp Eq} = +10.00\,\text{D} + \frac{-6.00\,\text{D}}{2} = +7.00\,\text{D}$$

A +7.00 D spherical lens gives a point image at the same position as the circle of least confusion given by the $+10.00 \bigcirc -6.00 \times 155$ spherocylindrical lens. In this sense, the $+10.00 \bigcirc -6.00 \times 155$ lens acts in a rough fashion like a +7.00 D spherical lens. Numerically, the spherical equivalent is also equal to the *mean dioptric power* of the spherocylindrical lens.

10.10 VIRTUAL LINE IMAGES

A toric wavefront that is converging in both principal meridians yields two real line images. Once the toric wavefront is past the second line image position, it is diverging in both meridians. An observer viewing the real line images as aerial images then has a diverging toric wavefront incident on his eye.

Exiting toric wavefronts can also be diverging in both principal meridians. These diverging toric wavefronts yield two virtual line images. To a downstream observer (Figure 10.25) it makes no difference optically whether the line images are virtual images or (real) aerial images. An exiting toric wavefront can also be diverging in one principal meridian while converging in the other. Such a wavefront yields one virtual line image and one real line image.

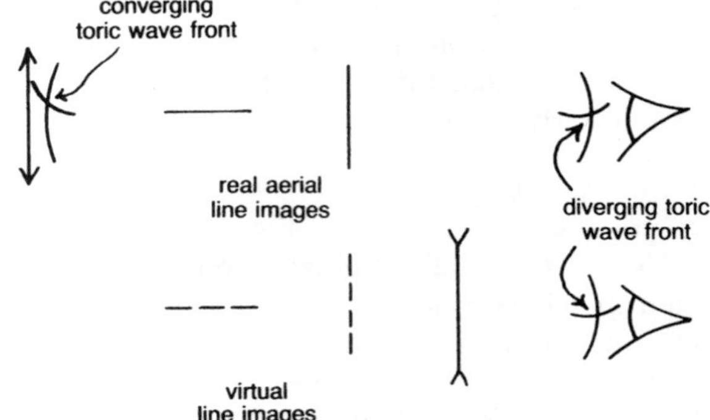

Figure 10.25 Converging toric wavefronts that form real aerial line images and then diverge to the eye compared to a spherocylindrical lens that forms two virtual line images and gives the same diverging toric wavefront incident on the eye.

Consider collimated light incident on a thin −5.00 ⊂ −3.00 × 180 spherocylindrical lens. The power cross representation for the exiting vergence is

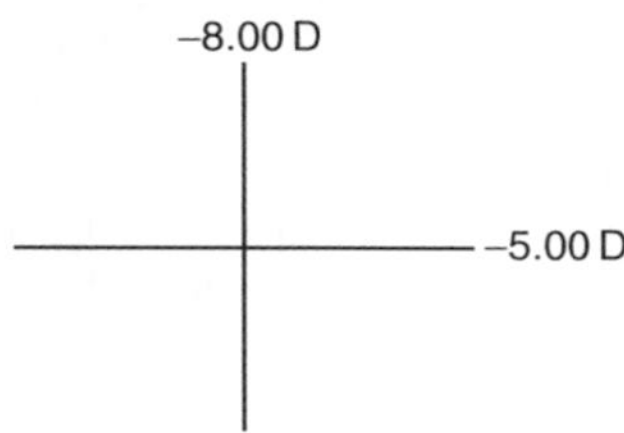

The resulting virtual line images are vertical at −20.0 cm and horizontal at −12.5 cm.

Consider the power cross analysis for a +6.00 × 180 lens with a point source 50 cm in front. From $V = P + U$,

V_y +6.00 D   −2.00 D

V_x = 0 + −2.00 D

or

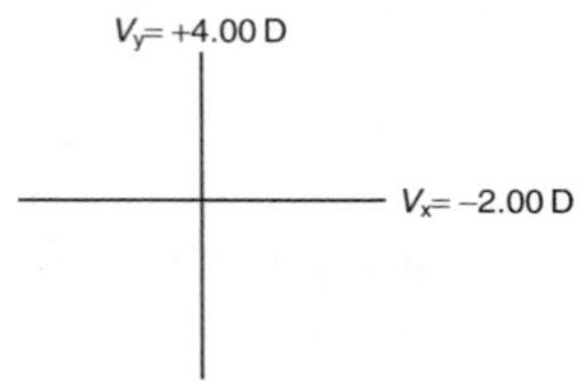

The vergence cross shows that the wavefront leaving the lens is toric with one converging meridian and one diverging meridian. As expected, the +4.00 D vergence in the vertical meridian gives a real horizontal line image at +25 cm. The −2.00 D vergence in the horizontal meridian gives a virtual vertical line image at −50 cm, the distance at which the original point source is located. Figure 10.26 shows the rays for the virtual line image.

When the object point for a plus cylindrical lens goes to optical infinity, the virtual line image also goes to optical infinity. Thus, a plus cylindrical lens with plane waves incident has a real line image parallel to the axis and at a finite distance from the lens, together with a virtual line image parallel to the power meridian at optical infinity.

Hence, every thin spherocylindrical lens with non-zero cylindrical power forms two perpendicular line

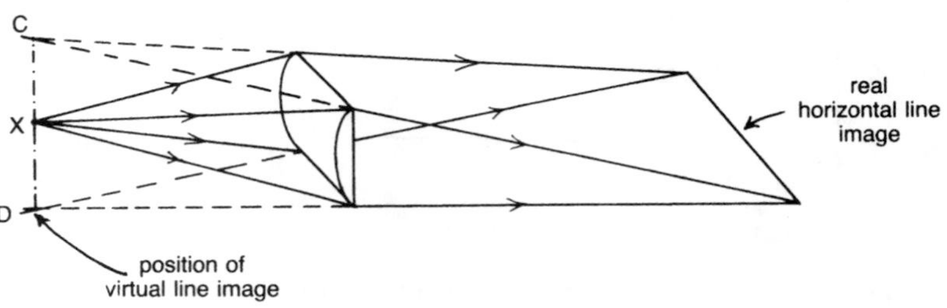

Figure 10.26 Real and virtual line images for a converging cylindrical lens.

images. The line images might both be real, both virtual, or one real and one virtual.

10.11 THROUGH A GLASS ASTIGMATICALLY

Suppose an unaccommodated emmetrope holds a +5.00 × 180 cylindrical lens directly in front of her eye and looks through it at a distant point source. What does the emmetrope see?

Before rushing to answer, let us first ask what an unaccommodated emmetrope would see through a +5.00 D spherical lens. By itself, the +5.00 D spherical lens forms a real point image at +20 cm. When held directly in front of the eye, the +5.00 D spherical lens pulls the eye's point image 5.00 D forward into the vitreous humor leaving a blur circle on the retina. Thus, the +5.00 D lens simulates 5 D of myopia. Note that the observer sees the blur circle, and not the point image (Figure 10.27a).

By itself, the power meridian of the +5.00 × 180 cylindrical lens forms a real horizontal line image. To analyze what the emmetrope will see through the lens, assume that the emmetropic eye has +60.00 D of power (spherical). Then we can represent the eye by the power cross

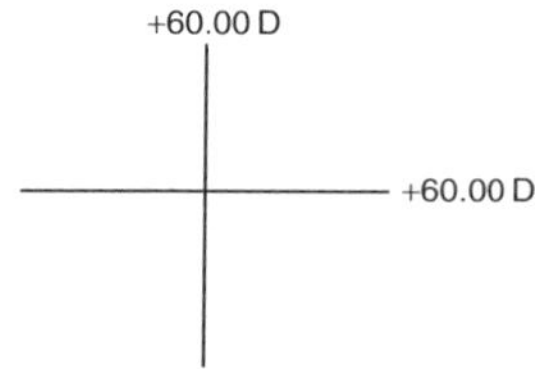

The +5.00 × 180 lens has a power cross of

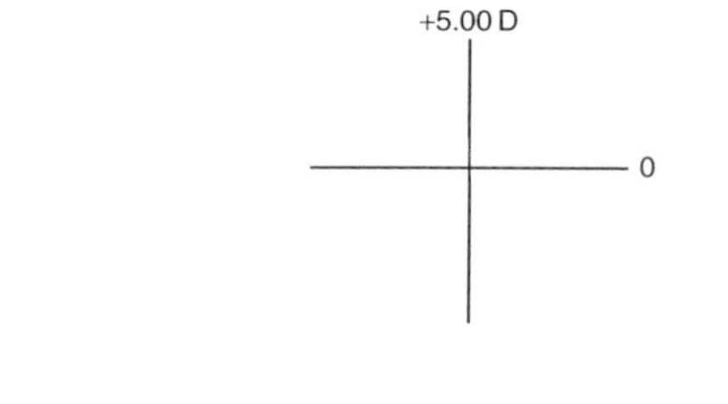

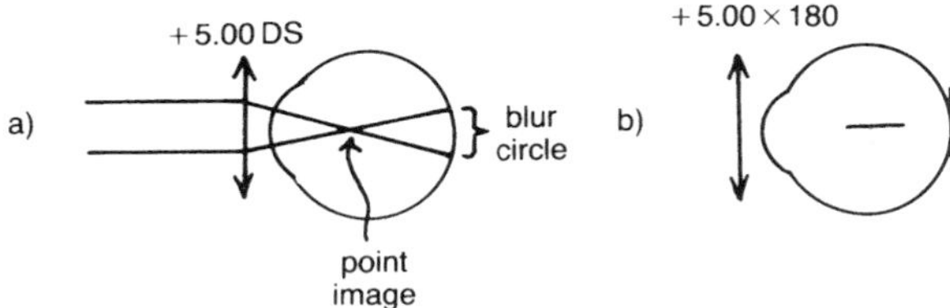

Figure 10.27 a, Observer viewing through a +5.00 D spherical lens; b, observer viewing through a +5.00 × 180 lens.

Neglecting effectivity, we can add the two power crosses to obtain

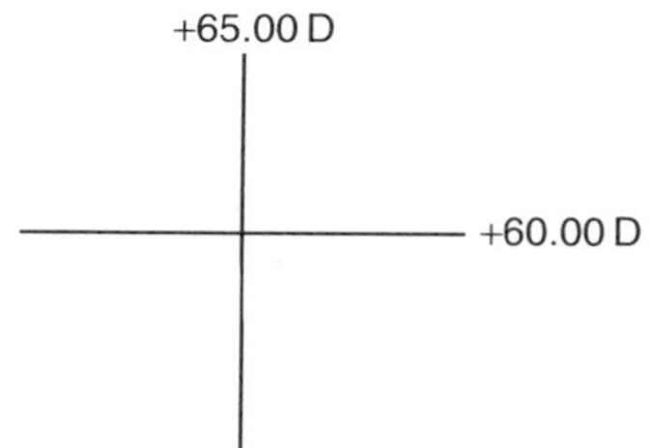

The +60.00 D of power in the horizontal meridian forms a vertical line image that is on the retina, while the +65.00 D of power in the vertical meridian forms a horizontal line image that is 5.00 D in front of the retina (i.e., in the vitreous). All the light in the single astigmatic bundle first goes through the horizontal line image and then goes through the vertical line. The person sees only what is on the retina, so the person sees a vertical line image.

It is instructive to consider an alternative explanation of this effect. When the emmetrope looks directly at the distant point source, there is a point image on the retina. We can think of this point image as two coincident perpendicular line images each of zero length. Now when the emmetrope looks through +5.00 × 180 lens at a distant point source, the +5.00 × 180 lens is responsible for horizontal lines and it pulls the horizontal line 5.00 D up into the vitreous while leaving the vertical line image on the retina. (Just as both line images in a conoid get shorter whenever the two lines are moved closer together, both line images get longer whenever the two lines are moved farther apart—even if only one line does the moving.)

Still another way to explain the effect of the emmetrope looking through the +5.00 × 180 lens is to consider that, for the distant point source, the lens by itself forms a real horizontal line image (20 cm behind the lens) and a virtual vertical line image that is at optical infinity. An unaccommodated emmetrope looking through the +5.00 × 180 cylindrical lens at the distance point source focuses on (or sees) the virtual vertical line image at optical infinity.

10.12 CLASSIFICATION AND CORRECTION OF ASTIGMATS

A central feature of the mathematical discipline of differential geometry is that over a small enough area any smooth surface can be approximated by a toric

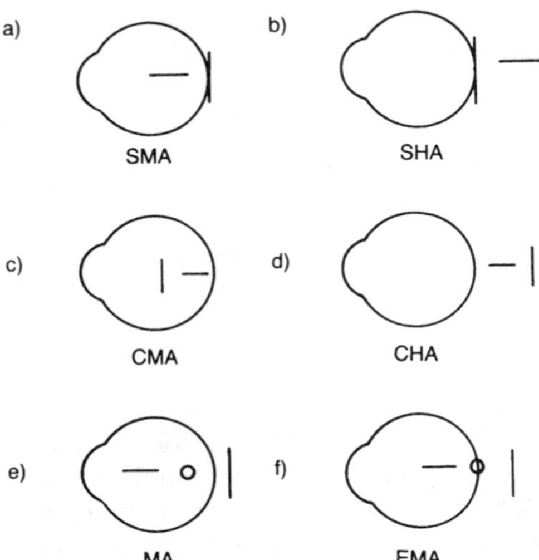

Figure 10.28 Classification of astigmatism.

surface. (Keep in mind that spherical and cylindrical surfaces are both special cases of toric surfaces.) The cornea is the major source of astigmatism in the human eye. This happens when the middle of the corneal surface is toric instead of spherical. Basically the cornea is trying to be spherical, but if it misses and is still smooth, then in most cases we can approximate the cornea by a toric surface. The crystalline lens is also a possible source of astigmatism in the eye.

When astigmatism is present, a conoid of Sturm is set up inside the eye. Astigmatism classification by power depends on where the conoid's line images are relative to the retina in the unaccommodated eye looking at a distant point source. The classifications are simple myopic, simple hyperopic, compound myopic, compound hyperopic, and mixed.

A simple myopic astigmat (SMA) has one line image on the retina and one in front of the retina (Figure 10.28a). A simple hyperopic astigmat (SHA) has one line image on the retina and one that wants to be formed behind the retina (Figure 10.28b). (We usually just say the second line image is behind the retina.)

A compound myopic astigmat (CMA) has both line images in front of the retina (Figure 10.28c). A compound hyperopic astigmat (CHA) has both line images behind the retina (Figure 10.28d).

A mixed astigmat (MA) has one line image in front of the retina and one line image behind the retina (Figure 10.28e). As a special case, an equal mixed astigmat (EMA) has each line image dioptrically the same distance from the retina, in which case the circle of least confusion is on the retina (Figure 10.28f).

Assuming that a typical emmetropic meridian has a power of +60.00 D, Figure 10.29 shows power crosses for the cases considered in Figure 10.28. Obviously, the SMA has one myopic and one emmetropic principal meridian (Figure 10.29a), the SHA has one hyperopic and one emmetropic principal meridian (Figure 10.29b), the CMA has two myopic principal meridians (Figure 10.29c), the CHA has two hyperopic principal meridians (Figure 10.29d), and a MA has one myopic and one hyperopic principal meridian (Figure 10.29e). In the EMA, the dioptric difference between the myopic meridian and the emmetropic meridian is equal in magnitude to the dioptric difference between the hyperopic meridian and the emmetropic meridian (Figure 10.29f).

Figure 10.29 Ocular power crosses and astigmatism classification.

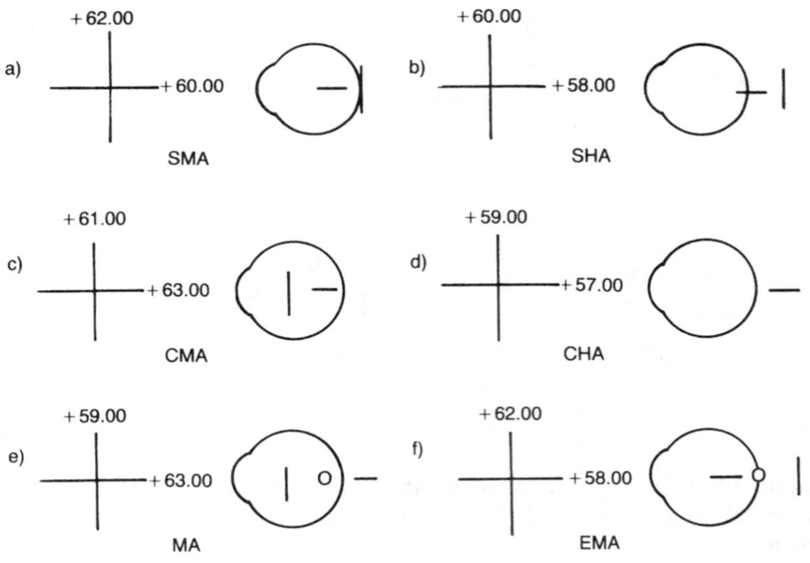

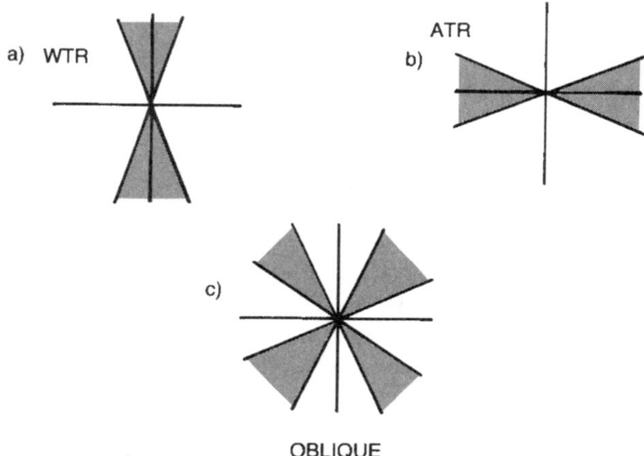

Figure 10.30 Classification by orientation of the major ocular meridian.

Astigmatism is also classified by orientation. The *major meridian* of the eye is the principal meridian with the most plus power. When the eye's major meridian is vertical or within 30° of vertical on either side, the astigmatism is called *with-the-rule* (WTR in Figure 10.30a). When the eye's major meridian is horizontal or within 30° of horizontal on either side, the astigmatism is called *against-the-rule* (ATR in Figure 10.30b). When the eye's major meridian is in either one of the remaining zones, the astigmatism is called *oblique* (Figure 10.30c). One oblique zone is centered on 45° and the other on 135°.

WTR is the most common type of astigmatism, and ATR is the next most common. As people age, WTR astigmatism tends to change to ATR astigmatism. Oblique astigmatism is the least common. In Figure 10.29, a, b, d and f are WTR, while c, and e are ATR.

In WTR astigmatism, the meridian of the eye with the most plus power (the major meridian) is within 30° of vertical. Thus a minus cylinder correction for WTR astigmatism must have its most minus power within 30° of vertical, which means that its axis meridian is within 30° of the horizontal meridian (e.g., −1.00 × 180, −1.00 × 22, −1.00 × 164). In summary: *In WTR astigmatism, it is the major meridian of the eye that is within 30° of vertical, while the minus cylinder axis meridian of the eye's correction is within 30° of horizontal.*

In ATR astigmatism, the meridian of the eye with the most plus power (the major meridian) is within 30° of horizontal. Thus a minus cylinder correction for ATR astigmatism must have its most minus power within 30° of horizontal, which means that its axis meridian is within 30° of the vertical (90) meridian (e.g., −1.00 × 90, −1.00 × 110, −1.00 × 75). In summary: *In ATR astigmatism, it is the major meridian of the eye that is within 30° of horizontal, while the minus cylinder axis meridian of the eye's correction is within 30° of vertical.*

A correction of −5.00 ⊂ −0.75 × 34 is for an oblique compound myopic astigmat. A correction of +0.50 ⊂ −1.00 × 90 is for an ATR EMA. Note that the spherical equivalent of a correction for an EMA is always zero.

EXAMPLE 10.10

When uncorrected and unaccommodated, Judge Belinda Smiley looks at a distant point source and sees a horizontal line. When a −3.50 D spherical lens is held directly in front of her unaccommodated eye, Belinda sees a vertical line. What type of astigmatism does Belinda have? What is her spherocylindrical prescription in minus cylinder form?

From the stated information, Belinda (uncorrected and unaccommodated) has a horizontal line image on her retina. When the −3.50 D spherical ens is added, it moves the horizontal line 3.50 D behind the retina. According to the stated information, with the −3.50 D lens in place, Belinda has a vertical line image on her retina. Figure 10.31a shows the line image locations with the −3.50 D lens in place. When the −3.50 D lens is removed, both line images moves forward 3.50 D, so the vertical line image would then be 3.50 D in front of Belinda's retina and the horizontal line returns to the retina (Figure 10.31b).

The lens needed to correct Belinda's vision must move the vertical line image 3.50 D back without moving the horizontal line image. This lens is a −3.50 × 90. Belinda is an ATR SMA.

We can also determine Belinda's correction from a power cross analysis. Assume that +60.00 D is emmetropic. Power in the vertical meridian forms horizontal line images. Since Belinda sees a horizontal line when uncorrected and unaccommodated, she must be emmetropic in the vertical meridian. Since power in the horizontal meridian forms vertical lines and Belinda sees a vertical line with the −3.50 D spherical

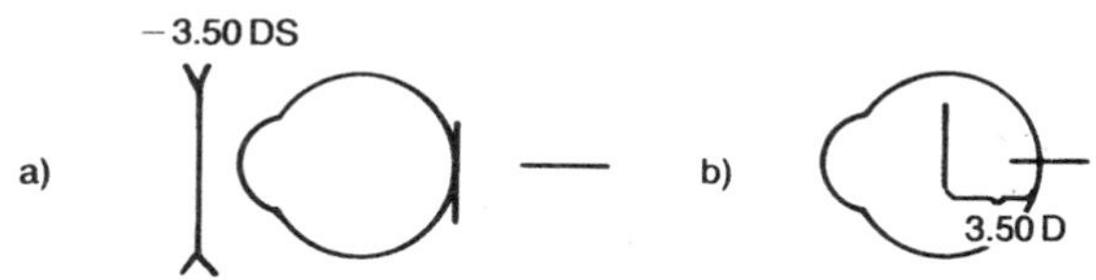

Figure 10.31 Line image locations for Belinda Smiley.

lens in place, her horizontal meridian must be myopic. A power cross for Belinda's eye is

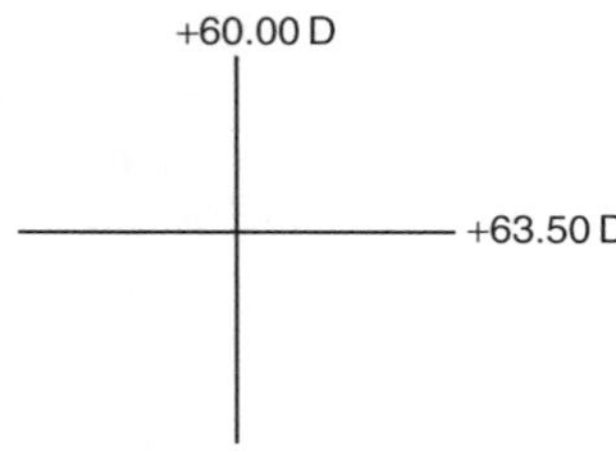

Neglecting effectivity, the correcting lens together with the eye must add to +60.00 D of power in both meridians, so the correcting lens power cross is

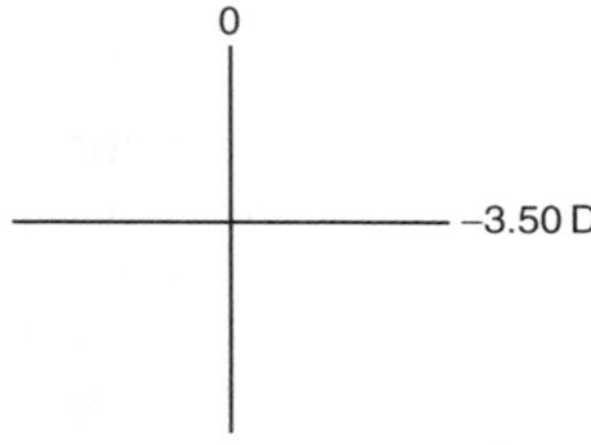

which is the power cross for a −3.50 × 90 cylindrical lens.

EXAMPLE 10.11

Dr. Ulysses Bonemeal looks at a distant point source through a +4.75 D spherical lens and sees a horizontal line image. When the +4.75 D lens is replaced by a +6.75 D spherical lens, Dr. Bonemeal sees a vertical line. Assuming no accommodation, what is Dr. Bonemeal's astigmatism classification and sphere-minus cylinder correction?

Since Dr. Bonemeal sees a horizontal line when the +4.75 D sphere is in place, the horizontal line image in Dr. Bonemeal's uncorrected eye must be 4.75 D behind the retina. Similarly, the vertical line image in Dr. Bonemeal's uncorrected eye must be 6.75 D behind the retina (Figure 10.32a).

Spherical lenses move both line images the same dioptric amount. When the +6.75 D spherical lens is in place, the vertical line image is on the retina and the horizontal line image is then 2.00 D in front of the retina (Figure 10.32b). Then a −2.00 × 180 lens moves the horizontal line back to the retina without moving the vertical line. This collapses the conoid and leaves a point image (Figure 10.32c). The sphere-minus cylinder correction is +6.75 ⊂ −2.00 × 180. Dr. Bonemeal is a WTR CHA.

Note that with the +4.75 D spherical lens in place, the horizontal line is on the retina and the vertical line is 2.00 D behind the retina. Then a +2.00 × 90 cylindrical lens would pull the vertical line forward and collapse the conoid. The resulting Rx, +4.75 ⊂ +2.00 × 90, is the transposition equivalent of the sphere-minus cylinder Rx. Note that both Dr. Bonemeal's sphere-minus cylinder correction and sphere-plus cylinder correction have the exact same power cross. Thus these two corrections are optically equivalent.

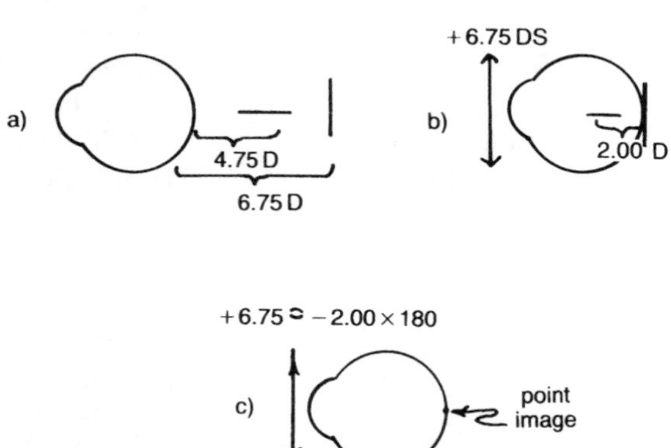

Figure 10.32 Line image locations for Dr. Bonemeal.

EXAMPLE 10.12

President Ann Hydrous needs a −5.00 ⊂ −1.00 ×144 distance vision correction. Classify Ann's astigmatism and show where her line images are when Ann is uncorrected and unaccommodated.

The power cross for Ann's correction is

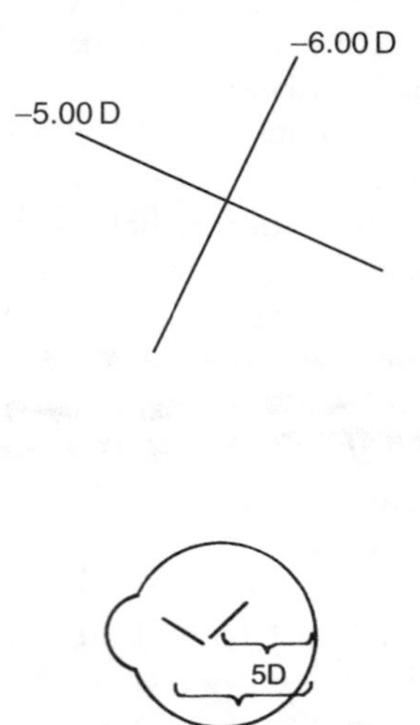

Figure 10.33 Line image locations for Ann Hydrous.

The major meridian is oblique, and Ann's correcting lens has minus power in both principal meridians. Ann is an oblique CMA.

We can work from the power cross to determine the line image location in the uncorrected eye. The 5.00 D in the 144 meridian means that in the uncorrected eye, a line image at 54 is 5.00 D in front of the retina. The −6.00 D in the 54 meridian means that in the uncorrected eye, a line image at 144 is 6.00 D in front of the retina (Figure 10.33).

EXAMPLE 10.13

Major Nancy Block-Head holds a +7.00 D spherical lens directly in front of her eye. With the spherical lens in place, Nancy can clearly see a grating target consisting of vertical lines when the target is 50 cm in front of the lens. When the target is rotated so that it consists of horizontal lines, Nancy can clearly see the chart when it is 33.3 cm in front of the lens. Assuming no accommodation, classify Nancy's astigmatism and give her correction in sphere-minus cylinder form.

For a single point source, power in the horizontal meridian forms vertical line images. The fact that the vertical lines are clear when the +7.00 D spherical lens is in place and the grating is at 50 cm ($U = -2.00$ D) indicates that the eye's horizontal meridian needs a +5.00-D vergence leaving the correcting lens (i.e., $V = P + U = +7.00\text{ D} - 2.00\text{ D} = +5.00\text{ D}$).

Power in the vertical meridian forms horizontal line images. The fact that the horizontal line images are clear when the +7.00 D spherical lens is in place and the grating is 33.3 cm away means that the eye's vertical meridian needs a +4.00 D vergence leaving the correcting lens (i.e., $V = P + U = +7.00\text{ D} + (-3.00\text{ D}) = +4.00\text{ D}$).

For distance vision, the power cross of the correction is

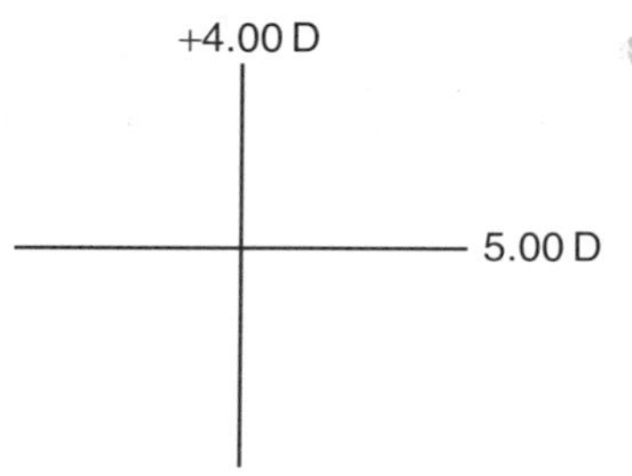

From the power cross, the correction is +5.00 ⊂ −1.00 × 180. Nancy is a WTR CHA.

EXAMPLE 10.14

The principal meridians of Duke Fred Overboot's eye are 55 and 145. In the 55 meridian, the power in Duke's eye is +62.00 D, while in the 145 meridian, the power is +58.00 D. The power cross for Duke's eye is

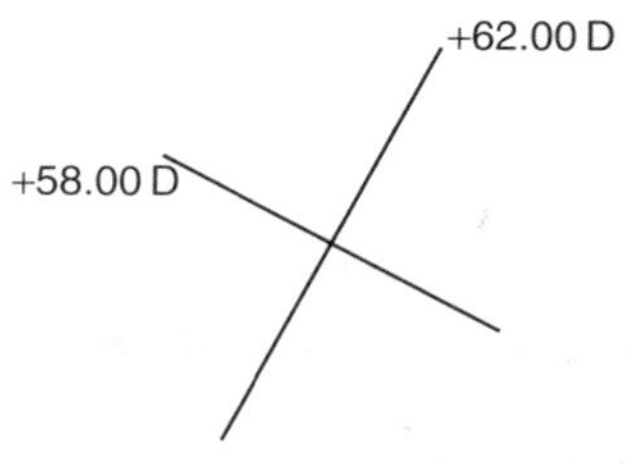

Assuming +60.00 D is emmetropic, what is the classification of Duke's astigmatism, and what is his correction?

The power cross for Duke's correction is

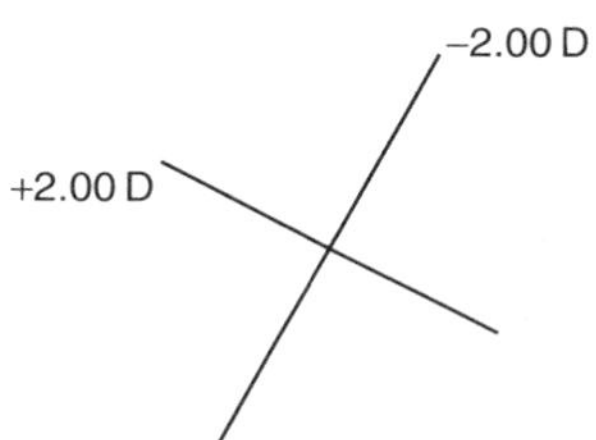

From the power cross, the correcting spherocylinder is +2.00 ⊂ −4.00 × 145. Duke is an oblique EMA.

10.13 THE CLOCK DIAL CHART

Extended targets are much easier to use clinically than point sources. We can use an extended target consisting of radial lines to check for the orientation of the principal meridians as well as the amount of astigmatism. Such a chart is called a clock dial chart (Figure 10.34). In situations where accommodation remains active, the clock dial chart is typically used as follows. The patient views the reasonably distant (i.e., 20 ft or 6 m) chart through a lens holder (usually a phoropter). Plus spherical lenses of increasing power are placed in

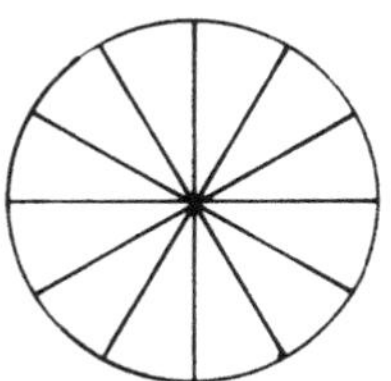

Figure 10.34 Clock dial chart.

the holder until the patient reports the chart is blurred, and the examiner is sure the patient's clear image is in front of the retina. In this case the patient is said to be *fogged*. In the fogged state, accommodation blurs the image more, and that presumably eliminates any stimulus to accommodate.

The examiner then decreases the plus spherical power (or adds minus spherical power), which moves the clear image back towards the retina. When the person has no astigmatism, all the radial lines clear up simultaneously. When the person has astigmatism, one of the radial lines clears first. At that point, one line image is on the retina and the other line image is in front of the retina, just as in simple myopic astigmatism. The examiner then starts adding minus cylindrical lenses of increasing power with the axis of the minus cylinder lined up perpendicularly to the clear line on the retina. This minus cylinder moves the other line back onto the retina collapsing the conoid.

In the clock dial procedure, the examiner must depend on the patient to tell him or her when the lines are clear. We call this a *subjective refraction* (dependent on the subject). There are also *objective refraction* procedures, such as retinoscopy or autorefraction, in which the information is gathered without depending on responses from the patient.

Consider Ella Mentary. Ella sits in front of a distant clock dial chart and is fogged. As the fog is decreased, Ella reports that a line at 63° comes clear first. The spherical power in place is +3.50 D. Minus cylinder axis 153 is then added to the sphere. Ella reports that all lines clear up when −0.75 D of cylindrical power is in place. Ella's Rx is +3.50 ⊂ −0.75 × 153.

Note that with this procedure, the Rx automatically comes out as a sphere-minus cylinder combination as opposed to a sphere-plus cylinder combination. The sphere-minus cylinder combination controls accommodation while the sphere-plus cylinder combination does not.

The standard coordinate system is set up in terms of the view of the examiner looking toward the patient (i.e., the contra-ocular view). However, the patient viewing the clock dial is looking in the other direction and would tend to set up a different coordinate system. To avoid this, we simply label the examiner's standard coordinate system as it would appear from the *ocular view* (Figure 10.35a). Recall that in the contra-ocular view, zero occurs on the right and the first quadrant angles are counter-clockwise up from the zero. In the ocular view, zero occurs on the left and the first quadrant angles are clockwise up from the zero.

You can investigate the two views by drawing a centered standard examiner's coordinate system on a sheet of paper (i.e., contra-ocular view), and then turn the paper over and draw a clock on the back side (the ocular view). Make one of the clock lines very dark (such as the 10–4 o'clock line). Then turn the paper around so that you are viewing the standard contra-ocular coordinate system. You can now identify the meridian that the dark clock line is parallel to. (It is the 30° meridian for the 10–4 o'clock line, the 60° meridian for the 11–5 o'clock line, the 120 meridian for the 1–7 o'clock line, and the 150 meridian for the 2–8 o'clock line).

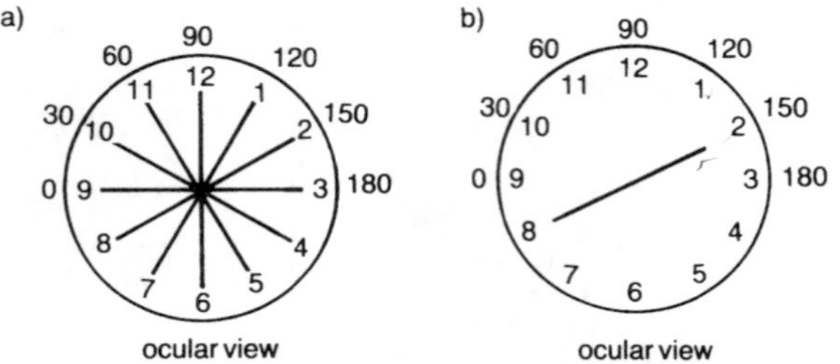

Figure 10.35 Ocular view of a clock dial.

EXAMPLE 10.15

Angela Basket-Case is fogged, and as the fog is reduced, the 11–5 o'clock line comes clear first. The spherical lens in place is −4.25 D. Then correctly oriented minus cylinders are added, and all lines come clear at a −1.25-D cylinder power. What is Angela's Rx in minus cylinder form?

From Figure 10.35b, the 11–5 o'clock line is the 60° line. The line image still in front of the retina is the 150° line. A −1.25 × 150 lens moves the 150 line back without moving the 60 line. This collapses the conoid and all lines clear. The Rx is −4.25 ⊂ −1.25 × 150.

For the minus cylinder refraction, one can derive a clinically used rule called the *rule of thirty*. As the fog is reduced with the spherical lenses, one of the clock lines clears first. According to the rule of thirty, take the smaller clock number of the first clear line (e.g., 5 in the 11–5 o'clock line), multiply it by 30°, and set the minus cylinder axis at the resulting angle (e.g., 5 times 30 = 150). Then add minus cylinder power until all lines are clear. (Note that the rule of thirty gives the minus cylinder axis of the correction in the previous example.)

10.14 JACKSON CROSS CYLINDER POWER REFINEMENT

Usually the clock dial test provides a first estimate of the spherocylindrical correction. Let's call this first estimate the tentative correction. (One could also obtain a tentative correction from other tests—such as retinoscopy or autorefraction.) The Jackson Cross Cylinder (JCC) is very useful for refining a tentative correction. Section 13.16 considers the JCC test for cylinder axis refinement. Here we consider the JCC test for the cylinder power refinement.

A JCC consists of a spherocylindrical lens with plus power in one principal meridian and minus power of equal magnitude in the other principal meridian (e.g., a +0.25 × 180 combined with −0.25 × 90, which can also be expressed as the sphere–cylinder combination +0.25 ⊂ −0.50 × 90). From Eqs. 10.5 or 10.6, the Sp Eq of JCC is zero.

EXAMPLE 10.16

Teddy Roosterbird is an emmetrope. Teddy looks through a +0.25 ⊂ −0.50 × 90 JCC (JCC #1) at a distant point source (left power cross below). When the JCC is flipped about a meridian 45° from the principal meridians, the power meridians exchange and the new parameters are +0.25 ⊂ −0.50 × 180 (JCC #2, right power cross below). Does flipping the JCC make any difference in the clarity of Teddy's retinal image?

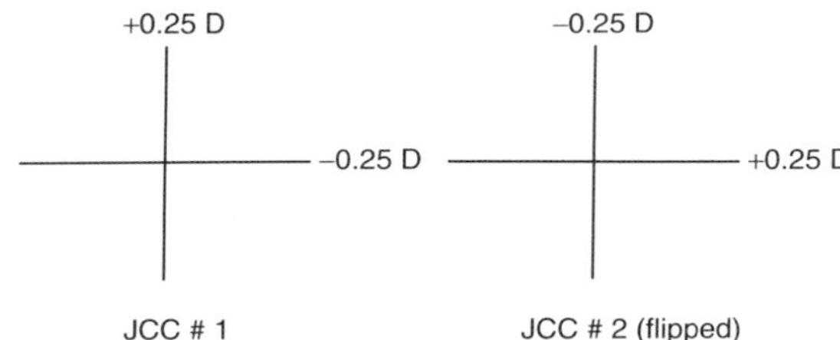

Together with the eye, JCC #1 sets up a conoid of Sturm in which the line image formed by the vertical meridian is pulled 0.25 D in front of the retina and the other line image is pushed 0.25 D behind the retina, leaving the circle of least confusion on the retina (Figure 10.36a). When the JCC is flipped (#2), the line images exchange positions, but the same circle of least confusion remains on the retina (Figure 10.36b). The circle of least confusion is a blur circle, so the JCCs blur Teddy's retina image, but the flips do not change the amount of blur. So for emmetropes, the flips do not change the clarity of the retinal image.

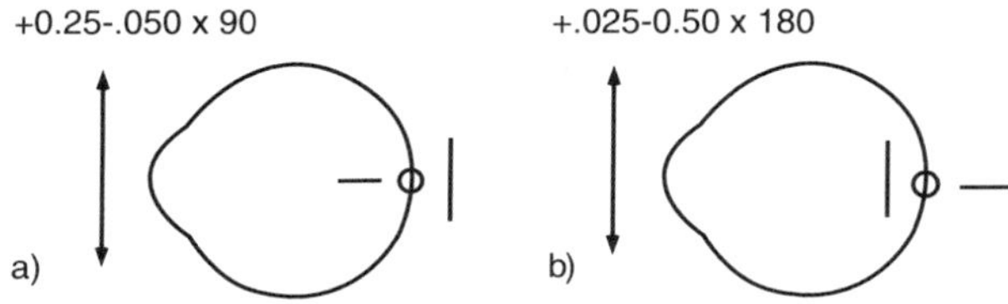

Figure 10.36 a, b, Flipped JCC positions for an emmetrope.

As Example 10.16 showed, a JCC placed in front of an emmetropic eye creates a conoid of Sturm inside the eye with the circle of least confusion on the retina. Flipping the JCC interchanges the powers in the principal meridians, but leaves the same circle of least confusion on the retina. The emmetrope then has no difference in clarity of the retinal image when the JCC is flipped. This is the endpoint of a JCC test for refinement (i.e., #1 is the same as #2).

Now consider Mr. U.R. Dippy who needs a −1.50 × 180 spectacle correction. In Dippy's uncorrected eye, the vertical line image is on the retina and the horizontal line image is 1.50 D in front of the retina (Figure 10.37a).

Suppose the cylinder power and axis in Dippy's tentative correction is only −0.50 × 180. This tentative correction leaves the horizontal line image 1.00 D in front of the retina, while the vertical line image is still on the retina (Figure 10.37b). We can improve Dippy's acuity under the circumstances by adding a −0.50 D spherical lens. The sphere moves both lines images back 0.50 D, which leaves the horizontal line 0.50 D in front of the retina, the vertical line 0.50 D behind the retina, and places the circle of least confusion on

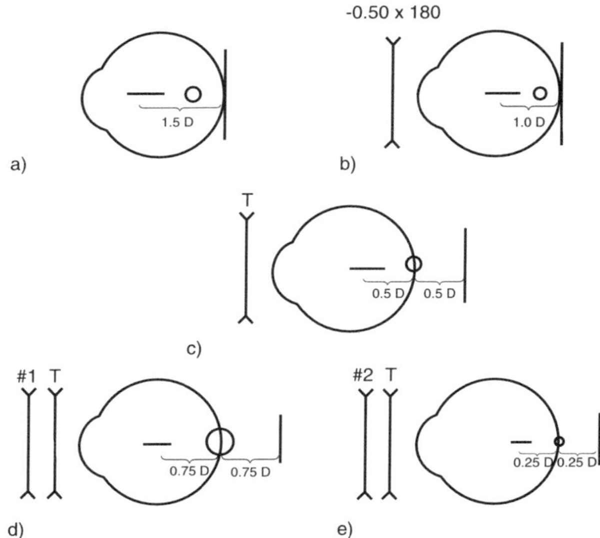

Figure 10.37 Line image positions for U.R. Dippy: a, uncorrected; b, with a −0.50×180 lens; c, with a tentative correction T of −0.50 ⊂ −0.50×180; d, with T and JCC #1 (+0.25 ⊂ −0.50×90); e, with T and JCC #2 (+0.25 ⊂ −0.50×180).

the retina. (The $-0.50 \bigcirc -0.50 \times 180$ lenses are labeled as lens *T* in Figure 10.37c).

Now suppose a $+0.25 \bigcirc -0.50 \times 90$ JCC (JCC #1) is placed over the $-0.50 \bigcirc -0.50 \times 180$ tentative correction T (Figure 10.37d). The power cross for the JCC is

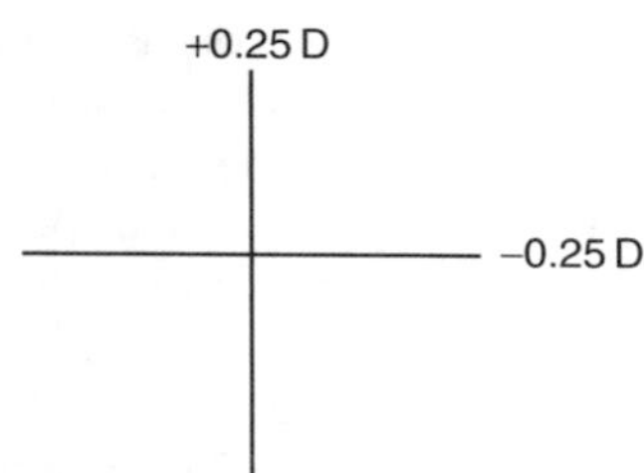

The +0.25 D power in the vertical meridian moves the horizontal line image to a location 0.75 D in front of the retina, while the −0.25 D of power in the horizontal meridian moves the vertical line image to a location 0.75 D behind the retina. Since the JCC has a spherical equivalent of zero, it does not change the location of the circle of least confusion. However, the circle gets larger (more blur) as the line images move farther away.

When the JCC is flipped to $+0.25 \bigcirc -0.50 \times 180$ (JCC #2), the powers interchange on the JCC principal meridians. Starting with the conoid in Dippy's eye with the tentative correction (Figure 10.37c), the −0.25 D of power in the vertical meridian moves the horizontal line image to a position 0.25 D in front of the retina, while the 0.25 D of power in the horizontal meridian moves the vertical line image to a position 0.25 D behind the retina. Dippy still has a circle of least confusion on the retina, but here the circle gets smaller (less blur) as the lines move closer to the retina. Dippy will report that #2 is better (less blurred) than #1. This tells us that we are not at the endpoint yet.

Furthermore since the JCC for choice #2 is $+0.25 \bigcirc -0.50 \times 180$, and the tentative correction of $-0.50 - 0.50 \times 180$ also has a minus cylinder axis of 180, we need to add minus cylinder axis 180 to improve the tentative correction. (If JCC#1 ($+0.25 \bigcirc -0.50 \times 90$) gave Dippy less blur than #2, we would need to remove some of the minus cylinder axis 180 from the tentative correction.)

Usually the changes are made in quarter-diopter steps. However, for illustration purposes, let's assume that -0.50×180 is added, which brings the new tentative correction to $-0.50 \bigcirc -1.00 \times 180$. In order to accurately repeat the JCC test, we need to keep a circle of least confusion on Dippy's retina. To do that, we need maintain a zero spherical equivalent in the lenses that are added. From Eq. 10.6,

$$\text{Sp Eq} = S + \frac{C}{2} = 0$$

gives

$$S = -\left(\frac{C}{2}\right)$$

So whenever we add $C = -0.50$ D of cylinder, we must also add $S = +0.25$ D of sphere power. This brings the improved tentative correction to $-0.25 \bigcirc -1.00 \times 180$.

Now we can repeat the JCC test with the improved correction. Eventually when we get to a correction of plano -1.50×180, JCC choices #1 and #2 will be equal, which is the endpoint. (If we go too far, and put in a -1.75×180 cylinder choice, then the JCC test will bring us back to a cylinder of -1.50×180).

In summary, *the JCC test assumes that a circle of least confusion (a blur circle) is on the patient's retina. In the JCC test for cylinder power, the principal meridians of the JCC are aligned with the principal meridians of the tentative correction. The JCC test has the patient compare two blurred images (#1 and #2). If the better choice (least blur) occurs when the JCC minus cylinder axis is aligned with the minus cylinder axis of the tentative correction, then we add minus cylinder power (and adjust spherical power by $S = -C/2$ to keep the spherical equivalent of the added lenses equal to zero). If the better choice (least blur) occurs when the JCC minus cylinder axis is 90° different from the minus cylinder axis of the tentative correction, then we subtract minus cylinder power (and adjust the spherical power accordingly).*

10.15 EFFECTIVITY AND SPHEROCYLINDRICAL LENSES

Due to vergence effectivity (Chapter 6), the correction at the cornea may have a different value than the correction at the spectacle plane. In the principal meridians of a toric wavefront, the vergence effectivity considerations are identical to those for a spherical wavefront. However, the work has now doubled since there are two principal meridians.

For a $S \bigcirc C \times \theta$ spherocylindrical lens, the powers in the principal meridians are S and $(S + C)$. These are the powers that must be used in the effectivity calculations. Note that C is the difference between the powers in the two meridians and cannot be used by itself in the effectivity calculations. (An apparent exception occurs when S is zero, in which case $S + C$ is equal to C.)

EXAMPLE 10.17

Harry Ape wears a $-9.00 \bigcirc -3.00 \times 180$ distance vision correction at a vertex distance of

13 mm. What is Harry's correction at the cornea?

The power cross for Harry's correction is

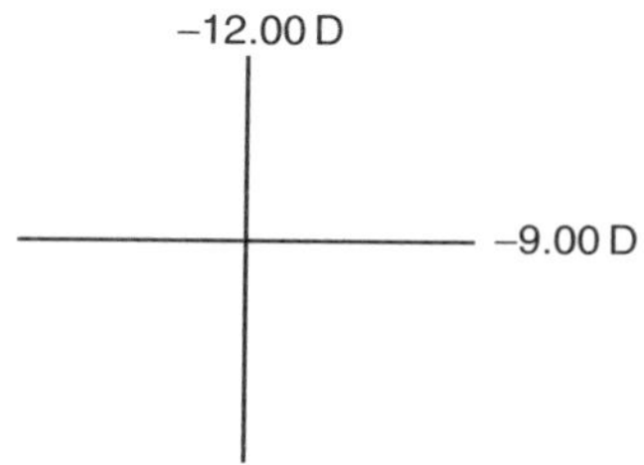

We then do the effectivity calculations in each meridian exactly as in Chapter 6. For the vertical meridian a −12.00 D wavefront traveling right has its center of curvature at 100/(12), or −8.33 cm. From the cornea, the center of curvature is −(8.33 + 1.3) cm or −9.63 cm. The vergence at the cornea is 100/(−9.63) cm or −10.38 D. The vergence changes show that the vertical meridian's diverging wavefront loses curvature as it moves from the spectacle plane to the cornea. The wavefront center of curvature in the vertical meridian is at the eye's far point for that meridian. The eye's vertical meridian is myopic and the far point is real. The same procedure for the horizontal meridian gives −8.06 D at the cornea (again, a loss in curvature). The horizontal meridian is also myopic and its far point is real and at the center of curvature of the wavefront in the horizontal meridian. The vergence cross at the cornea is

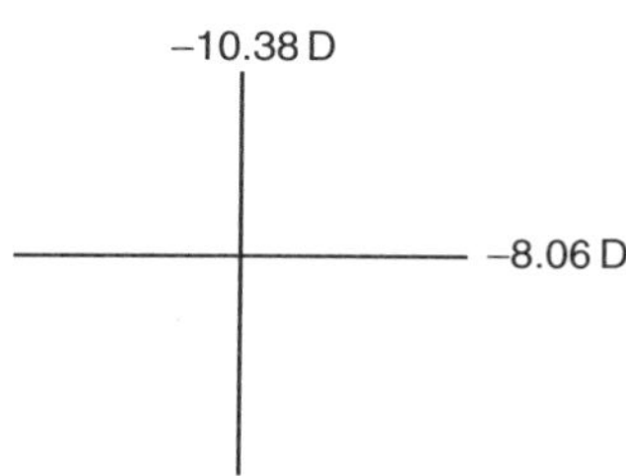

From the vergence cross, Harry's Rx at the cornea is −8.06 ⊂ −2.32 × 180.

Note that the minus cylinder axis did not change. Also, note that the effectivity calculations were done for the −12.00 D and −9.00 D principal meridian powers, and not for the −3.00 D cylinder power. If you use a −3.00 D in the spectacle plane, the result at the cornea is −2.89 D, which does not equal the −2.32 D of cylinder power in the answer.

EXAMPLE 10.18

Ms. Furri Ape has a +15.00 ⊂ −5.00 × 146 correction at the cornea. What is Furri's spectacle correction at an 11 mm vertex distance?

The power cross of the correction at the cornea is

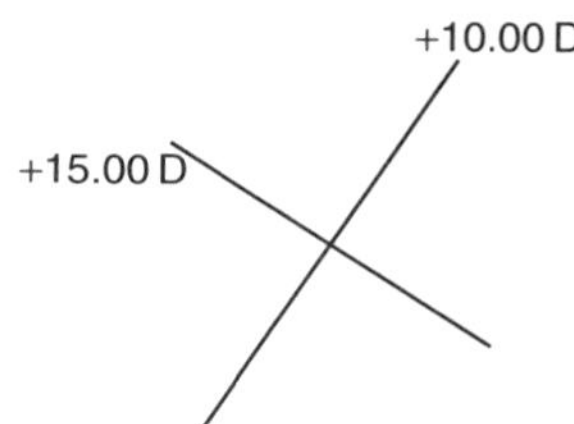

For the 146 meridian, the center of curvature of the wavefront is 100/(+15 D), or +6.67 cm. Clearly, the 146 meridian of the eye is hyperopic and the far point is virtual. From the center of curvature, the spectacle plane is +(6.67 + 1.1) cm, or +7.77 cm. The power in the 146 meridian of the spectacle plane is 100/(+7.77 D), or +12.88 D. A converging wavefront moving from the spectacle plane to the cornea gains curvature, and +12.88 D at the spectacle plane compared to +15.00 D at the cornea is consistent with this.

The same procedure for the 56 meridian gives a power of +9.01 D in the spectacle plane. The resulting power cross in the spectacle plane is

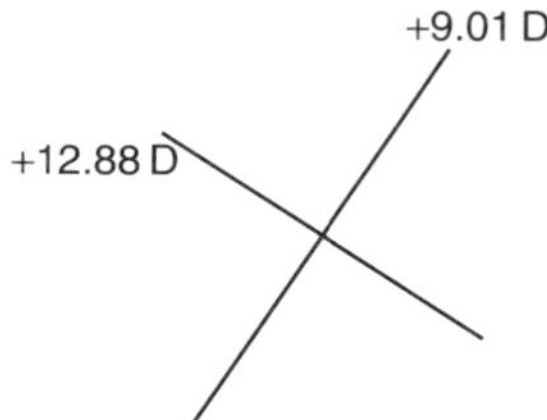

The spectacle Rx is +12.88 ⊂ −3.87 × 146. (Again, the minus cylinder axis is the same, and the −5.00 D of cylinder power cannot be used directly.)

10.16 ACCOMMODATION AND SPHEROCYLINDRICAL CORRECTIONS

As discussed in Chapter 6, vergence effectivity also influences the ocular accommodative demand. A spectacle corrected hyperope has to accommodate more than a spectacle corrected myope viewing the same object at the same distance. Because of vergence effectivity, a spectacle corrected astigmat may have different ocular accommodative demands in the principal meridians. Since accommodation is spherical, this means that the astigmatism at near would no longer be completely corrected.

EXAMPLE 10.19

Cornelius (Corny) Hooper wears a distance vision $+13.00 \bigcirc -9.00 \times 180$ spectacle correction at a 12 mm vertex distance. How much uncorrected astigmatism does Corny have when threading a needle held 14.29 cm in front of his lens?

We need the ocular accommodative demand A_o in each principal meridian. The approximation, Eq. 6.15, will be accurate enough for this example:

$$A_o = A_s\ (1 + 2dP_s)$$

where A_s is the spectacle accommodative demand, and P_s is the power. Here,

$$A_s = -U_s = -100/(-14.29)\,\text{cm} = +7.00\,\text{D}$$

The power cross for the correction is

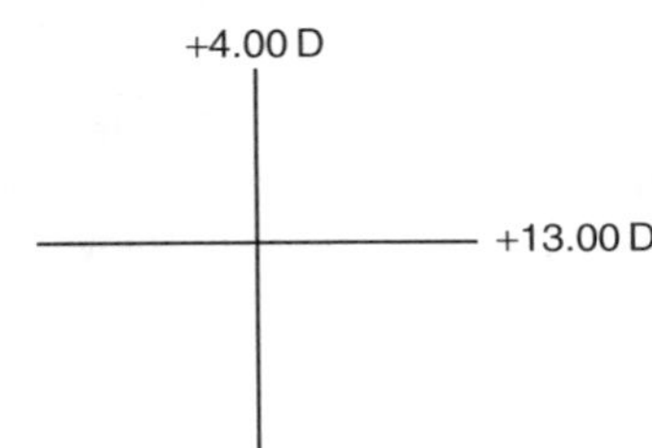

Then the accommodative demand for each principal meridian is

A_o = +7.00 D [1 + (2*0.012 m*4.00 D] = +7.67 D

A_o = +7.00 D [1 + (2*0.012 m*13.00 D] = +9.18 D

The ocular accommodative demand in the vertical meridian is 7.67 D, while the accommodative demand in the horizontal meridian is 9.18 D. The difference in the accommodative demands between the principal meridians is 1.51 D. Corny will have 1.51 D of uncorrected astigmatism when looking through his distance correction at the needle held 14.29 cm from the lens. If Corny accommodates +9.18 D, the vertical line image in each conoid will be on the retina. If Corny accommodates +7.67 D, the horizontal line image in each conoid will be on the retina. If Corny accommodates dioptrically halfway in-between (i.e., +8.43 D), the circle of least confusion in each conoid would be on the retina.

The difference in the ocular accommodative demand for the different principal meridians is significant only for high astigmats. If this difference is bothering a patient, they may need a spectacle correction for near that is different from their spectacle correction for distance. (Toric contact lenses may avoid this problem.) Fortunately, in most astigmats the amount of astigmatism is low (3.00 D or less), and the difference is insignificant.

PROBLEMS

1. A point source is located 25 cm in front of a $+6.00 \times 180$ cylindrical lens. Where is the real line image? What is its orientation?
2. A point source is located 50 cm in front of a $+4.50 \bigcirc +3.00 \times 90$ spherocylindrical lens. Find the line image positions and specify the orientations. Also, find the position of the circle of least confusion.
3. Specify the power cross for a $+5.75 \bigcirc -3.25 \times 64$ lens. Also, specify the spherical equivalent and the equivalent sphere-plus cylinder combination.
4. Each of the following patients has horizontal and vertical principal meridians. The eye is represented by a thin spherocylindrical lens in air located 16.67 mm in front of the screen (retina). For a distant point source, specify the part of the conoid on the retina for the uncorrected eye, classify the astigmatism, and specify the correction as a sphere-minus cylinder combination. You may neglect any vertex distance effects.
   a. Susan Vos—vertical power +62.00 D, horizontal power +60.00 D.
   b. Al Hoot—vertical power +62.00 D, horizontal power +58.00 D.
   c. Sammy Bavis—vertical power +58.00 D, horizontal power +56.00 D.
   d. Bonnie Arden—vertical power +58.00 D, horizontal power +60.00 D.
   e. Henry Kissing—vertical power +64.00 D, horizontal power +62.00 D.
   f. Wayne Pork—vertical power +54.00 D, horizontal power +59.00 D.
5. For each of the patients in the previous problem, specify what lines on a clock dial would appear darkest (least blurred) through a $+2.00 \times 180$ combined with a -2.00×90.
6. Express the correction for each of the patients in the problem #4 as a sphere-plus cylinder combination.

7. Computerina Smith has a $-4.50 \bigcirc +2.50 \times 110$ spectacle correction. What is Computerina's correction expressed as a sphere-minus cylinder combination.
8. Specify the sphere-minus cylinder combination that is equivalent to -0.25×180 combined with $+0.25 \times 90$.
9. When looking at a distant point source through a -5.00 D spherical lens, Gerald Weakman (unaccommodated) clearly sees a line parallel to the 54 meridian. When looking through a -3.00 D spherical lens, Gerald clearly sees a line at 144. What is Gerald's correction in minus cylinder form?
10. Mickey Rookie (unaccommodated) looks at a distant point source through a $+2.00$ D spherical lens and sees a clear line parallel to the 135 meridian. When Mickey looks through a -1.00 D spherical lens, he sees a clear line parallel to the 45 meridian. What is Mickey's correction in minus cylinder form?
11. Joyce Jinked (unaccommodated) looks at a distant point source through a -4.50 D spherical lens and reports that the 11–5 o'clock line is clear. When Joyce looks through a -2.50 D spherical lens, she reports that the 2–8 o'clock line is clear. What is Joyce's correction in minus cylinder form?
12. Kevin Wallflower (unaccommodated) looks at a distant point source through a $+2.25$ D spherical lens and reports that the 10–4 o'clock line is clear. When Kevin looks through a $+3.25$ D spherical lens, he reports that the 1–7 o'clock line is clear. What is Kevin's correction in minus cylinder form?
13. When uncorrected, Kevin Wallflower of the previous problem looks at the distant clock dial chart. What accommodation would make all lines equally visible?
14. June Tucks has a $-7.25 \bigcirc -4.50 \times 15$ spectacle correction at a 13 mm vertex distance. What is June's correction at the cornea?
15. Jermaine Bugle has a $+11.75 \bigcirc -4.00 \times 56$ correction at the cornea. What is Jermaine's spectacle correction at a 12 mm vertex distance?
16. Clem Obtuse has a $+11.00 \bigcirc -7.00 \times 180$ spectacle correction worn at a 13 mm vertex distance. For a thin lens eye model, use the ocular accommodative demand approximation to find A_o in each principal meridian when Clem views an object 17.4 cm from his spectacle lens. Since accommodation is spherical, how much uncorrected astigmatism does Clem have when viewing the near object through his spectacles?

CHAPTER 11

Prisms

11.1 INTRODUCTION

Figure 11.1a is a cross-sectional view of a glass plate with parallel sides. Plane waves pass through the plate without a change in vergence. When a collimated pencil is incident at an angle *i*, the beam emerges at an angle *i* but is displaced from the original path.

Figure 11.1 a, Plane waves traveling through a flat glass slab; b, plane waves bent toward the base of a prism; c, virtual image appears deviated toward the apex; d, dispersion.

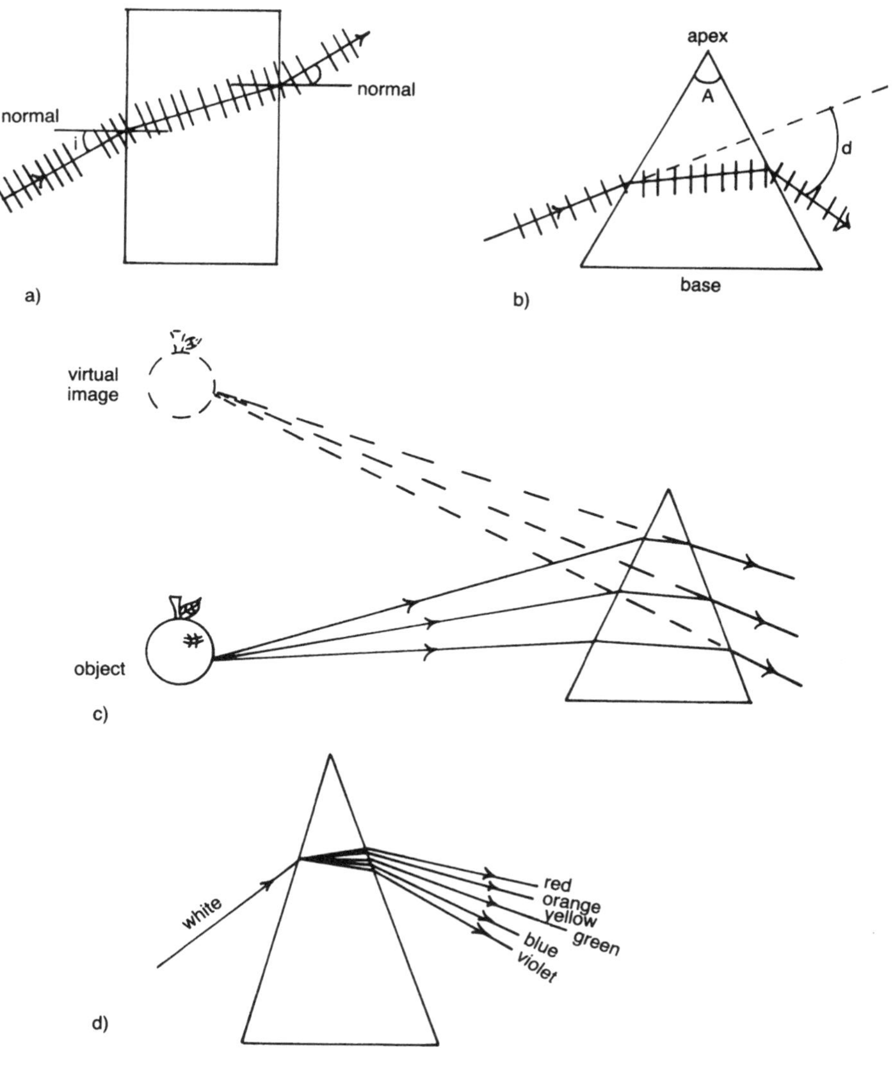

Figure 11.1b shows a cross-sectional view of a piece of glass in which the sides are inclined at an angle A. In optics, this general shape is called a prism. The *apex* of the prism is the point at which the sides meet, and the angle A is called the *apex angle*. The *base* of the prism is the side opposite the apex. Plane waves pass through the prism without a change in vergence. However, the prism changes the direction of travel, and deviates (bends) a collimated pencil through an angle d towards the base.

Figure 11.1c shows a (near) apple in front of a prism. For the bundle of rays shown, the prism deviates each ray towards the base. As a result, the rays leaving the prism appear to be diverging from a point that is displaced in the direction of the apex. In effect, the prism forms a virtual image that is displaced in the direction of the apex. The fact that a prism (in air) deviates light toward its base while the virtual image appears deviated toward the apex is crucial to the understanding of prism theory. A quick sketch, such as Figure 11.1c, helps keep the relationship clear.

If the rays in Figure 11.1c are reversed, then converging light traveling left is incident on the prism. In this case, the prism has a virtual object (the "old" virtual image) and a conjugate real image (the old object), and the prism deviates the real image toward the base.

When white light is incident on a thick prism, the short wavelengths are deviated more than the long wavelengths (Figure 11.1d). This is the phenomenon

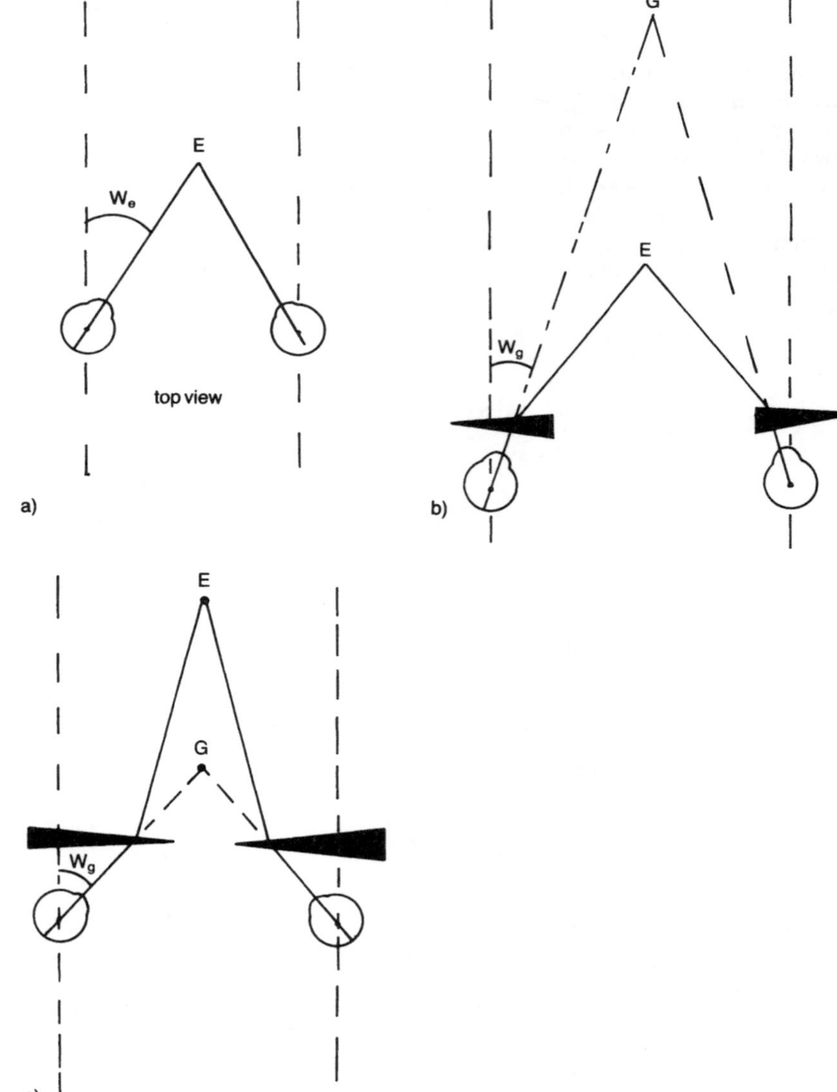

Figure 11.2 a, Convergence demand with object point at E; b, with base in prisms, eyes do not need to converge as much; c, with base out prisms, eyes have to converge more.

of dispersion and results in a rainbow-like spectrum. For thin prisms, the amount of dispersion is small.

The fovea is the small area on the human retina with the highest density of cones. In order for a person to resolve detail in the object, the conjugate retinal image must be on the fovea. This is normally achieved when the person looks directly at the object.

For humans to enjoy the full benefits of binocular vision, the two eyes must both look at the object so that the conjugate retinal image of each eye is on the fovea. Consider an emmetrope looking at a centrally located near object (point *E* in Figure 11.2a). Not only does the ciliary muscle have to provide the needed accommodation, but the extra-ocular muscles also have to correctly aim each eye. Relative to the straight-ahead position, the demand on each eye is to turn through the angle w_e. Problems in the extra-ocular muscle system can cause stress (itching, burning, tearing), or even double vision (when the eyes do not aim at the same point).

Prisms are tools that help us diagnose and solve problems with the extra-ocular muscle system. The so-called base in prisms shown in Figure 11.2b can help a convergence insufficiency problem by bending the rays so that the eyes only need to converge (turn in) to point *G* (instead of to *E*). Relative to the straight ahead position, the demand for point *G* is the angle w_g, which is less than the demand w_e for point *E* without the prisms. So base in prisms reduce the convergence demand, and can help a person with a convergence insufficiency problem achieve stress free binocular vision.

When the brain sends the involuntary neural signal to accommodate, it also sends a neural signal to the extra-ocular muscles to converge (turn in) the two eyes. This may result in an over-convergence problem. Consider Figure 11.2c. Suppose that when the person accommodates for point *E*, the innervation causes the eyes to converge towards point *G*. Then the extra-ocular muscles would try to pull the eyes back towards point *E* resulting in stress on the binocular neuromuscular system. The base out prisms in Figure 11.2c enables this person to image point *E* on both foveae even though the eyes are converging towards point *G*. This helps the person achieve stress free binocular vision.

11.2 TOTAL INTERNAL REFLECTION

Before we launch into prism theory, we need to again consider Snell's law and an associated effect called total internal reflection. For light incident on an interface between medium's n_1 and n_2, Snell's law is

$$n_1 \sin\theta_i = n_2 \sin\theta_r \tag{11.1}$$

When light is initially in the lower index medium, the ray bends (is refracted) towards the normal (Figure 11.3a). When the light is initially in the higher index medium, the ray bends away from the normal (Figure 11.3b). In both cases, a percentage of the incident light is reflected at the surface. For paraxial rays, Fresnel's law (Eq. 14.2) gives the percentage reflected, typically about 4% to 8%. For non-paraxial rays, the percentage reflected increases as a function of the incident angle. For light initially in the lower index medium, the percentage reflected approaches 100% at grazing incidence.

For light in the higher index medium, the percentage reflected as a function of the incident angle approaches 100% much quicker. Here the boundary angle for 100% reflection occurs when the angle of refraction θ_r is 90° (Figure 11.4). The *critical angle* θ_c is the incident angle θ_i for which θ_r is 90°. For light in the higher index medium, any incident angle greater than the critical angle θ_c, results in 100% reflection. This effect is called *total internal reflection*.

The critical angle for an interface can be found from Snell's law. When θ_r equals 90°, θ_i equals the critical angle θ_c, and

$$n_1 \sin\theta_c = n_2 \sin(90°)$$

Figure 11.3 Snell's law.

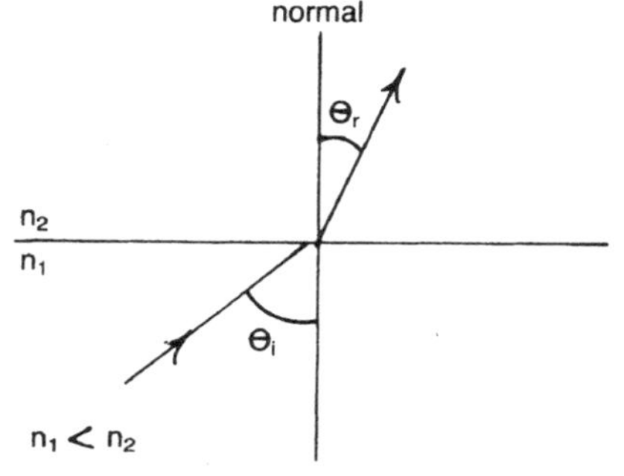

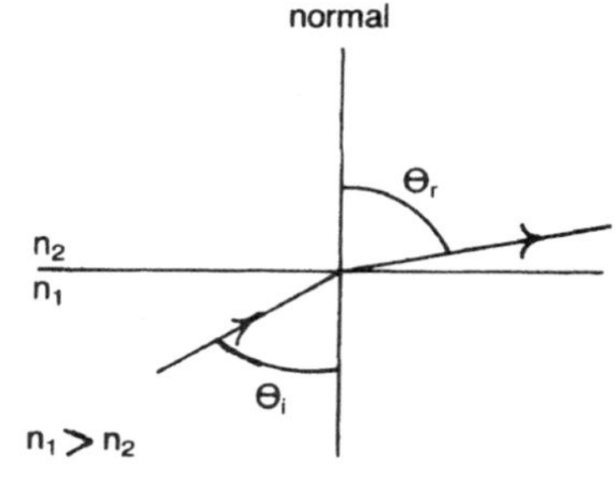

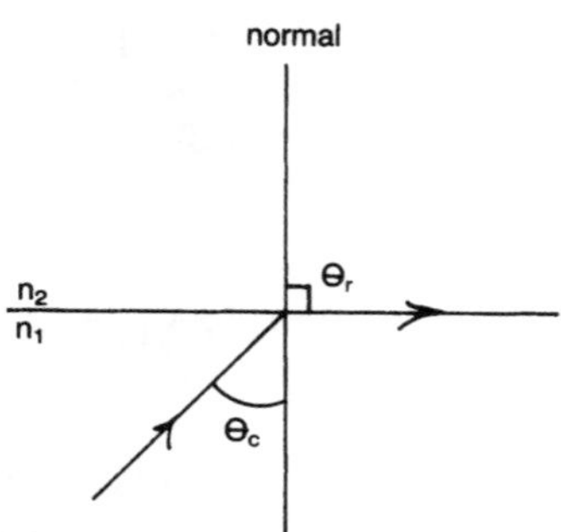

Figure 11.4 The critical angle.

Since the sine of 90° is +1, it follows that

$$\sin\theta_c = n_2/n_1 \quad (11.2)$$

For light in glass ($n = 1.50$) incident on a glass–air boundary, the critical angle is given by

$$\sin\theta_c = 1.00/1.50 = 0.67$$

or

$$\theta_c = 41.8°$$

Any light in the glass incident on the surface at an angle greater than 41.8° undergoes total internal reflection. In effect, this light is trapped in the glass—at least at this surface.

The higher the index of a medium in air, the smaller the critical angle. For light in diamond ($n = 2.4$) incident on a diamond–air interface, the critical angle is only 24.6°. For light in water incident on a water–air surface, the critical angle is 48.7°.

When the air is replaced by a medium, the critical angle changes. For light in glass ($n = 1.50$) incident on a glass–water ($n = 1.33$) interface, Eq. 11.2 gives

$$\sin\theta_c = 1.33/1.50 = 0.89$$
$$\theta_c = 62.4°$$

Thus, changing the second medium can thwart total internal reflection at certain angles.

The sine function has a maximum value of 1. In refraction angle computations with Snell's law, a computed sine greater than 1 indicates that the ray undergoes total internal reflection.

EXAMPLE 11.1

What is the angle of refraction for light in diamond ($n = 2.4$) incident on a diamond–air surface at a 35° incident angle?

From Snell's law,

$$2.4\sin(35°) = 1.0\sin\theta_r$$

or

$$\sin\theta_r = 1.38$$

Since the sine function cannot be greater than 1, this ray undergoes total internal reflection and there is no angle of refraction.

The aqueous humor flow in the eye is such that the aqueous is completely replaced every 4 h. The aqueous drains through the trabecular meshwork that is located at the angle made by the iris and the sclera. If this angle closes up, the aqueous flow is impeded, and the pressure inside the eye rises (a condition called glaucoma). This can eventually lead to retinal damage, tunnel vision, and even blindness. However, one cannot see the anterior chamber angle of a patient's eye because the light coming from the angle undergoes total internal reflection at the cornea (Figure 11.5a). This problem is solved by the use of special contact lenses placed on the eye. The index of the contact lens is higher than that of the eye, so total internal reflection can no longer occur, and the light escapes into the contact lens. A Koeppe lens allows direct viewing, while a Goldman lens incorporates a mirror and allows indirect viewing (Figures 11.5b and c).

Small fibers of glass or plastic are used to pipe light around corners. Fibers with diameters in the micron region work by total internal reflection (Figure 11.6a).

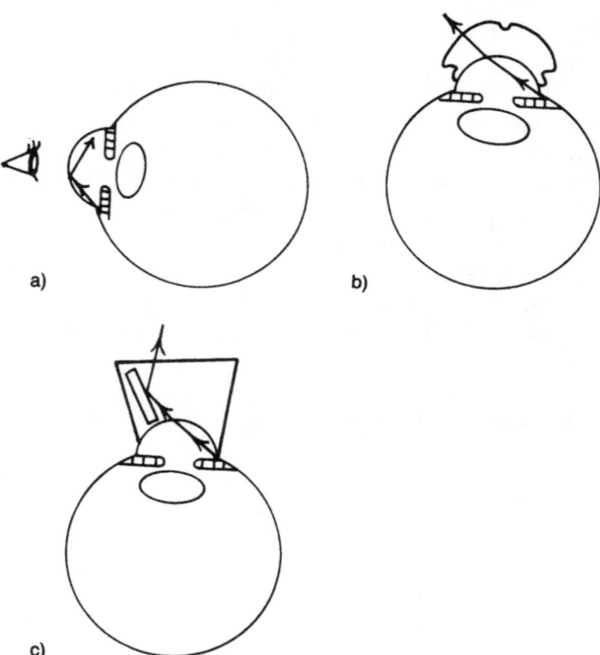

Figure 11.5 a, Total internal reflection from the anterior chamber angle; b, a Koeppe lens; c, a Goldman lens.

Figure 11.6 a, Total internal reflection in an optical fiber; b, a step index fiber; c, curved ray in a gradient index fiber.

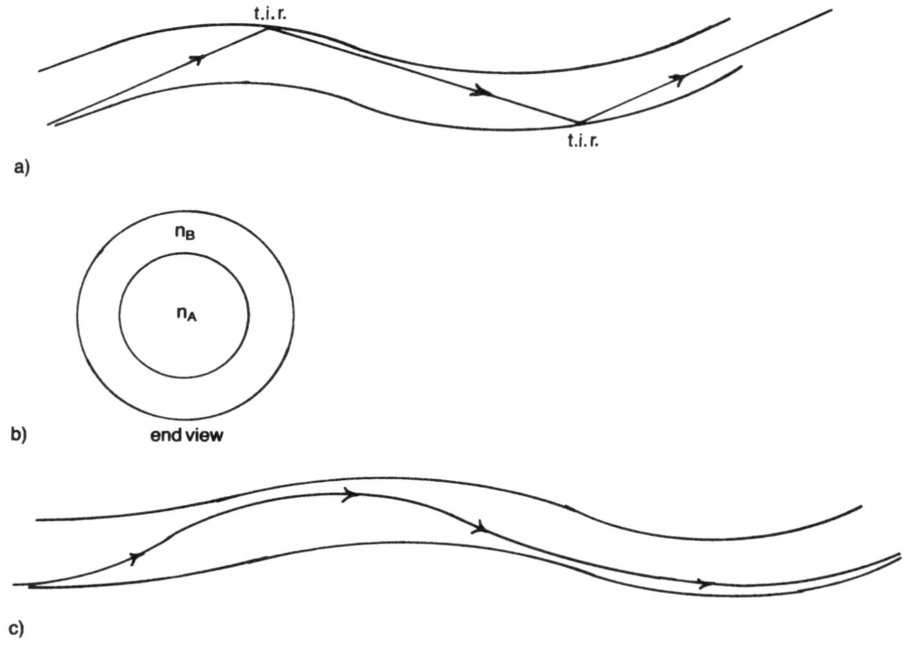

When the fiber is bent, the light hits the sides, but the incident angles are greater than the critical angle. Hence, total internal reflection occurs and the light remains trapped in the fiber. For fibers with micron diameters, the corners can be surprisingly sharp before any light leaks out.

Dust or scratches on the surface can frustrate the total internal reflection and cause leakage from a fiber. To combat this, the fibers are either a step index fiber or a gradient index fiber. In the step index fiber, an internal fiber is surrounded by an outer fiber with a lower index (Figure 11.6b). Similarly, in the gradient index fiber, the index of refraction is highest in the middle and lowest at the edge. The gradient index actually causes a curved ray path. When the ray wanders toward the edge, the gradient index causes it to curve back toward the middle (Figure 11.6c).

An *endoscope* is a fiber optics instrument that enables people to see around multiple bends and into dark cavities (Figure 11.7). Some of the fibers in the endoscope carry light down into the cavity to illuminate the object of regard. Other fibers carry the diffusely reflected light back to the observer. Endoscopes have made it possible to examine the insides of stomachs, bladders, etc., without having to surgically cut them open.

The light transported by fiber optics bundles can carry much more information than electrical signals transported by copper wire. The copper wires used for telephone communications in large cities need to be enormous in size. The smaller fiber optics bundles have replaced many of these enormous copper cables.

Total internal reflection is involved in the physical phenomenon called *tunneling*. Consider light in glass. When the light is totally internally reflected, a light wave with an exponentially decaying amplitude actually penetrates for a short distance (several wavelengths) into the lower index media. Even though this wave penetrates into the lower index medium, the energy carried by the exponentially decaying wave propagates circularly back into the glass and becomes part of the reflected beam. When a second

Figure 11.7 Schematic representation of an endoscope.

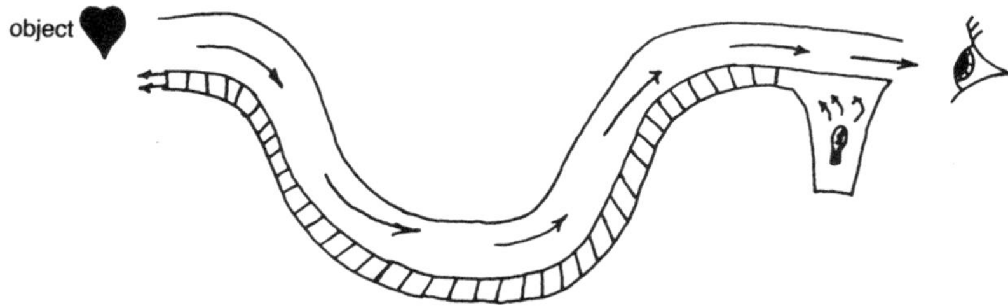

piece of glass is slowly brought closer to the first piece, it encounters the exponentially decaying wave before it touches the first piece of glass. Then the flow lines change and some light will enter the second piece even though contact is not yet established. It appears that the light that should have been trapped in the first piece of glass has tunneled across the air gap. Of course, once contact is established between the two pieces of glass, the total internal reflection condition is removed, and the light is transmitted.

The phenomenon of tunneling also shows up in quantum mechanics. Ordinarily, alpha particles are trapped or bound in an atomic nucleus by the nuclear forces. The strange thing about alpha decay is that the alpha particles appear to escape the nucleus even though they do not have enough energy to cross the nuclear energy gap. The quantum mechanical explanation is that the alpha particles have an exponentially decaying wavefunction that extends out into the gap even when the alpha particle is trapped inside the nucleus. If the gap is narrow enough, the alpha particles can tunnel across the gap and escape in a manner analogous to the light above.

11.3 DEVIATION BY A THICK PRISM

Figure 11.8a shows a thick prism. A *principal section* of the prism is the section that contains the normals of both the front and the back surfaces. Figure 11.8b shows a cross-sectional view of a principal section of a thick prism with index n_2 and apex angle A. The media in front of and behind the prism have respective indices of n_1 and n_2.

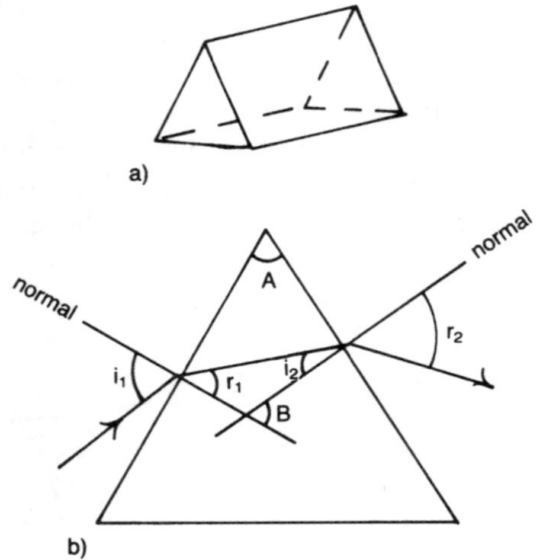

Figure 11.8 a, A thick prism; b, principal section of a thick prism.

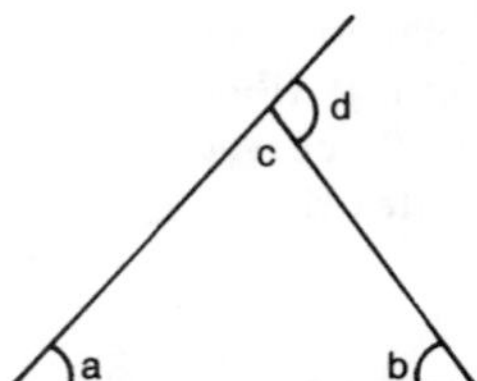

Figure 11.9 External angle d is the sum of the two opposite internal angles a and b.

Light incident on the prism is refracted at the first surface and again at the second surface. The deviation angle d for a ray incident on the prism at an incident angle of i_1 can be found by successively applying Snell's law at the surfaces.

The derivation of an equation for the deviation angle uses a geometry theorem, which says that the exterior angle of a triangle equals the sum of the two opposite interior angles, or from Figure 11.9,

$$a + b = d$$

It is easy to prove this theorem. The three angles inside a triangle add to 180°, or

$$a + b + c = 180^\circ$$

In Figure 11.9, c and d are supplementary angles that add to 180°. I.e.,

$$c + d = 180^\circ$$

We can subtract the above two equations to obtain

$$a + b - d = 0$$

or

$$a + b = d$$

The derivation also uses another geometry theorem that states angles with perpendicular sides are equal. In Figure 11.8b, angle B (made by the normals) has sides that are perpendicular to the sides of angle A; therefore, A and B are equal angles.

For the ray in Figure 11.8b, the incident and refraction angles at the first surface are i_1 and r_1, respectively. At the second surface, the incident and refraction angles are i_2 and r_2. Snell's law at the first surface is

$$n_1 \sin i_1 = n_2 \sin r_1 \tag{11.3}$$

Snell's law at the second surface is

$$n_2 \sin i_2 = n_3 \sin r_2 \tag{11.4}$$

The normals to each surface intersect, making the angle B. Since the normals are perpendicular to the sides, B is equal to A. B is the external angle to the triangle made by the two normals and the ray crossing the interior of the prism. The two opposite interior angles are r_1 and i_2.
Therefore,

$$i_2 + r_1 = B$$

and since A equals B,

$$i_2 = A - r_1 \tag{11.5}$$

Given the incident angle i_1, we can then apply Eqs. 11.3, 11.5, and 11.4 in sequence to obtain r_2.

Figure 11.10 shows the deviation angle between the incident ray and the emerging ray. The ray extensions and the internal ray form a triangle for which d is the external angle, while s_1 and s_2 are the two opposite internal angles. Thus,

$$d = s_1 + s_2$$

Now,

$$i_1 = s_1 + r_1$$

and

$$r_2 = s_2 + i_2$$

We can solve the above two equations for s_1 and s_2 and then substitute the results into the equation for d to obtain

$$d = i_1 + r_2 - A \tag{11.6}$$

Given the incident angle i_1 we can find the angle of refraction r_2 from Eqs. 11.3 through 11.5, and then compute the deviation angle d from Eq. 11.6.

If the ray is reversed, it retraces the same path back through the prism and has the same deviation angle. For the reversed ray, r_2 is the initial incident angle and i_1 is the final angle of refraction. Simply exchanging i_1 and r_2 in Eq. 11.6 algebraically confirms that the angle of deviation is the same for the reversed ray.

In computing the deviation d, we need to distinguish between a ray incident on the base side of the normal versus a ray incident on the apex side of the normal. When the ray is incident on the base side of the normal i_1 is positive (Figure 11.10). The sign convention for r_2 is the same as that for i_1 (since the reversed ray has an incident angle r_2).

It follows from Snell's law (Eq. 11.3) that r_1 and i_1 always have the same sign. Therefore, when i_1 is positive, so is r_1, and when i_1 is negative so is r_1. This means that r_1 is positive when the internal ray leaving the first surface is on the apex side of the normal (Figure 11.10). When the internal ray leaving the first surface is on the base side of the normal, r_1 is negative (Figure 11.11a).

It follows from Snell's law (Eq. 11.4) that i_2 and r_2 always have the same sign. Thus the angle i_2 is positive when the ray incident on the second surface is on the apex side of the normal (Figure 11.11a), and negative when the incident ray is on the base side of the normal (Figure 11.11b). Note that the angles r_1 and i_2 are related by reversibility.

The deviation angle d is positive when the bend is toward the base and negative when the bend is toward the apex. The above sign conventions and the successive use of Eqs. 11.3, 11.5, 11.4, and 11.6 constitute a four-step method for finding the deviation angle d of a thick prism.

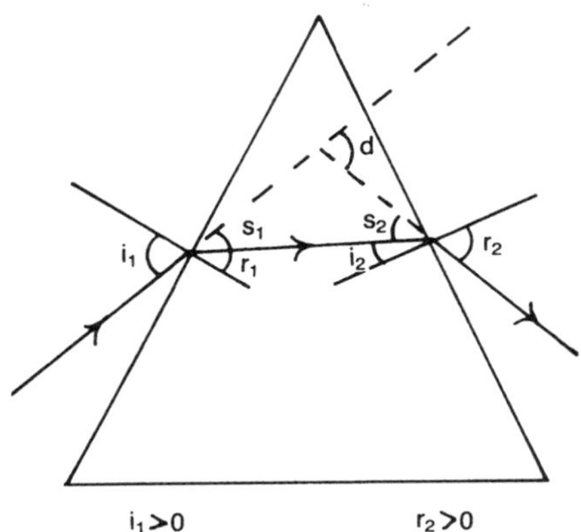

Figure 11.10 Thick prism with a deviation angle d.

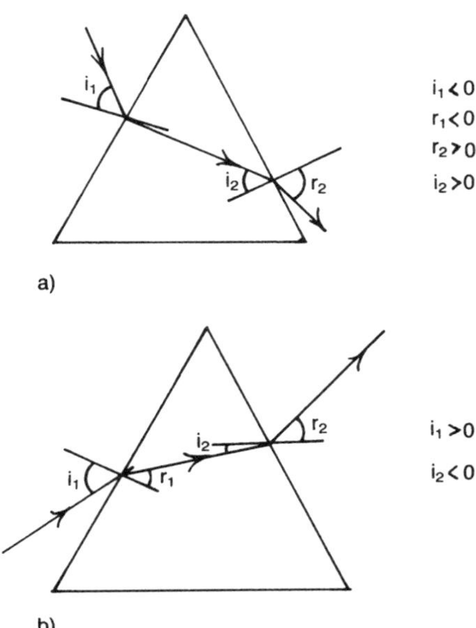

Figure 11.11 Sign convention.

EXAMPLE 11.2a

A flint glass ($n = 1.617$) prism in air has a 50° apex angle. What is the deviation for a ray with an incident angle of 70° on the base side of the normal?

From Eq. 11.3,

$$1.00 \sin(+70°) = 1.617 \sin r_1$$
$$\sin r_1 = 0.940/1.617 = 0.581$$

and

$$r_1 = 35.53°$$

From Eq. 11.5,

$$i_2 = 50° - 35.53° = +14.47°$$

From Eq. 11.4,

$$1.617 \sin(+14.47°) = 1.00 \sin r_2$$
$$\sin r_2 = 0.404$$

and

$$r_2 = 23.83°$$

From Eq. 11.6,

$$d = +70° + 23.83° - 50° = +43.83°$$

The prism bends this ray 43.83° toward the base. By reversibility, a ray with an incident angle of 23.83° will have a 70° final angle of refraction and a 43.83° deviation angle.

EXAMPLE 11.2b

What is the deviation angle for a ray that has grazing incidence on the base side of the normal?

In this case i_1 is +90° and the four-step method gives:

$$1.00 \sin(+90°) = 1.617 \sin r_1$$
$$\sin r_1 = 1/1.617 = 0.618$$

and

$$r_1 = +38.20°$$

(As an aside, note that 38.20° is the critical angle for light in a medium of 1.617 incident on a glass–air interface. Why?)

From Eq. 11.5,

$$i_2 = 50° - 38.20° = +11.8°$$

Then,

$$1.617 \sin(+11.8°) = 1.00 \sin r_2$$
$$\sin r_2 = 0.331$$
$$r_2 = +19.31°$$

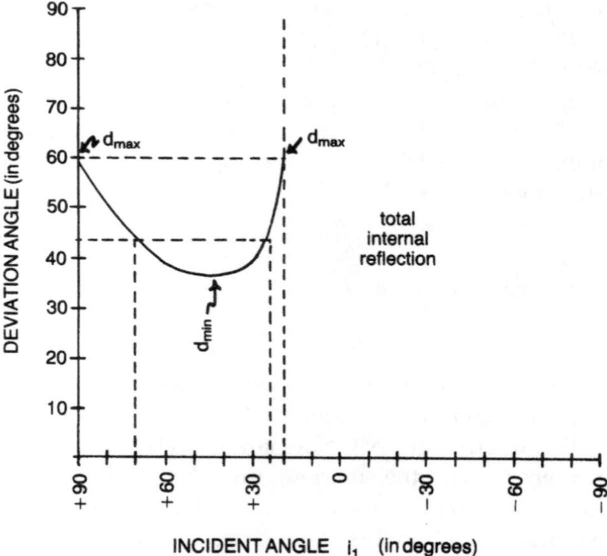

Figure 11.12 Deviation for a prism of index 1.617 and apex angle 50°.

and

$$d = +90° + 19.31° - 50° = 59.31°$$

Since grazing incidence gives the largest incident angle possible, the 59.31° deviation is the *maximum deviation* that this prism gives. By reversibility, the 59.31° maximum deviation will also occur for an incident angle of 19.31°.

Figure 11.12 shows a plot of the deviation angle versus the incident angle for this prism. The graph has a distorted U shape. At +90° the deviation angle is the 59.31° maximum. Note that at an incident angle of +19.31° the deviation angle is again 59.31°. Similarly, from Example 11.2a, incident angles of 70° or 23.83° both give a 43.83° deviation.

Starting at +90°, as the incident angle is decreased the deviation falls to a minimum and then rises back to the maximum at an incident angle of 19.31°. For incident angles of less than 19.31° (including incident angles above the normal), total internal reflection occurs at the second interface (Figure 11.13).

EXAMPLE 11.2c

For the same prism, what is the deviation angle for an incident angle of 10° on the base side of the normal?

From the four-step method,

$$1.00 \sin(+10°) = 1.617 \sin r_1$$
$$\sin r_1 = 0.107$$

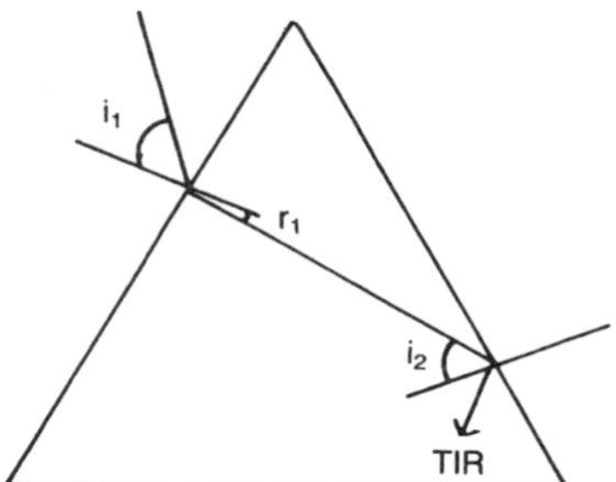

Figure 11.13 Total internal reflection at the prism's back surface.

or

$$r_1 = +6.17°$$

Then,

$$i_2 = 50° - 6.17° = +43.84°$$

and

$$1.617 \sin(+43.84) = 1.00 \sin r_2$$
$$\sin r_2 = 1.12$$

The sine function cannot be greater than +1, so the above equation says the incident angle of 43.84° is greater than the critical angle and total internal reflection occurs.

Figure 11.14 shows the deviation angle as a function of the incident angle for a prism of index 1.523 and apex angle 26°. Again, the shape is that of a distorted U. The maximum deviation is 40.72°, and occurs for incident angles of either +90° or −23.28°. The minimum deviation is 14.07°, and the deviation at normal incidence ($i_1 = 0$) is 15.89°. Total internal reflection occurs for incident angles i_1 to the right of −23.28°, which means the rays are incident on the apex side of the normal at angles greater than 23.28° in magnitude. The figures for an incident angle of −15° are worked out in the following example.

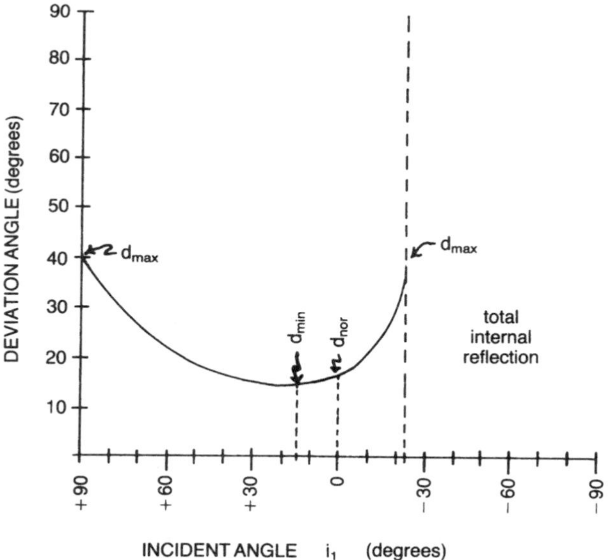

Figure 11.14 Deviation for a prism of index 1.523 and apex angle 26°.

EXAMPLE 11.3

Find the deviation angle for a ray incident at −15° on a prism ($n = 1.523$) with a 26° apex angle.

From the four-step method:

$$1.00 \sin(-15) = 1.523 \sin r_1$$
$$\sin r_1 = -0.170$$
$$r_1 = -9.78°$$

Then,

$$i_2 = 26° - (-9.78°) = +35.78°$$

and

$$1.523 \sin(+35.78°) = 1.00 \sin r_2$$

So

$$r_2 = 62.94°$$

and

$$d = (-15°) + 62.94° - 26° = 21.94°$$

Whenever the prism is the higher index media, such as a glass or plastic prism in air, the deviation is towards the base of the prism ($d > 0$). When the prism is the lower index media, such as a prism shaped air cavity in a piece of glass, the prism deviation is toward the apex ($d < 0$).

11.4 MINIMUM DEVIATION

The graph of the deviation of a thick prism as a function of the incident angle has the distorted U shape. Each deviation angle is given by two incident angles, and the two incident angles are connected by reversibility (when one is i_1 the other is r_2). Near the minimum the two connected angles (i_1 and r_2) are almost numerically equal.

At the minimum, the two connected angles are numerically equal ($i_1 = r_2$). For a prism in air ($n_1 = n_3 = 1$), this occurs when the internal ray crossing the

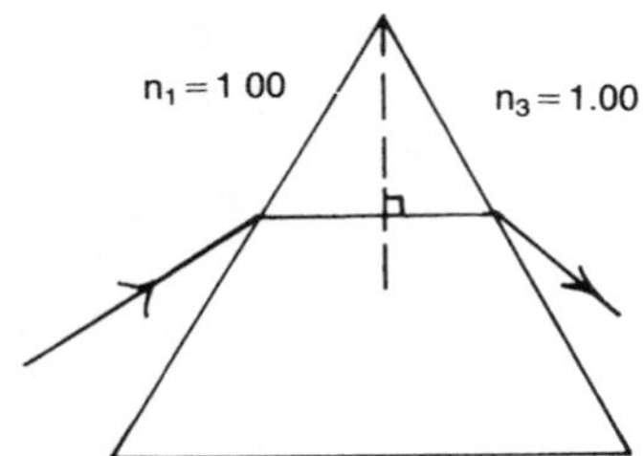

Figure 11.15 Minimum deviation ray.

prism is perpendicular to the bisector of the apex angle (Figure 11.15). In this case, the four-step method for the deviation simplifies to one equation.

For i_1 equal to r_2 Eq. 11.6 gives

$$d_{\min} = 2r_2 - A$$

or

$$r_2 = \frac{A + d_{\min}}{2}$$

From Snell's law, it is easy to show that the internal angles r_1 and i_2 are equal. Then from Eq. 11.5,

$$i_2 = \frac{A}{2}$$

Finally, Eq. 11.4 gives

$$n_2 \sin\left(\frac{A}{2}\right) = 1.00 \sin\left(\frac{A + d_{\min}}{2}\right)$$

which is typically written as

$$n_2 = \frac{\sin\left(\frac{A+d_{\min}}{2}\right)}{\sin\left(\frac{A}{2}\right)} \tag{11.7}$$

Equation 11.7 represents a classical method to determine the refractive index of a material. A prism with a known apex angle is made from the material. Then the minimum deviation angle is measured, and the index is calculated from Eq. 11.7.

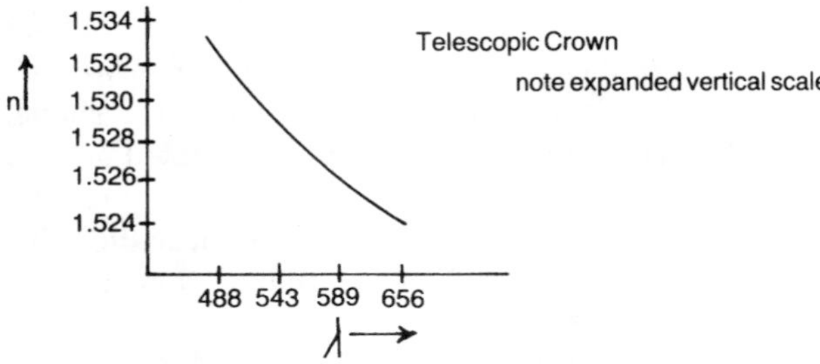

Figure 11.16 Index of refraction for telescopic crown glass as a function of incident light wavelength.

The minimum deviation angle is actually slightly different for each wavelength of incident light (dispersion). Then from Eq. 11.7, the refractive index n_2 of the prism is a function of the wavelength of the incident light. Figure 11.16 is a graph of the refractive index of telescopic crown glass as a function of the incident wavelength. So far we have been neglecting this slight dependence. The index dependence on wavelength is responsible for chromatic aberration of lenses and prisms. Chromatic aberration is treated in Chapter 20.

EXAMPLE 11.4

What is the minimum deviation angle for a prism with a 60° apex angle and index of 1.31?

Note that $\sin[(A + d_{\min})/2]$ is not equal to $\sin(A/2) + \sin(d_{\min}/2)$. Therefore, one technique to minimize computational mistakes is to rename the argument of the sine function in the numerator of Eq. 11.7. For example, let

$$q = (A + d_{\min})/2$$

Then Eq. 11.7 becomes

$$n_2 = \frac{\sin q}{\sin(A/2)}$$

or

$$\sin q = 1.31\ \sin(30°) = 0.655$$
$$q = 40.9°$$

Then we can solve for $d_{\min}$ as follows:

$$q = 40.9° = \frac{A + d_{\min}}{2}$$

or

$$A + d_{\min} = 81.8°$$
$$d_{\min} = 21.8° \cong 22°$$

Ice crystals that form in the atmosphere have a six-sided symmetry that is characteristic of their crystal lattice (Figure 11.17a). When light passes through the section of the crystal shown, the crystal acts like a prism with a 60° apex angle. The index of the ice crystals is 1.31. The previous example used the numbers for an ice crystal, and the minimum deviation angle was about 22°.

For a collection of randomly oriented ice crystals, all incident angles would be present. In the vicinity of maximum deviation, the deviation angles change very quickly with the incident angle (for example, see Figure 11.12). In the vicinity of minimum deviation, the deviation angles change slowly with the incident

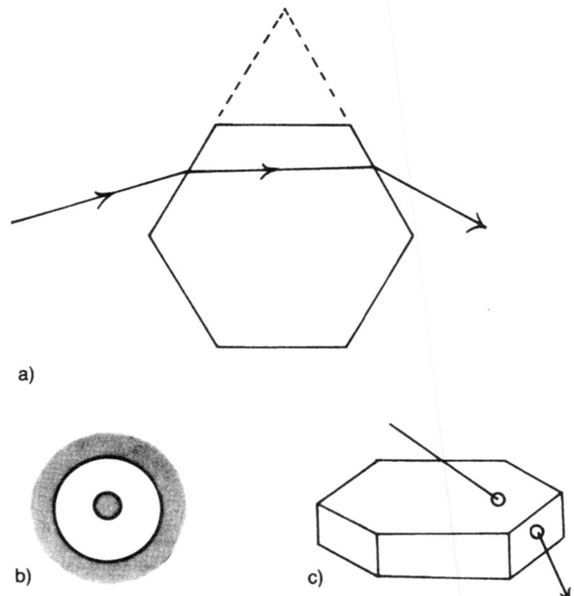

Figure 11.17 a, Prism effect of an ice crystal. Dashed lines show effective 60° apex angle; b, 22° halo; c, ray path for 90° apex angle.

angle. Because of this, the light is concentrated at or near the 22° minimum deviation angle. The visual result is the surprisingly common 22° ice crystal halo (Figure 11.17b). The 22° halo is frequently visible when looking at the sun or a full moon through thin cirrus clouds and sometimes visible when ice crystals are present without any noticeable clouds.

Consider looking through a bunch of ice crystals at either the rising or setting sun. When the ice crystals are shaped flat like a plate, they fall slowly through calm air just like leaves. In this case the majority of the crystals are aligned horizontally and the deviated light is concentrated at 22° horizontally from the sun. These are the sundogs of folklore. The sundogs are sometimes present together with the entire 22° halo, and at other times are visible even when the rest of the halo is not.

Since the ice crystals have some depth, it is also possible for a ray to enter a horizontal surface and leave a vertical surface (Figure 11.17c). In this case the crystal acts like a prism with a 90° apex angle. The minimum deviation angle for a 90° ice crystal ($n = 1.31$) prism is 46°. Though it is less common than the 22° halo, the 46° halo is occasionally observed and has been photographed. (For even more fascinating ice crystal halos see "Rainbows, Halos, and Glories" by Robert Greenler, Cambridge University Press, 1980; or "Color and Light in Nature" by David Lynch and William Livingston, Cambridge University Press, 1995.)

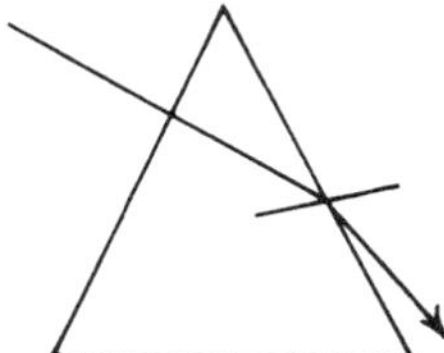

Figure 11.18 Ray path for normal incidence.

11.5 DEVIATION AT NORMAL INCIDENCE

The four-step method also simplifies when a ray is incident normally on a prism ($i_1 = 0$). In this case, the ray bends (refracts) only at the second surface (Figure 11.18). From Eq. 11.6,

$$d_{\text{nor}} = r_2 - A$$

or

$$r_2 = d_{\text{nor}} + A$$

From Eq. 11.5,

$$i_2 = A$$

Then Eq. 11.4 gives

$$n_2 \sin A = \sin (A + d_{\text{nor}})$$

which is typically written

$$n_2 = \frac{\sin (A + d_{\text{nor}})}{\sin A} \tag{11.8}$$

Equation 11.8 gives the deviation for normal incidence. It is similar in form to Eq. 11.7 for minimum deviation. By reversibility, Eq. 11.8 also gives the deviation for normal emergence ($r_2 = 90°$).

EXAMPLE 11.5

What is the deviation at normal incidence for a plastic ($n = 1.44$) prism with a 20° apex angle?

Just as for minimum deviation, we can minimize the possibility of a computational error by letting

$$q = A + d_{\text{nor}}$$

Then from Eq. 11.8,

$$\sin q = 1.44 \sin (20°) = 0.493$$
$$q = 29.5°$$

and

$$d_{\text{nor}} = q - A = 9.5°$$

EXAMPLE 11.6
What is the deviation for normal incidence for a flint glass ($n = 1.617$) prism with a 50° apex angle?

Just as in the preceding example, let

$$q = A + d_{nor}$$

Then,

$$\sin q = 1.617 \sin 50°$$

or

$$\sin q = 1.239$$

The sine function cannot be greater than 1, so total internal reflection occurs at the back surface. The deviation for this prism was plotted in Figure 11.12, and indeed, that graph shows that total internal reflection occurs for all incident angles less than +19.3°.

11.6 THICK PRISM COMPARISONS

Figure 11.19 is a plot of the deviation angle versus the incident angle for a series of prisms with the same index (1.50) but different apex angles. Each U-shaped curve is marked with the corresponding apex angle. As the apex angle increases, the (distorted) U-shaped plot moves up and to the left. This indicates a smaller range of incident angles for which light can get through the prism.

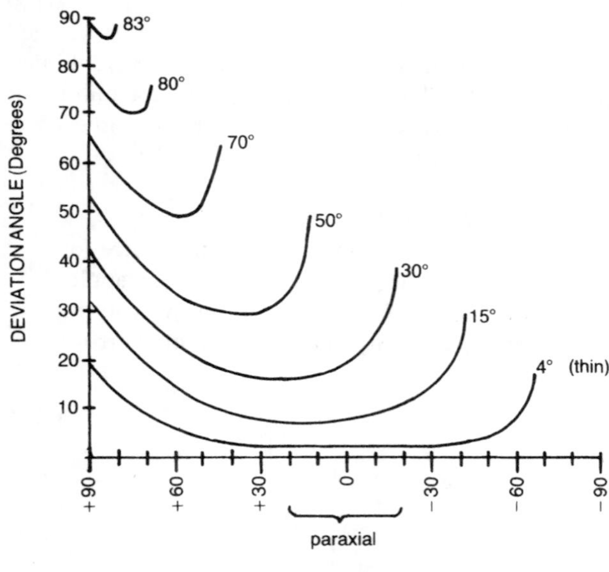

Figure 11.19 Deviation angles for a series of apex angles.

Eventually, an apex angle is reached for which only one ray will get through the prism. For larger apex angles, all light is totally internally reflected. In this case, a solution for d_{min} from Eq. 11.7 results in

$$n_2 \sin(A/2) > 1$$

The apex angle that lets only one ray through the prism can be found from

$$n_2 \sin(A/2) = 1$$

or

$$\sin(A/2) = 1/n_2$$

A comparison with Eq. 11.2 shows that $A/2$ equals the critical angle θ_c. Therefore, when the apex angle equals twice the critical angle, only one ray gets through the prism.

As the apex angle decreases, the (distorted) U-shaped plot moves down and to the right and flattens out. The minimum deviation angle eventually approaches the deviation at normal incidence. For an apex angle of zero, the deviation plot gives a straight line at zero for all incident angles.

For a fixed apex angle, increasing the refractive index increases the prismatic deviation. This would also make the U-shaped plot move up and to the left.

11.7 THIN PRISMS

Thin prisms are prisms with small apex angles and a negligible thickness across the interior of the prism (Figure 11.20a). For thin prisms, the U-shaped deviation plot is very flat on the bottom (as shown by the bottom curve in Figure 11.19). In particular, for all paraxial rays (i.e., rays for which $|i_1|$ is much smaller than 20°), the deviation angle is approximately a constant.

For paraxial incidence on thin prisms, we could determine the effectively constant deviation from Eq. 11.8 for normal incidence, but since the angles

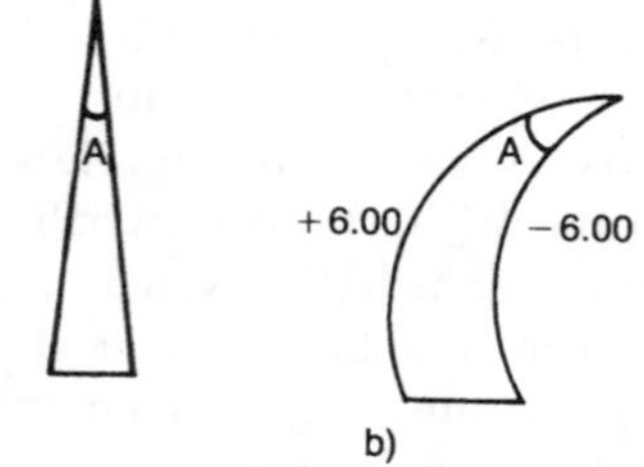

Figure 11.20 a, Thin prism with plane sides; b, thin prism with spherical sides.

involved are small, we can simplify further with a small angle approximation.

The small angle approximation consists of replacing the sine function by the angles expressed in radians. Let c be the conversion factor for degrees to radians, then Eq. 11.8 gives

$$n_2 = \frac{(A+d)c}{Ac}$$

The conversion factor c cancels out, and it follows that

$$d = (n_2 - 1)A \qquad (11.9)$$

For a thin prism in air, Eq. 11.9 shows that the paraxial deviation depends only on the prism's refractive index n_2 and apex angle A, and that increasing either n_2 or A increases the deviation angle d. Since the paraxial deviation is also the minimum deviation, Eq. 11.9 can also be derived from the minimum deviation equation (Eq. 11.7).

EXAMPLE 11.7a

What is the paraxial thin prism deviation for an ophthalmic crown glass prism ($n = 1.523$) with a 6° apex angle?

From Eq. 11.9,

$$d = (0.523)6^\circ = 3.1^\circ$$

EXAMPLE 11.7b

What is the paraxial thin prism deviation for a high index plastic ($n = 1.71$) prism with a 6° apex angle?

From Eq. 11.9,

$$d = (0.71)6^\circ = 4.3^\circ$$

EXAMPLE 11.7c

For a plastic ($n = 1.44$) prism with a 20° apex angle, the exact deviation at normal incidence was 9.5° (see Example 11.5). What does the thin prism approximation give?

From Eq. 11.9,

$$d = (0.44)20^\circ = 8.8^\circ$$

This is a 7% error, which is not bad since the 20° apex angle is pushing the limits of the paraxial region.

Figure 11.20b shows a prism (apex angle A) in bent form. The front surface is a +6.00 D spherical surface, while the back surface is a −6.00 D surface. For a thin prism, the dioptric power is the sum of the surface powers, and is still zero. The prismatic deviation is still given by Eq. 11.9.

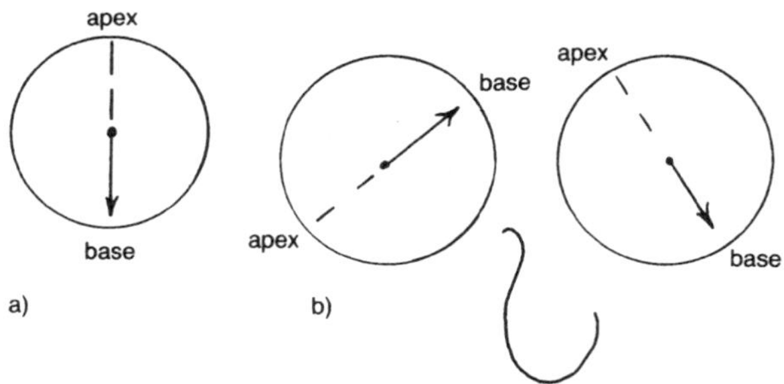

Figure 11.21 Base directions (contra-ocular view).

11.8 OPHTHALMIC BASE DIRECTIONS

The meridian occupied by a principal section of a prism is called the *base–apex meridian*. The orientation of an ophthalmic prism is specified by the direction of the base in the base–apex meridian (Figure 11.21a). A base down (BD) prism deviates the light vertically down, while a base up (BU) prism deviates the light vertically up. The nose is used as a horizontal reference. A base in (BI) prism deviates the light horizontally in toward the nose, while a base out (BO) prism deviates the light out away from the nose.

To specify oblique base–apex meridians, we use the cylinder axis coordinate system. Figure 11.21b is a contra-ocular view of a prism in front of each eye. For the right eye, a prism that deviates the light up and in along the 30° meridian is called a BU and in at 30 (BU & I @ 30). For the left eye, a prism that deviates the light down and out along the 120° meridian is called a BD and out at 120° (BD & O @ 120).

The above system is a redundant system in that the parameters are over-specified; however, it is a good system to use while learning. Note that strictly speaking, a BD prism is a BD @ 90, while a BI prism is a BI @ 180. Similar statements hold for BU and BO.

In the over-specified system, some prism base directions are not allowed. For the right eye, we can have a BU & I @ 45 or a BD & O @ 45, but we cannot have a BU & O @ 45 or a BD & I @ 45. Because of this we could, for the right eye, just specify a prism @ 45 with a BU component, i.e., a BU @ 45. The latter is a less redundant system. A third system is to specify the prism base directions by a 360° system (Figure 11.22). For the right eye, a BD & O @ 45 would then simply be a base @ 225, etc.

Remember that the virtual image formed by a prism appears deviated toward the apex. For example,

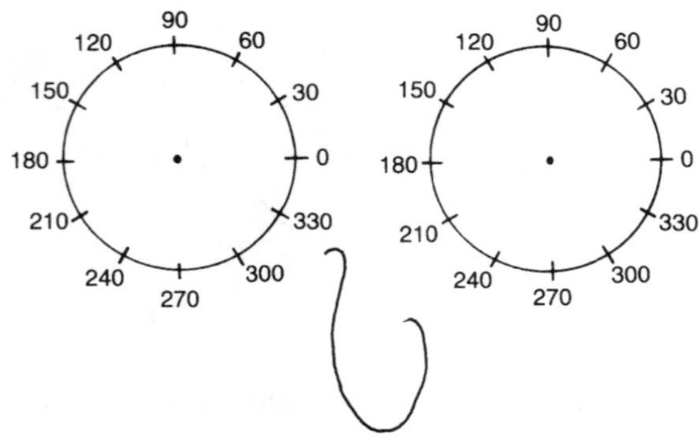

Figure 11.22 Coordinate system (contra-ocular).

a candle appears to be deviated down when looking through a BU prism.

11.9 PRISM-DIOPTERS

For paraxial purposes, we can classify thin prisms by their deviation angles. One measurement method uses a well-defined light beam (a laser beam works great) incident normally at a marked position on a flat surface such as a wall. Then the thin prism is inserted in the beam at a distance of 100 cm from the wall. The deviated beam now hits the wall at a distance y away from the initial spot (Figure 11.23). Given the distance y in centimeters, the deviation angle is found from

$$\tan d = y/100\,\text{cm}$$

For thin prisms, it turns out to be convenient to use the distance y directly in rating the prisms. In this sense, we consider the distance y at the fixed distance of 100 cm as a measure of the deviation power of the prism. By analogy to lenses, we refer to y as the (deviation) power of the prism in prism-diopters. Let Z designate the prism-diopter value. Then,

$$Z = 100 \tan d \tag{11.10}$$

where the 100 actually stands for 100 cm.

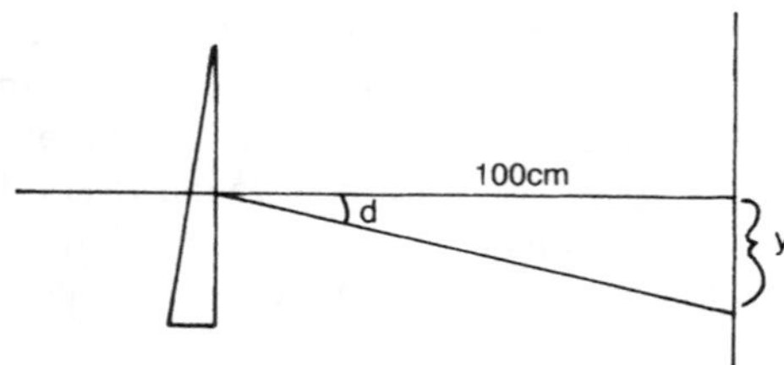

Figure 11.23 Linear versus angular deviation.

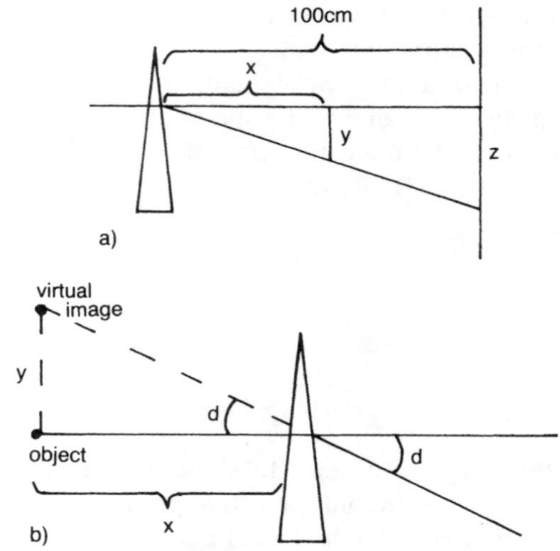

Figure 11.24 a, Similar triangles for prism-diopter values; b, location of virtual image.

The prism-diopter unit is represented by the Greek capital letter Δ used as a superscript. A 3^{Δ} prism shifts a beam 3 cm on a wall 100 cm from the prism. A 7^{Δ} prism shifts a beam 7 cm on a wall 100 cm from the prism, etc.

Suppose the wall is not 100 cm from the prism. Then the prism-diopter value is found by a simple similar triangle ratio (Figure 11.24a). If the deviation is y on a wall a distance x from the prism, then

$$\frac{Z}{100} = \frac{y}{x} \tag{11.11}$$

EXAMPLE 11.8a

On a wall 40 cm from the prism, the prism shifts the light down 20 mm. What is the power of the prism?

20 mm is 2 cm. From Eq. 11.11, the power is

$$\frac{Z}{100} = \frac{2\,\text{cm}}{40\,\text{cm}}$$

which gives

$$Z = 5^{\Delta}$$

For a prism of power Z, the shift is Z cm at 100 cm. For a closer distance, the shift is less than Z, and for a wall farther away the shift is greater than Z.

EXAMPLE 11.8b

A CR-39 plastic ($n = 1.50$) prism has a 6° apex angle. What is the power of the prism?

From Eq. 11.9,

$$d = (0.50)6^\circ = 3^\circ$$

Then from Eq. 11.9,

$$Z = 100 \tan 3^\circ = 5.2^\Delta$$

We can also use Eq. 11.11 to determine the location of the prism's virtual image. Since the prism has zero dioptric power, the image distance is equal to the object distance. The object point in Figure 11.24b is a distance x from the prism, and the virtual image is a distance y above the object point. Equation 11.11 then relates x and y to the prism power Z.

11.10 THIN PRISM COMBINATIONS

When the deviation angle is small,

$$\tan d = d \text{ (expressed in radians)}$$

Then from Eq. 11.10,

$$Z = 100d \text{ (in radians)}$$

Consider two thin prisms, both BD, held together. The first prism deviates the light down by an angle d_1, and the second prism deviates the light down further by an angle d_2 (Figure 11.25). The resultant deviation is the sum:

$$d_r = d_1 + d_2$$

Then,

$$100d_r = (100d_1) + (100d_2)$$

or

$$Z_r = Z_1 + Z_2 \qquad (11.12)$$

Equation 11.12 says that prism-diopters are additive for small deviation angles (i.e., in the paraxial region). For example, a 3^Δ BD prism combined with a 4^Δ BD prism is equivalent to a single 7^Δ BD prism. Essentially, this means that, on the wall at 100 cm, the 3^Δ BD prism deviates the light 3 cm down, and the 4^Δ BD deviates the light 4 more cm down. Therefore, the resultant deviation is 7 cm down.

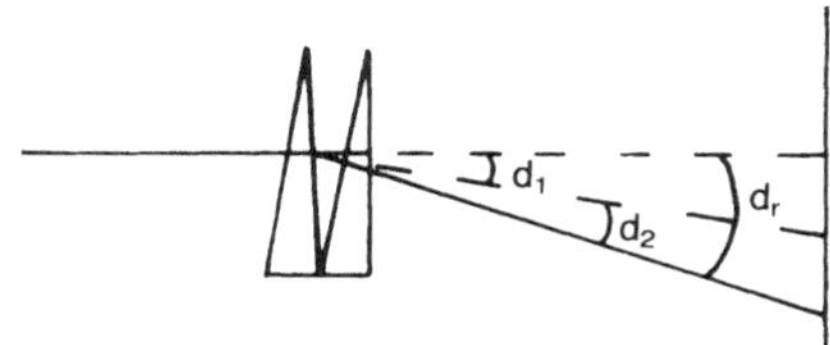

Figure 11.25 Thin prism combination.

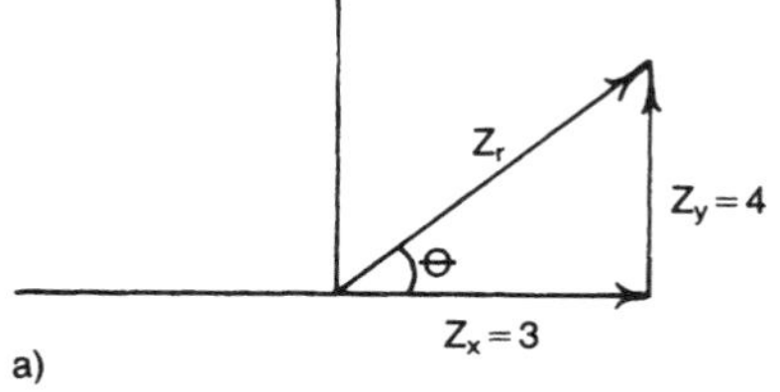

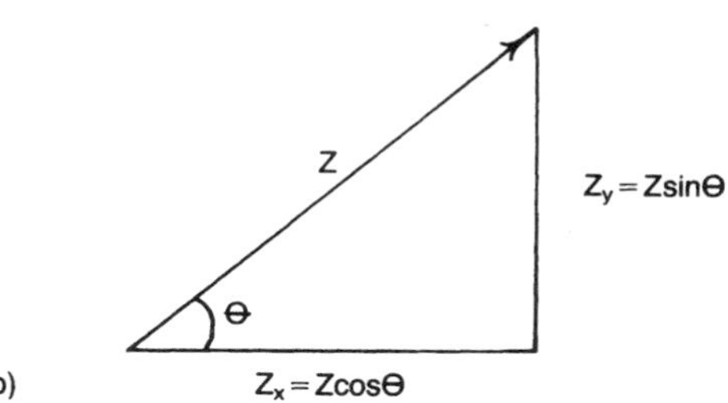

Figure 11.26 a, Horizontal and vertical prism combination; b, resolution into components.

By the same reasoning, prism-diopters subtract when the base directions are opposite. For example, a 3^Δ BD prism combined with a 4^Δ BU prism is equivalent to a single 1^Δ BU prism. Essentially, this means that, on the wall at 100 cm, the 3^Δ BD prism deviates the light 3 cm down, and the 4^Δ BU prism deviates the light 4 cm back up. Therefore, the resultant deviation is 1 cm up.

Suppose a 3^Δ BI prism is combined with a 4^Δ BU prism. For the wall at 100 cm, the 3^Δ BI deviates the light 3 cm horizontally in, while the 4^Δ BU deviates the light 4 cm up (Figure 11.26a). The Pythagorean theorem gives the magnitude of the resultant deviation:

$$\sqrt{(3)^2 + (4)^2} = 5$$

Thus, a single 5^Δ prism oriented correctly gives the same resultant deviation. If the prisms are held in front of the right eye,

$$\tan\theta = \frac{4}{3}$$

and

$$\theta = 53.1^\circ$$

Thus, for the right eye, the single prism equivalent to a 3^Δ BI combined with a 4^Δ BU is a 5^Δ BU & I @ 53.1.

The above process is just vector addition. So for paraxial incidence on thin prisms, prism-diopters add vectorally. The above equations are formalized as

$$Z_r = \sqrt{(Z_x)^2 + (Z_y)^2} \qquad (11.13)$$

and

$$\tan\theta = \frac{Z_y}{Z_x} \quad (11.14)$$

While Eq. 11.14 sometimes returns the standard meridian angle, at other times it returns the supplementary angle. A quick graph enables you to tell the difference. In fact, you can estimate the magnitude of all the parameters from a quick graph.

The oblique vector in Figure 11.26b represents a prism of power Z. The horizontal and vertical components of this prism are found by drawing perpendiculars to the horizontal and vertical axis. The magnitude of the components can also be estimated from the graph, or found from the equations

$$Z_x = Z\cos\theta \quad Z_y = Z\sin\theta \quad (11.15)$$

EXAMPLE 11.9a

Find the single prism equivalent to a 2^Δ BI combined with a 5^Δ BU in front of the left eye.

Figure 11.27 is the quick graph. An estimate of the result from the graph is 5.5^Δ BU & I @ 120. Equation 11.13 gives

$$Z_r = \sqrt{(2)^2 + (5)^2} = 5.4^\Delta$$

In this case, Eq. 11.14 gives the supplementary angle:

$$\tan\theta = \frac{5}{2}$$
$$\theta = 68^\circ$$

In standard notation, the angle is 180 − 68 or 112.

The single equivalent prism is 5.4^Δ BU & I @ 112. Note that the simple guess from the graph was not quite right, but it supplied a tremendous amount of intuition about the correct answer.

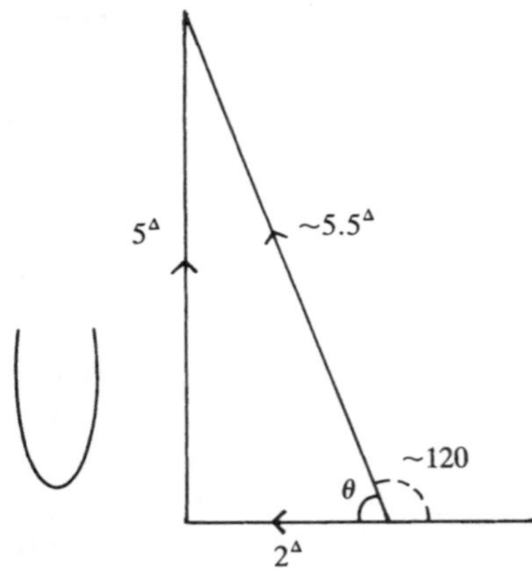

Figure 11.27 Quick graph for 2^Δ BI combined with 5^Δ BU in front of a left eye.

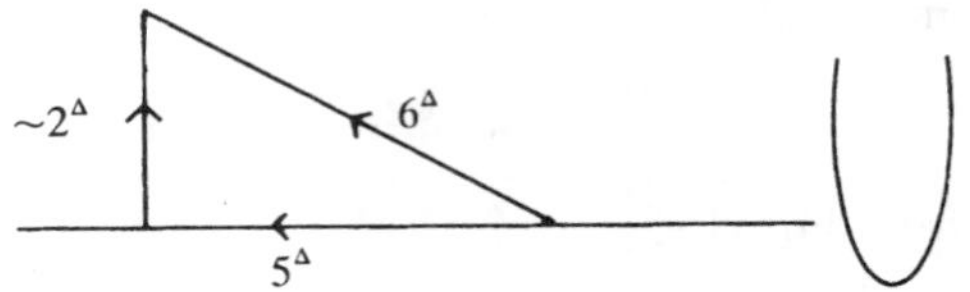

Figure 11.28 Quick graph for 5^Δ BO combined with 2^Δ BU in front of a right eye.

EXAMPLE 11.9b

A 6^Δ BU & O @ 154 is placed in front of a patient's right eye. What are the horizontal and vertical components of the prism?

Figure 11.28 is the quick graph. The estimates from the graph are 5^Δ BU and 2^Δ BO. In terms of the supplementary angle, Equation 11.15 gives

$$Z_x = 6\cos 26 = 5.4^\Delta \text{ BO}$$
$$Z_y = 6\sin 26 = 2.6^\Delta \text{ BU}$$

The graph and the estimates should be made quickly. These provide the intuition about the exact answer.

Z_r and θ are the polar coordinates of the prism power, while Z_x and Z_y are the rectangular coordinates of the prism power. In mathematical language, Example 11.9a is a rectangular to polar conversion, while Example 11.9b is a polar to rectangular conversion. Hand-held scientific calculators have buttons that automatically calculate the conversion of rectangular coordinates to polar coordinates, or vice versa!

When two oblique thin prisms are combined, the prism powers add vectorally (paraxial approximation). Again, the result may be estimated by a quick graph. One method of computing the result is to resolve each prism into its horizontal and vertical components. Then the horizontal components are added together to give the resultant horizontal component, and the vertical components are added together to give the resultant vertical component. If need be, the components can be recombined to give the parameters of the resultant prism. (This method corresponds to clinical procedure, where the clinician usually works and thinks in terms of the horizontal and vertical components.)

EXAMPLE 11.9c

For the left eye, a 7^Δ BD & I @ 35 is combined with a 3^Δ BO. What single prism is equivalent to the combination?

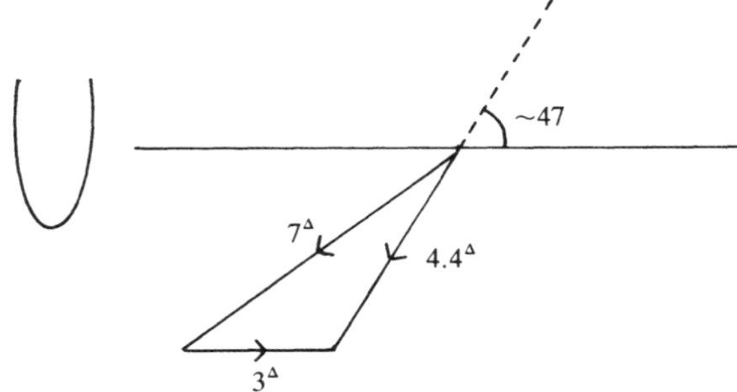

Figure 11.29 Quick graph for 7Δ BD & I @ 35 combined with 3Δ BO in front of the a left eye.

Figure 11.29 is the quick graph. From the graph, an estimate for the answer is 4.4Δ BD & I @ 47.

For the calculated value, first find the horizontal and vertical components for the 7Δ BU & I @ 35 prism. From Equation 11.15,

$$Z_x = 7^\Delta \cos 35 = 5.7^\Delta \text{ BI}$$
$$Z_y = 7^\Delta \sin 35 = 4.0^\Delta \text{ BD}$$

The 3Δ BO has a zero vertical component, so the resultant components are:
horizontal,

$$5.7^\Delta \text{ BI} + 3^\Delta \text{ BO} = 2.7^\Delta \text{ BI}$$

vertical,

$$4.0^\Delta \text{ BD} + 0 = 4.0^\Delta \text{ BD}$$

From Eqs. 11.13 and 11.14, the parameters of the single prism are:

$$Z_r = \sqrt{(2.7)^2 + (4.0)^2} = 4.9^\Delta$$
$$\theta = \tan^{-1}\left(\frac{4.0}{2.7}\right) = 56^\circ$$

or

$$Z_r = 4.9^\Delta \text{ BD } \& \text{ I @ } 56$$

It is important to emphasize that prism-diopters are additive only for thin prisms (small deviation angles) in the paraxial region. In some strabismus cases, prisms of fairly high prism-diopter ratings are used clinically. These prisms are not additive (i.e., a 30Δ prism combined with a 50Δ prism is not equal to an 80Δ prism). Also since the deviation angle is dependent on the incident angle for thick prisms, the way the prism is held in front of the patient is important (i.e., the front side of the prism normal to the incident light versus the back side of the prism normal to the patient's line of sight versus symmetrically splitting the difference).

11.11 CENTRADS

Prism-diopters are additive only for small angles. On the other hand, the deviation angles are always additive. An angle is defined as an arc length on a circle divided by the circle's radius. It follows that the arc lengths are additive.

The centrad is a measure of prism power that is equal to an arc length deviation. To measure centrads, one can place a prism at the center of curvature of a sphere that is 100 cm in radius. Then the arc length deviation y_c produced by the prism on the sphere is measured (Figure 11.30a). This deviation in centimeters is called the centrad rating of the prism. For example, a 1 centrad prism gives a 1 cm arc length deviation on the screen. A 2 centrad prism gives a 2 cm arc length, etc. Centrads are directly proportional to the deviation angle.

For small deviation angles, the arc length deviation y_c is approximately equal to the deviation y on the flat wall (Figure 11.30b). Thus, for small values, centrads and prism-diopters are essentially equal. However, for large values, the arc length deviation differs from the deviation on a flat wall, so the centrad value differs from the prism-diopter value.

The fact that centrads are additive is an advantage over prism-diopters. However, for the larger deviation

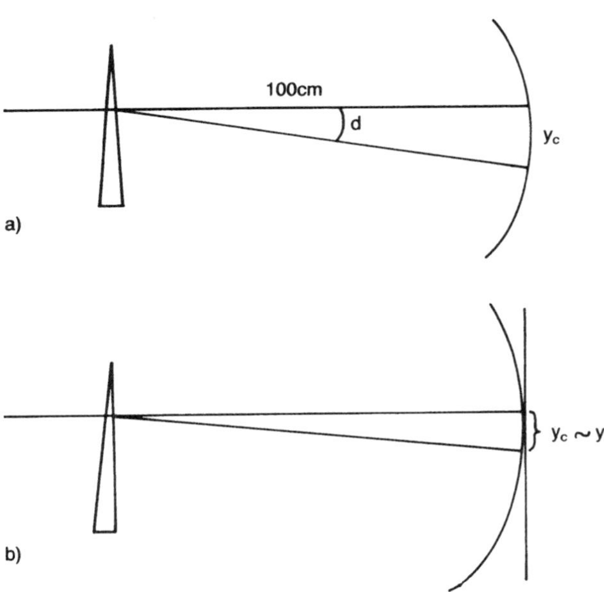

Figure 11.30 a, Arc length for centrad values; b, equivalence of small arc length and linear deviations.

values (where the biggest differences would occur), the deviation angle is a function of the incident angle, so that a single unit (such as the centrad) may not adequately describe the prism. Nevertheless, centrads are used in the "graphical analysis" of binocular vision.

11.12 THE RISLEY PRISM

A pair of counter-rotating prisms can be used to generate continuously varying prism power. Consider two combined BD prisms each of power Z. The resultant prism power is 2Z BD, which is the maximum power obtainable from the combination (Figure 11.31a). When the prisms are counter-rotated through an angle a_{max} from the maximum position (Figure 11.31b), the horizontal components are equal in magnitude and opposite in direction. So the resultant prism is still BD (i.e., BD @ 90) as shown in Figure 11.31c. Each prism has a vertical component of

$$Z_y = Z\cos a_{max}$$

and the sum of the vertical components gives the resultant:

$$Z_r = 2\,Z\cos a_{max} \qquad (11.16)$$

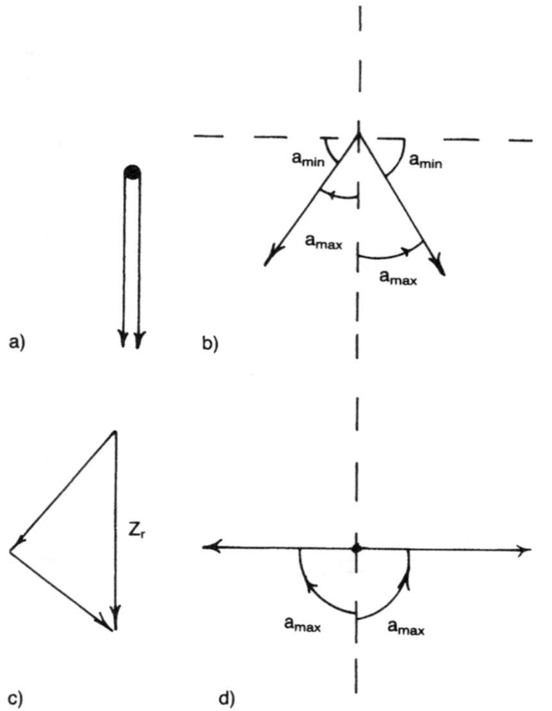

Figure 11.31 Risley prism component vectors: a, maximum setting; b, intermediate setting; c, resultant prism for *b*; d, zero setting.

EXAMPLE 11.10a
Each component of a Risley prism is a 10^{Δ} prism. The Risley is set so that both prisms are BD. What is the maximum prism power? What is the power when they are counter-rotated by 45° from the maximum?

The maximum is 2Z or 20^{Δ} BD.
For a counter-rotation of 45° from the maximum,

$$Z_r = 2(10^{\Delta})\cos 45° = 14.1^{\Delta}\text{ BD}$$

The minimum (zero) occurs when one prism is base left and the other is base right (Figure 11.31d). For each component, the angle of rotation a_{min} specified from the minimum position is the complement of a_{max} (Figure 11.31b), i.e.,

$$a_{min} + a_{max} = 90°$$

Therefore,

$$\cos a_{max} = \sin a_{min}$$

and we can write the Risley equation as

$$Z_r = 2\,Z\sin a_{min} \qquad (11.17)$$

EXAMPLE 11.10b
The Risley prism of the previous example is initially set at zero. Then a 15° counter-rotation is made. What is the prism power?

$$Z_r = 2(10)\sin 15 = 5.2^{\Delta}\text{ BD}$$

Since a counter-rotation of 15° from the minimum is equal to a counter-rotation of 75° from the maximum, we could solve the above problem as

$$Z_r = 2(10)\cos 75 = 5.2^{\Delta}\text{ BD}$$

We can rotate the Risley clockwise or counterclockwise to obtain other base directions. For example, one might start with both components BI, and then counter-rotate.

11.13 PRISM EFFECTIVITY

Consider an object point located straight ahead of an eye. When this object point is viewed through a prism, it appears deviated toward the apex of the prism. Hence, the eye must turn to keep the conjugate image point on the fovea. The amount the eye needs to turn is referred to as the effect of the prism on the eye.

Figure 11.32a is a thin prism with a deviation angle *d*. To see the virtual image formed by the prism, the

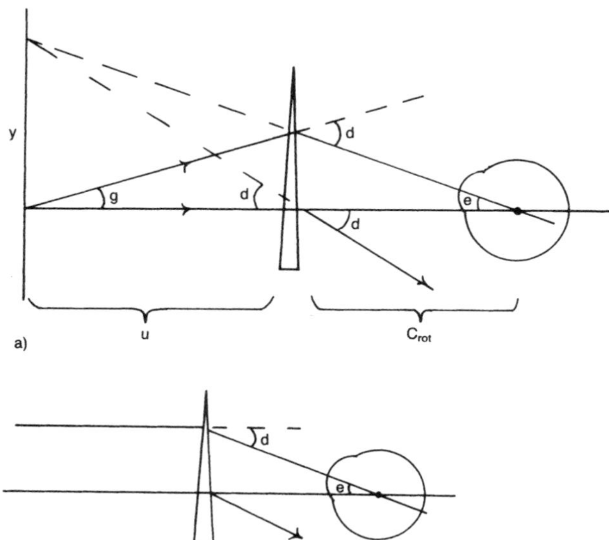

Figure 11.32 a, Prism effectivity ($e < d$) for a near object in front of a thin prism with deviation angle d; b, prism effectivity for a distant object ($e = d$).

eye rotates through the angle e about its center of rotation, which is typically about 13.5 mm behind the cornea.

The ray coming down the axis is bent down by the angle d and misses the eye. The backwards extension of the outgoing ray passes through the virtual image point, which is a distance y above the object point. The ray traveling upward at an angle g to the axis is bent down again by the angle d, and when extended passes through the eye's center of rotation. The angle e is the angle that the eye must rotate in order to image the object point on the fovea. This ray path, together with the straight ahead axis, forms a triangle for which d is an external angle with g and e as the two opposite internal angles. Thus,

$$g + e = d$$

and we see that d is greater than e.

In Figure 11.32a, the object point is a distance u from the prism, and the virtual image is a distance y above the object point. From the triangle involving the object point, the straight-ahead ray to the prism, and the image point,

$$\tan d = \left|\frac{y}{u}\right| = \frac{y}{-u}$$

or

$$y = -u \tan d$$

Let c_{rot} be the distance from the prism to the eye's center of rotation. Since $|u| = -u$

$$\tan e = \frac{y}{-u + c_{rot}}$$

The above two equations give

$$\tan e = \frac{-u \tan d}{-u + c_{rot}}$$

or

$$\tan e = \frac{\tan d}{1 - (c_{rot}/u)}$$

The prism has zero dioptric power, so

$$V = U = 1/u$$

and then,

$$\tan e = \frac{\tan d}{1 - c_{rot} V}$$

We can multiply both sides by 100 and let

$$Z_e = 100 \ \tan e \tag{11.18}$$

where Z_e is the prism-diopter value corresponding to the angle the eye turns through. Then,

$$Z_e = \frac{Z}{1 - c_{rot} V} \tag{11.19}$$

Equation 11.19 is the prism effectivity equation for a prism of power Z placed a distance c_{rot} from the center of rotation of the eye. The vergence V is the vergence leaving the prism. (The equation is written in terms of the vergence V instead of the incidence vergence U because in the next chapter, prism-lens combinations, it generalizes in that form.)

EXAMPLE 11.11a

An 8^{Δ} BD prism is held 20 cm in front of the center of rotation of Mr. Vul Gar's eye. Vul Gar looks through the prism at an object that is 2 m in front of the prism. How much does Vul Gar's eye have to turn to see the object? (That is, what is the effective prism power?)

From Eq. 11.19,

$$Z_e = \frac{8^{\Delta}\ \text{BD}}{1 - (0.20\ \text{m})(-0.5\ \text{D})} = \frac{8^{\Delta}\ \text{BD}}{1.10} = 7.3^{\Delta}\ \text{BD}$$

The BD means the apparent object is deviated up, and so Vul Gar's eye must turn up. However, it turns up by 7.3^{Δ} as opposed to 8^{Δ}. From Eq. 11.18, the angle e is

$$e = \tan^{-1}(7.3^{\Delta}/100) = 4.2^{\circ}$$

EXAMPLE 11.11b

As Vul Gar continues to hold the prism 20 cm in front of his eye's center of rotation, he walks forward until the prism is 25 cm from the object. Now what is the effective prism power?

$$Z_e = \frac{8^{\Delta}\ \text{BD}}{1 - (0.20\,\text{m})(-4.0\,\text{D})} = \frac{8^{\Delta}\ \text{BD}}{1.80} = 4.4^{\Delta}\ \text{BD}$$

The BD prism means that the object appears deviated up. As Vul Gar walks toward the object, the effective prism power changed from 7.3^{Δ} to 4.4^{Δ}. This is a noticeable effect as the object actually appears to move down as Vul Gar approaches it.

As a person looking through a prism backs away from the object, the effective prism power increases. For an object at optical infinity, $V = U = 0$, and Eq. 11.19 gives

$$Z_e = Z$$

This means that for a distant object the angle e the eye turns through equals the deviation angle d of the prism. Figure 11.32b shows the ray diagram. The incident rays are all parallel, and are all deviated by the angle d. For the ray that passes through the eye's center of rotation, angle e and angle d are opposite internal angles between two parallel lines, and are equal. Compared to the above two examples, when a person looks through an 8^{Δ} prism at a distant object, the effective power of the prism is 8^{Δ}.

EXAMPLE 11.11c

Ms. Deci Mal is wearing 7^{Δ} BU prism in a spectacle frame with a 12 mm vertex distance. Deci Mal looks at an object that is 33.3 cm from the prism. How much and in what direction does the eye turn?

The center of rotation is typically 13.5 mm behind the cornea, so

$$c_{\text{rot}} = 12 + 13.5 = 25.5\,\text{mm}$$

Here,

$$V = U = -3\,\text{D}$$

From Eq. 11.19,

$$Z_e = \frac{7^{\Delta}\ \text{BU}}{1 - (0.0255)(-3\,\text{D})} = \frac{7^{\Delta}\ \text{BU}}{1.077} = 6.5^{\Delta}\ \text{BU}$$

The eye turns down through an angle corresponding to 6.5 prism-diopters.

For a prism in the spectacle plane, the distance c_{rot} expressed in meters is small. In this case, we could use the standard approximation:

$$\frac{1}{1-x} \approx 1 + x \quad \text{when } x \text{ is small}$$

For Eq. 11.19, the approximation gives

$$Z_e \approx Z(1 + c_{\text{rot}}V) \tag{11.20}$$

Equation 11.20 shows that the difference between Z_e and Z increases with an increase in the distance c_{rot} between the prism and the eye's center of rotation, as well as with an increase in the magnitude of the vergence V. Clinically, the difference is frequently small enough to be neglected.

11.14 FRESNEL PRISMS

Figure 11.33a shows a collimated bundle of rays incident on a prism. Each ray in the bundle is deviated through an angle d by the prism. Even though a ray near the apex passes through a thin part of the prism, it has the same deviation as a ray that passes through a thicker part.

A Fresnel prism is a collection of prism sections from the apex area (Figure 11.33b). A ray traveling through any section is deviated by the angle d. However, the composite prism remains thin everywhere. Note that a "thin" prism has a small apex angle. A Fresnel prism in which the sections have large apex angles would act like a thick prism even though the actual thickness of the Fresnel remains small.

The boundary lines between the different sections of a Fresnel prism are perpendicular to the base-apex meridian. Figure 11.33c shows front and side views of a BD Fresnel prism.

Fresnel prisms can be made out of glass, hard plastic, or flexible polyvinyl membranes (about 1 mm thick). The flexible membrane Fresnel prisms adhere to spectacle lenses, and have ophthalmic uses for temporary corrections or for high prism powers.

Light is scattered at the section boundaries of a Fresnel prism. This scattered light causes a reduction in contrast, and hence, some loss of acuity compared to a regular prism.

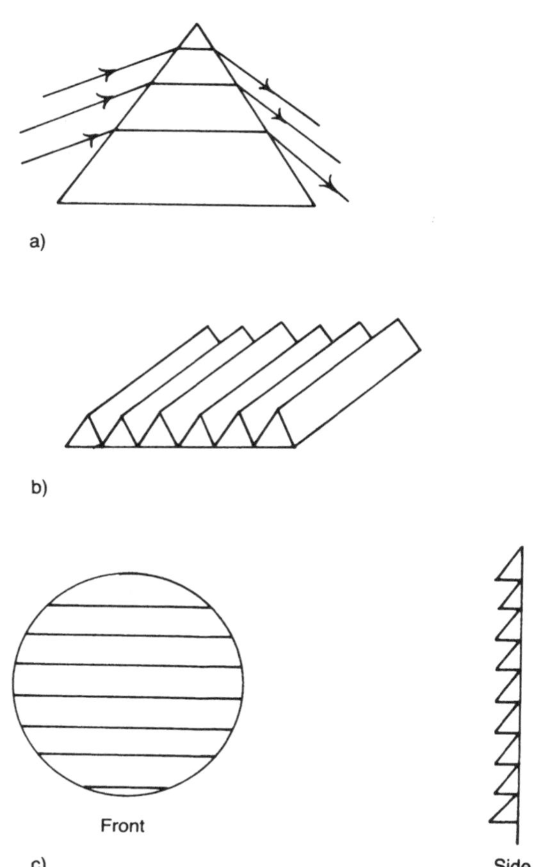

Figure 11.33 a, Independence of deviation angle for different ray paths; b, Fresnel prism; c, front and side views of base down Fresnel prism.

11.15 REFLECTING PRISMS

The internal reflections inside a prism are sometimes beneficial in optical system design. The simplest example is the right angle prism. Light enters the prism normal to the first surface. The light undergoes total internal reflection at the side opposite the right angle. In Figure 11.34, the light exits the prism at the bottom. The total deviation is 90°. The internal reflection gives a left–right inversion just like that of a flat mirror. So when the object is the palm of a right hand, the prism's virtual image is the palm of a left hand.

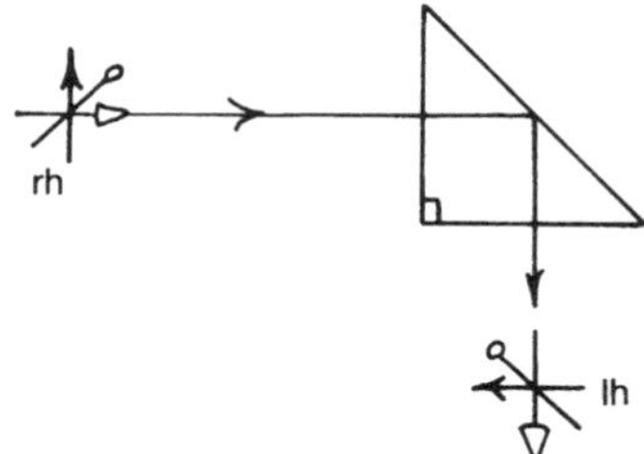

Figure 11.34 Right angle deviation by total internal reflection.

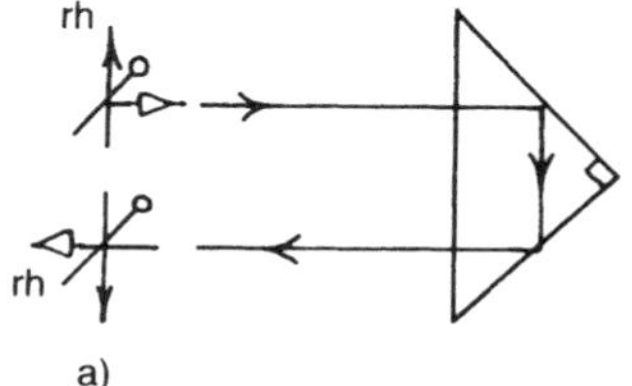

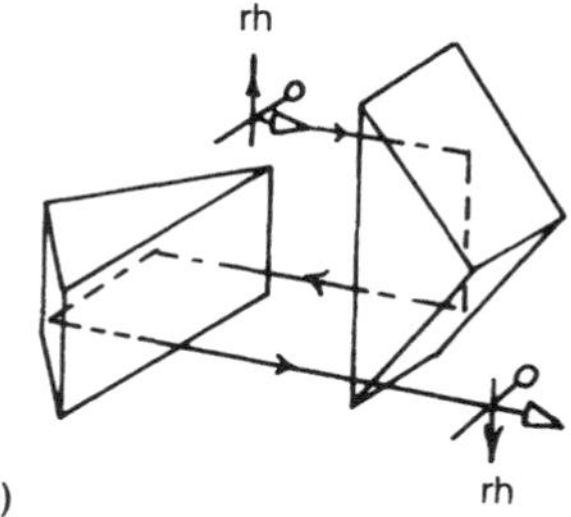

Figure 11.35 a, Porro prism as a retroreflector; b, double Porro prism erecting system.

A Porro prism is a right angle prism that is turned around so that the light enters the side opposite the right angle (Figure 11.35a). The light then undergoes two total internal reflections inside the prism and reemerges, traveling back toward the incident direction (i.e., the total deviation angle is 180°). Thus, the Porro prism can be used as a retroreflector. For example, the reflectors on bicycles are made up of many little Porro prisms.

Each reflection in the Porro prism introduces a left–right inversion, and two inversions cancel each other. The geometry also causes the image to be flipped in one meridian. So when the object for a Porro prism is an erect right hand, the virtual image is an inverted right hand. Common binoculars consist of a Keplerian telescope with a double Porro prism erecting system (Figure 11.35b). One prism flips the vertical meridian, while the other prism flips the horizontal meridian. The emergent beam, while traveling in the same direction as the incident beam, is offset relative to the incident beam. An actual Porro prism may have some truncated edges to reduce size and weight.

A Penta prism deviates the light 90° without introducing a left–right inversion (Figure 11.36). In the Penta prism, the two internal reflections are not total, so those sides must be silvered. The Penta prism is used in small rangefinders and in single lens reflex cameras.

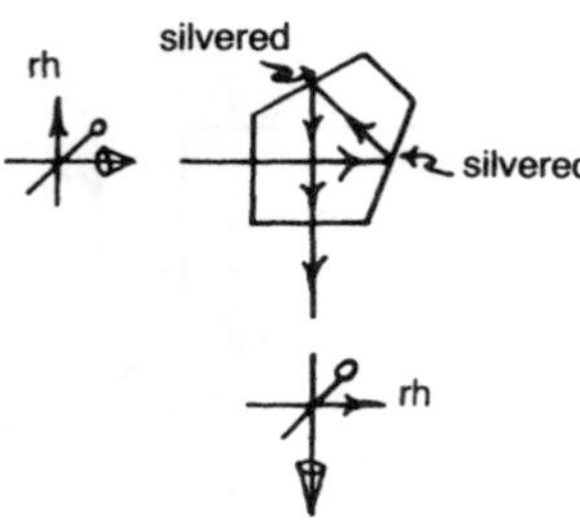

Figure 11.36 Penta prism.

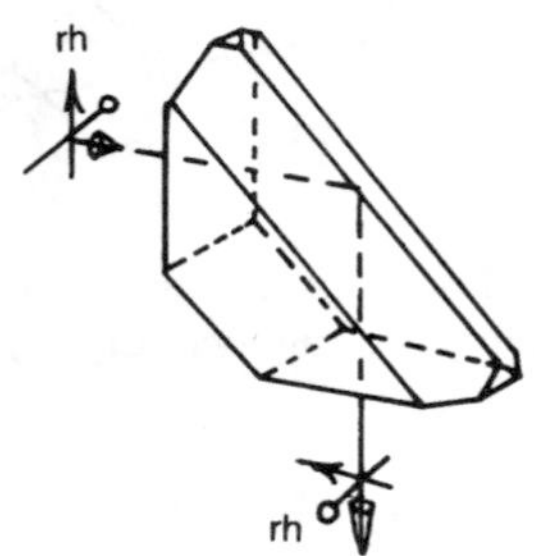

Figure 11.37 Amici prism.

The Amici prism is a truncated right angle prism with a roof section added onto the side opposite the right angle (Figure 11.37). Normally in a single reflection, a right hand is imaged as a left hand. For an object that is a right hand, the roof section of the Amici prism provides a left–right flip, so that the image is also a right hand.

Sometimes it is desirable to invert an image in all meridians without having the offset that the double Porro prisms introduce. One means of doing this is with the Abbe prism (Figure 11.38). A beam undergoes three reflections in an Abbe prism and emerges parallel to the incident beam. For the orientation shown in Figure 11.38, the three reflections provide the inversion, while the roof section provides the left–right flip. For an object that is an erect right hand, the resulting image is an inverted right hand. The angular

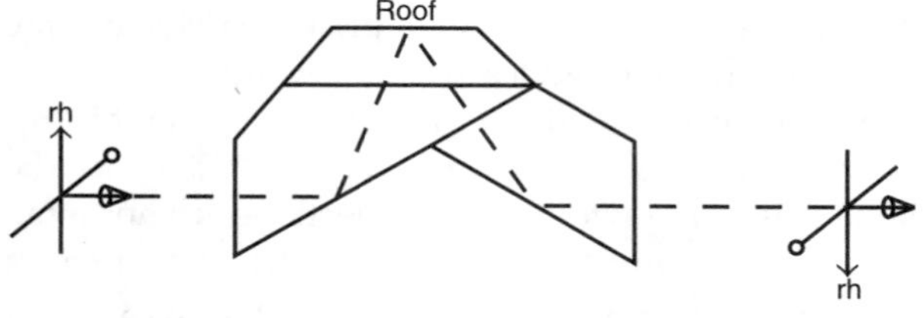

Figure 11.38 Side view of an Abbe prism.

tolerances on the roof are very precise, so the Abbe and the Amici prisms are difficult to manufacture.

There are also a number of other reflecting prisms. Some erect, some displace, some introduce left–right inversions, some serve as beam splitters, and some serve as polarizers.

PROBLEMS

1. A glass ($n = 1.617$) prism has a 40° apex angle. What is the deviation angle for light incident below the normal at an incident angle of 90° (grazing incidence)? At 60°? At 45°? At 23.145°? What is the angle of minimum deviation? What happens to light incident normally on the prism?
2. What is the critical angle for light in plastic with a 1.57 refractive index?
3. What is the deviation at normal incidence for light incident on prism of index 1.63 and apex angle 29°? What is the minimum deviation angle?
4. A prism with a 60° apex angle has a minimum deviation of 58°. What is the refractive index of the prism?
5. A thin prism has an index of 1.53 and an apex angle of 5.4°. What is the deviation angle and prism-diopter rating?
6. What linear deviation does a 6.7^{Δ} prism give on a wall 40 cm from the prism?
7. A prism gives a 13.2 cm linear deviation on a wall 330 cm from the prism. What is the prism-diopter value?
8. Two thin prisms have an apex angle of 6.8°. One has a 1.49 index, and the other a 1.58 index. What is the difference in prism-diopter values?
9. A 3.2^{Δ} BD prism is combined with a 4.7^{Δ} BU prism. What single prism is equivalent to the result?
10. A 3.2^{Δ} BD prism is combined with a 4.7^{Δ} BD prism. What single prism is equivalent to the result?
11. For the right eye, a 3.2^{Δ} BD prism is combined with a 4.7^{Δ} BO prism. What single prism is equivalent to the result?
12. For the left eye, a 2.7^{Δ} BD prism is combined with a 5.3^{Δ} BO prism. What single prism is equivalent to the result?
13. What are the horizontal and vertical components of a 6^{Δ} BU & I @ 122 prism. Which eye must this prism be for?
14. What are the horizontal and vertical components of a 7^{Δ} BD & O @ 25 prism. Which eye must this prism be for?
15. What single prism is equivalent to a 4^{Δ} BU & O @ 64 prism combined with a 5^{Δ} BD prism?
16. Jeremy Walk holds an 8^{Δ} prism 10 cm in front of his cornea (11.3 cm in front of his center of rotation) and looks at an object 32 cm from the prism. How much does he turn his eye (in prism-diopters)? For a distant object?
17. Nancy Dragon wears a 10^{Δ} BO prism at a 12 mm vertex distance. Nancy's entrance pupil is 3 mm

from her cornea, and Nancy's center of rotation is 13 mm from her cornea. When Nancy looks at an object 40 cm straight ahead of her lenses, how much does she turn her eye (in prism-diopters)?

18. A Risely prism consists of two 10^{Δ} components. What is the resultant prism power when each prism is counter-rotated 25° from the zero position? When each prism is counter-rotated 30° from the maximum position?

CHAPTER 12

Prism Properties of Lenses

12.1 PRENTICE'S RULE

Figure 12.1 shows parallel rays (from a distant axial point source) incident on a thin plus lens of dioptric power P. The lens converges the light and all the image space rays converge to the secondary focal point F_2. The incident ray that is farther from the axis has the larger deviation angle (d_2). The incident ray that is closer to the axis has the smaller deviation angle (d_1). In order to deal with prism–lens combinations, we use the ray deviation angles to assign different prism powers and base directions to each individual position on the lens.

Figure 12.2 shows an off-axis ray incident on a thin lens of dioptric power P. The ray leaves the axial object point (which is a distance u from the lens), hits the lens at a perpendicular distance h from the optical axis of the lens, is deviated through an angle d by the lens, and then travels to the conjugate image point (which is a distance v from the lens). The object and image space parts of this ray form two sides of a triangle, and the optical axis forms the third side.

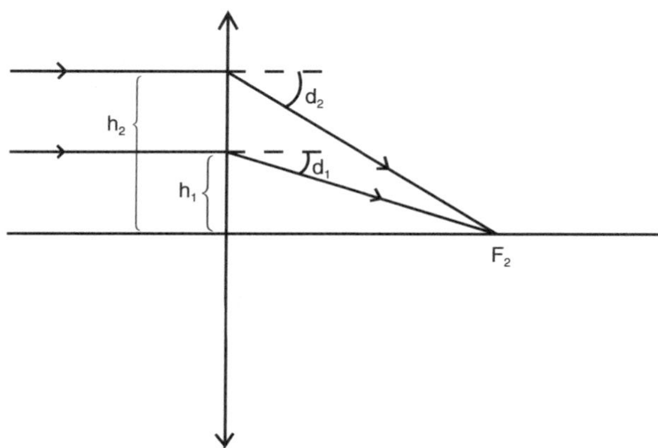

Figure 12.1 Deviation angles for two parallel rays incident on a plus thin lens.

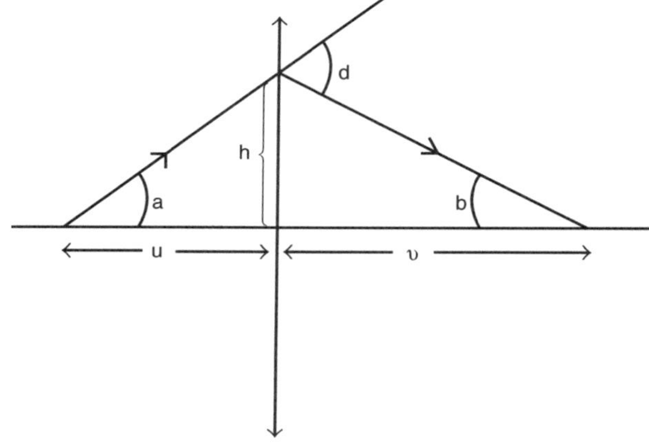

Figure 12.2 Deviation angle d for a ray incident at a distance h from the optical center on a thin lens of power P.

The deviation angle d is the external angle of this triangle. The two opposite internal angles are: the angle a formed at the object point by the object space ray and the optical axis, and the angle b formed at the image point by the image space ray and the optical axis. From the theorem (see Section 11.3) that the external angle of a triangle is equal to the two opposite internal angles,

$$|d| = |b| + |a|$$

The small angle approximations are good for paraxial rays. Therefore,

$$a \approx \tan a = h/|u|$$

and

$$b \approx \tan b = h/|v|$$

Then,

$$|d| = \frac{h}{|v|} + \frac{h}{|u|}$$

In general, we need to distinguish between a ray that is bent towards the axis (like the ray in Figure 12.2), and a ray that is bent away from the axis (see Figure 12.4b). We will assign a minus sign for the ray that bends towards the axis, and a plus sign for the ray that bends away from the axis. In Figure 12.2, the object distance u is a negative number, so when we remove the absolute value signs,

$$-d = \frac{h}{v} + \frac{h}{-u}$$

or in terms of vergences

$$-d = Vh - Uh = (V - U)h$$

Since $V = P + U$,

$$d = -Ph \qquad (12.1)$$

where d is in radians, P in diopters, and h in meters.

For small (paraxial) deviation angles

$$Z = 100 \tan d \approx 100d$$

When we multiply sides of Eq. 12.1 by 100, we obtain

$$100d = -(100)Ph$$

or

$$Z = -Ph \quad \text{where } h \text{ is in cm} \qquad (12.2)$$

Equation 12.2 is called *Prentice's rule*. It states that for a thin lens of dioptric power P, we can associate a different prism power Z with each point on the lens (the individual points being a distance h from the optical center of the lens). Dimensionally, when a distance is multiplied by a dioptric power, the distance usually needs to be expressed in meters. Prentice's rule is an exception because prism-diopters are dimensionally equal to centimeters.

In Eq. 12.2, h is a directed distance from the optical center to the point under consideration. The signs for a horizontal or vertical h value can be determined from a standard contra-ocular coordinate system in front of each eye (Figure 12.3). For example, when a ray hits 2 cm above the optical center, $h = +2$ cm. When the ray hits 2 cm below the optical center $h = -2$ cm. For the *right* eye, a ray hitting 3 cm out from the optical center gives $h = -3$ cm. For the *left* eye, a ray hitting 3 cm out from the optical center gives $h = +3$ cm.

We can determine the signs for a horizontal or a vertical base direction from the same coordinate system. We assign BU as positive and BD as negative. For the right eye, BI is positive while BO is negative (e.g., 3^{Δ}BO $= -3^{\Delta}$, while 3^{Δ}BI $= +3^{\Delta}$). The BI and BO signs are reversed for the left eye (e.g., 5^{Δ}BO $= +5^{\Delta}$, while 5BI $= -5^{\Delta}$).

A spherical lens is symmetric about its optical axis. For a plus spherical lens, the thickest part of the lens occurs at the optical center (Figure 12.4a). The associated prism base directions point toward the optical center, and a ray passing through bends toward the optical center. The arrows in Figure 12.4c represent the base directions. For example, at a point above the

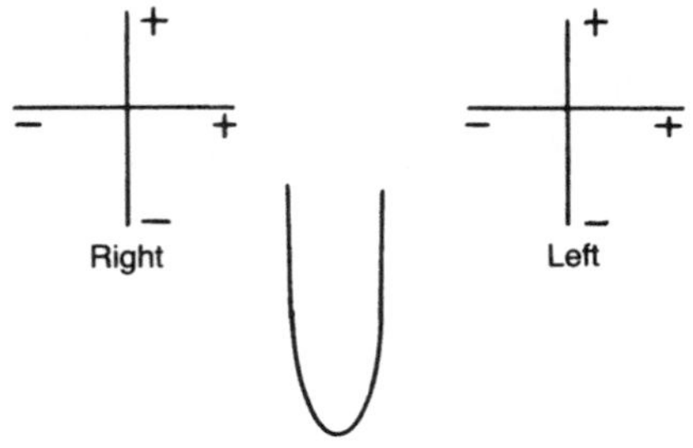

Figure 12.3 Plus-minus sign conventions for h (contra-ocular view).

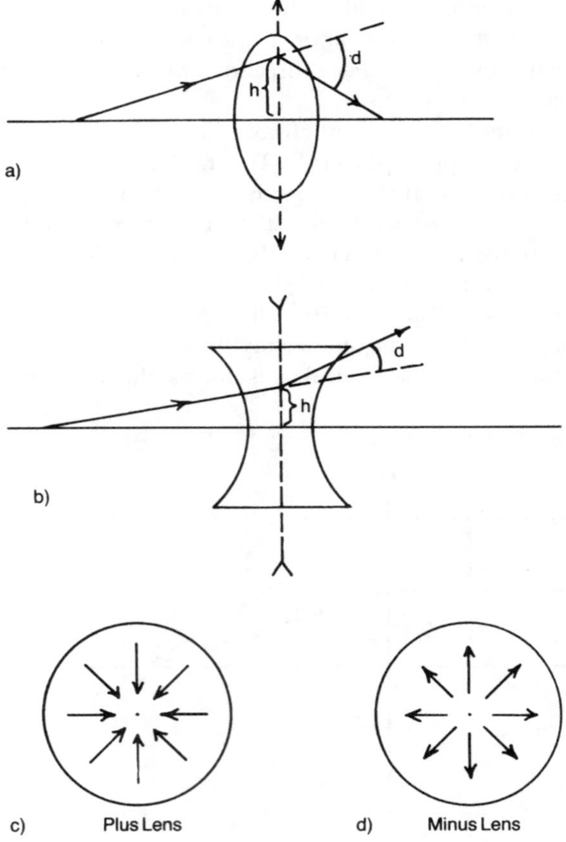

Figure 12.4 a, Deviation by plus lens; b, deviation by minus lens; c, base directions for plus spherical lens; d, base directions for minus spherical lens.

optical center ($h > 0$) on the plus lens ($P > 0$), Eq. 12.2 gives a BD result ($Z < 0$).

For a minus spherical lens, the thinnest part of the lens occurs at the optical center. The associated prism base directions point away from the optical center, and a ray passing through bends away from the optical center (Figures 12.4b and d). For example, at a point above the optical center ($h > 0$) on the minus lens ($P < 0$), Eq. 12.2 gives a BU result ($Z > 0$).

EXAMPLE 12.1a
What is the prism power and base direction at a point 15 mm above the optical center on a +4.00 D lens?

Here $h = +1.5$ cm. From Eq. 12.2,

$$Z = -(+4.00\,\text{D})(+1.5\,\text{cm}) = -6^{\Delta}$$

or

$$Z = 6^{\Delta}\text{BD}$$

The thickest part of the lens (at the optical center) is below the point under consideration and the thinnest part (the edge) is above, so it makes sense that the prism is BD.

EXAMPLE 12.1b
For the same lens, what is the prism power and base direction at a point 5 mm below the optical center?

Here $h = -0.5$ cm. From Eq. 12.2,

$$Z = -(+4.00\,\text{D})(-0.5\,\text{cm}) = +2^{\Delta}$$

or

$$Z = 2^{\Delta}\text{BU}$$

In this case, the thickest part of the lens is above the point, so it makes sense that the prism is BU. This point on the lens is closer to the optical center than the point in part a, so it also makes sense that the magnitude of the prism here is less than the magnitude in part a.

EXAMPLE 12.2a
Given a −15.00 D lens in front of the left eye, what is the prism power and base direction at a point 6 mm in from the optical center.

This is for the left eye, so from the coordinate system (Figure 12.3), $h = -0.6$ cm. From Eq. 12.2,

$$Z = -(-15.00\,\text{D})(-0.6\,\text{cm}) = -9^{\Delta}$$

For the left eye, minus prism is BI, so

$$Z = 9^{\Delta}\text{BI}$$

The BI is consistent with the fact that the thinnest part of the lens (the optical center) is out from the point under consideration.

EXAMPLE 12.2b
Given a −7.00 D lens in front of the right eye, what is the prism power and base direction at a point 12 mm in from the optical center.

This is for the right eye, so from the coordinate system (Figure 12.3), $h = +1.2$ cm. From Eq. 12.2,

$$Z = -(-7.00\,\text{D})(+1.2\,\text{cm}) = +8.4^{\Delta}$$

For the right eye, plus prism is BI, so

$$Z = +8.4^{\Delta}\text{BI}$$

The BI is consistent with the fact that the thinnest part of the lens (the optical center) is out from the point under consideration.

For a spherical lens, the prism base directions lie on radial lines that pass through the optical center (Figures 12.4c and d). For any point on the lens, the magnitude of the prism power can be obtained without worrying about the plus-minus signs, i.e.,

$$|Z| = |Ph| \quad \text{where } h \text{ is in cm} \qquad (12.3)$$

Then the base direction can be determined by checking where the optical center is relative to the point under consideration.

EXAMPLE 12.3
What is the prism power and base direction at a point 12 mm up and out from the optical center along the 128 meridian on a −3.00 D lens in front of the right eye?

From Eq. 12.3,

$$|Z| = |(-3.00\,\text{D})(1.2\,\text{cm})| = +3.6^{\Delta}$$

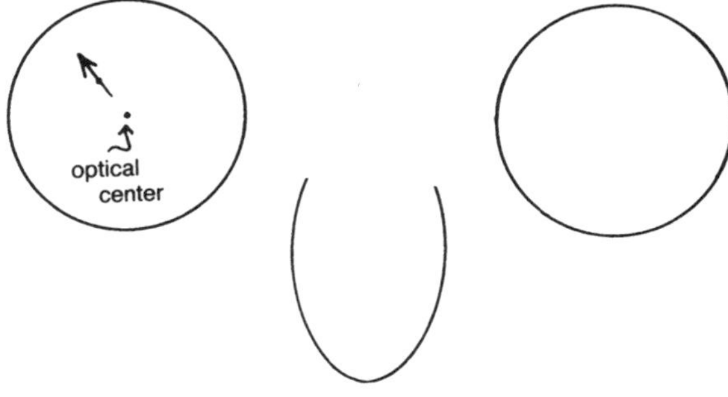

Figure 12.5 Prism at a point up and out from the optical center of a minus lens.

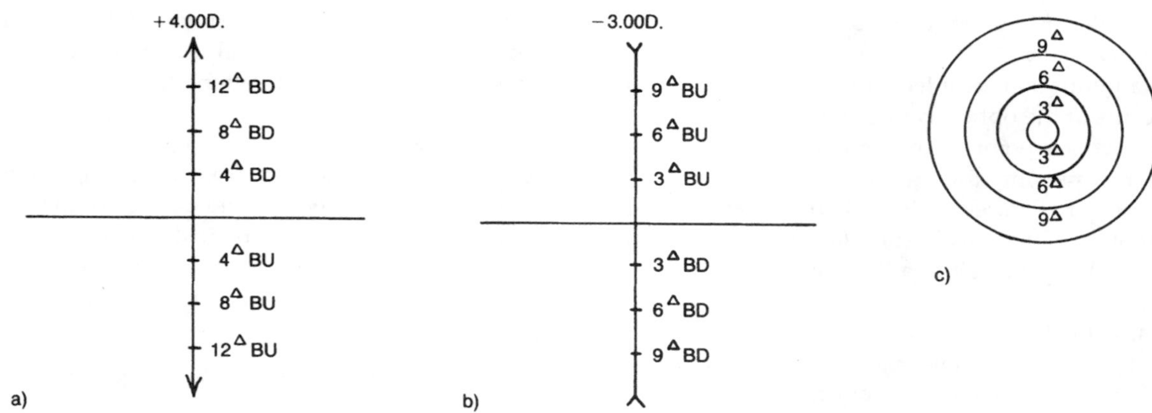

Figure 12.6 a, Prism powers and base directions for 1-cm steps on a +4.00-D lens; b, same for a −3.00-D lens; c, isoprism curves.

For the −3.00 D lens, the base directions point along the meridian and directly away from the optical center (Figure 12.5). So,

$$Z = 3.6^{\Delta}\text{BU} \ \& \ \text{O}@128$$

We can consider a thin spherical lens as a field of radial prism powers. Those points close to the optical center have small prism-diopter values, while those points far from the optical center have large prism-diopter values. Figure 12.6a shows some values for the +4.00 D lens, while Figure 12.6b shows some values for the −3.00 D lens. Figure 12.6c shows that the iso-prism curves on a spherical lens are circular and centered on the optical center of the lens. This is a manifestation of the rotational symmetry of a spherical lens about its optical axis.

12.2 PRISM–LENS COMBINATIONS

Consider a thin 2^{Δ}BU prism combined with the +4.00 D thin lens (Figure 12.7). The +4.00 D lens has the variable prism field given by Prentice's rule (Figure 12.6a). Each point on the prism has 2^{Δ}BU. To find the composite prism field, we vectorially add the prisms at each corresponding point.

For example, at a point 10 mm above the optical center, the prism from the lens is 4^{Δ}BD and when we add the 2^{Δ}BU from the prism, the resultant prism is 2^{Δ}BD. At a point 5 mm above the optical center of the original +4.00 D lens, the prism from the lens is 2^{Δ}BD and when we add the 2^{Δ}BU from the prism, the resultant prism is 0. At the optical center of the original +4.00 D lens, the resultant prism is 2^{Δ}BU (i.e., $0 + 2^{\Delta}$BU). At a point 5 mm below the optical center

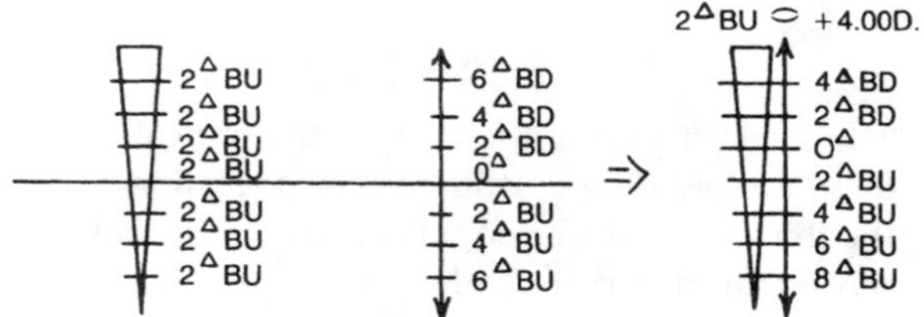

Figure 12.7 Prism–lens combination.

of the +4.00 D lens, the resultant prism power is 4^{Δ}BU (i.e., 2^{Δ}BU + 2^{Δ}BU).

A comparison of the resultant prism-diopter values of the combination to those of the original +4.00 D thin lens shows that the prism-diopter values for the combination are identical to the prism field of a +4.00 D thin lens that has been shifted (decentered) up by 5 mm. Thus, *a decentered thin spherical lens is equivalent to a thin prism–lens combination.*

Figure 12.8a shows three centered lenses. The optical axis of the system passes through the optical center of each lens. Assume that the middle (centered) lens is the +4.00 D lens. When a 2^{Δ}BU prism is placed against the +4.00 D lens, it shifts the prism field at each point by 2^{Δ}BU. In particular, the straight line that passes through the optical centers of the first and third lenses now passes through a point on the prism–lens combination that has prism power of 2^{Δ}BU (Figure 12.8b). We can achieve the same shift in prism values without using the prism by simply taking the original centered +4.00 D lens and decentering it up by 5 mm (Figure 12.8c).

For an uncorrected ametropic eye looking straight ahead at a distant object, the point at which the line of sight intersects the spectacle plane is called the Distance Reference Point (labeled DRP in Figure 12.9).

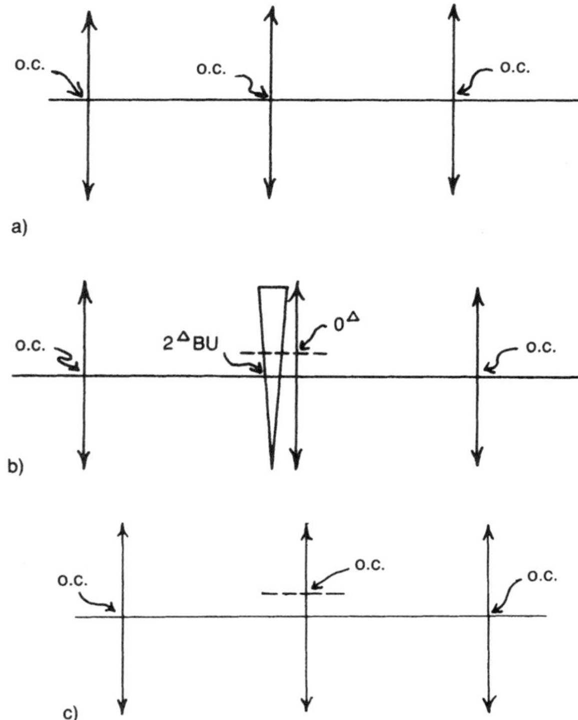

Figure 12.8 a, Three centered lenses; b, base up prism combined with middle lens. The numbers are the resultant prism powers at the indicated positions; c, same effect achieved by decentering middle lens up.

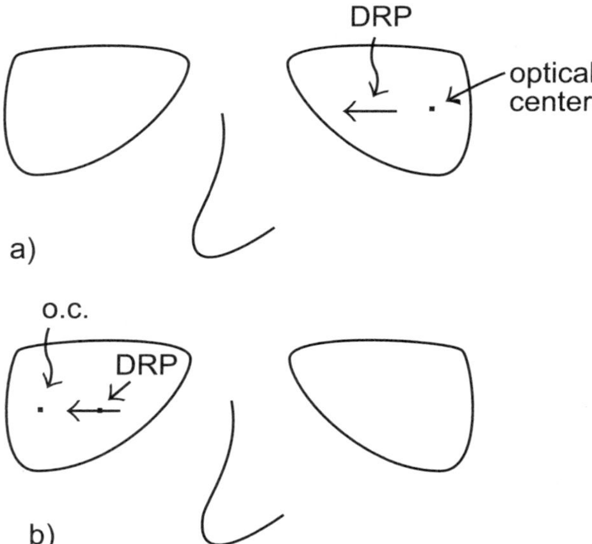

Figure 12.9 a, Outward decentration for minus lens; b, outward decentration for plus lens.

When there is no prism prescribed, the spectacle lens is placed in a frame so that its optical center is at the DRP. When the spectacle Rx is a prism–lens combination, the prism field of the lens is shifted, and the resultant prism power at the DRP is the prism power called for in the Rx. It may be possible to incorporate this prism power simply by decentering the lens relative to the DRP.

We can use the coordinate system in Figure 12.3 for horizontal and vertical decentrations. As a directed distance, the amount of decentration (DEC) is opposite in sign to the h value in Prentice's rule. For example, decentering a lens down (DEC < 0) causes the line of sight to pass through a point above the optical center ($h > 0$). Thus,

$$h = -\text{DEC}$$

and from Prentice's rule,

$$Z = P(\text{DEC}) \quad \text{where DEC is in cm} \qquad (12.4)$$

For a plus spherical lens ($P > 0$), DEC has the same sign as Z, so the decentration is always in the same direction as the prism base. For a minus spherical lens ($P < 0$), DEC is opposite in sign to Z, so the decentration direction is always in the opposite direction to the prism base direction.

EXAMPLE 12.4

Cilia Peach-Seed's left Rx is -7.00 D combined with 3^{Δ}BI. What decentration relative to the DRP gives the correct prism power?

The lens is minus, and so (according to the above stipulation) we expect the decentration to be out. From the coordinate system for the left eye (Figure 12.3),

$$Z = -3^{\Delta}$$

From Eq. 12.4,

$$-3^{\Delta} = (-7.00\text{ D})(\text{DEC})$$
$$\text{DEC} = +0.43\text{ cm} = 4.3\text{ mm out}$$

The prism base directions point directly away from the optical center (thinnest point) on a minus lens. In Figure 12.9a, the DRP has BI prism, so the optical center of the -7.00 D lens must be out from the DRP. This verifies that the decentration was out. Clinically, decentrations are specified in mm to the nearest mm, so the clinical answer is 4 mm out.

EXAMPLE 12.5

Jimmie B. Headed has a $+6.00$ D lens for the right eye that is decentered 8 mm out relative to the DRP. What prism does the decentration give?

The lens is plus, so we expect the prism to be BO. From the coordinate system for Jimmie's right eye,

$$\mathrm{DEC} = -0.8\,\mathrm{cm}$$

From Eq. 12.4,

$$Z = (+6.00\,\mathrm{D})(-0.8\,\mathrm{cm}) = -4.8^{\Delta}$$

or

$$Z = 4.8^{\Delta}\mathrm{BO}$$

In Figure 12.9b, the optical center of the +6.00 D lens is out from the DRP. The prism base directions point toward the optical center on a plus lens, so the prism at the DRP is BO, which confirms the calculated base direction.

While a decentered lens is equivalent to a prism–lens combination, the combination can also be made by molding or grinding (surfacing) the lens material. Figure 12.10a shows a thin BD ophthalmic prism with a +7.00 D front surface and a −7.00 D back surface. Figure 12.10b shows a +4.00 D thin lens of the same material with a +7.00 D front surface and a −3.00-D back surface. The prism and the lens could be glued together to give the prism–lens combination (Figure 12.10c). Figure 12.10d shows the single solid combination achieved by molding or grinding the lens material. In the solid combination, the front surface power is +7.00 D and the back surface power is −3.00 D.

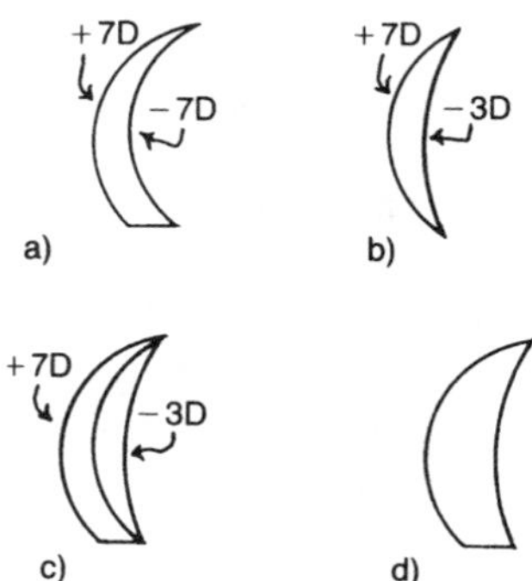

Figure 12.10 **a, Prism with −7.00 D back surface; b, lens with +7.00 D front surface; c, prism–lens combination; d, solid prism–lens combination made by prism surfacing the lens.**

12.3 PRISM IN CYLINDRICAL LENSES

A thin cylindrical lens does not have a unique optical center. Instead, each power meridian cross section has an optical center (Figure 12.11a). The line containing these optical centers is perpendicular to the power meridian cross sections, or parallel to the cylinder axis. For a plus cylindrical lens, the optical center line lies along the thickest part of the lens (Figure 12.11b). For a minus cylindrical lens, the optical center line lies along the thinnest part of the lens (Figure 12.11c).

A cylindrical lens bends rays only in the direction of the power meridian. The associated field of prism powers has the base directions aligned with the power meridian and perpendicular to the axis. The base directions point toward the optical center line on a plus cylinder and away from the optical center line on a minus cylinder. The arrows in Figure 12.12 show the base directions for a plus cylindrical lens with a horizontal axis meridian and a vertical power meridian. This lens bends the rays vertically (up or down) but not horizontally.

Consider a point *B* that is a perpendicular distance h_p from the optical center line of a cylindrical lens of

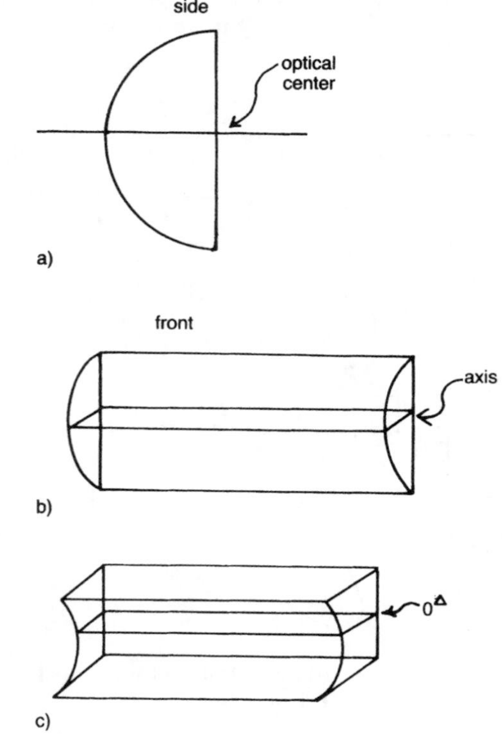

Figure 12.11 **a, Side view of a plus cylindrical lens; b, front view of a plus cylinder lens; c, minus cylinder lens.**

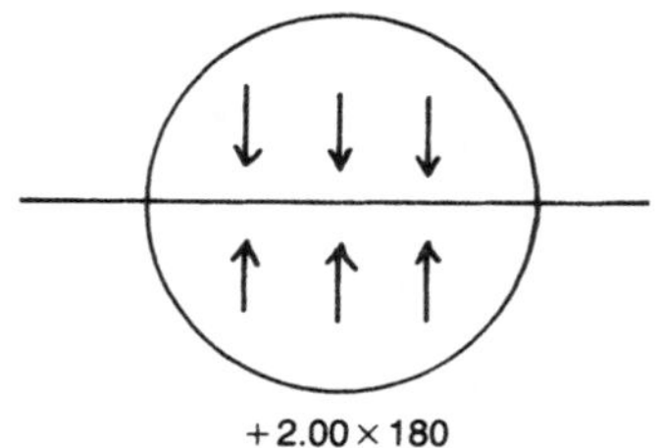

Figure 12.12 Prism base directions on a +2.00×180.

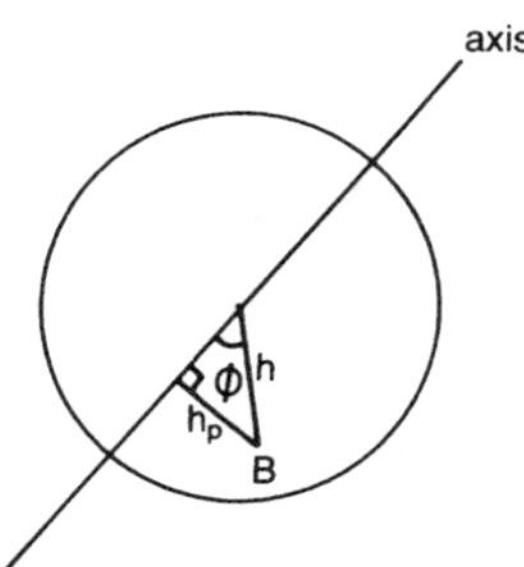

Figure 12.13 Parameters to determine prism power on a cylindrical lens.

power C (Figure 12.13). Since the distance h_p is aligned with the power meridian, it can be used in Prentice's rule to give

$$Z = -Ch_p \quad \text{where } h_p \text{ is in cm} \qquad (12.5)$$

EXAMPLE 12.6
What is the prism power at a point 11 mm vertically down from the optical center line of a −3.00 × 180 lens?

From Eq. 12.5,

$$Z = -(-3.00\,\text{D})(-1.1\,\text{cm}) = -3.3^{\Delta}$$

or

$$Z = 3.3^{\Delta}\text{BD}$$

(See Figure 12.11c for a base direction check.)

EXAMPLE 12.7
What is the prism power at a point 20 mm in from the optical center line of a +4.00 × 90 lens in front of the right eye?

From Eq. 12.5,

$$Z = -(+4.00\,\text{D})(+2.0\,\text{cm}) = -8.0^{\Delta}$$

or

$$Z = 8.0^{\Delta}\text{BD}$$

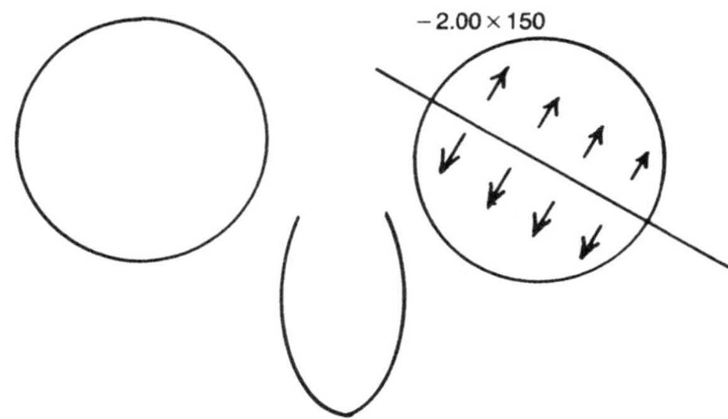

Figure 12.14 Prism base directions for a −2.00×150 in front of the left eye.

We can figure out the prism base directions on any cylindrical lens by considering the angular location of the power meridian. For example, on a −2.00 × 150 lens, the base directions lie along the 60 meridian (which is the power meridian) and point away from the optical center line. When the lens is in front of the left eye and we are considering a point below the optical center line, the base is BD & I @ 60 (Figure 12.14). For a point above the optical center line, the prism base is BU & O @ 60. These are the only two possible base directions for the −3.00 × 150 spectacle lens in front of the left eye.

Since the base directions are easy to obtain, we can put Eq. 12.5 in absolute values to obtain the magnitude of the prism power:

$$|Z| = |Ch_p| \quad \text{where } h_p \text{ is in cm} \qquad (12.6)$$

In Figure 12.13, point B is a distance h from the optical center line. From the triangle, the perpendicular distance h_p to the optical center line is given by

$$h_p = h \sin\phi$$

where ϕ is the acute angle that the directed distance h makes with the optical center line. From Eq. 12.6,

$$|Z| = |Ch \sin\phi| \quad \text{where } h \text{ is in cm} \qquad (12.7)$$

EXAMPLE 12.8
Zelmo Corkscrew's left spectacle lens is −5.00× 60. When Zelmo reads, his line of sight passes through a point 12 mm below the optical center line. What is the prism power at that point?

The base direction is BD & O @ 150 (Figure 12.15). For a 60° axis, and a vertical h, the angle ϕ is 30°. From Eq. 12.7,

$$|Z| = |(-5.00\,\text{D})(1.2\,\text{cm})(\sin 30°)|$$
$$= |(-5.00\,\text{D})(1.2\,\text{cm})(0.50)| = 3.0^{\Delta}$$

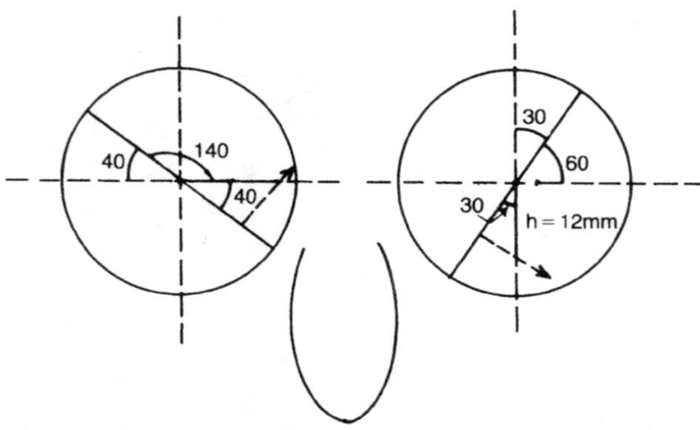

Figure 12.15 For left lens, prism at a point 12 mm down from the axis of a -5.00×60 lens. For right lens, prism at a point 6 mm in from the axis of a -4.00×140.

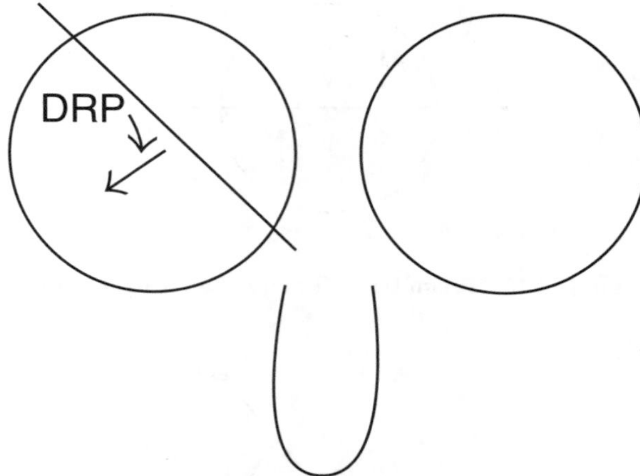

Figure 12.16 A -4.00×135 decentered in.

So,

$$Z = 3.0^{\Delta}\text{BD \& O@150}$$

EXAMPLE 12.9

Zelmo's right spectacle lens is -4.00×140. What is the prism at a point 6 mm in from the optical center line?

From Figure 12.15, the base direction is BU & I @ 50, and the angle ϕ is 40°. From Eq. 12.7,

$$|Z| = |(-4.00\,\text{D})(0.6\,\text{cm})(\sin 40°)| = 1.5^{\Delta}$$

So,

$$Z = 1.5^{\Delta}\text{BU \& I@50}$$

When a cylindrical lens is decentered relative to the DRP, the prism base directions at the DRP are aligned with the power meridian of the cylinder. This severely limits the prism base directions that can be obtained by decentration of a cylindrical lens. Consider an Rx for the right eye of -4.00×135 combined with some prism. Decentration of the cylindrical lens can give either BU & I @ 45 or BD & O @ 45. Figure 12.16 shows an "in" decentration relative to the DRP that results in BD& O @ 45 at the DRP. In particular, decentration of the -4.00×45 cannot give a BD prism (which is really a BD @ 90) or a BO prism (which is really a BO @ 180).

The only cylindrical lenses that can give BU or BD by decentration are those with a vertical power meridian (i.e., a 180 axis meridian). The only cylindrical lenses that can give BI or BO are those with a horizontal power meridian (i.e., a 90 axis meridian). On the other hand, any prism base direction can be molded or ground (surfaced) into a lens.

In the clinic, the horizontal prism testing is done separately from the vertical prism testing. Chapter 13 gives specific procedures for dealing with the horizontal and vertical components in any spherocylindrical lens.

12.4 ROTATIONAL DEVIATIONS BY A CYLINDRICAL LENS

Consider an emmetrope viewing a distant line through a cylindrical lens. Not only will the distant line have an astigmatic blur, but it also might appear to be rotated. We can use the prism power in the cylinder to qualitatively explain the apparent rotation.

Figure 12.17a shows an ocular view of a distant vertical line viewed through a -3.00×135. The prism at point A has its base direction up and to the left along the power meridian, so a point viewed through A would appear to be at A', which is down and to the right along the power meridian (i.e., toward the apex). There is zero prism power at B, so a point viewed through B would not appear deviated. The prism at C has its base down and to the right, so an object viewed through C would appear to be at C' which is up and to the left along the power meridian. We can find the apparent position of the vertical line by connecting A', B, and C'. The line appears to be rotated clockwise.

Figure 12.17b shows a distant horizontal line viewed through the same minus cylinder lens. The prism at point D has its base down and to the right along the power meridian, so a point viewed through D would appear to be at D', which is up and to the left along the power meridian (i.e., in the direction of the apex). Again, there is zero prism at B, so a point viewed through B does not appear deviated. At E, the prism base is up and to the left, so a point viewed

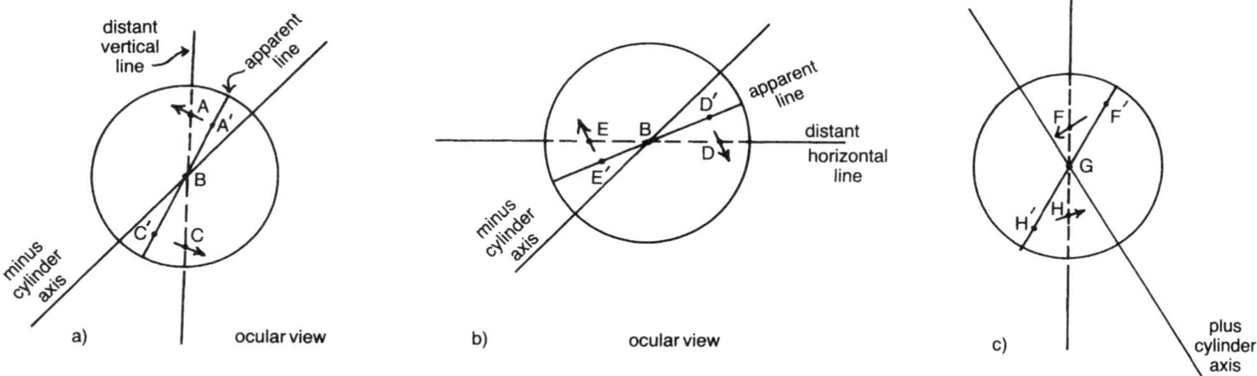

Figure 12.17 a, Ocular view of apparent rotation of a vertical line by a minus cylinder; b, ocular view of apparent rotation of a horizontal line by the same cylinder; c, plus cylinder lens giving same rotation as a.

through E appears at E', which is down and to the right. The apparent position of the vertical line is found by connecting D', B, and E'. The line appears to be rotated counter-clockwise.

The fact that the two lines appear to be rotated in opposite directions is called the *scissors effect*. Any lens with cylindrical power gives a scissors effect whenever the object lines are not aligned with the principal meridians. When the object lines are aligned with the principal meridians, there is no rotational deviation.

By transposition, the minus cylinder axis 135 in Figures 12.17a and b is equivalent to a spherical lens combined with a plus cylinder axis 45. Since the sphere has rotational symmetry, it does not contribute to rotational deviations. Therefore, the plus cylinder axis 45 lens must give the same rotational deviations as the minus cylinder axis 135 lens. Figure 12.17c shows a distant vertical line viewed through a plus cylinder axis 45 lens (ocular view). The prism base at point F is down and to the left along the power meridian, and a point viewed through F appears to be at F', which is up and to the right along the power meridian (i.e., toward the apex). There is zero prism at G, so a point viewed through G does not appear deviated. The prism at H is up and to the right, so a point viewed through H appears at H', which is down and to the left. The apparent line is found by connecting F', G, and H'. Indeed, the vertical line appears to be rotated clockwise (as in Figure 12.17a). You should repeat the argument for the horizontal line.

Note that when the above plus cylinder originally had a vertical axis and then was rotated counter-clockwise, the distant vertical line appeared to rotate clockwise (against rotation). When a minus cylinder (Figure 12.17a) originally has a vertical axis and then is rotated clockwise, the distant vertical line appears to also rotate clockwise (with rotation). As general rule: *the plus cylinder axis meridian of a lens gives against rotations, while the minus cylinder axis meridian of the lens gives with rotations.*

By transposition any lens with cylindrical power has both a plus and a minus cylinder axis meridian. So both rotations occur simultaneously. In other words, the lines appear to open and close like a scissors as the lens is rotated.

12.5 MOTIONS OF HAND NEUTRALIZATION

In a spherocylindrical correction for a compound hyperopic astigmat, both principal meridians have plus power; while in the correcting lens for a compound myopic astigmat, both principal meridians have minus power. We can use the with and against *rotations* of the previous section to find the principal meridians. Then we can use another type of movement, with and against *motion*, to determine if the power in a principal meridian is plus or minus.

Consider a vertical principal meridian. An observer can determine whether the power in that meridian is plus or minus by holding the lens close to her eye, and moving the lens up or down. A real object observed through the lens appears to move in the same direction when the lens is diverging (a phenomenon called *with motion*) and in the opposite direction when the lens is converging (*against motion*). The latter motions assume that the lens is held close to the eye. In particular, if converging light emerges from the lens, it is assumed that the light is still converging when incident on the eye. (In other words, the latter motions assume that a physically real aerial image is not formed between the lens and the observer's eye.)

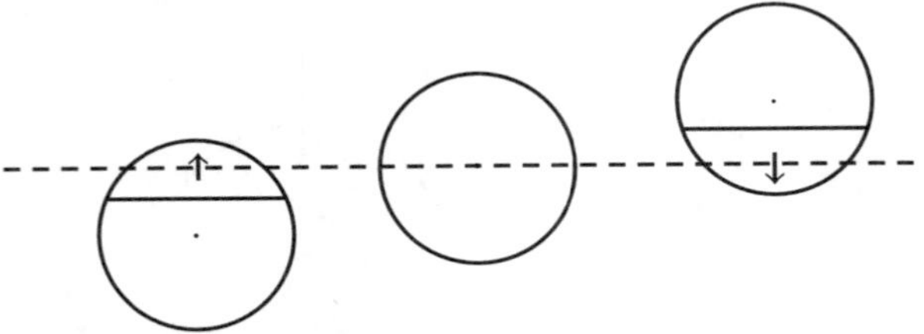

Figure 12.18 Representation of three frames of a motion picture sequence showing with motion for a minus lens. The dashed line is a distant horizontal object. The solid line shows the apparent location of the line as seen through the lens. The left to right sequence shows the change in the apparent line as the lens is moved up.

The prism power in a lens provides a simple way to understand the motions. For a vertical principal meridian with minus power, the prism bases directions point away from the optical center. Figure 12.18 shows three successive frames of a motion picture. The dashed line represents a distant horizontal line, while the solid line represents the apparent position of the horizontal line as seen through the lens. When the person looks through a point on the lens above the optical center, he is looking through a base up prism point, and the line appears to be deviated down (Figure 12.18 left). When the lens is raised so that the person is looking through the optical center, the prism power is zero and the apparent line is not deviated (Figure 12.18 center). When the lens is further raised so the person is looking through a point below the optical center, the prism is base down, and the line appears to be deviated up (Figure 12.18 right). So as the lens was raised, the apparent object position went from down to up, or went *with* the motion of the lens.

For plus power in the vertical meridian, the base directions point toward the optical center, and a similar analysis gives *against motion* provided the eye is immediately behind the lens. A plano lens (zero dioptric power) gives no motion.

The with and against motions form the basis of hand neutralization. In hand neutralization, a known trial lens is combined with an unknown ophthalmic lens. When the resultant power is plus, the combination gives against motion. When the resulting power is minus, the combination gives with motion. When the resulting power is zero, the combination gives no motion. The power of a thin unknown lens is then equal in magnitude but opposite in sign to that of the trial lens that neutralizes the motion.

Thick lenses provide a slight complication in the analysis. When the second lens neutralizes the first lens, it is the back vertex power of the first lens that is equal in magnitude but opposite in sign to the neutralizing power of the second lens.

Ophthalmic lenses usually have a bent form (concave back surface), and a trial lens placed against the back gives an air gap. To avoid errors introduced by the air gap, the trial lens is placed against the front of the unknown ophthalmic lens. In this case, the unknown lens parameter determined by hand neutralization is the neutralizing power (or front vertex) as opposed to the back vertex power (which is the parameter specified in the Rx).

12.6 MOTIONS OF THE RETINOSCOPE REFLEX

Retinoscopy is an objective refraction technique in which the examiner shines a spot or streak of light into the patient's eye, and then looks through a peephole in the retinoscope at the light (the reflex) coming back out of the patient's pupil. (Recall that objective refraction does not rely on subjective responses from the patient: i.e., the patient does not need to say anything.) During retinoscopy, the examiner holds the retinoscope at some distance from the patient's eye, places lenses (perhaps in a phoropter) in front of the patient's eye, and observes the reflex through these lenses. The spot or streak of incident light illuminates the patient's retina, and the illuminated area acts like a secondary spot or streak source for the reflex. The examiner scans the spot or streak across a principal meridian of the patient's eye and watches the "with" or "against" motion of the reflex in the patient's pupil. (Streak retinoscopes are easier to use clinically than spot retinoscopes, so the following discussion is in terms of streaks.)

The with and against motions of the retinoscopy reflex as seen through the peephole differ from the with and against motions of hand neutralization. In hand neutralization, the examiner looks through a lens or lenses at a *distant* object and then moves the lenses back and forth along a principal meridian. The endpoint is zero observed motion of the apparent distant object. In retinoscopy, the examiner, viewing through the peephole, looks through the refraction lenses and the patient's eye at the retinal streak acting as a *near* secondary object, and then scans the streak across a principal meridian. The endpoint occurs when very fast motion of the reflex (essentially a flash) is observed in the patient's pupil.

You can simulate the observation part of retinoscopy by holding a high plus spherical lens at about half of an arm's length from your eye, and looking through it at a pen or pencil held a short distance from the lens. (The high plus lens represents the patient's eye, and the pen or pencil represents the streak on the patient's retina.) Hold the pencil vertical and move it horizontally left and right so that it scans across the horizontal meridian of the lens. The apparent pencil that you see through the lens is a simulation of the reflex. If you first hold the pen or pencil quite close to the lens, you will see with motion of the simulated reflex. If you then hold the pen or pencil a full arm's length away, while the lens is still at a half arm's length, you will see against motion of the reflex. You can adjust the distance of the pen or pencil from the lens to find the reversal point between the with and against motion. As you get closer to the reversal point, the observed reflex motion gets faster. At the reversal point, an infinitely fast reflex motion, essentially an off-on "flash," is observed. The flash is sometimes described as "neither with nor against motion."

When the patient is an emmetrope, the far point of the patient's eye is at optical infinity. When the patient is a spherical ametrope, the far point of the patient's eye is closer than optical infinity (real for myopes and virtual for hyperopes). When the patient is astigmatic, there is a different far point for each principal meridian. A lens placed in front of the patient's eye changes the location of the point conjugate to the patient's retina. When the patient's accommodation is relaxed, we can refer to this conjugate point as the far point of the lens–eye system. The retinoscopy endpoint flash occurs when this far point is coincident with the retinoscope peephole.

When the examiner scans the incident streak across a principal meridian, the reflex shows either with or against motion depending on where the far point for that meridian is located relative to the retinoscope peephole. The examiner can change the observed reflex motion by either changing the lenses in the spectacle plane, or perhaps by changing the distance between the retinoscope and the patient's eye. As the far point moves farther away from the retinoscope peephole, the reflex moves slower. As the far point comes closer to the retinoscope peephole, the reflex moves faster (just as it does for the pencil simulation). When the far point moves past the peephole, the reflex motion changes from one motion to the opposite motion (e.g., with to against or vice versa). When the far point is at the retinoscope peephole, the reflex motion is infinitely fast, and the examiner sees only the apparent off-on flash of the reflex in the patient's pupil (i.e., the examiner sees neither a with nor an against motion).

On retinoscopes, there are several settings for the incident streak of light (e.g., plane mirror retinoscopy versus convex mirror retinoscopy). The examiner can vary these settings to change the motion on one side of the endpoint from with to against or vice versa. Here we discuss only the light coming out of the patient's pupil, and derive an equation for the motion of the reflex relative to the motion of the streak across the retina. (The resulting motions are consistent with plane mirror retinoscopy.)

Figure 12.19a shows a ray diagram of a vertical principal meridian for a low myope's eye. The screen S represents the retina, and the thin lens E represents the refracting elements of the patient's eye and any lens in front of the eye. (For simplicity, we are neglecting the vertex distance of any lenses in front of the patient's eye and placing them directly at the position of E.) The length of the eye is represented by the distance u. Power in a vertical principal meridian is responsible for imaging horizontal lines, so the streak on the retina is horizontal at a vertical distance O above the eye's optical axis. (The distance O acts like an object size.) The rays leaving the eye are converging and the streak is imaged at a vertical distance I from the axis in the far point plane FP, which is behind the retinoscope peephole R. (The distance I acts like an image size.) The far point plane is a distance v from the thin lens representing the eye.

The examiner looks through the retinoscope peephole at the reflex as it appears in the patient's pupil. The retinoscope peephole is a distance t, taken to be positive, from the thin lens E. We'll call t the working distance. The solid ray in Fig 12.19a passes through the center of the peephole and, as viewed through the peephole, the reflex appears to the examiner to be located in the pupil at a distance h above the optical axis.

The triangle involving the optical axis, the side I, and the ray through the center of the peephole is similar to the triangle involving the optical axis (segment of length t), the side h, and the same ray. From the base to height ratios of these similar triangles,

$$\frac{h}{t} = \frac{-I}{v - t}$$

We can solve for h, and then divide both the numerator and the denominator by t and v to obtain

$$h = \frac{-I(1/v)}{(1/t) - (1/v)}$$

Let

$$V = \frac{1}{v}$$

where V is the vergence leaving E, and let

$$T = \frac{1}{t}$$

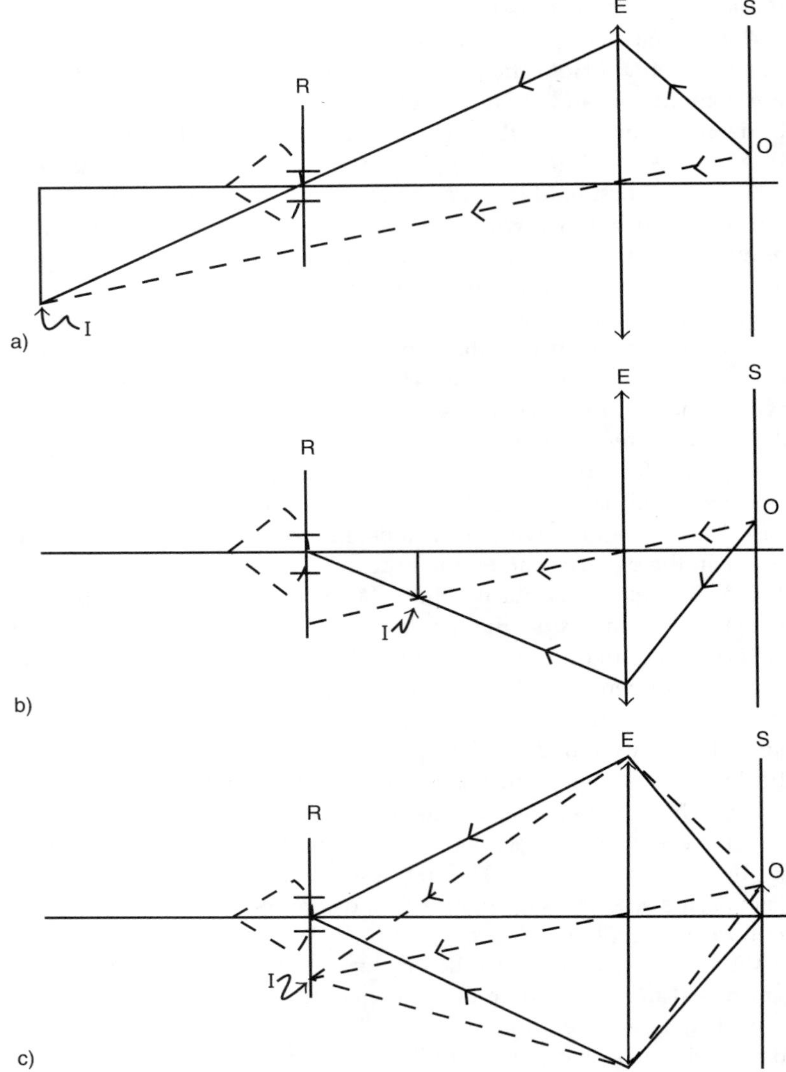

Figure 12.19 Retinoscopy Rays. Patient's eye is on the right (represented by *E* and *S*). *O* is the location of the retinoscope streak on the patient's retina. In each case, the image *I* of the streak occurs in the far point plane of the patient's eye. The examiner looks through the retinoscope peephole, which is at *R*, at the patient's eye and sees the retinoscope reflex at the vertical distance h in the patient's pupil. a, The far point plane (*I*) is farther from the patient's eye than the peephole. b, The far point plane (*I*) is closer to the patient's eye than the peephole. c, The far point plane (*I*) is at the peephole plane. In c, the solid lines are a bundle of rays for an on-axis streak, while the dashed lines are a bundle of rays for an off-axis streak.

where T is the dioptric location of the peephole, or the dioptric working distance. Then combine the above three equations to obtain

$$h = \frac{-VI}{T - V}$$

The definition of the lateral magnification m gives

$$I = mO$$

Since $m = U/V$, where U is the vergence of the light incident on lens E (i.e., $U = 1/u$, where u is the reduced length of the eye model, or the distance from E to S), we have

$$I = \frac{U}{V}O = \frac{-|U|}{V}O$$

Substitution into the equation for h gives

$$h = \frac{|U|O}{T - V}$$

When the streak is scanned across the retina, O changes and so does h. The derivative of O with respect to time is the speed O' of the scan across the retina. The derivative of h with respect to time is the speed h' of the reflex across the pupil. Differentiation of the above equation gives

$$h' = \frac{|U|O'}{T - V}$$

For simplicity, let

$$K' = |U|O'$$

Then,

$$h' = \frac{K'}{T - V} \tag{12.8}$$

For a fixed scan speed O', K' is a constant directly proportional to O'. Equation 12.8 gives the reflex speed h' relative to K'.

The derivation is general, so it applies to high myopes, emmetropes, and hyperopes (as well as low myopes). The following are some numerical examples for a 50 cm working distance (i.e., the retinoscope is held 50 cm from the lens E). Then $t = 50\,\text{cm}$, and $T = 2\,\text{D}$.

For an uncorrected 4 D myope, $V = +4\,\text{D}$, and

$$h' = \frac{K'}{2\,\text{D} - 4\,\text{D}} = \frac{K'}{-2\,\text{D}}$$

The minus sign indicates that the reflex motion across the pupil is against (opposite of) the scan motion across the retina. Here the far point is 25 cm (i.e., 100/4 D) from the eye, so it is in front of the retinoscope peephole (Figure 12.19b, note that h is below the axis even though O is above the axis).

For an uncorrected 3 D myope, $V = +3\,\text{D}$, and

$$h' = \frac{K'}{2\,\text{D} - 3\,\text{D}} = \frac{K'}{-1\,\text{D}}$$

which says that the reflex motion is "against" and twice as fast as that for the 4 D myope. Here the far point is 33 cm (i.e., 100/3 D) from the eye, so it is still in front of the retinoscope peephole, but it is closer to it than in the 4 D myope case. (On the distorted circle representation of Section 6.10, the far point is moving clockwise around the circle.)

For an uncorrected 2 D myope, $V = +2\,\text{D}$, and

$$h' = \frac{K'}{2\,\text{D} - 2\,\text{D}} = \frac{K'}{0}$$

This is the endpoint infinitely fast motion (flash) of the reflex. Here the far point is at the retinoscope peephole (i.e., at 100/2 D or 50 cm). Figure 12.19c shows this case. Note that when O is zero, it is imaged in the retinoscope peephole (solid rays) and it appears to the examiner that the entire pupil of the patient is filled with light. When the steak is moved a distance O above the axis (dashed rays), all the rays go to the I position, and so none of them go through the peephole. Here the entire pupil appears black. Thus as the steak is scanned, the entire pupil is black, except when the flash (entire pupil bright) occurs.

For an uncorrected 1 D myope, $V = +1\,\text{D}$, and

$$h' = \frac{K'}{2\,\text{D} - 1\,\text{D}} = \frac{K'}{+1\,\text{D}}$$

The plus sign indicates that the reflex motion across the pupil is with (same direction as) the scan motion across the retina. Here the far point is 100 cm (i.e., 100/4 D) from the eye, so it is behind the retinoscope peephole (Figure 12.19a).

For an emmetrope, $V = 0\,\text{D}$, and

$$h' = \frac{K'}{2\,\text{D} - 0} = \frac{K'}{+2\,\text{D}}$$

which says that the reflex motion is still "with" and twice as slow as the 1 D myope case. Here the far point is at optical infinity, so it is (much) farther behind the retinoscope peephole than in the 1 D myope case. (On the distorted circle representation of Section 6.10, the far point, moving clockwise and behind the peephole, has advanced to optical infinity.)

For an uncorrected 1 D hyperope, $V = -1\,\text{D}$, and

$$h' = \frac{K'}{2\,\text{D} - (-1\,\text{D})} = \frac{K'}{+3\,\text{D}}$$

which says that the reflex motion is "with" and even slower. (On the distorted circle representation of Section 6.10, the far point, moving clockwise and behind the peephole, has now advanced past optical infinity and is in the virtual part of the circle.)

The examiner can change lenses in front of the eye to change the vergence V in Equation 12.8. Thus by changing lenses, the examiner can make the far point of the lens–eye system coincident with the peephole, which gives the endpoint flash.

Suppose a lens of power P_w is in front of the eye (power P_e) at the endpoint. Here the vergence V coming out of the lens equals the dioptric working distance T, or

$$V = (P_w + P_e) + U = T$$

The distance vision correction in this principal meridian is the lens (power P_c) that gives $V = 0$ (i.e., the reversed situation to normal distance vision). In this situation,

$$V = (P_c + P_e) + U = 0$$

Subtraction of the above two equations gives

$$T = P_w - P_c$$

or

$$P_c = P_w - T \tag{12.9}$$

In other words, *to get the distance vision correction P_c in a principal meridian, subtract the dioptric working distance T from the power P_w of the endpoint lens.*

As an example, suppose the endpoint flash occurs with a $P_w = -5.00\,D$ lens in front of the eye (power P_e). For a 50 cm working distance, $T = +2.00\,D$. So Eq. 12.9 gives

$$P_c = -5.00\,D - 2.00\,D = -7.00\,D$$

Here the power of the distance vision correction is 2 D more minus (or less plus) than the endpoint lens.

For a second example, assume the endpoint lens in front of the eye is +3.00 D. Then for the 50 cm working distance Eq. 12.9 gives

$$P_c = +3.00\,D - 2.00\,D = +1.00\,D$$

When the eye is astigmatic, each principal meridian needs to be scoped, and the two results are the power cross values for the correction. When the lenses placed in front of the eye are in the spectacle plane and the working distance is figured from the spectacle plane, then the spectacle correction at that vertex distance is the final result of the retinoscopy.

The cylindrical component of an astigmatic eye can cause rotational deviations of the type discussed in Section 12.4. In streak retinoscopy, the examiner locates the principal meridians of the patient's eye by looking at the rotational deviation of the streak reflex relative to the incident streak (Figure 12.20). The reflex streak is aligned with the incident streak only in the principal meridians. When the incident streak is not aligned with a principal meridian of the patient's eye, the reflex is not aligned with the incident streak. The examiner locates the principal meridians by rotating the incident streak clockwise or counter-clockwise until alignment with the reflex is attained.

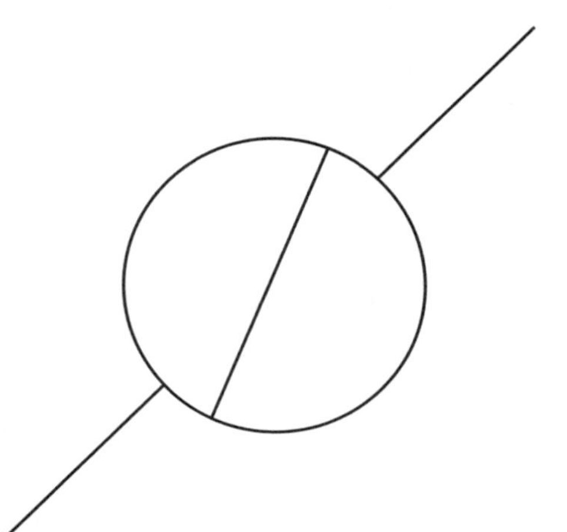

Figure 12.20 Appearance of reflex when the retinoscope streak is not aligned with a principal meridian.

Once the principal meridians are located, the examiner turns the streak so that it is perpendicular to the principal meridian being examined, and then scans the streak back and forth across that meridian. (For example, to examine a vertical principal meridian, the streak is horizontal and is scanned up and down across the vertical meridian.) Once the endpoint lens is found for that meridian, the examiner rotates the streak 90°, and then finds the endpoint for the other principal meridian.

12.7 FRESNEL LENSES

Figure 12.21a shows a -2.00×180 cylindrical lens. The prism base directions all point away from the optical center line. Along a line 1 cm above the optical center line, the prism power is 2^{Δ}BU, while along a line 2 cm above the optical center line the prism power is 4^{Δ}BU (Figure 12.21b). Here the iso-prism contour curves are lines that are parallel to the optical center line (in other words parallel to the axis meridian).

Section 11.14 discussed Fresnel prisms. We can make a Fresnel equivalent to a -2.00×180 cylindrical lens by again using prism sections. The sections all run horizontal, and Prentice's rule for the cylinder gives the prism power for each section (Figure 12.21c). For

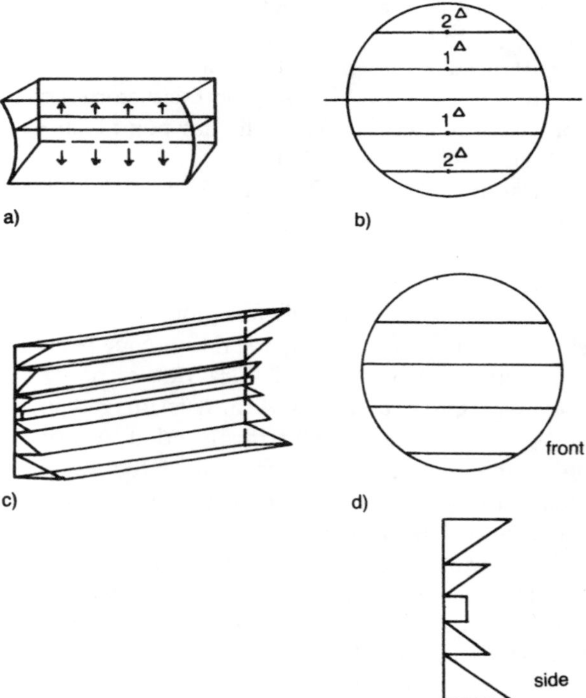

Figure 12.21 a, −2.00×180 lens; b, isoprism lines; c, Fresnel lens; d, Fresnel lens—front and side views.

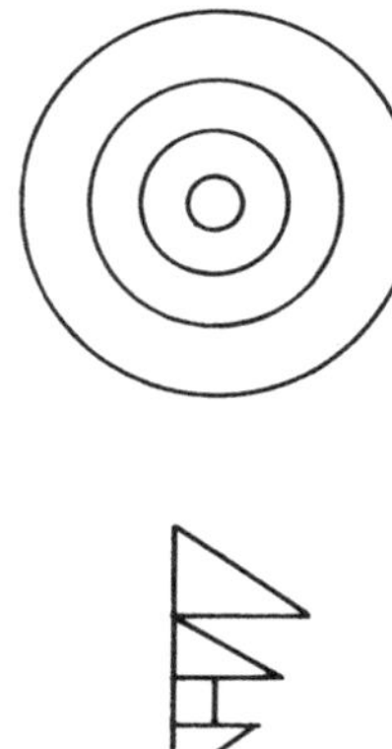

Figure 12.22 Front and side views of a Fresnel spherical lens.

the Fresnel minus cylinder lens, the prism base directions point away from the optical center line (Figure 12.21d shows front and side views). For a Fresnel plus cylinder, the prism sections would again be parallel to the optical center line, but the prism base directions would point towards the optical center line.

A Fresnel spherical lens can be made in a similar manner. On a spherical lens, the iso-prism contour curves are circular and centered on the optical center. Therefore, the prism sections are annular sections with their prism power given by Prentice's rule. Figure 12.22 shows front and side views for a plus spherical Fresnel lens.

One advantage of a Fresnel lens is that they can be made with a large diameter. Augustin–Jean Fresnel originally invented this type of lens for lighthouses that needed large diameter plus collimating lenses. The weight and thickness in regular spherical lenses were prohibitive, but the Fresnel lenses solved this problem.

A common contemporary use of a large diameter Fresnel plus lens is in the overhead projector. Plus Fresnel lenses are also used in car and truck headlights, and in some traffic light signal covers. Large diameter Fresnel minus lenses are commonly used in the back windows of motor-homes or large vans to increase the driver's field of view when backing up.

Soft polyvinyl membrane Fresnel lenses and prisms have special ophthalmic uses. One example is very high prism powers in the Rx. If needed, scissors can be used to cut a soft Fresnel membrane to a desired shape. When a wet soft Fresnel membrane is placed on a spectacle lens and the water squeezed out, the membrane (usually) adheres to the lens. If needed, the membrane can later be removed by immersing the lens in water. Thus for a stroke victim who has lost vision in their temporal field, a BO Fresnel prism might be placed over the temporal half of a lens as an aid. The BO prism deviates the image nasally towards the apex, which may bring it into the person's field of view. The Fresnel prism does not cover the nasal part of the lens, so the field through that part appears at its normal position. Fresnel lenses and/or prisms can also be used for temporary corrections, such as after surgery.

12.8 PRISM EFFECTIVITY WITH THIN LENSES

Section 11.13 discussed prism effectivity with thin prisms only. This section considers prism effectivity with thin lenses and/or thin prism–lens combinations. (The effect of lens thickness is addressed later in Section 18.13.)

Figure 12.23 shows a corrected hyperope viewing an off-axis object point through a decentered spherical lens. As measured at the DRP, the object point makes an angle c with the straight-ahead line. The prism at the DRP produces a deviation angle d, and in order to image the object on the fovea the eye rotates through an angle e around its center of rotation. The distance from the spectacle plane to the center of rotation is c_{rot}.

Figure 12.23 Prism effectivity ($e \neq d$) for a decentered thin lens and an object point that subtends angle c at the DRP.

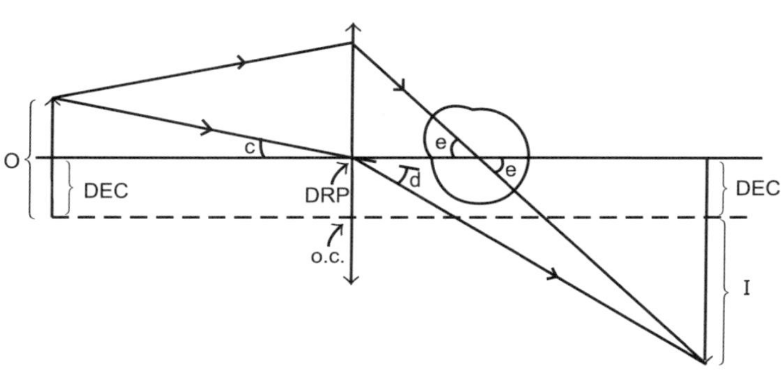

From the triangle involving the object, and the DRP, we obtain

$$|\tan c| = \frac{O - |\text{DEC}|}{|u|}$$

or

$$O = |u||\tan c| + |\text{DEC}|$$

From the triangle involving the center of rotation of the eye and the spectacle lens image point, we obtain

$$|\tan e| = \frac{|I| + |\text{DEC}|}{v - c_{\text{rot}}}$$

Since

$$|I| = |mO| = \frac{v}{|u|}O$$

it follows that

$$|I| = \frac{v}{|u|}(|u||\tan c| + |\text{DEC}|)$$

or

$$|I| = v|\tan c| + \frac{v}{|u|}|\text{DEC}|$$

Then,

$$|\tan e| = \frac{v|\tan c| + \frac{v}{|u|}|\text{DEC}| + |\text{DEC}|}{v - c_{\text{rot}}}$$

We can factor |DEC| out of the common terms, and divide both the numerator and denominator by v to obtain

$$|\tan e| = \frac{|\tan c| + |\text{DEC}|\left(\frac{1}{|u|} + \frac{1}{v}\right)}{1 - \frac{c_{\text{rot}}}{v}}$$

Since $|u| = -u$, $U = 1/u$, $V = 1/v$, and $P = V - U$,

$$|\tan e| = \frac{|\tan c| + |\text{DEC}|P}{1 - c_{\text{rot}}V}$$

Dimensionally, DEC is in meters in the above equation. We can multiply both sides by 100 to obtain

$$|100\tan e| = \frac{|100\tan c| + |\text{DEC(in cm)}|P}{1 - c_{\text{rot}}V}$$

The term on the right in the numerator is Prentice's rule for the prism Z in the Rx. The term on the left in the numerator is a prism-diopter expression for the angle c. Let

$$Z_c = 100\tan c$$

Then,

$$|Z_e| = \frac{|Z_c| + |Z|}{1 - c_{\text{rot}}V}$$

In this derivation, the prism Z makes the object look even farther away from the straight-ahead line, so Z_c and Z add. When the prism makes the object point appear to be closer to the straight-ahead line (or even past it on the opposite side), then Z_c and Z subtract.

Base direction assignments for Z_e were previously discussed in Section 11.13. Just as for Z_e, when the object point is "in" from the straight-ahead direction, a BO direction is assigned to Z_c. Similarly, when the object point is "up" from the forward direction, a BD direction is assigned to Z_c, etc. In other words, a BI assignment for Z_c means that the eye has to turn out to see the object (i.e., image it on the fovea), a BU assignment for Z_c means the eye has to turn down to see the object, etc.

In general, Z_c and Z act like vectors, so we can remove the absolute value signs if we consider the sum in the numerator as a vector sum:

$$Z_e = \frac{\vec{Z}_c + \vec{Z}}{1 - c_{\text{rot}}V} \tag{12.10}$$

Equation 12.10 is the general (paraxial) prism effectivity equation for thin lenses.

For a straight-ahead object point $Z_c = 0$, and Equation 12.10 simplifies to

$$Z_e = \frac{Z}{1 - c_{\text{rot}}V}$$

When there is only a prism in the spectacle plane, $V = U$, and the above equation is identical to Eq. 11.19. When there is both dioptric power and prism power, then $V = P + U$, and the denominator depends on the dioptric power.

12.8.1 Examples for $Z_c = 0$

EXAMPLE 12.10a

Michael Bolteater wears an Rx of +13.00 D combined with 6^{Δ} BD at a vertex distance of 12.5 mm. How much does Michael's eye turn when viewing a distant bolt that is straight ahead?

The center of rotation of the eye is typically 13.5 mm behind the eye, so

$$c_{\text{rot}} = 12.5\,\text{mm} + 13.5 = 26\,\text{mm} = 0.026\,\text{m}$$

For the distant bolt, $U = 0$, and $V = P$. Then Eq. 12.10 gives

$$Z_e = \frac{6^{\Delta}\text{BD}}{1 - (0.026\,\text{m})(+13.00\,\text{D})}$$

or

$$Z_e = \frac{6^{\Delta}\text{BD}}{0.66} = 9.1^{\Delta}\text{BD}$$

If Bolteater's correction consisted of only a 6^{Δ}BD prism (i.e., zero dioptric power P), then Z_e would equal 6^{Δ} and his eye needs to turn up to image the object on the fovea. With the +13.00 D lens combined with the 6^{Δ}BD, the prism makes the eye turn up, and then the additional base down prism that the plus lens provides above its optical center causes the eye to turn up even more (so Z_e is 9.1^{Δ} versus 6^{Δ}).

EXAMPLE 12.10b

Suppose Michael Bolteater walks toward the bolt until it is 25 cm from the spectacle plane. Then how much must his eye turn?

Recall that for a prism only, the nearer the object is to the prism, the smaller Z_e becomes. (In fact for a zero object distance in Section 11.13, $Z_e = 0$.) Therefore, we might expect a smaller Z_e than in part a.

Here $U = -4$ D, and $V = +13.00\,\text{D} + (-4.00\,\text{D}) = +9.00$ D. Equation 12.10 gives

$$Z_e = \frac{6^{\Delta}\text{BD}}{1 - (0.026\,\text{m})(+9.00\,\text{D})} = \frac{6^{\Delta}\text{BD}}{0.77} = 7.8^{\Delta}\text{BD}$$

Indeed the effective prism power decreases as Michael approaches the bolt.

EXAMPLE 12.11

Chuck Creampuff wears an Rx of −13.00 D combined with 6 BD at a vertex distance of 12.5 mm. How much does Chuck's eye turn when viewing a distant cream pie that is straight ahead?

The center of rotation of the eye is typically 13.5 mm behind the eye, so

$$c_{\text{rot}} = 12.5\,\text{mm} + 13.5 = 26\,\text{mm} = 0.026\,\text{m}$$

For the distant pie, $U = 0$, and $V = P$. Then Eq. 12.10 gives

$$Z_e = \frac{6^{\Delta}\text{BD}}{1 - (0.026\,\text{m})(-13.00\,\text{D})}$$

or

$$Z_e = \frac{6^{\Delta}\text{BD}}{1.34} = 4.5^{\Delta}\text{BD}$$

If Creampuff's correction was only 6^{Δ}BD (i.e., zero dioptric power P), then Z_e would equal 6^{Δ} and his eye needs to turn up to image the object on the fovea. With the −13.00 D combined with the 6^{Δ}BD, the prism makes the eye turn up, but then the base up prism that the minus lens provides above its optical center counteracts some of the base down prism effect (so Z_e is 4.5^{Δ} versus 6^{Δ}).

12.8.2 Examples for $Z = 0$

EXAMPLE 12.12a

Caryn High-Brow has an Rx of +8.00 D for each eye. The vertex distance is 10 mm. The distance between the centers of rotation of Caryn's left and right eyes is 64 mm. Caryn holds a book 40 cm from the spectacle plane. How much must Caryn turn her left eye to see the detail in a centrally located letter that is 40 cm from the spectacle plane?

The centrally located letter is 3.2 cm from the straight-ahead direction (Figure 12.24a). The angle c is the angle that the letter subtends at the DRP of the spectacle lens. So,

$$Z_c = 100 \tan c = 100\left(\frac{3.2\,\text{cm}}{40\,\text{cm}}\right) = 8.0^{\Delta}\text{BO}$$

Since Caryn has a plus lens, the rays bend toward the optical center, and Figure (12.24a) shows that Z_e should be greater than Z_c. For the 40 cm object distance,

$$V = (+8.00\,\text{D}) + (-2.50\,\text{D}) = +5.50\,\text{D}$$
$$c_{\text{rot}} = 10\,\text{mm} + 13.5\,\text{mm} = 23.5\,\text{mm} = 0.0235\,\text{m}$$

Since there is no prism in the Rx, $Z = 0$, and from Eq. 12.10,

$$Z_e = \frac{8^{\Delta}\text{BO}}{1 - (0.0235\,\text{m})(+5.50\,\text{D})} = \frac{8^{\Delta}\text{BO}}{0.87} = 9.2^{\Delta}\text{BO}$$

EXAMPLE 12.12b

Suppose Caryn can accommodate enough to see the detail in the letter without her lenses. Then how much must she turn her eye?

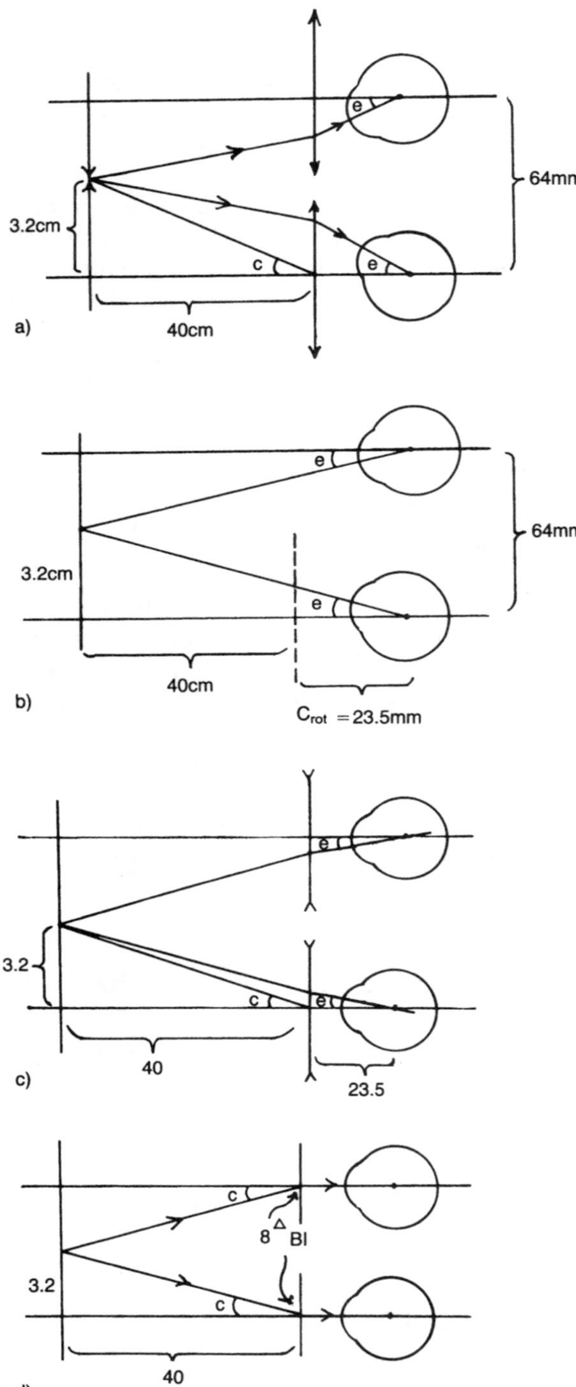

Figure 12.24 Prism effectivity or convergence demands; a, plus lenses; b, no lenses; c, minus lenses; d, base in prisms that neutralize the convergence demand.

The angle c is still measured from the spectacle plane, but now $P = 0$. Therefore, $V = U = -2.50\,\text{D}$, and

$$Z_e = \frac{8^{\Delta}\text{BO}}{1 - (0.0235\,\text{m})(-2.50\,\text{D})}$$

$$= \frac{8^{\Delta}\text{BO}}{1.059} = 7.6^{\Delta}\text{BO}$$

Without her glasses Caryn turns her eye through an angle corresponding to 7.6^{Δ}BO.

Note from Figure 12.24b, with no lens in place, we can find the tangent of e directly:

$$\tan e = \frac{3.2\,\text{cm}}{40\,\text{cm} + 2.35\,\text{cm}} = 0.076$$

So

$$Z_e = 100 \tan e = 7.6^{\Delta}\text{BO},$$

which agrees with the results from the prism effectivity equation.

In the above example, Caryn is a hyperope. When Caryn wears a contact lens correction, the contact lens moves with the eye. Thus to see the detail in the centrally located letter, Caryn's contact corrected eye needs to turn the same 7.6^{Δ} that it turns with no lenses on. This amount is less than the 9.2^{Δ} needed when Caryn is spectacle corrected.

In general, to see the detail in a centrally located near object point (i.e., to place the retinal image on the fovea), a spectacle corrected hyperope has to converge the eye more than when contact corrected. This correlates with the fact that a spectacle corrected hyperope has a larger retinal image size than the same hyperope corrected with contact lenses (Section 6.19). When the retinal image size is larger, the eye needs to turn more to image an off-axis point on the fovea, and vice versa.

EXAMPLE 12.13

Rebecca Ratchet has an Rx of −8.00 D for each eye. The vertex distance is 10 mm. The distance between the centers of rotation of Rebecca's left and right eyes is 64 mm. Rebecca holds a book 40 cm from the spectacle plane. How much must Rebecca turn her left eye to view a centrally located letter that is 40 cm from the spectacle plane?

From Figure 12.24c,

$$Z_c = \tan c = 100\left(\frac{3.2\,\text{cm}}{40\,\text{cm}}\right) = 8.0^{\Delta}\text{BO}$$

Since Rebecca has a minus lens, the rays bend away from the optical center, and Figure 12.24c shows that Z_e should be less than Z_c. For the 40 cm object distance,

$$V = (-8.00\,\text{D}) + (-2.50\,\text{D}) = -10.50\,\text{D}$$

$$c_{\text{rot}} = 10\,\text{mm} + 13.5\,\text{mm} = 23.5\,\text{mm} = 0.0235\,\text{m}$$

Since there is no prism in the Rx, $Z = 0$, and from Eq. 12.10,

$$Z_e = \frac{8^{\Delta}\text{BO}}{1 - (0.0235\,\text{m})(-10.50\,\text{D})}$$

$$= \frac{8^{\Delta}\text{BO}}{1.25} = 6.4^{\Delta}\text{BO}$$

The 64 mm distance between Rebecca's eyes is the same as the 64 mm distance between Caryn's eyes of the previous example. Therefore to see the detail in a centrally located letter with either no lenses in front of her eye or with contact lenses on, Rebecca's eye needs to turn the same 7.6^{Δ} as Caryn's eye. For Rebecca, the myope, this amount is larger than the 6.4^{Δ} needed when she is spectacle corrected.

In general, *to see a centrally located near object point, a spectacle corrected myope has to converge the eye less than a contact corrected myope.* This correlates with the fact that a spectacle corrected myope has a smaller retinal image size than the same myope corrected with contact lenses (Section 6.19). When the retinal image size is smaller, the eye needs to turn less to image an off-axis point on the fovea.

When a person with good binocular vision looks at a relatively localized object, each eye images the object on the foveal area, and the brain fuses the two images so that the person perceives a single object in three dimensional space. If this person holds a strong enough vertical prism in front of one eye, fusion is broken and the person has double vision (i.e., perceives two objects that are vertically displaced from each other). Typically a vertical prism as weak as 2^{Δ} is strong enough to do this. In such a case, we say the person has a *vertical prism imbalance* between the two eyes.

When a spectacle corrected person reads, they often look through points on their lenses that are below the optical center. A spectacle corrected person with significantly different Rxs for the two eyes (called *anisometropia*) will experience a vertical prism imbalance when looking through the lenses at positions below the optical center, and so may have complaints of double vision while reading. A way to correct this, especially for bifocal or progressive add wearers, is to incorporate extra vertical prism into the reading area (lower portion) of at least one of the lenses. *Reverse slab prism* incorporates extra base down prism into the reading area. In *slab-off prism*, the lens undergoes special surfacing that incorporates extra base up prism into the reading area. Lenses with reverse slab or slab-off prism may have two optical centers and are called *bicentric* lenses.

EXAMPLE 12.14

Nico Time has a right eye (OD) spectacle Rx of +2.50 D and a left eye spectacle Rx of +6.50 D. For each eye, the distance c_{rot} from the spectacle lens to the eye's center of rotation is 27 mm. A single distant object is located 20.3° below the straight-ahead line. If Nico Time keeps his head straight, how much must he turn each eye in order to image the object on the fovea?

Here $c = 20.3°$ and

$$Z_c = 100 \tan c = 37.0^{\Delta}\text{BU}$$

Since Nico's lenses are plus, we expect that that Z_e will be greater than Z_c, and further we expect that Z_e will be greater for the left eye than for the right eye. For the distant object, $U = 0$, and $V = P$. Since there is no prism in the Rx, $Z = 0$, and from Eq. 12.10 for the right eye,

$$Z_e = \frac{37^{\Delta}\text{BU}}{1 - (0.027\,\text{m})(+2.50\,\text{D})}$$

$$= \frac{37^{\Delta}\text{BU}}{0.933} = 39.7^{\Delta}\text{BU}$$

For the left eye,

$$Z_e = \frac{37^{\Delta}\text{BU}}{1 - (0.027\,\text{m})(+6.50\,\text{D})}$$

$$= \frac{37^{\Delta}\text{BU}}{0.825} = 44.9^{\Delta}\text{BU}$$

Here Nico needs to turn his right eye 39.7^{Δ} down, while his left eye needs to turn 44.9^{Δ} down. The vertical difference in the Z_e values for the right versus the left eye is 5.2^{Δ}, and Nico has a significant vertical prism imbalance.

Nico (previous example) could avoid the vertical prism imbalance by dropping his chin, so that he is looking through each spectacle lens at the vertical level of the optical center. On the other hand, we could minimize the vertical prism imbalance in the lower portion of the lens by making the right lens a slab-off lens or by making the left lens a reverse slab lens. We can use Eq. 12.10 to figure the prism Z that would completely eliminate the vertical prism imbalance. (The result is 4.8^{Δ} slab-off for the right lens or 4.3^{Δ} reverse slab for the left lens.) However, clinically even if the VPI is completely eliminated for one position, it will not be completely eliminated for a different vertical position. Furthermore the VPI does not need to be completely eliminated. It just needs to be brought below a certain level. This minimization is usually done by an approximation of the following type.

The object was 20.3° below the straight-ahead direction. A straight line from the eye's center of rotation to the object will pass through the spectacle plane at a distance h_y below the optical center, where,

$$\tan 20.3^\circ = \frac{|h_y|}{27\,\text{mm}}$$

This gives a $|h_y|$ of 10.0 mm. At a point 10.0 mm below the optical center, the prism on Nico's right lens is 2.5^ΔBU (from Prentice's rule) and the prism on Nico's left lens is 6.5^ΔBU. The difference is 4.0^Δ, and this is frequently used as a sufficiently close approximation for the slab-off or reverse slab prism. (In Nico's case, Eq. 12.10 shows that a 4^Δ reverse slab on the left lens leaves a 0.3^Δ vertical prism imbalance, while a 4^Δ slab-off on the right lens leaves a 0.9^Δ vertical prism imbalance.)

12.8.3 Examples for Non-zero Z and Z_c

EXAMPLE 12.15a

Suppose Caryn High-Brow in Example 12.12a also has 3^Δ BI prism in her Rx. If all other parameters are the same, how much must Caryn turn her eye to see the detail in a centrally located letter?

From Example 12.12a, $Z_c = 8^\Delta\text{BO}, c_{rot} = 0.0235$ mm, and $V = +5.50$ D. The 3^ΔBI prism makes the centrally located letter appear closer to the straight-ahead position, so we expect a subtractive effect in the numerator. From Eq. (12.10),

$$Z_e = \frac{8^\Delta\text{BO} + 3^\Delta\text{BI}}{1 - (0.0235\,\text{m})(+5.50\,\text{D})} = \frac{5^\Delta\text{BO}}{0.87} = 5.7^\Delta\text{BO}$$

EXAMPLE 12.15b

Suppose Caryn's prism is 3^ΔBO (instead of the 3^ΔBI above). If all other parameters are the same, how much must Caryn turn her eye to see the centrally located letter?

From Example 12.12a, $Z_c = 8^\Delta\text{BO}$, $c_{rot} = 0.0235$ mm, and $V = +5.50$ D. The 3^ΔBO prism makes the centrally located letter appear farther from the straight-ahead position. Again this affects the numerator of Eq. 12.10,

$$Z_e = \frac{8^\Delta\text{BO} + 3^\Delta\text{BO}}{1 - (0.0235\,\text{m})(+5.50\,\text{D})} = \frac{11^\Delta\text{BO}}{0.87} = 12.6^\Delta\text{BO}$$

EXAMPLE 12.15c

What prism would Caryn need to make the centrally located letter look straight-ahead?

Here we need Z_e to equal zero. From the previous parts, Z_c is 8^ΔBO. Then from Eq. 12.10, Z must be 8^ΔBI in order to make the numerator zero. So an 8^ΔBI prism makes the object appear straight-ahead (Figure 12.24d).

PROBLEMS

1. George Jones wears a −8.00 D spectacle correction. George looks through the lenses at a point 7 mm above the optical center. What is the prism power and base direction at this point on the lenses?
2. Sally Smith wears +5.00 D spectacles. When Sally reads she converges her eyes and looks down so that her line of sight passes through the lens at a point 8 mm and 3 mm in from the optical center. What is the prism power and base direction at this point on the lens?
3. Peter Smith wears +7.00 D spectacles. Peter looks 6 mm up and in with his right eye along a line 30° with the horizontal. What is the prism power and base direction at the point on the lens that Peter looks through?
4. Michael O'Rielly has an Rx of OD −4.00 D combined with 3^ΔBI; OS −5.00 D combined with 3^ΔBI. What decentration relative to the DRP will result in the proper Rx?
5. Patricia O'Rielly has an Rx of OD +6.00 D combined with 4^ΔBU. What decentration relative to the DRP will result in the proper Rx?
6. A −4.50 D lens is decentered 8 mm in from the DRP. What is the prism in the Rx?
7. A +3.00 D lens is decentered 4 mm up from the DRP. What is the prism in the Rx?
8. Mickey Corlione wears an OS spectacle lens of −2.00 × 40.
   a. What is the prism power and base direction at a point 10 mm vertically down from the axis?
   b. What is the prism power and base direction at a point 10 mm horizontally in from the axis?
9. a. Can a −8.00 × 90 OD lens be decentered to give 3^ΔBI in the Rx? If so, how much?
   b. Can a −8.00 × 180 OD lens be decentered to give 3^ΔBI in the Rx? If so, how much?
   c. Can a −8.00 × 150 OD lens be decentered to give 3^ΔBI in the Rx? If so, how much?
10. Claudine Longneck's spectacle Rx is: OD 10^ΔBI, OS 10^ΔBI. Assume the center of rotation of Longneck's eye is 25 mm behind the spectacle plane.
    a. When Claudine looks at a distant object, how much and in what direction does her eye turn?
    b. When Claudine looks at a book 20 cm in front of the prisms, how much and in what direction does her eye turn?

11. Briget Barbot is aphakic. Briget's Rx is +13.00 combined with 6^{Δ}BI at a 14 mm vertex distance. When Briget looks straight through her lenses at a distant object, how much and in what direction must she turn her eye? (Assume the center of rotation of Briget's eye is 13 mm behind the cornea.)
12. For near vision Briget Barbot wears +15.50 D lenses combined with 6^{Δ}BI at a 14-mm vertex distance. The +15.50 D lenses, which have +2.50 D more plus than her distance vision lenses, enable Briget to read a book 40 cm in front of the lenses. Assume the horizontal distance between the centers of rotation of Briget's eyes is 62 mm, and that her eye's center of rotation is 13 mm behind the cornea. How much must she converge her eyes to read a centrally located letter in the book that is 40 cm from her lenses?
13. a. Compare the answer for problem no. 12 to the answer than one would get for Briget wearing only +15.50 D lenses and nothing else (i.e., no prism).
    b. Compare the answers above to the answers that one would obtain prior to cataract surgery (i.e., assume Briget wore no correction prior to surgery).
14. For the right eye, Remi Korsokov has a spectacle correction of −8.50 D combined with 9^{Δ}BD at a 12 mm vertex distance. Remi is looking a book that is 42 cm from his spectacle lenses and looks at a letter that is 2 cm vertically below the straight-ahead direction. How much in prism-diopters does Remi have to turn his eye to image the letter on his fovea, and does Remi have to turn his eye up or down? (Assume that the center of rotation of Remi's eye is 13.5 mm behind his cornea.) Also, what much must Remi's eye turn in degrees?

CHAPTER 13

Prism and Dioptric Power in Off-Axis Meridians

13.1 CURVATURE AND TORSION

Curvature has been an important component in the optics of the previous chapters. In particular, Eq. 7.20 showed that the dioptric power of a SSRI equals the product of the refractive index difference times the curvature of the surface.

In general, a curve in three dimensional space is completely specified at each point by two parameters—its curvature and its torsion. Curvature can be defined as the rate at which a curve changes its direction in a plane. *Torsion is defined as the rate at which the curve twists out of a plane.* An example of a curve with both a non-zero curvature and a non-zero torsion is a circular helix, such as the curve formed by the thread on a bolt. The non-zero torsion means that the helix does not stay in a single plane, and this property enables us to screw the bolt in or out. Conversely, the torsion is zero for a curve that stays in a single plane. For example, the torsion at any point on a circle or an ellipse is zero.

Consider a curve on a cylinder such that at each point the curve makes an angle ϕ with the axis meridian. To learn about the torsion of this curve, draw a vertical line on a flat sheet of paper, and then a diagonal line that makes a 45° angle with the vertical line. Now curve the paper around so that it makes a cylinder with the vertical line on the axis meridian, and note that the diagonal curve does not stay in a single plane but instead spirals up and around the cylinder (Figure 13.1). This diagonal curve on the surface of the cylinder is actually a circular helix that has a constant, non-zero torsion. The vertical line in the axis meridian of this cylinder does not twist and so has zero torsion. A curve in the other principal meridian (horizontal) also does not twist and has zero torsion.

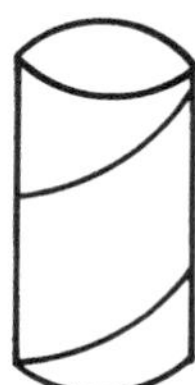

Figure 13.1 The helix that makes a constant angle with the axis meridian.

Similarly, on a torus, a curve that makes a constant angle with a principal meridian also spirals around the torus and does not stay in a single plane. So an off-axis meridian of a toric interface, defined by a constant angle with a principal meridian, has a non-zero torsion. The curves that specify the principal meridians of a torus are circles that stay in a single plane, and so the principal meridians have zero torsion.

Since there is zero torsion in the principal meridians of a toric interface, Chapter 10 dealt only with the dioptric power due to the curvature of those meridians. We will now call this the curvital component of the dioptric power. When we deal with off-axis meridians, the torsion is non-zero, and hence there is also a dioptric power component due to the torsion. For the off-axis meridians of spherocylindrical interfaces and lenses, both the curvital component and the torsional component of the dioptric power contribute to the optical effects.

13.2 STENOPEIC SLITS

Consider a $+5.00 \bigcirc -3.00 \times 90$ spherocylindrical lens. For a distant point source, this lens creates a conoid of Sturm with a horizontal line image at 20 cm and a vertical line image at 50 cm. When a square aperture with horizontal and vertical sides is placed against the lens, the cross sections of the conoid are rectangular. As a function of the distance from the lens, the rectangles initially converge faster vertically (5.00 D) than horizontally (2.00 D) and so form the horizontal line image first and the vertical line image second (Figure 13.2a). For the single point source, all of the light in the conoid first passes through the horizontal line image and then through the vertical line image.

Clinical trial lens sets contain a slit aperture called a stenopeic slit. The stenopeic slit is used to isolate a single meridian of an eye. We can use a thin vertical stenopeic slit to isolate the vertical principal meridian of the $+5.00 \bigcirc -3.00 \times 90$ lens. Neglecting diffraction, the light that passes through the vertical slit stays in the vertical meridian and converges to form a point image at 20 cm. Similar to the cases in Chapter 10, this point image is just one of the points that make up the horizontal line image in the conoid. For a thin horizontal stenopeic slit in front of the $+5.00 \bigcirc -3.00 \times 90$ lens, the light that passes through the slit stays in the horizontal meridian and converges to form a point image at 50 cm. This point image is just one of the points that make up the vertical line image in the conoid.

Note that the ray on the upper right corner (marked J in Figure 13.2) moves down and to the left as it passes through the conoid. Similarly, the ray on the lower left corner moves up and to the right as it passes through the conoid. When a stenopeic slit is oriented diagonally to expose the 45 meridian of the $+5.00 \bigcirc -3.00 \times 90$ spherocylindrical lens, these rays form the end rays of a sheet of light that twists around clockwise (as viewed from the lens) as it moves through the conoid. In Figure 13.2b, the diagonals in the rectangular cross sections show the orientation of the twisting sheet of light as it moves through the conoid, and the letter J follows the path of the ray that starts at the upper right corner. In particular, the sheet twists around so that it is aligned with the horizontal line image when it passes through that position (20 cm from the lens), and then continues to twist so that it is aligned with the vertical line image when it passes through that position (50 cm from the lens). At a large distance from the lens (not shown in Figure 13.2b), the rotating sheet approaches the initial 45° orientation. Thus the sheet makes one complete twist as it passes through the conoid. Note also that the twisting sheet of light does not converge to form a point image anywhere in the conoid.

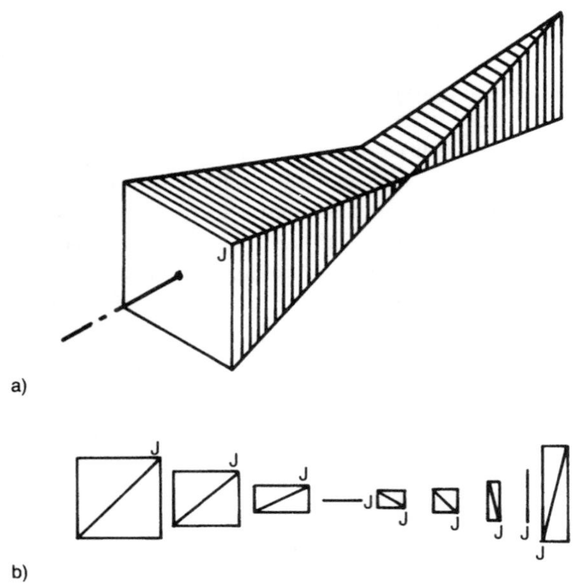

Figure 13.2 a, Conoid of Sturm for a square aperture. J marks the ray in the upper right corner; b, cross sections showing the twisting sheet of light.

When the diagonal slit is set to expose the 135 meridian, we get a twisting sheet of light that rotates counter-clockwise as viewed from the lens. This sheet of light twists around and is horizontal when it passes through the horizontal line image position at 20 cm behind the lens and is vertical when it passes through the vertical line image position at 50 cm behind the lens.

In general, when a stenopeic slit exposes a principal meridian (or an on-axis meridian) of a spherocylindrical lens, the light stays in that meridian and converges to form a point image. When the stenopeic slit exposes a non-principal meridian (or an off-axis meridian), the light forms a twisting sheet as it passes through the conoid. The light twists in such a manner as to pass through both line images in the conoid. Actually, the twisting sheet of light was already present in the conoid before the slit was introduced. The stenopeic slit simply blocks the other rays so that the twisting sheet is readily apparent.

The underlying geometric basis for the varying behavior of the isolated sheets of light is the fact that the off-axis (or non-principal) meridians of a toric interface have non-zero torsion, while the principal meridians have zero torsion. The torsional component of the dioptric power causes the off-axis sheets to twist as they move through the conoid, while the principal meridian sheets do not twist.

13.3 CURVATURE AND LENS CLOCK READINGS

Consider a plus cylinder axis 90 lens with a convex cylindrical front surface and a plano back surface

(Figure 13.3a). The principal meridians of this lens are the horizontal and vertical meridians. The vertical meridian of the front cylindrical surface is flat (or plano), while the horizontal meridian is circular with a radius of curvature r_p. The center thickness of this lens is equal to the sagitta s of the power meridian for a chord length $2h_p$, where h_p is the horizontal distance from the lens center to the edge. As applied to the power meridian, the sagittal approximation (Eq. 7.6) gives

$$s = \frac{h_p^2}{2r_p}$$

(Recall that we used the sagittal approximation in the Chapter 7 derivation of $V = P + U$.)

The diagonal curve shown in Figure 13.3a is for an off-axis meridian that makes an angle ϕ with the axis meridian. This off-axis meridian has the same sagitta s as the principal meridian. The chord length of the off-axis (or oblique) meridian is $2h_{ob}$ across the back surface of the lens. (Figure 13.3b shows the chord lengths across the back surface of the lens.) For a small enough h_{ob}, the sagittal approximation as applied to this off-axis meridian is

$$s = \frac{h_{ob}^2}{2r_{ob}}$$

where r_{ob} is radius of curvature of the off-axis meridian at the vertex of the surface.

We can set the right hand sides of the above two equations equal to each other to obtain

$$\frac{h_{ob}^2}{2r_{ob}} = \frac{h_p^2}{2r_p}$$

From the triangle involving the angle ϕ in Figure 13.3b,

$$\sin\phi = \frac{h_p}{h_{ob}}$$

We can solve the sine equation for h_p and substitute the result into the previous equation to obtain

$$\frac{h_{ob}^2}{r_{ob}} = \frac{h_{ob}^2 \sin^2\phi}{r_p}$$

or

$$\frac{1}{r_{ob}} = \frac{\sin^2\phi}{r_p}$$

Then,

$$R_{ob} = R_p \sin^2\phi \qquad (13.1)$$

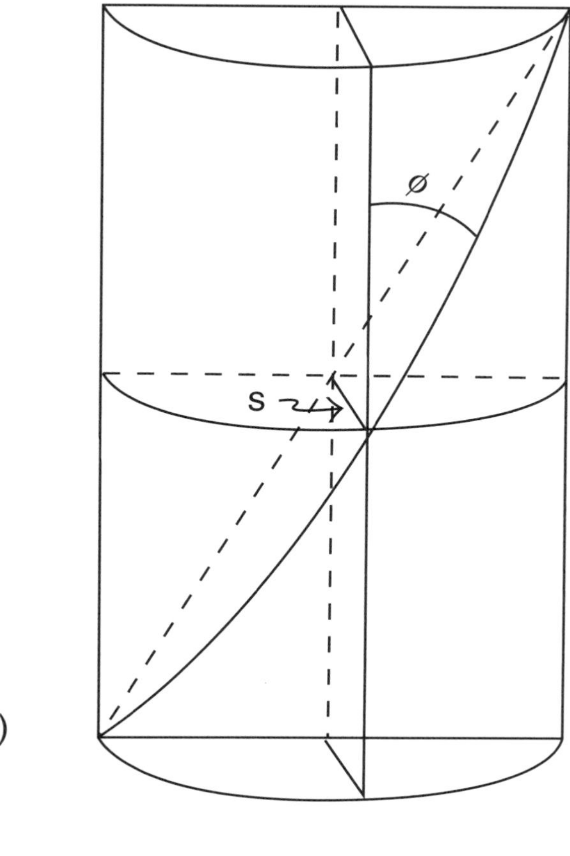

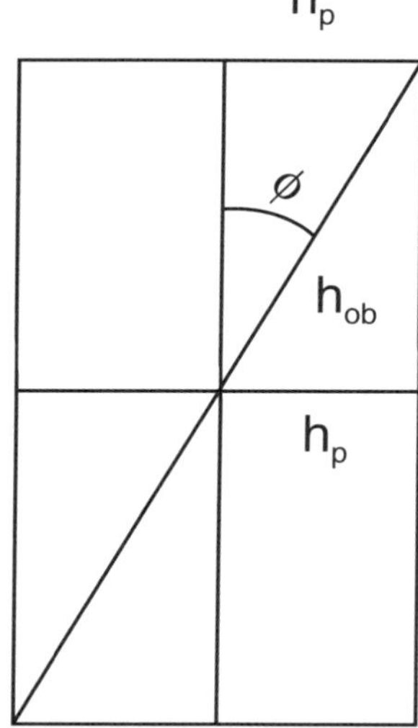

Figure 13.3 a, Plus cylinder lens with a center thickness *s*. Here *s* is the sagitta for both the power meridian and for the oblique meridian that makes an angle ϕ with the axis meridian; b, the chord lengths on the back surface.

where $R_{ob} = 1/r_{ob}$ and is the curvature of the off-axis meridian that makes the angle ϕ with the axis, and $R_p = 1/r_p$ is the curvature of the power meridian. Equation 13.1 indicates that the curvature of a cylindrical surface as a function of the angle ϕ varies like the sine-squared of ϕ.

For a cylindrical interface, the cylinder power C equals

$$C = (n_2 - n_1)R_p$$

where n_1 is the index of the medium in front of the lens, and n_2 is the index of the lens. Similarly the dioptric power curvital component P_m in meridian m that make an angle ϕ with the axis is given by

$$P_m = (n_2 - n_1)R_{ob}$$

Then from the above three equations,

$$P_m = C\sin^2\phi \qquad (13.2)$$

We frequently say that a lens clock measures curvature, although it actually measures a sagitta (Section 7.16). When the legs of a lens clock are aligned with the meridian m, the lens clock dial is calibrated to directly give the dioptric power curvital component P_m in that meridian for the assumed indices $n_2 = 1.53$ and $n_1 = 1.00$. Equation 13.2 shows that the lens clock readings on a cylindrical surface vary like the sine-squared of the angle ϕ with the axis.

In a 30-60-90 right triangle, the length of the side opposite the 30° angle equals 1/2 the length of the hypotenuse. So for a hypotenuse of length 2, the side opposite the 30° angle has length 1, and by the Pythagorean Theorem the side adjacent to the 30° angle has a length equal to $\sqrt{3}$ (Figure 13.4b). It follows that $\sin 30° = 1/2$ and so $\sin^2 30° = 1/4$. Similarly $\sin^2 60° = \sqrt{3}/2$, and so $\sin^2 60° = 3/4$. In a 45-45-90 right triangle where the sides opposite to the 45° angles have each has a length of 1, the Pythagorean Theorem gives a length of $\sqrt{2}$ for the hypotenuse (Figure 13.4a). Therefore, $\sin 45° = 1/\sqrt{2}$, and so $\sin^2 45° = 1/2$.

Now consider a $+8.00 \times 90$ cylindrical front surface ($n = 1.53$). A lens clock reads zero in the plano vertical meridian, and +8.00 D in the horizontal power meridian. We can use Eq. 13.2 to get the lens clock reading in the other meridians.

For the 60 meridian:

$$\begin{aligned} P_m &= (+8.00\,\text{D})\sin^2(60 - 90) \\ &= (+8.00\,\text{D})\sin^2(-30) \\ &= (+8.00\,\text{D})(1/4) = +2.00\,\text{D} \end{aligned}$$

Similarly, the lens clock reads +2.00 D in the 120 meridian.

For the 45 meridian:

$$\begin{aligned} P_m &= (+8.00\,\text{D})\sin^2(45 - 90) \\ &= (+8.00\,\text{D})\sin^2(-45) \\ &= (+8.00\,\text{D})(1/2) = +4.00\,\text{D} \end{aligned}$$

Similarly, the lens clock reads +4.00 D in the 135 meridian, and +6.00 D in both the 30 and in the 150 meridians.

Figure 13.5 shows how the lens clock readings vary on the $+8.00 \times 90$ cylindrical surface as a function of the angle ϕ. Note that the 45 and 135 meridians are exactly halfway between the principal meridians, and the +4.00 D lens clock reading in either of those meridians is exactly halfway between the powers in the principal meridians (i.e., 0 D and 8 D). The variation in P_m is slowest near the principal meridians and fastest at the midway meridians (i.e., $\phi = \pm 45°$).

On a cylindrical surface of power C, the maximum and minimum values for P_m are the powers in the principal meridians, which are 0 and C respectively. A spherical surface of power S has the same curvature in all meridians, so P_m equals S in all meridians.

A derivation similar to that for a cylindrical surface shows that on a toric surface of parameters $S \bigcirc C \times \theta$

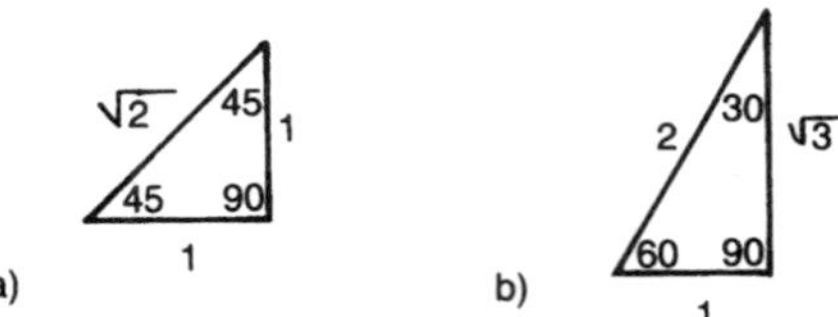

Figure 13.4 a, 45-45-90 right triangle; b, 30-60-90 right triangle.

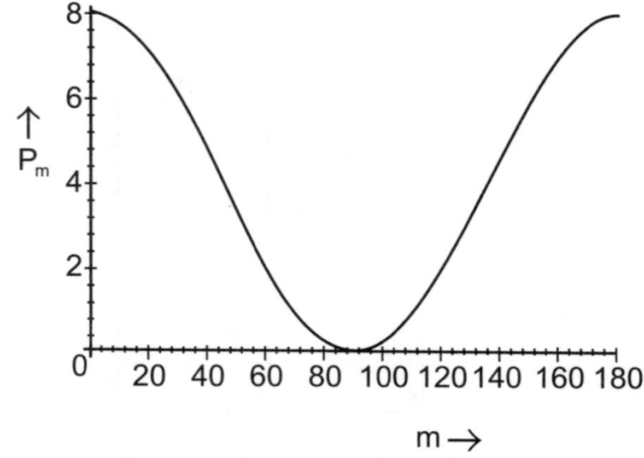

Figure 13.5 Dioptric power curvital component P_m for the meridians m of a +8.00×90 surface. (Here $\phi = m - \theta$, where θ is the cylinder axis.)

the dioptric power curvital component in the meridian m is given by

$$P_m = S + C\sin^2\phi \qquad (13.3)$$

where ϕ is the angle with the axis meridian θ (i.e., $\phi = m - \theta$). The maximum and minimum readings on this surface occur in the principal meridians and are S (for $\phi = 0$) and $S + C$ (for $\phi = \pm 90°$). Equation 13.3 also shows that P_m equals $S + (C/2)$ for a meridian m that is halfway between the principal meridians (i.e, $\phi = \pm 45°$).

EXAMPLE 13.1

For a $-2.00 \subset -5.00 \times 120$ toric surface ($n = 1.53$), what are the lens clock readings in the principal meridians, in the meridians halfway between the principal meridians (75 and 165), in the horizontal meridian, and in the vertical meridian?

The principal meridians are the 120 and 30 meridians. The power in the 120 meridian is -2.00 D, and that is what the lens clock reads on the 120 meridian. The power in the 30 meridian is -7.00 D, and that is what the lens clock reads on the 30 meridian.

For the midway meridians (75 or 165), we expect the lens clock reading to be -4.50 D, which halfway between -2.00 D and -7.00 D. From Eq. 13.3 for the 165 meridian:

$$\begin{aligned} P_m &= -2.00\,\text{D} + (-5.00\,\text{D})\sin^2(165 - 120) \\ &= -2.00\,\text{D} + (-5.00\,\text{D})\sin^2(45) \\ &= -2.00\,\text{D} + (-2.50\,\text{D}) = -4.50\,\text{D} \end{aligned}$$

as expected.

The vertical meridian is closer to the 120 meridian than to the 30 meridian, so we expect the lens clock reading in the vertical meridian to be closer to -2.00 D than to -7.00 D. For the vertical meridian:

$$\begin{aligned} P_m &= -2.00\,\text{D} + (-5.00\,\text{D})\sin^2(120 - 90) \\ &= -2.00\,\text{D} + (-5.00\,\text{D})\sin^2(30) \\ &= -2.00\,\text{D} + (-1.25\,\text{D}) = -3.25\,\text{D} \end{aligned}$$

which agrees with the expectations.

The horizontal meridian is closer to the 30 meridian than to the 120 meridian, so we expect the lens clock reading in the horizontal meridian to be closer to -7.00 D than to -2.00 D. For the horizontal meridian:

$$\begin{aligned} P_m &= -2.00\,\text{D} + (-5.00\,\text{D})\sin^2(120 - 180) \\ &= -2.00\,\text{D} + (-5.00\,\text{D})\sin^2(-60) \\ &= -2.00\,\text{D} + (-3.75\,\text{D}) = -5.75\,\text{D} \end{aligned}$$

which agrees with the expectations. Figure 13.6a shows a plot of these lens clock readings (the curvital component of the power) on the meridians of this interface.

For a toric surface, it turns out that the sum of the dioptric power curvital components in any two perpendicular meridians is equal to a constant called Euler's constant E. We can prove this as follows. Let q be the meridian that is perpendicular to meridian m, and let

$$E = P_m + P_q$$

Then from Eq. 13.3,

$$E = [S + C\sin^2\phi] + [S + C\sin^2(\phi \pm 90)]$$

But $\sin^2(\phi \pm 90) = \cos^2\phi$, so

$$E = [S + C\sin^2\phi] + [S + C\cos^2\phi]$$

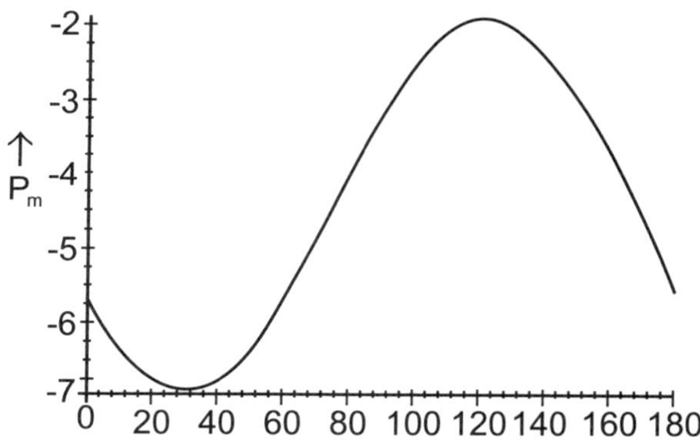

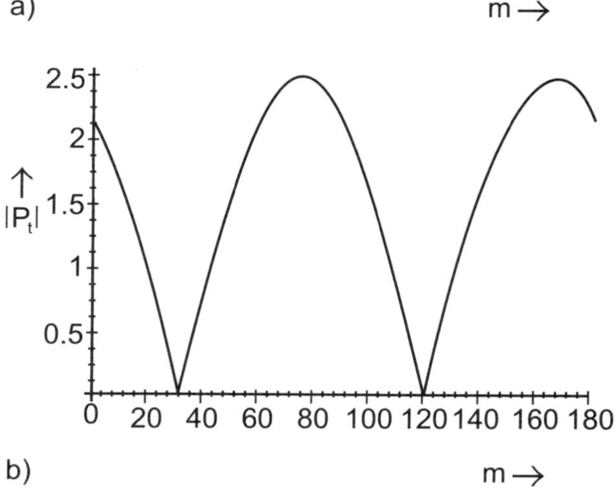

Figure 13.6 **a, Lens clock readings (or dioptric power curvital components) on a $-2.00 \subset -5.00 \times 120$ toric surface; b, magnitude of the dioptric power torsional component for the same surface.**

or

$$E = 2S + C(\sin^2\phi + \cos^2\phi)$$

Since $\sin^2\phi + \cos^2\phi = 1$, it follows that

$$E = 2S + C \tag{13.4}$$

which completes the proof.

For the $-2.00 \subset -5.00 \times 120$ surface, Eq. 13.4 gives

$$E = 2(-2.00\,\text{D}) + (-5.00\,\text{D}) = -9.00\,\text{D}$$

We can check this by adding the P_m values in perpendicular meridians. From the values in Example 13.1, the sum of the lens clock readings in the 120 and 30 principal meridians is

$$E = -2.00\,\text{D} + (-7.00\,\text{D}) = -9.00\,\text{D}$$

Similarly from Example 13.1, the sum of the lens clock readings in the vertical and horizontal meridians is

$$E = -3.25\,\text{D} + (-5.75\,\text{D}) = -9.00\,\text{D}$$

Finally from Example 13.1, the sum of the lens clock readings in the 75 and 165 meridians is

$$E = -4.50\,\text{D} + (-4.50\,\text{D}) = -9.00\,\text{D}$$

So the results from Example 13.1 all check.

13.4 TORSIONAL COMPONENT OF DIOPTRIC POWER

To get the curvital component of the dioptric power for an interface, we multiplied the curvature by the index difference (i.e., $n_2 - n_1$). Similarly, we can get the torsional component of the dioptric power of an off-axis meridian by multiplying the torsion in that meridian by the index difference. For a toric interface with parameters $S \subset C \times \theta$, the magnitude of the torsional component P_t of the dioptric power in a meridian m that makes an angle ϕ with the axis meridian θ is given by

$$|P_t| = |C \sin\phi \cos\phi| \tag{13.5}$$

(Section 13.6 contains a derivation of the sine times cosine dependence.)

The principal meridians occur at $\phi = 0$ and $\phi = 90°$. Since $\sin 0° = 0$ and $\cos 90° = 0$, Equation 13.5 shows that P_t is zero for the principal meridians. The off-axis meridian that is farthest away from a principal meridian is that for which $\phi = \pm 45°$. Since both sin 45° and cos 45° equal $1/\sqrt{2}$, $|P_t| = |C/2|$ for $\phi = \pm 45°$, and this is the largest value that $|P_t|$ obtains.

Again consider the $-2.00 \subset -5.00 \times 120$ toric interface (see Example 13.1). The magnitude of the torsional component $|P_t|$ is 0 in the principal meridians (30 and at 120). $|P_t|$ is one half of the cylinder power (i.e., 5.00 D/2) or 2.50 D in the 75 or 165 meridians that are midway between the principal meridians. For the horizontal meridian, $\phi = 180° - 120° = 60°$, and

$$\begin{aligned}|P_t| &= |(-5.00\,\text{D}) \sin 60° \cos 60°| \\ &= |(-5.00\,\text{D})(0.87)(0.50)| = 2.17\,\text{D}\end{aligned}$$

For a toric interface, the magnitude of the dioptric power torsional components is equal in any two perpendicular meridians. This occurs because

$$|\sin(\phi \pm 90°)\cos(\phi \pm 90°)| = |\sin\phi\cos\phi|$$

For example, $|P_t|$ for the $-2.00 \subset -5.00 \times 120$ toric interface is 2.17 D for the vertical meridian (i.e, $\phi = 90° - 120° = -30°$ in Eq. 13.5), which is the same result obtained above for the horizontal meridian. Figure 13.6b shows a plot of $|P_t|$ for the meridians on this interface.

13.5 ISOTHICKNESS CURVES

A spherical plus lens is thickest at the optical center and then gets thinner for positions away from the optical center. Away for the optical center on the lens, there are positions that have the same thickness. These positions can be connected together with a curve called an *isothickness curve*. The isothickness curves for a spherical lens are circular and centered on the optical center. The prism base directions on a spherical lens lie along radial lines emanating from the optical center. Thus the prism base directions for the spherical lens are perpendicular (or orthogonal) to the isothickness curves.

The isothickness curves for a cylindrical lens are straight lines that are parallel to the optical center line, which is parallel to the axis meridian (Figure 13.7). The prism base directions on a cylindrical lens are always aligned with the power meridian, which is perpendicular to the optical center line. Thus, the prism base directions for a cylindrical lens are also perpendicular to the isothickness curves.

It turns out that, excluding the optical center, *the prism base direction at a point on a spherocylindrical lens is perpendicular to the isothickness curve at that point and points towards the thicker part of the lens.* Therefore the isothickness curves of a spherocylindrical lenses pro-

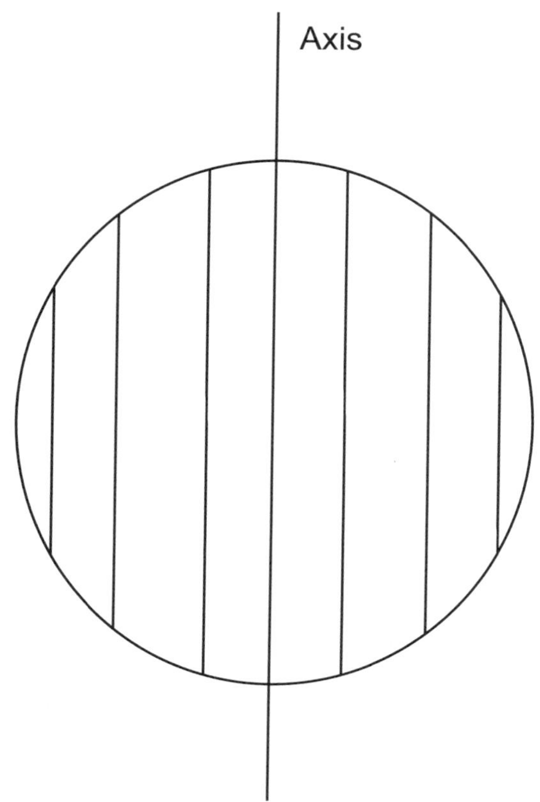

Figure 13.7 Isothickness curves and prism base directions for a plus cylinder with a vertical axis meridian.

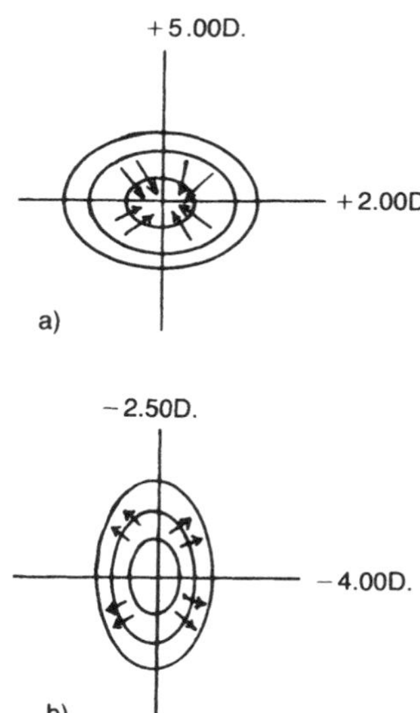

Figure 13.8 Isothickness curves and prism base directions: a, +5.00 ⊃ −3.00 × 90 lens; b, −2.50 ⊃ −1.50 × 90 lens.

vide intuition about the prism base directions at various points on the lens.

For a +5.00 ⊃ −3.00 × 90 lens, the power in the vertical meridian is +5.00 D, and the power in the horizontal meridian is +2.00 D. The thickest point on the lens is at the optical center. The thickness decreases for points progressively farther away from the optical center. The decrease in thickness is faster along the +5.00 D vertical meridian than along the +2.00 D horizontal meridian. So the thinnest points on the lens are the top and bottom edges in the vertical meridian. The left and right (or nasal and temporal) edges in the horizontal meridian are thicker than the edges in the vertical meridian. It follows that the edges in the horizontal meridian have a thickness that is equal to the vertical meridian thickness somewhere between the optical center and the vertical edge. In particular, the thickness at the horizontal edge equals the vertical meridian thickness about 0.4 (i.e., 2.00 D/5.00 D) of the way along the vertical meridian.

We can proceed meridian by meridian to find all the points on the lens with the same thickness as the horizontal edge. In the paraxial approximation, all the points with the same thickness on this lens lie on a horizontally oriented ellipse. Thus the isothickness curves for the +5.00 ⊃ −3.00 × 90 lens are sets of horizontally oriented ellipses (Figure 13.8a). At any point on the lens, the prism base direction is directed inward (since the optical center is the thickest point), and is perpendicular to the elliptical isothickness curve at that point. Along a principal meridian, the prism base directions are aligned with the meridian and point directly towards the optical center of the lens. For a non-principal or off-axis meridian, the prism directions are not aligned with the meridian and do not point *directly* toward the optical center. (It is the dioptric power torsional component that deviates the prism base direction so that it does not point directly toward the optical center.)

The isothickness curves for a spherocylindrical lens are ellipses as long as the power in both principal meridians has the same sign (i.e., both plus or both minus). The ellipses have their major axis aligned with the meridian in which the power is least in magnitude. For example, the principal meridian powers for a −2.50 ⊃ −1.50 × 90 are −2.50 D vertically and −4.00 D horizontally. In this case, the optical center is the thinnest point on the lens, and the thickness increases slower in the vertical meridian and faster in the horizontal meridian. The nasal and temporal edges in the horizontal meridian are the thickest points on the lens. The top and bottom edge thickness in the vertical meridian is less than that at the horizontal edges. It follows that the thickness at the top vertical edge will be equal to the thickness in the horizontal meridian about 0.63 (i.e., 2.50 D/4.00 D) of the way along the horizontal meridian, and the isothickness ellipses are vertically oriented (Figure 13.8b).

The prism base directions are perpendicular to the elliptical isothickness curves and for the $-2.50 \bigcirc -1.50 \times 90$ lens always point outward towards the edges, which are thicker than the optical center. For a principal meridian, the prism base directions are aligned with the meridian and point directly away from the optical center. For an off-axis meridian, the prism base directions are not aligned with the meridian and do not point *directly* away from the optical center.

When the powers in the principal meridians have opposite signs, the isothickness curves are not elliptical. Consider a $+3.00 \bigcirc -5.00 \times 90$ lens. In the vertical meridian, the power is +3.00 D, and the thickness is a maximum at the optical center. In the horizontal meridian, the power is −2.00 D and the thickness is a minimum at the optical center. So starting at the optical center, the lens gets thinner vertically and thicker horizontally. For such a lens, there is some off-axis meridian m for which the thickness does not change. For a thin spherocylindrical lens with parameters $S \bigcirc C \times \theta$, the meridian with no thickness change is the meridian with a zero dioptric power curvital component P_m.

For the $+3.00 \bigcirc -5.00 \times 90$ thin lens, we can find the meridians with no thickness change by setting P_m in Eq. 13.3 equal to zero. Then,

$$0 = +3.00\,\mathrm{D} + (-5.00\,\mathrm{D})\sin^2\phi$$

$$\sin^2\phi = \frac{-3.00\,\mathrm{D}}{-5.00\,\mathrm{D}} = 0.60$$

$$\sin\phi = \pm 0.77$$

and

$$\phi = \pm 50.8^\circ$$

Since $\phi = m - \theta$, the two meridians with no thickness change are given by $m = \theta + \phi$. For this lens, $m = 90 + 50.8 = 140.8$, and $m = 90 - 50.8 = 39.2$. The isothickness curves are straight lines along the 39.2 and 140.8 meridians.

For the $+3.00 \bigcirc -5.00 \times 90$ lens, the isothickness curves between these straight lines are hyperbolas that are asymptotic to the straight lines (Figure 13.9a). The principal meridians of the lens are the axes of the hyperbolas, so the vertex of each hyperbola occurs in a principal meridian, and the hyperbolas are symmetric relative to each principal meridian. The minus power gives one set of hyperbolas and the plus power gives the other set of hyperbolas. At any point on the lens, the prism base directions are perpendicular to the isothickness curves and point towards the thicker part of the lens. This is true for positions along the straight asymptotic lines as well as for positions along the hyperbolas.

The remaining parts of Figure 13.9 shows the effect on the isothickness curves of reducing the cylinder power, while keeping the sphere power and cylinder axis constant. As the cylinder power is smoothly reduced from −5.00 D to −3.25 D to −3.00 D, the isothickness hyperbolas smoothly change into straight horizontal lines (Figure 13.9a, then b, then c). When the cylinder power is smoothly changed changes from −3.00 D to −1.50 D, the straight-line isothickness curves change smoothly to horizontally oriented ellipses (Figure 13.9c, then d).

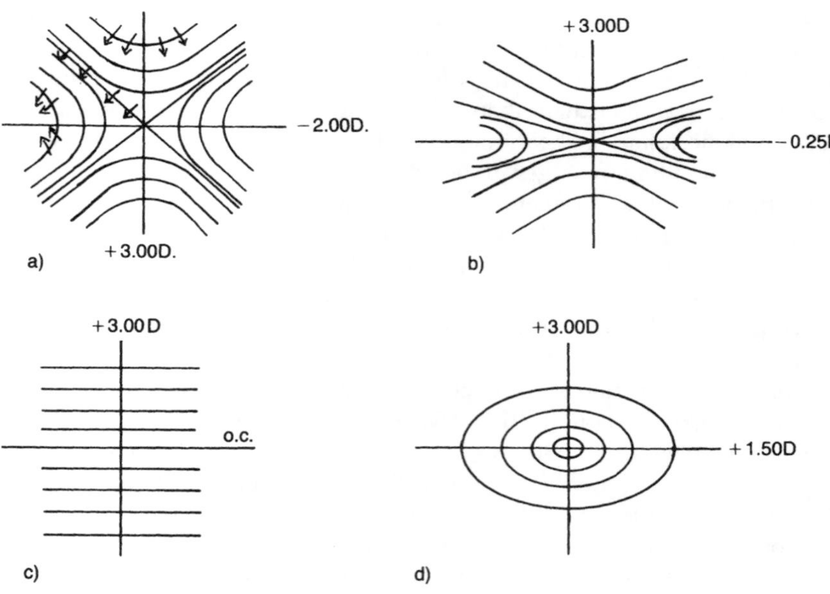

Figure 13.9 a, Isothickness curves and prism base directions for a $+3.00 \bigcirc -5.00 \times 90$ lens; b, $+3.00 \bigcirc -3.25 \times 90$; c, $+3.00 \bigcirc -3.00 \times 90$ or by transposition a $+3.00 \times 180$; d, $+3.00 \bigcirc -1.50 \times 90$.

It is helpful to remember that on a centered cylindrical lens with a round shape, the plus cylinder axis meridian always has the thickest edge while the minus cylinder axis meridian always has the thinnest edge. One way to remember this is to just think of elementary minus and plus cylinder lenses (see Figure 12.11). It turns out that on any centered spherocylindrical lens with a round shape as viewed from the front, the minus cylinder axis meridian always has the thinnest edge and the plus cylinder axis meridian always has the thickest edge.

In summary: For a spherocylindrical lens, the isothickness curves are either circles, ellipses, hyperbolas, or straight lines. Given the power cross of the lens, it is relatively easy to make a quick estimate of the isothickness curves. Since the prism base directions on the lens are always perpendicular to the isothickness curves, the curves supply us with intuition about the prism base directions on a lens.

13.6 MATRIX FORM OF PRENTICE'S RULE

The human visual system is neurologically wired to treat horizontal and vertical eye movements differently. Hence, in the clinic, the horizontal prism measurements (Z_x) are made separately from the vertical prism measurements (Z_y). This occurs even when the principal meridians of the eye are not horizontal and vertical. Therefore for a thin spherocylindrical lens with parameters $S \bigcirc C \times \theta$, it is useful to have an equation that directly gives Z_x and Z_y at any position H on the lens.

When one buys multiple items at a grocery store, it is much easier to transport the items by placing them in a bag or a basket. Similarly in math, it is much easier to work with multiple numbers by placing them in "bags" called matrices. Basic matrix algebra (appendix B) is fairly simple to learn and provides a tool that has helped clarify a number of concepts in the optics of astigmatism. This section contains a derivation of the matrix form of Prentice's Rule that gives Z_x and Z_y at a position H specified by its horizontal and vertical components h_x and h_y on a spherocylindrical lens. (The next section, 13.7, contains examples and discussion.)

Consider a $S \bigcirc C \times \theta$ spherocylindrical lens where θ is a first quadrant angle. Label the first quadrant principal meridian u and the second quadrant principal meridian v. Then the power cross orientation is

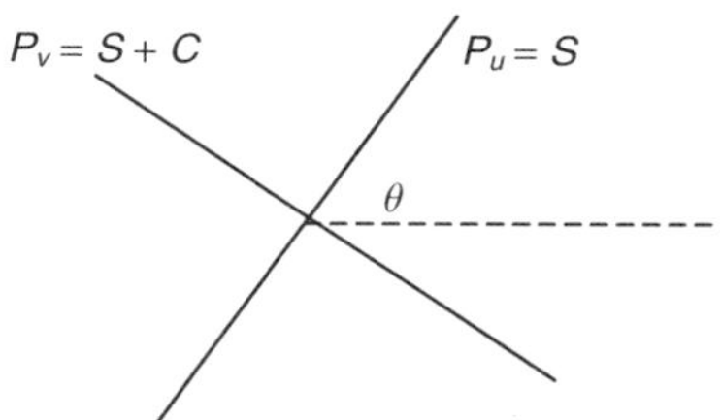

In the principal meridians, the respective power are

$$P_u = S \quad \text{and} \quad P_v = S + C \tag{13.6}$$

Prentice's Rule (Eq. 12.2) applies separately to each principal meridian. So

$$Z_u = -P_u h_u = -S h_u$$

and

$$Z_v = -P_v h_v = -(S + C) h_v$$

where h_u is a distance in cm from the optical center in the principal meridian u, and h_v is a distance in cm from the optical center in the principal meridian v. Z_u is the prism power component along the u meridian, and Z_v is the prism power component along the v meridian. We can write the above two Prentice's Rule equations as one matrix equation:

$$\begin{pmatrix} Z_u \\ Z_v \end{pmatrix} = -\begin{pmatrix} S & 0 \\ 0 & S+C \end{pmatrix} \begin{pmatrix} h_u \\ h_v \end{pmatrix} \tag{13.7}$$

The top matrix multiplication gives Prentice's Rule for the principal meridian u, and the bottom matrix multiplication gives it for the other principal meridian v.

Let $\mathbf{h}_{uv}$ be the column matrix (vector)

$$\mathbf{h}_{uv} = \begin{pmatrix} h_u \\ h_v \end{pmatrix} \tag{13.8}$$

and $\mathbf{Z}_{uv}$ be the column matrix (vector)

$$\mathbf{Z}_{uv} = \begin{pmatrix} Z_u \\ Z_v \end{pmatrix} \tag{13.9}$$

Then Eq. 13.7 can be written as,

$$\mathbf{Z}_{uv} = -\mathbf{P}_{uv} \mathbf{h}_{uv} \tag{13.10}$$

where,

$$\mathbf{P}_{uv} = \begin{pmatrix} S & 0 \\ 0 & S+C \end{pmatrix} \tag{13.11}$$

The distances h_u and h_v are the components of an off-axis point H on the lens as expressed in a u-v

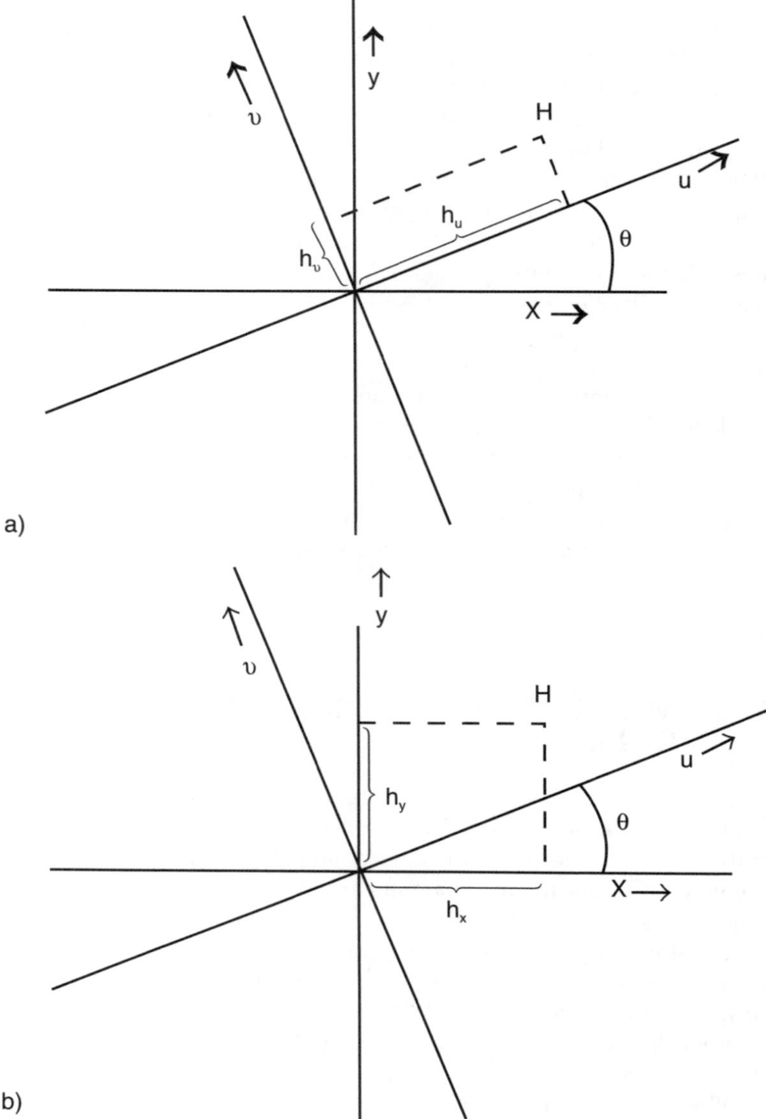

Figure 13.10 **The x-y coordinate system is horizontal and vertical while the u-v coordinate system is aligned with the principal meridians of a spherocylindrical lens with a first quadrant cylinder axis θ: a, the coordinates h_u and h_v of the point H in the u-v system; b, the coordinates h_x and h_y of the same point H in the x-y system.**

coordinate system that is aligned with the principal meridians (Figure 13.10a). The same point H also has components h_x and h_y as expressed in a horizontal (x) and vertical (y) coordinate system (Figure 13.10b). The standard analytical geometry relations between the two sets of coordinates for the same point H are

$$h_u = (\cos\theta)h_x + (\sin\theta)h_y \tag{13.12}$$

and

$$h_v = (-\sin\theta)h_x + (\cos\theta)h_y \tag{13.13}$$

Define the column matrix **h** as

$$\mathbf{h} = \begin{pmatrix} h_x \\ h_y \end{pmatrix} \tag{13.14}$$

Then we can write the two standard coordinate relations (13.12 and 13.13) as a single matrix equation

$$\mathbf{h}_{uv} = \mathbf{Gh} \tag{13.15}$$

where **G** is the rotation matrix given by

$$\mathbf{G} = \begin{pmatrix} \cos\theta & \sin\theta \\ -\sin\theta & \cos\theta \end{pmatrix} \tag{13.16}$$

Define the column matrix (vector) **Z** as

$$\mathbf{Z} = \begin{pmatrix} Z_x \\ Z_y \end{pmatrix} \tag{13.17}$$

The rotation matrix **G** also relates the components Z_u and Z_v of the prism **Z** as expressed in the principal meridians to the components Z_x and Z_y of the same prism **Z** as expressed in the horizontal and vertical coordinate system: i.e.,

$$\mathbf{Z}_{uv} = \mathbf{GZ} \tag{13.18}$$

We can substitute Eqs. 13.15 and 13.18 into 13.10 to obtain

$$\mathbf{GZ} = -\mathbf{P}_{uv}\mathbf{Gh} \tag{13.19}$$

The inverse of the rotation matrix **G** is

$$\mathbf{G}^{-1} = \begin{pmatrix} \cos\theta & -\sin\theta \\ \sin\theta & \cos\theta \end{pmatrix} \tag{13.20}$$

We can multiply both sides of Eq. 13.19 from the left by the inverse matrix to obtain

$$\mathbf{G}^{-1}\mathbf{GZ} = \mathbf{G}^{-1}(-\mathbf{P}_{uv})\mathbf{Gh}$$

The product of the inverse matrix times the matrix equals the unit matrix (i.e., $\mathbf{G}^{-1}\mathbf{G} = \mathbf{U}$) and the product of a unit matrix times a matrix equals the matrix itself (i.e., $\mathbf{UZ} = \mathbf{Z}$). So the left side of the above equation equals **Z**. We can group the middle terms on the right side to obtain

$$\mathbf{Z} = -(\mathbf{G}^{-1}\mathbf{P}_{uv}\mathbf{G})\mathbf{h}$$

which can be written as

$$\mathbf{Z} = -\mathbf{Ph} \tag{13.21}$$

where **P** is a 2 × 2 matrix given by

$$\mathbf{P} = \mathbf{G}^{-1}\mathbf{P}_{uv}\mathbf{G} \tag{13.22}$$

We can explicitly represent the elements of **P** as

$$\mathbf{P} = \begin{pmatrix} P_x & P_t \\ P_t & P_y \end{pmatrix} \tag{13.23}$$

Then for h_x and h_y in cm, Eq. 13.21 can be explicitly written as

$$\begin{pmatrix} Z_x \\ Z_y \end{pmatrix} = -\begin{pmatrix} P_x & P_t \\ P_t & P_y \end{pmatrix}\begin{pmatrix} h_x \\ h_y \end{pmatrix} \tag{13.24}$$

We can substitute Eqs. 13.11, 13.16 and 13.20 into Eq. 13.22, algebraically multiply the matrices, and compare to the results to Eq. 13.23 to obtain the equations

$$P_x = S + C\sin^2\theta \tag{13.25}$$

$$P_y = S + C\cos^2\theta \tag{13.26}$$

and

$$P_t = -C\sin\theta\cos\theta \tag{13.27}$$

Equation 13.21 is the matrix form of Prentice's Rule and was first derived by William Long. It is particularly useful since it deals with the horizontal and vertical prism components even when the principal meridians of the lens are not horizontal and vertical. *For a spherocylindrical lens, the 2 × 2 matrix* **P** *is the dioptric power matrix as expressed in a horizontal and vertical coordinate system.*

13.7 PRISM IN SPHEROCYLINDRICAL LENSES

The previous section gave a derivation of the matrix form of Prentice's Rule. The main results are summarized here. The horizontal and vertical prism components, Z_x and Z_y, at a point H (specified by the horizontal and vertical components h_x and h_y of the distance from the optical center to H) on a thin $S \bigcirc C \times \theta$ spherocylindrical lens are related by the matrix equation

$$\mathbf{Z} = -\mathbf{Ph} \tag{13.21}$$

where **Z** is the 2 × 1 column matrix

$$\mathbf{Z} = \begin{pmatrix} Z_x \\ Z_y \end{pmatrix} \tag{13.9'}$$

h is the 2 × 1 column matrix

$$\mathbf{h} = \begin{pmatrix} h_x \\ h_y \end{pmatrix} \tag{13.8'}$$

and **P** is the 2 × 2 matrix

$$\mathbf{P} = \begin{pmatrix} P_x & P_t \\ P_t & P_y \end{pmatrix} \tag{13.23}$$

The elements of **P** are given by

$$P_x = S + C\sin^2\theta \tag{13.25}$$

$$P_y = S + C\cos^2\theta \tag{13.26}$$

and

$$P_t = -C\sin\theta\cos\theta \tag{13.27}$$

For a $S \bigcirc C \times \theta$ spherocylindrical lens, **P** is the 2 × 2 dioptric power matrix as expressed in a horizontal and vertical coordinate system. In the matrix: P_x is the dioptric power curvital component in the horizontal meridian, and P_y is the dioptric power curvital component in the vertical meridian. The cosine squared appears in the equation for P_y because $\cos^2\theta = \sin^2(\theta \pm 90°)$.

The lower left P_t is the dioptric power torsional component in the horizontal meridian, while the upper right P_t is the dioptric power torsional component in the vertical meridian. Equation 13.23 shows that the torsional component in the horizontal meridian equals the torsional component in the vertical meridian. P_t has a definite sign in the dioptric power matrix. The cosine is positive for a first quadrant θ (i.e., $\theta < 90°$) and negative for a second quadrant θ (i.e., $\theta > 90°$). For a minus cylinder, C is negative. It then follows from Eq. 13.27 that *for a minus cylinder first quadrant axis, P_t is always positive; while for a minus cylinder second quadrant axis, P_t is always negative.*

The equations in Sections 13.3 and 13.4 for the dioptric power curvital and torsional components in the meridian m contained the angle ϕ with the axis meridian (i.e., $\phi = m - \theta$). The horizontal meridian, usually designated the 180 meridian, is the same as the $m = 0$ meridian. Therefore $|\phi| = |m - \theta| = |\theta|$, and so only the cylinder axis θ appears in Eqs. 13.25 through 13.27. If we had picked a coordinate system other than horizontal and vertical, then the angle ϕ would appear in the equations.

We can also explicitly write out the matrix elements in Eq. 13.21 to get

$$\begin{pmatrix} Z_x \\ Z_y \end{pmatrix} = -\begin{pmatrix} P_x & P_t \\ P_t & P_y \end{pmatrix}\begin{pmatrix} h_x \\ h_y \end{pmatrix} \tag{13.24}$$

Figure 12.3 of the last chapter gives the plus-minus signs for the horizontal and vertical components of **Z** and **h**.

EXAMPLE 13.2

Example 12.8 computed the prism at a point 12 mm below the optical center line in Zelmo Corkscrew's left spectacle Rx of -5.00×60. Check if the matrix form of Prentice's Rule give the same prism.

Here $h_x = 0$ and $h_y = -1.2$ cm (Figure 12.3). Also $S = 0$, $C = -5.00$ D, and $\theta = 60°$. From Eqs. 13.25 through 13.27,

$$P = \begin{pmatrix} -3.75\,\text{D} & +2.17\,\text{D} \\ +2.17\,\text{D} & -1.25\,\text{D} \end{pmatrix}$$

Then from Eq. 13.24,

$$\begin{pmatrix} Z_x \\ Z_y \end{pmatrix} = -\begin{pmatrix} -3.75\,\text{D} & +2.17\,\text{D} \\ +2.17\,\text{D} & -1.25\,\text{D} \end{pmatrix}\begin{pmatrix} 0 \\ -1.2\,\text{cm} \end{pmatrix}$$

A common mistake is to forget the minus sign in the above equation. We can avoid this mistake by multiplying each element of the **h** matrix by the minus sign as the first step in the procedure. Then,

$$\begin{pmatrix} Z_x \\ Z_y \end{pmatrix} = \begin{pmatrix} -3.75\,\text{D} & +2.17\,\text{D} \\ +2.17\,\text{D} & -1.25\,\text{D} \end{pmatrix}\begin{pmatrix} 0 \\ +1.2\,\text{cm} \end{pmatrix}$$

and

$$\begin{pmatrix} Z_x \\ Z_y \end{pmatrix} = \begin{pmatrix} +2.6^{\Delta} \\ -1.5^{\Delta} \end{pmatrix} = \begin{pmatrix} 2.6^{\Delta} & \text{BO} \\ 1.5^{\Delta} & \text{BD} \end{pmatrix}$$

Here the horizontal component of the prism is 2.6^{Δ} BO, while the vertical component is component is 1.5^{Δ} BD. From the procedures of Section 11.10, these horizontal and vertical prism components give a resultant prism of 3.0^{Δ}BD & O @ 150, which checks with Example 12.8.

EXAMPLE 13.3

Myra Dell-Shrimpsky has a $+3.00 \bigcirc -6.00 \times 122$ spectacle correction for his left eye. When Dell-Shrimpsky reads, she looks through the lens at a point 9 mm down and 3 mm in from the optical center of the lens. What are the prism components at this point?

Let us first check the isothickness curves to develop some intuition about the answer. Since one power is plus and the other is minus, the isothickness curves are hyperbolas. The methods of the Section 13.5 show that the straight line boundaries are 45° away from the principal meridians. The isothickness curves are shown in Figure 13.11. From these curves, the prism base components at the reading center are up and in.

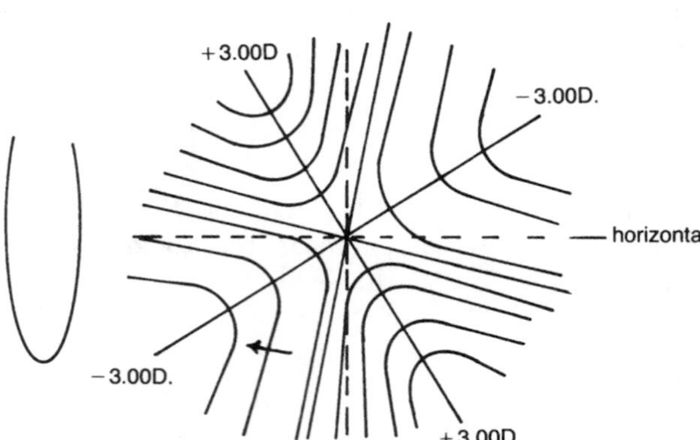

Figure 13.11 Isothickness curves for a +3.00 ⊂−6.00 ×122 lens. Prism base directions at indicated position.

Here $h_x = -0.3\,\text{cm}$ and $h_y = -0.9\,\text{cm}$ (i.e, see Figure 12.3). Also $S = +3.00\,\text{D}$, $C = -6.00\,\text{D}$, and $\theta = 122°$. From Eqs. 13.25 through 13.27,

$$P = \begin{pmatrix} -1.32\,\text{D} & -2.70\,\text{D} \\ -2.70\,\text{D} & +1.32\,\text{D} \end{pmatrix}$$

Then from Eq. 13.24,

$$\begin{pmatrix} Z_x \\ Z_y \end{pmatrix} = -\begin{pmatrix} -1.32\,\text{D} & -2.70\,\text{D} \\ -2.70\,\text{D} & +1.32\,\text{D} \end{pmatrix}\begin{pmatrix} -0.3\,\text{cm} \\ -0.9\,\text{cm} \end{pmatrix}$$

Again to prevent errors, first bring the minus sign inside the **h** matrix:

$$\begin{pmatrix} Z_x \\ Z_y \end{pmatrix} = \begin{pmatrix} -1.32\,\text{D} & -2.70\,\text{D} \\ -2.70\,\text{D} & +1.32\,\text{D} \end{pmatrix}\begin{pmatrix} +0.3\,\text{cm} \\ +0.9\,\text{cm} \end{pmatrix}$$

Then,

$$\begin{pmatrix} Z_x \\ Z_y \end{pmatrix} = \begin{pmatrix} -2.8^{\Delta} \\ +0.4^{\Delta} \end{pmatrix} = \begin{pmatrix} 2.8^{\Delta} & \text{BI} \\ 0.4^{\Delta} & \text{BU} \end{pmatrix}$$

The horizontal component is 2.8^{Δ} BI while the vertical component is 0.4^{Δ} BU. The up and in directions agree with the isothickness curves.

EXAMPLE 13.4

Ms. Selma Nella has a $-2.00 \bigcirc -5.00 \times 50$ spectacle correction for the right eye. When Selma Nella looks through the lens at a point 11 mm down and 4 mm in from the optical center, what prism components occur at that point?

Here for each lens, $S = -2.00\,\text{D}$, $C = -5.00\,\text{D}$, and $\theta = 50°$. From Eqs. 13.25 through 13.27,

$$P = \begin{pmatrix} -4.93\,\text{D} & +2.46\,\text{D} \\ +2.46\,\text{D} & -4.07\,\text{D} \end{pmatrix}$$

For the right lens: $h_x = +0.4\,\text{cm}$ and $h_y = -1.1\,\text{cm}$ (see Figure 12.3). From Eq. 13.24,

$$\begin{pmatrix} Z_x \\ Z_y \end{pmatrix} = -\begin{pmatrix} -4.93\,\text{D} & +2.46\,\text{D} \\ +2.46\,\text{D} & -4.07\,\text{D} \end{pmatrix}\begin{pmatrix} +0.4\,\text{cm} \\ -1.1\,\text{cm} \end{pmatrix} = \begin{pmatrix} -4.93\,\text{D} & +2.46\,\text{D} \\ +2.46\,\text{D} & -4.07\,\text{D} \end{pmatrix}\begin{pmatrix} -0.4\,\text{cm} \\ +1.1\,\text{cm} \end{pmatrix}$$

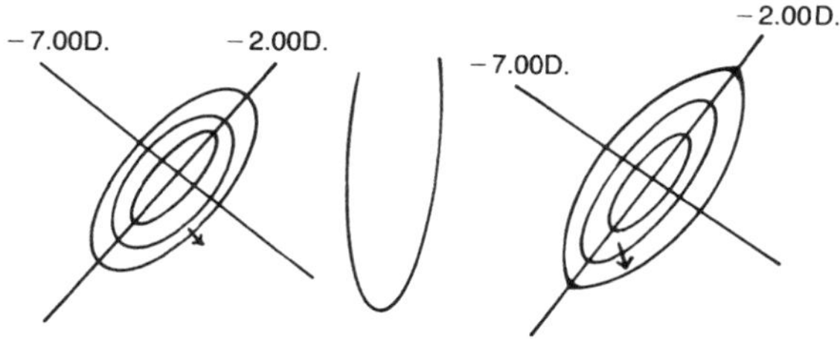

Figure 13.12 Isothickness curves and prism base directions at indicated positions on a −2.00 ⊂ −5.00 × 90 lens.

and

$$\begin{pmatrix} Z_x \\ Z_y \end{pmatrix} = \begin{pmatrix} +4.7^{\Delta} \\ -5.5^{\Delta} \end{pmatrix} = \begin{pmatrix} 4.7^{\Delta} & \text{BI} \\ 5.5^{\Delta} & \text{BD} \end{pmatrix}$$

As shown in Figure 13.12, the isothickness curves are elliptical, and the base down and in components are consistent with the curves. (Figure 13.12 also shows the prism base directions at a point that is down and in from the optical center of a $-2.00 \bigcirc -5.00 \times 50$ lens in front of the left eye.)

The algebraic matrix multiplications in Eq. 13.24 give

$$Z_x = -P_x h_x - P_t h_y \tag{13.28}$$

and

$$Z_y = -P_t h_x - P_y h_y \tag{13.29}$$

Consider a point H that is along the horizontal meridian of the spherocylindrical lens. Then $h_y = 0$, and the above equations reduce to

$$Z_x = -P_x h_x$$

and

$$Z_y = -P_t h_x$$

These equations show that the dioptric power curvital component P_x in the horizontal meridian results in the horizontal prism component Z_x. In other words, P_x bends rays only horizontally. On the other hand, P_t results in the vertical prism component Z_y. In other words, the dioptric power torsional component P_t in the horizontal meridian bends the rays vertically (or perpendicular to the meridian). Thus when the horizontal meridian is isolated by a stenopeic slit, it is P_t that causes the rays to bend out of the horizontal meridian and results in the twisting sheet of light. Similarly, we can isolate the vertical meridian and make a similar argument.

In general, an off-axis meridian of a spherocylindrical lens has two components of the dioptric power, the curvital component and the torsional component. The dioptric power torsional component refracts (bends) rays in a direction perpendicular (or orthogonal) to the meridian. Thus from a meridional point of view, it is the dioptric power torsional component that is responsible for the rotational deviations discussed in Section 12.4. In the off-axis meridian, the curvital component of the power refracts rays in the same direction as the meridian.

For spherocylindrical lenses with axis 90 or 180, Eq. 13.27 gives $P_t = 0$. Then Eqs. 13.28 and 13.29 reduce to

$$Z_x = -P_x h_x$$

while

$$Z_y = -P_y h_y$$

Here the horizontal and vertical meridians are the principal meridians. A ray hitting the lens in the horizontal meridian has $h_y = 0$, and thus $Z_y = 0$. Thus the ray stays in the horizontal meridian and is bent by an amount indicated by Z_x. A similar argument exists for the vertical meridian. Thus when we isolate a principal meridian with a stenopeic slit, the sheet of light that passes through the slit stays in that meridian (i.e., has no twist). Note also that for a spherical lens, $C = 0$, and thus P_t is zero for all meridians.

An instructive case occurs when a meridian of a spherocylindrical lens has a dioptric power curvital component that is zero, while the torsional component is non-zero. In such a meridian, all of the refraction comes from the torsional component and rays are bent in a direction perpendicular to the meridian. The following is a numerical example.

EXAMPLE 13.5

Scott Bushsnake has a $+2.00 \bigcirc -8.00 \times 120$ spectacle correction for his left eye. What is the prism at a point 12 mm vertically below the optical center?

From Eqs. 13.25 through 13.27,

$$P = \begin{pmatrix} -4.00\,\text{D} & -3.46\,\text{D} \\ -3.46\,\text{D} & 0.00\,\text{D} \end{pmatrix}$$

Here the curvital component P_y is zero, while the torsional component P_t is -3.46 D. For $h_y = -1.2$ cm, Prentice's rule gives

$$\begin{pmatrix} Z_x \\ Z_y \end{pmatrix} = -\begin{pmatrix} -4.00\,\text{D} & -3.46\,\text{D} \\ -3.46\,\text{D} & 0 \end{pmatrix}\begin{pmatrix} 0 \\ -1.2\,\text{cm} \end{pmatrix}$$

$$= \begin{pmatrix} -4.2^{\Delta} \\ 0 \end{pmatrix} = \begin{pmatrix} 4.2^{\Delta}\ \text{BI} \\ 0 \end{pmatrix}$$

So for Scott's left eye, the prism at a point 12 mm vertically below the optical center is 4.2^{Δ} BI, which is purely horizontal and is entirely due to the torsional component P_t. The isothickness curves for this lens are hyperbolic (Figure 13.13). From Eq. 13.3, the straight-line boundaries are 30° on either side of the axis (i.e., at 90 and 150). At 12 mm below the optical center, the isothickness curve is a straight vertical line with the thicker part of that lens on the side toward the nose. This confirms that the prism at the point vertically below the optical center is BI. (Figure 13.13 also shows that on a point that is 11 mm down and 5 mm in from the optical center, the isothickness curves indicate that the prism at that point has both a BD component and a BI component.)

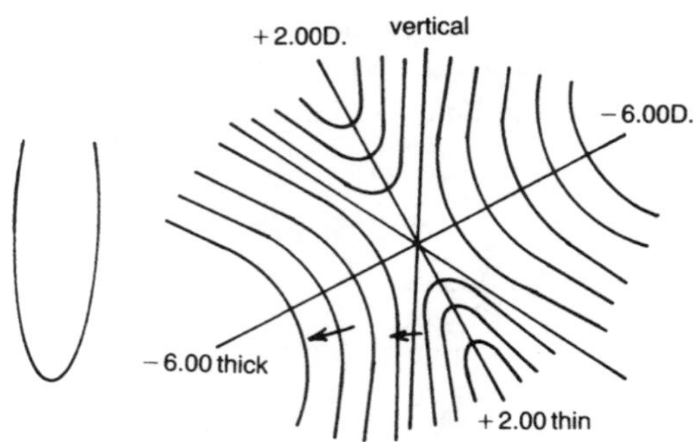

Figure 13.13 Isothickness curves for a lens with a vertical dioptric power curvital component equal to zero. Prism base directions at indicated positions.

13.8 MATRIX PROPERTIES AND EXPANDED POWER CROSSES

For a thin $S \bigcirc C \times \theta$ spherocylindrical lens, Eq. 13.23 gives the dioptric power matrix **P** as expressed in a horizontal and vertical coordinate system:

$$\mathbf{P} = \begin{pmatrix} P_x & P_t \\ P_t & P_y \end{pmatrix}$$

In matrix theory the element P_x is the first row-first column element (or the 11 element), and the element P_y is the second row-second column element (or the 22 element). The upper right P_t is the first row-second column element (or the 12 element), while the lower left P_t is the second row-first column element (or the 21 element). The 11 and 22 elements are called the *diagonal elements*, while the 12 and 21 elements are called the off-diagonal elements. Therefore the dioptric power curvital components P_x and P_y are diagonal elements, while the equal torsional components P_t are the *off-diagonal elements*. A matrix with equal off-diagonal elements is called a *symmetric matrix*. Equation 13.23 shows that the dioptric power matrix for a thin spherocylindrical lens is a symmetric matrix.

The trace τ of a matrix is the sum of the diagonal elements. For the dioptric power matrix **P**,

$$\tau = P_x + P_y \tag{13.30}$$

For a toric interface, the sum of the dioptric power curvital components from any two perpendicular meridians equals Euler's constant E (Section 13.3). Similarly we can substitute Eqs. 13.25 and 13.26 into Eq. 13.30 to show that the trace of **P** equals Euler's constant E, or

$$\tau = E = 2S + C \tag{13.31}$$

The trace depends only on S and C, and does not depend on the cylinder axis θ. Note also that from Eq. 10.6, the Sp Eq of the spherocylindrical lens equals 1/2 the trace, or

$$\text{SpEq} = S + \frac{C}{2} = \frac{\tau}{2} \tag{13.32}$$

For $\theta = 90$ or 180, the horizontal and vertical meridians are the principal meridians, and the torsional component P_t equals zero. For a $+5.00 \bigcirc -3.00 \times 180$, we can write an expanded power cross for the horizontal and vertical meridians that shows both the curvital components of the power together with the zero torsional components as:

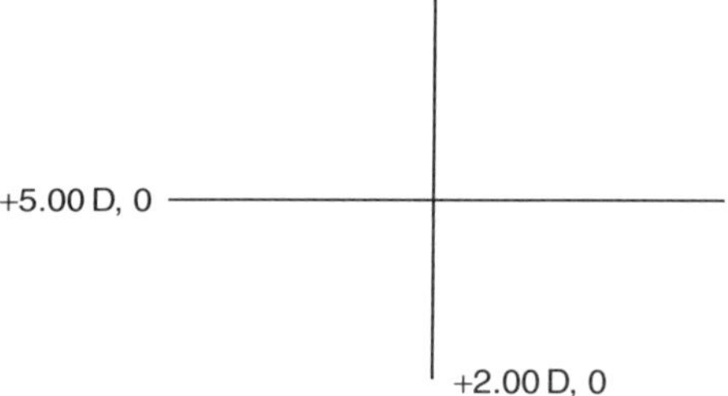

Here Eqs. 13.25 through 13.27 give

$$\mathbf{P} = \begin{pmatrix} +5.00\,\text{D} & 0 \\ 0 & +2.00\,\text{D} \end{pmatrix}$$

The matrix **P** is just a formal way of writing the expanded power cross. Recall that the transposed form of $+5.00 \bigcirc -3.00 \times 180$ is $+2.00 \bigcirc +3.00 \times 90$, and both forms give the same power cross. Similarly we can use $+2.00 \bigcirc +3.00 \times 90$ in Eqs. 13.25 through 13.27 to get the same **P**.

From Eq. 13.30, the trace of the above matrix is

$$\tau = +5.00\,\text{D} + (+2.00\,\text{D}) = +7.00\,\text{D}$$

From Eq. 13.31, we can also check that the trace equals Euler's constant for the $+5.00 \bigcirc -3.00 \times 180$:

$$E = 2(+5.00\,\text{D}) + (-3.00\,\text{D}) = +7.00\,\text{D}$$

which is equal to τ.

When the above lens is rotated by 30° to get $+5.00 \bigcirc -3.00 \times 30$, the principal meridians are 30 and 120. For the dioptric power matrix **P** as expressed in the horizontal and vertical meridians, Eqs. 13.25 through 13.27 give

$$\mathbf{P} = \begin{pmatrix} +4.25\,\text{D} & +1.30\,\text{D} \\ +1.30\,\text{D} & +2.75\,\text{D} \end{pmatrix}$$

Note that as the lens rotated from axis 180 to 30: the dioptric power curvital component P_x in the horizontal meridian changed from +5.00 D to +4.25 D, the dioptric power curvital component P_y in the vertical meridian changed from +2.00 D to +2.75 D, and the dioptric power torsional components in both meridians changed from 0 to +1.30 D. The matrix **P** is equivalent to putting the dioptric power curvital and torsional components on the expanded power cross.

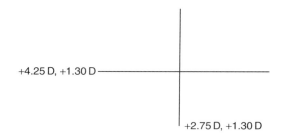

By transposition, the $+5.00 \bigcirc -3.00 \times 30$ lens is optically the same as a $+2.00 \bigcirc +3.00 \times 120$ lens. For either of these forms, Eqs. 13.25 through 13.27 give the same dioptric power matrix **P**.

From Eq. 13.30, the trace of the above matrix **P** is

$$\tau = +4.25\,\text{D} + (+2.75\,\text{D}) = +7.00\,\text{D}$$

which equals Euler's constant E for the $+5.00 \bigcirc -3.00 \times 30$ lens.

A +5.00 D spherical lens has a +5.00 D dioptric power curvital component and a zero torsional component in all meridians, including the horizontal and vertical meridians. Here $S = +5.00$ D, $C = 0$, and Eqs. 13.25 through 13.27 give

$$\mathbf{P} = \begin{pmatrix} +5.00\,\text{D} & 0 \\ 0 & +5.00\,\text{D} \end{pmatrix}$$

as expected.

13.9 DECENTRATION WITH SPHEROCYLINDRICAL LENSES

In some spherocylindrical Rx's, horizontal and/or vertical prism can be obtained by decentration relative to the DRP. For a spherocylindrical lens, the matrix version of Prentice's rule is

$$\mathbf{Z} = -\mathbf{Ph}$$

Let DEC be a 2×1 decentration matrix where

$$\mathbf{DEC} = \begin{pmatrix} \mathrm{DEC}_x \\ \mathrm{DEC}_y \end{pmatrix}$$

DEC_x is the horizontal decentration component and DEC_y is the vertical decentration component each relative to the DRP. Then, as in the derivation of Eq. 13.4,

$$\mathbf{DEC} = -\mathbf{h}$$

and

$$\mathbf{Z} = \mathbf{P}\ \mathbf{DEC} \tag{13.33}$$

We can multiply both sides from the left by the inverse of **P** to obtain

$$\mathbf{DEC} = \mathbf{P}^{-1}\mathbf{Z} \tag{13.34}$$

Since **P** is a 2×2 matrix: the inverse of **P** is found by exchanging the diagonal elements, changing the sign of the off-diagonal elements, and dividing by the determinant δ, where δ is the product of the diagonal elements minus the product of the off-diagonal elements, or

$$\delta = P_x P_y - P_t P_t \tag{13.35}$$

So given

$$\mathbf{P} = \begin{pmatrix} P_x & P_t \\ P_t & P_y \end{pmatrix} \tag{13.36}$$

the inverse matrix is given by

$$\mathbf{P}^{-1} = \frac{1}{\delta}\begin{pmatrix} P_y & -P_t \\ -P_t & P_x \end{pmatrix} \tag{13.37}$$

For a $S \bigcirc C \times \theta$ spherocylindrical lens, the determinant is independent of the cylinder axis θ. In fact, one can substitute Eqs. 13.25 through 13.27 into 13.35 to show that the determinant is equal to the product of the powers in the two principal meridians, or

$$\delta = S(S + C) \tag{13.38}$$

The discussion in Section 12.3 showed that an arbitrary prism cannot be obtained by decentering a cylindrical lens (i.e., sphere power $S = 0$). For such a cylindrical lens, the determinant δ is zero, and the regular inverse matrix does not exist.

EXAMPLE 13.6

In Example 13.5, Scott Bushsnake had a $+2.00 \bigcirc -8.00 \times 120$ spectacle Rx (left eye). Suppose Scott's Rx also calls for a 3^Δ BU prism. What decentration (relative to the DRP) will give the prism?

From Example 13.5, the dioptric power matrix is

$$\mathbf{P} = \begin{pmatrix} -4.00\,\mathrm{D} & -3.46\,\mathrm{D} \\ -3.46\,\mathrm{D} & 0.00\,\mathrm{D} \end{pmatrix}$$

From Eq. 13.35, the determinant is

$$\begin{aligned} \delta &= (-4.00\,\mathrm{D})(0.00\,\mathrm{D}) - (-3.46\,\mathrm{D})(-3.46\,\mathrm{D}) \\ &= -12.00\,\mathrm{D}^2 \end{aligned}$$

(Note that the principal meridian powers are +2.00 D and −6.00 D, and their product also equals δ.) Then from Eq. 13.37 for the inverse matrix:

$$\mathbf{P}^{-1} = \frac{1}{-12.00\,\mathrm{D}^2}\begin{pmatrix} 0.00\,\mathrm{D} & +3.46\,\mathrm{D} \\ +3.46\,\mathrm{D} & -4.00\,\mathrm{D} \end{pmatrix}$$

The prism matrix is

$$\mathbf{Z} = \begin{pmatrix} Z_x \\ Z_y \end{pmatrix} = \begin{pmatrix} 0 \\ +3^\Delta \end{pmatrix}$$

Then,

$$\begin{aligned} \mathbf{DEC} &= \mathbf{P}^{-1}\mathbf{Z} \\ \begin{pmatrix} \mathrm{DEC}_x \\ \mathrm{DEC}_y \end{pmatrix} &= \frac{1}{-12.00}\begin{pmatrix} 0.00 & +3.46 \\ +3.46 & -4.00 \end{pmatrix}\begin{pmatrix} 0 \\ +3^\Delta \end{pmatrix} \\ &= \frac{1}{-12.00}\begin{pmatrix} +10.39 \\ -12.00 \end{pmatrix} = \begin{pmatrix} -0.87\,\mathrm{cm} \\ +1.0\,\mathrm{cm} \end{pmatrix} \end{aligned}$$

This is for the left lens, so the decentration that gives the prism is 8.7 mm in and 10 mm up from the DRP. (For clinical purposes, decentrations

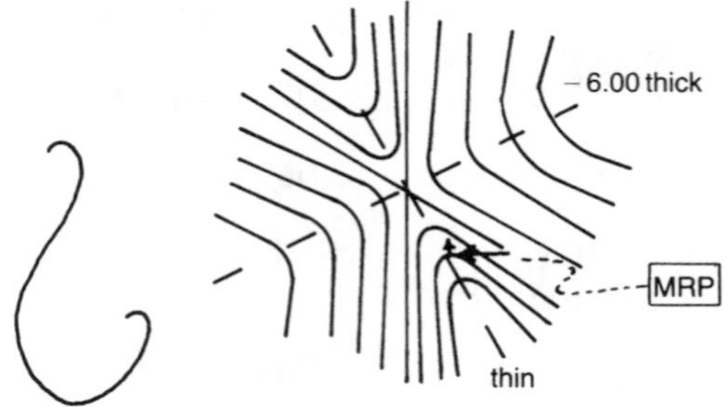

Figure 13.14 Lens that has been decentered up and in relative to the MRP. (The MRP is now referred to as the DRP.)

are rounded off to the nearest millimeter.) Figure 13.14 shows the isothickness curves for the decentered lens. The prism at the DRP is BU. Note that even though only vertical prism was called for in the Rx, the decentration has both horizontal and vertical components.

EXAMPLE 13.7

Ruby Rose has a right Rx of $-7.00 \bigcirc -3.00 \times 35$ combined with 5^{Δ} BI combined with 2^{Δ} BD. What decentration relative to the DRP gives the prism?

From Eqs. 13.25 through 13.27,

$$\mathbf{P} = \begin{pmatrix} -7.99\,\text{D} & +1.41\,\text{D} \\ +1.41\,\text{D} & -9.01\,\text{D} \end{pmatrix}$$

From Eq. 13.35, the determinant is

$$\begin{aligned} \delta &= (-7.99\,\text{D})(-9.01\,\text{D}) - (+1.41\,\text{D})(+1.41\,\text{D}) \\ &= +70.00\,\text{D}^2 \end{aligned}$$

(Note that the principal meridian powers are -7.00 D and -10.00 D, and their product also equals δ.) From Eq. 13.37, the inverse matrix is

$$\mathbf{P}^{-1} = \frac{1}{+70.00\,\text{D}^2}\begin{pmatrix} -9.01\,\text{D} & -1.41\,\text{D} \\ -1.41\,\text{D} & -7.99\,\text{D} \end{pmatrix}$$

This is the right lens, so the prism matrix is

$$\mathbf{Z} = \begin{pmatrix} Z_x \\ Z_y \end{pmatrix} = \begin{pmatrix} +5^{\Delta} \\ -2^{\Delta} \end{pmatrix}$$

Then,

$$\mathbf{DEC} = \mathbf{P}^{-1}\mathbf{Z}$$

$$\begin{aligned} \begin{pmatrix} \text{DEC}_x \\ \text{DEC}_y \end{pmatrix} &= \frac{1}{+70.00}\begin{pmatrix} -9.01 & -1.41 \\ -1.41 & -7.99 \end{pmatrix}\begin{pmatrix} +5^{\Delta} \\ -2^{\Delta} \end{pmatrix} \\ &= \frac{1}{+70.00}\begin{pmatrix} -42.25 \\ +8.93 \end{pmatrix} = \begin{pmatrix} -0.60\,\text{cm} \\ +0.13\,\text{cm} \end{pmatrix} \end{aligned}$$

The decentration that gives the prism is 6 mm out and 1.3 mm up from the DRP. (You can check the isothickness curves for consistency.)

13.10 PRISM FOR COMBINED SPHEROCYLINDRICAL LENSES

When two thin spherocylindrical lenses are combined with their principal meridians aligned, the powers in the respective principal meridians are additive. When the principal meridians of the two lenses are obliquely crossed (i.e., not aligned), the powers in the respective principal meridians are not additive. A consideration of the resultant prism power for two combined thin spherocylindrical lenses leads to the fact that the dioptric power matrices for thin spherocylindrical lenses are additive even when the principal meridians of the two lenses are obliquely crossed. This section contains a derivation of the matrix additivity property. Section 13.12 contains numerical examples.

Consider the combination of two centered thin obliquely crossed spherocylindrical lenses with respective parameters $S_1 \bigcirc C_1 \times \theta_1$ and $S_2 \bigcirc C_2 \times \theta_2$. Prentice's Rule for each lens is

$$\mathbf{Z}_1 = -\mathbf{P}_1\mathbf{h}_1 \quad \text{and} \quad \mathbf{Z}_2 = -\mathbf{P}_2\mathbf{h}_2$$

When a ray is incident on the first lens at the position indicated by the matrix $\mathbf{h}_1$, it experiences the prism $\mathbf{Z}_1$. This emergent ray is immediately incident on lens 2, so

$$\mathbf{h}_2 = \mathbf{h}_1$$

Then the prism experienced by the ray at the second lens is

$$\mathbf{Z}_2 = -\mathbf{P}_2\mathbf{h}_1$$

The two prism powers are vectorally additive, which is the same as adding the matrices. So the total or resultant prism power experienced by the ray is

$$\mathbf{Z}_r = \mathbf{Z}_1 + \mathbf{Z}_2$$

When we substitute in the Prentice's Rule expression into the sum equation, we get

$$\mathbf{Z}_r = (-\mathbf{P}_1\mathbf{h}_1) + (-\mathbf{P}_2\mathbf{h}_1)$$

or

$$\mathbf{Z}_r = -(\mathbf{P}_1 + \mathbf{P}_2)\mathbf{h}_1$$

This can be written as

$$\mathbf{Z}_r = -\mathbf{P}_r\mathbf{h}_1 \qquad (13.39)$$

where,

$$\mathbf{P}_r = \mathbf{P}_1 + \mathbf{P}_2 \qquad (13.40)$$

Equations 13.39 and 13.40 show that at every point the combination of the two thin spherocylindrical lens gives the same prism as a single thin spherocylindrical lens which has a dioptric power matrix $\mathbf{P}_r$, where $\mathbf{P}_r$ is the sum of the matrices for the individual lenses. In other words, *the single thin spherocylindrical lens with a dioptric power matrix* $\mathbf{P}_r$ *is optically equivalent to the combination of the two obliquely crossed thin spherocylindrical lenses, and* $\mathbf{P}_r$ *is the sum of the dioptric power matrices of the two spherocylindrical lenses.*

13.11 FINDING $S \bigcirc C \times \theta$ FROM THE DIOPTRIC POWER MATRIX

For the combination of two obliquely crossed thin spherocylindrical lenses, the previous section showed that the dioptric power matrices are additive, and that the resultant matrix is the dioptric power matrix of the single spherocylindrical lens that is equivalent to the obliquely crossed combination. In this event, we need to know how to get the spherocylindrical parameters $S \bigcirc C \times \theta$ from the resultant dioptric power matrix.

First let us look at the case for a spherical lens of dioptric power S. The matrix for a spherical lens is easy to recognize, since it has zero torsional components P_t and curvital components (P_x and P_y) that are both equal to S. The matrix for a +5.00 D spherical lenses is given at the end of Section 13.8.

Next let us look at the case for a spherocylindrical lens with axes 90 or 180. The dioptric power matrix for this lens has zero torsional components P_t and unequal curvital components P_x and P_y. So for a matrix with this pattern, the principal meridians of the lens are horizontal and vertical. Then we can simply put P_x and P_y on a power cross and determine the spherocylindrical parameters $S \bigcirc C \times \theta$ from the power cross.

Now consider the general case for a spherocylindrical lens that has non-zero torsional components P_t in its dioptric power matrix **P**. Given

$$\mathbf{P} = \begin{pmatrix} P_x & P_t \\ P_t & P_y \end{pmatrix}$$

then Eq. 13.30 for the trace gives

$$\tau = P_x + P_y$$

and Eq. 13.35 for the determinant gives

$$\delta = P_x P_y - P_t P_t$$

The trace τ and the determinant δ of **P** depend only on the sphere power S and cylinder power C. Specifically Eq. 13.31 gives

$$\tau = 2S + C$$

while Eq. 13.38 gives

$$\delta = S(S + C)$$

We can solve the trace equation for the sphere power S to get

$$S = \frac{\tau - C}{2} \tag{13.41}$$

We can substitute Eq. 13.41 into the determinant equation to get

$$\begin{aligned} \delta &= \left(\frac{\tau - C}{2}\right)\left(\frac{\tau - C}{2} + C\right) \\ &= \left(\frac{\tau - C}{2}\right)\left(\frac{\tau + C}{2}\right) \\ &= \left(\frac{\tau^2 - C^2}{4}\right) \end{aligned}$$

Then we can solve for C to obtain:

$$C = \pm\sqrt{\tau^2 - 4\delta} \tag{13.42}$$

Given C from Eq. 13.42 and then S from Eq. 13.41, we can find the cylinder axis from

$$\tan\theta = \frac{S - P_x}{P_t} \tag{13.43}$$

or

$$\theta = \tan^{-1}[(S - P_x)/P_t] \tag{13.44}$$

You can verify Eq. 13.43 using Eqs. 13.25 through 13.27. For a first quadrant cylinder axis, Eq. 13.44 returns the axis θ directly. For a second quadrant cylinder axis, Eq. 13.44 returns the negative angle θ_m shown in Figure 13.15. Then θ in standard axis notation is found by adding 180 degrees to θ_m.

The plus or minus sign in Eq. 13.42 is an arbitrary choice and determines whether the resulting spherocylindrical parameters will be in plus or minus cylinder form. The plus or minus cylinder answers are related by transposition.

EXAMPLE 13.8

Given the dioptric power matrix,

$$\mathbf{P} = \begin{pmatrix} -0.73\,\text{D} & -1.68\,\text{D} \\ -1.68\,\text{D} & +0.23\,\text{D} \end{pmatrix}$$

find the minus cylinder S, C, and θ.

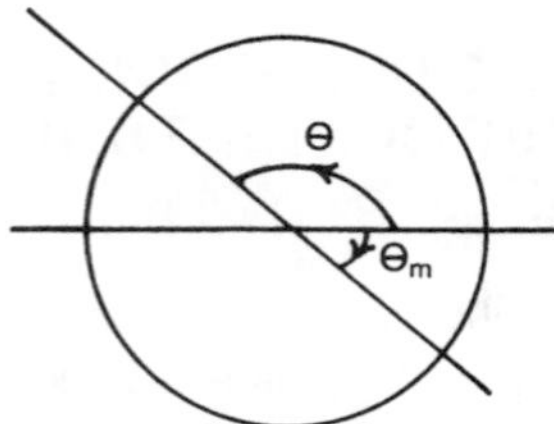

Figure 13.15 Relation of negative angle θ_m to the standard axis notation θ.

The torsional component P_t is negative, so the minus cylinder axis must be a second quadrant angle. From Eq. 13.30, the trace is

$$\tau = -0.73\,\text{D} + 0.23\,\text{D} = -0.50\,\text{D}$$

From Eq. 13.35, the determinant is

$$\delta = (-0.73\,\text{D})(+0.23\,\text{D}) - (-1.68\,\text{D})^2 = -2.99\,\text{D}^2$$

Then from Eq. 13.42,

$$C = -\sqrt{(-0.50\,\text{D})^2 - 4(-2.99\,\text{D}^2)} = -3.49\,\text{D}$$

From Eq. 13.41,

$$S = \frac{-0.50\,\text{D} - (-3.49\,\text{D})}{2} = \frac{+2.99\,\text{D}}{2} = +1.50\,\text{D}$$

Equation 13.43 then gives

$$\tan\theta = \frac{1.50 - (-0.73)}{-1.68} = -1.33$$

or

$$\theta = \tan^{-1}(-1.33) = -53^\circ$$

In standard axis notation,

$$\theta = -53 + 180 = 127$$

The answer is $+1.50 \bigcirc -3.49 \times 127$, which has the expected second quadrant axis.

If one chooses the plus sign in Eq. 14.41 for C, the resulting spherocylindrical parameters are $-1.99 \bigcirc +3.49 \times 37$. This is just the transposed form of $+1.50 \bigcirc -3.49 \times 127$.

EXAMPLE 13.9

Given the dioptric power matrix,

$$P = \begin{pmatrix} -9.66\,\text{D} & +1.12\,\text{D} \\ +1.12\,\text{D} & -6.34\,\text{D} \end{pmatrix}$$

find the minus cylinder S, C, and θ.

Since the torsional component P_t is positive, the minus cylinder axis must be a first quadrant angle. From Eq. 13.30, the trace is

$$\tau = -9.66\,\text{D} + (-6.34\,\text{D}) = -16.00\,\text{D}$$

From Eq. 13.35, the determinant is

$$\delta = (-9.66\,\text{D})(-6.34\,\text{D}) - (+1.12\,\text{D})^2 = +59.99\,\text{D}^2$$

Then from Eq. 13.42,

$$C = -\sqrt{(-16.00\,\text{D})^2 - 4(+59.99\,\text{D}^2)} = -4.00\,\text{D}$$

From Eq. 13.41,

$$S = \frac{-16.00 - (-4.00)}{2} = \frac{-12.00}{2} = -6.00\,\text{D}$$

Equation 13.43 then gives

$$\tan\theta = \frac{-6.00 - (-9.66)}{+1.12} = +3.27$$

or

$$\theta = \tan^{-1}(-3.27) = 73^\circ$$

The answer is $-6.00 \bigcirc -4.00 \times 73$, which has the expected first quadrant axis.

Again if one chose the plus sign for the cylinder, the calculated results would come out at $-10.00 \bigcirc +4.00 \times 163$, which is just the transposed form of $-6.00 \bigcirc -4.00 \times 73$.

13.12 COMBINING OBLIQUELY CROSSED SPHEROCYLINDRICAL LENSES

Consider two thin spherocylindrical lenses in contact. When the principal meridians of two lenses are aligned, we can add the powers in the respective principal meridians (as considered in Chapter 10).

EXAMPLE 13.10

A -3.00×60 lens is combined with a -4.00×150 lens. What are the spherocylindrical parameters of the single lens that is equivalent to the combination?

The principal meridians of these two lenses are aligned, and so we can add the respective powers. Figure 13.16 shows the power cross addition. The answer is $-3.00 \bigcirc -1.00 \times 150$.

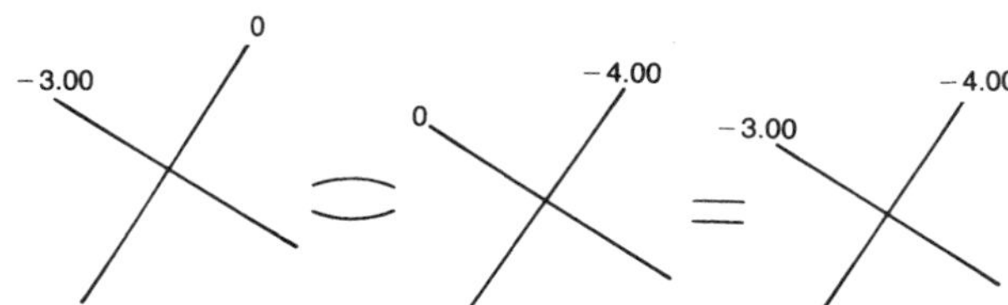

Figure 13.16 Power cross addition for aligned lenses.

When the principal meridians of the two spherocylindrical lenses in contact are obliquely crossed (i.e. not aligned), then the powers in the principal meridians are not additive. Equations 13.39 and 13.40 shows that is a single spherocylindrical lens with a dioptric power $\mathbf{P}_r$ is optically equivalent to the combination, where $\mathbf{P}_r$ equals the sum of the dioptric power matrices of the individual lenses. This is formally equivalent to respectively adding the dioptric power curvital and torsional components in the horizontal meridians of the two lenses and then respectively adding the dioptric power curvital and torsional components in the vertical meridians of the two lenses. In the following discussion, the single lens equivalent to the combination is referred to as the resultant lens.

EXAMPLE 13.11

The -3.00×60 lens in the previous example is rotated 30° to -3.00×90. The two lenses in contact are then -3.00×90 and -4.00×150. What are the resultant spherocylindrical parameters?

These two lenses are obliquely crossed, and from Eq. 13.40 the dioptric power matrices add.

Lens	*Matrix*
-3.00×90	$\begin{pmatrix} -3.00\,\text{D} & 0 \\ 0 & 0 \end{pmatrix}$
	+
-4.00×150	$\begin{pmatrix} -1.00\,\text{D} & -1.73\,\text{D} \\ -1.73\,\text{D} & -3.00\,\text{D} \end{pmatrix}$
Resultant	$\begin{pmatrix} -4.00\,\text{D} & -1.73\,\text{D} \\ -1.73\,\text{D} & -3.00\,\text{D} \end{pmatrix}$

From the resultant matrix, Eqs. 13.30 and 13.35 give the trace and determinant:

$$\tau = -4.00\,\text{D} + (-3.00\,\text{D}) = -7.00\,\text{D}$$

$$\delta = (-4.00\,\text{D})(-3.00\,\text{D}) - (-1.73\,\text{D})^2 = +9.01\,\text{D}^2$$

Then Eqs. 13.41 through 13.43 give the spherocylindrical parameters.

$$C = -\sqrt{(-7.00\,\text{D})^2 - 4(+9.01\,\text{D}^2)} = -3.60\,\text{D}$$

$$S = \frac{-7.00\,\text{D} - (-3.60\,\text{D})}{2} = -1.70\,\text{D}$$

$$\tan\theta = \frac{-1.70\,\text{D} - (-4.00\,\text{D})}{-1.73\,\text{D}} = 1.33$$

or

$$\theta = -53^\circ$$

In standard axis notation,

$$\theta = -53 + 180 = 127$$

The resultant lens is $-1.70 \bigcirc -3.60 \times 127$.

If the -3.00 cylindrical lens in the previous two examples was rotated to -3.00×150 and then combined with the -4.00×150 lens, the resultant lens is -7.00×150 (i.e., zero sphere). When the two lenses were perpendicularly crossed in Example 13.10, the resultant lens was $-3.00 \bigcirc -1.00 \times 150$. For the obliquely crossed intermediate case (Example 13.11), we would expect the sphere and cylinder powers to lie between the perpendicularly crossed case and the axes aligned case. The result for the intermediate obliquely crossed case was $-1.70 \bigcirc -3.60 \times 127$. Indeed the sphere power lies between zero and -3.00 D, while the cylinder power lies between -7.00 D and -1.00 D.

Several rules can be developed to help judge whether the final answer for the single lens equivalent to the obliquely crossed combination makes sense or not. The first rule concerns the additivity of the Sp Eq. Whenever two matrices add, it is easy to show that the traces also add. Equation 13.32 showed that the trace τ equals 1/2 of the Sp Eq. Since the traces add, the Sp Eq also add. In other words: *For any two thin spherocylindrical lenses in contact, even obliquely crossed, the Sp Eq of the resultant thin lens is equal to the sum of the Sp Eq of the individual lenses.*

From Eq. 13.32,

$$\text{Sp Eq} = S + \frac{C}{2}$$

For the above example, the Sp Eq of the -3.00×90 lens is -1.50 D, while the Sp Eq of the -4.00×150 lens is -2.00 D. Then from the sum rule, the Sp Eq of the resultant lens must be

$$\text{Sp Eq} = -1.50\,\text{D} + (-2.00\,\text{D}) = -3.50\,\text{D}$$

From the computed sphere and cylinder powers for the resultant lens,

$$\text{Sp Eq} = -1.70 + \frac{-3.60}{2} = -3.50\,\text{D}$$

which checks.

The second rule concerns the resultant cylinder axis. The rule can be stated either in terms of plus or minus cylinder axes. Consider the two minus cylinder axes of the obliquely crossed lenses. One of the angles between the two minus cylinder axes is an acute angle (less than 90°) such as angle w in Figure 13.17a. The rule is that the minus cylinder axis of the resultant lens always lies in the interval occupied by this acute

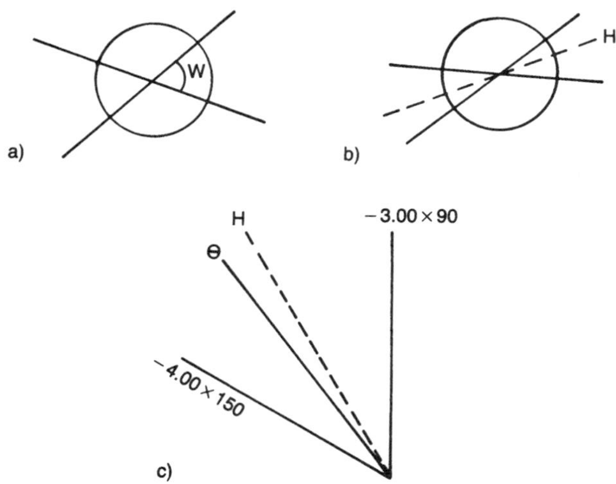

Figure 13.17 a, The acute angle w between two obliquely crossed minus cylinder axis meridians; b, the midway meridian H; c, the resultant minus cylinder axis θ is tilted from H toward the minus cylinder axis meridian of the lens with the most cylinder power.

angle. Furthermore, when the minus cylinder powers of the two obliquely crossed lenses are equal, the resultant minus cylinder axis lies exactly in the middle of the interval occupied by the acute angle (H in Figure 13.17b). When one of the minus cylinder powers is greater in magnitude than the other minus cylinder power, the resultant minus cylinder axis is closer to the axis of the stronger cylinder. This is like a tug-of-war, and the amount closer depends on the difference in the powers.

We can restate the second rule in terms of plus cylinder axes: For two obliquely crossed plus cylinder lenses, the resultant plus cylinder axis lies in the interval occupied by the acute angle between the plus cylinder axes, and is closer to the axis of the stronger cylinder (like a tug-of-war). If the two cylinder powers are equal, the resultant axis is exactly halfway between the two axes of the obliquely crossed lenses (across the acute angle). In cases where one lens is expressed as a plus cylinder and the other as a minus cylinder, we need to transpose one of the lenses to get either both as minus cylinders or both as plus cylinders.

In Example 13.11, the obliquely crossed lenses were −3.00 × 90 and −4.00 × 150. The interval occupied by the 60° acute angle between the axes is from 90 to 150. According to the second rule: if the two cylinder powers were equal, then the resultant axis would be exactly halfway in between or 120 (H in Figure 13.17c). Since the powers are not equal, the resultant minus cylinder axis θ is closer to the axis of the −4.00 × 150, so θ must lie between 120 and 150. The calculated minus cylinder axis was 127, and is consistent with the "tug-of-war" between the −4.00 × 150 versus the −3.00 × 90.

EXAMPLE 13.12

A −8.00 ⊂ −2.00 × 22 lens is combined with a −1.00 ⊂ −5.00 × 72. First, find the Sp Eq of the resultant lens and estimate the minus cylinder axis of the resultant lens. Then calculate the resultant lens parameters.

Rule one states that the Sp Eq add.

Lens	*Sp Eq*
−8.00 ⊂ −2.00 × 22	−9.00 D
	+
−1.00 ⊂ −5.00 × 72	−3.50 D
Resultant Sp Eq	−12.50 D

We don't know the resultant spherocylindrical parameters yet, but the Sp Eq of the resultant lens is −12.50 D.

The acute angle interval between the two minus cylinder axes is 50° (i.e., from meridian 22 to 72). Rule two states that if the cylinder powers were equal, the resultant minus cylinder axis would be exactly halfway between, or at meridian 47. The −5.00 × 72 wins the tug-of-war with the −2.00 × 22, so the resultant minus cylinder axis must lie between 47 and 72. From the tug-of-war idea, let us guess that the resultant minus cylinder axis is around 60. We do not know if that is correct, but we have some intuition that tells us whether or not the calculated answer makes sense.

To calculate the resultant lens parameters, we add the dioptric power matrices for each lens.

Lens	*Matrix*
−8.00 ⊂ −2.00 × 22	$\begin{pmatrix} -8.28\,D & +0.70\,D \\ +0.70\,D & -9.72\,D \end{pmatrix}$
	+
−1.00 ⊂ −5.00 × 72	$\begin{pmatrix} -5.52\,D & +1.47\,D \\ +1.47\,D & -1.48\,D \end{pmatrix}$
Resultant lens	$\begin{pmatrix} -13.80\,D & +2.17\,D \\ +2.17\,D & -11.20\,D \end{pmatrix}$

From the sum matrix, the trace and determinant are:

$$\tau = (-13.803) + (-11.197) = -25.00\,D$$

$$\delta = (-13.803)(-11.197) - (2.164)^2 = +149.85\,D^2$$

From Eq. 13.41 through 13.43:

$$C = -\sqrt{(-25.00\,\text{D})^2 - (4)(+149.85\,\text{D}^2)}$$
$$= -5.06\,\text{D}$$
$$S = \frac{-25.00\,\text{D} - (-5.06\,\text{D})}{2} = -9.97\,\text{D}$$
$$\tan\theta = \frac{-9.97\,\text{D} - (-13.80\,\text{D})}{+2.16\,\text{D}} = +1.76$$

or

$$\theta = \tan^{-1}(+1.76) = 60.5°$$

The resultant lens parameters are $-9.97 \bigcirc -5.06 \times 60.5$.

The axis agrees well with the initial estimate of 60. From Eq. 13.32, the Sp Eq of the resultant lens is

$$\text{Sp Eq} = -9.97 + \frac{-5.06}{2} = -12.50\,\text{D}$$

which also agrees with the initial estimate.

13.13 OVER-REFRACTION

Over-refraction consists of performing a clinical refraction while the person is wearing a spectacle or contact lens. The over-refraction lens determines what additional power that person needs. For generality, we will call the spectacle or contact lens that is being worn the *tentative correction*. Then the combination of the tentative correction and the over-refraction lens gives the Rx. In general, the tentative correction and the over-refraction lens may be obliquely crossed. Then, assuming thin lenses and neglecting the distance between the lenses,

$$\mathbf{P}_{rx} = \mathbf{P}_{tent} + \mathbf{P}_{over} \tag{13.45}$$

where $\mathbf{P}_{over}$ is the dioptric power matrix of the over-refraction lens, $\mathbf{P}_{tent}$ is the dioptric power matrix of the tentative correction, and $\mathbf{P}_{rx}$ is the dioptric power matrix of the Rx. Similarly, the Sp Eq sum rule gives

$$\text{Sp Eq}_{rx} = \text{Sp Eq}_{tent} + \text{Sp Eq}_{over} \tag{13.46}$$

EXAMPLE 13.13

Consider an aphake who is wearing a $+15.00 \bigcirc -3.00 \times 170$ spectacle lens. An over-refraction shows that he needs an additional $-0.50 \bigcirc -0.50 \times 150$ lens. Neglecting the vertex distance (and assuming thin lenses), what is the patient's new Rx?

Here the $+15.00 \bigcirc -3.00 \times 170$ spectacle lens is the tentative correction and is obliquely crossed with the over-refraction lens. Before solving the matrices let us first make expectations about the Sp Eq and the resultant cylinder axis. Equation 13.46 gives:

Lens	*Sp Eq*
$+15.00 \bigcirc -3.00 \times 170$	+13.50 D
	+
$-0.50 \bigcirc -0.50 \times 150$	−0.75 D
Resultant Sp Eq	+12.75 D

To estimate the resultant axis: the acute angle between the two minus cylinder axes is 20° (from 150 to 170). If the cylinder powers were equal, the resultant cylinder axis θ would be at 160. Here the -3.00×170 wins the tug-of-war with the -0.50×150, so θ must lie between 160 and 170. Since the −3.00 D is quite a bit stronger than the −0.50 D, let us estimate 166 for θ.

From Eq. 13.45, the matrix calculations are:

Lens	*Matrix*
$+15.00 \bigcirc -3.00 \times 170$	$\begin{pmatrix} +14.91\,\text{D} & -0.51\,\text{D} \\ -0.51\,\text{D} & +12.09\,\text{D} \end{pmatrix}$
	+
$-0.50 \bigcirc -0.50 \times 150$	$\begin{pmatrix} -0.63\,\text{D} & -0.22\,\text{D} \\ -0.22\,\text{D} & -0.88\,\text{D} \end{pmatrix}$
$\mathbf{P}_{rx}$	$\begin{pmatrix} +14.29\,\text{D} & -0.73\,\text{D} \\ -0.73\,\text{D} & +11.21\,\text{D} \end{pmatrix}$

From the resultant matrix, the trace and determinant are

$$\tau = +14.29\,\text{D} + 11.21\,\text{D} = +25.50\,\text{D}$$
$$\delta = (+14.29\,\text{D})(+11.21\,\text{D}) - (-0.3)^2 = 159.80\,\text{D}^2$$

From Eqs. 13.41 through 13.43:

$$C = -\sqrt{(25.50\,\text{D})^2 - (4)(159.90\,\text{D}^2)} = -3.40\,\text{D}$$
$$S = \frac{+25.50 - (-3.40)}{2} = +14.45\,\text{D}$$
$$\tan\theta = \frac{+14.45 - 14.29}{-0.73} = -0.23$$
$$\theta = \tan^{-1}(-0.23) = -12.7°$$

In standard axis notations, the minus cylinder axis is $-12.7 + 180 = 167.3°$.

Based on the estimate of 166° for the axis, the calculated value of 167.3 makes intuitive sense. From Eq. 13.32, the Sp Eq of the resultant lens is:

$$\text{Sp Eq} = S + \frac{C}{2}$$

$$= +14.45 + \frac{(-3.40)}{2} = +12.75\,\text{D}$$

which also agrees with the expectations. To the nearest quarter diopter, the new Rx is $+14.50 \bigcirc -3.50 \times 167$ compared to the $+15.00 \bigcirc -3.00 \times 170$ that the aphake was wearing.

EXAMPLE 13.14

Attorney James Baked-Goods has an Rx at the cornea of $-4.00 \bigcirc -2.00 \times 90$. Baked-Goods is wearing a contact lens fit on K (i.e., no tears lens effect), and an over-refraction results in a $+0.45 \bigcirc -0.90 \times 128.5$ over-refraction lens. Neglecting vergence effectivity, what are the spherocylindrical parameters of the contact lens that the patient is wearing?

Here the "unknown" contact lens on the eye functions like the tentative Rx. Then from Eq. 13.45,

$$\mathbf{P}_{\text{tent}} = \mathbf{P}_{\text{rx}} - \mathbf{P}_{\text{over}}$$

Similarly from Eq. 13.46,

$$\text{Sp Eq}_{\text{tent}} = \text{Sp Eq}_{\text{rx}} - \text{Sp Eq}_{\text{over}}$$

We can solve these equations for the spherocylindrical parameters of the tentative lens (i.e., the contact lens). Let us first look at the Sp Eq expectations. The Sp Eq of the $-4.00 \bigcirc -2.00 \times 90$ Rx is -3.00 D, while the Sp Eq of the $+0.45 \bigcirc -0.90 \times 128.5$ over-refraction lens is zero. Then from the above equation, the Sp Eq of the tentative lens is also -3.00 D. We don't yet know the spherocylindrical parameters of the tentative lens, but we do know that its Sp Eq has to be -3.00 D.

The matrix equation for $\mathbf{P}_{\text{tent}}$ gives:

Lens	*Matrix*
$-4.00 \bigcirc -2.00 \times 90$	$\begin{pmatrix} -6.00\,\text{D} & 0 \\ 0 & -4.00\,\text{D} \end{pmatrix}$
	−
$+0.45 \bigcirc -0.90 \times 128.5$	$\begin{pmatrix} -0.10\,\text{D} & -0.44\,\text{D} \\ -0.44\,\text{D} & +0.10\,\text{D} \end{pmatrix}$
$\mathbf{P}_{\text{tent}}$	$\begin{pmatrix} -5.90\,\text{D} & +0.44\,\text{D} \\ +0.44\,\text{D} & -4.10\,\text{D} \end{pmatrix}$

From Eqs. 13.41 through 13.43, the spherocylindrical parameters for the tentative lens (i.e., the contact lens) are $-4.00 \bigcirc -2.00 \times 77$. From the Rx, the contact lens was supposed to have parameters $-4.00 \bigcirc -2.00 \times 90$. Here the sphere and cylinder powers of the contact lens are correct, but when placed on the eye the contact lens has incorrectly rotated 13° to from axis 90 to axis 77.

In the above example, the tentative lens (the contact lens) had the correct sphere and cylinder power, the Sp Eq of the tentative lens equaled the Sp Eq of the Rx (both -3.00 D), and the Sp Eq of the over-refraction lens was zero. In general, the Sp Eq sum rule shows that whenever the tentative lens has the correct sphere and cylinder power but is not oriented at the correct axis, the over-refraction lens has to have a zero Sp Eq. From Section 10.4, a spherocylindrical lens with a zero Sp Eq is a Jackson Cross Cylinder (JCC). Therefore, *when the tentative correction has the proper sphere and cylinder power but does not have the correct cylinder axis θ (i.e. differs from the correction only by a clockwise or counter-clockwise orientation), the over-refraction lens is a JCC.*

For a distant point source, the proper spherocylindrical correction in front of an astigmatic eye collapses the conoid of Sturm inside the eye and results in a point image on the retina. If the correction is then rotated clockwise or counter-clockwise, this results in a new conoid of Sturm in the eye. This new conoid is the same conoid that exists when a tentative correction has the correct sphere and cylinder power but does not have the correct cylinder axis. Here the zero Sp Eq of the over-refraction lens means that the circle of least confusion of the new conoid stays on the retina, which is characteristic of an equal mixed astigmatism (EMA) situation. In other words, in the new conoid created by rotating a correction, one line image moves in front of the retina, the other line image wants to move behind the retina by the same dioptric distance, and the circle of least confusion stays on the retina.

In the situation of the above two paragraphs, we also need to consider the cylinder axis of the over-refraction lens. Assume that a tentative lens has spherocylindrical parameters $S \bigcirc C \times \theta$, and that S and C are correct but the minus cylinder axis θ differs slightly from the correct minus cylinder axis. In this case, perhaps surprisingly, the minus cylinder axis of the over-refraction lens differs by about 45° from θ. We'll illustrate this with the following example.

Ms. Cran Berry's Rx is $+5.00 \bigcirc -3.00 \times 10$, and she is wearing a $+5.00 \bigcirc -3.00 \times 180$ tentative lens. These two lenses are obliquely crossed. When we solve Eq. 13.45 for the over-refraction dioptric power matrix, we get

$$\mathbf{P}_{\text{over}} = \mathbf{P}_{\text{rx}} - \mathbf{P}_{\text{tent}} \qquad (13.47)$$

Before solving the matrix equation, let us first estimate the axis of the over-refraction lens. We can start by symbolically representing the problem as

$$[\text{over-refraction lens}] = [+5.00 \bigcirc -3.00 \times 10] - [+5.00 \bigcirc -3.00 \times 180]$$

To make the axis estimation, we need to be adding two obliquely crossed lenses not subtracting them. We can achieve this by bringing the minus sign inside the second brackets, in which case

$$[\text{over-refraction lens}] = [+5.00 \bigcirc -3.00 \times 10] + [-5.00 \bigcirc +3.00 \times 180]$$

Now we are adding a minus cylinder lens and a plus cylinder lens, but for the axis estimation we need the cylinder powers to have the same sign. We can achieve this by transposing the second lens to get

$$[\text{over-refraction lens}] = [+5.00 \bigcirc -3.00 \times 10] + [-2.00 \bigcirc -3.00 \times 90]$$

Now we can estimate the minus cylinder axis of the over-refraction lens from the combination of the -3.00×10 and the -3.00×90. The acute angle between the axis is the 80° angle between 90 and 10. The cylinder powers are equal, so the "estimated" axis must be exactly halfway between 90 and 10, which is the 50 meridian.

In summary, Cran Berry's tentative correction had a minus cylinder axis 10, which was a little off. The resulting (exactly) estimated minus cylinder axis of the over-refraction lens is 50, which is 40° different from 10, and is consistent with the "about" 45° statement.

We can use Eq. 13.47 to verify the axis estimate.

Lens	*Matrix*
$+5.00 \bigcirc -3.00 \times 10$	$\begin{pmatrix} -4.91\,\text{D} & +0.51\,\text{D} \\ +0.51\,\text{D} & -2.09\,\text{D} \end{pmatrix}$
	$-$
$+5.00 \bigcirc -3.00 \times 180$	$\begin{pmatrix} +5.00\,\text{D} & 0 \\ 0 & +2.00\,\text{D} \end{pmatrix}$
$\mathbf{P}_{\mathbf{over}}$	$\begin{pmatrix} -0.09\,\text{D} & +0.51\,\text{D} \\ +0.51\,\text{D} & +0.09\,\text{D} \end{pmatrix}$

Then from Eqs. 13.41 through 13.43, the spherocylindrical parameters of the over-refraction lens are $+0.52 \bigcirc -1.04 \times 50$. The over-refraction lens has a Sp Eq of zero (as expected) and a minus cylinder axis of 50 (as expected).

Similarly in Example 13.14, the (originally unknown) contact lens was the tentative lens and had a slightly incorrect minus cylinder axis of 77. The over-refraction lens has a minus cylinder axis of 128.5, which is 41.5° away from 77. Had the contact lens minus cylinder axis been even closer to the minus cylinder axis of the Rx, the difference would be even closer to 45°.

13.14 THE VECTOR ADDITION METHOD

Besides the dioptric power matrix method, there are other methods for solving the obliquely crossed lens problem. One of the other methods is a vector addition approach.

The vector addition approach can be derived from the additivity of the dioptric power matrices as follows. For a spherocylindrical lens with parameters $S \bigcirc C \times \theta$, Eqs. 13.23 together with 13.25 through 13.27 give

$$\mathbf{P} = \begin{pmatrix} S + C\sin^2\theta & -C\sin\theta\cos\theta \\ -C\sin\theta\cos\theta & S + C\cos^2\theta \end{pmatrix}$$

From trigonometry,

$$\sin^2\theta = \frac{1 - \cos 2\theta}{2}$$

and

$$\sin\theta\cos\theta = \frac{\sin 2\theta}{2}$$

Note that the argument of the sine and cosine on the right side of the above two equations is 2 times the cylinder axis θ. We can substitute the above two trigonometry equations into the matrix equation for $\mathbf{P}$ to obtain

$$\mathbf{P} = \begin{pmatrix} S + \frac{C}{2} - \frac{C\cos 2\theta}{2} & -\frac{C\sin 2\theta}{2} \\ \frac{-C\sin 2\theta}{2} & S + \frac{C}{2} + \frac{C\sin 2\theta}{2} \end{pmatrix}$$

We can then rewrite the right hand side of this equation as the matrix sum

$$\mathbf{P} = \text{Sp Eq}\begin{pmatrix} 1 & 0 \\ 0 & 1 \end{pmatrix} + \frac{1}{2}\begin{pmatrix} -C\cos 2\theta & -C\sin 2\theta \\ -C\sin 2\theta & +C\cos 2\theta \end{pmatrix} \quad (13.48)$$

The addition of the dioptric power matrices meant that the three elements, P_x, P_y, and P_t, are respectively additive. In the above equation for $\mathbf{P}$, the matrix on the far right has only two independent numbers: $C\cos 2\theta$ and $C\sin 2\theta$. The third independent number is the Sp Eq. Thus, the addition of the dioptric power matrices

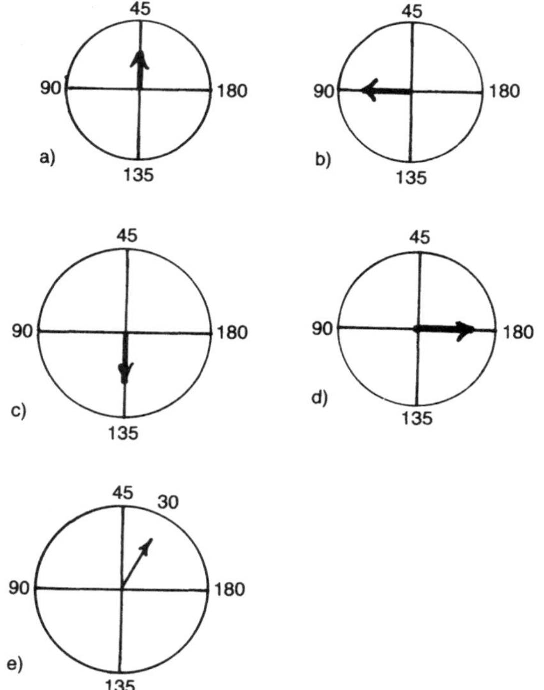

Figure 13.18 Vector representations of cylinder power and axis (double-angle plots): a, +2.00×45; b, +2.00×90; c, +2.00×135 (or −2.00×45); d, +2.00×180; c, +2.00×30.

also means that the three numbers Sp Eq, $C \cos 2\theta$, and $C \sin 2\theta$ are respectively additive.

We discussed the additivity of the Sp Eq in Section 13.12. The new information is that the two numbers, $C \cos 2\theta$ and $C \sin 2\theta$, are also additive. The latter two numbers act like the components of a vector of length C and direction 2θ. The additivity of the components means that the cylinders satisfy vector addition rules provided the angles used are 2 times the cylinder axis (i.e., 2θ). This vector addition can be represented graphically using a coordinate system in which the angles are doubled.

Figure 13.18a shows such a double-angle coordinate system. The vector representing a +2.00 × 45 lens is plotted at 90° (i.e., the vector points straight up). The vector representing a +2.00 × 90 lens is plotted at 180° (i.e., pointing left in Figure 13.18b). The vector representing a +2.00 × 135 lens is plotted at 270° (or straight down in Figure 13.18c). The vector representing a +2.00 × 180 lens is plotted at 360° (or right in Figure 13.18d). The vector representing +2.00 × 30 lens is plotted at 60° (Figure 13.18e).

The vector for a minus cylindrical lens points in the opposite direction relative to the vector for a plus cylindrical lens with the same axis. For example, the vector for a +2.00 × 45 lens points up, and so the vector for a −2.00 × 45 lens points down. Note that the vector pointing down also represents a +2.00 × 135 cylindrical lens. This is a manifestation of the standard transposition properties (since a −2.00 × 45 lens transposes to a −2.00 ◯ +2.00 × 135 lens). Remember that the vector is representing only the cylinder power and axis. The Sp Eq contains the spherical power.

On a double-angle plot, the obliquely crossed cylinder powers add vectorally to give the resultant cylinder power and axis. Then the Sp Eq sum gives the resultant sphere power.

EXAMPLE 13.15

Consider a +4.00 × 50 combined with a +3.00 × 90. What single spherocylindrical lens is equivalent to the combination?

In Figure 13.19, the +4.00 × 50 is plotted @ 100°, the +3.00 × 90 is plotted @ 180° (i.e., to the left). The vector sum algebra is the same as for adding prisms (Section 11.10). The vector sum gives a vector of length 5.40 @ 134°. Since this is a double-angle plot, the cylinder power and axis of the single spherocylindrical lens that is equivalent to the combination is +5.40 × 67. The resultant sphere value can then be computed from the fact that the Sq Eq add to +3.50 D. I.e.,

$$\text{Sp Eq} = S + \frac{C}{2}$$

gives

$$+3.50 = S + (5.40/2)$$

and

$$S = +0.80\,\text{D}$$

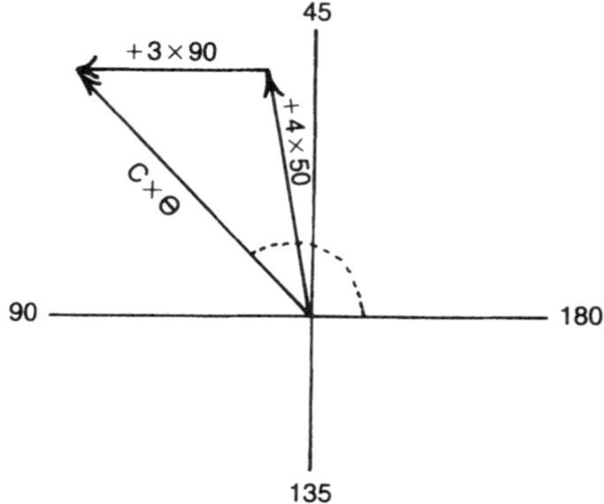

Figure 13.19 Vector sum for cylinder power (double angle plot).

Thus, the single lens equivalent to the combination has spherocylindrical parameters $+0.80 \bigcirc +5.40 \times 67$. (You can also obtain these results by adding the dioptric power matrices.)

A nice feature of the double-angle vector addition method for obliquely crossed lenses is that one can make a quick graphical sketch to estimate the resultant cylinder power and axis (as in Figure 13.19).

13.15 THE RESIDUAL REFRACTIVE ERROR

Recall that the thin lens and screen eye model for the typical unaccommodated emmetrope was a +60.00 D thin lens located 16.67 mm in front of the screen that represents the retina. Now consider an unaccommodated eye model with a +62.00 D thin lens still located 16.67 mm in front of the screen (retina). This eye model represents a 2.00 D myopic eye. In other words, the +62.00 D lens has 2.00 D too much plus, or has a refractive error of +2.00 D. The correction at the cornea neutralizes the refractive error, and the Rx is −2.00 D. Note that the refractive error has a dioptric power that is opposite in sign to the Rx.

Now suppose that a tentative lens of −1.50 D is placed at the cornea of the 2.00 D myopic eye. These are spherical lenses, so the matrix Eq. 13.47 reduces to the spherical powers, and

$$P_{over} = P_{rx} - P_{tent}$$
$$= -2.00\,\text{D} - (-1.50\,\text{D}) = -0.50\,\text{D}$$

The −1.50 D lens corrects 1.50 D of the +2.00 D refractive error so there is still a +0.50 error left. Let us call this the residual refractive error. In this case, the over-refraction lens (−0.50 D) neutralizes the residual refractive error (+0.50 D). Note that the over-refraction lens has a dioptric power that is opposite in sign to the power of the residual refractive error.

We can rewrite the above equation in the terms of the errors to get

$$-P_{res} = -P_{err} - P_{tent}$$

or

$$P_{res} = P_{err} + P_{tent}$$

where P_{res} is the dioptric power of the residual error and P_{err} is the dioptric power of the refractive error.

In cases of astigmatism, the tentative lens may be incorrect in cylinder axis as well as in sphere and cylinder powers. In general then the tentative lens can be obliquely crossed with the refractive error. Here the dioptric power matrices are additive, or

$$\mathbf{P}_{res} = \mathbf{P}_{err} + \mathbf{P}_{tent} \tag{13.49}$$

In the case of spherical ametropes (i.e., no astigmats), when the tentative lens is close to the correction, it almost neutralizes the refractive error and the dioptric power of the residual refractive error is small. Now consider the case of astigmats where the tentative correction has the correct sphere and cylinder power but has a slightly incorrect cylinder axis θ. Here we expect the residual refractive error to have small dioptric parameters (i.e., sphere and cylinder power). However, as discussed in Section 13.13, the cylinder axis of the over-refraction lens is about 45° away from θ.

The double-angle vector addition method of the previous section gives a pictorial representation of the origins of the "about" 45° difference. In Figure 13.20, the vector **A** pointing up and to the right represents the cylinder power and axis of the refractive error. The vector for the correction should have the same length and point in the opposite direction (along the dashed line), and in that case the two vectors would add to give a zero residual error vector. Now suppose the correction is rotated to a slightly different axis θ so that its vector **B** points straight down. The rotated lens is now the tentative correction. The vector sum of the refractive error **A** and the tentative correction **B** gives the vector **E** for the residual refractive error. Figure 13.20 graphically shows that the vector

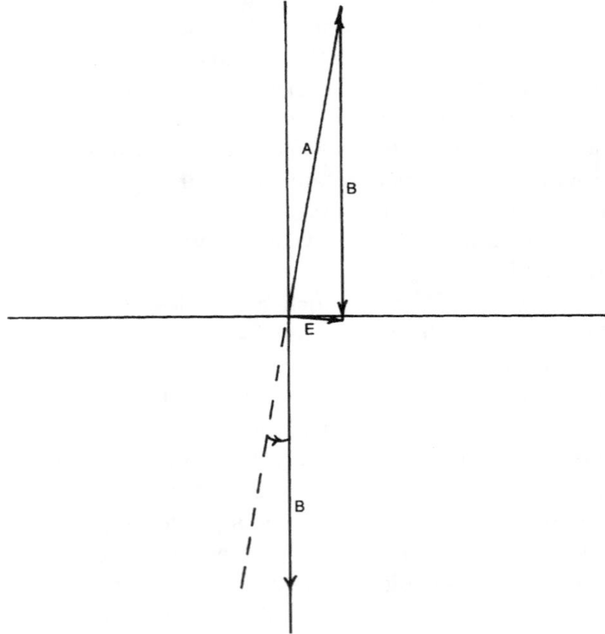

Figure 13.20 A is the refractive error, B is the tentative correction, and E is the residual refractive error.

E is almost perpendicular to the vector **B**. Since this is a double-angle plot, this means that the axis of the residual refractive error is about 45° (i.e., one half of 90°) from the axis of lens **B**. As the tentative lens (represented by vector **B**) is rotated to the correct axis, the residual refractive error vector **E** shrinks to zero length but on the double-angle plot continually gets closer to being perpendicular to the vector **B** while shrinking.

13.16 AXIS REFINEMENT WITH A JCC

Consider a +0.25 ◯ −0.50 × 180 JCC. On a phoropter, the JCC lens can be rotated clockwise or counterclockwise (e.g., a 17° rotation gives +0.25 ◯ −0.50 ×17). The JCC can also be flipped about a meridian that is 45° away from a principal meridian. The flip simply exchanges the powers in the principal meridians. When flipped, a +0.25 ◯ −0.50 × 180 JCC becomes a +0.25 ◯ −0.50 × 90 JCC.

For a tentative correction determined in some manner (clockdial, retinoscopy, auto-refraction, old Rx, etc.), Section 10.14 discussed the Jackson Cross Cylinder (JCC) test for refining the cylinder power. For a distant point source, Example 10.16 showed that when a JCC is placed in front of an emmetropic eye it creates a conoid of Sturm in the eye with the circle of least confusion on the retina. When the JCC is flipped, the line images change positions, but the circle of least confusion remains on the retina and remains the same size. Thus the endpoint of a JCC refinement test occurs when the flips give no difference in blur.

The JCC tests are very efficient when the tentative spherocylindrical parameters are close to the Rx. As discussed in previous sections when the tentative cylinder axis θ is close to the actual Rx, an over-refraction lens will have an axis that is about 45° from θ. Another way of saying this is that the axis of the residual refractive error is about 45° from θ. The JCC test for axis refinement depends on this "about" 45° difference.

When the tentative cylinder power and/or minus cylinder axis θ are not quite right, a conoid of Sturm still exists in the patient's eye. The tentative spherical lens power is then adjusted to give the best acuity for a letter chart. This adjustment places the circle of least confusion on the retina. Then for axis refinement, a JCC is placed in front of the tentative correction with the minus cylinder axis of the JCC 45° away from θ (e.g., for a tentative correction of −1.50 × 80, the JCC is placed at a minus cylinder axis of either 35 or 125).

Since the JCC has a zero Sp Eq, it leaves the circle of least confusion on the patient's retina. The JCC is then flipped (i.e., if position #1 is +0.25 ◯ −0.50 × 35, the flipped position #2 is +0.25 ◯ −0.50 × 125). The circle of least confusion remains on the retina during the flip. In one of these flipped positions, the JCC neutralizes part of the residual refractive error, which make the circle of least confusion smaller. In the other flipped position the JCC increases the residual refractive error, which makes the circle of least confusion larger.

The patient looks through the lenses at an extended target (probably letters) and reports which flipped position gives the better image. The better image corresponds to the flipped position that results in the smaller circle of least confusion on the patient's retina. The minus cylinder axis of the tentative lens is then rotated a little bit toward the minus cylinder axis of the JCC position that gives the clearest image. The JCC is then readjusted so that its minus cylinder axis is again 45° from the minus cylinder axis of the newly oriented tentative lens, and the process is repeated. The process continues until the flipped positions give equally blurred results (i.e., one is not better than the other). This endpoint occurs when the size of the circle of least confusion is unchanged during a flip. The "tentative" cylinder axis at the endpoint is the refined or improved cylinder axis of the correction.

In the axis refinement process, the JCC and the tentative correction lens are obliquely crossed lenses. The theory of the refinement process can be demonstrated graphically with the vector addition approach. Consider a person with a refractive error of +2.00 × 80 (i.e., he or she needs a correction of −2.00 × 80). Suppose the tentative correction given is a −1.50 × 90. In Figure 13.21a, **A** is the vector for the refractive error and **B** is the vector for the −1.50 × 90 lens. The residual refractive error is the vector sum **E** of the refractive error and the tentative correction. (The matrix equations give +0.78 × 59.5 as the cylindrical parameters of the residual refractive error.)

A +0.25 ◯ −0.50 × 45 JCC is now placed in front of the correcting lens. The JCC together with the residual refractive error give the effective refractive error for the patient's vision through the JCC and the tentative correction. On a double-angle plot, the vector for the minus cylinder axis 45 JCC points down, while the vector for the flipped position (minus cylinder axis 135) points up. Figure 13.21b shows the vector sum #1 of the residual refractive error **E** combined with the JCC minus cylinder axis 45 and the vector sum #2 for **E** combined with the flipped JCC (i.e., minus cylinder axis 135). The vector sum #1 for the JCC pointing down is smaller in magnitude than the vector sum #2 for the JCC pointing up. The smaller magnitude #1 means that the effective refractive error is less, and the patient has a smaller circle of least confusion on the retina. Here position #1 occurs for the JCC minus

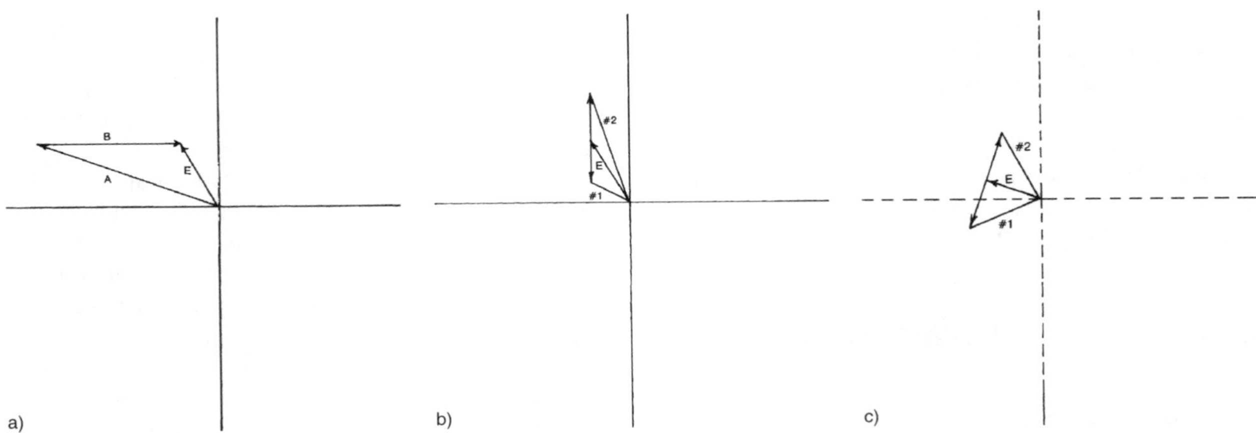

Figure 13.21 a, A is the refractive error, B is the tentative correction, and E is the residual refractive error; b, #1 and #2 are the vector sums of the residual refractive error with the two flipped positions of the JCC; c, same as the previous part for the correct cylinder axis.

cylinder axis 45, and the patient will report #1 is better than #2. Once the patient reports #1 as better, the examiner moves the tentative axis of the correction from 90 a little bit toward 45.

Suppose the tentative axis is now rotated to 80. The refractive error is still $+2.00 \times 80$ and now the tentative correction is -1.50×80. Here the principal meridians are aligned, and the residual refractive error is simply $+0.50 \times 80$, which is represented by vector **E** in Figure 13.21c. The JCC positions now have minus cylinder axis 35 (#1) and minus cylinder axis 125 (#2), and on the double-angle plot the JCC vectors are perpendicular to the residual refractive error vector **E**. The vector sums #1 and #2 represent the resultant refractive error through the JCC and the tentative correction. Here the #1 and #2 vector sums are equal in magnitude, which means that the circle of least confusion on the retina stays the same size when the JCC is flipped. Thus, the patient reports that the two positions are equal (actually equally blurred). Since we have equality, the minus cylinder axis 80 is the refined axis of the correction.

In summary, the endpoint of the test occurs when the axis of the tentative correcting lens is the correct axis of the Rx. In this case, the JCC vector is perpendicular to the residual refractive error vector **E**, and the two JCC flipped positions give the same length for the resultant vectors #1 and #2 that represent the resultant refractive error with the JCC in place over the tentative correction. This means that the circle of least confusion on the patient's retina is unchanged in size when the JCC is flipped. Here the patient reports that #1 and #2 result in equal images (actually equally blurred). When the tentative axis is not correct, the vector for the JCC is not perpendicular to the residual refractive error vector, and then one of the JCC positions gives a shorter sum (either #1 or #2). The circle of least confusion on the patient's retina is smaller for the shorter sum, and the patient reports that choice results in a better (less blurred) image. The tentative minus cylinder axis of the correction is then rotated a little bit toward the better minus cylinder JCC axis and the process is repeated. A tremendous advantage of the JCC process is that the cylinder axis can be refined even when the cylinder power is not quite correct. Once the axis refinement is made, then the cylinder power can be refined (as discussed in Section 10.14).

13.17 THE VERGENCE MATRIX

The generalization of the dioptric power for a toric surface is the 2×2 dioptric power matrix **P**. Similarly, the generalization of the vergence for a toric wavefront is a 2×2 vergence matrix **V**.

Consider a toric wavefront with spherocylindrical vergence parameters $S_v \bigcirc C_v \times \theta_v$. Then the vergence matrix is obtained with equations analogous to 13.25 through 13.29:

$$\mathbf{V} = \begin{pmatrix} V_x & V_t \\ V_t & V_y \end{pmatrix}$$

where,

$$V_x = S_v + C_v \sin^2 \theta_v$$

$$V_y = S_v + C_v \cos^2 \theta_v$$

$$V_t = -C_v \sin \theta_v \cos \theta_v$$

Here V_x is directly related to the horizontal curvature of the toric wavefront, V_y is directly related to the vertical curvature, and V_t is directly related to the wavefront torsion in the horizontal and in the vertical meridians. Given the matrix **V**, the spherocylindrical parameters can be extracted from the same trace and determinant equations that work for the dioptric power matrix **P**.

Consider a toric wavefront incident on a toric surface (or thin spherocylindrical lens). The matrices are additive even when the wavefront and the surface are obliquely crossed, i.e.,

$$\mathbf{V} = \mathbf{P} + \mathbf{U} \tag{13.50}$$

where **U** is the 2 × 2 vergence matrix for the incident wavefront **V** is the 2 × 2 matrix for the emergent wavefront, and **P** is the 2 × 2 matrix for the surface.

EXAMPLE 13.16

A +4.00 × 45 thin lens is 10 cm in front of a +5.00 × 90 thin lens. What are the back vertex power spherocylindrical parameters for this system? What are the neutralizing (or front vertex) power spherocylindrical parameters for this system?

The back vertex power is the vergence leaving the back of the system when plane waves are incident on the front. For incident plane waves, the front surface creates a cylindrical wavefront with principal meridians at 45 and 135. There is zero vergence in the 45 meridian, and this vergence does not change as the wave propagates downstream to the second lens. There is +4.00 D vergence in the 135 meridian. The radius of curvature of the wavefront in the 135 meridian is 25 cm (i.e., 100/4.00 D), and 10 cm downstream the wave has a radius curvature of 15 cm (i.e., 25 − 10) in the 135 meridian, or a vergence of +6.67 D. Thus a cylindrical wavefront of vergence +6.67 × 45 is incident on the +5.00 × 90 lens. The vergence equations give the vergence matrix **U** of

$$\mathbf{U} = \begin{pmatrix} +3.33\,\text{D} & -3.33\,\text{D} \\ +3.33\,\text{D} & +3.33\,\text{D} \end{pmatrix}$$

The dioptric power matrix for the +5.00 × 90 lens is

$$\mathbf{P} = \begin{pmatrix} +5.00\,\text{D} & 0 \\ 0 & 0 \end{pmatrix}$$

The back vertex dioptric power matrix $\mathbf{P_v}$ equals **V**, and Eq. 13.50 gives

$$\mathbf{P_v} = \begin{pmatrix} +8.33\,\text{D} & -3.33\,\text{D} \\ +3.33\,\text{D} & +3.33\,\text{D} \end{pmatrix}$$

Then from the trace and determinant equations (i.e., 13.30, 13.35, and 13.41 through 13.43), the back vertex power spherocylindrical parameters are +1.67 ⬭ +8.33 × 63.4.

We can find the front vertex or neutralizing power by reversing the light and considering plane waves incident on the +5.00 × 90 lens. Then the neutralizing dioptric power is equal to the vergence that emerges from the +4.00 × 45 lens. For the reversed light, a +5.00 × 90 cylindrical wave leaves the +5.00 × 90 lens, and from downstream vergence changes this wave has a vergence of +10.00 × 45 when it hits the +4.00 × 45 lens. Then,

$$\mathbf{U} = \begin{pmatrix} +10.00\,\text{D} & 0 \\ 0 & 0 \end{pmatrix}$$

The dioptric power matrix for the +4.00 × 45 lens is

$$\mathbf{P} = \begin{pmatrix} +2.00\,\text{D} & -2.00\,\text{D} \\ -2.00\,\text{D} & +2.00\,\text{D} \end{pmatrix}$$

Then Eq. 13.50 gives a neutralizing dioptric power matrix of

$$\mathbf{P_n} = \mathbf{V} = \begin{pmatrix} +12.00\,\text{D} & -2.00\,\text{D} \\ -2.00\,\text{D} & +2.00\,\text{D} \end{pmatrix}$$

From $\mathbf{P_n}$, the neutralizing power spherocylindrical parameters are +1.61 ⬭ +10.77 × 79.1. Note that the principal meridians are not the same for the front and back vertex powers.

For the horizontal meridian, Eq. 13.50 shows that curvital components are additive,

$$V_x = P_x + U_x$$

and that the torsional components are additive,

$$V_t = P_t + U_t$$

So the torsional vergence component behaves exactly as the curvital vergence component. The vertical meridian components behave in the same way.

13.18 AVERAGE STRENGTH OF A SPHEROCYLINDRICAL LENS

In situations where the values of an entity are sometimes positive and sometimes negative, an average magnitude of the values independent of the plus-minus sign is obtained by first squaring the values, adding the squares, dividing the sum by the number of values, and then taking the square root. This is called a root-mean-square average. An example is the common 110 volts of alternating current electricity, where the 110 is a root-mean-square average of the voltage. The voltage itself changes sinusoidally back and forth from +156 volts to −156 volts.

Some statistical studies on refractive error and its correction use an average strength of the spherocylindrical lens to refract light (or bend light rays) independent of the direction of the refraction or bending. In such a case, the appropriate average is a root-mean-square average.

Consider a circle of semidiameter h centered on the optical center of a spherocylindrical lens. We first want to find the root-mean-square average of the prism power around this circle. The number of radians in a full circle is 2π. We can track the points around the circle by the angle ϕ (in radians) with the horizontal. In other words the polar coordinates of a point on the circle are h and ϕ. The horizontal and vertical coordinates of a point on the circle are then

$$h_x = h\cos\phi \quad \text{and} \quad h_y = h\sin\phi$$

Let Z_ϕ be a function that equals the prism power in each small angular increment $d\phi$ around the circle. The total number of angular increments around the circle is 2π radians. In the limit of very small increments, the sum in the root-mean-square average becomes a calculus integral, and

$$Z^2_{\text{rms}} = \frac{1}{2\pi}\int_0^{2\pi} Z^2_\phi d\phi \qquad (13.51)$$

where Z_{rms} is the root-mean-square average of the prism power around the circle.

Equations 13.28 and 13.29 give the horizontal and vertical prism components of Z_ϕ. I.e.,

$$Z_x = -P_x h_x - P_t h_y$$

and

$$Z_y = -P_t h_x - P_y h_y$$

Then,

$$Z^2_\phi = Z^2_x + Z^2_y$$

Combining the above 5 equations gives

$$Z^2_{\text{rms}} = \frac{1}{2\pi}\int_0^{2\pi} [(P^2_x + P^2_t)h^2\cos^2\phi + (P^2_t + P^2_y)h^2\sin^2\phi + 2(P_x + P_y)P_t h^2\cos\phi\sin\phi]d\phi$$

We can bring the common factor h^2 outside the integral and note that

$$\frac{1}{2\pi}\int_0^{2\pi}\cos^2\phi d\phi = \frac{1}{2\pi}\int_0^{2\pi}\sin^2\phi d\phi = \frac{1}{2}$$

and

$$\frac{1}{2\pi}\int_0^{2\pi}\cos\phi\sin\phi d\phi = 0$$

Then evaluation of the integral results in

$$Z^2_{\text{rms}} = \frac{h^2}{2}[(P^2_x + P^2_t) + (P^2_t + P^2_y)]$$

or

$$Z^2_{\text{rms}} = \frac{h^2}{2}(P^2_x + 2P^2_t + P^2_y)$$

Taking the square root gives

$$Z_{\text{rms}} = h\sqrt{\frac{P^2_x + 2P^2_t + P^2_y}{2}} \qquad (13.52)$$

Let us define an average dioptric strength of the lens by

$$P_{\text{strength}} = \sqrt{\frac{P^2_x + 2P^2_t + P^2_y}{2}} \qquad (13.53)$$

Then Eq. 13.52 becomes

$$Z_{\text{rms}} = hP_{\text{strength}} \qquad (13.54)$$

which is a Prentice's Rule type equation that relates the root-mean-square prism average and the dioptric average dioptric strength. Equation 13.54 (or 13.52) gives the root-mean-square prism average around any circle of radius h on the lens characterized by P_{strength}. In this sense, P_{strength} is a dioptric value that represents the lens's average strength to refract light (bend rays) independent of the direction of the bending.

Equation 13.52 gives P_{strength} in terms of the curvital and torsional components of the dioptric power matrix as expressed in a horizontal and vertical coordinate system. We can substitute Eqs. 13.25 through 13.27 for the elements into Eq. 13.52, and do some algebra to obtain

$$P_{\text{strength}} = \sqrt{\frac{S^2 + (S+C)^2}{2}} \qquad (13.55)$$

Equations 13.53 and 13.55 give the same value for P_{strength}. Equation 13.55 shows that we can get P_{strength}

by squaring the dioptric powers in the principal meridians, adding them together, dividing by 2, and then taking the square root. Equation 13.55 also explicitly shows that P_{strength} does not depend on the cylinder axis θ.

As an example, consider a $+4.00 \bigcirc -8.00 \times 120$ lens. (This is a JCC lens that corrects equal mixed astigmatism.) The dioptric power matrix for this lens is

$$\mathbf{P} = \begin{pmatrix} -2.00\,\text{D} & -3.46\,\text{D} \\ -3.46\,\text{D} & +2.00\,\text{D} \end{pmatrix}$$

Equation 13.53 gives

$$P_{\text{strength}} = \sqrt{\frac{(-2.00\,\text{D})^2 + 2(-3.46\,\text{D})^2 + (+2.00\,\text{D})^2}{2}}$$
$$= 4.00\,\text{D}$$

When we rotate this lens to $+4.00 \bigcirc -8.00 \times 135$,

$$\mathbf{P} = \begin{pmatrix} 0 & -4.00\,\text{D} \\ -4.00\,\text{D} & 0 \end{pmatrix}$$

Then,

$$P_{\text{strength}} = \sqrt{\frac{(0)^2 + 2(-4.00\,\text{D})^2 + (0)^2}{2}}$$
$$= 4.00\,\text{D}$$

Note that the average strength of this JCC is 4.00 D independent of θ. We can also confirm this from Eq. 13.55 for any $+4.00 \bigcirc -8.00 \times \theta$ lens, or

$$P_{\text{strength}} = \sqrt{\frac{(+4.00)^2 + (+4.00 - 8.00)^2}{2}} = 4.00\,\text{D}$$

Note from Eq. 13.32, that the Sp Eq of this JCC is 0 (as it is for any JCC). Therefore P_{strength} and the Sp Eq supply different information about the dioptric properties of the lens.

When the lens is a spherical lens only, $C = 0$, and Eq. 13.55 gives

$$P_{\text{strength}} = |S|$$

as one might expect. This corresponds to the fact that the prism power has the same magnitude at all points around a circle of semidiameter h centered on the optical center, and the spherical lens has the same power S in all meridians around the circle. Therefore the average strength in magnitude of the lens to refract light (bend rays) is $|S|$.

When the lens is a cylindrical lens, $S = 0$ and Eq. 13.55 gives

$$P_{\text{strength}} = \frac{|C|}{\sqrt{2}}$$

Here around a centered circle on the cylindrical lens, the prism values vary from a maximum (given by $|Z| = |Ch|$) in the principal power meridian to a minimum of zero in the axis meridian, and the average strength of the lens to refract light (bend rays) is $|C|$ divided by the square root of 2. Thus for a -5.00×180 cylindrical lens,

$$P_{\text{rms}} = \frac{|5.00\,\text{D}|}{\sqrt{2}} = 3.54\,\text{D}$$

Note that from Eq. 13.32 the Sp Eq of this lens is −2.50 D.

In matrix theory, the norm of a matrix $\mathbf{P}$, represented as $||\mathbf{P}||$, is the square root of the sum of the squares of the individual elements. For the dioptric power matrix $\mathbf{P}$ given by Eq. 13.23,

$$||\mathbf{P}|| = \sqrt{P_x^2 + P_t^2 + P_t^2 + P_y^2}$$

or

$$||\mathbf{P}|| = \sqrt{P_x^2 + 2P_t^2 + P_y^2} \qquad (13.56)$$

Therefore,

$$||\mathbf{P}|| = \frac{P_{\text{strength}}}{\sqrt{2}} \qquad (13.57)$$

The norm $||\mathbf{P}||$ has sometimes been called the "cylinder equivalent dioptric strength," while P_{strength} has been called the "sphere equivalent dioptric strength."

13.19 THREE DIMENSIONAL DIOPTRIC POWER REPRESENTATIONS

The spherocylindrical parameters $S \bigcirc C \times \theta$ of a collection of lenses are not directly additive. Therefore the many statistical analyses of astigmatic refractive errors and spherocylindrical dioptric power parameters carried out in terms of the S, C, and θ parameters are not based on firm mathematical principles and have questionable validity.

The dioptric power matrix is the underlying basis for a three dimensional mathematically sound statistical analysis of astigmatic refractive errors and spherocylindrical dioptric power parameters. In the three dimensional analysis, the spherocylindrical parameters are represented by a vector in a three dimensional space. Since the dioptric power matrix for a thin lens only has three independent parameters, one set of components for a three dimensional representation is a vector with components P_x, P_t, and P_y. These three components are orthogonal or perpendicular to each other in the three dimensional space. The vector **H** introduced by W.F. Harris has a length that corresponds to the norm of **P** given by Eq. 13.56. The **H** vector has coordinates h_x, h_y, and h_t, where h_t is a scaled torsional component of length equal to $\sqrt{2}P_t$, while h_x equals P_x and h_y equals P_y.

There are a number of other three dimensional representations for the dioptric power. For a sphero-cylindrical lens with parameters $S \bigcirc C \times \theta$, we again start with the dioptric power matrix **P**. We can rewrite Eq. 14.38 for **P** as

$$\mathbf{P} = \text{Sp Eq}\begin{pmatrix} 1 & 0 \\ 0 & 1 \end{pmatrix} + \text{P}_0\begin{pmatrix} +1 & 0 \\ 0 & -1 \end{pmatrix} + \text{P}_{45}\begin{pmatrix} 0 & +1 \\ +1 & 0 \end{pmatrix} \tag{13.58}$$

where,

$$P_0 = -\frac{1}{2}C\cos 2\theta \tag{13.59}$$

and

$$P_{45} = -\frac{1}{2}C\sin 2\theta \tag{13.60}$$

The matrix

$$\begin{pmatrix} 1 & 0 \\ 0 & 1 \end{pmatrix}$$

is the matrix for a +1.00 D sphere, and has a norm of 1. The matrix

$$\begin{pmatrix} +1 & 0 \\ 0 & -1 \end{pmatrix}$$

is the matrix for a $+1.00 \bigcirc -2.00 \times 180$ JCC, and has a norm of 1. The matrix

$$\begin{pmatrix} 0 & +1 \\ +1 & 0 \end{pmatrix}$$

is the matrix for a $+1.00 \bigcirc -2.00 \times 45$ JCC, and also has a norm of 1.

It follows from Eq. 13.58 that we can set up a vector space with basis vectors that represent the +1.00 D sphere, the $+1.00 \bigcirc -2.00 \times 180$ JCC, and the $+1.00 \bigcirc -2.00 \times 45$ JCC. In this space, the components of the vector representing the dioptric power are Sp Eq, P_0, and P_{45}. Similar to the double-angle vectors in Section 13.14, P_0 and P_{45} lens are represented by vectors that are perpendicular to each other. These two vectors define the plane of astigmatism. The three dimensional representation is then obtained by letting a vector perpendicular to the astigmatism plane represent the Sp Eq. Harris calls the Sp Eq component the *nearest equivalent sphere*, the P_0 component, the *ortho-astigmatism* component, and the P_{45} component the *oblique astigmatism* component. The length of the vector with components Sp Eq, P_0, and P_{45} equals the norm $||\mathbf{P}||$ of the dioptric power matrix **P**. (Recall also that Equation 13.57 relates the norm of **P** to the average dioptric strength of the lens.)

(An article with many references to papers on the matrix and vector analysis of astigmatism is: Harris WF. Astigmatism. *Ophthal Physiol Opt* 2000; 11–30.)

PROBLEMS

1. Consider a $+5.00 \bigcirc -4.00 \times 125$ toric interface. As a function of meridians on this surface, what are the maximum and minimum dioptric power curvital components? What is the dioptric power curvital component for the 160 meridian on this interface? As a function of meridians on this surface, what are the maximum and minimum magnitudes of the dioptric power torsional components? What is the magnitude of the dioptric power torsional component in the 160 meridian?
2. Consider a $-2.00 \bigcirc -5.00 \times 115$ toric interface. As a function of meridians on this surface, what are the maximum and minimum dioptric power curvital components? What is the dioptric power curvital component for the 70 meridian on this toric interface? As a function of meridians on this surface, what are the maximum and minimum magnitudes of the dioptric power torsional components? What is the magnitude of the torsional component in the 70 meridian?
3. Find the dioptric power matrix for the following lens:

   a. $+1.00 \bigcirc -4.00 \times 90$.
   b. $+1.00 \bigcirc -4.00 \times 120$.
   c. $+1.00 \bigcirc -4.00 \times 60$.
   d. $+1.00 \bigcirc -4.00 \times 135$.
   e. $+1.00 \bigcirc -4.00 \times 45$.

   Also, a plus torsional component corresponds to a minus cylinder first quadrant axis, and a minus torsional component corresponds to a minus cylinder second quadrant axis. Are the torsional component signs in the dioptric power matrices for parts b–e consistent with this?

4. For each of the lenses in the previous problem find the trace and determinant of the dioptric power matrix.
5. The following dioptric power matrix is equivalent to a power cross with horizontal and vertical principal meridians.

$$\begin{pmatrix} -3.50\,\text{D} & 0 \\ 0 & -5.50\,\text{D} \end{pmatrix}$$

Write the power cross, and from it write down the spherocylindrical parameters in minus cylinder form of the lens corresponding to the matrix.

6. Given the following dioptric power matrices, find the spherocylindrical parameter of the lens in minus cylinder form.

a. $\begin{pmatrix} +0.53\,\text{D} & -1.29\,\text{D} \\ -1.29\,\text{D} & -2.53\,\text{D} \end{pmatrix}$

b. $\begin{pmatrix} -0.84\,\text{D} & +1.35\,\text{D} \\ +1.35\,\text{D} & -2.16\,\text{D} \end{pmatrix}$

c. $\begin{pmatrix} +11.00\,\text{D} & -2.00\,\text{D} \\ -2.00\,\text{D} & +11.00\,\text{D} \end{pmatrix}$

7. What single thin lens is equivalent to a −3.50 × 60 thin lens combined with a −6.25 × 20 thin lens?

8. A patient is wearing a +12.00 ⊂ −3.00 × 110 lens. An over-refraction shows that the patient needs an additional +0.50 ⊂ −1.00 × 135. Assuming thin lenses and neglecting the distance between the lenses, what is the patient's Rx?

9. Kevin Soupy's eye is modeled by two thin lenses in air in front of a screen (the retina). The first thin lens represents the cornea and the second thin lens represents the crystalline lens. In this model, there is no space between the thin lens representing the cornea and the thin lens representing the crystalline lens. The cornea is represented by a thin +45.00 ⊂ −4.00 × 90 lens, while the crystalline lens is represented by a +18.00 ⊂ −3.00 × 135 lens. What are the spherocylindrical parameters of Soupy's eye? (In other words, what single lens is equivalent to the combination?) FYI, the dioptric power matrix for a +18.00 ⊂ −3.00 × 135 lens is

$$\begin{pmatrix} +16.50\,\text{D} & -1.50\,\text{D} \\ -1.50\,\text{D} & +16.50\,\text{D} \end{pmatrix}$$

10. A cornea is represented by a +44.00 ⊂ +3.00 × 180 lens. The crystalline lens is represented by a +19.00 ⊂ +2.00 × 65 lens. The reduced distance between the cornea and crystalline lens is 4.5 mm, and the reduced distance between the crystalline lens and the retina is 15.0 mm. What correction (minus cylinder form) does this eye need at the cornea?

11. From the Sp Eq sum rule, what is the Sp Eq of the resultant of a −5.00 ⊂ −2.00 × 170 combined with a −2.00 ⊂ −4.00 × 124?

12. A +5.00 ⊂ −3.50 × 70 is combined with a spherocylindrical lens of unknown parameters. For a distant point source, the combination forms a conoid of Sturm with a horizontal line image 12.50 cm behind the lenses and a vertical line image 18.18 cm behind the lenses. What are the spherocylindrical parameters of the unknown lens (in minus cylinder form)?

13. Miss Take has an Rx at the cornea of −4.00 ⊂ −2.00 × 180. A rigid contact lens of unknown parameters is placed on the eye. An over-refraction shows that Miss Take needs an additional +0.45 ⊂ −0.90 × 141.5. What are the parameters of the contact lens? How does the contact lens differ from the Rx? With the contact lens on the eye, what part of the conoid of Sturm is on the retina?

14. Mr. Fic Shun needs a correction of −3.00 × 80. Fic Shun is given a tentative correction of −3.00 × 90. An over-refraction is done over the tentative lens. What are the principal meridians of the over-refraction lens? (Note, from the axis estimation rules, that you can answer this without using the matrices.)

15. What does a lens clock read on the 50 meridian of a +5.00 ⊂ −4.00 × 10 plastic ($n = 1.53$) surface?

16. What is the average dioptric strength (magnitude) of a +2.00 ⊂ −6.00 × 146 lens? What is Sp Eq of this lens?

17. What is the average dioptric strength (magnitude) of a +7.00 ⊂ −3.00 × 35 lens? What is Sp Eq of this lens?

18. A spherocylindrical lens has a dioptric power matrix of

$$P = \begin{pmatrix} -1.00\,\text{D} & +5.00\,\text{D} \\ +5.00\,\text{D} & 0.00\,\text{D} \end{pmatrix}$$

From the matrix, what is the average dioptric strength (magnitude) of this lens, and what is the Sp Eq of the lens?

CHAPTER 14

Reflection

14.1 MIRRORS AND OTHER REFLECTING INTERFACES

Chapters 4 through 13 treated image formation by refraction. Images are also formed by reflection. The reflection may be from metallic surfaces that reflect most of the incident light, or the reflection may be from dielectric surfaces, such as glass, which reflect only a small percentage of the incident light.

The law of reflection states that

$$\theta_i = \theta_s \tag{14.1}$$

where θ_i and θ_s, are the angles of incidence and reflection, respectively (Figure 14.1). The media involved influence the percentage of light reflected, but the geometry of Eq. 14.1 is independent of the media.

This chapter covers paraxial image formation by spherical and/or plane mirrors. A convex metallic surface diverges light, so that a diverging mirror is also referred to as a convex mirror (Figure 14.2a). Thus, *for reflection the word convex is associated with divergence, whereas for lenses (refraction) the word convex is associated with convergence.* A concave metallic surface converges light, so that a converging mirror is also referred to as a concave mirror (Figure 14.2b). Thus, *for reflection the word concave is associated with convergence, whereas for lenses (refraction) the word concave is associated with divergence.*

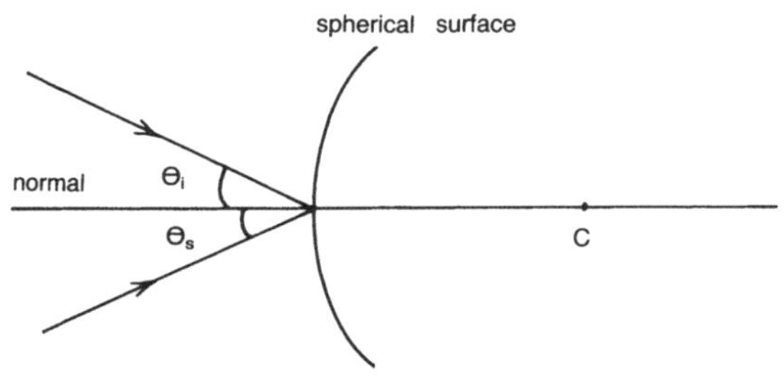

Figure 14.1 Ray reflection at spherical surface.

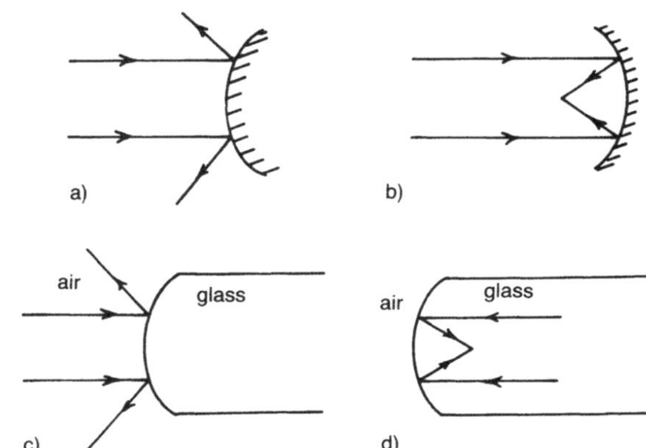

Figure 14.2 a, Divergence by reflection from a convex silvered mirror; b, convergence by reflection from a concave silvered mirror; c, divergence by reflection of light incident in air; d, convergence by reflection of light incident in glass.

An air–glass single spherical refracting interface (SSRI) convex with respect to the lower index medium converges the transmitted light no matter which way the light travels through the interface. The same interface can either diverge or converge the reflected light depending on which way the incident light is traveling. The interface diverges the reflected light incident from the air side, but converges the reflected light incident from the glass side (Figures 14.2c and d). Thus, we need to take the direction of propagation into account in deciding whether a particular spherical interface acts like a converging or a diverging mirror.

When light in a transparent medium of refractive index n_1 is incident on a transparent medium of refractive index n_2 the percentage of light $R_{\%}$ that is paraxially reflected is given by Fresnel's law:

$$R_{\%} = \left(\frac{n_2 - n_1}{n_2 + n_1}\right)^2 100\% \tag{14.2}$$

The refractive indices n_1 and n_2 can be exchanged in Eq. 14.2 without changing the value of $R_{\%}$. This means that the percentage of light reflected at an interface is the same no matter which medium the light is initially in.

Fresnel's law for paraxial light reflected from an interface between two transparent media can be derived from Maxwell's classical electromagnetic equations. As such, $R_{\%}$ is a fundamental electromagnetic property of the materials involved. This chapter treats only the paraxial situation, but you should be aware that the percent reflection increases outside the paraxial region.

EXAMPLE 14.1

Light in air is paraxially incident on an air-CR-39 plastic ($n = 1.498$) interface. What percentage of the incident light is reflected?

From Eq. 14.2,

$$R_{\%} = \left(\frac{1.498 - 1.000}{1.498 + 1.000}\right)^2 100\%$$
$$= \left(\frac{0.498}{2.498}\right)^2 100\%$$
$$= (0.040)100\% = 4.0\%$$

Since 4.0% of the incident light is reflected at the air–glass interface, 96.0% of the incident light is transmitted through the interface and refracted. The percent reflected is independent of which medium the light is initially in. So if the light is reversed and is incident on the air–glass interface from the glass side, then again 4.0% of the incident light is reflected.

EXAMPLE 14.2

Light is paraxially incident on a water ($n = 1.333$)–ophthalmic crown glass ($n = 1.523$) interface. What percent of the incident light is reflected?

$$R_{\%} = \left(\frac{1.523 - 1.333}{1.523 + 1.333}\right)^2 100\%.$$
$$= (0.067)^2 100\% = 0.4\%$$

Only 0.4% of the incident light is reflected at the water–glass interface, so 99.6% is transmitted.

From Fresnel's law, the percentage of light reflected at an interface between two transparent media depends on the difference in refractive indices. The higher the difference, the larger the percent reflection, and vice versa. The percentage reflected at an air–water ($n = 1.33$) interface is 2.0%, while the percentage reflected at an air–diamond ($n = 2.4$) interface is 17.0%. The first example above showed that a CR-39 spectacle lens interface in air reflects 4.0%. For spectacles in air, a polycarbonate ($n = 1.586$) interface reflects 5.1%, while a high index glass interface ($n = 1.9$) reflects 9.6%.

A 2%, 3%, or 4% reflection is a small percentage. However, the incident luminance may be high enough so that these small percentages are significant (e.g., 4% of 4 million dollars is $160,000.) Also, according to Steven's power law, the suprathreshold subjective sensation of brightness in the human visual system under normal illumination is proportional to the cube root of the luminance. In other words, when the incident luminance is 100 units, 4% reflection gives a luminance of 4 units. However, the subjective human sensation of brightness for the two luminances is respectively proportional to $100^{1/3}$, which is 4.64, and $4^{1/3}$, which is 1.59. Thus the relative subjective brightness of the reflected light to the incident light is 1.59/4.64, which is 0.34. So even though the reflected luminance is only 4% of the incident luminance, the reflected light gives a relative subjective brightness response that is 34% of that given by the incident luminance. Similarly a 0.5% reflection gives a relative subjective brightness response that is 17% of the response given by the incident light.

A lens has two interfaces, and some light is reflected at each interface. A first approximation to the total percent reflection by the lens is just twice that reflected at each interface. A more accurate calculation takes into account the fact that not all the incident light gets to the second interface, and a still more accurate calculation would take into account multiple reflections back and forth across the interior of the lens.

EXAMPLE 14.3

Taking into account only single reflections, what percent of the incident light is transmitted by a CR-39 plastic spectacle lens ($n = 1.498$) in air?

From Example 14.1, 4.0% is reflected at each surface. Therefore, 96.0% of the incident light is transmitted through each surface (Figure 14.3). As a first guess, since the lens has two surfaces,

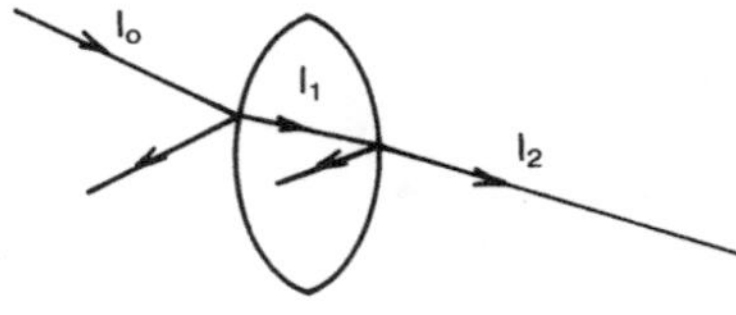

Figure 14.3 Reflection losses for a ray passing through a lens.

we would expect the lens to lose 8.0% due to reflection (i.e., 2 times 4.0%). For a more accurate calculation, let I_0, I_1, and I_2 be the intensity of the light, respectively, incident on the first surface, transmitted through the first surface and incident on the second surface, and transmitted through the second surface (Figure 14.3). The transmittance factor at the first surface is 0.960, or

$$I_1 = 0.960\ I_0$$

The transmittance factor at the second surface is again 0.960, or

$$I_2 = 0.960\ I_1$$

so that

$$I_2 = (0.960)(0.960)I_0$$

or

$$I_2 = 0.922\ I_0$$

Thus, the transmittance factor for both surfaces is 0.922, or 92.2% of the light incident on the lens is transmitted through it. The other 7.8% is lost by reflection. The 7.8% differs only slightly from the first guess of 8.0%. For interfaces with a higher percent reflection the first guess is not as close to the answer, whereas for interfaces with a lower percent reflection the first guess is better.

14.2 FOCAL POINTS

This book uses a sign convention in which the positive direction is the direction that the light is traveling when it leaves the system. For refraction systems the outgoing direction is the same as the incident direction, but for single reflection systems the outgoing direction is opposite to the incident direction. Even for reflection, we will continue to take the positive direction as the direction that the outgoing light is traveling.

Consider parallel light incident from the right on a spherical concave mirror. The mirror converges the light, and a real image point is formed at the secondary focal point F_2 (Figure 14.4a). The reflected light is traveling to the left, which is then the positive direction. Similar to lenses and refracting interfaces, the directed distances (focal lengths, radii of curvature, image and object distances) are distances from the reflecting interface or mirror to the position involved.

Figure 14.4b isolates some incident paraxial rays. In the paraxial diagram, the spherical mirror appears flat

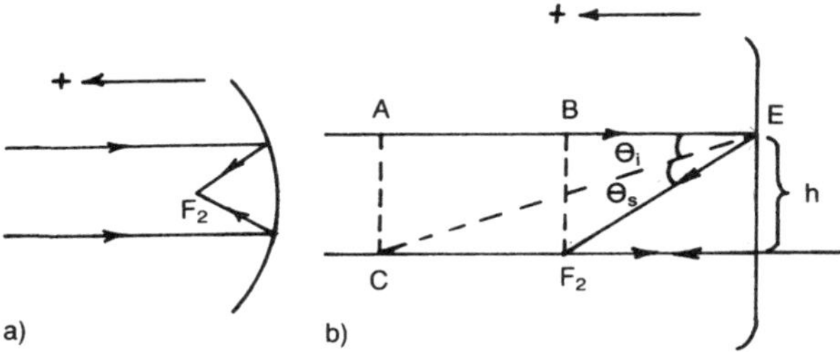

Figure 14.4 a, Actual rays associated with the (secondary) focal point; b, scaled ray.

because the vertical scale is expanded. The ray that travels along the optical axis (through the center of curvature C) is incident normally on the mirror and has a zero angle of incidence. From Eq. 14.1 the angle of reflection is also zero, and the reflected ray travels in the opposite direction back along the optical axis.

The off-axis ray hits the mirror at point E, a vertical distance h from the axis, and makes the angle θ_i with the normal (which passes through C). The reflected ray makes angle θ_s with the normal, and passes through F_2. Vertical lines have been drawn though C and F_2, and these lines intersect the off-axis ray at the points A and B, respectively.

For paraxial rays, the small angle approximations are valid. Then from the triangle AEC,

$$\theta_i \approx \tan\theta_i = \frac{h}{r} \tag{14.3}$$

where r is the radius of curvature of the mirror. From the triangle BEF_2

$$\theta_i + \theta_s \approx \tan(\theta_i + \theta_s) = \frac{h}{f_2} \tag{14.4}$$

where f_2, is the secondary focal length of the mirror.

From Eq. 14.1, θ_i and θ_s are equal, so Eq. 14.4 becomes

$$2\theta_i = \frac{h}{f_2} \tag{14.5}$$

Then from Eqs. 14.3 and 14.5,

$$f_2 = \frac{r}{2} \tag{14.6}$$

Equation 14.6 shows that the secondary focal length is one half the radius of curvature, or F_2 is halfway between the center of curvature C and the mirror. Equation 14.6 follows directly from the law of reflection, and is independent of the medium in front of the mirror. Even if the medium in front of the mirror is changed, f_2 remains the same. Equation 14.6 also holds for diverging mirrors, in which case F_2 is virtual.

EXAMPLE 14.4a

A concave mirror in air has a radius of curvature of 20 cm. Where is the image conjugate to a distant object?

The concave mirror is a converging mirror. The image conjugate to a distant object is at the secondary focal plane (by definition). From Eq. 14.6, the secondary focal plane is 10 cm in front of the mirror. In Figure 14.4, the positive direction is to the left, so

$$r = +20\,\text{cm} \quad \text{and} \quad f_2 = +10\,\text{cm}$$

Thus the image would be visible on a small screen held 10 cm in front of the mirror.

EXAMPLE 14.4b

Suppose the converging mirror in Example 14.4a was on the *Titanic*. What happened to the secondary focal point of the mirror as the ship sank, and the room flooded with water ($n = 1.33$)?

The law of reflection, Eq. 14.1, is independent of the media involved. Because of this, Eq. 14.6 is also independent of the media involved. As the room filled with water, the radius of curvature r remained +20 cm, the secondary focal length f_2 remained +10 cm, and F_2 remained in the same location relative to the mirror.

EXAMPLE 14.5

A convex mirror has a radius of curvature of 100 cm. What is the secondary focal length of the mirror (Figure 14.5)?

The convex mirror is a diverging mirror. In Figure 14.5, the reflected light is traveling left, so the positive direction is to the left. Then,

$$r = -100\,\text{cm}$$

and from Eq. 14.6,

$$f_2 = -50\,\text{cm}$$

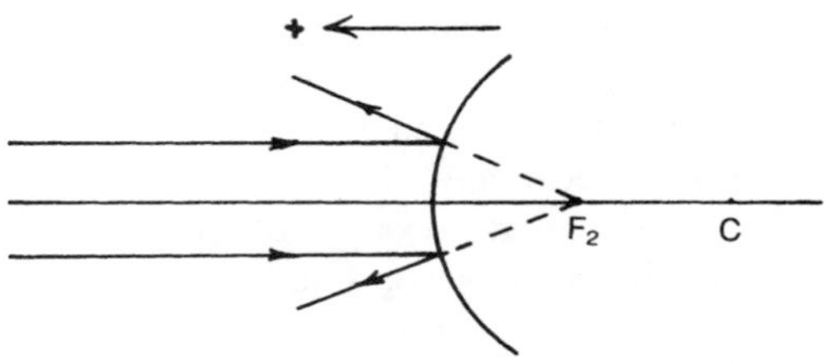

Figure 14.5 Paraxial rays associated with the (secondary) focal point of a diverging (convex) mirror.

For incoming plane waves, a virtual image would be formed 50 cm behind the mirror. An observer looking at the mirror would see the virtual image.

Let us apply the principle of reversibility to the case where plane waves are incident on the converging mirror. In Figure 14.4a, we would reverse the arrows on the rays. The reversed rays are diverging from the point marked F_2, would reflect off the mirror, and leave parallel to each other. This means that the point marked F_2 is also the primary focal point F_1 of the mirror. Refracting interfaces and lenses always had their primary and secondary focal points on opposite sides, but for a mirror the primary and secondary focal points coincide at the same point. For this reason, the subscripts on the focal points for a mirror are usually dropped:

$$F = F_2 = F_1$$

and

$$f = f_2 = f_1 = \frac{r}{2} \tag{14.7}$$

EXAMPLE 14.6

Where must an object be placed in order for a converging mirror with a 20 cm radius of curvature to form an image at optical infinity?

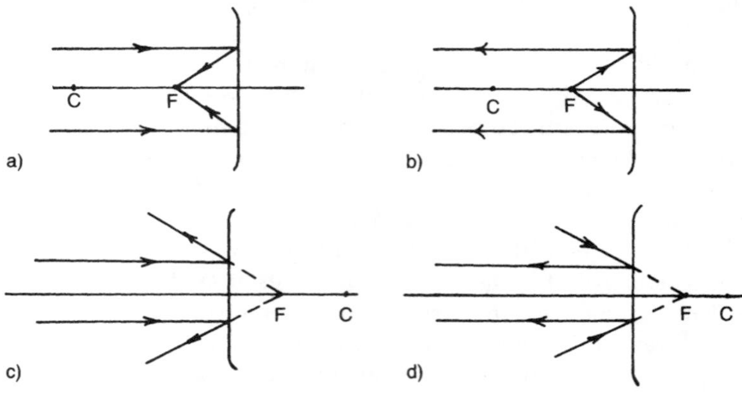

Figure 14.6 Predictable rays: a, b, converging (concave) mirror; c, d, diverging (convex) mirror.

The object must be placed at the primary focal point, which like the secondary focal point, is located halfway between the mirror and the radius of curvature. Here,

$$r = +20\,\text{cm} \quad \text{and} \quad f = f_1 = +10\,\text{cm}$$

You should compare this answer to that in Example 14.4a.

Once the focal point is known, then any ray incident parallel to the axis is predictable, and passes out through F for converging mirrors (Figure 14.6a), or appears to be coming from F for diverging mirrors (Figure 14.6c). Any incident ray either coming from F for converging mirrors or pointing toward F for diverging mirrors is predictable, and leaves the mirror parallel to the axis (Figures 14.6b and d).

14.3 RAY DIAGRAMS AND THE NODAL RAY

The third predictable ray is the nodal ray, and it is associated with the center of curvature C of the mirror. Any ray through C for a converging mirror or pointing toward C for a diverging mirror is normal to the mirror's surface, and has an incident angle of zero. From Eq. 14.1, the reflected angle is also zero, and the reflected ray travels back along the path of the incident ray (Figure 14.7). On a ray diagram, the only change needed is to reverse the direction of the arrow. Since this reflected ray is not bent up or down at the reflection, it is considered the nodal ray, and the nodal point for the mirror is the center of curvature C. (Remember that the nodal point for an SSRI was also at its center of curvature.)

Consider a converging (concave) mirror with a real object located outside C. The focal point is located halfway between C and the mirror. The incident ray traveling parallel to the axis reflects at the mirror and then travels through F (Figure 14.8a). The incident ray that passes through F reflects at the mirror and comes out parallel to the axis. The two reflected rays are converging and indicate that a small, inverted real image is formed between C and F. The third predictable ray is drawn from the object through C to the mirror (Figure 14.8b). This ray also passes through the conjugate point because when it reflects at the mirror

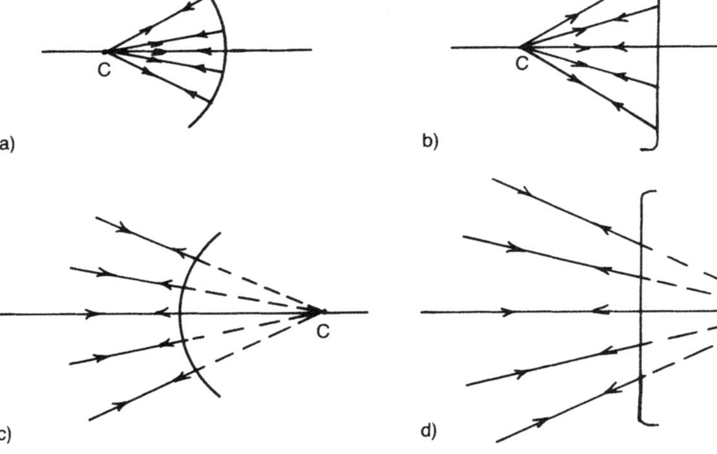

Figure 14.7 Object point at a mirror's center of curvature: a, converging mirror-actual; b, converging mirror-scaled; c, diverging mirror-actual; d, diverging mirror-scaled.

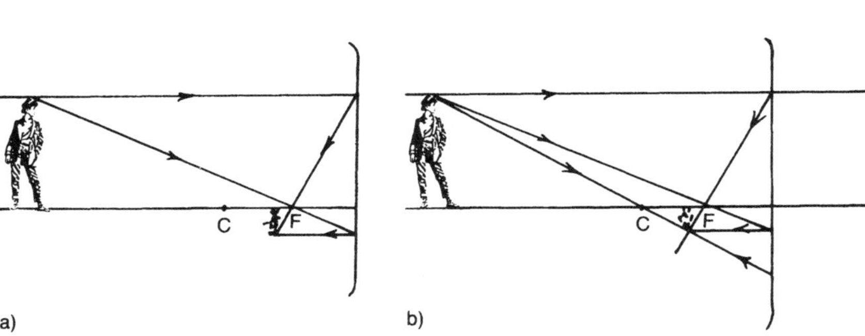

Figure 14.8 a, Two predictable rays for object outside C; b, nodal ray.

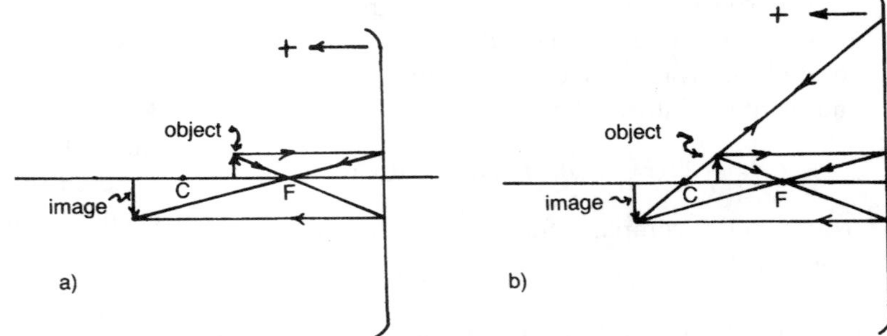

Figure 14.9 a, Two predictable rays for object between *C* and *F*; b, nodal ray.

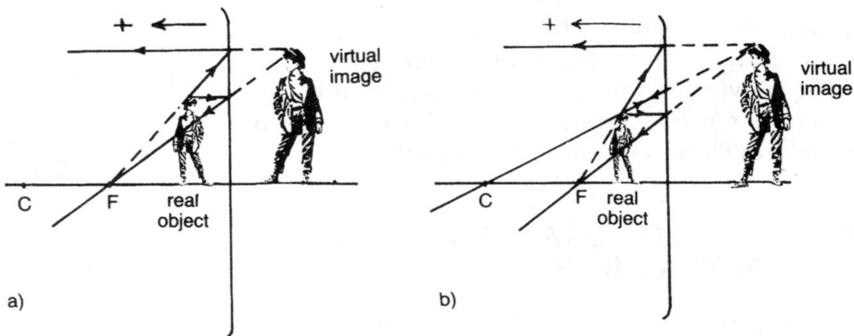

Figure 14.10 a, Two predictable rays for object inside *F*; b, nodal ray.

it comes straight back along itself. An observer looking in the mirror would see the small, inverted image. In fact, because the object is a person, the person sees his or her own reflected image as inverted and smaller.

The real object is now placed between *C* and *F*. Again, the incident parallel ray reflects and passes through *F*, and the incident ray through *F* reflects and comes out parallel (Figure 14.9a). The two reflected rays indicate that the outgoing light is converging and a larger, inverted real image is formed outside of *C*. The nodal ray, drawn through *C* to the mirror and then back along itself, also passes through the conjugate image point (Figure 14.9b).

Next, the real object is moved inside of *F*. The incident parallel ray again reflects and passes through *F*, and the incident ray that appears to be coming from *F* reflects and goes out parallel to the axis (Figure 14.10a). The two outgoing rays indicate that the reflected light is diverging and the image is virtual. The virtual image is located by extending the outgoing rays backwards until they intersect. The virtual image is erect and larger than the object. When the object is a person, that person will see his/her own erect and larger image in the mirror. This is the principle of cosmetic and shaving mirrors. The nodal ray is drawn from the object to the mirror so that it appears to be coming from *C*, and it reflects directly back along itself (Figure 14.10b). When the reflected ray is extended backwards, it also passes through the virtual image point. The virtual image point is just the center of curvature of the diverging wavefront that is physically leaving the mirror, so the image space medium is the medium in front of the mirror even though the virtual image location is behind the mirror.

Now, consider an object in the center of curvature plane, and remember that *F* is exactly halfway between *C* and the mirror. The ray incident parallel to the axis reflects and passes through *F*, while the ray incident through *F* reflects and comes out parallel to the axis. The two outgoing rays intersect at the center of the curvature plane, and an inverted real image is formed there (Figure 14.11). The inverted real image is the same size as the object ($m = -1$). Note *C* is at 2*F*,

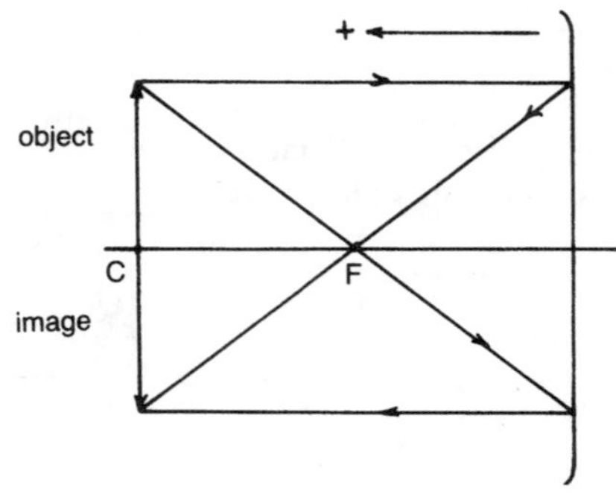

Figure 14.11 Object in the center of curvature plane.

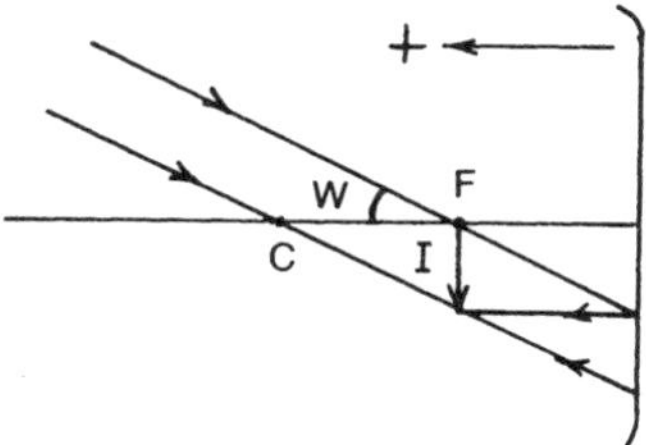

Figure 14.12 Predictable rays for extend object at optical infinity.

and is the symmetry point for the mirror. It is not possible to draw the nodal ray for this case.

Next, consider an object at optical infinity. The off-axis incident rays are parallel to each other, but not to the axis (Figure 14.12). Two of the rays are predictable: the one through *F*, which comes out parallel to the axis; and the one through *C*, which comes directly back along itself. The two reflected rays intersect in the (secondary) focal plane forming a small, inverted image there. Note from Figure 14.12 that the size *I* of the image can be found from the subtended angle *w* and the incident ray through *F* (i.e., $|I| = f \tan w$).

When the real object is placed in the focal plane, the ray diagram is essentially the reverse of Figure 14.12. The incident ray parallel to the axis reflects and goes out through *F* (Figure 14.13a). The incident ray that appears to be coming from *C* reflects and goes back out through *C*. The two outgoing rays are parallel to each other, so the conjugate image is at optical infinity. In this case it is not possible to draw an incident ray through *F*.

Actually, a fourth ray is easy to draw for each of the mirror cases. The fourth ray is a ray from the object drawn to the place where the optical axis intersects the mirror (i.e., the vertex or pole of the mirror). The outgoing ray is drawn by making the reflected angle θ_s equal to the incident angle θ_i (Figure 14.13b). Even on a quick freehand sketch, one can draw this ray fairly accurately.

Finally, consider a virtual object. In this case, converging light is incident on the converging mirror so the reflected light is even more convergent. The incident

Figure 14.13 a, Two predictable rays for extended object in the focal plane; b, another predictable ray.

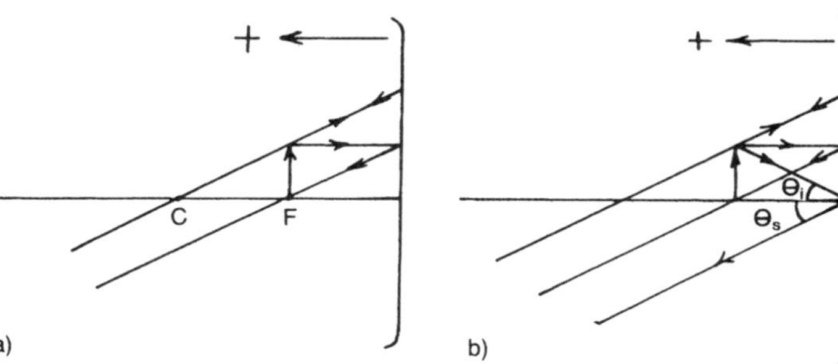

Figure 14.14 a, Converging light incident on a converging mirror; b, two predictable rays; c, the nodal ray.

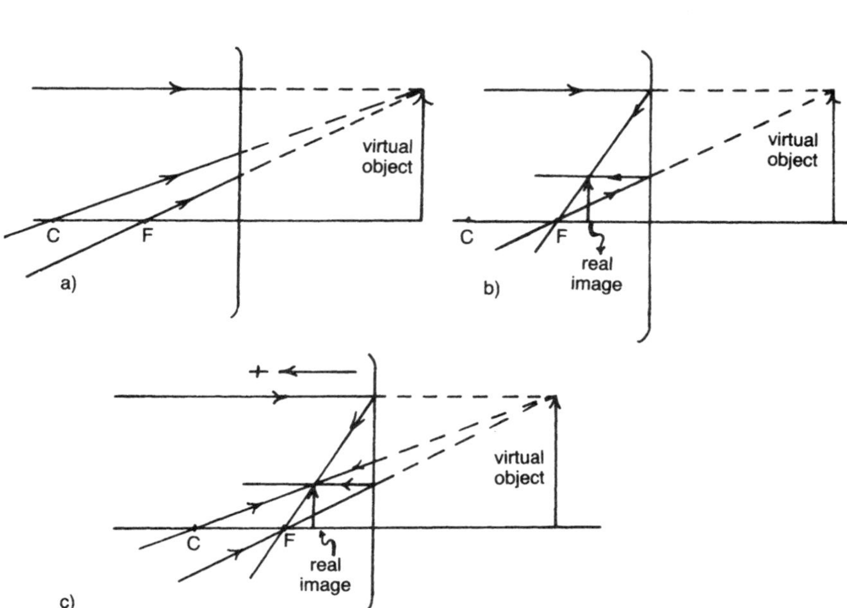

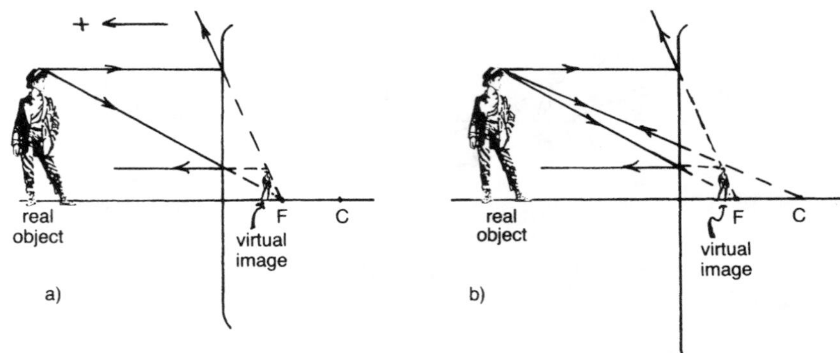

Figure 14.15 a, Two predictable rays for a real object in front of a diverging mirror; b, the nodal ray.

rays all point towards the virtual object point (Figure 14.14a). The ray parallel to the axis reflects and goes through *F* (Figure 14.14b). The incident ray that passes through *F* reflects and comes out parallel to the axis. The two reflected rays show that the outgoing light is converging, and a smaller, erect, real image is formed between *F* and the mirror. The third predictable ray is incident through *C*, and the reflected ray passes through the image point and then back through *C* (Figure 14.14c).

Now consider a diverging (convex) mirror. The focal point *F* is a virtual point, and is still halfway

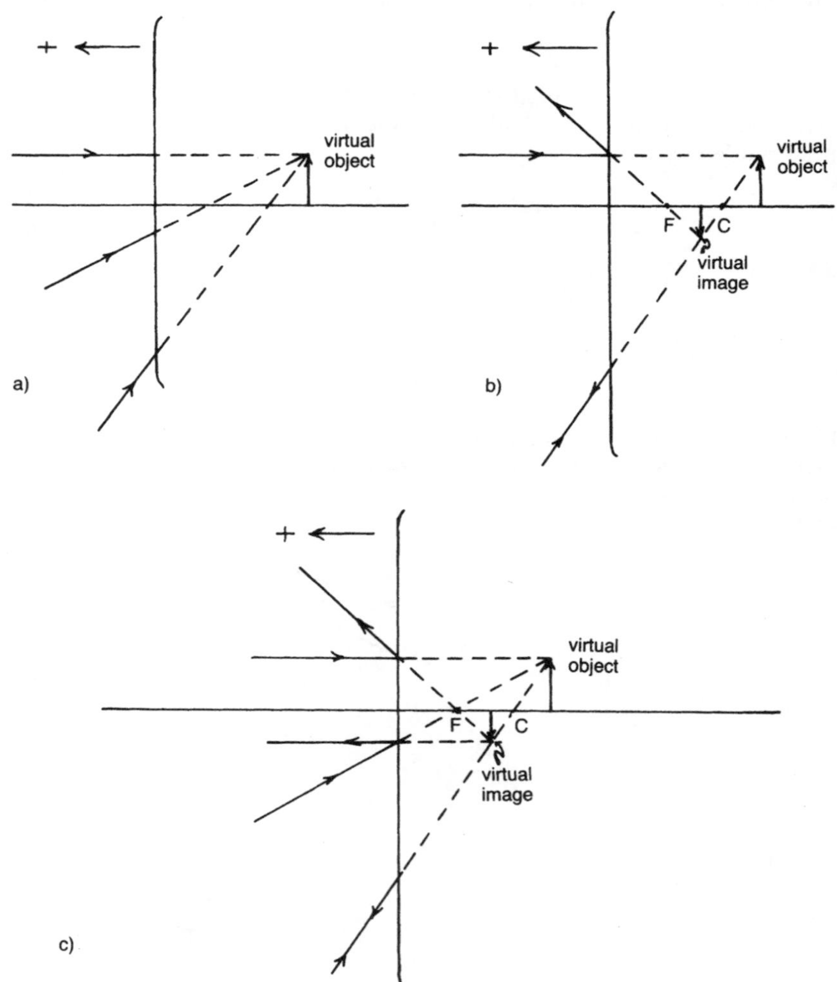

Figure 14.16 a, Incident converging light giving virtual object outside *C*; b, two predictable rays; c, third predictable ray.

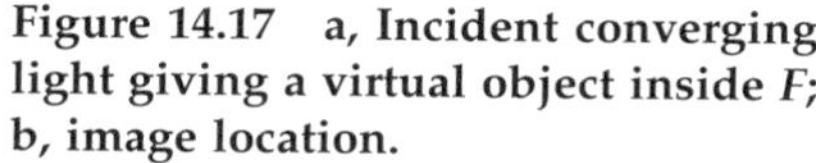
Figure 14.17 a, Incident converging light giving a virtual object inside F; b, image location.

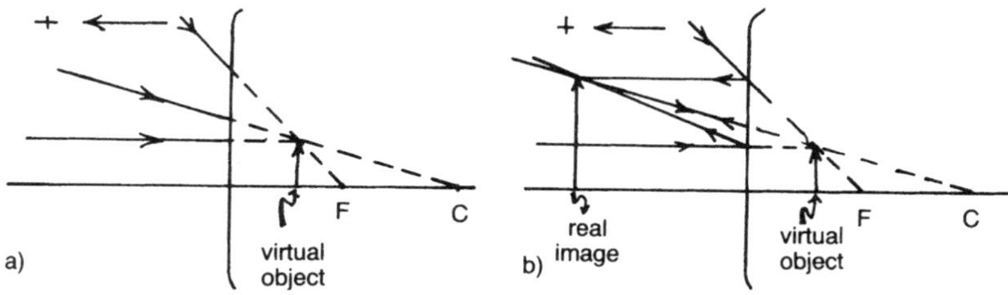

Figure 14.18 a, Incident converging light giving a virtual object in the focal plane; b, predictable rays.

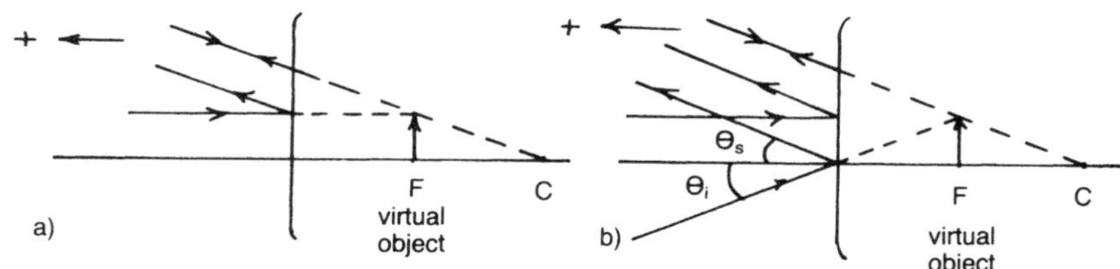

between the center of curvature C and the mirror. The predictable rays associated with F are shown in Figures 14.6c and d. The nodal ray is shown in Figure 14.7d.

Figure 14.15a shows a real object in front of the diverging mirror. The incident ray parallel to the axis reflects at the mirror, and the outgoing ray appears to be coming from F. The incident ray that points toward F reflects at the mirror, and the outgoing ray is parallel to the axis. The two outgoing rays are diverging, and their extensions backwards intersect at the virtual image location. The virtual image is smaller and erect. The nodal ray is drawn from the object toward C, and its extension also passes through the virtual image point (Figure 14.15b). (This type of mirror gives a large field of view, and is used as a car passenger side mirror or as a security mirror in stores.)

Figure 14.16a shows a virtual object located farther away than C. The incident rays all point toward the virtual object point. The incident ray parallel to the axis reflects at the mirror, and the outgoing ray appears to be coming from F (Figure 14.16b). The incident ray that points toward C reflects, and the outgoing ray goes straight back along the path of the incident ray. The two outgoing rays are diverging, and their extensions give a virtual image that is smaller and inverted relative to the virtual object. The third predictable ray points towards F, as well as towards the object. The outgoing ray is parallel to the axis, and its extension backwards passes through the virtual image point (Figure 14.16c).

In Figure 14.17a, the virtual object is between F and the mirror. Again, all the incident rays point toward the object. The incident ray parallel to the axis reflects, and the outgoing ray appears to be coming from F (Figure 14.17b). The incident ray pointing toward F

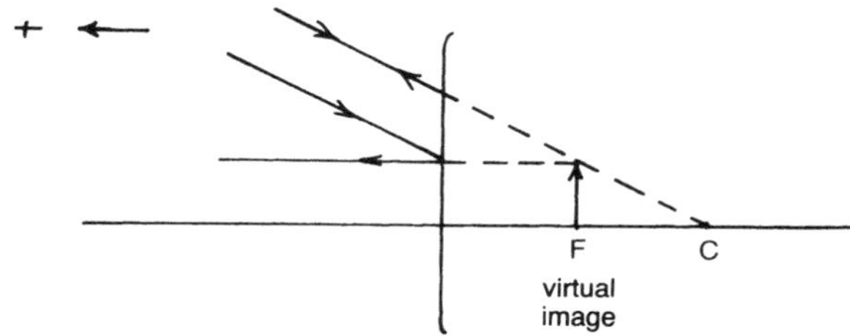

Figure 14.19 Ray diagram for incident parallel rays from a distant off-axis object.

reflects, and the outgoing ray is parallel to the axis. The nodal ray points toward C (as well as toward the virtual object), and reflects straight back. The outgoing rays indicate that the reflected light is converging, and a larger, erect real image is formed.

Now consider a virtual object in the focal plane. All the incident rays point toward the virtual object. The nodal ray points toward C, and the outgoing ray goes straight back along the path of the incident ray (Figure 14.18a). The incident ray parallel to the axis reflects, and the outgoing ray appears to be coming from F. The two outgoing rays are parallel to each other, indicating that the reflected light consists of plane waves. In this case, it is not possible to draw an incident ray pointing toward the off-axis object point and also toward F. However, the fourth predictable ray, the one incident at the vertex of the mirror, can be drawn, and the outgoing ray is parallel to the other outgoing rays (Figure 14.18b).

Finally, Figure 14.19 shows parallel light from a distant off-axis object point incident on the diverging mirror. The ray pointing toward C reflects and goes back out along the incident path. The incident ray pointing toward F reflects, and the outgoing ray is parallel to the axis. The two outgoing rays are diverging, and their backward extensions locate the virtual image, which is in the (secondary) focal plane.

14.4 VERGENCE EQUATIONS

The vergence equations for reflection from a spherical surface can be obtained from the sagittal approximation, from the law of reflection, or as a special modification of the single spherical refracting interface equations. The latter method is used here. The vergence equations for a SSRI are:

$$V = P + U \tag{14.8}$$

where,

$$U = \frac{n_1}{u} \tag{14.9}$$

$$V = \frac{n_2}{v} \tag{14.10}$$

$$P = \frac{n_2 - n_1}{r} \tag{14.11}$$

$$P = \frac{n_2}{f_2} \tag{14.12}$$

and

$$P = -\frac{n_1}{f_1} \tag{14.13}$$

The lateral magnification equations are:

$$m = \frac{U}{V} \tag{14.14}$$

or

$$m = \frac{n_1 v}{n_2 u} \tag{14.15}$$

These equations can be modified to describe image formation by reflection by making specific selections for the indices n_1 and n_2. Assume that the refractive index in front of the reflecting surface is n. In the reflection process, the light is always in this medium, but the reflected light and the incident light travel in opposite directions. Therefore, let

$$n_2 = +n \quad \text{and} \quad n_1 = -n \tag{14.16}$$

where the minus sign describes the change in direction that occurs at the reflection. (Other choices are possible, but no matter what choice is made a minus sign needs to be introduced to describe the reflection.) Equation 14.8 remains the same, while Eq. 14.11 becomes

$$P = \frac{+n - (-n)}{r}$$

or

$$P = \frac{2n}{r} \tag{14.17}$$

Equation 14.17 describes the converging or diverging power of a spherical interface as a result of reflection. The power P in Eq. 14.17 is referred to as the *reflecting power* or as the *catoptric power*. (The word catoptric comes from *katoptrikos*, the Greek word for mirror.) The catoptric power acts exactly like dioptric power in that it is measured in diopters, and in that it is positive for converging power and negative for diverging power.

When Eqs. 14.12, 14.16, and 14.17 are combined, the result is

$$\frac{2n}{r} = \frac{+n}{f_2}$$

or

$$f_2 = \frac{r}{2}$$

which is just Eq. 14.6. Note that while Eq. 14.17 for P depends on n, the relationship between the focal length and the radius of curvature of the mirror is independent of n, and the focal point for reflection is always halfway between the center of curvature and the mirror. We can also derive Eq. 14.6 by combining the primary focal length equation, 14.13, with Eqs. 14.16 and 14.17.

14.5 IMAGING EXAMPLES IN AIR

EXAMPLE 14.7

A real object is 50 cm in front of a concave mirror with a radius of curvature of 20 cm. Where is the conjugate image? Is it real or virtual, erect or inverted, larger or smaller?

Assume the object is in air unless otherwise specified. A concave mirror is a converging

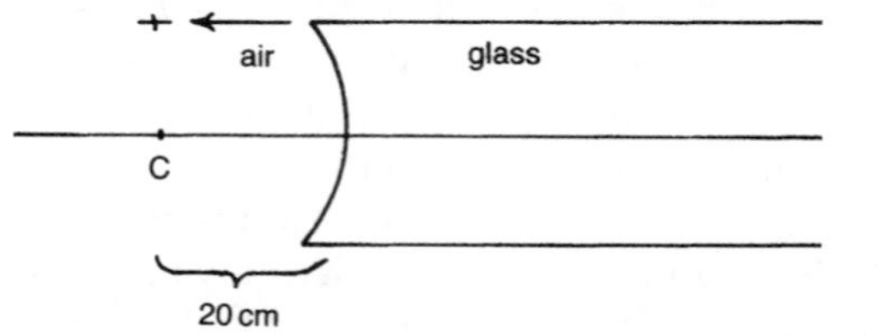

Figure 14.20 Outgoing direction for light in air reflecting off a spherical air–glass interface.

mirror, and P must be positive. In Figure 14.20, the outgoing light travels left, so r is positive. From Eq. 14.15,

$$P = \frac{2(1.00)(100\,\text{cm/m})}{+20\,\text{cm}} = \frac{200}{+20} = +10.00\,\text{D}$$

Alternatively, we could use Eq. 14.6 to find f,

$$f = \frac{r}{2} = \frac{+20\,\text{cm}}{2} = +10\,\text{cm}$$

and then use Eq. 14.12 to find P:

$$P = \frac{100\,\text{cm/m}}{+10\,\text{cm}} = +10.00\,\text{D}$$

Draw a quick ray diagram, and make your guesses at the answers. Your ray diagram should resemble Figure 14.8.

When a real object is 50 cm in front of any system, the incident light is diverging and the incident vergence U is -2.00 D. i.e.,

$$|U| = \left|\frac{100\,\text{cm/m}}{50\,\text{cm}}\right| = 2.00\,\text{D}$$

and since the light is diverging,

$$U = -2.00\,\text{D}$$

Then, from Eq, 14.8,

$$V = P + U = +10.00\,\text{D} + (-2.00\,\text{D}) = +8.00\,\text{D}$$

and from Eq. 14.10 and 14.16,

$$v = \frac{+n}{V} = \frac{100}{+8.00\,\text{D}} = +12.5\,\text{cm}$$

The outgoing light is converging, and the image is real and located 12.5 cm in front of the mirror. From Eq. 14.14, the lateral magnification is

$$m = \frac{U}{V} = \frac{-2\,\text{D}}{+8\,\text{D}} = -0.25$$

so the image is inverted and considerably smaller than the object (in agreement with the ray diagram).

The above example shows that if you think in terms of vergences, you really do not need to worry about the signs of the object distance u and the image distance v.

For completeness, let us consider the object distance. The positive direction is to the left, so

$$u = +50\,\text{cm}$$

which feels wrong based on our refraction intuition. However, Eqs. 14.9 and 14.16 give

$$U = \frac{n_1}{u} = \frac{-n}{u} = \frac{-(1.00)100\,\text{cm/m}}{+50\,\text{cm}}$$

or

$$U = \frac{-100}{+50} = -2.00\,\text{D}$$

Our intuition in terms of the vergences is unchanged. Diverging light still has a minus vergence, and converging light a positive vergence. Therefore, you should check the vergences instead of the object and image distances to see whether your answers make sense sign-wise.

EXAMPLE 14.8

A real object is 16.66 cm in front of the same mirror used in Example 14.7. Where is the conjugate image? Is it real or virtual, erect or inverted, larger or smaller?

Be sure to draw your own quick ray diagram and guess the answers before calculating. Figure 14.9 is the ray diagram that roughly fits this situation.

The light incident on the mirror is still diverging, and the incident vergence U is 6.00 D. i.e.,

$$|U| = \left|\frac{100}{16.67}\right| = 6.00\,\text{D}$$

and since the light is diverging,

$$U = -6.00\,\text{D}$$

Then,

$$V = P + U = +10.00\,\text{D} + (-6.00\,\text{D}) = +4.00\,\text{D}$$

and

$$v = \frac{+n}{V} = \frac{100}{+4.00\,\text{D}} = +25.0\,\text{cm}$$

The light leaving the mirror is converging so the image is real and the image 25 cm in front of the mirror. The lateral magnification is

$$m = \frac{U}{V} = \frac{-6\,\text{D}}{+4\,\text{D}} = -1.5$$

so the image is inverted and larger than the object.

Again, the sign of U is chosen because the incident light is diverging, as opposed to using the sign of the object distance u. For completeness,

$$u = +16.67\,\text{cm}$$

and

$$U = \frac{n_1}{u} = \frac{-n}{u} = \frac{-100}{+16.67} = -6.00\,\text{D}$$

EXAMPLE 14.9
The real object is placed 5 cm in front of the same mirror. Where is the conjugate image? Is it real or virtual, erect or inverted, larger or smaller?

From your quick ray diagram, what are your guesses? Figure 14.10 is the corresponding diagram.

The magnitude of the incident vergence is 20 D (i.e., 100/5). Since the incident light is diverging, the vergence is

$$U = -20.00\,\text{D}$$

Then,

$$V = P + U = +10.00\,\text{D} + (-20.00\,\text{D}) \\ = -10.00\,\text{D}$$

and

$$v = \frac{+n}{V} = \frac{100}{-10.00\,\text{D}} = -10.0\,\text{cm}$$

The outgoing light is diverging, so the image is virtual and located 10 cm behind the mirror. The lateral magnification is

$$m = \frac{U}{V} = \frac{-20\,\text{D}}{-10\,\text{D}} = +2$$

The image is erect and twice as large as the object. (This is the cosmetic or shaving mirror example.)

EXAMPLE 14.10
Consider the same mirror with a virtual object located 20 cm behind the mirror. Where is the conjugate image? Is it real or virtual, erect or inverted, larger or smaller?

From your quick ray diagram, what are your guesses? Figure 14.14 is the corresponding diagram. The incident light is converging and the magnitude of the incident vergence is 5 D (i.e., 100/20). Then,

$$U = +5.00\,\text{D}$$
$$V = P + U = +10.00\,\text{D} + 5.00\,\text{D}$$

and

$$V = +15.00\,\text{D}$$

The outgoing light is converging, so the image is real and located 6.67 cm (i.e., 100/15) in front of the mirror. The lateral magnification is

$$m = \frac{U}{V} = \frac{+5\,\text{D}}{+15\,\text{D}} = +0.33$$

so the image is erect and smaller than the object.

For completeness, the object distance is negative in this case, or

$$u = -20\,\text{cm}$$

Then from

$$U = \frac{n_1}{u}$$

$$U = \frac{(-1.00)(100\,\text{cm/m})}{-20\,\text{cm}} = \frac{-100}{-20} = +5.00\,\text{D}$$

EXAMPLE 14.11
A real object is 40 cm in front of a convex mirror with a radius of curvature of 25 cm. Where is the conjugate image? Is it real or virtual, erect or inverted, larger or smaller?

Be sure to draw a quick ray diagram, and make your estimate for the answer. The ray diagram in Figure 14.15 roughly matches this situation.

A convex mirror is a diverging mirror so P must be negative. In Figure 14.15, the outgoing light travels left, so r is negative. From Eq. 14.15,

$$P = \frac{2(1.00)(100\,\text{cm/m})}{-25\,\text{cm}} \\ = \frac{200}{-25} = -8.00\,\text{D}$$

Alternatively, we could use Eq. 14.6 to find f,

$$f = \frac{r}{2} = \frac{-25\,\text{cm}}{2} = -12.5\,\text{cm}$$

and then use Eq. 14.12 to find P,

$$P = \frac{100\,\text{cm/m}}{-12.5\,\text{cm}} = -8.00\,\text{D}$$

When a real object is 40 cm in front of any system, the incident light is diverging and the incident vergence U is −2.50 D, i.e.,

$$|U| = \left|\frac{100\,\text{cm/m}}{40\,\text{cm}}\right| = 2.50\,\text{D}$$

and since the light is diverging

$$U = -2.50\,\text{D}$$

Then,

$$V = P + U = -8.00\,\text{D} + (-2.50\,\text{D})$$

and

$$V = -10.5\,\text{D}$$

The outgoing light is diverging, and the image is virtual and located 9.52 cm behind the mirror (i.e., 100/10.5 D). From Eq. 14.14, the lateral magnification is

$$m = \frac{U}{V} = \frac{-2.50\,\text{D}}{-10.5\,\text{D}} = +0.24$$

so the image is erect and considerably smaller than the object (in agreement with the ray diagram). Again, this example shows that if you think in terms of vergences, you really do not need to worry about the signs of the object distance u and the image distance v.

EXAMPLE 14.12

Consider the same diverging mirror with a virtual object located 20 cm behind the mirror. Where is the conjugate image? Is it real or virtual, erect or inverted, larger or smaller?

From your quick ray diagram, what are your guesses? The incident light is converging and the magnitude of the incident vergence is 5.00 D (i.e., 100/20, or see Example 14.10). Then,

$$U = +5.00\,\text{D}$$
$$V = P + U = -8.00\,\text{D} + (+5.00\,\text{D})$$

and

$$V = -3.00\,\text{D}$$

The outgoing light is diverging, so the image is virtual and located 33.33 cm (i.e., 100/3) behind the mirror. The lateral magnification is

$$m = \frac{U}{V} = \frac{+5\,\text{D}}{-3\,\text{D}} = -1.66$$

The image is inverted and larger than the object.

EXAMPLE 14.13

A real object in air is 50 cm to the left of a −2.50 D single spherical refracting interface between air and glass ($n = 1.50$). 4% of the incident light reflects at the interface. Where is the reflected image? Is it real or virtual, erect or inverted, larger or smaller?

From the refraction information, the radius of curvature r of the interface is

$$r = \frac{(1.50 - 1.00)100\,\text{cm/m}}{-2.50\,\text{D}} = \frac{50}{-2.50\,\text{D}} = -20\,\text{cm}$$

While the interface diverges the refracted light, it converges the reflected light so the catoptric (reflecting) power of the interface must be positive. For the reflected light, the outgoing direction is opposite to that of the refracted light (Figure 14.20), and the sign of r needs to be changed: $r = +20$ cm.

The catoptric power of the interface is then

$$P = \frac{2n}{r} = \frac{2(1.00)100\,\text{cm/m}}{+20\,\text{cm}} = +10.00\,\text{D}$$

The remainder of the problem is identical to Example 14.7, and the reflected image is real and located 12.5 cm to the left of the interface. The lateral magnification is −0.25. Note that the reflected light never enters the glass and the refractive index of the glass is not used in the reflection calculation.

14.6 IMAGING EXAMPLES FOR $n \neq 1$

EXAMPLE 14.14

Consider the preceding example (14.13) again. The real object is 50 cm in front of the air–glass interface, which has a radius of curvature of magnitude 20 cm. Suddenly, a flood fills the room with water ($n = 1.333$). Now where is the reflected image? What is the lateral magnification? There are at least three ways to solve the problem.

Method 1

Since the law of reflection and the interface's center of curvature do not depend on the index, the ray diagram is unchanged by the water, and one can solve the problem as if air was still present. This is exactly the solution of the previous example. The image is still real and formed 12.5 cm in front of the mirror. The lateral magnification is still −0.25.

Method 2

The solution can also be worked out in the actual system. Here, for the reflected light

$$n = 1.333 \quad \text{and} \quad r = +20\,\text{cm}$$

Then,

$$P = \frac{2n}{r} = \frac{266.6}{+20} = +13.33\,\text{D}$$

The light incident on the mirror is diverging, and the incident vergence U is negative. Then,

$$u = +50\,\text{cm}$$
$$U = \frac{n_1}{u} = \frac{-n}{u}$$
$$= \frac{-133}{+50} = -2.66\,\text{D}$$
$$V = P + U = +13.33\,\text{D} + (-2.66\,\text{D})$$

and

$$V = +10.67\,\text{D}$$

The light leaving the mirror is converging, so the image is real and in the water in front of the mirror. The image distance is

$$v = \frac{n_2}{V} = \frac{+n}{V}$$
$$= \frac{+133}{10.67\,\text{D}} = +12.5\,\text{cm}$$

The lateral magnification is

$$m = \frac{U}{V} = \frac{-2.66\,\text{D}}{+10.67\,\text{D}} = -0.25$$

These answers agree with those of method 1.

Method 3

The third method is to reduce the system. There is no advantage to reducing the system for a single mirror, but in mixed lens–mirror systems there is an advantage. *The dioptric and/or catoptric power in the reduced system has to be the same as in the actual system*, so from method 2, the reflecting power is +13.33 D. The reduced object distance is 50/1.333 or 37.51 cm. A real object in air 37.51 cm from a surface gives an incident vergence on the surface of −2.67 D. Then,

$$V = P + U = +13.33\,\text{D} + (-2.67\,\text{D})$$
$$= +10.66\,\text{D}$$

Note that the vergences in the reduced system are the same as those in the actual system (except for possible numerical round-off differences). Then,

$$\bar{v} = \frac{100}{+10.66\,\text{D}} = +9.38\,\text{cm}$$

The image space index is water, so the actual image distance is

$$v = (1.333)(9.38\,\text{cm}) = +12.5\,\text{cm}$$

The lateral magnification is still given by U/V, and equals −0.25. Again, these answers are the same as those in methods 1 and 2.

EXAMPLE 14.15

A thick polycarbonate lens ($n = 1.58$) has a front surface dioptric power of +10.00 D, a back surface dioptric power of −3.00 D, and a central thickness of 3.16 cm (Figure 14.21a). You stand 50 cm from the front surface of the lens, and can see your own reflected images from the front and back surfaces of the lens. Describe the location and size of these images.

For the Image Formed by Reflection from the Front Surface

From the refraction information, the radius of the front surface is

$$r = \frac{(1.58 - 1.00)100\,\text{cm/m}}{+10.00\,\text{D}}$$
$$= \frac{+58}{+10} = +5.8\,\text{cm}$$

The front surface of the lens is convex and acts like a diverging mirror. Therefore, the catoptric power is negative. With the sign convention for the reflected light,

$$r = -5.8\,\text{cm}$$

and

$$P = \frac{2n}{r} = \frac{200}{-5.8\,\text{cm}} = -34.48\,\text{D}$$

Then,

$$U = -2.00\,\text{D}$$
$$V = P + U = -34.48\,\text{D} + (-2.00\,\text{D})$$
$$= -36.48\,\text{D}$$
$$v = \frac{100}{-36.48\,\text{D}} = -2.74\,\text{cm}$$

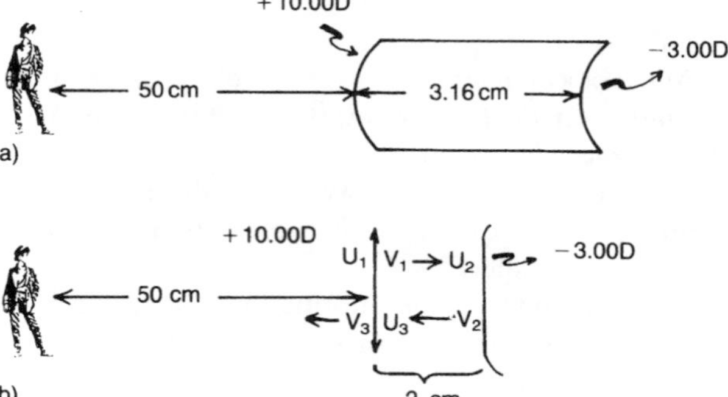

Figure 14.21 a, Geometry for an observer to view his or her own reflected images off the front and back surfaces of the lens; b, reduced system.

and

$$m = \frac{U}{V} = \frac{-2.00\,\text{D}}{-36.48\,\text{D}} = +0.0548$$

The reflected image is virtual, erect, much smaller, and located 2.74 cm behind the front surface.

For the Image Formed by Reflection from the Back Surface

Here the light has to pass through the front surface, reflect off the back surface, and pass back out through the front surface.

For the positive direction specified by the direction of the refracted light, the back surface radius of curvature is

$$r = \frac{-58}{-3} = +19.33\,\text{cm}$$

The back surface of the lens acts like a diverging mirror for the light incident in the glass, so the catoptric power must be negative. With the positive direction specified by the reflected light, $r = -19.33\,\text{cm}$,

$$P = \frac{2n}{r} = \frac{2(1.58)100\,\text{cm/m}}{-19.33\,\text{cm}}$$

and

$$P = \frac{316}{-19.33\,\text{cm}} = -16.34\,\text{D}$$

The reduced thickness of the lens is 2.00 cm (i.e., 3.16 cm/1.58). The reduced system consists of a real object 50 cm in front of a +10.00 D lens that is 2 cm in front of a −16.34 D mirror (Figure 14.21b). Then starting with the +10.00 D lens,

$$U_1 = -2.00\,\text{D}$$
$$V_1 = +8.00\,\text{D}$$
$$\bar{v} = +12.50\,\text{cm}$$
$$\bar{u} = +12.50\,\text{cm} - 2.00\,\text{cm} = +10.50\,\text{cm}$$
$$U_2 = \frac{100}{+10.50\,\text{cm}} = +9.52\,\text{D}$$

So far, the sign convention for the light that traveled through the +10.00 D lens has been used. The converging light gained vergence (from +8.00 D to +9.52 D) as it traveled from the lens to the mirror. Then,

$$V_2 = -16.34\,\text{D} + 9.52\,\text{D} = -6.82\,\text{D}$$

Now use the plus direction for the reflected light, and

$$\bar{v}_2 = \frac{100}{-6.82\,\text{D}} = -14.66\,\text{cm}$$
$$\bar{u}_3 = -(14.66 + 2)\,\text{cm} = -16.66\,\text{cm}$$
$$U_3 = \frac{100}{-16.66\,\text{cm}} = -6.00\,\text{D}$$

The diverging light lost vergence (from −6.82 D to −6.00 D) as it crossed back from the mirror to the lens. At the lens,

$$V_3 = +10.00\,\text{D} + (-6.00\,\text{D}) = +4.00\,\text{D}$$

and

$$v_3 = \bar{v}_3 = \frac{100}{+4.00\,\text{D}} = +25\,\text{cm}$$

The total lateral magnification is

$$m = m_1 m_2 m_3$$
$$= \left(\frac{-2.00\,\text{D}}{+8.00\,\text{D}}\right)\left(\frac{+9.52\,\text{D}}{-6.82\,\text{D}}\right)\left(\frac{-6.00\,\text{D}}{+4.00\,\text{D}}\right)$$
$$= (-0.25)(-1.40)(-1.50) = -0.52$$

So the image is real, inverted, about one half the size, and located 25 cm in front of the +10.00 D surface.

EXAMPLE 14.16

A thin −4.00 D CR-39 lens ($n = 1.50$) has a +4.00 D front surface and a −8.00 D back surface. A distant object is in front of the lens. Find the image formed by the light that reflects from the back surface of the lens and comes back out the front.

First, we need to find the catoptric power of the back surface. The light incident on the back surface is in the CR-39, and the back surface diverges the reflected light. For the positive direction specified by the transmitted light, the radius of curvature is given by

$$r = \frac{n_2 - n_1}{P}$$
$$= \frac{-50}{-8} = +6.25\,\text{cm}$$

The plus direction is opposite for the reflected light, so

$$r = -6.25\,\text{cm}$$

Then,

$$P = \frac{2n}{r} = \frac{2(1.50)100\,\text{cm/m}}{(-6.25\,\text{cm})}$$
$$= \frac{300}{-6.25} = -48.00\,\text{D}$$

Since the lens is thin, no significant vergence changes occur across the interior of the lens, and it follows that we can simply add the dioptric powers to get the total dioptric power. The light goes through the front surface first, is reflected, and then goes back out through the front surface. The total dioptric power is

$$P_t = (+4.00\,\text{D}) + (-48.00\,\text{D}) + (+4.00\,\text{D}) = -40.00\,\text{D}$$

The image is at the secondary focal point for the catadioptric system or

$$f = \frac{100}{-40.00\,\text{D}} = -2.5\,\text{cm}$$

The image for the light that passes through the front surface, reflects off the back surface, and comes back through the front surface is virtual and located 2.5 cm behind the lens.

14.7 THROUGH A GLASS DARKLY

Consider Emmy, an emmetrope, standing in front of her cosmetic (converging) mirror. When Emmy is far away from the mirror, the reflected light forms a real image at F. The light then diverges away from F and returns to Emmy. The diverging wavefronts become plane waves by the time they reach her. Emmy can then clearly see her reflected image, which is inverted and smaller, without accommodating.

As Emmy walks toward the mirror's center of curvature C, her inverted reflected image moves out toward C and gets larger. To see it clearly, Emmy needs to accommodate. At some point prior to Emmy reaching C, she will run out of accommodation. Emmy's view of her large, inverted reflected image then starts blurring. As Emmy moves from the first blur position to C, her view of the reflected image blurs out completely. (To simulate this condition, hold this book against your face. Are the letters clear or blurred?)

As Emmy moves from C toward F, the reflected image moves from C toward infinity. The reflected light going into Emmy's eye is now converging. The object for Emmy's eye is virtual, and Emmy is completely fogged like an uncorrected high myope viewing a distant object. As the reflected image approaches optical infinity, the wavefronts entering Emmy's eye become flatter and the fog decreases. Eventually, Emmy begins to see a blurred, erect, and large reflected image.

Why erect? Emmy is a real object for the mirror. The mirror's image is real and inverted. The inverted image is a virtual object for Emmy's eye. The real image formed by Emmy's eye is erect relative to her eye's virtual object. Thus, Emmy's blurred retinal image is erect relative to the virtual object, or inverted relative to the mirror's real object which is herself. Emmy perceives inverted retinal images as erect. (Note that your retinal image of these letters is inverted, but you perceive the letters as erect.)

When Emmy reaches F, plane waves leave the mirror. Then, without accommodating, Emmy can see her erect and magnified reflected image clearly. As Emmy starts to move from F toward the mirror, the light leaving the mirror starts to diverge. Emmy now needs to accommodate to see her erect (and large) reflected image clearly.

At some point Emmy uses all of her accommodation, and her reflected image starts to blur again. As Emmy's nose swoops in toward the mirror, her virtual reflected nose also swoops in toward the mirror. As Emmy's nose meets the mirror, her virtual nose meets her real nose (i.e., an object distance of zero gives an image distance of zero). However, unless Emmy's nose is very long, she cannot clearly see the meeting. (You should be able to draw ray diagrams for each of the above situations.)

EXAMPLE 14.16a

Emmy's cosmetic mirror is a +4.00 D mirror. What is Emmy's accommodative demand when she stands 100 cm from the mirror?

For the mirror, $f = +25\,\text{cm}$, and $r = +50\,\text{cm}$. When Emmy is 100 cm in front of the mirror, the vergence U incident on the mirror is -1 D. Then,

$$V = P + U = +4.00\,\text{D} + (-1.00\,\text{D}) = +3.00\,\text{D}$$

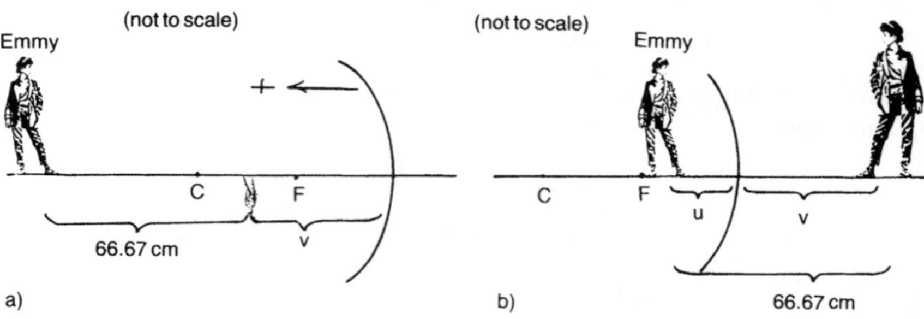

Figure 14.22 a, Emmy outside C; b, Emmy inside F.

and

$$v = +33.33\,\text{cm}$$

The light leaving the mirror converges to form a real aerial image 33.33 cm in front of the mirror and then diverges away from that position and is incident on Emmy's eye (Figure 14.22a). Thus the reflected image is 66.67 cm from Emmy, and the diverging light incident on Emmy's eye has a vergence of −1.50 D. Since Emmy is emmetropic, her accommodative demand is +1.50 D.

EXAMPLE 14.16b

Besides the 100 cm of the previous example, at what other distance would Emmy have an accommodative demand of 1.50 D?

Let us think a little before calculating. Figure 14.22a shows the situation of the previous example. The reflected image is 66.67 cm from Emmy's eye. The other possible case occurs when Emmy is closer than *F* and the image is virtual (Figure 14.22b). A guess might be 20 cm.

We could check the 20 cm guess by calculating the accommodative demand, and then modify the guess if needed. This is essentially an iteration procedure, which with a calculator can be fairly fast. Alternatively, from Figure 14.22b,

$$-66.67\,\text{cm} = v - u$$

or

$$v = -66.67\,\text{cm} + u$$

Let us work in terms of vergences, and for a mirror

$$U = \frac{n_1}{u} = \frac{-1}{u}$$

Diopters are the reciprocal of meters, so convert 66.67 cm to 2/3 m. Then,

$$\begin{aligned} v &= -\frac{2}{3} - \frac{1}{U} \\ &= \frac{2U+3}{-3U} \end{aligned}$$

$$V = \frac{n_2}{v} = \frac{+1}{v} = \frac{-3U}{2U+3}$$

From

$$\begin{aligned} V &= P + U \\ \frac{-3U}{2U+3} &= 4 + U \\ -3U &= (2U+3)(4+U) \\ &= 8U + 12 + 2U^2 + 3U \end{aligned}$$

and

$$2U^2 + 14U + 12 = 0$$

The standard quadratic equation solution gives

$$\begin{aligned} U &= \frac{-14 \pm \sqrt{14^2 - (4)(2)(12)}}{2(2)} \\ &= \frac{-14 \pm 10}{4} \end{aligned}$$

The two solutions are:

$$U = -1\,\text{D} \quad \text{and} \quad U = -6\,\text{D}$$

The −1 D solution gives the 100 cm distance of the previous example. The −6 D solution specifies that when Emmy is 16.67 cm in front of the mirror, her accommodative demand is +1.50 D. (Note the closeness of the initial guess made before calculating.)

14.8 UNIT LATERAL MAGNIFICATION AND THE RADIUSCOPE

Cases in which the lateral magnification is equal to plus or minus one are of special interest. For a mirror (just as for a thin lens or an SSRI), when the object distance goes to zero, the image distance goes to zero, and the lateral magnification is +1.

For a mirror, 2*F* coincides with the center of curvature *C*. An object at *C* results in an image at *C*, and a lateral magnification of −1. Figure 14.11 shows the ray diagram for converging mirrors and Figure 14.23 shows the ray diagram for a diverging mirror. For the diverging mirror, an object and image at *C* are both virtual. Thus, the center of curvature *C* of a mirror serves both as the nodal point and as the symmetry points.

The *radiuscope* (optical microspherometer) is an ophthalmic instrument that uses both the +1 and −1

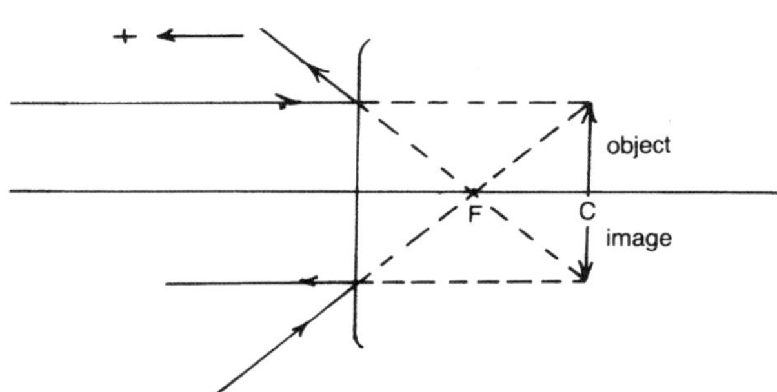

Figure 14.23 A virtual object in the center of curvature plane.

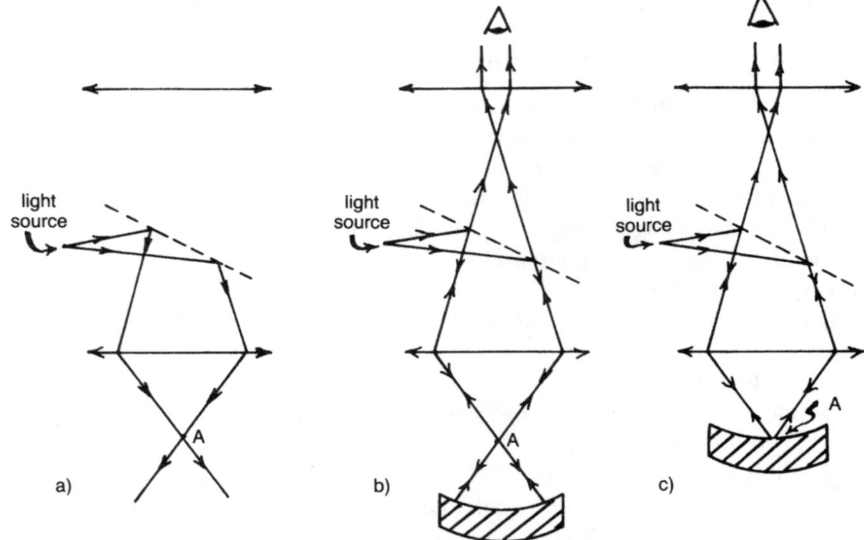

Figure 14.24 Radiuscope: a, illumination system; b, setting for a clear image; c, the other setting for a clear image.

cases. The radiuscope measures the radius of curvature of the central part of a back contact lens surface. The radiuscope works by first forming a target image at point A as shown in Figure 14.24a. The light that formed the target image is traveling away from the radiuscope and does not return unless reflected off something.

The contact lens is oriented so that its back surface faces the radiuscope. Some of the light traveling away from the radiuscope reflects at the back surface of the contact lens and returns to the radiuscope. An observer looking in the radiuscope can clearly see the reflected image of the target when the reflected image is also formed at A; otherwise, the observer sees a blurred image of the target. The reflected image is clear at two different locations of the radiuscope from the contact lens. The first (Figure 14.24b) is when the point A is at the center of curvature of the back surface of the contact lens. Then the reflected image is also at A and is the same size as the target image (but inverted). The second is when the point A is at the back surface of the contact lens (Figure 14.24c). Then the target image constitutes an object at zero distance for the back surface of the lens. The reflected image is also at A (zero image distance) and is the same size as the target image (erect this time). Dust or scratches on the contact lens surface are also clear in position two.

The distance the radiuscope moves between the two clear images is just the radius of curvature of the back surface of the contact lens. For example, suppose one starts with the radiuscope relatively far away from the contact lens. The image that the observer sees is blurred. The radiuscope is then moved toward the contact lens until the observer's image clears (Figure 14.24b). The distance measuring dial is then set to zero. Now the radiuscope is moved closer to the contact lens. The observed image first blurs and then comes clear again (Figure 14.24c). The distance on the measuring dial (i.e., the distance between the two clear image positions) is the radius of curvature of the contact lens' back surface.

14.9 KERATOMETRY

Another ophthalmic instrument that uses reflected light is the keratometer (ophthalmometer). We use the keratometer to determine the radius of curvature r of the anterior surface of the cornea. The keratometer works by using a prism doubling procedure to measure the size I of the reflected image. The reflected image size I is then used to determine r. The anterior surface of the cornea acts like a diverging mirror, so the reflected image is virtual and erect (Figure 14.15).

EXAMPLE 14.17

The keratometer target (called a mire) is 7 cm from the cornea. The mire is 5 cm in size, and the measured size of the reflected image is 2.45 mm. What is the corneal radius of curvature?

The lateral magnification is

$$m = \frac{I}{O} = \frac{+0.245\,\text{cm}}{+5\,\text{cm}} = +0.0490$$

The target is real and 7 cm from the cornea, so the light incident on the cornea has a vergence U of -14.29 D. Then from Eq. 14.14,

$$V = \frac{U}{m} = \frac{-14.29\,\text{D}}{+0.0490} = -291.63\,\text{D}$$

From Eq. 14.8,

$$P = V - U = (-291.63\,\text{D}) - (-14.29\,\text{D})$$
$$= -277.34\,\text{D}$$

and from Eq. 14.17,

$$r = \frac{2n}{P} = \frac{2000\,\text{mm/m}}{-277.34\,\text{D}} = -7.21\,\text{mm}$$

The radius r was read off the scale on the original keratometers. The newer keratometers have been modified to give a refractive power reading for the cornea. The cornea has a refractive index of about 1.376 and about a −5 D back interface with the aqueous humor. Assuming a lower refractive index for the cornea compensates for the negative back surface. The assumed index is 1.3375. The plus direction for the refracted light is opposite that of the reflected light so that r is now +7.21 mm. Then,

$$P = \frac{(1.3375 - 1.0000)1000\,\text{mm/m}}{7.21\,\text{mm}}$$
$$= \frac{+337.5}{+7.21} = +46.81\,\text{D}$$

The +46.81 D, or its approximation due to the instrument tolerances, is then read directly off the keratometer scale.

The keratometer dioptric readings are referred to as the K readings. When a contact lens, as in Sections 9.7 and 9.8, is fit with the same back surface radius as the cornea, the fit is described as *on K*. When the contact lens is fit with a smaller back surface radius of curvature (higher curvature) than the cornea, the fit is described as *steeper than K*. When the contact lens is fit with a larger radius of curvature (smaller curvature) than the cornea, the fit is described as *flatter than K*.

In the older keratometer, the mires were located farther away from the patient's cornea. Then, due to the high catoptric power of the cornea, the reflected image was formed essentially at the focal point ($r/2$), and the calculations shown in Example 14.17 could be simplified (see problem 14.14). However, use of the simplification for the close object distances of contemporary keratometers can lead to significant error.

Exact ray tracing shows that the keratometer samples only a small area of the central cornea. Various other instruments and target configurations (Placido's disk, keratoscopes, corneal topographers) exist that use reflection information to determine the shape and/or refraction characteristics of larger areas of the cornea.

14.10 PLANE MIRRORS

Plane or flat mirrors are special cases of spherical mirrors. As the radius of curvature r of a spherical mirror gets longer and longer, the mirror gets flatter and flatter. A plane mirror has a radius of curvature r of infinity and a curvature R of zero. The plane mirror has zero catoptric power. Therefore,

$$V = P + U$$

gives

$$V = U$$

Then from Eqs. 14.9, 14.10, and 14.16,

$$v = -u$$

From Eq. 14.14 the lateral magnification is +1. So the image is located the same distance away from the plane mirror as the object, but on the opposite side. The image is erect and the same size as the object. We can construct ray diagrams for plane mirrors by using the law of reflection, Eq. 14.1.

EXAMPLE 14.18

An uncorrected 3.00 D ocular hyperope stands 25 cm in front of her bathroom (flat) mirror. What is the hyperope's accommodative demand A_o when looking at her reflected image?

The ray diagram is shown in Figure 14.25a. One ray is incident normal to the surface and reflects straight back along the path of the incident ray. A second ray is incident at a particular incident angle θ, and the outgoing ray also makes an angle of θ with the normal. The reflected image is virtual and located 25 cm behind the mirror.

The reflected image is 50 cm from the hyperope's eye, so the light incident on the eye has a vergence $U_x = -2.00$ D. U_{fp} for the hyperope is +3.00 D. Then from Eq. 6.7,

$$A_o = U_{fp} - U_x$$
$$A_o = +3.00\,\text{D} - (-2.00\,\text{D}) = +5.00\,\text{D}$$

What is the smallest plane mirror in which you can see your whole body? The answer is one half

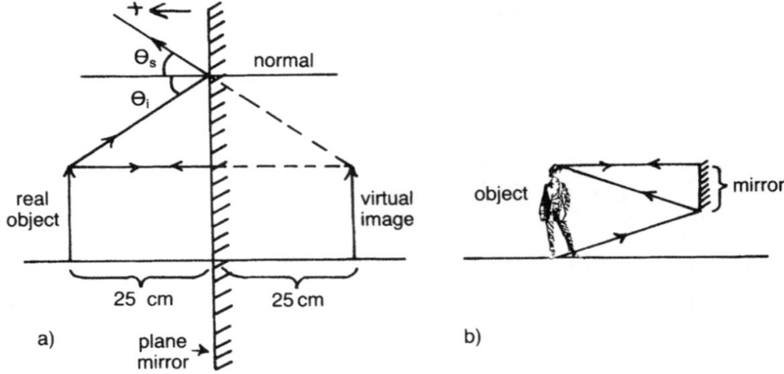

Figure 14.25 a, Plane mirror image; b, minimum size to see all of self in a plane mirror.

of your height. The reasoning is shown in Figure 14.25b. For simplicity, the eye is shown on top of the head. The top ray is normal to the surface and reflects directly back. The bottom ray originates at the foot and obeys the law of reflection. From the law of reflection and a little trigonometry, one can show that the normal for the bottom ray bisects the person, so the mirror's size is equal to one half the person's height. The argument is easily adjusted for an eye that is not on the top of the head, and the answer remains one half the person's height.

14.11 LEFT–RIGHT INVERSION

When you stand in front of your bathroom mirror, your reflected image is virtual and erect. However, when you hold your right hand up, the reflected image holds its left hand up. In short, your bathroom mirror images your right hand as a left hand and vice versa. Historically, the mirror's image was said to be perverted. A contemporary description is that the mirror's image is *reversed in handedness*.

Spherical mirrors with real objects also give reversed virtual images. In contrast, when a thin lens forms a virtual image of a real object, the image is erect and no reversal in handedness occurs. Catadioptric systems, including prisms, can be designed to maintain the same handedness or to reverse it.

14.12 GHOST IMAGES AND PARTIALLY SILVERED MIRRORS

The light that is reflected at lens surfaces can form images that were not intended to be there. These images are called ghost images. Figure 14.26a shows the reflections that give one of the ghost images for people wearing spectacle corrections. This ghost image involves a reflection from the back surface of the lens followed by a reflection from the front surface. This particular ghost image sometimes bothers speakers who are trying to look at their audience, and instead they see the ghost image of the overhead lights.

Figure 14.26b shows another ghost image that occurs for spectacle wearers. This ghost image is of an object behind and to the side of the person and involves a single reflection at the back surface. For distant objects, I can see this ghost image clearly. It enables me to spy on people or objects behind me while I am looking the other way.

There are a number of other possible ghost images for spectacle lenses (see the problems). Ghost images are sometimes visible on developed camera pictures and in ophthalmic instruments.

The appearance of the ghost images together with the desired image was due to the fact that a certain percentage of the light is reflected at an interface and a certain percent is transmitted. Partially silvered mirrors are frequently used to superimpose two images,

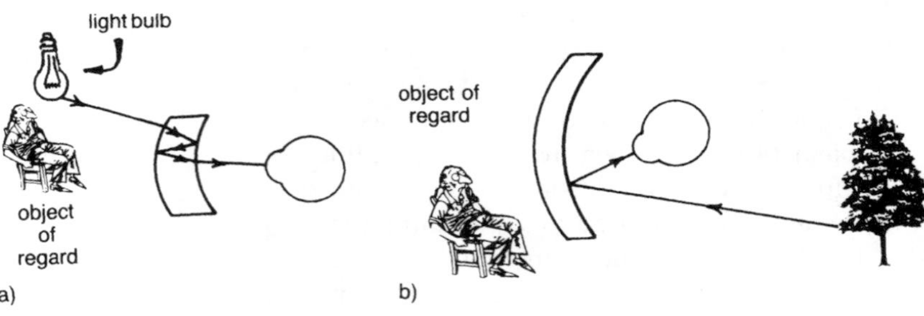

Figure 14.26 a, Ray path for reflected (ghost) image of light bulb superimposed on object of regard; b, ray path for reflected (ghost) image of tree superimposed on object of regard.

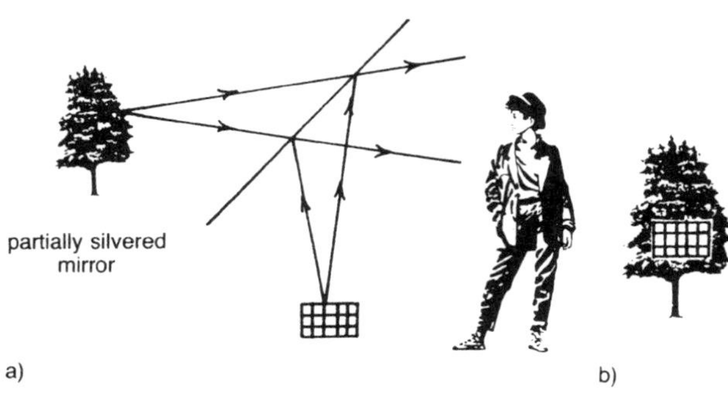

Figure 14.27 a, Ray paths for a partially silvered mirror; b, appearance of superimposed images.

as shown in Figure 14.27a. The appearance to an observer is shown in Figure 14.27b. Since the two objects are in different places they can be manipulated separately. This concept is very useful for gathering information about the human visual system.

14.13 EQUIVALENT MIRRORS

The reflected image from the anterior corneal surface is used in keratometry. The reflected images from the front and back surface of the crystalline lens provide information about the accommodation mechanism of the lens in the living human eye. These reflected images from the eye are called the *Purkinje–Sanson images*.

The light involved in the reflected images from the crystalline lens must pass through the cornea, reflect and then pass back out through the cornea. Therefore, both refraction and reflection are involved, and the system is a catadioptric system.

When there is a single reflecting surface behind a number of refracting surfaces, we can find a single mirror that is equivalent to the catadioptric system. The equivalent mirror concept simplifies the repeated analysis of data from such systems including those that form the Purkinje–Sanson images.

Two parameters that specify the equivalent mirror are its position H and its power P_e. The position H of the equivalent mirror is the apparent position of the reflecting surface as seen through the refracting surfaces. Since the equivalent mirror must give the same images as the actual system, the focal point of the equivalent mirror must be at the focal point F of the actual system. The focal length f_e of the equivalent mirror is then the directed distance HF where the plus direction is the direction of the reflected light, and

$$P_e = \frac{+n_i}{f_e} \tag{14.18}$$

where n_i is the image space index. The equivalent mirror parameters can also be found in a reduced system, and then

$$P_e = 1/\bar{f}_e \tag{14.19}$$

EXAMPLE 14.19

A +6.00 D thin lens is located 5 cm to the left of a −4.00 D mirror. What is the position and power of the equivalent mirror?

Let us first find the focal point F of the system since F is also the focal point of the equivalent mirror. Consider plane waves incident from the left on the +6.00 D lens (Figure 14.28a). Then the vergence leaving the lens is +6.00 D, and the image distance is 16.67 cm. The converging wavefronts gain curvature as they travel the 5 cm to the mirror, and the vergence incident on the mirror is +8.57 D (i.e., 100/11.67 cm). The mirror has a power of −4.00 D, so the vergence leaving the mirror is +4.57 D. The converging wavefronts gain curvature again as they travel back toward the lens, and the vergence incident on the lens from the right is +5.93 D (i.e., 100/16.88 cm). The vergence leaving the +6.00 D lens is then +11.93 D, and the focal point is 8.38 cm to the left of the lens (i.e., 100/11.93 D).

The position H of the equivalent mirror is the apparent position of the actual mirror as seen through the lens, so we consider the mirror as a real object for the lens. In Figure 14.28b the plus direction is to the left. For the lens,

$$u = -5\,\text{cm} \quad \text{and} \quad U = -20.00\,\text{D}$$

Then,

$$\begin{aligned} V &= P + U \\ &= +6.00\,\text{D} + (-20.00\,\text{D}) = -14.00\,\text{D} \end{aligned}$$

and

$$v = -7.14\,\text{cm}$$

The image of the mirror is virtual and is located 7.14 cm to the right of the lens. This is the position H of the equivalent mirror.

The focal length f_e of the equivalent mirror is the distance HF, with the plus direction being that of the reflected light or left in Figure 14.28b. So,

$$f_e = +(8.38\,\text{cm} + 7.14\,\text{cm}) = +15.52\,\text{cm}$$

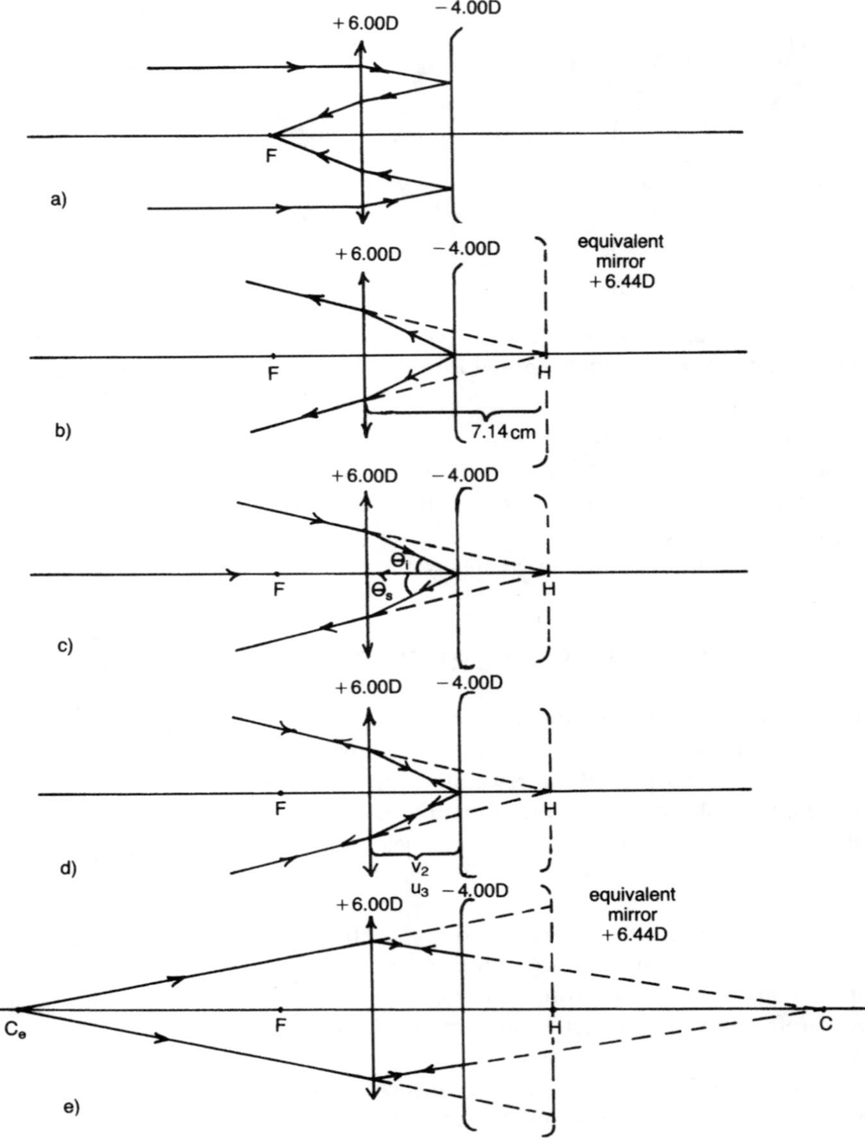

Figure 14.28 A +6.00 D lens in front of a −4.00-D mirror: a, incident parallel rays and focal point for the system; b, the mirror as an object for the lens gives the equivalent mirror location *H*; c, d, two incident rays converging toward the axial point *H* give the conjugate image at *H*; e, Ray paths for object at the center of the curvature of the equivalent mirror.

Then,

$$P_e = \frac{100}{+15.52\,\text{cm}} = +6.44\,\text{D}$$

The single mirror equivalent to the lens–mirror system has a power of +6.44 D and is located 7.14 cm to the right of the +6.00 D lens position.

For the same object, the single equivalent mirror in the above example gives the same final image and total lateral magnification as the actual lens–mirror system. If an object is placed at the position *H*, it has a zero object distance for the equivalent mirror, and thus the image distance should be zero and the lateral magnification +1.

Figure 14.28c shows two incident rays converging toward the axial point on *H* of the actual system in the above example. One of the rays is incident along the axis, and travels back along the axis when exiting. Since *H* is conjugate to the mirror, the incident off-axis ray bends at the lens and goes to the vertex of the mirror. There, it reflects according to Eq. 14.1 and is incident on the lens again. When this ray leaves the lens, it again has to be pointing away from *H* (just as in Figure 14.28b). So, the conjugate image for the actual system is indeed at *H*.

Figure 14.28d shows two off-axis rays incident towards *H*. It is easy to prove that for the actual system, the total lateral magnification is +1. Let U_1 be the vergence initially incident on the lens and V_1 be the vergence initially leaving the lens. Then the lateral magnification m_1, of the lens is

$$m_1 = \frac{U_1}{V_1}$$

The image of the lens is at the mirror, so the mirror's object and image distances are zero, and the lateral magnification of the mirror m_2 is +1. Let U_3 be the vergence of the light incident on the lens from the back side and V_3 be the light leaving the lens. This time the lateral magnification m_3 for the lens is

$$m_3 = \frac{U_3}{V_3}$$

The total lateral magnification m_t is

$$m_t = m_1 m_2 m_3$$

According to Figure 14.28d, the initial image distance for the lens v_1 is equal in magnitude to the object distance u_3. This, together with the fact that the light initially leaving the lens is converging while the light incident on the lens from the back side is diverging, means that U_3 is equal to $-V_1$. It follows from the vergence equation for the lens that V_3 is equal to $-U_1$. Then,

$$m_t = \left(\frac{U_1}{V_1}\right)(+1)\left(\frac{U_3}{V_3}\right)$$
$$= \left(\frac{U_1}{V_1}\right)\left(\frac{-V_1}{-U_1}\right) = +1$$

Another characteristic of an equivalent mirror, as with any mirror, is that the symmetry points coincide at its center of curvature C_e. The radius of curvature r_e of the equivalent mirror is the distance HC_e, and is equal to twice the equivalent focal length f_e. An object in the actual system at a position coinciding with C_e must be conjugate to itself and have a lateral magnification of −1.

EXAMPLE 14.20

For the lens–mirror system in the previous example, use the actual system to verify that an object at the center of curvature C_e of the equivalent mirror results in a conjugate image at C_e with a −1 total lateral magnification.

In the previous example, f_e was +15.52 cm. Then,

$$r_e = 2f_e = +31.04\,\text{cm}$$

So C_e is 31.04 cm to the left of H, or 23.90 cm to the left of the +6.00 D lens (Figure 14.28e). An object at this position is a real object for the actual system, and

$$u_1 = -23.90\,\text{cm}$$

Then,

$$U_1 = -4.18\,\text{D} \quad \text{and} \quad V_1 = +1.82\,\text{D}$$

giving

$$v_1 = +55\,\text{D} \quad \text{and} \quad u_2 = +50\,\text{cm}$$

Then for the −4.00 D mirror,

$$U_2 = +2.00\,\text{D} \quad \text{and} \quad V_2 = -2.00\,\text{D}$$

Since the light has reflected, the plus direction is now to the left. Then,

$$v_2 = -50\,\text{cm} \quad \text{and} \quad u_3 = -55\,\text{cm}$$

giving

$$U_3 = -1.82\,\text{D} \quad \text{and} \quad V_3 = +4.18\,\text{D}$$

The light leaving the lens is converging and

$$v_3 = +23.90\,\text{cm}$$

So the final image is at the same position as the object. The total lateral magnification is given by

$$m_t = m_1 m_2 m_3$$
$$= \left(\frac{-4.18\,\text{D}}{+1.82\,\text{D}}\right)\left(\frac{+2.00\,\text{D}}{-2.00\,\text{D}}\right)\left(\frac{-1.82\,\text{D}}{+4.18\,\text{D}}\right) = -1.00$$

which checks. Note from u_1, v_1, and u_2 (or from Figure 14.28e) that C_e is conjugate to the center of curvature C of the actual mirror.

The relationship discussed in Example 14.20 can be used to experimentally find the unknown radius of curvature of a diverging mirror. A known plus lens of high enough power is placed a distance d in front of the diverging mirror. An object is placed in front of the lens, and the object distance is adjusted until the light that passes through the lens, reflects off the mirror, and comes back out through the lens forms an inverted image at the same location as the object (i.e., $m_t = -1$). From Figure 14.28e, the image formed by the lens is at the center of curvature of the mirror. So one can locate the mirror's center of curvature by removing the mirror, and finding the real image formed by the lens.

EXAMPLE 14.21

A +5.00 D lens is placed 8 cm in front of a diverging mirror of unknown power. When an object is placed 28.0 cm in front of the lens, the light that passes through the lens, reflects off the mirror, passes back through the lens, and forms an inverted image of the same size in the object plane (like Figure 14.28e). What is the radius of curvature and catoptric power of the mirror? In this case, the lens's image is formed at the center of curvature of the mirror. Experimentally, one could simply remove the mirror and find the lens's image on a screen. Here we'll calculate where the lens's image is. For the lens,

$$u = -28.0\,\text{cm} \quad \text{gives} \quad U = -3.57\,\text{D}$$

Then,

$$V = P + U = +5.00\,\text{D} + (-3.57\,\text{D}) = +1.43\,\text{D}$$

and

$$v = +69.9\,\text{cm}$$

This image is at the mirror's center of curvature, so one can get the magnitude of the mirror's radius of curvature by subtracting d, the distance between the lens and the mirror:

$$|r| = v - d = +69.9\,\text{cm} - 8.0\,\text{cm} = 61.9\,\text{cm}$$

For the mirror's sign convention,

$$r = -61.9\,\text{cm}$$

and

$$P = \frac{2n}{r} = \frac{200}{-61.9\,\text{cm}} = -3.23\,\text{D}$$

(Note in this case, the object 28.0 cm in front of the lens is at the center of curvature C_e of the single equivalent mirror.)

EXAMPLE 14.22

Find the equivalent mirror for a −5.00 D thin lens located 8 cm to the left of a +10.00 D mirror.

First, find the focal point of the system by considering plane waves incident from the left (Figure 14.29a). Then the vergence leaving the lens is −5.00 D. The diverging wavefronts lose curvature as they cross the 8 cm to the mirror, and the vergence incident on the mirror is −3.57 D. The mirror has a power of +10.00 D, so the vergence leaving it is +6.43 D. The converging wavefronts gain vergence as they travel back to the lens, and the light incident on the lens from the back has a vergence of +13.24 D. The light leaving the −5.00 D lens has a vergence of +8.24 D, and the image (which is at F) is real and located 12.14 cm to the left of the lens.

To find the location H of the equivalent mirror, take the mirror as a real object for the −5.00 D lens. The mirror is 8 cm from the lens, so the light incident on the lens has a vergence of −12.5 D, and the light leaving the lens has a vergence of −17.5 D. The image is virtual and located 5.71 cm to the right of the lens (Figure 14.29b).

The distance HF is the equivalent focal length. So from Figure 14.29b,

$$f_e = +(12.14\,\text{cm} + 5.71\,\text{cm}) = +17.85\,\text{cm}$$

and

$$P_e = \frac{100}{+17.85\,\text{cm}} = +5.60\,\text{D}$$

The equivalent mirror is a +5.60 D mirror located 5.71 cm to the right of the lens.

As a check, let us see whether C_e is conjugate to the center of curvature C of the actual mirror. The actual mirror had a power of +10.00 D, and from Eq. 14.17, r is +20 cm. So C is 20 cm to the left of the mirror or 12 cm to the left of the lens. For the equivalent mirror,

$$r_e = 2f_e = +35.70\,\text{cm}$$

and C_e is located 35.70 cm left of H, or 29.99 cm left of the −5.00 D lens.

For the actual system an object point 29.99 cm left of the −5.00 D lens gives an incident vergence of −3.33 D, and the vergence leaving is −8.33 D. The image is virtual, located 12 cm to the left of the lens, and thus is at C. So everything checks. When the rays from C_e are drawn all the way through the actual system, they come right back to C_e (Figure 14.29c).

EXAMPLE 14.23

Consider the following eye model (Figure 14.30a). The cornea is a +43.00 D SSRI between air and the aqueous ($n = 1.336$). The crystalline lens ($n = 1.416$) has a central thickness of 3.6 mm, a front surface that is a +8.00 D SSRI with the aqueous and a back surface that is a +13.33 D SSRI with the vitreous ($n = 1.336$). The front surface of the crystalline lens is located

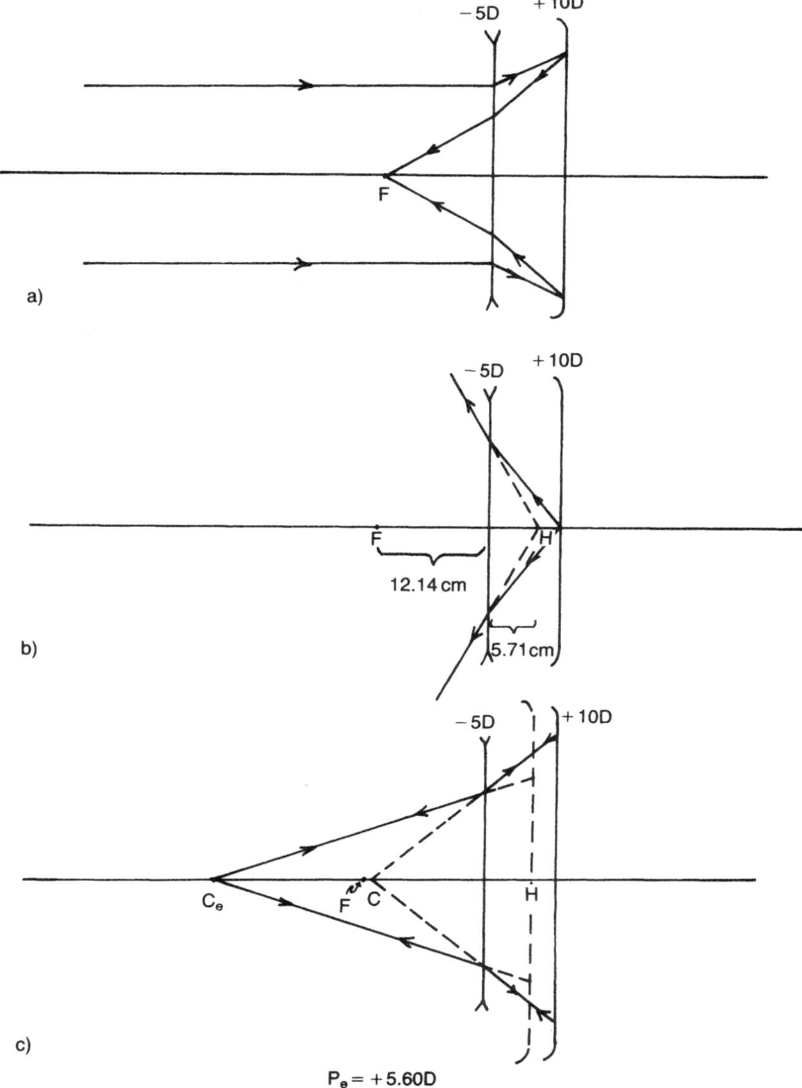

Figure 14.29 **A −5.00 D lens in front of a +10.00 D mirror: a, incident parallel rays showing focal point for the system; b, Location *H* of the equivalent mirror; c, ray paths for an object at the center of curvature of the equivalent mirror.**

3.6 mm behind the cornea. The fourth Purkinje–Sanson image is the image formed by the light that reflects off the back surface of the crystalline lens and comes back out of the eye. This light first passes through the cornea, and then the front surface of the crystalline lens, then reflects, and passes back through the two refracting surfaces again. By using the techniques of this section, we can show that the equivalent mirror for the catadioptric system that forms the fourth Purkinje–Sanson image is a +346.15 D mirror located 6.874 mm behind the corneal location. Where is the fourth Purkinje–Sanson image for a penlight held 5 cm in front of the cornea? What is the lateral magnification?

This question can be answered either from the actual catadioptric system (which involves four refractions and a reflection calculation), or from the equivalent mirror (which involves only one reflection calculation). Let us use the equivalent mirror.

The penlight is 5 cm in front of the cornea, or 5.6874 cm in front of the equivalent mirror. Both the object and image space are air. The vergence that would be incident on the equivalent mirror is then −17.58 D, and the vergence, leaving it is

$$V = +346.15\,\text{D} + (-17.58\,\text{D}) = +328.57\,\text{D}$$

The image distance is

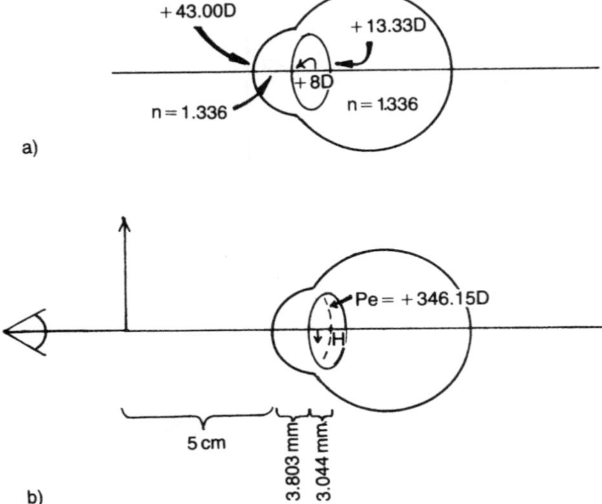

Figure 14.30 a, Eye model; b, equivalent mirror for the fourth Purkinje–Sanson image.

$$v = \frac{1000\,\text{mm/m}}{+328.57\,\text{D}} = +3.044\,\text{mm}$$

and the lateral magnification is

$$m = \frac{U}{V} = \frac{-17.58\,\text{D}}{+328.57\,\text{D}} = -0.054$$

The fourth Purkinje–Sanson image is inverted and considerably smaller than the penlight. The image is formed 3.044 mm in front of the equivalent mirror position, or 3.803 mm behind the cornea (Figure 14.30b). Think of the light leaving the equivalent mirror as converging to the real image position and then diverging away. The light at the position corresponding to the cornea is then diverging. In the actual system the final image formed by the last corneal refraction is virtual and identical in position and size to the equivalent mirror image.

If you wish, you can check the results by doing the four refraction and one reflection calculation of the actual system.

PROBLEMS

1. A concave (converging) spherical mirror has a 25 cm radius of curvature. Locate the conjugate image, specify whether it is real or virtual, and give the lateral magnification for the following objects:

   a. real object, 50 cm from the mirror.
   b. real object, 25 cm from the mirror.
   c. real object, 18 cm from the mirror.
   d. real object, 10 cm from the mirror.
   e. virtual object, 50 cm from the mirror.

2. A convex (diverging) spherical mirror has a 20 cm radius of curvature. Find the conjugate image, specify whether it is real or virtual, and give the lateral magnification for the following objects:

   a. real object, 50 cm from the mirror.
   b. real object, 15 cm from the mirror.
   c. virtual object, 5 cm from the mirror.
   d. virtual object, 15 cm from the mirror.
   e. virtual object, 20 cm from the mirror.
   f. virtual object, 50 cm from the mirror.

3. A person stands 50 cm in front of the bathroom mirror. Where is the conjugate image? What is the lateral magnification? How much must an emmetrope accommodate to clearly see his or her image in the mirror?
4. A +9.00 D lens is 10 cm in front of a diverging mirror of unknown power. When a real object is placed 20 cm in front of the +9.00 D lens, the light travels through the lens, reflects from the mirror, travels back through the lens, and forms an image in the same plane as the original real object. The image is inverted and has the same size as the object. What is the radius of curvature and the dioptric power of the mirror?
5. A convex mirror has a 32 cm radius of curvature. What is the dioptric power and focal length of the mirror in air? What is the dioptric power and focal length of the mirror in water ($n = 1.33$)? Compare your results.
6. A thin biconvex glass ($n = 1.50$) lens has a front surface refracting power of +3.00 D and a back surface refracting power of +2.00 D. When plane waves are incident on the front, find the resulting image for the light that passes through the front surface, reflects internally at the back surface, and passes back through the front. What would be the dioptric power of a single mirror that would give the same image position?
7. What percent of the incident light is reflected at an air–highlite ($n = 1.70$) glass interface? Taking surface reflections into account, what percent of the incident light is transmitted through a highlite glass lens in air?
8. Plane waves in air are incident on a −5.50 D refracting surface ($n = 1.50$). Where is the image for the light that is reflected?
9. A real object in air is located 20 cm in front of a +45.00 D cornea ($n = 1.3375$). What percent of the incident light is reflected? Where is the image for the reflected light? Is the image real or virtual, erect or inverted? What is the lateral magnification?
10. A real object 12.0 cm in size is located 20 cm from a cornea ($n = 1.3375$). The reflected image has a size of 2.10 mm. What is the corneal radius of curvature?

What is the refracting power of the cornea? What is the keratometer reading for this cornea?

11. An emmetrope stands 14 cm from a concave mirror with a 40 cm radius of curvature. What ocular accommodative demand does the emmetrope have when viewing his or her own image?
12. An uncorrected 6.00 D hyperope stands 25 cm from a concave mirror with a 16 cm focal length. What is the ocular accommodative demand for the hyperope to see his or her own image?
13. A keratometer reads +44.50 D on the front surface of a contact lens ($n = 1.49$). What is the true power of the contact lens surface? What is its radius of curvature?
14. Assume that the mires of an (old) keratometer are far enough away from the cornea that the reflected image is effectively formed at the focal point of the cornea acting as a convex mirror. With this assumption, derive that the $|r| = |(2uI)/O|$, where r is the corneal radius of curvature, u is the distance from the cornea to the mires, O is the size of the mires, and I is the reflected image size. (Note: in contemporary keratometers, this is not a good assumption.)

CHAPTER 15

The Gauss System

15.1 INTRODUCTION

Consider a focal system of many centered spherical interfaces or lenses. For such a system, we can always find an object (it could be real or it could be virtual) such that the conjugate image is erect and the same size as the object (i.e., the total lateral magnification m_t is $+1$). Note that the object, whether real or virtual, is always in object space; and the image, whether real or virtual, is always in image space. The Gauss system takes advantage of the particular object–image conjugate pair with unit lateral magnification and enables us to get from the multisurface system's object space to the system's image space in one step (e.g., one $V = P + U$ type equation). For the special conjugate pair with $m_t = +1$, the paraxial object location is called the primary principal plane, and the paraxial image location is called the secondary principal plane. The dioptric power that is used in the one-step connection between object space and image space is called the equivalent dioptric power P_e. Sections 15.2 through 15.5 give a ray trace development of the principal planes and their properties. Section 15.6 gives the $V = P + U$ Gauss system equations.

15.2 THE SECONDARY PRINCIPAL PLANE

Consider plane waves traveling along the optical axis incident on a system of centered refracting interfaces. The image point is the secondary focal point F_2 of the system. The incident rays are parallel to the axis. The rays can be traced through each interface, and the result is a zigzag path through the system. The exiting rays either point toward F_2 (if F_2 is real) or point away from F_2 (if F_2 is virtual).

Figure 15.1a shows the zigzag paraxial ray trace for a system with a real F_2. A ray bends at each internal interface in the system. (The internal interfaces are not shown, but their locations can be determined from the ray trace.) In object space, the incident rays are parallel to the axis. In image space, the outgoing rays leave the back of the system and pass through F_2. The object and image space rays can be extended forward and backward. At some point, the object space ray or its extension intersects the image space ray or its extension (e.g., point A, Figure 15.1b).

Figure 15.1c shows two paraxial rays incident parallel to the axis. The image space rays both pass through F_2. There is an intersection point for each of the incident rays. The two intersection points lie in a plane, marked H_2, which is perpendicular to the optical axis. It turns out that, for a given system, all of the intersection points for incident paraxial rays parallel to the axis lie in the same plane. The plane H_2 containing these intersection points is called the *secondary principal plane*. The point at which the optical axis passes through H_2 is called the *secondary principal point*.

The zigzag ray paths through a system determine the position of the secondary focal point F_2, and F_2 is thus a characteristic of the system. The zigzag ray paths through a system also determine the location of the secondary principal plane H_2, and H_2 is also a characteristic of the system.

In general, H_2 might be in front of, inside, or behind the system (Figures 15.1c, 15.2 and 15.3). In each case, H_2 is the intersection plane for the incoming rays parallel to the axis and the outgoing rays that pass through F_2. The point A on H_2, is the intersection point for the top incident ray. Note that H_2 is a geometric concept (the set of intersection points) and that, in general, nothing physically real exists at the H_2 position.

Figure 15.4 shows the zigzag paraxial ray trace (solid lines) for two rays parallel to the axis incident on a system with a virtual F_2. The image space rays appear to be coming from F_2. For each incident ray, there is an intersection point between the object space ray (or its extension) and the corresponding image

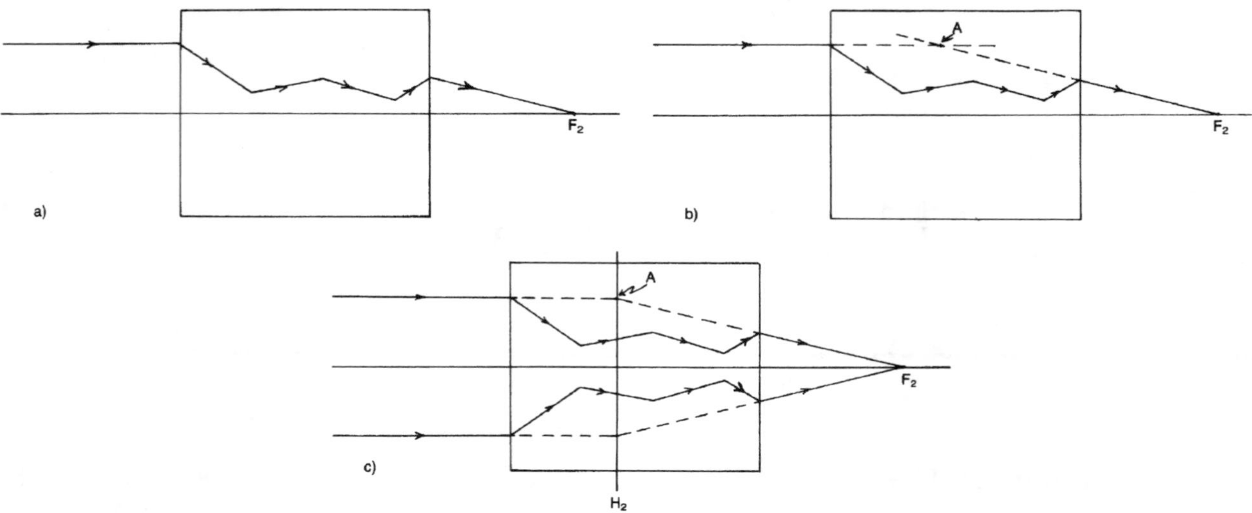

Figure 15.1 a, Zigzag paraxial ray path through a multi-interface system; b, *A* is the intersection point between the object and image space rays; c, the intersection plane H_2 for a series of incident rays parallel to the axis.

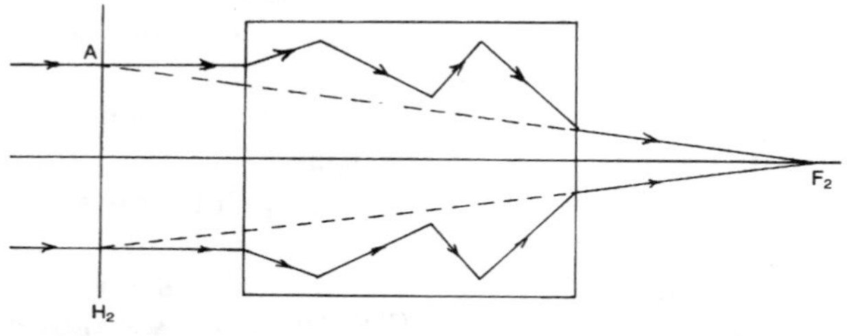

Figure 15.2 Secondary principal plane (intersection plane) in front of a system.

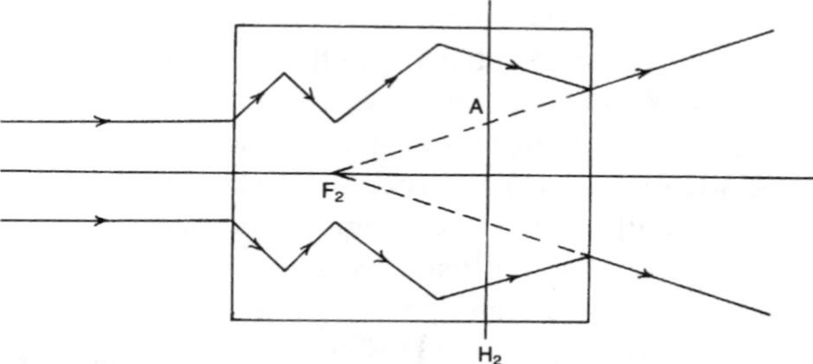

Figure 15.4 Secondary principal plane and virtual secondary focal point.

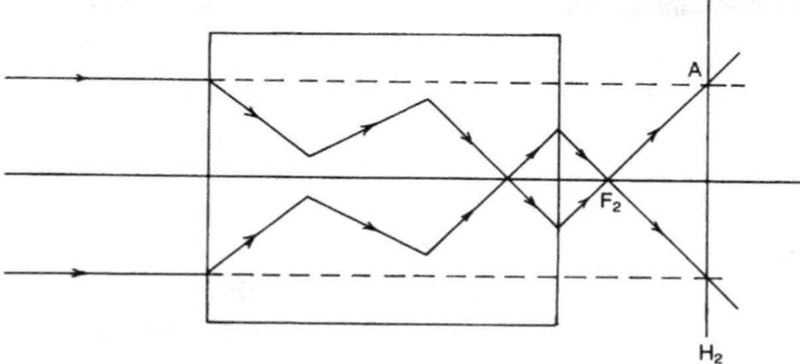

Figure 15.3 Secondary principal plane behind a system.

space ray (or its extension). Point *A* is the intersection point for the top ray. Again, all of the intersection points lie in the secondary principal plane H_2.

How is the secondary principal plane H_2 useful? When we know the locations of H_2 and F_2, then we can take an incident ray parallel to the axis and immediately draw the exiting ray without having to follow all the internal zigzags throught the system. For example, Figure 15.5a shows H_2 and F_2 for a system. The individual interfaces, which determine the locations, are not shown. The incident ray parallel to the axis is extended, and the extension reaches H_2 at the point labeled *A*. Since H_2 is the intersection point between the object and image space ray, the exiting (image space) ray must lie along the line from *A* to F_2 (Figure 15.5b). The line from *A* to F_2, hits the back of the system at the point *B*. We do not know the actual zigzag path of the ray through the system, but we do know that the actual image space ray travels from *B* to F_2. All of the image space rays can be constructed in the same manner (Figure 15.5c).

Figure 15.6 shows a system with H_2 in front of it and F_2 behind it. The object space rays are incident parallel to the axis. The top incident ray intersects H_2 at point *A*. The image space ray again lies on the line from *A* to F_2, and this line hits the back of the system at point *B*. We do not know the actual zigzag path of the ray through the system, but we do know that the

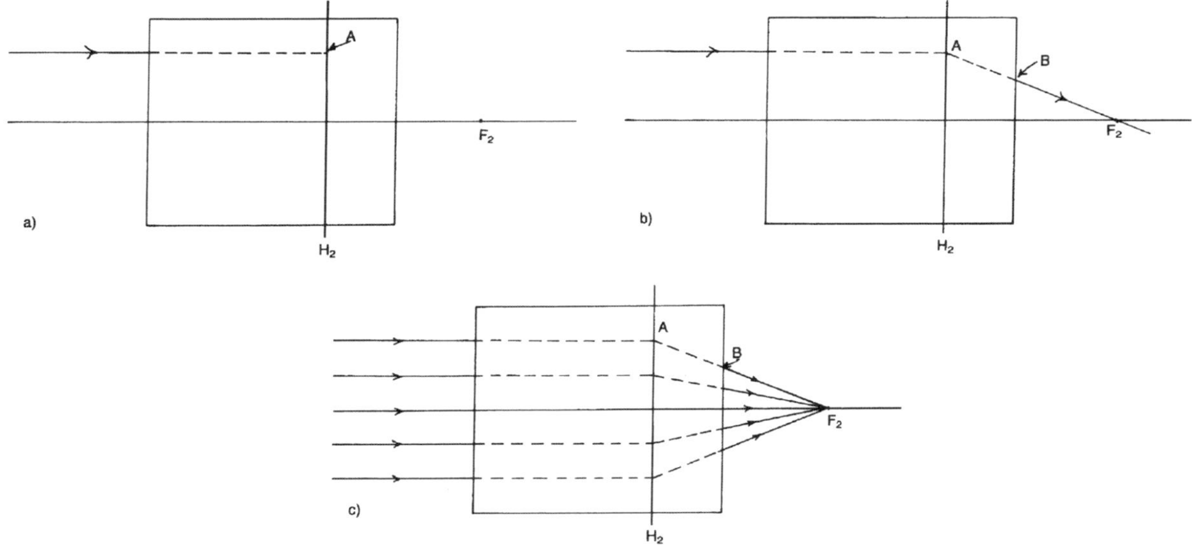

Figure 15.5 **a, Object space ray extension for a system with a known H_2 and F_2; b, image space ray must lie on line connecting A and F_2. Ray actually emerges from system at B; c, Multiple image and object space rays.**

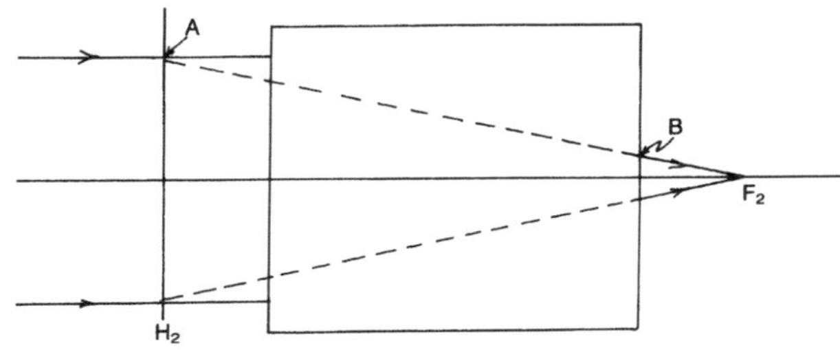

Figure 15.6 **Object and image rays for secondary principal plane in front of the system.**

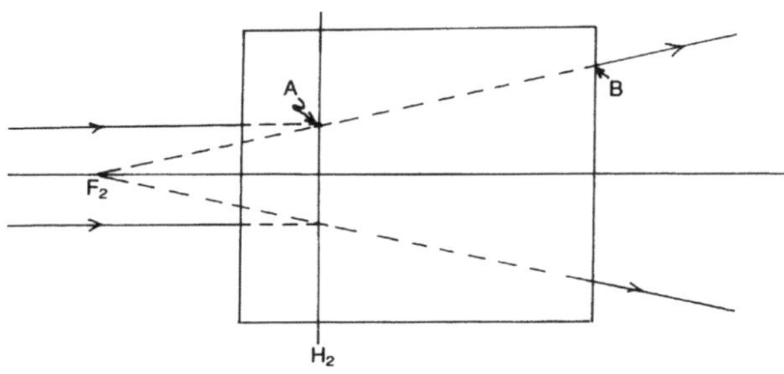

Figure 15.7 **Rays for a virtual secondary focal point.**

actual exiting ray travels from B to F_2. The path of the bottom incident ray is constructed similarly.

Figure 15.7 shows the construction for a case in which F_2 is virtual and H_2, is somewhere inside the system. The top incident ray (parallel to the axis) is extended, and the extension intersects H_2 at point A. The exiting ray must lie along the line that contains both A and F_2, and this line hits the back of the system at B. We do not know the actual zigzag path of the ray through the system, but we do know that the actual exiting ray leaves B and appears to be coming from F_2. The path of the bottom ray is constructed similarly.

15.3 THE PRIMARY PRINCIPAL PLANE

Consider a point source at the primary focal point F_1 for a system of centered refracting interfaces. The waves leaving the system are plane waves traveling along the optical axis. Figure 15.8a shows the paraxial ray diagram for a system with a real F_1. The rays that originate at F_1, zigzag through the system and leave parallel to the optical axis.

Both the incident and the exiting rays can be extended forward or backward. At some point, the incident ray or its extension intersects the exiting ray or its extension. Point E in Figure 15.8b is the intersection point for the top incident ray. The bottom incident ray also has an intersection point, and the two intersection points lie in the plane labeled H_1, which is perpendicular to the axis. It turns out that, for all of the incident paraxial rays associated with F_1, the intersection points lie in the same plane. The plane H_1 containing these intersection points is called the *primary principal plane*. The point at which the optical axis passes through H_1, is called the *primary principal point*.

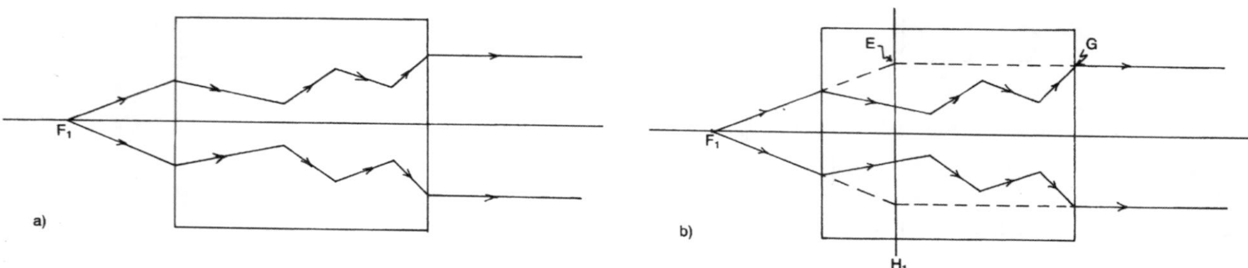

Figure 15.8 a, Zigzag paraxial ray path for an object point at the primary focal point of a multisurface system; b, for the top ray, E is the intersection point between the object space and image space ray, and G is where the ray actually leaves the system. The primary principal plane H_1 is the plane containing the respective intersection points.

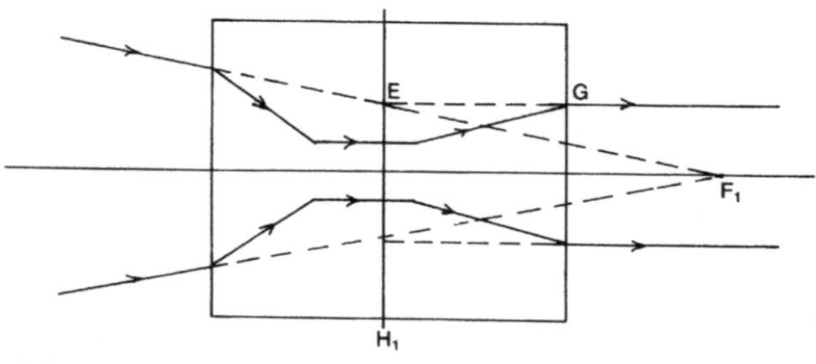

Figure 15.9 Primary principal plane for a virtual primary focal point.

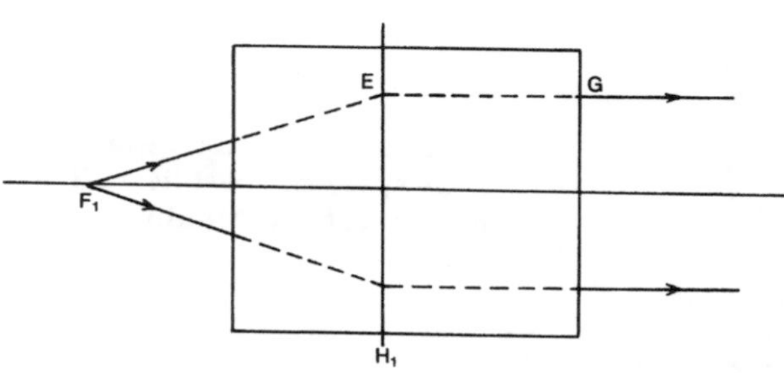

Figure 15.10 Object and image space rays.

Figure 15.9 shows the paraxial ray diagram for a system with a virtual F_1. The incident rays that point toward F_1 zigzag through the system and leave parallel to the optical axis. In Figure 15.9, the point E is the intersection point between the extension of the top object space ray and the extension of the corresponding image space ray. All of the intersection points between the object space rays associated with F_1 and the corresponding image space rays parallel to the axis lie in the primary principal plane H_1.

In general, the primary principal plane H_1 can be in front of, coincident with, or behind H_2. The individual interfaces in the system determine the location of F_1, and F_1 is thus a characteristic of the system. The individual interfaces in the system also determine the location of H_1 and thus H_1 is a characteristic of the system. When the location of H_1 and F_1 are known, then for an object space ray associated with F_1 we can immediately determine the actual path of the image space ray that is parallel to the axis without having to follow the zigzag path of the ray through the system.

Figure 15.10 shows a system with a real F_1 and an H_1 located inside the system. The top incident ray originates at F_1, and its extension intersects H_1 at point E. The outgoing ray must lie along the line that is parallel to the optical axis and passes through E. This

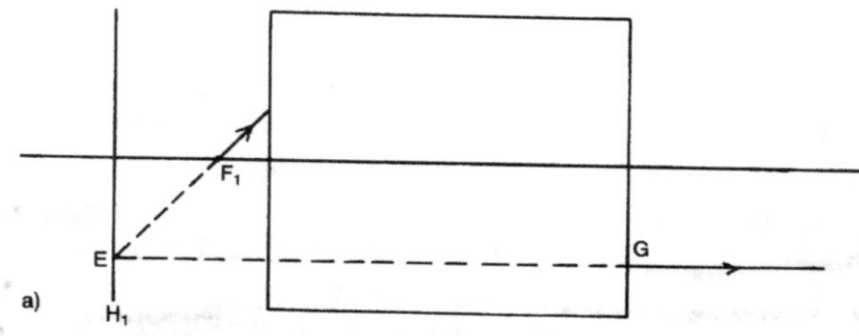

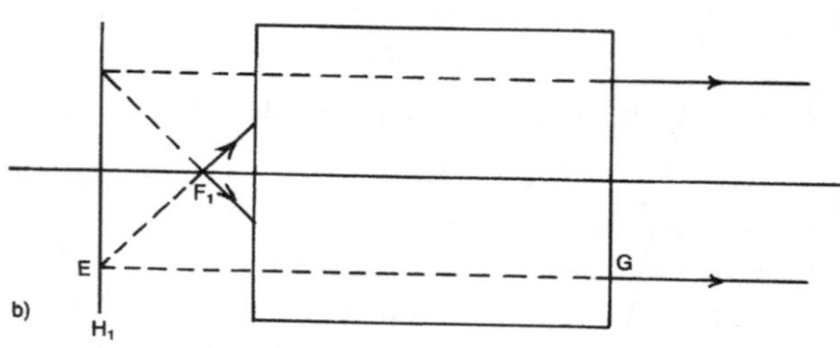

Figure 15.11 a, E is the intersection point for the object and image space rays; G is where the ray actually leaves the system; b, second ray.

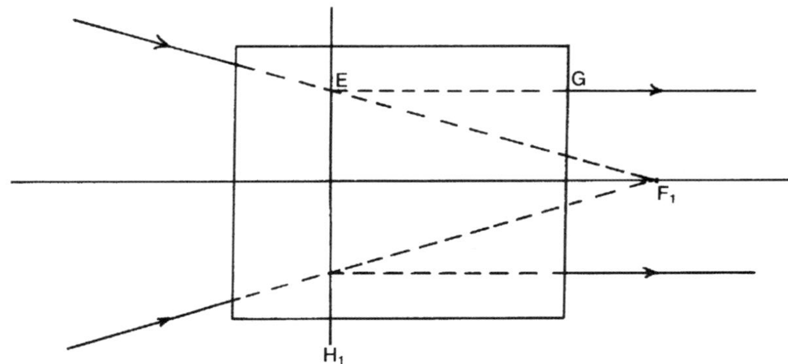

Figure 15.12 Ray prediction for virtual primary focal point.

line hits the back surface of the system at G. We do not know the actual zigzag path of the ray through the system, but we do know that the actual image space ray leaves G parallel to the axis.

Figure 15.11a shows a system with H_1 in front of a real F_1. The incident ray from F_1 can be extended backwards until it intersects H_1 at E. The image space ray must lie on a line passing through E and parallel to the axis. This line hits the back of the system at G. We do not know the actual zigzag path of the ray through the system, but we do know that the actual image space ray leaves G parallel to the axis. The path of the second ray is found similarly (Figure 15.11b).

Figure 15.12 shows a system with H_1 inside the system and F_1 (virtual) behind the system. The top incident ray points toward F_1 and intersects H_1 at point E. The outgoing ray must lie along the line that passes through point E and is parallel to the axis. This line hits the back surface of the system at G. We do not know the actual zigzag path of the ray through the system, but we do know that the actual outgoing ray leaves G parallel to the axis.

15.4 RAY DIAGRAMS

For a given system, the principal planes together with the focal points provide us with two predictable rays. Consider a system with real focal points and the principal planes located inside the system (Figure 15.13). Remember that the positions of the focal points and the principal planes are determined by the interfaces in the system.

A real object of size O is located outside F_1 at a distance of u_1 from the front surface of the system. One of the predictable rays is incident parallel to the axis, and the outgoing ray must pass through F_2. The intersection plane for this ray or its extension is the secondary principal plane H_2. The extension of the ray incident parallel to the axis intersects H_2 at A. The outgoing ray must lie along the line AF_2, and this line hits the back surface of the system at B. We do not know the actual zigzag path of the ray through the system, but we do know that the actual outgoing ray leaves the system at B and passes through F_2.

The other incident predictable ray passes through F_1, and the outgoing ray must be parallel to the axis. The intersection plane for these rays or their extensions is the primary principal plane H_1. The incident ray passes through F_1 and its extension intersects H_1 at point E. The outgoing ray must lie along a line parallel to the axis and passing through E. This line hits the back surface of the system at G. We do not know the actual zigzag path of the rays through the system, but

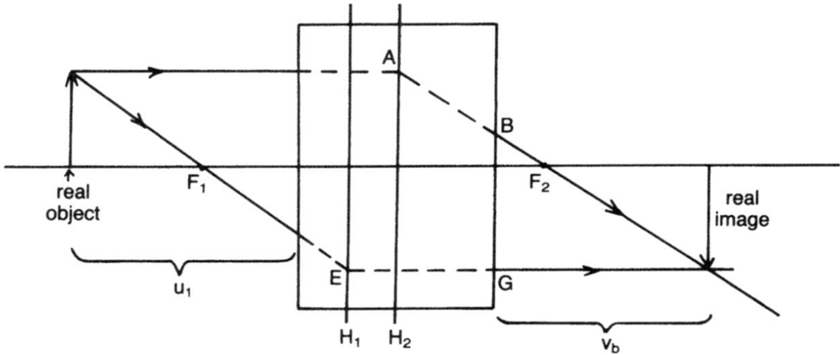

Figure 15.13 Real image by use of principal planes.

we do know that the actual outgoing ray leaves G parallel to the axis.

The two actual exiting rays tell us that the image space light is converging and a real image of size I is formed at a distance of v_b from the back surface of the system. We do not know what the light inside the system is doing, but we do know that the light leaving the system is converging.

Figure 15.14 shows another system with real focal points. H_1 and H_2 are inside the system with H_2 in front of H_1. A real object is inside F_1 at a distance u_1 from the front surface of the system. Again, the extension of the ray incident parallel to the axis intersects H_2 at A. The exiting ray must lie along the line AF_2, and the actual exiting ray leaves the system at B. When extended, the incident ray that appears to be coming from F_1 intersects H_1 at E. The exiting ray lies on the line parallel to the axis that passes through E, and the actual exiting ray leaves the system at G. The two actual exiting rays indicate that the image space light is diverging. The virtual image is located by extending the actual outgoing rays back until they intersect each other. The virtual image is erect, larger (size I), and located a distance v_b from the back surface of the system.

Figure 15.15 shows a system with virtual focal points. H_1 and H_2 are located in front of the system. A virtual object of size O is located behind the system at a distance of u_1 from the front surface. The two predictable incident rays are converging and both point toward the virtual object point. The incident ray parallel to the axis intersects H_2 at A. The exiting ray must lie along the line AF_2, and the actual exiting ray leaves the system at B and appears to he coming from F_2. The incident ray that is pointing toward F_1 intersects H_1 at E. The exiting ray must lie along the line parallel to the axis and passing through E, and the actual ray leaves the system at G. The two exiting rays indicate that the actual light leaving the system is diverging. The image is virtual and located by extending the two exiting rays backward until they intersect each other. The image is inverted and the same size as the object.

15.5 CONJUGACY OF THE PRINCIPAL PLANES

Figure 15.16 shows a system with real focal points. The primary principal plane H_1 is in front of the system, and the secondary principal plane H_2 is inside the system. A real object happens to be at the same position as H_1. The extension of the incident ray parallel to the axis intersects H_2 at A. The outgoing ray lies along the line AF_2 and leaves the system at B.

The ray incident on the system that appears to be coming from F_1 intersects H_1 at E, which is the same point as the top of the object. The outgoing ray lies on the line through E that is parallel to the axis, and the actual ray leaves the system at G. Since E coincides with the top of the object and the line through E and G

Figure 15.14 Virtual image location.

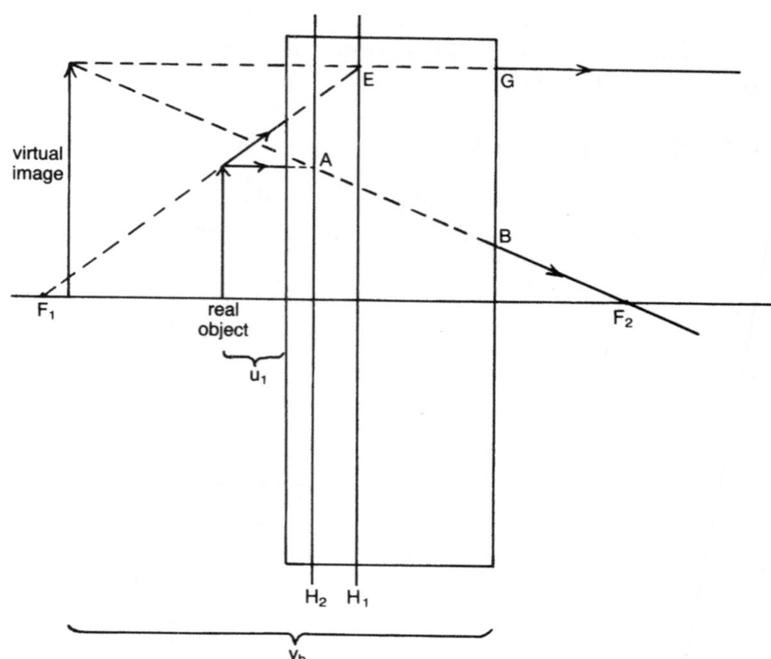

Figure 15.15 Image location for virtual object.

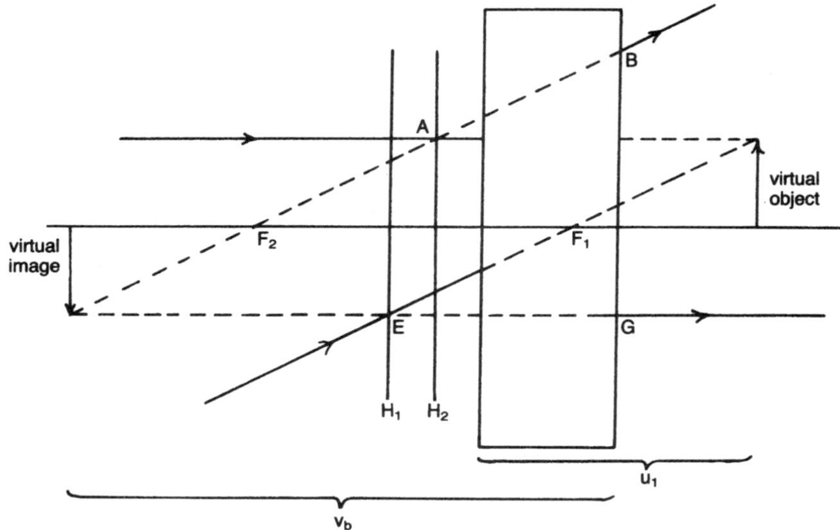

must pass through the conjugate image, the image is erect and the same size as the object.

The two outgoing rays indicate that the light leaving the system is diverging. The image is virtual and located by extending the outgoing rays backward until they intersect each other. In this case, the intersection occurs at the point A on H_2 (See Figure 15.16). So for an object at H_1, the conjugate image is at H_2. This image is erect and the same size as the object, so the total lateral magnification m_t for the system is +1.

We can construct similar ray diagrams for other systems, and an object at H_1 is always conjugate to an image at H_2 with a lateral magnification of +1. Therefore, we say that H_1 and H_2 are unit conjugate planes. Note that for light going in the same direction, an object at H_2 does not give an image at H_1 (Figure 15.17).

In the previous section, we learned how to predict the path of two special rays. In general, we can use the conjugacy of the principal planes to trace the path of any image space ray corresponding to an object space ray. Consider the system in Figure 15.18a. The focal points are real, and the principal planes are inside the system. A real object is located outside F_1 and the conjugate real image, found by tracing the two predictable rays, is real and located outside F_2. A third incident ray, when extended, hits the point K on H_1. We know that the corresponding image space ray must pass through the bottom image point. We also know that an object point at K on H_1 is conjugate to an image point at L on H_2 with a lateral magnification of +1. Therefore, L and K are the same perpendicular distance from the axis, and can be connected by a line parallel to the axis (Figure 15.18b). Since L is conjugate to K, the image space ray must lie on the line that connects L and the bottom of the image, and this line hits the back surface of the system at M. We do not

Figure 15.16 Object at H_1 gives erect image of the same size at H_2.

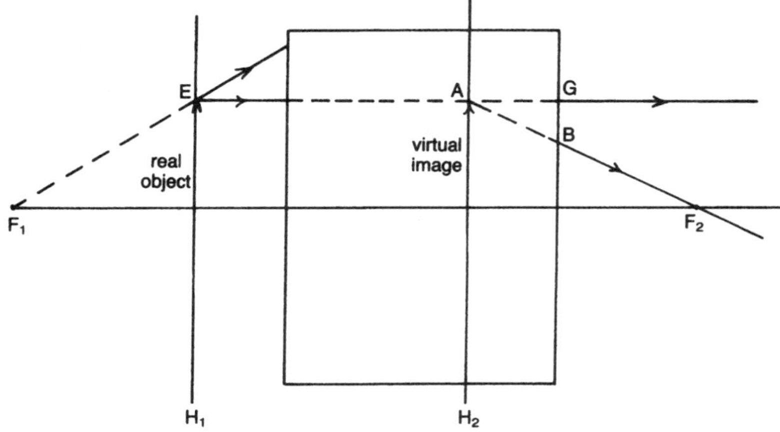

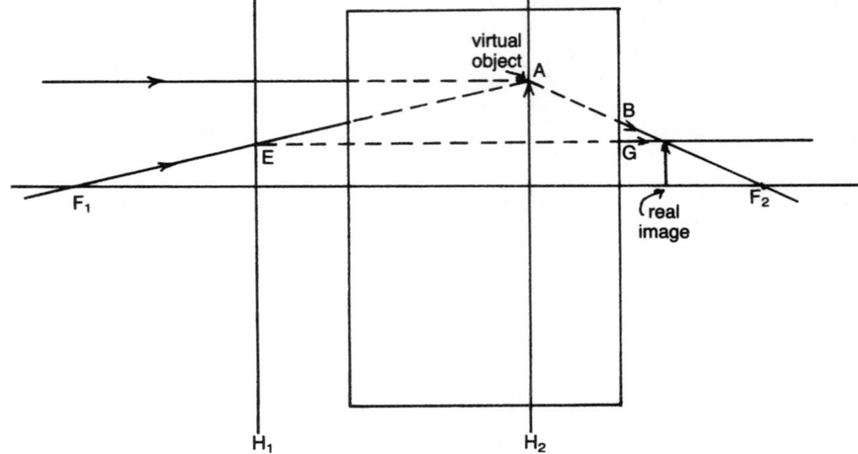

Figure 15.17 Object at same location as the secondary principal plane.

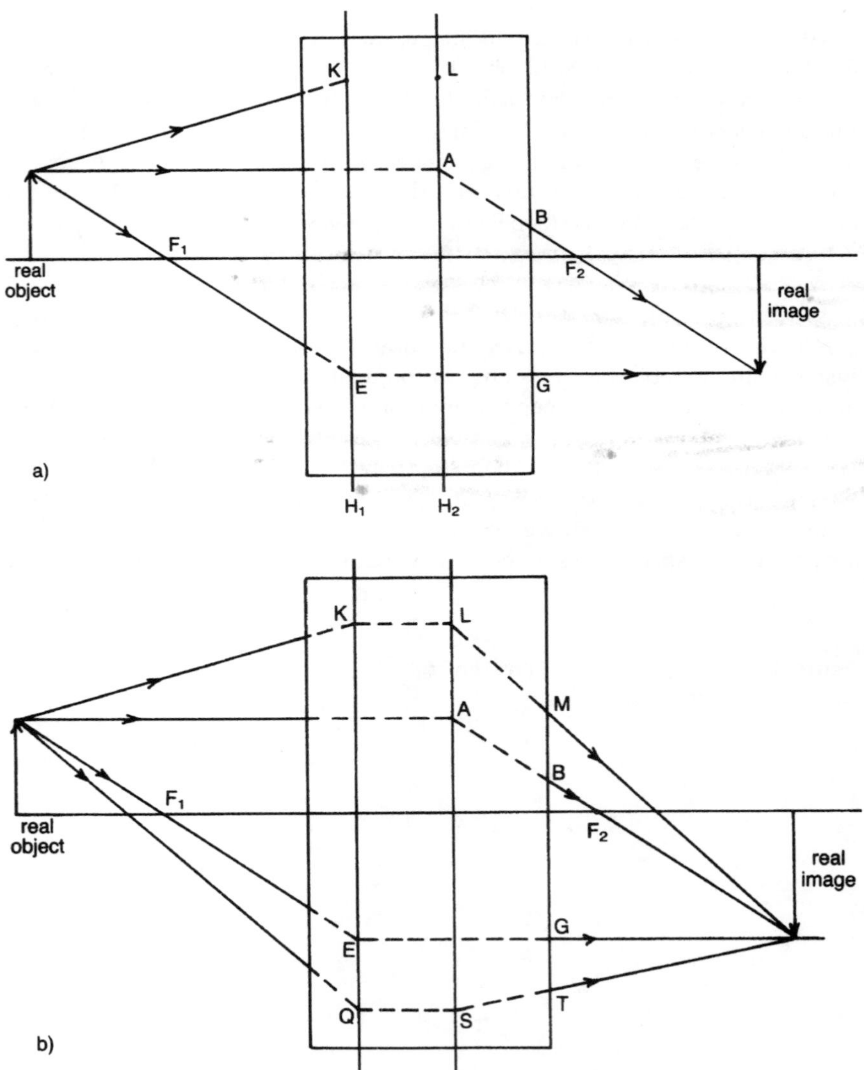

Figure 15.18 a, Object space ray intersecting primary principal plane at *K*. Image space ray must leave the secondary principal plane at the same height (*L*); b, other rays.

know the ray path inside the system, but we do know that the actual image space ray leaves the system at M and travels to the image point.

The same procedure can be used for any other ray. The bottom ray in Figure 15.18b is an example. The incident ray is extended until it hits point Q on H_1. Then we go across parallel to the axis to point S on H_2. The exiting ray must lie on the line from S to the bottom image point, and the actual ray leaves the back of the system at T.

The general rule is that once an object space ray or its extension hits a point on the primary principal plane H_1, a line parallel to the optical axis is drawn from that point to a point on the secondary principal plane H_2, and the corresponding image space ray lies on the line that includes the point on H_2 and the image point. Note that in the previous figures that the two predictable rays also follow this rule.

15.6 VERGENCE EQUATIONS

Figure 15.18b is a ray diagram in which all of the object space rays and their extensions are straight until they hit the primary principal plane H_1, and all image space rays and their extensions are straight once they leave the secondary principal plane H_2. Figure 15.18b resembles a SSRI ray diagram except that the interface is peeled into two layers, H_1 and H_2. H_1 interacts with the incident rays and is thus the object space layer, while H_2 interacts with the exiting rays and is thus the image space layer.

We can imagine the incident (object space) wavefronts propagating all the way to H_1, and we can compute the (reduced) vergence U_{H_1} that they would have there:

$$U_{H_1} = \frac{n_o}{u_{H_1}} \tag{15.1}$$

where u_{H_1} is the object distance measured from H_1, and n_o is the object space index.

Similarly, we can imagine the exiting (image space) wavefront propagating away from H_2, and we can compute the (reduced) vergence V_{H_2} that they would have there:

$$V_{H_2} = \frac{n_i}{v_{H_2}} \tag{15.2}$$

where v_{H_2} is the image distance measured from H_2, and n_i is the image space index.

As suggested by the ray diagrams, the incident and exiting vergences are related by an equation that has the same form as the SSRI vergence equation, namely,

$$V_{H_2} = P_e + U_{H_1} \tag{15.3}$$

where P_e is called the equivalent dioptric power of the system. (Equation 15.3 is derived in Chapter 16, Section 16.12.)

The name equivalent dioptric power refers to the fact that the system is acting like an SSRI of dioptric power P_e between mediums of refractive indices n_o and n_i. Just as for an SSRI, Eq. 15.3 enables us to get from the object space to the image space in one step without having to do the calculations for all the internal interfaces. In fact, the refractive indices for the mediums inside the system do not appear in Eq. 15.3.

In Section 8.9, we discussed the back vertex power P_v and the neutralizing power P_n for a system. For plane waves incident on the system, P_v is the vergence of the wavefront leaving the system's back vertex. For plane waves leaving the system, P_n is equal in magnitude but opposite in sign to the vergence incident on the system's front vertex. P_v and P_n provide information only in their respective plane wave situations, and hence are not true dioptric powers in a $V = P + U$ sense. On the other hand, Eq. 15.3 is good for any incident or exiting vergence, and thus P_e functions as a true dioptric power.

It turns out that the total lateral magnification m_t, defined as the ratio of the system's image size I to the system's object size O, is given by

$$m_t = \frac{U_{H_1}}{V_{H_2}} \tag{15.4}$$

EXAMPLE 15.1

A multiple interface system with air ($n = 1.00$) in front and water ($n = 1.33$) behind has a central thickness of 10 cm and an equivalent dioptric power of +9.00 D. The primary focal point is located 5.11 cm in front of the system's front surface, and the secondary focal point is located 12.78 cm behind the system's back surface. The primary principal plane is located 6 cm behind the front surface, and the secondary principal plane is located 8 cm behind the front surface (or 2 cm in front of the back surface). A real object is located 19 cm from the front surface of the system. Where is the conjugate image? What is the total lateral magnification?

Figure 15.19a shows the ray diagram for the situation. For the calculations, $n_o = 1.00$ and $n_i = 1.33$. The real object is 19 cm from the front surface, or 25 cm from H_1. Therefore,

$$U_{H_1} = -25\,\text{cm}$$

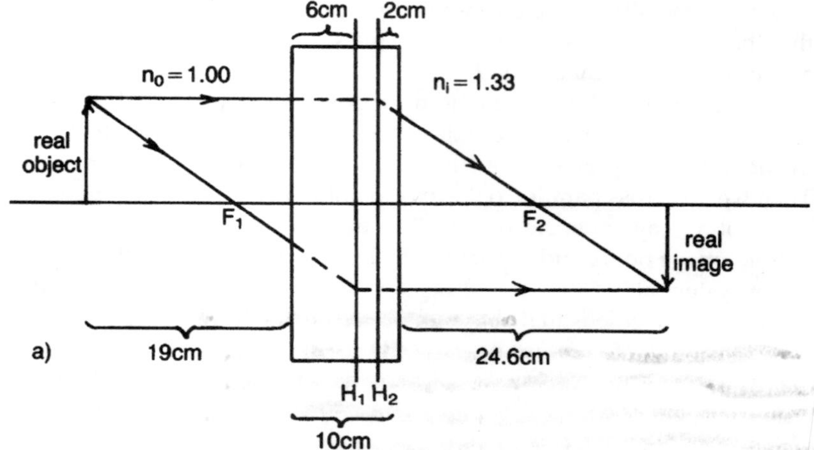

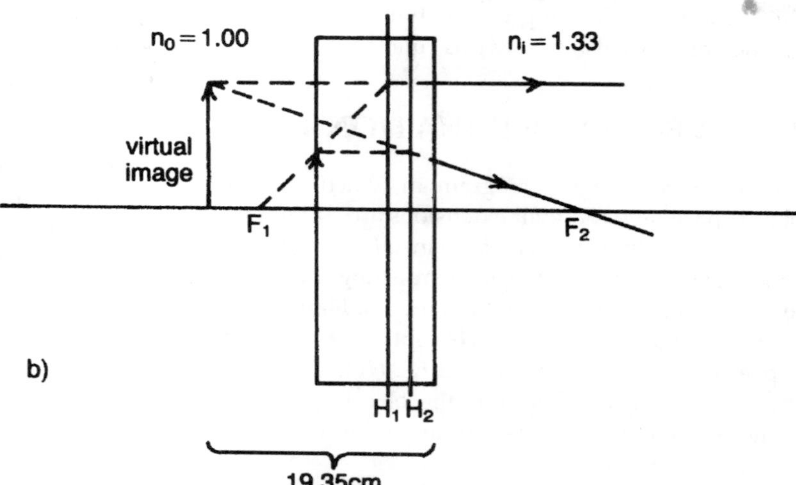

Figure 15.19 a, Predictable rays to locate a real image; b, predictable rays to locate a virtual image.

The incident light is diverging and in air. We are pretending that this incident light goes all the way to H. From Eq. 15. 1,

$$U_{H_1} = \frac{100}{-25\,\text{cm}} = -4.00\,\text{D}$$

Then,

$$V_{H_2} = P_e + U_{H_1}$$

gives

$$V_{H_2} = +9.00\,\text{D} + (-4.00\,\text{D}) = +5.00\,\text{D}$$

We are pretending the light leaving H_2 is converging and in the image space medium, water. From Eq. 15.2,

$$v_{H_2} = \frac{133}{+5.00\,\text{D}} = +26.6\,\text{cm}$$

The image is located +26.6 cm from H_2, or +24.6 cm from the back surface of the system. From Eq. 15.4,

$$m_t = \frac{-4.00\,\text{D}}{+5.00\,\text{D}} = -0.8$$

The calculated results agree with the ray diagram.

EXAMPLE 15.2

The object in the previous example is moved against the front surface of the system. Where is the conjugate image? What is the total lateral magnification?

Figure 15.19b shows the ray diagram. The real object is 6 cm in front of H_1. Therefore,

$$u_{H_1} = -6\,\text{cm}$$

As far as H_1, is concerned, the incident light is diverging and in air. Here we are pretending that this light goes all the way to H_1. From Eq. 15.1,

$$U_{H_1} = \frac{100}{-6\,\text{cm}} = -16.67\,\text{D}$$

Then,

$$V_{H_2} = P_e + U_{H_1}$$

gives

$$V_{H_2} = +9.00\,\text{D} + (-16.67\,\text{D}) = -7.67\,\text{D}$$

We are pretending the light leaving H_2 is diverging and in the image space medium, water. From Eq.15.2,

$$v_{H_2} = \frac{133}{-7.67\,\text{D}} = 17.35\,\text{cm}$$

The image is virtual and located -17.35 cm from H_2, or -19.35 cm from the back surface of the system (Figure 15.19b). From Eq. 15.4,

$$m_t = \frac{-16.67\,\text{D}}{-7.67\,\text{D}} = +2.17$$

The image is erect and a little over two times larger than the object.

15.7 POWER AND FOCAL LENGTH RELATIONS

Consider plane waves incident on the system along the optical axis. The image is located at the system's secondary focal point. Then,

$$U_{H_1} = 0 \quad \text{and} \quad v_{H_2} = f_2$$

It follows from Eqs. 15.2 and 15.3 that

$$P_e = \frac{n_i}{f_2} \tag{15.5}$$

where f_2 is the distance from H_2 to F_2 and is called the *secondary equivalent focal length*.

Remember that the distance from the back vertex L_b of the system to F_2 is called the back focal length f_b, and Eq. 8.8 was

$$P_v = \frac{n_i}{f_b} \tag{15.6}$$

For incident plane waves, we can consider a hypothetical image space wavefront that is either propagating from H_2 to L_b or from L_b to H_2, depending on which one is downstream. The vergence of the image space wavefront at H_2 is P_e, and at L_b the vergence of the image space wavefront P_v. So P_e and P_v are related by vergence effectivity in the image space.

When the object is placed at F_1 of the system, plane waves leave the back of the system. Then,

$$V_{H_2} = 0 \quad \text{and} \quad u_{H_1} = f_1$$

It follows from Eqs. 15.1 and 15.3 that

$$P_e = -\frac{n_o}{f_1} \tag{15.7}$$

where f_1 is the distance from H_1 to F_1 and is called the *primary equivalent focal length*.

Remember that the distance from the front vertex of the system to F_1 is called the front focal length f_f, and Eq. 8.9 was

$$P_n = -\frac{n_o}{f_f} \tag{15.8}$$

For plane waves leaving the system, the vergence of the wavefront incident on the system's front vertex L_1 is $-P_n$, and the vergence of the wavefront hypothetically incident on H_1 is $-P_e$. We can consider the incident object space wavefront as propagating either from L_1 to H_1 or from H_1 to L_1 depending on which one is downstream. So $-P_n$ and $-P_e$ are related by vergence effectivity in the object space.

From Eqs. 15.5 and 15.7, the primary and secondary equivalent focal lengths are related by

$$\frac{f_2}{n_i} = -\frac{f_1}{n_o} \tag{15.9}$$

Note that when the object space index n_o equals the image space index n_i, f_1 and f_2 are equal in magnitude but opposite in sign.

EXAMPLE 15.3

A multiple interface system with an equivalent dioptric power of $+5.00$ D has water ($n = 1.33$) in front of it and air ($n = 1.00$) behind it. The system is 10 cm thick, its primary principal plane is located 5 cm behind the front surface of the system, and its secondary principal plane is located 7 cm in front of the back surface of the system (Figure 15.20). Find the back vertex power and the neutralizing power.

Here $n_o = 1.33$, and $n_1 = 1.00$. For incident plane waves,

$$U_{H_1} = 0$$

and

$$V_{H_2} = P_e + U_{H_1} = +5.00\,\text{D}$$

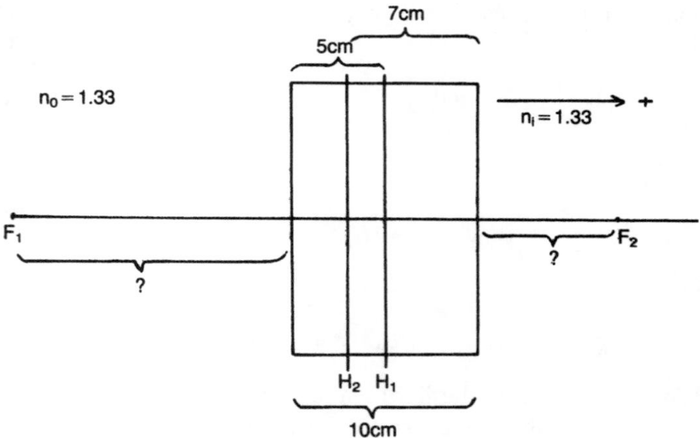

Figure 15.20 System with +5.00-D equivalent dioptric power.

H_2 is 7 cm in front of the system's back surface L_b. To get the back vertex power, we can imagine a +5.00 D wavefront in the image space medium (air in this case) propagating 7 cm downstream. From downstream vergence effectivity relations, the vergence of the wavefront at L_b is +7.69 D, and P_v is thus 7.69 D. On a more formal basis, the calculations are:

$$f_2 = \frac{n_i}{P_e} = \frac{100}{+500\,\text{D}} = +20.00\,\text{cm}$$

$$f_b = +(20.00 - 7.00)\,\text{cm} = +13.00\,\text{cm}$$

$$P_v = \frac{n_i}{f_b} = \frac{100}{+13.00\,\text{cm}} = +7.69\,\text{D}$$

Now consider an object at F_1 so that plane waves leave the back of the system. Then,

$$P_n = -U_1$$

where U_1 is the vergence incident on the system's front surface. For plane waves leaving,

$$V_{H_2} = 0$$

and from Eq. 15.3,

$$U_{H_1} = -5.00\,\text{D}$$

H_1 is 5 cm behind the system's front vertex L_1. So the wavefront incident on L_1 is upstream from H_1, and if allowed to propagate in the object space medium (water in this case), gets to H_1 with a vergence of −5.00 D. From upstream vergence effectivity relations, the wavefront at L_1 has a vergence of −6.16 D. The system can neutralize a vergence of −6.16 D incident on its front surface, so P_n is +6.16 D. On a more formal basis, the calculations are:

$$f_1 = \frac{n_o}{P_e} = \frac{133}{-5.00\,\text{D}} = -26.6\,\text{cm}$$

$$f_f = -(26.6 - 5.00)\,\text{cm} = -21.6\,\text{cm}$$

$$P_n = \frac{n_o}{f_f} = \frac{133}{-21.6\,\text{cm}} = +6.16\,\text{D}$$

As shown, we can find the vertex powers if we know the equivalent power and the principal plane locations. Conversely, when we know P_e, P_v, and P_n, we can find the principal plane locations. An easy way to find H_2 is to picture a trip from the system's back vertex to H_2 by way of F_2. In terms of directed distances,

$$L_bH_2 = L_bF_2 + F_2H_2$$
$$= L_bF_2 - H_2F_2$$

or

$$L_bH_2 = f_b - f_2 \tag{15.10}$$

Equations 15.5 and 15.6 give the focal lengths needed for Eq. 15.10. To find H_1, picture a trip from the system's front surface L_1 to H_1 via F_1. In terms of directed distances,

$$L_1H_1 = L_1F_1 + F_1H_1$$
$$= L_1F_1 - H_1F_1$$

or

$$L_1H_1 = f_f - f_1 \tag{15.11}$$

Equations 15.7 and 15.8 give the focal lengths needed in Eq. 15.11.

EXAMPLE 15.4

A multi-interface system has air in front ($n = 1.00$) and water ($n = 1.33$) behind. The central thickness of the system is 4 cm. P_e, P_v, and P_n are -10.88 D, -11.83 D, and -6.97 D, respectively. Where are the principal planes?

Let us think a little before calculating. For incident plane waves the vergence leaving H_2 is -10.88 D, and these wavefronts lose vergence as they propagate downstream. However, the back vertex power is -11.83 D, so the back vertex L_b must be upstream from H_2.

For Eq. 15.10 we need f_b and f_2:

$$f_2 = \frac{n_i}{P_e} = \frac{133}{-10.88\,\text{D}} = -12.22\,\text{cm}$$

$$f_b = \frac{n_i}{P_v} = \frac{133}{-11.83\,\text{D}} = -11.24\,\text{cm}$$

Then,

$$L_bH_2 = f_b - f_2$$

$$= -11.24\,\text{cm} - (-12.22\,\text{cm}) = +0.98\,\text{cm}$$

The secondary principal plane is 0.98 cm behind the back vertex of the system. This agrees with our expectations that L_b must be upstream from H_2.

Again, let us think about the primary principal plane location before calculating for the primary principal plane. For plane waves leaving, the vergence of the object space wavefront at H_2 must be $+10.88$ D, and the vergence of the wavefront incident on the system must be $+6.97$ D. The converging wavefronts gain vergence, so H_1 must be downstream from the front vertex L_1.

For Eq. 15.11, we need f_f and f_1:

$$f_f = -\frac{n_o}{P_n} = \frac{-100}{-6.97\,\text{D}} = +14.35\,\text{cm}$$

$$f_1 = -\frac{n_o}{P_e} = \frac{-100}{-10.88\,\text{D}} = +9.19\,\text{cm}$$

Then,

$$L_1H_1 = f_f - f_1$$

$$= 14.35\,\text{cm} - 9.19\,\text{cm} = +5.16\,\text{cm}$$

The primary principal plane is $+5.16$ cm behind the front vertex of the system, which agrees with our expectations that H_1 must be downstream from L_1. In this case, the principal plane locations are quite close together (Figure 15.21).

15.8 SYSTEMS IN AIR

When the system is in air, both the object space index n_o and the image space index n_i are equal to 1.00. The indices of 1 simplify the calculations, and from Eq. 15.9, the primary and secondary equivalent focal lengths become equal in magnitude but opposite in sign. In this case, we can think of the system as being equivalent to a single thin lens, except the thin lens has been peeled into two layers. The object space layer is at H_1, while the image space layer is at H_2. The object space layer H_1 interacts with the incident light, while the image space layer H_2 interacts with the exiting light. In practice, H_1 may be in front of, coincident with, or behind H_2, but in any event, the incident light is referenced to H_1 and the exiting light to H_2.

EXAMPLE 15.5

A 15 cm thick system with air on both sides has an equivalent dioptric power of $+4.50$ D. The primary principal plane is located 5 cm in front of the front vertex of the system, and the secondary principal plane is located 8 cm in front of the front vertex. A real object is 49.44 cm from the front vertex of the system. Where is the conjugate image? What is the lateral magnification?

To draw a ray diagram, we need to locate the focal points. From Eq. 15.5,

$$f_2 = \frac{n_i}{P_e} = \frac{100}{+4.50\,\text{D}} = +22.22\,\text{cm}$$

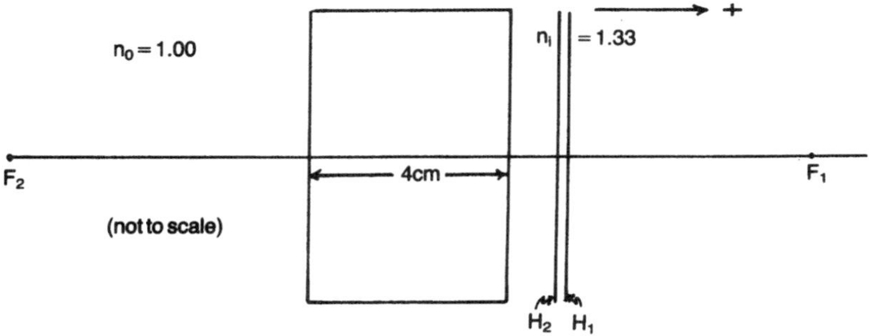

Figure 15.21 System with −10.88 D equivalent dioptric power.

and from Eq. 15.7,

$$f_1 = -\frac{n_o}{P_e} = \frac{100}{+4.50\,\text{D}} = -22.22\,\text{cm}$$

From Eq. 15.11,

$$f_f = L_1H_1 + f_1$$
$$= -5\,\text{cm} + (-22.22\,\text{cm}) = -27.22\,\text{cm}$$

So F_1, is 27.22 cm from the system's front vertex. H_2 is 8 cm in front of L_1, or 23 cm in front of the back vertex L_b. From Eq. 15.10,

$$f_b = L_bH_2 + f_2$$
$$= -23\,\text{cm} + 22.22\,\text{cm} = -0.78\,\text{cm}$$

So F_2 is 0.78 cm in front of the system's back vertex. Figure 15.21 shows the ray diagram.

The real object is 49.44 cm from the front vertex, or 44.44 cm in front of H_1. So,

$$u_{H_1} = -44.44\,\text{cm}$$

and

$$U_{H_1} = \frac{100}{-44.44\,\text{cm}} = -2.25\,\text{D}$$

Then,

$$V_{H_2} = P_e + U_{H_1}$$

gives

$$V_{H_2} = +4.50\,\text{D} + (-2.25\,\text{D}) = +2.25\,\text{D}$$

and

$$v_{H_2} = \frac{100}{+2.25\,\text{D}} = +44.44\,\text{cm}$$

The image is located 44.44 cm behind H_2. Since H_2 is 23 cm in front of L_b, the image is real and located 21.44 cm behind L_b. From Eq. 15.4, the lateral magnification is

$$m = \frac{U_{H_1}}{V_{H_2}} = \frac{-2.25\,\text{D}}{+2.25\,\text{D}} = -1$$

15.9 THE SYMMETRY POINTS

Previously, we saw that the symmetry points $2F_1$ and $2F_2$ gave a lateral magnification of −1. In the above example, the total lateral magnification is −1, the object distance as measured from H_1 (−44.44 cm) is twice the primary equivalent focal length (−22.22 cm), and the image distance as measured from H_2 is twice the secondary equivalent focal length. Hence, we can identify $2F_1$ and $2F_2$ as the symmetry points for the Gauss system, provided that by $2F_1$ and $2F_2$ we mean that

$$u_{H_1} = 2f_1 \quad \text{and} \quad v_{H_2} = 2f_2 \qquad (15.12)$$

The above equations give the symmetry points even when the object and image space indices differ from 1. Thus, $2F_1$ and $2F_2$ are the symmetry points in all cases. Figure 15.15 is a ray diagram for a symmetry point case in which the equivalent dioptric power is negative.

EXAMPLE 15.6

Where are the symmetry points for the system in Example 15.1?

From example 15.1, $n_o = 1.00$, $n_i = 1.33$, and $P_e = +9.00$ D. So,

$$f_2 = \frac{n_i}{P_e} = \frac{133}{+9.00\,\text{D}} = +14.78\,\text{cm}$$

and

$$f_1 = -\frac{n_o}{P_e} = \frac{-100}{+9.00\,\text{D}} = -11.11\,\text{cm}$$

For the symmetry points

$$u_{H_2} = 2f_1 = 2(-11.11\,\text{cm}) = -22.22\,\text{cm}$$

and

$$v_{H_2} = 2f_2 = 2(+14.78\,\text{cm}) = +29.56\,\text{cm}$$

You may verify that the total lateral magnification is −1.

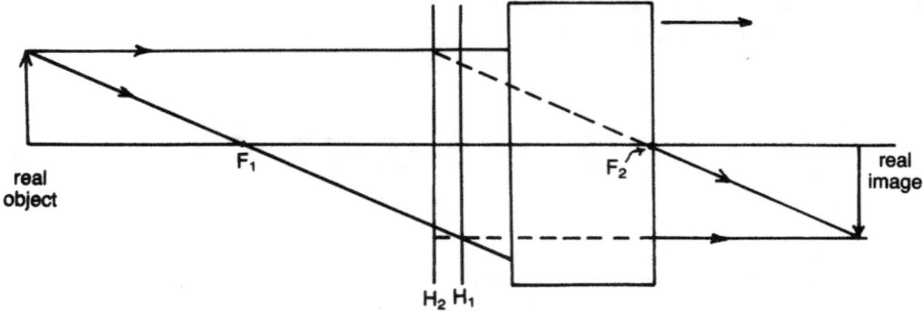

Figure 15.22 Inverted image that is the same size as the object.

15.10 REDUCED SYSTEMS

For a reduced system, the object and image space indices are both 1. Furthermore, the dioptric powers and vergences in the reduced system must equal those in the actual system. Then from Eqs. 15.1 through 15.9, the reduced distances are as follows:

15.10.1 Object Space Distances

$$\bar{u}_{H_1} = \frac{u_{H_1}}{n_o} \tag{15.13}$$

$$\bar{f}_1 = \frac{f_1}{n_o} \tag{15.14}$$

$$\bar{f}_f = \frac{f_f}{n_o} \tag{15.15}$$

From Eq. 15.11,

$$\overline{L_1H_1} = \bar{f}_f - \bar{f}_1 \tag{15.16}$$

We can substitute Eqs. 15.14 and 15.15 into 15.16 to show that

$$\overline{L_1H_1} = \frac{L_1H_1}{n_o} \tag{15.17}$$

Equation 15.17 shows that the directed distance L_1H_1 acts like an object space distance.

15.10.2 Image Space Distances

$$\bar{v}_{H_2} = \frac{v_{H_2}}{n_i} \tag{15.18}$$

$$\bar{f}_2 = \frac{f_2}{n_i} \tag{15.19}$$

$$\bar{f}_b = \frac{f_b}{n_i} \tag{15.20}$$

Then from Eq. 15.10,

$$\overline{L_bH_2} = \bar{f}_b - \bar{f}_2 \tag{15.21}$$

We can substitute Eqs. 15.19 and 15.20 into 15.21 to show that

$$\overline{L_bH_2} = \frac{L_bH_2}{n_i} \tag{15.22}$$

Equation 15.22 shows that the directed distance L_bH_2 acts like an image space distance. The vergence and dioptric power equations are:

$$V_{H_2} = 1/\bar{v}_{H_2} \tag{15.23}$$

$$U_{H_1} = 1/\bar{u}_{H_1} \tag{15.24}$$

$$P_e = 1/\bar{f}_2 = -1/\bar{f}_1 \tag{15.25}$$

$$P_v = 1/\bar{f}_b \quad \text{and} \quad P_n = -1/\bar{f}_f \tag{15.26}$$

Equations 15.13 through 15.26 enable us to work in a reduced system when advantageous to do so.

EXAMPLE 15.7a

A 21 cm glass ($n = 1.500$) rod with spherical surfaces has ethyl alcohol ($n = 1.362$) in front and water ($n = 1.333$) behind. The respective dioptric powers of the front and back interfaces are −6.00 D and +6.00 D. The equivalent dioptric power of the system is +5.040 D. When reduced, the system is represented by lenses L_1 and L_b representing the rod's front and back interfaces, separated by reduced central thickness of 14 cm. In the reduced system, the primary principal plane is 2.667 cm behind L_b and the secondary principal plane is 16.667 cm behind L_b (Figure 15.23a). Find the focal points in the reduced system.

From Eq. 15.25, the equivalent focal lengths are:

$$\bar{f}_2 = \frac{1}{P_e} = \frac{100}{+5.040\text{ D}} = +19.841\text{ cm}$$

and

$$\bar{f}_1 = -19.841\text{ cm}$$

From Eq. 15.22,

$$\bar{f}_b = \overline{L_bH_2} + \bar{f}_2$$
$$= +16.667\text{ cm} + 19.841\text{ cm} = +36.508\text{ cm}$$

H_1 is 2.667 cm behind L_b or 16.667 cm behind L_1. From Eq. 15.17,

$$\bar{f}_f = \overline{L_1H_1} + \bar{f}_1$$
$$= +16.667\text{ cm} + (-19.841\text{ cm}) = -3.174\text{ cm}$$

EXAMPLE 15.7b

For the previous example, find the principal planes and the focal points in the actual system.

From Example 15.7a, $\bar{f}_f = 3.174$ cm and $\bar{f}_b = 36.508$ cm. From Eq. 15.15,

$$f_f = n_o\bar{f}_f$$
$$= (1.362)(-3.174\text{ cm}) = -4.323\text{ cm}$$

From Eq. 15.20,

$$f_b = n_i\bar{f}_b$$
$$= (1.333)(+36.508\text{ cm}) = +48.665\text{ cm}$$

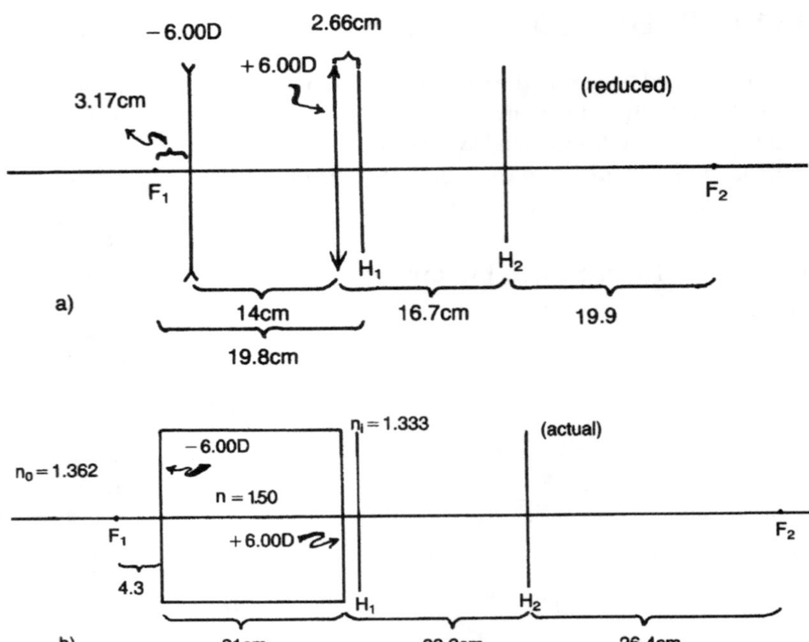

Figure 15.23 a, Reduced system; b, actual system.

From Eq. 15.17,

$$L_1H_1 = n_o\overline{L_1H_1}$$
$$= (1.362)(+16.667\,\text{cm}) = +22.700$$

From Eq. 15.22,

$$L_bH_2 = n_i\overline{L_bH_2}$$
$$= (1.33)(+16.667\,\text{cm}) = +22.217\,\text{cm}$$

Figure 15.23b shows the actual system.

15.11 THE NODAL POINTS

Consider Figure 15.18b, which is a diagram for an actual system. A number of the top rays are bent down by the system, and a number of the bottom rays are bent up by the system. Somewhere in the middle there must be a ray that does not bend, although it may be displaced due to the fact that H_1 and H_2 are not at the same position. The ray that does not bend is the nodal ray.

The outgoing nodal ray is always parallel to the incident nodal ray (Figure 15.24). The point at which the incident nodal ray or its extension hits the optical axis is called the *primary nodal point* N_1. The point at which the exiting nodal ray or its extension hits the axis is called the *secondary nodal point* N_2. As shown, the nodal points do not have to coincide with the principal points.

Figure 15.25 shows an actual ray diagram for incident plane waves. The two incident rays are parallel to each other and both make an angle w with the axis. One is the nodal ray and the other passes through F_1. Since plane waves are incident on the system, the image is in the secondary focal plane.

The exiting nodal ray, being parallel to the incident nodal ray, makes the same angle w with the axis. The incident nodal ray or its extension intersects H_1 at a distance g above the axis, so the exiting nodal ray or its

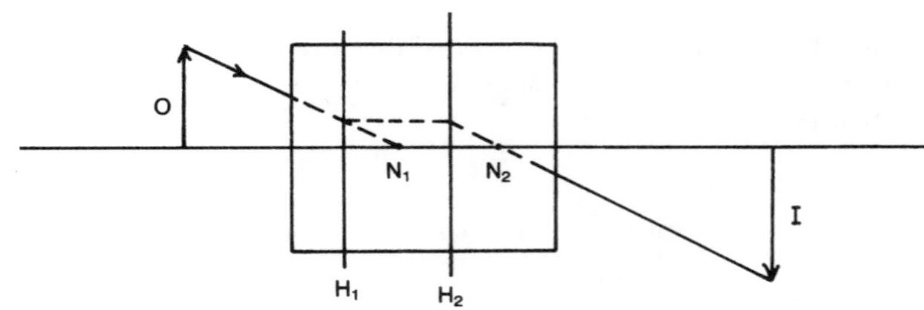

Figure 15.24 Primary and secondary nodal points.

Figure 15.25 Predictable rays for incident plane waves from an off-axis object point.

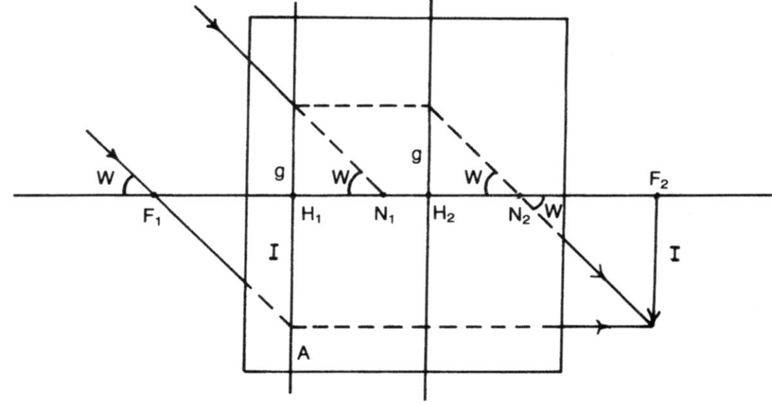

extension has to leave H_2, at the same distance g above the axis. Then from the triangles involving H and N,

$$\tan w = \frac{g}{H_1N_1} \quad \text{and} \quad \tan w = \frac{g}{H_2N_2}$$

It follows that the displacement H_1N_1 equals the displacement H_2N_2. Frequently the subscripts are dropped with the understanding that

$$HN = H_1N_1 = H_2N_2 \tag{15.27}$$

From the triangle involving N_2 and the image of size I (which is negative),

$$I = -N_2F_2 \tan w \tag{15.28}$$

For the incident ray through F_1 the exiting ray is parallel to the axis, leaves H_1 at point A, and passes through the image point. Consequently, the distance along H_1 from the axis to A is equal to the image size I. Then from the triangle involving H_1, A, and F_1,

$$I = f_1 \tan w \tag{15.29}$$

Note that we can use either Eq. 15.28 or Eq. 15.29 to calculate the image size for a distant object that subtends the angle w. In particular, f_1 is quickly determined from the equivalent dioptric power, and so, Eq. 15.29 is easy to use. From Eqs. 15.28 and 15.29,

$$F_1 = -N_2F_2 \tag{15.30}$$

From the figure,

$$N_2F_2 = H_2F_2 - HN$$

or

$$N_2F_2 = f_2 - HN$$

It follows from Eq. 15.30 and the above equation that

$$HN = f_1 + f_2 \tag{15.31}$$

Equation 15.31 indicates that the displacement of the nodal points from the principal planes is equal to the sum of the primary and secondary equivalent focal lengths.

The nodal point of an SSRI is at the center of curvature of the SSRI. In other words, the nodal point for an SSRI is displaced from the interface by the distance r where r is the interface's radius of curvature. From Eq. 7.25 for an SSRI,

$$r = f_1 + f_2$$

Equations 15.31 and 7.25 are clearly analogous.

Equations 15.5 and 15.7 can be substituted into Eq. 15.31 with the result that

$$HN = \frac{n_i - n_o}{P_e} \tag{15.32}$$

Equation 15.32 is analogous to the familiar SSRI equation

$$r = \frac{n_2 - n_1}{P}$$

The analogous equations reemphasize the fact that the system acts like an SSRI of power P_e between the object space medium (index n_o) and the image space medium (index n_i).

Because of the SSRI analogy, it is easy to decide which way the nodal points are displaced away from the principal planes. We simply think of which way the corresponding SSRI would be curved. Consider a multi-interface system with a positive equivalent dioptric power separating water on the left from air on the right. The corresponding SSRI between water and air has a positive P, and is convex to the lower index medium, so C is to the left of the interface

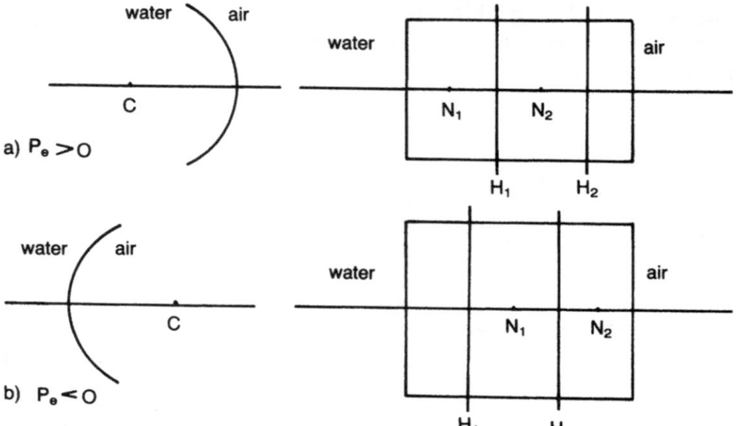

Figure 15.26 SSRI analogy for nodal point displacement: a, positive equivalent power; b, negative equivalent power.

(Figure 15.26a). Consequently, the nodal points for the multi-interface system are displaced to the left (i.e., toward the water). When the equivalent dioptric power is negative, the displacement is the other way (i.e., toward the air as shown in Figure 15.26b).

When the object and image spaces have the same refractive index, then HN is zero and the nodal points coincide with the principal points. In a reduced system, the object and image space indices are both one. Therefore, in a reduced system, the nodal points are at the principal points.

EXAMPLE 15.8

When we look at an object, the cornea and crystalline lens of the eye constitute a refracting system between air (the object space medium) and the eye's vitreous humor (the image space medium). In Gullstrand's #1 schematic eye, the equivalent power is +58.64 D, the primary and secondary principal planes are, respectively, 1.348 mm and 1.602 mm behind the front surface of the cornea. Where are the nodal points of the eye relative to the principal planes? (The vitreous index is 1.336).

First, let us think about which way we expect the displacement to be. A positive SSRI between air and vitreous would have a center of curvature in the vitreous, so the displacement should be toward the vitreous (Figure 15.27).

From Eq. 15.32,

$$HN = \frac{(1.336 - 1.000)1000\,\text{mm/m}}{+58.64\,\text{D}}$$
$$= \frac{336}{+58.64\,\text{D}} = +5.730\,\text{mm}$$

The nodal points are displaced 5.73 mm from the principal planes toward the vitreous. Then N_1 and N_2 are, respectively, 7.078 mm and 7.332 mm behind the anterior cornea. In Gullstrand's #1 eye, the posterior surface of the crystalline lens is 7.2 mm behind the anterior cornea, so the nodal points straddle this surface. It is interesting to note that a small posterior cataract in the nodal point region is much more detrimental to vision than a large cataract elsewhere in the crystalline lens. This is because such a cataract sits directly on the visual axis and scatters light along the nodal ray path back toward the fovea when a person tries to look at an object. A cataract, even a larger one, that is located elsewhere in the crystalline lens, scatters light but not necessarily toward the foveal area.

Figure 15.28a shows two nodal rays, one traveling slightly downward and one traveling slightly upward. Consider a virtual point source located at N_1. The incident rays in Figure 15.28a are two of the object space rays for this virtual object point. The exiting rays in Figure 15.28a are the corresponding image space rays, and they show that the conjugate image is virtual and located at N_2. We can repeat this type of diagram for any system, so that an object at N_1 is always conjugate to an image at N_2. For an extended object at N_1, the lateral magnification is n_o/n_i. (You can verify the lateral magnification for the conjugate nodal planes by

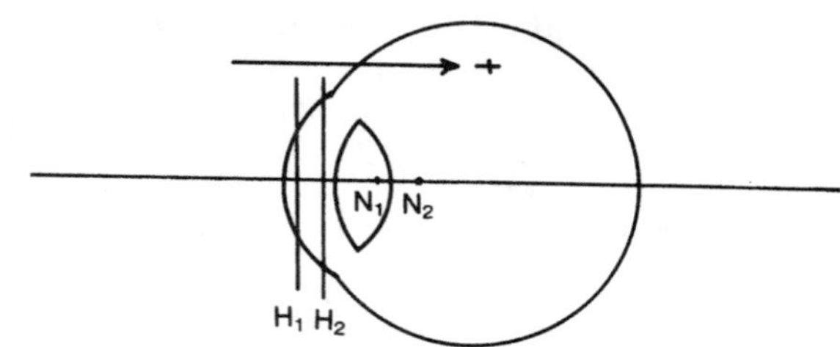

Figure 15.27 Principal planes and nodal points for the eye.

Figure 15.28 Object at primary nodal plane: a, axial rays; b, off-axis rays.

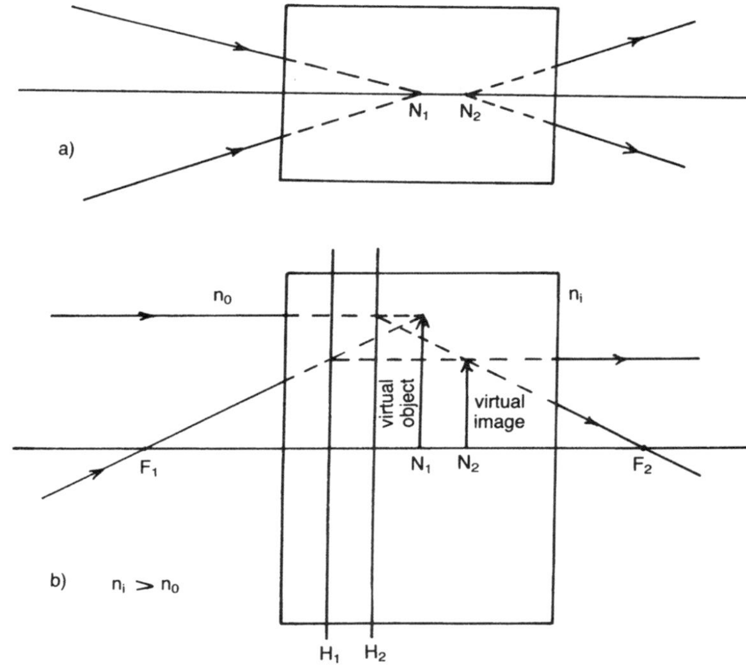

using Eqs. 15.1, 15.2, 15.4, and 15.27.) The nodal point case is analogous to an SSRI when the object is at the center of curvature *C*. Figure 15.28b shows an extended ray diagram for an object for a system with a positive P_e, and n_i greater than n_o.

15.12 THE CARDINAL POINTS AND REVERSIBILITY

The following points are collectively called the *cardinal points* of a system: the primary and secondary focal points (F_1 and F_2), the primary and secondary principal points (H_1 and H_2), the primary and secondary nodal points (N_1 and N_2), and the primary and secondary symmetry points ($2F_1$ and $2F_2$—where the doubling is done with the equivalent focal lengths). When the direction of light through a system is reversed, each pair of cardinal points stays in the same place but exchanges roles (i.e., F_1 and F_2 exchange roles, H_1 and H_2 exchange roles, N_1 and N_2 exchange roles, and $2F_1$ and $2F_2$ exchange roles). Figure 15.29a shows the cardinal points for light traveling right, and Figure 15.29b shows the same system for light traveling left.

Figure 15.29 a, Gauss parameters for light traveling right; b, same system for light traveling left.

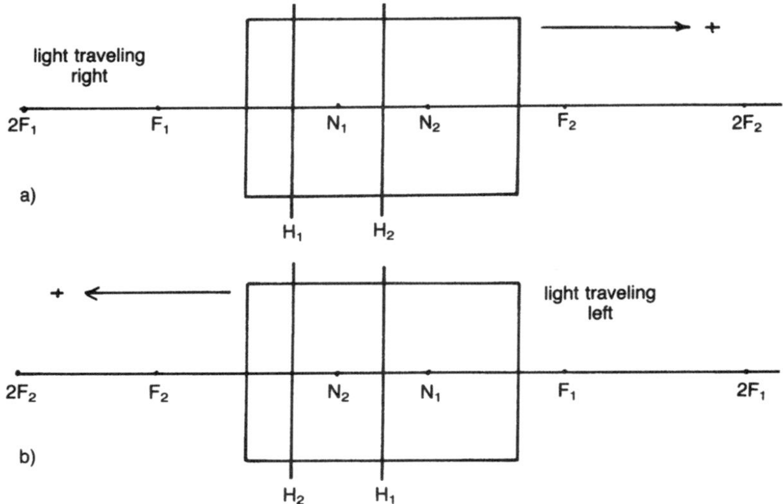

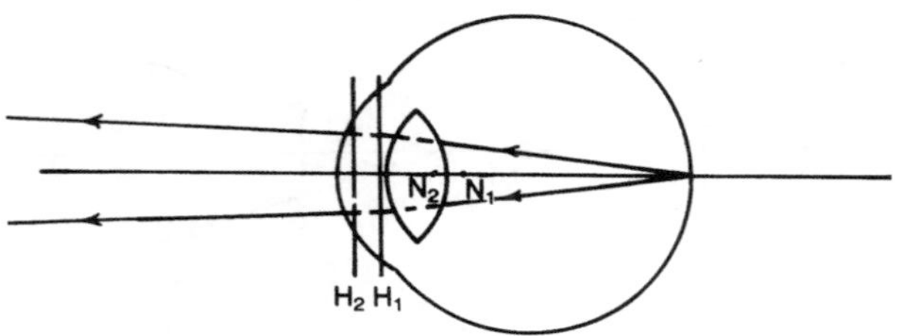

Figure 15.30 Retina as the object.

EXAMPLE 15.9

Gullstrand's #1 schematic eye (used in Example 15.8) is a model of the typical human eye. In Gullstrand's #1 eye, the retina is located 24.0 mm from the anterior corneal surface. Where is the far point for Gullstrand's #1 schematic eye?

The far point is conjugate to the retina, and we could find it by using the image distance and working backwards. Alternatively, we can consider light coming out of the eye (i.e., reversed), which is the situation when doing ophthalmoscopy or retinoscopy.

For light going into the eye, the equivalent dioptric power, principal plane locations, and refractive indices are given in Example 15.8 and shown in Figure 15.27. Figure 15.30 shows the schematic eye for light coming out, in which case H_1 and H_2 have exchanged roles. Thus, the reversed H_1 is 1.602 mm behind the cornea, or 22.398 mm from the retina. For the reversed light,

$$n_o = 1.336 \quad \text{and} \quad n_i = 1.000$$

From Eq. 15.1,

$$U_{H_1} = \frac{1336}{-22.398\,\text{mm}} = -59.65\,\text{D}$$

The equivalent dioptric power does not change, and from Eq. 15.3,

$$V_{H_2} = +58.65\,\text{D} + (-59.65\,\text{D}) = -1.00\,\text{D}$$

The light leaving Gullstrand's #1 eye is diverging, and the image is virtual. As referenced to the principal planes, the typical eye is 1 D hyperopic.

From Eq. 15.2,

$$v_{H_2} = \frac{100}{-1.00\,\text{D}} = -100\,\text{cm}$$

For the reversed light, H_2 is 1.348 mm behind the anterior cornea, so the far point is 101.35 cm from the cornea. It is interesting to note that for people aged 35 or younger, a 1 D hyperope has accommodation to spare and essentially functions the same as an emmetrope.

EXAMPLE 15.10

Consider an axial myopic eye with refracting interfaces the same as those in Gullstrand's #1 eye, but with a lengthened vitreous chamber so that the distance from the anterior cornea to the retina is 30 mm. Find the distance vision contact correction for the myopic eye.

As compared to Example 15.9, the only change is the axial length. So for the reversed situation (light coming out of the eye), the retina is 28.398 cm from H_1, (i.e., 30 − 1.602). Then,

$$U_{H_1} = \frac{1336}{-28.398\,\text{mm}} = -47.05\,\text{D}$$

$$V_{H_2} = +58.64\,\text{D} + (-47.05\,\text{D}) = +11.59\,\text{D}$$

$$v_{H_2} = \frac{100}{+11.59\,\text{D}} = +8.63\,\text{cm}$$

The eye is 11.59 D myopic as measured at the principal planes. The far point is real and 8.63 cm in front of the reversed H_2 or 8.49 cm in front of the cornea. The contact correction needed is then −11.77 D (i.e., 100 divided by −8.49).

15.13 SSRI AND THIN LENS AS A GAUSS SYSTEM

Consider an SSRI as the system. Where are the principal planes? Figure 15.31 shows a standard paraxial

Figure 15.31 Principal planes for an SSRI.

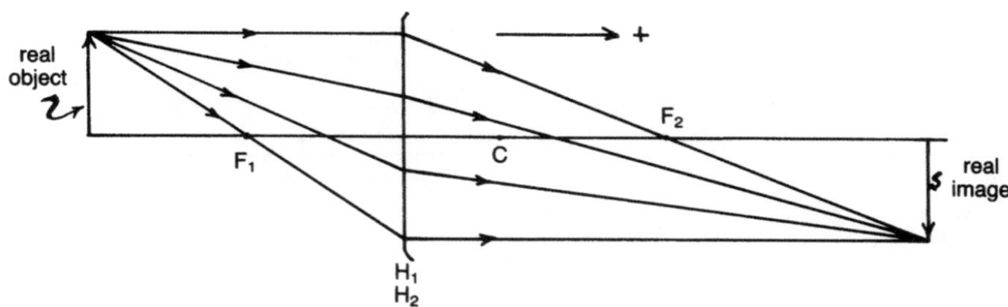

Figure 15.32 Principal planes for a thin lens.

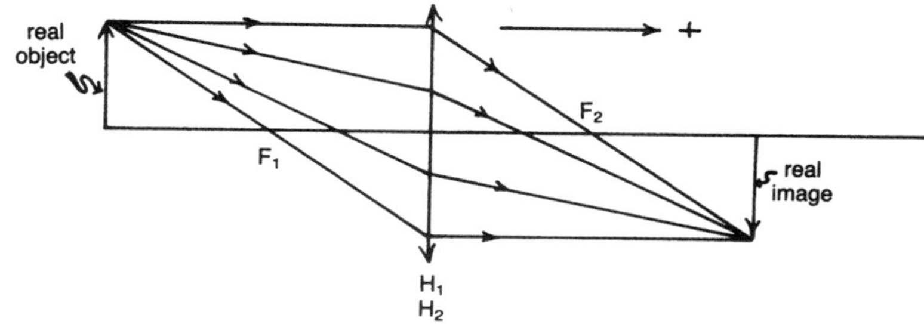

ray diagram for a converging SSRI. The rays bend (are refracted) only at the interface, so the object and image space intersection points occur only at the interface. Hence, the principal points H_1 and H_2 coincide at the vertex of the interface. This is consistent with the fact that for an SSRI, an object distance of zero gives an image distance of zero and a lateral magnification of +1. For the SSRI, the nodal points are displaced from the principal planes, and they are both coincident with C, the center of curvature of the interface.

For a thin lens in air, a standard ray diagram, such as Figure 15.32, shows that the object and image space intersection points occur in the plane of the lens. Thus, H_1 and H_2 are both in the plane of the lens. Since the object and image space indices are the same ($n = 1$), the nodal points are not displaced and both N_1 and N_2 are located at the optical center of the lens.

15.14 NEWTON'S EQUATION

Newton's equation (Section 9.9) can also be applied to a Gauss system. Figure 15.33 shows a Gauss system ray diagram. The image is a distance x' (i.e., the extra-focal image distance) from F_2, while the object is a distance x (i.e., the extra-focal object distance) from F_1. For the incident ray through F_1, the exiting ray leaves parallel to the axis at a distance I from the axis. The triangle involving the incident ray, the object, and the extra-focal distance x is similar to the triangle involving the incident ray, the primary equivalent focal length f_1, and H_1. Then,

$$\frac{O}{x} = \frac{-I}{f_1}$$

or

$$m_t = \frac{I}{O} = \frac{-f_1}{x} \tag{15.33}$$

The incident ray parallel to the axis is a distance O from the axis, and the exiting ray passes through F_2. The triangle involving the exiting ray, the secondary equivalent focal length f_2, and H_2 is similar to the triangle involving the exiting ray, the extra-focal distance x', and the image. Then,

$$\frac{O}{f_2} = \frac{-I}{x'}$$

or

$$m_t = \frac{I}{O} = \frac{-x'}{f_2} \tag{15.34}$$

Equations 15.33 and 15.34 can be combined to give

$$x\,x' = f_1\,f_2 \tag{15.35}$$

In terms of the vergences at the focal points, Eq. 15.35 becomes

$$X\,X' = -(P_e)^2 \tag{15.36}$$

Figure 15.33 Newton's parameters for a thick system. The extra-focal image distance x' is the directed distance from F_2 to the image. The extra-focal object distance x is the directed distance from F_1 to the object.

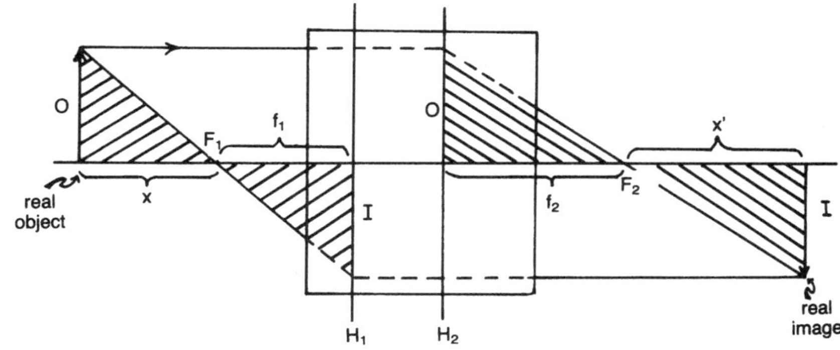

Note that the focal lengths that appear in Equations 15.33 through 15.35 are the primary and secondary equivalent focal lengths (f_1 and f_2), and not the front and back focal lengths (f_f or f_b). Equation 15.33, 15.34, or 15.36 can be used directly to determine the equivalent power of a system even when the principal plane location is not yet known.

EXAMPLE 15.11a

Consider an 8 cm thick multilens system in air. For a distant object, the system forms an real image 12 cm behind the back vertex. When a real object placed 20 cm from the front vertex of the system, the system forms a conjugate real image 18.67 cm behind the back vertex with a lateral magnification of −0.667. What is the equivalent dioptric power of the system? Where is the secondary principal plane?

For the extrafocal image distance:

$$x' = +18.67\,\text{cm} - 12\,\text{cm} = +6.67\,\text{cm}$$

From Eq. 15.34,

$$f_2 = \frac{-x'}{m} = \frac{-6.67\,\text{cm}}{-0.667} = +10.0\,\text{cm}$$

Then Eq. 15.5 gives

$$P_e = \frac{100}{+10.0\,\text{cm}} = +10.0\,\text{D}$$

From Eq. 15.10,

$$L_bH_2 = +12.0\,\text{cm} - 10.0\,\text{cm} = +2\,\text{cm}$$

or the secondary principal plane is located 2 cm behind the system's back vertex.

EXAMPLE 15.11b

If the primary focal point of the same system is 3 cm in front of the front vertex, where is the primary principal plane?

Here the front focal length f_f is −3 cm. From Example 15.11a, the secondary focal length f_2 is +10.00 cm and Eq. 15.7 gives $f_1 = -10.0\,\text{cm}$. Then from Eq. 15.11,

$$L_1H_1 = -3.0\,\text{cm} - (-10.0\,\text{cm}) = +7.0\,\text{cm}$$

So the primary principal plane is 7.0 cm behind the system's front vertex.

15.15 THE NODAL SLIDE

The nodal slide is an apparatus that is used to measure the location of a system's nodal points. For a system in air, the nodal points are at the principal planes, which are then located by this method.

Assume the system has a horizontal optical axis. The method consists of rotating the system back and forth around a vertical axis and observing the effects on the image. Typically, the image moves back and forth on the image screen. However, the speed of movement of the image varies depending on the point of rotation. At some point, the image remains stationary during the rotation. This is the end point of the method.

Figure 15.34a shows a light from a distance axial object point, in which case the image is at F_2, Figure 15.34b shows the system rotated about some point R. The image space nodal ray is displaced down relative to the object space nodal ray. The conjugate image

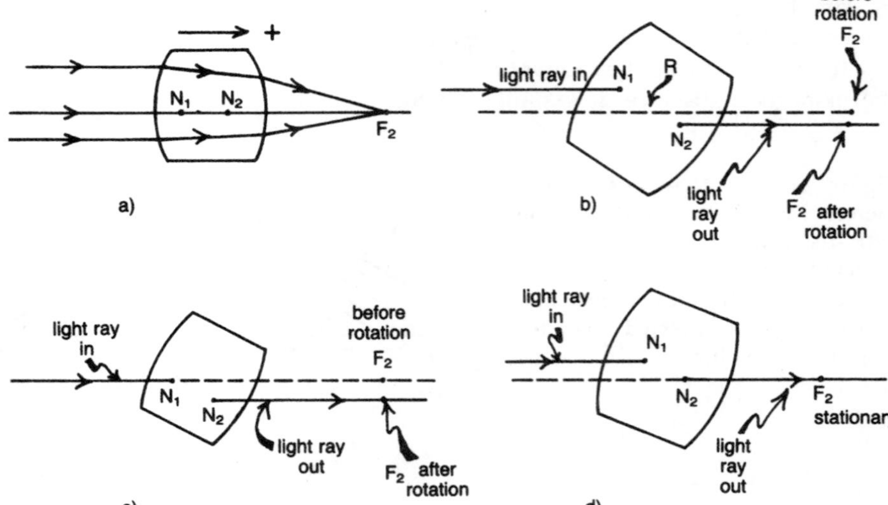

Figure 15.34 a, Rays from a distant axial object point; b, system rotated around point R; c, system rotated around primary nodal point; d, stationary image for system rotated around the secondary nodal point.

point lies on the nodal ray, so the conjugate image is displaced down relative to the unrotated lens in Figure 15.34a. Figure 15.34c shows the results of a rotation around the primary nodal point N_1. The nodal ray is traced, and again the image is displaced down relative to Figure 15.34a. Figure 15.34d shows the results for a rotation around the secondary nodal point N_2. Here, the image point has not moved relative to that of Figure 15.34a, and thus, the image is stationary for rotations around N_2.

When the light through the system is reversed, then F_1 and F_2 trade places. H_1 and H_2 trade places, and N_1 and N_2 trade places. The principal of reversibility applied to the situation of Figure 15.34d shows that for an object at F_1, the conjugate image at optical infinity is stationary for rotations around N_1. In summary, for an object at optical infinity, the stationary point is at N_2. For an object at F_1, the stationary point is N_1. As an object is moved from optical infinity to F_1 the stationary point moves from N_2 to N_1.

The easiest way to use a nodal slide is with a distant object (or a collimated source). The stationary point procedure then determines the location of N_2. As opposed to using an object at F_1 to find N_1, it is easier to just turn the nodal slide around so that the light from the distant object is now passing backwards through the system. We can then determine N_2 for the reversed situation by the stationary point procedure, but the reversed N_2 is just the N_1 of the original system. Thus the nodal slide determines the location of both N_1 and N_2 of the original system.

15.16 THICK LENSES

As shown, the equivalent power of a system can be found by using Eqs. 15.34 and 15.5. However, it would be useful to be able to find the equivalent power directly from the individual powers and (reduced) distances in the system. The modern procedure for doing this is a simple method that utilizes matrices, and is covered in Chapter 16. For two surface systems, there is a simple equation for P_e. A geometric derivation is given below, and a derivation using matrices is given in Chapter 16.

A thick lens has two refracting surfaces. When reduced, the thick lens is represented by two separated thin lenses. Therefore, the equations below apply to either two separated thin lenses or to a thick lens.

First let us review the procedure for finding the back vertex power P_v of a thick lens. The back vertex power is just the vergence leaving the back surface when plane waves are incident on the front surface.

EXAMPLE 15.12

An 11.4 mm thick ophthalmic crown ($n = 1.523$) spectacle lens has a front surface power of +16.00 D and a back surface power of −2.00 D. What is the back vertex power of the lens?

$$\bar{d} = \frac{d}{n} = \frac{1.14\,\text{cm}}{1.523} = 0.75\,\text{cm}$$

Let

$$U_1 = 0$$

Then,

$$V_1 = P_1 + U_1 = +16.00\,\text{D}$$
$$\bar{v}_1 = \frac{100}{+16.00\,\text{D}} = +6.25\,\text{cm}$$
$$\bar{u}_2 = +6.25\,\text{cm} - 0.75\,\text{cm} = +5.50\,\text{cm}$$
$$U_2 = \frac{100}{+5.50\,\text{D}} = +18.18\,\text{D}$$
$$V_2 = P_2 + U_2 = -2.00\,\text{D} + (18.18\,\text{D})$$
$$P_v = V_2 = +16.18\,\text{D}$$

Now consider the procedure algebraically (instead of numerically). We want to determine the back vertex power of a lens with a refractive index n, a central thickness d, a front surface power P_1, and a back surface power P_2. The reduced system, shown in Figure 15.35a, consists of two thin lenses of dioptric powers P_1 and P_2 separated by the reduced thickness $\bar{d}$ (which equals d/n). For plane waves incident on the front, the vergence leaving the front surface equals P_1, and the downstream vergence effectivity (equation 6.9) gives the vergence U_2 incident on the back surface:

$$U_2 = \frac{P_1}{1 - \bar{d}P_1}$$

Then $V = P + U$ for the second surface gives

$$P_v = P_2 + \frac{P_1}{1 - \bar{d}P_1}$$

or

$$P_v = \frac{P_2(1 - \bar{d}P_1) + P_1}{1 - \bar{d}P_1}$$

and

$$P_v = \frac{P_1 + P_2 - \bar{d}P_1P_2}{1 - \bar{d}P_1} \tag{15.37}$$

We need Eq. 15.37 for the deviation of Eq. 15.40.

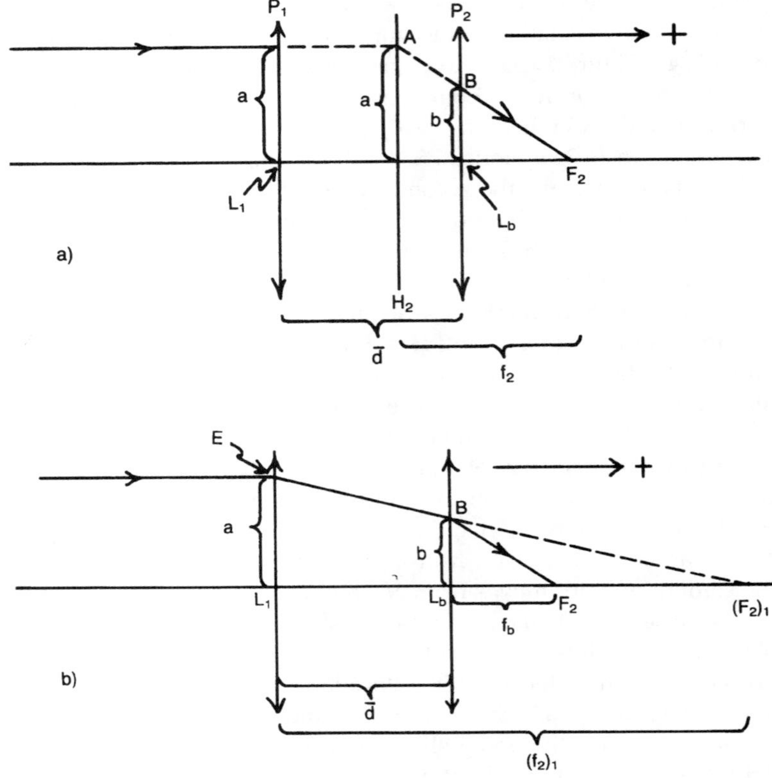

Figure 15.35 a, Secondary principal plane for two lens system; b, actual ray path for two lens system.

Figure 15.35a shows the secondary principal plane and an incoming ray parallel to and at a distance a above the axis. The secondary principal point is labeled H_2. The point A on the secondary principal plane is the intersection point between the extensions of the object space ray and the image space ray. The actual image space ray leaves the back surface at point B and travels to the system's F_2. The distance from the axis to A is a, and the distance from the axis to B is b. The triangles AH_2F_2 and BL_bF_2 are similar. It follows that

$$\frac{a}{f_2} = \frac{b}{f_b}$$

and it then follows that

$$\frac{a}{b} = \frac{P_v}{P_e} \tag{15.38}$$

Figure 15.35b shows the actual ray path. The points L_1 and L_b are the vertex points of the first and second surface, respectively. The incident ray is parallel to and at a distance a from the axis, and hits the first surface at point E. The ray leaving the first surface points toward the secondary focal point $(F_2)_1$ of surface 1 and hits the second surface at B. The image space ray goes from B to the system's F_2. The triangles $EL_1(F_2)_1$ and $BL_b(F_2)_1$ are similar. It follows that

$$\frac{a}{(f_2)_1} = \frac{b}{(f_2)_1 - \bar{d}}$$

$$aP_1 = \frac{b}{(1/P_1) - \bar{d}}$$

$$\frac{a}{b} = \frac{1}{1 - \bar{d}P_1}$$

The combination of Eq. 15.38 with the above equation gives

$$P_v = \frac{P_e}{(1 - \bar{d}P_1)} \tag{15.39}$$

Then by comparing Eqs. 15.39 and 15.37, we obtain

$$P_e = P_1 + P_2 - \bar{d}P_1P_2 \tag{15.40}$$

Equation 15.40 gives the equivalent dioptric power of a thick lens directly in terms of the surface powers and reduced central thickness. Equation 15.40 is a linear equation as a function of the reduced thickness $\bar{d}$. Therefore, a plot of P_e

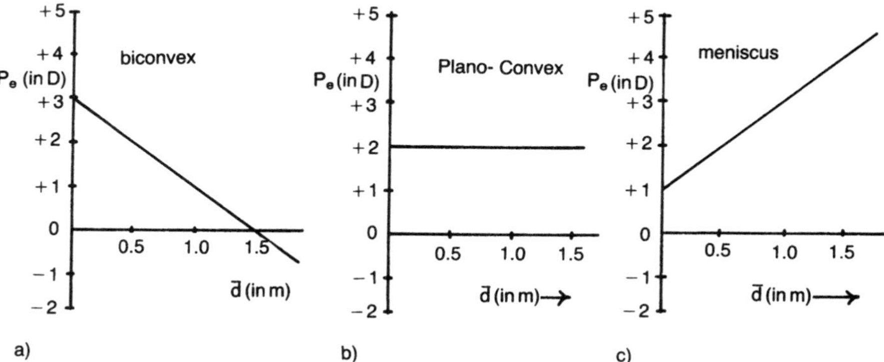

Figure 15.36 Equivalent dioptric power as a function of thickness: a, biconvex lens; b, planoconvex lens; c, meniscus lens.

as a function of $\bar{d}$ is a straight line with an intercept equal to the sum of the surface powers and a slope equal to −1 times the product of the surface powers. For a biconvex or biconcave lens, the slope is negative (Figure 15.36a). For a planoconvex or planoconcave lens, there is a zero slope (Figure 15.36b); and for a meniscus lens the slope is positive (Figure 15.36c).

Equation 15.39 gives a connection between P_v and P_e. By reversibility, there must be a similar connection between P_n and P_e:

$$P_n = \frac{P_e}{1 - \bar{d}P_2} \tag{15.41}$$

In Eqs. 15.39 through 15.41, the reduced distance $\bar{d}$ is always positive and dimensionally has to be in meters (since it is multiplying diopters).

Note from the derivation of Eq. 15.37, that the denominator of Eq. 15.39 for the back vertex power comes from the downstream vergence equation for the lens' first surface (power P_1.) For the reversed light case, the denominator of Eq. 15.41 comes from the downstream vergence equation for the lens' back surface (power P_2).

When the reduced central thickness $\bar{d}$ goes to zero, the lens becomes thin. For a thin lens, Eqs. 15.39 and 15.41 show that the back vertex power and the neutralizing power are both equal to the equivalent power. Equation 15.40 shows that the thin lens equivalent power is equal to the sum of the surface powers, or the equivalent power just equals the thin lens power.

EXAMPLE 15.13

What is the equivalent power and neutralizing power for the lens in Example 15.12? Also use Eq. 15.39 to verify the back vertex power obtained in Example 15.12.

From Example 15.12,

$$P_1 = +16.00\,\text{D} \quad P_2 = -2.00\,\text{D}$$

and

$$\bar{d} = 7.5\,\text{mm} = 0.0075\,\text{m}$$

From Eq. 15.40,

$$\begin{aligned} P_e &= +16.00\,\text{D} + (-2.00\,\text{D}) \\ &\quad - (0.0075\,\text{m})(+16.00\,\text{D})(-2.00\,\text{D}) \\ &= +14.00\,\text{D} - (-0.24\,\text{D}) = +14.24\,\text{D} \end{aligned}$$

The sum of the surface powers is +14.00 D, and the thickness term contributed 0.24 D more.

From Eq. 15.41,

$$\begin{aligned} P_n &= \frac{+14.24\,\text{D}}{1 - (0.0075\,\text{m})(-2.00\,\text{D})} \\ &= \frac{+14.24\,\text{D}}{1.015} = +14.03\,\text{D} \end{aligned}$$

To verify the back vertex power, Eq. 15.39 gives

$$\begin{aligned} P_v &= \frac{+14.24\,\text{D}}{1 - (0.0075\,\text{m})(+16.00\,\text{D})} \\ &= \frac{+14.24\,\text{D}}{0.880} = +16.18\,\text{D} \end{aligned}$$

which agrees with Example 15.12.

Figure 15.37 shows a plot of the equivalent dioptric power, back vertex power, and neutralizing power as a function of reduced thickness for a lens with a front surface power of +10.00 D and a back surface power of +5.00 D. This graph of the equivalent power is linear with a negative slope and a power of +15.00 D for zero thickness. The reduced distance that gives zero equivalent power is found from Eq. 15.40:

$$P_e = 0 = P_1 + P_2 - \bar{d}P_1P_2$$

$$0 = +15.00\,\text{D} - \bar{d}(+50.00\,\text{D}^2)$$

Figure 15.37 Graph of power parameters for a lens as a function of thickness.

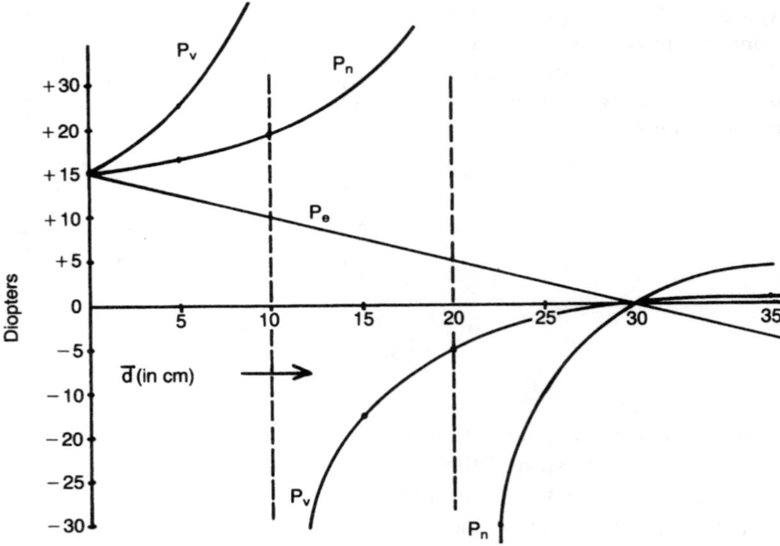

or

$$\bar{d} = \frac{+15.00}{+50.00} = 0.30\,\text{m} = 30\,\text{cm}$$

The back vertex power is equal to the vergence leaving the back surface when plane waves are incident on the front surface. In Figure 15.37, the back vertex power is +15.00 D at zero thickness and then starts to increase as the thickness increases. This increase occurs because of the vergence gain of the converging light across the interior of the lens. At a reduced thickness of 10 cm, the image from the +10.00 D front surface is formed at the back surface and the back vertex power goes to infinity. For a reduced thickness just greater than 10 cm, the image for the +10.00 D front surface is formed just in front of the back surface. The light diverges away from the internal image position, and highly divergent light is incident on the back surface. The back vertex power is then a large negative number indicating that highly divergent light leaves the back surface of the lens. As the thickness is increased further, the diverging wavefronts incident on the second surface become flatter, and the light leaving becomes less divergent. Eventually, the vergence incident on the +5.00 D back surface is −5.00 D, resulting in plane waves leaving the lens and a back vertex power of zero. As is evident from Eq. 15.39, the zero back vertex power occurs at the same distance (30 cm) that gives zero equivalent dioptric power. As the reduced thickness is increased past 30 cm, the light incident on the back surface has a vergence that is negative but smaller in magnitude than 5.00 D, so the light leaving the back of the lens becomes convergent again. Eventually, the lens is so thick that the wavefronts coming from the internal image become plane waves before they are incident on the +5.00 D back surface. In the limit of infinite thickness, the back vertex power goes to +5.00 D.

By reversibility, a similar argument can be made for the neutralizing power. Note that when the equivalent power is zero, the neutralizing power also equals zero. A system with an equivalent power of zero is called an *afocal system*. Afocal systems neither converge nor diverge light, but they do affect magnification. As discussed in Chapter 17, telescopic systems focused for emmetropes are afocal systems.

15.17 SPECIAL THICK LENS EXAMPLES

EXAMPLE 15.14

Verify that the equivalent dioptric power given in Example 15.7a is correct.

From Example 15.7a, $P_1 = -6.00\,\text{D}$, $P_2 = +6.00\,\text{D}$, and $\bar{d} = 21\,\text{cm}/1.5 = 14\,\text{cm} = 0.14\,\text{m}$. From Eq, 15.40,

$$\begin{aligned} P_e &= -6.00\,\text{D} + 6.00\,\text{D} \\ &\quad - (0.14\,\text{m})(-6.00\,\text{D})(+6.00\,\text{D}) \\ &= 0 - (-5.040\,\text{D}) = +5.040\,\text{D} \end{aligned}$$

which agrees. Note that here the entire contribution to the equivalent power comes from the thickness term.

EXAMPLE 15.15

Small plastic ($n = 1.49$) spheres mounted on the end of a pencil are useful in visual testing of small children. For paraxial viewing through a sphere of diameter 2 cm, what is P_e, P_v, and P_n? Where are the principal points?

Let us first find the surface power of the sphere. The radius of curvature is 1 cm. Then for the front surface,

$$P_1 = \frac{n_2 - n_1}{r} = \frac{+49}{+1} = +49.00\,\text{D}$$

The sphere has the same surface power all around, so the back surface power P_2 is also +49.00 D. Then,

$$\bar{d} = \frac{2\,\text{cm}}{1.49} = 1.34\,\text{cm} = 0.0134\,\text{m}$$

From Eq. 15.40,

$$\begin{aligned} P_e &= +49.00\,\text{D} + 49.00\,\text{D} \\ &\quad - (0.0134\,\text{m})(+49.00\,\text{D})(+49.00\,\text{D}) \\ &= +98.00\,\text{D} - 32.23\,\text{D} = +65.77\,\text{D} \end{aligned}$$

From Eq. 15.39,

$$\begin{aligned} P_v &= \frac{+65.77\,\text{D}}{1 - (0.0134)(+49.00\,\text{D})} \\ &= \frac{+65.77\,\text{D}}{0.342} = +192.16\,\text{D} \end{aligned}$$

Since the sphere is perfectly symmetrical, P_n should equal P_v, and indeed Eq. 15.42 gives $P_n = +192.16$ D.

For the Principal Points

From Eqs. 15.5 through 15.8,

$$f_2 = \frac{100}{+65.77\,\text{D}} = +1.52\,\text{cm} \quad f_1 = -1.52\,\text{cm}$$

$$f_b = \frac{100}{192.16\,\text{D}} = +0.52\,\text{cm} \quad f_f = -0.52\,\text{cm}$$

From Eqs. 15.10 and 15.11,

$$L_bH_2 = +0.52\,\text{cm} - 1.52\,\text{cm} = -1.00\,\text{cm}$$
$$L_1H_1 = -0.52\,\text{cm} - (-1.52\,\text{cm}) = +1.00\,\text{cm}$$

Since the radius of the sphere is 1 cm, the principal points coincide at the center of the sphere (Figure 15.38a). Since the object and image space indices are equal, the nodal points are at the principal points and hence at the center of the sphere. We can verify this by noting that any incident ray pointing toward the center of the sphere is incident normally on the sphere and does not bend. These rays travel straight through the center of the sphere, are incident normally on the back side, and again do not bend (Figure 15.38b).

Note that for paraxial imaging, we can computationally replace the sphere by a +65.77 D thin lens located at the position occupied by the sphere's center. This makes the analysis of the sphere's optics particularly straightforward.

EXAMPLE 15.16

Consider a thick lens with a convex front surface and a plane back surface (Figure 15.39a). Where are the principal planes located?

Here $P_2 = 0$ and

$$P_e = P_1 + P_2 - \bar{d}P_1P_2 = P_1$$

Then,

$$P_v = \frac{P_e}{1 - \bar{d}P_1}$$

becomes

$$P_v = \frac{P_1}{1 - \bar{d}P_1}$$

For plane waves incident on the front, the vergence leaving the front is equal to P_1, and the above equation is just the downstream vergence equation for the reduced distance $\bar{d}$. Since the back surface is plane, the exiting vergence (which is the back vertex power) equals the vergence of the light incident on the back surface.

Since the back surface is plano, when we reverse the light and consider plane waves

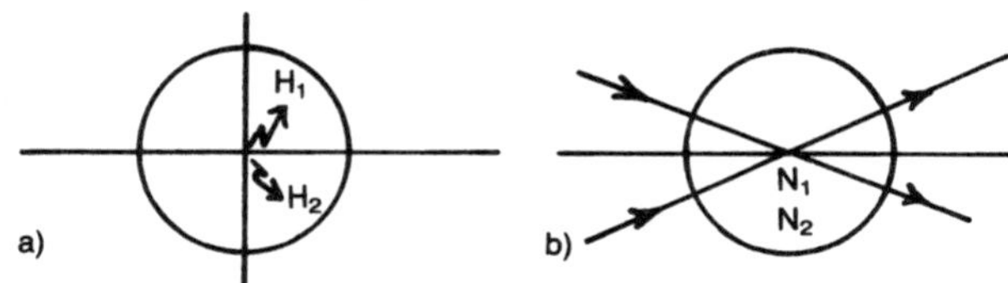

Figure 15.38 Transparent Sphere: a, principal planes; b, nodal rays.

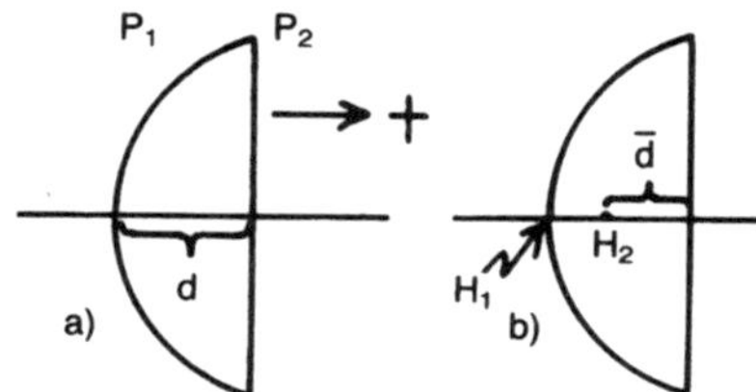

Figure 15.39 a, Planoconvex thick lens; b, principal points.

incident on the back surface, the plane waves proceed through and are incident on the front surface. The emerging light then has a vergence equal to P_1, and P_n equals P_1. Indeed, here Eq. 15.41 gives

$$P_n = \frac{P_e}{1 - \bar{d}P_2} = \frac{P_1}{1 - 0} = P_1$$

For the Principal Plane Locations
From Eqs. 15.10, 15.7, and 15.8,

$$\begin{aligned} L_bH_2 &= f_b - f_2 \\ &= \frac{1}{P_v} - \frac{1}{P_e} \\ &= \frac{1 - \bar{d}P_1}{P_1} - \frac{1}{P_1} = -\bar{d} \end{aligned}$$

From Eqs. 15.10, 15.5, and 15.6,

$$\begin{aligned} L_1H_1 &= f_f - f_1 \\ &= -\frac{1}{P_n} + \frac{1}{P_e} \\ &= -\frac{1}{P_1} + \frac{1}{P_1} = 0 \end{aligned}$$

For the given thick lens, H_1 is at the vertex of the front surface, which is the only surface with a non-zero dioptric power (Figure 15.39b). H_2 is in front of the back surface by the reduced thickness of the lens. In this example, the image space is air, so n is 1. If n_i differs from 1, then the above derivation gives

$$L_bH_2 = -n_i\bar{d}$$

Note that the image space index n_i is different from the index of the lens material.

15.18 SUMMARY OF THE IMPORTANT EQUATIONS

15.18.1 General

$$V_{H_2} = P_e + U_{H_1} \quad (15.3)$$

$$U_{H_1} = \frac{n_o}{u_{H_1}} \quad (15.1)$$

$$V_{H_2} = \frac{n_i}{v_{H_2}} \quad (15.2)$$

$$m_t = \frac{U_{H_1}}{V_{H_2}} \quad (15.4)$$

For incident plane waves, Eqs. 15.3 and 15.2 give

$$P_e = \frac{n_i}{f_2} \quad (15.5)$$

From the back vertex power definition,

$$P_v = \frac{n_i}{f_b} \quad (15.6)$$

For plane waves leaving, Eqs. 15.3 and 15.1 give

$$P_e = \frac{n_o}{f_1} \quad (15.7)$$

From the neutralizing power definition

$$P_n = \frac{n_o}{f_f} \quad (15.8)$$

A trip from the back of the system to F_2, and then to H_2 results in

$$L_bH_2 = f_b - f_2 \quad (15.10)$$

A trip from the front of the system to F_1, and then to H_1 results in

$$L_1H_1 = f_f - f_1 \quad (15.11)$$

The nodal points are displaced away from the principal planes by

$$HN = \frac{n_i - n_o}{P_e} \quad (15.32)$$

All object space distances are reduced with n_o, and all image space distances are reduced with n_i.

15.18.2 For Thick Lenses (or Two Thin Lenses)

$$P_e = P_1 + P_2 - \bar{d}P_1P_2 \quad (15.40)$$

$$P_v = \frac{P_e}{1 - \bar{d}P_1} \quad (15.39)$$

$$P_n = \frac{P_e}{1 - \bar{d}P_2} \quad (15.41)$$

PROBLEMS

1. An optical system in air has an 11 cm central thickness. The primary principal plane is 3 cm behind the front surface, and the secondary principal plane is 6 cm in front of the back surface. If the back focal length is 5 cm, what is the equivalent dioptric power?

What is the neutralizing power? What is the back vertex power? For a real object 20 cm from the front surface of the system, where is the conjugate image relative to the back surface? What is the lateral magnification?

2. An optical system in air has a 7 cm central thickness and a +6.50 D equivalent power. When a real object is placed 14 cm in front of the system, its conjugate image is erect, the same size as the object and located 3 cm in front of the back surface. (It is a virtual image.) For a real object located 40 cm in front of the system, where is the conjugate image relative to the back surface? What is the lateral magnification?
3. An optical system with air in front and water ($n = 1.33$) behind has 6 cm central thickness. The equivalent power is +5.00 D, the primary principal plane is 8 cm behind the first surface, and the secondary principal plane is 3 cm in front of the back surface. For a real object in air 21 cm from the front surface, where is the conjugate image relative to the back surface? What is the lateral magnification ? Where are the nodal points for this system?
4. An optical system in air has a 20 cm central thickness. The neutralizing power is −10.36 D, the equivalent power is +6.05 D, and the back vertex power is +7.06 D. Find the primary and secondary focal points and the primary and secondary principal planes.
5. An eye has a 21 mm cornea-to-retina distance and a +59.00 D equivalent power. The primary principal plane is 1 mm behind the cornea, and the secondary principal plane is 2 mm behind the cornea. The vitreous has a 1.336 index. What distance vision spectacle correction is needed at a 10 mm vertex distance?
6. An emmetropic eye has a vitreous of index 1.336, a +62.00 D equivalent power, a primary principal plane located 1.3 mm behind the cornea, and a secondary principal plane located 1.9 mm behind the cornea. What is the cornea-to-retina length? Where are the nodal points? What is the retinal image size (in microns) for a distance object that subtends an angle of $5'$?
7. A 12 cm thick glass ($n = 1.63$) rod has air in front and water ($n = 1.33$) behind. The front air–glass interface has a power of +5.00 D. The back glass–water interface has a power of +3.00 D. Find the neutralizing, back vertex, and equivalent dioptric powers. Find the principal planes and the nodal points.
8. It is desired to use a plastic ($n = 1.44$) sphere for clinic testing with many patients. The sphere has a radius of 10 mm. What is the equivalent power? Where are the principal planes for the sphere?
9. An 8 mm thick ophthalmic crown ($n = 1.523$) spectacle lens has a +14.00 D front surface and a −3.00 D back surface. What is the equivalent power, the neutralizing power, and the back vertex power? Where are the principal planes?
10. An optical system in air has a 14 cm central thickness. The front focal length is −8 cm and the back focal length is +4 cm. A real object is located 20 cm from the front vertex, and an inverted real image 2.70 times larger than the object is formed on a screen behind the system. What is the equivalent power? Where must the screen be placed?
11. Example 15.16 dealt with a thick lens that had a spherical front surface and a plano back surface. Derive similar equations for the principal plane locations for a lens with a plano front surface and a spherical back surface.

CHAPTER 16

System Matrices

16.1 THE TRANSLATION MATRIX

This chapter considers reduced centered refraction systems. Such systems are equivalent to a system of thin lenses in air. A centered system is one that has a common optical axis for all lenses (or interfaces) in the system. For the following algebraic derivations, all angles are expressed in radians and all distances are expressed in meters.

Assume that the horizontal line in Figure 16.1a is the optical axis. A ray at a particular point relative to the optical axis can be quantitatively described by two parameters: the (reduced) angle q that the ray makes with the optical axis, and the perpendicular distance h of the point from the optical axis. To define the plus–minus signs, let the h values be positive for distances above the axis and negative for distances below the axis, and let the angles be positive when they are above the horizontal (as in Figure 16.1a) and negative when they are below the horizontal (as in Figure 16.1b).

In Figure 16.1a, two planes perpendicular to the axis are separated by a reduced distance $\bar{d}$ (expressed in meters). The ray in Figure 16.1a is propagating from the point A on the first plane to the point B on the second plane. The ray parameters at the first plane are q_1 and h_1. At the second vertical plane, the ray parameters are q_2 and h_2. Because of the law of rectilinear propagation

$$q_2 = q_1 \tag{16.1}$$

From Figure 16.1a,

$$w = h_2 - h_1$$

and

$$h_2 - h_1 = \bar{d} \tan q_1 \tag{16.2}$$

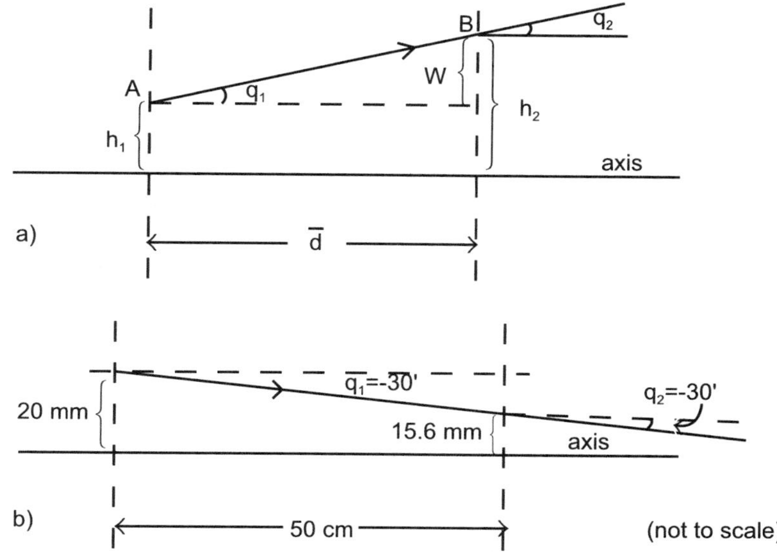

Figure 16.1 Paraxial ray parameters for translation.

For paraxial rays and q_1 in radians, the small angle approximation gives

$$h_2 - h_1 = \bar{d}q_1$$

or

$$h_2 = h_1 + \bar{d}q_1 \tag{16.3}$$

Equations 16.1 and 16.3 can be written as one matrix equation.

$$\begin{pmatrix} q_2 \\ h_2 \end{pmatrix} = \begin{pmatrix} 1 & 0 \\ \bar{d} & 1 \end{pmatrix} \begin{pmatrix} q_1 \\ h_1 \end{pmatrix} \tag{16.4}$$

The top matrix multiplication gives Eq. 16.1, and the bottom matrix multiplication gives Eq. 16.3.

The 2×2 matrix in Eq. 16.4 is called the translation matrix **T**, i.e.

$$\mathbf{T} = \begin{pmatrix} 1 & 0 \\ \bar{d} & 1 \end{pmatrix} \tag{16.5}$$

where $\bar{d}$ is in meters. Then Eq. 16.4 can be written as

$$\begin{pmatrix} q_2 \\ h_2 \end{pmatrix} = \mathbf{T} \begin{pmatrix} q_1 \\ h_1 \end{pmatrix}$$

When $\bar{d}$ is zero in Eq. 16.5, **T** equals the unit matrix **1**:

$$\mathbf{T} = \mathbf{1} = \begin{pmatrix} 1 & 0 \\ 0 & 1 \end{pmatrix}$$

EXAMPLE 16.1

A point source in air is located 20 mm vertically above an optical axis. A ray traveling slightly downward leaves the point source and makes an angle of 30′ with the axis. Determine the ray parameters at the point source and at a distance that is 50 cm along the axis from the point source.

The ray is traveling downward so the angle is negative, and

$$30' = 0.5^\circ = 8.73 \times 10^{-3}\,\text{rad}$$

So,

$$q_1 = -8.73 \times 10^{-3}\,\text{rad}$$

The point source is 20 mm or 0.020 m above the axis, and so

$$h_1 = +0.020\,\text{m}$$

Thus,

$$\begin{pmatrix} q_1 \\ h_1 \end{pmatrix} = \begin{pmatrix} -8.73 \times 10^{-3}\,\text{rad} \\ +0.020\,\text{m} \end{pmatrix}$$

The translation matrix for 50 cm is

$$\mathbf{T} = \begin{pmatrix} 1 & 0 \\ 0.50\,\text{m} & 1 \end{pmatrix}$$

The ray parameters 50 cm downstream are

$$\begin{pmatrix} q_2 \\ h_2 \end{pmatrix} = \begin{pmatrix} 1 & 0 \\ 0.50\,\text{m} & 1 \end{pmatrix} \begin{pmatrix} -8.73 \times 10^{-3}\,\text{rad} \\ +2.00 \times 10^{-2}\,\text{m} \end{pmatrix}$$

$$= \begin{pmatrix} -8.73 \times 10^{-3}\,\text{rad} \\ +1.56 \times 10^{-2}\,\text{m} \end{pmatrix}$$

At 50 cm downstream, the ray is 15.6 mm above the axis.

16.2 THE REFRACTION MATRIX

Reduced refraction systems consist of a series of thin lenses. Figure 16.2 shows a ray being refracted at a distance h from the optical axis of a thin lens of dioptric power P. The incident ray parameters are q_1 and h_1 while the outgoing ray parameters are q_2 and h_2. The ray is not displaced at the lens, and thus,

$$h_2 = h_1 = h \tag{16.6}$$

When refracted, the ray is bent down through the angle d. The incident ray leaves the axial object point at the angle q_1. The outgoing ray passes through the conjugate image point at the angle b. The optical axis, incident ray, and exiting ray make a triangle with internal angles q_1, b, and q. The angle d is an external angle to this triangle. The external angle of a triangle is equal to the sum of the two opposite internal angles (see Sections 11.3 and 12.1). Here this theorem gives

$$|d| = q_1 + b$$

Because the bend is down, let d be a negative angle. Then,

$$d = -q_1 - b$$

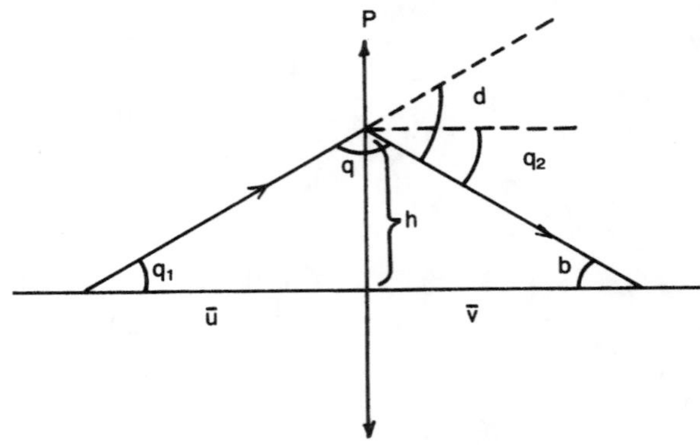

Figure 16.2 Paraxial ray parameters for refraction.

From Figure 16.2, the angle q_2 equals $-b$, so

$$d = q_2 - q_1$$

From Eq. 12.1,

$$d = -Ph \tag{16.7}$$

where h is in meters, P is in diopters, and d is in radians. Equation 12.1 or 16.7 is mathematically equivalent to Prentice's rule, which is given in Eq. 12.2. It follows from the above two equations that

$$q_2 = q_1 - Ph \tag{16.8}$$

Equations 16.6 and 16.8 can be written as:

$$\begin{pmatrix} q_2 \\ h_2 \end{pmatrix} = \begin{pmatrix} 1 & -P \\ 0 & 1 \end{pmatrix} \begin{pmatrix} q_1 \\ h_1 \end{pmatrix} \tag{16.9}$$

The top matrix multiplication gives Eq. 16.8, while the bottom matrix multiplication gives Eq. 16.6. The 2×2 matrix in Eq. 16.9 is called the refraction matrix **R**, i.e.,

$$\mathbf{R} = \begin{pmatrix} 1 & -P \\ 0 & 1 \end{pmatrix} \tag{16.10}$$

Then Eq. 16.9 can be written as

$$\begin{pmatrix} q_2 \\ h_2 \end{pmatrix} = \mathbf{R} \begin{pmatrix} q_1 \\ h_1 \end{pmatrix}$$

When P is zero in Eq. 16.10, then R equals the unit matrix **1**:

$$\mathbf{R} = \mathbf{1} = \begin{pmatrix} 1 & 0 \\ 0 & 1 \end{pmatrix}$$

EXAMPLE 16.2

A ray leaves an axial point source 25 cm from a +6 D lens and hits the lens 12 mm below the optical center. What are the ray parameters when it leaves the lens?

From the fact that the +6 D lens has BU prism below its optical center, we expect that the lens bends the ray up. The angle that the ray makes with the axis is

$$q_1 \sim \tan q_1 = \frac{-1.2\,\text{cm}}{25\,\text{cm}} = -4.8 \times 10^{-2}\,\text{rad}$$

From Eq. 16.9,

$$\begin{pmatrix} q_2 \\ h_2 \end{pmatrix} = \begin{pmatrix} 1 & -6\,\text{D} \\ 0 & 1 \end{pmatrix} \begin{pmatrix} -4.8 \times 10^{-2}\,\text{rad} \\ -1.2 \times 10^{-2}\,\text{m} \end{pmatrix}$$

$$= \begin{pmatrix} +2.40 \times 10^{-2}\,\text{rad} \\ -1.2 \times 10^{-2}\,\text{m} \end{pmatrix}$$

Since q_2 is a positive angle, the ray leaving the lens is traveling upward, which agrees with the expectations.

16.3 THE SYSTEM MATRIX

Consider a system consisting of two lenses separated by a reduced distance $\bar{d}$. For a ray incident on the system with parameters q_1 and h_1 the ray parameters when it leaves the first lens are

$$\begin{pmatrix} q_2 \\ h_2 \end{pmatrix} = \mathbf{R_1} \begin{pmatrix} q_1 \\ h_1 \end{pmatrix}$$

where $\mathbf{R_1}$ is the refraction matrix for the first lens. The ray then travels across the distance between the lenses, and is incident on the second lens with parameters q_3 and h_3 where,

$$\begin{pmatrix} q_3 \\ h_3 \end{pmatrix} = \mathbf{T_1} \begin{pmatrix} q_2 \\ h_2 \end{pmatrix}$$

and $\mathbf{T_1}$ is the translation matrix for the distance $\bar{d}$. Next the ray is refracted by the second lens, and the outgoing ray has parameters q_4 and h_4 where,

$$\begin{pmatrix} q_4 \\ h_4 \end{pmatrix} = \mathbf{R_2} \begin{pmatrix} q_3 \\ h_3 \end{pmatrix}$$

We can combine the above three matrix equations to obtain

$$\begin{pmatrix} q_4 \\ h_4 \end{pmatrix} = \mathbf{R_2 T_1 R_1} \begin{pmatrix} q_1 \\ h_1 \end{pmatrix} \tag{16.11}$$

The product of the refraction and translation matrices is a 2×2 matrix called the system matrix **S**, i.e.,

$$\mathbf{S} = \mathbf{R_2 T_1 R_1} \tag{16.12}$$

Then,

$$\begin{pmatrix} q_4 \\ h_4 \end{pmatrix} = \mathbf{S} \begin{pmatrix} q_1 \\ h_1 \end{pmatrix} \tag{16.13}$$

Let's label the elements of the system matrix **S** by the row number–column number convention:

$$\mathbf{S} = \begin{pmatrix} s_{11} & s_{12} \\ s_{21} & s_{22} \end{pmatrix} \tag{16.14}$$

The system matrix is a single 2×2 matrix that relates the parameters of the ray incident on the front of the system to the parameters of the ray leaving the back of the system. Insofar as it relates the incident (or object space) ray to the exiting (or image space) ray, the system matrix performs the same task as the Gauss system.

EXAMPLE 16.3

A system consists of a +4.00 D thin lens 10 cm in front of a −3.00 D thin lens. What is the system matrix **S**?

The distance must be expressed in meters. Then from Eqs. 16.5, 16.10, and 16.13,

$$\mathbf{S} = \begin{pmatrix} 1 & +3\,\mathrm{D} \\ 0 & 1 \end{pmatrix} \begin{pmatrix} 1 & 0 \\ 0.1\,\mathrm{m} & 1 \end{pmatrix} \begin{pmatrix} 1 & -4\,\mathrm{D} \\ 0 & 1 \end{pmatrix}$$
$$= \begin{pmatrix} 1 & +3\,\mathrm{D} \\ 0 & 1 \end{pmatrix} \begin{pmatrix} 1 & -4\,\mathrm{D} \\ 0.1\,\mathrm{m} & 0.6 \end{pmatrix}$$
$$= \begin{pmatrix} 1.3 & -2.2\,\mathrm{D} \\ 0.1\,\mathrm{m} & 0.6 \end{pmatrix}$$

In the refraction matrix, P is expressed in diopters. In the translation matrix, $\bar{d}$ is expressed in meters. Then from the matrix multiplications, s_{11} and s_{22} are dimensionless, s_{12} is in diopters, and s_{21} is in meters.

If the system consists of one lens of dioptric power P, then $\mathbf{S}$ is equal to the refraction matrix $\mathbf{R}$ of that lens, and s_{12} is equal to $-P$. If the system consists of an empty tube of length $\bar{d}$, then $\mathbf{S}$ is equal to the translation matrix $\mathbf{T}$ for the tube length and s_{21} is equal to $\bar{d}$.

EXAMPLE 16.4

An axial object point is 40 cm from the front of the two-lens system in the last example. A ray leaves the object point and hits the +4.00 D lens 14 mm above the axis. What are the ray parameters as it leaves the back lens?

Here h_1 is +0.014 m, and

$$q_1 \sim \tan q_1 = \frac{+1.4\,\mathrm{cm}}{40\,\mathrm{cm}} = 3.5 \times 10^{-2}\,\mathrm{rad}$$

From Eq. 16.13,

$$\begin{pmatrix} q_b \\ h_b \end{pmatrix} = \begin{pmatrix} 1.3 & -2.2\,\mathrm{D} \\ 0.1\,\mathrm{m} & 0.6 \end{pmatrix} \begin{pmatrix} +3.5 \times 10^{-2}\,\mathrm{rad} \\ +1.4 \times 10^{-2}\,\mathrm{m} \end{pmatrix}$$
$$= \begin{pmatrix} +1.47 \times 10^{-2}\,\mathrm{rad} \\ +1.19 \times 10^{-2}\,\mathrm{m} \end{pmatrix}$$

Suppose the reduced system consists of three separated lenses. Following exactly the same procedure used to derive Eq. 16.12, we can show that the system matrix is given by

$$\mathbf{S} = \mathbf{R}_3\mathbf{T}_2\mathbf{R}_2\mathbf{T}_1\mathbf{R}_1 \qquad (16.15)$$

where $\mathbf{R}_1$, $\mathbf{R}_2$, and $\mathbf{R}_3$ are the respective refraction matrices for the first, second, and third lens, $\mathbf{T}_1$ is the translation matrix for the reduced distance between the first and second lens, and $\mathbf{T}_2$ is the translation matrix for the reduced distance between the second and third lens.

For k lenses, the system matrix is

$$\mathbf{S} = \mathbf{R}_k\mathbf{T}_{k-1}\mathbf{R}_{k-1}\ldots\mathbf{T}_2\mathbf{R}_2\mathbf{T}_1\mathbf{R}_1 \qquad (16.16)$$

Since matrix multiplication is not commutative, the order of the product is very important. The refraction matrix for the first lens always appears on the right because, as shown in Eq. 16.11, it is the first matrix to operate on the incident ray parameters.

Since in general, the system matrix performs the same task as the Gauss system, and since s_{12} has the dimension of diopters, you might have made an educated guess that $-s_{12}$ is the equivalent dioptric power P_e of the system. If so, you are correct. The proof follows.

Figure 16.3 is a diagram of the reduced system showing a ray incident parallel to the axis. The ray can be extended in until it intersects the secondary principal plane H_2. The distance from H_2 to F_2 is the reduced secondary equivalent focal length $\bar{f}_2$. The exiting ray or its extension leaves the intersection point on H_2 pointing toward F_2 of the system. For the incident ray, the angle q_1 with the axis is zero. For the exiting ray, the angle with the axis is q_b, and the small angle tangent approximation results in

$$q_b = -\frac{h_1}{\bar{f}_2}$$

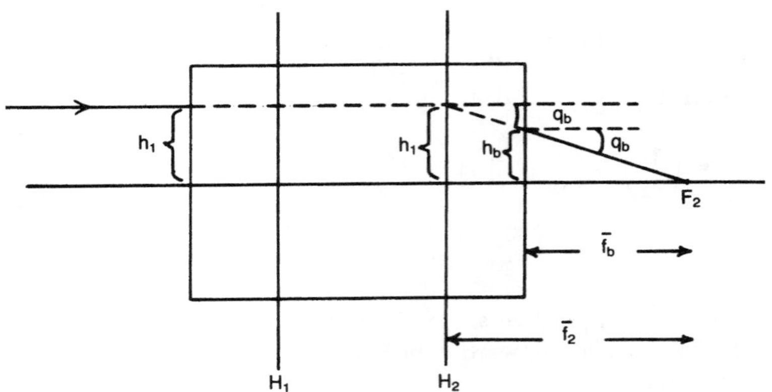

Figure 16.3 Ray incident parallel to the axis.

where the minus sign is introduced because q_b is negative. P_e is reciprocally related to $\bar{f}_2$ so

$$q_b = -P_e h_1 \tag{16.17}$$

Now the system matrix **S** relates the parameters q_1 and h_1 of the ray incident on the front of the system to the parameters q_b and h_b of the ray incident on the back of the system:

$$\begin{pmatrix} q_b \\ h_b \end{pmatrix} = \mathbf{S}\begin{pmatrix} q_1 \\ h_1 \end{pmatrix} \tag{16.18}$$

or

$$\begin{pmatrix} q_b \\ h_b \end{pmatrix} = \begin{pmatrix} s_{11} & s_{12} \\ s_{21} & s_{22} \end{pmatrix}\begin{pmatrix} q_1 \\ h_1 \end{pmatrix} \tag{16.19}$$

Since q_1 is zero, the top matrix multiplication gives

$$q_b = s_{12} h_1 \tag{16.20}$$

A comparison of Eqs. 16.17 and 16.20 shows that

$$s_{12} = -P_e \tag{16.21}$$

In Figure 16.3, F_2 is a distance $\bar{f}_b$ from the back of the system. The exiting ray parameters at the back of the system are q_b and h_b. Then from the tangent of q_b, and the small angle tangent approximation,

$$q_b = -\frac{h_b}{\bar{f}_b}$$

P_v is reciprocally related to f_b, so

$$q_b = -h_b P_v$$

or

$$P_v = -\frac{q_b}{h_b}$$

Since q_1 is zero, the bottom matrix multiplication in Eq. 16.19 gives

$$h_b = s_{22} h_1$$

The above two equations together with Eqs. 16.20 and 16.21 give

$$P_v = \frac{P_e}{s_{22}} \tag{16.22}$$

Similarly,

$$P_n = \frac{P_e}{s_{11}} \tag{16.23}$$

EXAMPLE 16.5

Find P_e, P_v, and P_n for the system in Example 16.3.

From Example 16.3,

$$\mathbf{S} = \begin{pmatrix} 1.3 & -2.2\,\text{D} \\ 0.1\,\text{m} & 0.6 \end{pmatrix}$$

Then from Eq. 16.21,

$$P_e = +2.2\,\text{D}$$

From Eq. 16.22,

$$P_v = \frac{+2.2\,\text{D}}{0.6} = +3.67\,\text{D}$$

From Eq. 16.23,

$$P_n = \frac{+2.2\,\text{D}}{1.3} = +1.69\,\text{D}$$

EXAMPLE 16.6

A system consists of a +3.00 D lens 5 cm in front of a −4.00 D lens, which in turn is 7 cm in front of a +6.00 D lens. Find P_e, P_v, and P_n.

The system matrix is

$$\begin{aligned} \mathbf{S} &= \begin{pmatrix} 1 & -6\,\text{D} \\ 0 & 1 \end{pmatrix}\begin{pmatrix} 1 & 0 \\ 0.07\,\text{m} & 1 \end{pmatrix}\begin{pmatrix} 1 & +4\,\text{D} \\ 0 & 1 \end{pmatrix} \\ &\times \begin{pmatrix} 1 & 0 \\ 0.05\,\text{m} & 1 \end{pmatrix}\begin{pmatrix} 1 & -3\,\text{D} \\ 0 & 1 \end{pmatrix} \\ &= \begin{pmatrix} 1 & -6\,\text{D} \\ 0 & 1 \end{pmatrix}\begin{pmatrix} 1 & +4\,\text{D} \\ 0.07\,\text{m} & 1.28 \end{pmatrix} \\ &\times \begin{pmatrix} 1 & -3\,\text{D} \\ 0.05\,\text{m} & 0.85 \end{pmatrix} \\ &= \begin{pmatrix} 0.40 & -4.87\,\text{D} \\ 0.13\,\text{m} & 0.88 \end{pmatrix} \end{aligned}$$

Then,

$$P_e = +4.87\,\text{D}$$

From Eq. 16.22,

$$P_v = \frac{+4.87\,\text{D}}{0.88} = +5.54\,\text{D}$$

From Eq. 16.23,

$$P_n = \frac{+4.87\,\text{D}}{0.40} = +12.29\,\text{D}$$

The first multiplications performed in a system matrix product are typically the **TR** products. Let

$$\mathbf{B} = \mathbf{TR}$$

Then,

$$\mathbf{B} = \begin{pmatrix} 1 & 0 \\ \bar{d} & 1 \end{pmatrix}\begin{pmatrix} 1 & -P \\ 0 & 1 \end{pmatrix} = \begin{pmatrix} 1 & -P \\ \bar{d} & 1-\bar{d}P \end{pmatrix} \quad (16.24)$$

If desired, B can be used as the building block matrix for a system. Note that when $\bar{d}$ is zero, **B** is equal to **R**. Conversely, when P is zero, **B** is equal to **T**. For a system of k lenses,

$$\mathbf{S} = \mathbf{B}_k\mathbf{B}_{k-1}\ldots\mathbf{B}_2\mathbf{B}_1, \quad (16.25)$$

where $\bar{d}$ is set equal to zero for $\mathbf{B_k}$.

The matrix multiplications are tedious when performed without automation. However the matrix multiplications are easy to program on either a personal computer or a hand held calculator. There are also computer software packages that automatically do matrix multiplications. In addition, there are fairly inexpensive hand-held scientific calculators that also have preprogrammed matrix multiplications.

16.4 DETERMINANT CONDITION

The determinant of a 2×2 matrix is the product of the diagonal elements minus the product of the off-diagonal elements. For the system matrix **S**,

$$\mathbf{S} = \begin{pmatrix} s_{11} & s_{12} \\ s_{21} & s_{22} \end{pmatrix} \quad (16.26)$$
$$\det \mathbf{S} = s_{11}s_{22} - s_{12}s_{21}$$

From Eq. 16.10, the determinant of the refraction matrix **R** is:

$$\det \mathbf{R} = (1)(1) - (-P)(0) = +1$$

From Eq. 16.5, the determinant of the translation matrix **T** is:

$$\det \mathbf{T} = (1)(1) - (0)(\bar{t}) = +1$$

There is a general matrix algebra theorem that states: Given square matrices **X**, **Y**, and **Z** where,

$$\mathbf{Z} = \mathbf{XY}$$

then

$$\det \mathbf{Z} = \det \mathbf{X} \det \mathbf{Y}$$

Let us apply this theorem to the building block matrix **B**, where,

$$\mathbf{B} = \mathbf{TR}$$

Then,

$$\det \mathbf{B} = \det \mathbf{T} \det \mathbf{R} = (+1)(+1) = +1$$

We can check this result by calculating the determinant of **B** directly from Eqs. 16.24 and 16.26:

$$\det \mathbf{B} = (1)(1-\bar{d}P) - (-P)(\bar{d}) = 1 - \bar{d}P + \bar{d}P = +1$$

The system matrix is a product of refraction and translation matrices. By the above theorem, the determinant of the system matrix must equal +1. I.e.,

$$\det \mathbf{S} = s_{11}s_{22} - s_{12}s_{21} = +1 \quad (16.27)$$

Thus, only three of the four elements of the system matrix are independent of each other. I.e., given any three elements, we can determine the fourth from Eq. 16.27.

We can use Eq. 16.27 as a check on our arithmetic in doing the matrix multiplications. Alternatively, given the dioptric power parameter P_e, P_v, and P_n, we can use Eq. 16.27 together with Eqs. 16.21, 16.22, and 16.23 to calculate the elements of **S**.

EXAMPLE 16.7

Does the system matrix of Example 16.3 satisfy the determinant condition?

The determinant of the matrix in Example 16.3 is

$$\det \mathbf{S} = (1.3)(0.6) - (-2.2)(0.1) = 0.78 + 0.22 = +1.00$$

So the answer is yes.

EXAMPLE 16.8

Does the system matrix of Example 16.6 satisfy the determinant condition?

To four digits the system matrix in Example 16.6 is

$$\mathbf{S} = \begin{pmatrix} 0.3960 & -4.8680 \\ 0.1340 & 0.8780 \end{pmatrix}$$

and

$$\det \mathbf{S} = (0.3960)(0.8780) - (-4.8680)(0.1340) = 0.3477 + 0.6523 = +1.000$$

which does satisfy the determinant condition.

However, when the system matrix is rounded to two digits, as in Example 16.6, then the arithmetic gives

$$\det \mathbf{S} = (0.40)(0.88) - (-4.87)(0.13) = 0.35 + 0.63 = +0.98$$

The difference between 0.98 and +1.000 is due to the error introduced in the numerical round-off.

EXAMPLE 16.9

A system has an equivalent dioptric power of −16.48 D, a back vertex power of −10.38 D, and a neutralizing power of −10.83 D. What is **S**?

From Eq. 16.21,

$$s_{12} = +16.48\,\text{D}$$

From Eq. 16.22,

$$s_{22} = \frac{P_e}{P_v} = \frac{-16.48\,\text{D}}{-10.38\,\text{D}} = +1.59$$

From Eq. 16.23,

$$s_{11} = \frac{P_e}{P_n} = \frac{-16.48\,\text{D}}{-10.83\,\text{D}} = +1.52$$

From Eq. 16.27,

$$(1.52)(1.59) - (+16.48\,\text{D})s_{21} = +1$$

and

$$s_{21} = \frac{2.42 - 1.00}{+16.48\,\text{D}} = 0.0862\,\text{m}$$

So,

$$\mathbf{S} = \begin{pmatrix} 1.52 & +16.48\,\text{D} \\ 0.0862\,\text{m} & 1.59 \end{pmatrix}$$

16.5 SUBSYSTEM MATRICES

In analyzing a system, we can break it up into two or more subsystems. Similarly, we can combine two or more systems together to make a larger system. In either event the total system matrix is equal to the product of the component system matrices. For example,

$$\mathbf{S_t} = \mathbf{S_2 S_1} \tag{16.28}$$

where $\mathbf{S_1}$ is the system matrix for the first subsystem and $\mathbf{S_2}$ is the system matrix for the second subsystem (Figure 16.4). Again the order of the multiplication is very important, and $\mathbf{S_1}$ is the system matrix for the component system that the light is incident on first.

Consider a system with a system matrix $\mathbf{S_a}$. Suppose we place a thin lens against the back of this system. What is the system matrix $\mathbf{S_t}$ for the combination? The system matrix for the thin lens is just the refraction matrix **R**. The light is first incident on the system and then on the thin lens. So Eq. 16.28 gives

$$\mathbf{S_t} = \mathbf{R\,S_a} \tag{16.29}$$

Conversely, if we place the lens against the front of the system, the total system matrix would be

$$\mathbf{S_t} = \mathbf{S_a\,R} \tag{16.30}$$

EXAMPLE 16.10a

Consider a system with a +8.80 D equivalent dioptric power, a +22.00 D back vertex power, and a +6.29 D neutralizing power, and a system matrix of

$$\mathbf{S_a} = \begin{pmatrix} 1.40 & -8.80\,\text{D} \\ 0.05\,\text{m} & 0.40 \end{pmatrix}$$

When a +5.00 D lens is placed against the back of the system, what is the equivalent dioptric power, back vertex power, and neutralizing power of the new system?

In this case, the back vertex power is easy to determine. When plane waves are incident on the front of a system, the vergence leaving the back of the system is the back vertex power. For the original system, the back vertex power is +22.00 D, and hence a wavefront of vergence +22.00 D would leave the original system and immediately hit the +5.00 D lens. The light leaving the +5.00 D lens then has a vergence of +27.00 D, which is the back vertex power for the new system.

We can determine the equivalent power and the neutralizing power of the new system by

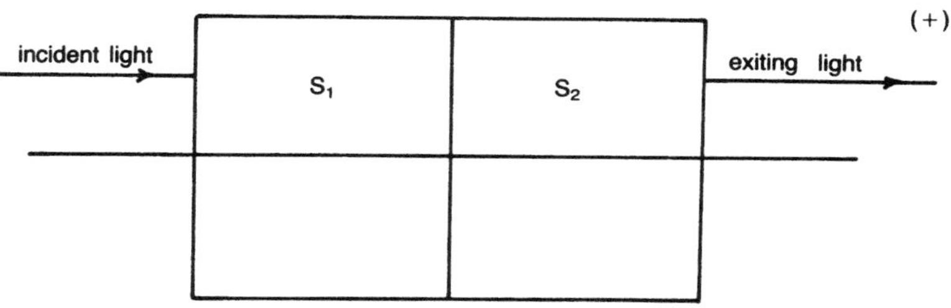

Figure 16.4 Subsystems 1 and 2.

first finding the new system matrix. From Eq. 16.29,

$$\mathbf{S}_t = \mathbf{RS}_a = \begin{pmatrix} 1 & -5\,\mathrm{D} \\ 0 & 1 \end{pmatrix} \begin{pmatrix} 1.40 & -8.80\,\mathrm{D} \\ 0.05\,\mathrm{m} & 0.40 \end{pmatrix}$$
$$= \begin{pmatrix} 1.15 & -10.8\,\mathrm{D} \\ 0.05\,\mathrm{m} & 0.40 \end{pmatrix}$$

From the system matrix, the equivalent power of the combination is +10.8 D. From Eq. 16.23,

$$P_n = \frac{+10.80\,\mathrm{D}}{1.15} = +9.39\,\mathrm{D}$$

As a numerical check, we can compute the new back vertex from the system matrix and see if it agrees with the +27.00 D computed above. From Eq. 16.22,

$$P_v = \frac{+10.80\,\mathrm{D}}{0.40} = +27.00\,\mathrm{D}$$

which agrees.

EXAMPLE 16.10b

When a −4.00 D lens is placed against the front of the original system used in Example 16.10a, what is the equivalent dioptric power, back vertex power and neutralizing power of the new combination?

In this case, the neutralizing power is easy to determine. The neutralizing power of the original system was +6.29 D. When we reverse the light and have plane waves incident on the back of the system, the vergence of the wavefront leaving the front vertex is +6.29 D. When the −4.00 D lens is placed against the front vertex, the +6.29 D vergence is incident on the −4.00 D lens, and the vergence leaving the lens is +2.29 D, which equals the neutralizing power of the new combination.

We can determine the equivalent power and the back vertex power of the new combination by first finding the new system matrix. From Example 16.10a,

$$\mathbf{S}_a = \begin{pmatrix} 1.40 & -8.80\,\mathrm{D} \\ 0.05\,\mathrm{m} & 0.40 \end{pmatrix}$$

From Eq. 16.30,

$$\mathbf{S}_t = \mathbf{S}_a\mathbf{R} = \begin{pmatrix} 1.40 & -8.80\,\mathrm{D} \\ 0.05\,\mathrm{m} & 0.40 \end{pmatrix} \begin{pmatrix} 1 & +4\,\mathrm{D} \\ 0 & 1 \end{pmatrix}$$
$$= \begin{pmatrix} 1.40 & -3.20\,\mathrm{D} \\ 0.05\,\mathrm{m} & 0.60 \end{pmatrix}$$

The equivalent power of the combination is +3.20 D. From Eq. 16.22,

$$P_v = \frac{+3.20\,\mathrm{D}}{0.60} = +5.33\,\mathrm{D}$$

As a numerical check, we can compute the neutralizing power from the new system matrix and see if it agrees with the +2.29 D computed above. From Eq. 16.23,

$$P_n = \frac{+3.20\,\mathrm{D}}{1.40} = +2.29\,\mathrm{D}$$

which agrees.

16.6 TWO LENS SYSTEMS

Consider two thin lenses of power P_1 and P_2 in contact with each other. We know from the previous chapters that the dioptric powers are additive for thin lenses in contact with each other, so that the combination just acts like one lens with a power of $P_1 + P_2$. The system matrix for the combination should also manifest the additivity relationship.

For the two thin lenses in contact with each other,

$$\mathbf{S} = \mathbf{R}_2\mathbf{R}_1,$$
$$= \begin{pmatrix} 1 & -P_2 \\ 0 & 1 \end{pmatrix} \begin{pmatrix} 1 & -P_1 \\ 0 & 1 \end{pmatrix}$$

The matrix multiplication gives:

$$\mathbf{S} = \begin{pmatrix} 1 & -(P_1 + P_2) \\ 0 & 1 \end{pmatrix}$$

Indeed, **S** has the form of a refraction matrix with the power given by the sum of P_1 and P_2.

EXAMPLE 16.11

A +3.00 D thin lens is held in contact with a +4.00 D thin lens. What is **S** for the two lenses?

We can either add the dioptric powers together to get +7.00 D, and then the system matrix is just a refraction matrix for a +7.00 D lens; or we can write down the system matrix for each lens and do the matrix multiplications.

$$\mathbf{S} = \mathbf{R}_2\mathbf{R}_1$$
$$= \begin{pmatrix} 1 & -4\,\mathrm{D} \\ 0 & 1 \end{pmatrix} \begin{pmatrix} 1 & -3\,\mathrm{D} \\ 0 & 1 \end{pmatrix}$$
$$= \begin{pmatrix} 1 & -7\,\mathrm{D} \\ 0 & 1 \end{pmatrix}$$

Consider the system matrix for either a thick lens or two separated thin lenses. The lens powers are P_1 and P_2, and the separation distance in the reduced system is $\bar{d}$ (Figure 16.5). From Eq. 16.12,

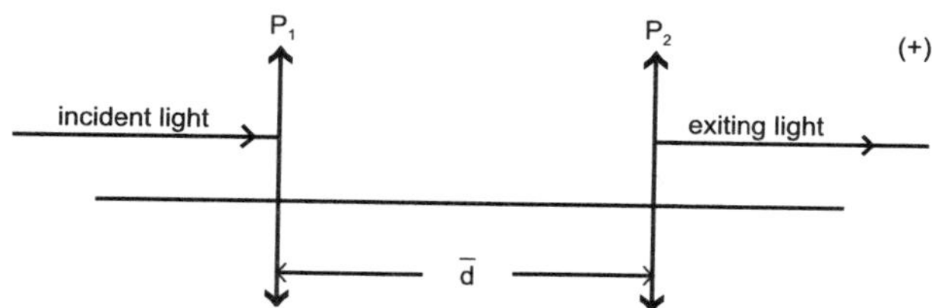

Figure 16.5 Two lens system.

$$\mathbf{S} = \mathbf{R}_2\mathbf{T}_1\mathbf{R}_1$$
$$= \begin{pmatrix} 1 & -P_2 \\ 0 & 1 \end{pmatrix}\begin{pmatrix} 1 & 0 \\ \bar{d} & 1 \end{pmatrix}\begin{pmatrix} 1 & -P_1 \\ 0 & 1 \end{pmatrix}$$
$$= \begin{pmatrix} 1 & -P_2 \\ 0 & 1 \end{pmatrix}\begin{pmatrix} 1 & -P_1 \\ \bar{d} & 1-\bar{d}P \end{pmatrix}$$
$$= \begin{pmatrix} 1-\bar{d}P_2 & -(P_1+P_2-\bar{d}P_2P_1) \\ \bar{d} & 1-\bar{d}P_1 \end{pmatrix}$$

From **S** and Eq. 16.21,

$$P_e = P_1 + P_2 - \bar{d}P_2P_1$$

which is identical in form to Eq. 15.40 for the equivalent dioptric power of a thick lens.

From **S** and Eq. 16.22,

$$P_v = \frac{P_e}{1-\bar{d}P_1}$$

which is identical in form to Eq. 15.39 for the back vertex power of a thick lens.

From **S** and Eq. 16.23,

$$P_n = \frac{P_e}{1-\bar{d}P_2}$$

which is identical in form to Eq. 15.41 for the neutralizing power of a thick lens.

EXAMPLE 16.12

A +3.00 D lens is located 10 cm in front of a +4.00 D lens. What is the system matrix, P_e, P_v, and P_n for the two lenses?

$$\mathbf{S} = \mathbf{R}_2\mathbf{T}_1\mathbf{R}_1$$
$$= \begin{pmatrix} 1 & -4\,\mathrm{D} \\ 0 & 1 \end{pmatrix}\begin{pmatrix} 1 & 0 \\ 0.1\,\mathrm{m} & 1 \end{pmatrix}\begin{pmatrix} 1 & -3\,\mathrm{D} \\ 0 & 1 \end{pmatrix}$$
$$= \begin{pmatrix} 1 & -4\,\mathrm{D} \\ 0 & 1 \end{pmatrix}\begin{pmatrix} 1 & -3\,\mathrm{D} \\ 0.1\,\mathrm{m} & 0.7 \end{pmatrix}$$
$$= \begin{pmatrix} 0.6 & -5.8\,\mathrm{D} \\ 0.1\,\mathrm{m} & 0.7 \end{pmatrix}$$

We can use the determinant condition, Eq. 16.27, to check the arithmetic:

$$\det \mathbf{S} = (0.6)(0.7) - (-5.8\,\mathrm{D})(0.1\,\mathrm{m})$$
$$= 0.42 + 0.58 = +1.00.$$

Then from Eqs. 16.21 through 16.23,

$$P_e = +5.8\,\mathrm{D},$$
$$P_v = \frac{+5.8\,\mathrm{D}}{0.7} = +8.29\,\mathrm{D}$$
$$P_n = \frac{+5.8\,\mathrm{D}}{0.6} = +9.68\,\mathrm{D}$$

16.7 THE OBJECT–IMAGE MATRIX

The box in Figure 16.6 represents the reduced system for a series of lenses with a front to back vertex system matrix $\mathbf{S_b}$. The system has a real object in front of it and a real image behind it. Conceptually, we can expand the system and consider it starting at the object plane and ending at the image plane. The system matrix for the expanded system is called an object–image matrix $\mathbf{S_{IO}}$. $\mathbf{S_{IO}}$ is related to $\mathbf{S_b}$ by

$$\mathbf{S_{IO}} = \mathbf{T}_v\mathbf{S_b}\mathbf{T}_u \qquad (16.31)$$

where $\mathbf{T}_u$ is the translation matrix for the distance from the object plane to the front vertex of the lens system and $\mathbf{T}_v$ is the translation matrix for the distance from the back vertex to the image plane.

The object–image matrix is still a 2 × 2 matrix; it is similar to Eq. 16.19 in that it relates the ray parameters (q_b, h_b) at the image plane to the ray parameters (q_1, h_1) at the object plane:

$$\begin{pmatrix} q_b \\ h_b \end{pmatrix} = \mathbf{S_{IO}}\begin{pmatrix} q_1 \\ h_1 \end{pmatrix}$$

or

$$\begin{pmatrix} q_b \\ h_b \end{pmatrix} = \begin{pmatrix} s_{11} & s_{12} \\ s_{21} & s_{22} \end{pmatrix}\begin{pmatrix} q_1 \\ h_1 \end{pmatrix}$$

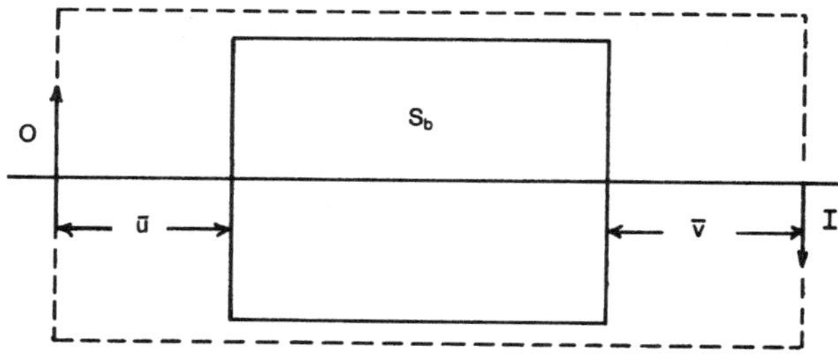

Figure 16.6 Expanded system—object to image.

The bottom matrix multiplication gives

$$h_b = s_{21}q_1 + s_{22}h_1$$

For a ray leaving the axial object point, h_1 is zero. The corresponding image space ray must go to the axial image point ($h_b = 0$) independent of the object space angle q_1. This means that s_{21} in the above equation must equal zero, and then

$$h_b = s_{22}h_1$$

For an off-axis object point, h_1 is the size of the object and h_b is the size of the image. The element s_{22} is just the total lateral magnification m. Hence,

$$\mathbf{S_{IO}} = \begin{pmatrix} s_{11} & s_{12} \\ 0 & m \end{pmatrix}$$

The determinant of any system matrix has to equal +1 (Eq. 16.26), so

$$\det \mathbf{S_{IO}} = s_{11}m - s_{12}0 = +1$$

and it follows that

$$s_{11} = \frac{1}{m} = m^{-1}$$

The element s_{12} is the equivalent dioptric power of the expanded system. However, multiplication by translation matrices does not change the equivalent power. Therefore, s_{12} is equal to the equivalent power P_e of the lens system. The object–image matrix can then be written as

$$\mathbf{S_{IO}} = \begin{pmatrix} m^{-1} & -P_e \\ 0 & m \end{pmatrix} \qquad (16.32)$$

EXAMPLE 16.13

Consider the two lens system used in the last example, namely, a +3.00 D lens 10 cm in front of a +4.00 D lens. The equivalent dioptric power of the two lenses is +5.80 D. A real object is one third of a meter from the first lens, and a conjugate real image is 25 cm behind the second lens. Find the object–image matrix and the lateral magnification.

From Example 16.12, the front to back vertex system matrix is

$$\mathbf{S_b} = \begin{pmatrix} 0.6 & -5.8\,\mathrm{D} \\ 0.1\,\mathrm{m} & 0.7 \end{pmatrix}$$

In the translation matrix $\mathbf{T}_u$, the distance is from the object to the lens, which is +1/3 m. This is opposite in sign to the object distance u for the first lens. Then from Eq. 16.31,

$$\mathbf{S_{IO}} = \begin{pmatrix} 1 & 0 \\ 0.25\,\mathrm{m} & 1 \end{pmatrix} \begin{pmatrix} 0.6 & -5.8\,\mathrm{D} \\ 0.1\,\mathrm{m} & 0.7 \end{pmatrix} \times \begin{pmatrix} 1 & 0 \\ 0.3333\,\mathrm{m} & 1 \end{pmatrix} = \begin{pmatrix} -1.33 & -5.8\,\mathrm{D} \\ 0 & -0.75 \end{pmatrix}$$

Then from Eq. 16.32, the lateral magnification m is −0.75. Note that the equivalent dioptric power in the object–image matrix, +5.80 D, is identical to the equivalent dioptric power of the two lens system.

When the image for one system becomes the object for a second system, the total object–image matrix is the product of the object–image matrices of the components. (Remember the first system goes on the right.) Therefore,

$$(\mathbf{S_{IO}})_t = (\mathbf{S_{IO}})_2(\mathbf{S_{IO}})_1$$

From the individual system matrices and the matrix multiplication, we obtain

$$(\mathbf{S_{IO}})_t = \begin{pmatrix} (m_1m_2)^{-1} & s_{21} \\ 0 & m_1m_2 \end{pmatrix}$$

The second row–second column element is the total lateral magnification, and the above matrix reconfirms that the total lateral magnification is the product of the individual lateral magnifications.

16.8 THE FRONT VERTEX TO SECONDARY FOCAL PLANE MATRIX

When the object or the image is at optical infinity, the object–image matrix loses its usefulness. For an object at optical infinity, the image is in the secondary focal plane. It then becomes useful to consider a system matrix for the components that start at the front vertex of the lens system and go to the secondary focal plane (Figure 16.7).

Consider a lens system with a front to back vertex system matrix $\mathbf{S_b}$. Then the front vertex to F_2 system matrix $\mathbf{S}_{1F}$ is given by

$$\mathbf{S}_{1F} = \mathbf{T}_F\mathbf{S_b}$$

where $\mathbf{T}_F$ is the translation matrix for the back focal length. $\mathbf{S}_{1F}$ is a 2 × 2 matrix that relates the ray parameters (q_1, h_1) at the front vertex to the ray parameters (q_b, h_b) in the secondary focal plane:

$$\begin{pmatrix} q_b \\ h_b \end{pmatrix} = \mathbf{S}_{1F}\begin{pmatrix} q_1 \\ h_1 \end{pmatrix}$$

Figure 16.7 **Expanded system—front vertex to secondary focal plane.**

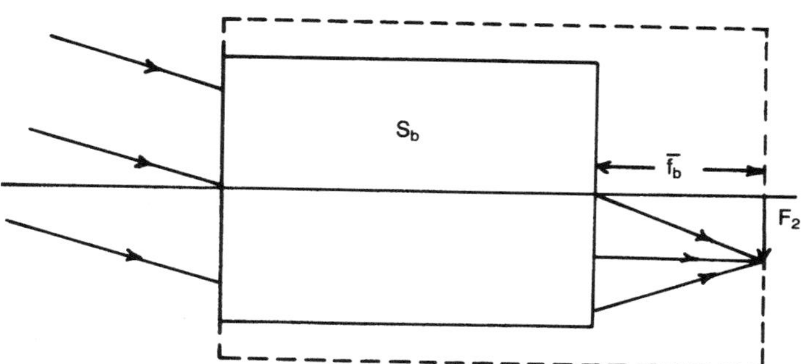

Since multiplication by a translation matrix does not change the equivalent dioptric power, s_{12} remains equal to $-P_e$ of the lens system.

In terms of the elements of $\mathbf{S}_{1F}$, the bottom matrix multiplication gives

$$h_b = s_{21}q_1 + s_{22}h_1$$

Consider an off-axis object point at optical infinity that subtends the angle q_1 at the front vertex of the system. Then all of the incident rays from the top object point are parallel to each other and have the same q_1 value. Each of these rays must go to the conjugate image point, which is at h_b, independent of point h_1 at which the ray hits the front vertex of the system. From the above equation, this means that s_{22} must be zero, and

$$h_b = s_{21}q_1$$

The form of the $\mathbf{S}_{1F}$ system matrix is:

$$\mathbf{S}_{1F} = \begin{pmatrix} s_{11} & -P_e \\ s_{21} & 0 \end{pmatrix}$$

where P_e is the equivalent power of the lens system. In this case, the determinant condition gives

$$\det \mathbf{S}_{1F} = s_{11}0 - (-P_e)(s_{21}) = +1$$

and it follows that

$$s_{21} = \frac{1}{P_e} = \bar{f}_2$$

EXAMPLE 16.14

Figure 16.8b shows a model of Gullstrand's #2 (simplified) schematic eye (unaccommodated). The cornea and aqueous are both considered to have a four thirds (i.e., 4/3) refractive index. The corneal power is +42.735 D. The anterior chamber containing the aqueous is 3.6 mm thick. The aqueous–crystalline lens interface has a power of +8.267 D. The crystalline lens is homogenous with a refractive index of 1.416 and a central thickness of 3.6 mm. The crystalline lens–vitreous interface has a power of +13.778 D, and the distance from this interface to the retina is 16.7 mm. The vitreous refractive index is 4/3. Find the cornea to retina system matrix, and determine the eye's equivalent dioptric power.

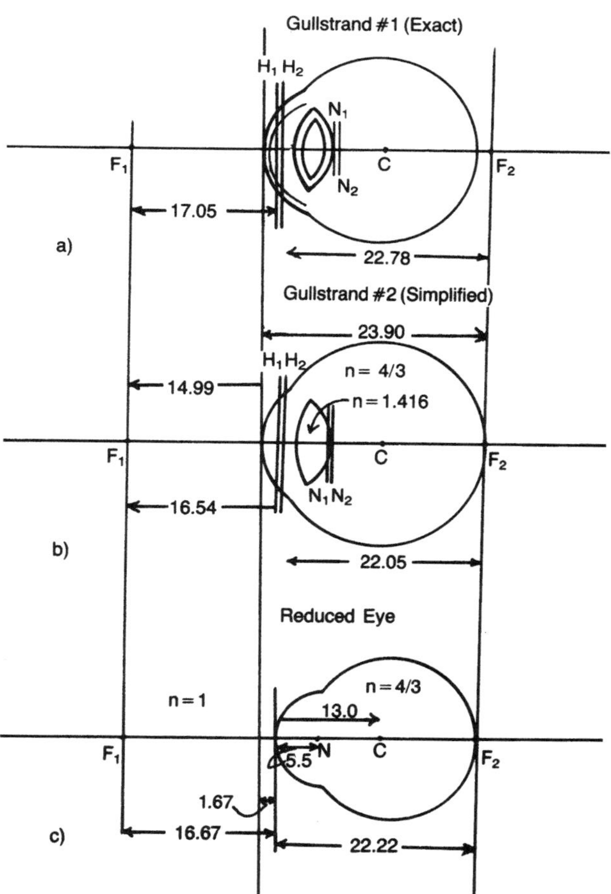

Figure 16.8 **Gullstrand's schematic eyes.**

The respective reduced distances for the anterior chamber, crystalline lens, and vitreous chamber are:

$$\bar{d}_1 = \frac{3.6\,\text{mm}}{1.333} = 2.700\,\text{mm}$$
$$\bar{d}_2 = \frac{3.6\,\text{mm}}{1.416} = 2.542\,\text{mm}$$
$$\bar{d}_3 = \frac{16.700\,\text{mm}}{1.333} = 12.525\,\text{mm}$$

The system matrix is given by:

$$\mathbf{S} = \mathbf{T}_3\mathbf{R}_3\mathbf{T}_2\mathbf{R}_2\mathbf{T}_1\mathbf{R}_1$$

where

$$\mathbf{R}_1 = \begin{pmatrix} 1 & -42.735\,\text{D} \\ 0 & 1 \end{pmatrix}$$
$$\mathbf{T}_1 = \begin{pmatrix} 1 & 0 \\ 0.002700\,\text{m} & 1 \end{pmatrix}$$
$$\mathbf{R}_2 = \begin{pmatrix} 1 & -8.267\,\text{D} \\ 0 & 1 \end{pmatrix}$$
$$\mathbf{T}_2 = \begin{pmatrix} 1 & 0 \\ 0.002542\,\text{m} & 1 \end{pmatrix}$$
$$\mathbf{R}_3 = \begin{pmatrix} 1 & -13.778\,\text{D} \\ 0 & 1 \end{pmatrix}$$
$$\mathbf{T}_3 = \begin{pmatrix} 1 & 0 \\ 0.012525\,\text{m} & 1 \end{pmatrix}$$

Performing these matrix multiplications by hand can be quite tedious. However, there are computer programs or relatively inexpensive handheld calculators that automatically perform the matrix multiplications. One just enters the numbers and presses the evaluate button, and (presto) the answer is

$$\mathbf{S} = \begin{pmatrix} 0.9062 & -60.48\,\text{D} \\ 0.01653\,\text{m} & 0 \end{pmatrix}$$

The equivalent dioptric power of the eye model is +60.48 D. As shown by the fact that s_{22} is zero, the secondary focal plane is at the retina, and the Gullstrand #2 schematic eye is emmetropic.

16.9 AMETROPIC EYES

When the eye is ametropic, the secondary focal point of the eye is not on the retina and the element s_{22} in the cornea to retina system matrix is not zero.

EXAMPLE 16.15

Consider an eye model with the same parameters used in the preceding example except that the vitreous chamber (the distance from the back of the crystalline lens to the retina) is 14 mm. Find the cornea to retina system matrix and the equivalent power of the eye.

The system matrix is given by:

$$\mathbf{S} = \mathbf{T}_3\mathbf{R}_3\mathbf{T}_2\mathbf{R}_2\mathbf{T}_1\mathbf{R}_1$$

The only change is in $\mathbf{T}_3$ since now

$$\bar{d}_3 = \frac{14\,\text{mm}}{1.333} = 10.500\,\text{mm}$$

The matrix multiplications give

$$\mathbf{S} = \begin{pmatrix} 0.9062 & -60.48\,\text{D} \\ 0.01471\,\text{m} & 0.1223 \end{pmatrix}$$

The equivalent dioptric power is still +60.48 D because the eye's refracting system (cornea and crystalline lens) is unchanged. The change in the vitreous chamber depth results in an ametropic eye, which is apparent from the non-zero s_{22} element.

Suppose we want a thin contact lens of power P_c placed on the cornea such that a distant object is imaged clearly on the retina of the unaccommodated eye. Assume the contact lens is fit on K (Section 14.9). Then the total system matrix $\mathbf{S}_t$ for the contact lens and eye should have a zero s_{22} element. The total system matrix is given by

$$\mathbf{S}_t = \mathbf{SR}$$

where $\mathbf{S}$ is the cornea to retina system matrix and $\mathbf{R}$ is the refraction matrix for the thin contact lens.

Let the elements of $\mathbf{S}_t$ be primed and those of $\mathbf{S}$ unprimed. Then,

$$\begin{pmatrix} s'_{11} & s'_{12} \\ s'_{21} & s'_{22} \end{pmatrix} = \begin{pmatrix} s_{11} & s_{12} \\ s_{21} & s_{22} \end{pmatrix} \begin{pmatrix} 1 & -P_c \\ 0 & 1 \end{pmatrix}$$

The matrix multiplication for s'_{22} gives

$$s'_{22} = (s_{21})(-P_c) + (s_{22})(1)$$

Since s'_{22} must equal 0, it follows that

$$P_c = \frac{s_{22}}{s_{21}} \tag{16.33}$$

In Eq. 16.33, s_{21} and s_{22} are elements of the cornea to retina system matrix, and P_c is the dioptric power of a distance vision thin contact lens correction.

EXAMPLE 16.16

Given the eye model and system matrix of Example 16.15, what contact lens correction is needed?

From the system matrix in the preceding example,

$$P_c = \frac{0.1223}{0.01470\,\text{m}} = +8.32\,\text{D}$$

We can check $\mathbf{S_t}$ by computing the matrix product for the contact lens to retina system (i.e., $\mathbf{S_t} = \mathbf{SR}$). The result is

$$\mathbf{S_t} = \begin{pmatrix} 0.9062 & -68.02\,\text{D} \\ 0.01470\,\text{m} & 0 \end{pmatrix}$$

The fact that s_{22} is zero verifies the dioptric power of the correction.

EXAMPLE 16.17

An eye model has a +47.50 D cornea, a 3.6 mm anterior chamber depth, a +8.00 D aqueous–crystalline lens interface, a 3.6 mm thick crystalline lens, a +14.00 D crystalline lens–vitreous interface, and a 17 mm vitreous chamber depth. The refractive index of the vitreous and the aqueous is 1.336, and the refractive index of the crystalline lens is 1.416. Find the cornea to retina system matrix and specify what contact correction the eye needs.

The respective reduced distances for the anterior chamber, crystalline lens, and vitreous chamber are:

$$\bar{d}_1 = \frac{3.6\,\text{mm}}{1.336} = 2.695\,\text{mm}$$

$$\bar{d}_2 = \frac{3.6\,\text{mm}}{1.416} = 2.542\,\text{mm}$$

$$\bar{d}_3 = \frac{17.\,\text{mm}}{1.336} = 12.72\,\text{mm}$$

The system matrix is given by

$$\mathbf{S} = \mathbf{T_3R_3T_2R_2T_1R_1}$$

where,

$$\mathbf{R_1} = \begin{pmatrix} 1 & -47.50\,\text{D} \\ 0 & 1 \end{pmatrix}$$

$$\mathbf{T_1} = \begin{pmatrix} 1 & 0 \\ 0.002695\,\text{m} & 1 \end{pmatrix}$$

$$\mathbf{R_2} = \begin{pmatrix} 1 & -8.00\,\text{D} \\ 0 & 1 \end{pmatrix}$$

$$\mathbf{T_2} = \begin{pmatrix} 1 & 0 \\ 0.002542\,\text{m} & 1 \end{pmatrix}$$

$$\mathbf{R_3} = \begin{pmatrix} 1 & -14.00\,\text{D} \\ 0 & 1 \end{pmatrix}$$

$$\mathbf{T_3} = \begin{pmatrix} 1 & 0 \\ 0.01272\,\text{m} & 1 \end{pmatrix}$$

The matrix multiplications give the cornea to retina system matrix.

$$\mathbf{S} = \begin{pmatrix} 0.9059 & -64.75\,\text{D} \\ 0.01671\,\text{m} & -0.09035 \end{pmatrix}$$

From Eq. 16.33,

$$P_c = \frac{-0.09035}{0.01671\,\text{m}} = -5.41\,\text{D}$$

16.10 THE GULLSTRAND #1 SCHEMATIC EYE

Example 16.14 referred to the Gullstrand #2 schematic eye. Allvar Gullstrand (1862–1930), a Swedish professor of ophthalmology, was one of the world's leading figures in the study of the eye as an optical instrument. Gullstrand developed new instrumentation to make measurements on living human eyes. Based on his measurements, Gullstrand developed some schematic representations of the typical or average living human eye. The models differ in complexity and are discussed below.

In the course of Gullstrand's work on the eye, he discovered a number of widespread misconceptions about image formation in general. Gullstrand worked hard to rectify these misconceptions, and his work included some very sophisticated mathematical analyses of image formation. As a result, he became highly regarded in the physics community, as well as in the ophthalmology community. (Incidentally, Gullstrand was an advocate of the vergence approach to visual optics.)

In both 1910 and 1911, Gullstrand was nominated for the Nobel prize in physics. In 1911, the original suggestion of the Physics Nobel prize committee was that Gullstrand be given the prize for his work on geometric optics. The Physiology and Medicine Nobel Prize committee had the same idea and independently recommended Gullstrand for the 1911 Nobel prize in medicine for his work on the dioptrics of the eye. Gullstrand declined the Physics Prize so that he could accept the Physiology and Medicine Nobel Prize.

Gullstrand's eye models are simplified in the sense that spherical surfaces are used and certain assumptions are made about the indices of refraction. Gullstrand's #1 schematic eye is shown in Figure 16.8a, and the corresponding data is in Table 16.1. In the #1 schematic eye, the cornea is given a uniform refractive index (1.376), which is different from that of the aqueous humor (1.336). The crystalline lens does not have a uniform refractive index, and this is modeled in the #1 eye by assigning a core with a 1.406 index, while the outer part of the lens is assigned a 1.386 index. The aqueous and vitreous humors are each assigned a 1.336 index.

Table 16.1 Gullstrand's #1 Schematic Eye

	Unaccommodated	*Maximum Accommodation*
Refractive index		
Cornea	1.376	1.376
Aqueous and vitreous	1.336	1.336
Lens	1.386	1.386
Equivalent core lens	1.406	1.406
Position (mm)		
Anterior corneal surface	0	0
Posterior corneal surface	+0.5	+0.5
Anterior lens surface	+3.6	+3.2
Equivalent core lens anterior surface	+4.146	+3.8725
Equivalent core lens posterior surface	+6.565	+6.5275
Posterior lens surface	+7.2	+7.2
Radius of curvature (mm)		
Anterior corneal surface	+7.7	+7.7
Posterior corneal surface	+6.8	+6.8
Anterior lens surface	+10.0	+5.33
Equivalent core lens anterior surface	+7.911	+2.655
Equivalent core lens posterior surface	−5.76	−2.655
Posterior lens surface	−6.0	− 5.33
Refracting power (D)		
Anterior corneal surface	+48.83	+48.83
Posterior corneal surface	−5.88	− 5.88
Anterior lens surface	+5.0	+9.375
Anterior core surface	+2.53	+7.53
Posterior core surface	+3.47	+7.53
Posterior lens surface	+8.33	+9.375
Corneal system		
Equivalent power (D)	+43.05	+43.05
Position primary principal point	−0.0496	−0.049
Position secondary principal point	−0.0506	−0.0506
Lens system		
Equivalent power (D)	+19.11	+33.06
Position primary principal point	+5.678	+5.145
Position secondary principal point	+5.808	+5.255
Complete optical system of eye		
Equivalent power (D)	+58.64	+70.57
Position primary principal point	+1.348	+1.772
Position secondary principal point	+1.602	+2.086
Position primary focal point	−15.707	−12.397
Position secondary focal point	+24.387	+21.016
Primary focal length	−17.055	−14.169
Secondary focal length	+22.785	+18.930
Position primary nodal point	+7.08	+6.53
Position fovea centralis	+23.9	+23.9
Position near point (mm)	—	−102.3

The cornea to retina system matrix for Gullstrand's #1 schematic eye is

$$\mathbf{S} = \begin{pmatrix} 0.921 & -58.64\,\mathrm{D} \\ 0.0168\,\mathrm{m} & 0.0169 \end{pmatrix}$$

From the system matrix and Eq. 16.33,

$$P_c = \frac{0.0169}{0.0168\,\mathrm{m}} = +1.01\,\mathrm{D}$$

So Gullstrand's #1 schematic eye is a 1 D hyperope.

Figure 16.8c shows the so-called reduced eye. This model is misnamed in the sense that a reduced system is an equivalent air system, and yet the reduced eye is really a single spherical refracting surface model of the eye. The reduced eye has an index of four thirds, an axial length of 22.22 mm, and a 60.00 D refracting surface. The location of the refracting surface roughly corresponds to the location of the principal planes in the #1 and #2 schematic eyes. The system matrix for the reduced eye is

$$\mathbf{S} = \mathbf{TR}$$
$$= \begin{pmatrix} 1.000 & -60.00\,\text{D} \\ 0.0166\,\text{m} & 0 \end{pmatrix}$$

From the zero two–two element, the reduced eye is emmetropic. The corresponding equivalent air system is the +60.00 D thin lens in air model that we have often used in previous chapters.

16.11 VERTEX VERGENCE RELATIONS

In Figure 16.6, u is the reduced distance from the front of the system to the object and v is the reduced distance from the back of the system to the image. The front-to-back vertex system matrix was $\mathbf{S_b}$, and from Eq. 16.31, the object–image matrix $\mathbf{S_{IO}}$ is

$$\mathbf{S_{IO}} = \begin{pmatrix} 1 & 0 \\ \bar{v} & 1 \end{pmatrix} \begin{pmatrix} s_{11} & s_{12} \\ s_{21} & s_{22} \end{pmatrix} \begin{pmatrix} 1 & 0 \\ -\bar{u} & 1 \end{pmatrix}$$

The matrix multiplications give

$$\mathbf{S_{IO}} = \begin{pmatrix} 1 & 0 \\ \bar{v} & 1 \end{pmatrix} \begin{pmatrix} s_{11} - s_{12}\bar{u} & s_{12} \\ s_{21} - s_{22}\bar{u} & s_{22} \end{pmatrix}$$
$$\mathbf{S_{IO}} = \begin{pmatrix} s_{11} - s_{12}\bar{u} & s_{12} \\ s'_{21} & \bar{v}s_{12} + s_{22} \end{pmatrix} \tag{16.34}$$

where,

$$s'_{21} = s_{11}\bar{v} - s_{12}\bar{v}\bar{u} + s_{21} - s_{22}\bar{u}$$

But from Eq. 16.32, s'_{21} equals zero. It then follows from the above equation that

$$s_{22}\bar{u} - s_{21} = (s_{11} - s_{12}\bar{u})\bar{v}$$

We can divide both sides of the above equation by $\bar{u}$ and by $\bar{v}$, and then substitute

$$U_1 = \frac{1}{\bar{u}} \text{ and } V_b = \frac{1}{\bar{v}}$$

where U_1 is the vergence of the light incident on the front vertex and V_b is the vergence of the light leaving the back vertex. The result is

$$V_b = \frac{-s_{12} + s_{11}U_1}{s_{22} - s_{21}U_1}$$

where the s's are the elements of the front-to-back vertex matrix $\mathbf{S_b}$. From Eq. 16.21,

$$P_e = -s_{12}$$

So,

$$V_b = \frac{P_e + s_{11}U_1}{s_{22} - s_{21}U_1} \tag{16.35}$$

Equation 16.35 is an equation that relates the vergence V_b of the light leaving the back vertex of the system to the vergence U_1 of the light incident on the front vertex of the system and to the matrix elements of the front-to-back vertex system matrix. Equation 16.35 is a little more complicated than the Gauss equation,

$$V_{H_2} = P_e + U_{H_1}$$

However, one can use Eq. 16.35 without needing to know the locations of the primary and secondary principal planes.

A comparison of Eqs. 16.32 and 16.34 provides equations for the total lateral magnification

$$m = \frac{s_{12}}{V_b} + s_{22} \tag{16.36}$$

or

$$\frac{1}{m} = s_{11} - \frac{s_{12}}{U_1} \tag{16.37}$$

In terms of the equivalent dioptric power, Eqs. 16.36 and 16.37 are, respectively,

$$m = -\frac{P_e}{V_b} + s_{22} \tag{16.38}$$

or

$$\frac{1}{m} = s_{11} + \frac{P_e}{U_1} \tag{16.39}$$

EXAMPLE 16.18

The system in Example 16.6 consisted of a +3.00 D lens 5 cm in front of a −4.00 D lens, which in turn was 7 cm in front of a +6.00 D lens. Use Eq. 16.35 to find the system's image conjugate to a real object 50 cm in front of the first lens. Use Eq. 16.39 to find the lateral magnification.

From Example 16.6, the front-to-back vertex system matrix is

$$\mathbf{S} = \begin{pmatrix} 0.40 & -4.87\,\text{D} \\ 0.13\,\text{m} & 0.88 \end{pmatrix}$$

The vergence incident on the first lens is

$$U_1 = -2.00\,\text{D}$$

From Eq. 16.35,

$$V_b = \frac{4.87\,\text{D} + (0.40)(-2.00\,\text{D})}{0.88 - (0.13\,\text{m})(-2.00\,\text{D})} = \frac{+4.07\,\text{D}}{1.14} = +3.57\,\text{D}$$

The light leaving the back of the system is converging, the image is real, and

$$\bar{v}_b = \frac{100}{+3.57\,\text{D}} = +28.0\,\text{cm}$$

From Eq. 16.39, the total lateral magnification is

$$m = \frac{-4.87\,\text{D}}{+3.57\,\text{D}} + 0.88 = -0.48$$

EXAMPLE 16.19

Does Eq. 16.23 for the neutralizing power follow from the front-to-back vertex vergence equation (Eq. 16.35)?

When plane waves leave the back of the system, the neutralizing power is equal to $-U_1$. For plane waves leaving

$$V_b = 0$$

and Eq. 16.35 gives

$$0 = \frac{P_e + s_{11}U_1}{s_{22} - s_1 U_1}$$

Then,

$$0 = P_e + s_{11}U_1$$

and

$$P_n = -U_1 = \frac{P_e}{s_{11}}$$

which agrees with Eq. 16.23.

16.12 DERIVATION OF THE GAUSS EQUATION

The Gauss equation is easily derived from the front-to-back vertex vergence equation. Recall that the primary principal plane H_1 is in object space, while the secondary principal plane H_2 is in image space. Recall also that an object at H_1 is conjugate to an image at H_2, where the image is erect and the same size as the object. When we pretend that the "front" of the system is H_1 and the "back" of the system is H_2, then because of the conjugacy of the principal planes, the vertex system matrix must have the form of an object–image matrix with a lateral magnification of +1. Thus,

$$\mathbf{S}_{\mathbf{H_2H_1}} = \begin{pmatrix} +1 & -P_e \\ 0 & +1 \end{pmatrix}$$

With the above vertex system matrix, Eq. 16.35 gives

$$V_b = \frac{P_e + (+1)U_1}{+1 - (0)U_1}$$

or

$$V_b = P_e + U_1$$

In this case, since the "back" is H_2 and the "front" is H_1, we can change the subscripts to obtain

$$V_{H_2} = P_e + U_{H_1}$$

The Gauss equation for the lateral magnification follows from Eq. 16.38 with s_{22} equal to +1.

$$m = -\frac{P_e}{V_b} + 1$$

The subscript change gives

$$m = -\frac{P_e}{V_{H_2}} + 1$$

Then for a common denominator,

$$m = \frac{-P_e + V_{H_2}}{V_{H_2}}$$

or

$$m = \frac{U_{H_1}}{V_{H_2}}$$

16.13 CONVERSION TO *abcd* NOTATION

Some authors use the letters *a*, *b*, *c*, and *d* to represent the elements of the system matrix **S**. In particular, Eq. 16.19 is sometimes written as

$$\begin{pmatrix} q_b \\ h_b \end{pmatrix} = \begin{pmatrix} d & c \\ b & a \end{pmatrix} \begin{pmatrix} q_1 \\ h_1 \end{pmatrix} \tag{16.40}$$

where,

$$\mathbf{S} = \begin{pmatrix} d & c \\ b & a \end{pmatrix} \tag{16.41}$$

The conversion equations between the notation in this chapter and the *abcd* notation is

$$a = s_{22} \tag{16.42}$$
$$b = s_{21} \tag{16.43}$$
$$c = s_{12} = -P_e \tag{16.44}$$

and

$$d = s_{11} \tag{16.45}$$

In terms of the *abcd* notation, Eq. 16.22 becomes

$$P_v = \frac{P_e}{a} = P_e a^{-1} \tag{16.46}$$

and Eq. 16.23 becomes

$$P_n = \frac{P_e}{d} = d^{-1} P_e \tag{16.47}$$

The origin of the *abcd* notation comes from writing the ray position on the top of the ray matrix and the ray angle on the bottom. Then the system matrix equations become

$$\begin{pmatrix} h_b \\ q_b \end{pmatrix} = \begin{pmatrix} a & b \\ c & d \end{pmatrix} \begin{pmatrix} h_1 \\ q_1 \end{pmatrix}$$

16.14 ASTIGMATIC SYSTEMS

A tremendous conceptual advantage of the system matrix approach is that it is easily extended to systems of centered spherocylindrical thin lenses or toric interfaces—even when the lenses are obliquely crossed. The system matrix for spherocylindrical lenses is a 4×4 matrix, where each 2×2 sub-block plays the same role as the individual elements in the preceding sections of this chapter. In particular, the 2×2 dioptric power matrix **P** (Chapter 13) plays the role that the spherical dioptric power P plays in systems of spherical lenses. The purpose of this section is to present a general sketch of some of the 4×4 results. Full details are contained in the references at the end of the chapter.

At a general point on a spherocylindrical lens with parameters S ⌒ C × θ, where θ is oblique, the lens has both a horizontal (Z_x) and a vertical (Z_y) prism component. Thus the lens bends rays both horizontally and vertically, and we need to keep track of the ray components in both the horizontal (x) and the vertical (y) meridians. At a plane that is perpendicular to the optical axis, the ray position has horizontal and vertical components h_x and h_y (as in Chapter 13), while the ray angle has horizontal and vertical components q_x and q_y.

At a $x'-y'$ plane that is a (reduced) distance $\bar{d}$ downstream from an initial plane, the ray has horizontal and vertical components q'_x, q'_y, h'_x, and h'_y. We can use Eqs. 16.6 and 16.8 to relate the horizontal components, and then use these equations again to relate the vertical components. The resulting four equations can be written as one matrix equation:

$$\begin{pmatrix} q'_x \\ q'_y \\ h'_x \\ h'_y \end{pmatrix} = \begin{pmatrix} 1 & 0 & 0 & 0 \\ 0 & 1 & 0 & 0 \\ \bar{d} & 0 & 1 & 0 \\ 0 & \bar{d} & 0 & 1 \end{pmatrix} \begin{pmatrix} q_x \\ q_y \\ h_x \\ h_y \end{pmatrix} \tag{16.48}$$

We can further write the incident ray matrix (on the right) in partitioned form as

$$\begin{pmatrix} q_x \\ q_y \\ h_x \\ h_y \end{pmatrix} = \begin{pmatrix} \mathbf{q} \\ \mathbf{h} \end{pmatrix} \tag{16.49}$$

where,

$$\mathbf{q} = \begin{pmatrix} q_x \\ q_y \end{pmatrix} \text{ and } \mathbf{h} = \begin{pmatrix} h_x \\ h_y \end{pmatrix} \tag{16.50}$$

We can also write similar equations for the emerging ray matrix (on the left in Eq. 16.46). Then Eq. 16.48 can be written as

$$\begin{pmatrix} \mathbf{q}' \\ \mathbf{h}' \end{pmatrix} = \mathbf{T} \begin{pmatrix} \mathbf{q} \\ \mathbf{h} \end{pmatrix} \tag{16.51}$$

where **T** is the translation matrix

$$\mathbf{T} = \left(\begin{array}{cc|cc} 1 & 0 & 0 & 0 \\ 0 & 1 & 0 & 0 \\ \hline \bar{d} & 0 & 1 & 0 \\ 0 & \bar{d} & 0 & 1 \end{array}\right) \tag{16.52}$$

The horizontal and vertical lines in this matrix indicate that we can write **T** in partitioned form as

$$\mathbf{T} = \left(\begin{array}{c|c} \mathbf{1} & \mathbf{0} \\ \hline \bar{\mathbf{d}} & \mathbf{1} \end{array}\right) \tag{16.53}$$

where **1** is the 2×2 unit matrix

$$\mathbf{1} = \begin{pmatrix} 1 & 0 \\ 0 & 1 \end{pmatrix}$$

0 is the 2×2 null (or zero) matrix

$$\mathbf{0} = \begin{pmatrix} 0 & 0 \\ 0 & 0 \end{pmatrix}$$

and

$$\bar{\mathbf{d}} = \begin{pmatrix} \bar{d} & 0 \\ 0 & \bar{d} \end{pmatrix}$$

Note the similarity between the partitioned form of the 4×4 translation matrix (Eq. 16.53), and the 2×2 translation matrix (Eq. 16.5) for a spherical system.

The translation matrix gets a ray from one plane to another. We also need a refraction matrix to get a ray through a thin spherocylindrical lens. (Remember that in a reduced system, a thin lens represents each single refracting surface.) At a thin lens, the horizontal and vertical position components of the ray do not change, so $h'_x = h_x$ and $h'_y = h_y$. The multiplications in the matrix form of Prentice's Rule in Chapter 13 give two equations that relate the horizontal and vertical ray angle components. The position and angle equations, a total of four, describe the effect of the spherocylindrical lens on the ray. Given the dioptric power matrix $\mathbf{P}$, where

$$\mathbf{P} = \begin{pmatrix} P_x & P_t \\ P_t & P_y \end{pmatrix}$$

these four equations can be written as one matrix equation:

$$\begin{pmatrix} q'_x \\ q'_y \\ h'_x \\ h'_y \end{pmatrix} = \begin{pmatrix} 1 & 0 & -P_x & -P_t \\ 0 & 1 & -P_t & -P_y \\ 0 & 0 & 1 & 0 \\ 0 & 0 & 0 & 1 \end{pmatrix} \begin{pmatrix} q_x \\ q_y \\ h_x \\ h_y \end{pmatrix} \tag{16.54}$$

In partitioned form, this equation becomes

$$\begin{pmatrix} \mathbf{q}' \\ \mathbf{h}' \end{pmatrix} = \mathbf{R} \begin{pmatrix} \mathbf{q} \\ \mathbf{h} \end{pmatrix} \tag{16.55}$$

where,

$$\mathbf{R} = \left(\begin{array}{cc|cc} 1 & 0 & -P_x & -P_t \\ 0 & 1 & -P_t & -P_y \\ \hline 0 & 0 & 1 & 0 \\ 0 & 0 & 0 & 1 \end{array}\right) \tag{16.56}$$

Again the horizontal and vertical lines suggest that

$$\mathbf{R} = \left(\begin{array}{c|c} \mathbf{1} & -\mathbf{P} \\ \hline \mathbf{0} & \mathbf{1} \end{array}\right) \tag{16.57}$$

where $\mathbf{1}$ is the 2×2 unit matrix, $\mathbf{0}$ is the 2×2 null matrix, and $\mathbf{P}$ is a 2×2 dioptric power matrix as expressed in a horizontal and vertical coordinate system. Note the similarity between the partitioned form of the 4×4 refraction matrix (Eq. 16.57) and the 2×2 refraction matrix (Eq. 16.10) for a spherical lens.

For combinations of spherocylindrical lenses, there is a 4×4 system matrix $\mathbf{S}$, which is just the product of the individual 4×4 refraction and translation matrices, i.e., for k separated spherocylindrical lenses,

$$\mathbf{S} = \mathbf{R}_k \mathbf{T}_{k-1} \mathbf{R}_{k-1} \ldots \mathbf{T}_2 \mathbf{R}_2 \mathbf{T}_1 \mathbf{R}_1 \tag{16.58}$$

Since the system matrix $\mathbf{S}$ is a 4×4 matrix, we can write its elements as

$$\mathbf{S} = \left(\begin{array}{cc|cc} s_{11} & s_{12} & s_{13} & s_{14} \\ s_{21} & s_{22} & s_{23} & s_{24} \\ \hline s_{31} & s_{32} & s_{33} & s_{34} \\ s_{41} & s_{42} & s_{43} & s_{44} \end{array}\right) \tag{16.59}$$

We can further write $\mathbf{S}$ in partitioned form (and in ABCD notation) as

$$\mathbf{S} = \left(\begin{array}{c|c} \mathbf{D} & \mathbf{C} \\ \hline \mathbf{B} & \mathbf{A} \end{array}\right) \tag{16.60}$$

where $\mathbf{D}$ is the 2×2 matrix consisting of the upper left sub-block, $\mathbf{C}$ is the 2×2 matrix consisting of the upper right sub-block, $\mathbf{B}$ is the 2×2 matrix consisting of the lower left sub-block, and $\mathbf{A}$ is the 2×2 matrix consisting of the lower right sub-block. The elements of $\mathbf{B}$ have units of length (meters), the elements of $\mathbf{C}$ have units of diopters, and the elements of $\mathbf{D}$ and $\mathbf{A}$ are unitless.

The 2×2 equivalent power matrix $\mathbf{P_e}$ of the system is

$$\mathbf{P_e} = -\mathbf{C} \tag{16.61}$$

which is analogous to Eq. 16.44 for a spherical system. The 2×2 back vertex power matrix $\mathbf{P_v}$ is given by

$$\mathbf{P_v} = \mathbf{P_e}\mathbf{A}^{-1} \tag{16.62}$$

which is analogous to the Eq. 16.46 for a spherical system. Similarly the 2×2 neutralizing power matrix $\mathbf{P_v}$ is given by

$$\mathbf{P_n} = \mathbf{D}^{-1}\mathbf{P_e} \tag{16.63}$$

which is analogous to Eq. 16.47 for a spherical system.

EXAMPLE 16.20

Example 13.16 considered a $+4.00 \times 45$ thin lens 10 cm in front of a $+5.00 \times 90$ thin lens. What is the 4×4 system matrix for this system? What is the 2×2 equivalent dioptric power matrix for the system, and do Eqs. 16.63 and 16.62 give the same 2×2 back and front vertex dioptric power matrices as Example 13.16?

From the dioptric power matrix for the $+4.00 \times 45$ lens (see Example 13.16) and Eq. 16.56

$$\mathbf{R}_1 = \left(\begin{array}{cc|cc} 1 & 0 & -2.00\,\text{D} & +2.00\,\text{D} \\ 0 & 1 & +2.00\,\text{D} & -2.00\,\text{D} \\ \hline 0 & 0 & 1 & 0 \\ 0 & 0 & 0 & 1 \end{array}\right)$$

Here $\bar{d} = 0.10\,\text{m}$, and from Eq. 16.52,

$$\mathbf{T_1} = \left(\begin{array}{cc|cc} 1 & 0 & 0 & 0 \\ 0 & 1 & 0 & 0 \\ \hline 0.10\,\text{m} & 0 & 1 & 0 \\ 0 & 0.10\,\text{m} & 0 & 1 \end{array}\right)$$

From the dioptric power matrix for the $+5.00 \times 90$ lens and Eq. 16.56,

$$\mathbf{R_2} = \left(\begin{array}{cc|cc} 1 & 0 & -5.00\,\text{D} & 0 \\ 0 & 1 & 0 & 0 \\ \hline 0 & 0 & 1 & 0 \\ 0 & 0 & 0 & 1 \end{array}\right)$$

From Eq. 16.58, the 4×4 system matrix is

$$\mathbf{S} = \mathbf{R_2 T_1 R_1}$$

It is quite tedious to carry out the 4×4 matrix multiplications by hand. However with a hand-held calculator or computer program that performs matrix multiplications, one simply fills in the numbers, pushes the evaluate button, and the program gives the answer as

$$\mathbf{S} = \left(\begin{array}{cc|cc} 0.50 & 0 & -6.00\,\text{D} & +1.00\,\text{D} \\ 0 & 1.00 & +2.00\,\text{D} & -2.00\,\text{D} \\ \hline 0.10\,\text{m} & 0 & 0.80 & 0.20 \\ 0 & 0.10\,\text{m} & 0.20 & 0.80 \end{array}\right)$$

From Eqs. 16.60 and 16.61, the 2×2 equivalent dioptric power matrix $\mathbf{P_e}$ is then

$$\mathbf{P_e} = \begin{pmatrix} +6.00\,\text{D} & -1.00\,\text{D} \\ -2.00\,\text{D} & +2.00\,\text{D} \end{pmatrix}$$

Note that the two torsional components of $\mathbf{P_e}$ (the 12 and 21 elements) are not equal to each other. In other words, $\mathbf{P_e}$ is asymmetric. This is discussed further in the next section.

From Eq. 16.60 and 16.62,

$$\mathbf{P_v} = \begin{pmatrix} +6.00\,\text{D} & -1.00\,\text{D} \\ -2.00\,\text{D} & +2.00\,\text{D} \end{pmatrix} \begin{pmatrix} 0.80 & 0.20 \\ 0.20 & 0.80 \end{pmatrix}^{-1}$$

$$= \begin{pmatrix} +6.00\,\text{D} & -1.00\,\text{D} \\ -2.00\,\text{D} & +2.00\,\text{D} \end{pmatrix} \begin{pmatrix} 1.33 & -0.33 \\ -0.33 & 1.33 \end{pmatrix}$$

and

$$\mathbf{P_v} = \begin{pmatrix} 8.33 & -3.33 \\ -3.33 & 3.33 \end{pmatrix}$$

The back vertex dioptric power matrix $\mathbf{P_v}$ is symmetric (equal torsional components) and agrees with that in Example 13.16.

From Eq. 16.60 and 16.62,

$$\mathbf{P_n} = \begin{pmatrix} 0.50 & 0 \\ 0 & 1.00 \end{pmatrix}^{-1} \begin{pmatrix} +6.00\,\text{D} & -1.00\,\text{D} \\ -2.00\,\text{D} & +2.00\,\text{D} \end{pmatrix}$$

$$= \begin{pmatrix} 2.00 & 0 \\ 0 & 1.00 \end{pmatrix} \begin{pmatrix} +6.00\,\text{D} & -1.00\,\text{D} \\ -2.00\,\text{D} & +2.00\,\text{D} \end{pmatrix}$$

and

$$\mathbf{P_n} = \begin{pmatrix} +12.00\,\text{D} & -2.00\,\text{D} \\ -2.00\,\text{D} & +2.00\,\text{D} \end{pmatrix}$$

The neutralizing (or front vertex) dioptric power matrix $\mathbf{P_n}$ is symmetric and also agrees with Example 13.16.

16.15 ASYMMETRIC EQUIVALENT DIOPTRIC POWER

Consider a system of two spherocylindrical lenses separated by the reduced distance $\bar{d}$. Here Eq. 16.58 gives the system matrix as

$$\mathbf{S} = \mathbf{R_2 T_1 R_1}$$

Just as Section 16.6 gave the equation for the spherical equivalent power of two separated lenses, the matrix multiplication of the above equation gives the 2×2 matrix equation

$$\mathbf{P_e} = \mathbf{P_1} + \mathbf{P_2} - \bar{d}\mathbf{P_2 P_1} \tag{16.64}$$

For two thin spherocylindrical lenses in contact, $\bar{d} = 0$, and Eq. 16.64 confirms that the dioptric power matrices are additive. However when $\bar{d}$ is not zero, the term with the matrix product $\mathbf{P_2 P_1}$ results in an asymmetric $\mathbf{P_e}$.

EXAMPLE 16.21:

Example 13.16 and the previous example considered a $+4.00 \times 45$ thin lens that is 10 cm in front of a $+5.00 \times 90$ thin lens. Does Eq. 16.64 give the same equivalent dioptric power matrix $\mathbf{P_e}$ as the system matrix in the previous example.

Here $\bar{d} = 0.10\,\text{m}$, the dioptric power matrix of the $+4.00 \times 45$ lens (see Example 13.16) is

$$\mathbf{P_1} = \begin{pmatrix} +2.00\,\text{D} & -2.00\,\text{D} \\ -2.00\,\text{D} & +2.00\,\text{D} \end{pmatrix}$$

and the dioptric power matrix for the $+5.00 \times 90$ lens is

$$\mathbf{P_2} = \begin{pmatrix} +5.00\,\text{D} & 0 \\ 0 & 0 \end{pmatrix}$$

Then from Eq. 16.64,

$$\mathbf{P_e}=\begin{pmatrix} +7.00\,\text{D} & -2.00\,\text{D} \\ -2.00\,\text{D} & +2.00\,\text{D} \end{pmatrix}-(0.10\,\text{m})\begin{pmatrix} +10.00\,\text{D} & -10.00\,\text{D} \\ 0 & 0 \end{pmatrix}$$

and

$$\mathbf{P_e}=\begin{pmatrix} +6.00\,\text{D} & -1.00\,\text{D} \\ -2.00\,\text{D} & +2.00\,\text{D} \end{pmatrix}$$

which is the same equivalent power matrix as in the preceding example.

The 2×2 vergence matrix of a toric wavefront is always symmetric. Hence the 2×2 back vertex power matrix $\mathbf{P_v}$ and 2×2 neutralizing power (or front vertex) matrix $\mathbf{P_n}$ are always symmetric. (They are in fact vergences.) However the previous two examples show that in general, the equivalent dioptric power matrix is asymmetric and contains four independent numbers. In other words,

$$\mathbf{P_e}=\begin{pmatrix} P_x & P_{12} \\ P_{21} & P_y \end{pmatrix} \qquad (16.65)$$

where $P_{12} \neq P_{21}$. (In vector space language, this means that for the asymmetric powers, we need a four dimensional dioptric power space.)

For a symmetric dioptric power matrix, we frequently used the three spherocylindrical parameters $S \bigcirc C \times \theta$ to describe the lens. For an asymmetric equivalent dioptric, we can use an asymmetric set of spherocylindrical parameters $S \bigcirc C \times \theta$: g, where g is the asymmetry parameter. To get the asymmetric spherocylindrical parameters, first set

$$P_t = \frac{P_{12}+P_{21}}{2} \qquad (16.66)$$

Then define the asymmetry parameter g such that

$$P_{12} = P_t + g \quad \text{and} \quad P_{21} = P_t - g \qquad (16.67)$$

The above four equations result in

$$\mathbf{P_e}=\begin{pmatrix} P_x & P_t \\ P_t & P_y \end{pmatrix}+g\begin{pmatrix} 0 & g \\ -g & 0 \end{pmatrix} \qquad (16.68)$$

or

$$\mathbf{P_e}=\begin{pmatrix} P_x & P_t \\ P_t & P_y \end{pmatrix}+\begin{pmatrix} 0 & 1 \\ -1 & 0 \end{pmatrix} \qquad (16.69)$$

Here the asymmetric dioptric power matrix has been separated into the sum of a symmetric matrix, which by itself has spherocylindrical parameters $S \bigcirc C \times \theta$, and an asymmetric matrix. Thus we can write the four numbers representing the asymmetric equivalent dioptric power $\mathbf{P_e}$ as $S \bigcirc C \times \theta$: g. For symmetric dioptric power, $g = 0$, and all we needed was just $S \bigcirc C \times \theta$.

EXAMPLE 16.22

Given the equivalent dioptric power matrix in the previous two examples, what are the asymmetric spherocylindrical parameters $S \bigcirc C \times \theta$: g?

Here,

$$\mathbf{P_e}=\begin{pmatrix} +6.00\,\text{D} & -1.00\,\text{D} \\ -2.00\,\text{D} & +2.00\,\text{D} \end{pmatrix}$$

Then Eq. 16.66 through 16.68 result in

$$\mathbf{P_e}=\begin{pmatrix} +6.00\,\text{D} & -1.50\,\text{D} \\ -1.50\,\text{D} & +2.00\,\text{D} \end{pmatrix}+\begin{pmatrix} 0 & +0.50\,\text{D} \\ -0.50\,\text{D} & 0 \end{pmatrix}$$

and

$$\mathbf{P_e}=\begin{pmatrix} +6.00\,\text{D} & -1.50\,\text{D} \\ -1.50\,\text{D} & +2.00\,\text{D} \end{pmatrix}+(+0.50\,\text{D})\begin{pmatrix} 0 & +1 \\ -1 & 0 \end{pmatrix}$$

The asymmetry parameter is +0.50 D. We can find $S \bigcirc C \times \theta$ (see Eqs. 13.41 through 13.43) from the symmetric matrix, and the total result for $S \bigcirc C \times \theta$: g is $+6.50 \bigcirc -5.00 \times 161.6$: $+0.50$, or in transposed form $+1.50 \bigcirc +5.00 \times 71.6$: $+0.50$.

It is also interesting to note that a lens with a symmetric dioptric matrix ($g = 0$) always has principal meridians that are 90° apart. For example, the symmetric matrix in this example corresponds to a lens with principal meridians of +6.50 D @ 161.6 and +1.50 D @ 71.6. For asymmetric equivalent power, the principal meridians are no longer 90° apart. For the asymmetric power in this example ($g = +0.50$ D), the principal meridian powers are +6.45 D @ 155.8 and +1.55 D @ 77.3. Here the principal meridians are 78.5° apart.

PROBLEMS

1. A +4.50 D lens is located 10 cm in front of a −4.50 D lens. Find the system matrix, the equivalent power, the back vertex power, and the neutralizing power.
2. A thin lens in air and screen eye model consists of a +58.00 D lens located 18 mm in front of the retina (screen). Find the system matrix for the eye and the (thin) contact correction.
3. A −8.00 D lens is located 6 cm in front of a +3.00 D lens. Find the system matrix, the equivalent power, the back vertex power, and the neutralizing power.
4. A +9.00 D lens is located 5 cm in front of a −4.00 D lens, which in turn is located 7 cm in front of a +6.00 D lens. Find the system matrix, the equivalent power,

the back vertex power, and the neutralizing power. Be sure to check the determinant of the system matrix.

5. The system matrix for a multiple lens system is

$$\mathbf{S} = \begin{pmatrix} 0.72 & -6.56\,\text{D} \\ 0.26\,\text{m} & 0.556 \end{pmatrix}$$

Find the back vertex power and the neutralizing power.

6. A +4.00 D lens is placed against the back of the system in problem no. 5. Find the new system matrix, the new equivalent power, the new back vertex power, and the new neutralizing power.
7. A −3.00 D lens is placed against the front of the system in problem no. 5. Find the new system matrix, the new equivalent power, the new back vertex power, and the new neutralizing power.
8. The equivalent power of a multiple lens system is +2.900 D. The back vertex power is +24.166 D and the front vertex power is −1.261 D. Find the system matrix.
9. Find the system matrix for three thin lenses in contact. According to the system matrix, are the dioptric powers of the three lenses additive?
10. A real object is 40 cm in front of a system with a system matrix of

$$\mathbf{S} = \begin{pmatrix} 0.400 & -6.480\,\text{D} \\ 0.120\,\text{m} & 0.556 \end{pmatrix}$$

Find the conjugate image and the lateral magnification.

11. Derive Eq. 16.22 for the back vertex power from the vertex vergence equation (Eq. 16.35).
12. The system in problem no. 10 is placed against the back vertex of the system in problem no. 5. What is the system matrix for the combination?
13. A reflection (catoptric power) matrix is identical in form to a refraction (dioptric power) matrix. Given this, consider the lens–mirror system in Example 14.19. Use the matrix-product method to find the system matrix. Your equivalent power from the system matrix should equal the power of the equivalent mirror. From the system matrix, find the back vertex and the neutralizing power of the lens–mirror system. (Your matrix product should correspond to the lens refraction, a translation over a positive distance to the mirror, the reflection by the spherical mirror, a translation over a positive distance back to the lens, and the second lens refraction.)
14. Given a system of separated spherocylindrical lenses with the asymmetric equivalent dioptric power

$$\mathbf{P_e} = \begin{pmatrix} -5.00\,\text{D} & +2.00\,\text{D} \\ +3.00\,\text{D} & -4.00\,\text{D} \end{pmatrix}$$

what are the four asymmetric spherocylindrical parameters?

CHAPTER 17

Angular Magnification

17.1 RELATIVE SIZE MAGNIFICATION

The foveal area of the human retina has the highest density of cones, and is the area that provides the best resolution of detail. The peripheral retina has a smaller density of cones, and provides much poorer resolution of detail. If a person's foveal area is impaired, the person will have decreased visual acuity even when the image is clear.

Increasing the size of the object can help a person with an impaired foveal area. This results in an increase in retinal image size, and enables the retina to obtain more information about the object's detail. For example, consider a person who holds a regular print book at 40 cm and has a retinal image size that is clear but too small for the detail to be resolved. The same person can perhaps hold a large print book at 40 cm and have a clear retinal image that is large enough for the detail to be resolved.

In the above situation, each book is held at 40 cm, each image is in focus on the retina, and the lateral magnification m of the observer's eye remains exactly the same when the books are switched. However, we are not so much interested in the lateral magnification as we are in the increase in the retinal image size. The ratio of the retinal image sizes is generically referred to as the *angular magnification* M. As shown below, the reason for the name is that the ratio of the retinal image sizes is equal to the ratio of the nodal angles subtended by the objects.

Figure 17.1 shows a thin lens in air eye model. The retina (screen) is a distance v_e from the lens. Figure 17.1a shows an object that has a nodal angle of w_1, and results in a retinal image size of I_1. Figure 17.1b shows a larger object at the same distance from the eye. The larger object has a nodal angle of w_2 and results in a retinal image size of I_2. From Figure 17.1a,

$$\tan w_1 = \frac{I_1}{v_e}$$

From Figure 17.1b,

$$\tan w_2 = \frac{I_2}{v_e}$$

By definition,

$$M = \frac{I_2}{I_1} \tag{17.1}$$

Since v_e is unchanged, it follows from the above three equations that

$$M = \frac{\tan w_2}{\tan w_1} \tag{17.2}$$

In paraxial cases, the tangent can be replaced by the angle, so

$$M = \frac{w_2}{w_1} \tag{17.3}$$

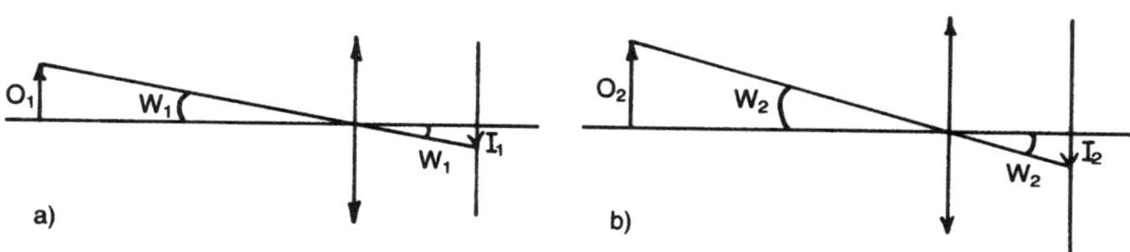

Figure 17.1 Relative size magnification.

Equation 17.3 is the mathematical statement that M is equal to the ratio of the subtended nodal angles.

EXAMPLE 17.1

Represent an unaccommodated emmetropic eye by a +60 D thin lens located 16.67 mm in front of a screen (the retina). For a set of letters located 40 cm from the lens, the ocular accommodative demand is 2.5 D and the lateral magnification is 16.67 mm/(−40 cm), which equals −0.042. What is the increase in retinal image size when viewing a 20/80 letter, which subtends an angle of 20′, as compared to viewing a 20/20 letter, which subtends an angle of 5′? What is the change in the lateral magnification?

From Eqs. 17.1 and 17.3,

$$M = \frac{20'}{5'} = 4\times$$

The retinal image size increases by a factor of 4. Since the object and image distances are unchanged, the lateral magnification is unchanged.

Angular magnification is conventionally labeled with an ×, although the × is a dimensionless unit. There are other ways of increasing an observer's retinal image size without physically changing the object size, and these are considered in the next sections. The angular magnification due to an object size change is sometimes called *relative size magnification*.

17.2 ANGULAR MAGNIFICATION WITHOUT A PHYSICAL SIZE CHANGE

A distant hot air balloon appears as a tiny shape in the sky. Even a visually normal person cannot make out the colorful pattern on the balloon because the retinal image of the balloon is too small. As the balloon drifts closer, the observer's retinal image of the balloon grows in size until the pattern is resolvable.

Alternatively, an observer can make out the pattern on the distant balloon by looking through a telescope. The telescope optically magnifies the image of the balloon, and the pattern then becomes resolvable. Similarly, when a near object is too small for resolution of the fine detail, a magnifying lens or a microscope can be used to increase one's retinal image size.

Thus, without changing the physical size of the object, people can increase their retinal image sizes either by bringing the object closer or by using a magnifying system, such as a converging lens, a telescope, or a microscope. Just as in relative size magnification, the increase is quantified by comparing the magnified retinal image size to the original unmagnified retinal image size. Again, the magnification of interest is not lateral magnification, which is a comparison of an image size to its conjugate object size, but rather is a comparison of one image size to another image size. As above, *angular magnification* is the generic name for the ratio of one retinal image size to another.

Figure 17.2 shows the comparison for an object at two different distances. The person's eye is represented by the thin lens and screen. The object has size O and is initially at position 1, which is a distance of u_1 from the eye. The conjugate image size, determined by the nodal ray, is I_e. When the object is moved in to position 2 (which is a distance u_2 from the eye) and the person accommodates appropriately, then the retinal image is clear and the size is I_m. The angular magnification M is specified by

$$M = \frac{I_m}{I_e} \tag{17.4}$$

The angles w_e and w_m subtended by the images at the nodal point of the lens are given by

$$\tan w_m = I_m / v_e$$

and

$$\tan w_e = I_e / v_e$$

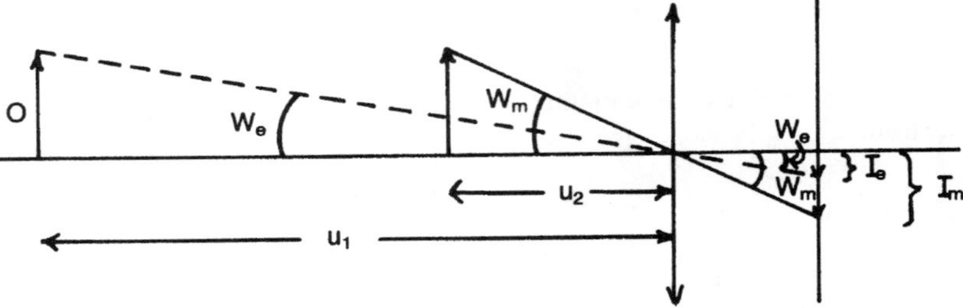

Figure 17.2 Relative distance magnification.

Figure 17.3 a, Unaided eye; b, eye aided by simple magnifier.

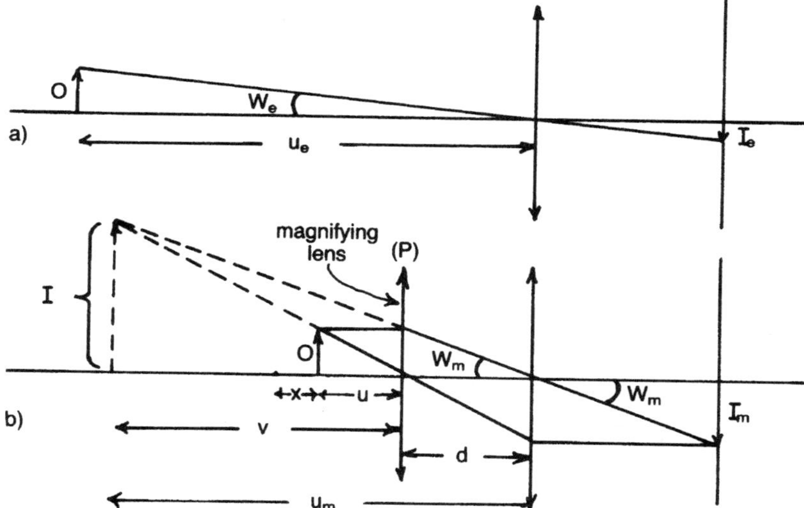

When accommodation occurs, the power of the lens changes but the lens–screen distance v_e remains the same. Then from the above three equations,

$$M = \frac{I_m}{I_e} = \frac{\tan w_m}{\tan w_e} \tag{17.5}$$

In the small angle approximation, which is accurate in the paraxial region, the tangents can be replaced by the angles and then

$$M = \frac{w_m}{w_e} \tag{17.6}$$

Equation 17.6 shows that the ratio of retinal image sizes is equal to the ratio of the nodal angles. In effect, one can increase (magnify) the retinal image size by increasing (magnifying) the angle of the nodal ray incident on the eye.

Figure 17.3 shows the situation for a person viewing a near object directly, and then viewing the near object through the magnifying lens. The retinal image size and the nodal angles are labeled the same as in Figure 17.2. Equations 17.4 through 17.6 again give the angular magnification.

It is important to note that angular magnification is always a comparison of one situation versus another. To emphasize this comparison, consider the relation between angular magnification and lateral magnification for the case in which the physical size of the object is unchanged. For the situation shown in Figure 17.3a, the lateral magnification m_1 for the direct viewing is defined as

$$m_1 = I_e/O$$

while the lateral magnification m_2 for the total magnifying lens–eye system (Figure 17.3b) is defined as

$$m_2 = I_m/O$$

Since the object size O is unchanged in the two different situations, one can use the above two equations together with Eq. 17.4 to obtain

$$M = \frac{m_2}{m_1} \tag{17.7}$$

Equation 17.7 shows that the angular magnification is equal to the ratio of the lateral magnifications, provided the object size remains unchanged.

In particular, the angular magnification M can be large even when the lateral magnification m_2 is small. In order for this to happen, m_1 has to be much smaller than m_2. Similarly, the angular magnification M can be small even when m_2 is large. This occurs whenever m_1 is much larger than m_2. Consequently, when dealing with angular magnification, it is important to keep the initial viewing conditions in mind.

(As an analogy, consider Pat and Mike, who have just returned from a casino each with \$3000. Are they happy or unhappy about their winnings? The answer depends on the initial amount that each went to the casino with. Pat went to the casino with \$65, while Mike went to the casino with \$9000. Even though both left the casino with \$3000, Pat is happy but Mike is not.)

17.3 RELATIVE DISTANCE MAGNIFICATION

As stated in Section 17.2, the retinal image size of an object can be increased by bringing the object closer to the eye. The angular magnification that results in this case is sometimes referred to as *relative distance magnification*.

In Figure 17.2, the object is originally at a distance u_1 from the eye, and then is moved in to a distance u_2 from the eye. In each case, the angle subtended by the object at the nodal point is equal to the angle subtended by the image at the nodal point. From the triangles involving the object,

$$\tan w_e = O/(-u_1)$$

and

$$\tan w_m = O/(-u_2)$$

Then from Eq. 17.5, the angular magnification equals the ratio of the object distances, or

$$M = \frac{(u_1)}{(u_2)} \tag{17.8}$$

Again, the angular magnification M is dimensionless but is conventionally labeled with an $\times$. For example, an angular magnification of $9\times$ indicates a ninefold increase in the retinal image size (or in the angle of the eye's nodal ray). Note that as the object is moved closer to the eye, the person's accommodative demand increases. The person's near point is the closest the object can get and still be seen clearly.

EXAMPLE 17.2

G.O. Student has her notes propped on her desk 100 cm from her eyes, and is having trouble reading the fine print. She then moves the notes in to 20 cm from her eyes. What angular magnification does G.O. achieve? (i.e., What is the increase in G.O.'s retinal image size?)

From Eq. 17.8,

$$M = \frac{(-100\,\text{cm})}{(-20\,\text{cm})} = +5\times$$

G.O.'s retinal image increases by a factor of 5 when the notes are moved in.

EXAMPLE 17.3

G.O.'s homework solutions are 25 cm in front of her eyes. What angular magnification does G.O. achieve when she brings the homework solutions in to 20 cm in from of her eyes?

From Eq. 17.8,

$$M = \frac{(-25\,\text{cm})}{(-20\,\text{cm})} = +1.25\times$$

In each of the above two examples, the object ended up 20 cm from the eye, but the angular magnification (or increase in retinal image size) is different because the starting conditions are different.

As a final note, it should be obvious that if the object is moved away from the eye instead of closer, the retinal image size will decrease and M will be less than one. For example, when the object at 20 cm is moved to 25 cm from the eye, the angular magnification due to the distance change is $0.80\times$. M less than one indicates a decrease in the retinal image size.

17.4 PLUS LENS AS A SIMPLE MAGNIFIER: INTUITIVE METHOD

When an object is placed inside the primary focal point of a plus (converging) lens, the conjugate image is virtual, erect, and larger. Thus, one can use a plus lens as a simple magnifying lens as shown in Figure 17.3.

In order to determine the angular magnification, we must first establish the initial conditions. Assume that initially the person directly views the object at a distance u_e in front of the eye (Figure 17.3a). The angle subtended by the object at the eye's nodal point is equal to the angle subtended by the retinal image at the nodal point, and both are labeled w. Then,

$$\tan w_e = O/(-u_e)$$

Figure 17.3b shows the person viewing the object through the magnifying lens. Note that the actual object to eye distance is different from u_e. The object is a distance of u in front of the magnifying lens, and the lens is a distance d in front of the eye. The virtual image (size I) is a distance of v from the magnifier and u_m from the eye. From the nodal ray for the eye,

$$\tan w_m = I/(-u_m)$$

From Eq. (17.5), the angular magnification M is then

$$M = \frac{I(u_e)}{O(u_m)}$$

I/O is the lateral magnification of the magnifier. Further, the ratio of the eye's object distances is just the angular magnification due to the distance changes (i.e. the relative distance magnification). Therefore, the total angular magnification M is equal to the product of the lateral magnification m_{lens} of the magnifying lens and the relative distance magnification M_{dis}, or

$$M = m_{lens} M_{dis} \tag{17.9}$$

EXAMPLE 17.4

Ranger Rick, an emmetrope, is examining a small insect 20 cm in front of his eye. Rick then uses a +20.00 D thin lens located 7 cm in front of his eye as a magnifier. Relative to the initial 20 cm viewing distance, what angular magnification does Rick achieve when he holds the insect 4.5 cm in front of the +20.00 D lens?

For the +20.00 D lens:

$$u_1 = -4.5\,\text{cm}$$
$$U_1 = \frac{100}{-4.5\,\text{cm}} = -22.22\,\text{D}$$

From $V = P + U$

$$V_1 = +20.00\,\text{D} + (-22.22\,\text{D}) = -2.22\,\text{D}$$

and

$$v_1 = -45.0\,\text{cm}$$

The lateral magnification for the lens is

$$m_{\text{lens}} = \frac{U_1}{V_1} = \frac{-22.22\,\text{D}}{-2.22\,\text{D}} = +10$$

The virtual image formed by the magnifying lens is 10 times larger than the insect. The virtual image is 45 cm from the magnifier, and the magnifier is 7 cm from Ranger Rick's eye, so the virtual image is 52 cm from his eye (i.e., 45 + 7). The object distance for Rick's eye is then

$$u_m = -52\,\text{cm}$$

The initial (direct) viewing distance was 20 cm, so the relative distance magnification is

$$M_{\text{dis}} = \frac{-20\,\text{cm}}{-52\,\text{cm}} = 0.38$$

The total angular magnification is

$$M = m_{\text{lens}} M_{\text{dis}} = (+10)(+0.38) = +3.8\times$$

When Ranger Rick uses the magnifying lens, the virtual image that he sees is actually 10 times larger than the insect but is also farther away than the object initially was. The angular magnification due to the distance change is 0.38 (a decrease). As a result, Ranger Rick increases his retinal image size by only a factor of 3.8 when using the +20.00 D magnifying lens under the specified conditions.

EXAMPLE 17.5

Paula Bear, an emmetrope, holds the fine print of a playbill program at a typical reading distance of 40 cm in front of her eye. Since she still cannot read the letters, Paula uses a +10.00 D thin lens as a magnifier. She holds the playbill 6 cm from the lens and the lens 4 cm from her eye. What angular magnification does Paula achieve?

For the lens:

$$u_1 = -6.00\,\text{cm}$$
$$U_1 = -16.67\,\text{D}$$
$$V_1 = +10.00 + (-16.67\,\text{D}) = -6.67\,\text{D}$$
$$v_1 = -15.00\,\text{cm}$$
$$m_{\text{lens}} = -16.67\,\text{D}/(-6.67\,\text{D}) = +2.5$$

The object distance for the eye is

$$u_m = -(15\,\text{cm} + 4\,\text{cm}) = -19\,\text{cm}$$

and the angular magnification due to distance changes is

$$M_{\text{dis}} = \frac{-40\,\text{cm}}{-19\,\text{cm}} = 2.105$$

The total angular magnification is

$$M = m_{\text{lens}} M_{\text{dis}} = (2.5)(2.105) = 5.26\times$$

17.5 PLUS LENS AS A COLLIMATING MAGNIFIER

As the object is moved closer to the primary focal point of the magnifying lens, the virtual image formed by the lens gets larger and moves farther away. Hence, the lateral magnification of the lens gets larger while the angular magnification due to the distance change gets smaller.

In the limit of the object going to the primary focal point, the lateral magnification m_{lens} goes to infinity and the angular magnification M_{dis} goes to zero. From Eq. 17.9, the total angular magnification M is then the product of infinity times zero, which is an indeterminate form. The value can be determined by numerically taking the limit. This involves calculating the result for a series of cases as the object is moved closer and closer to the primary focal point.

Consider a person viewing an object 10 cm in front of his eye. The person then takes a +20.00 D magnifying lens and holds the lens 3 cm in front of his eye. The object is originally placed 4 cm in front of the lens and then moved closer and closer to the primary focal point (which is 5 cm in front of the lens). The calculations are done as in Examples 17.4 and 17.5; Table 17.1 shows the results.

Table 17.1 Numerical Limit for Angular Magnification

u (cm)	v_1 (cm)	m_{lens}	M_{dis}	M
−4.00	−20	5	4.35×10^{-1}	2.17
−4.50	−45	10	2.08×10^{-1}	2.08
−4.90	−245	50	4.03×10^{-2}	2.02
−4.99	−2495	500	4.00×10^{-3}	2.00
−5.00	∞	∞	0	?

Note that in Table 17.1, m_{lens} steadily increases while M_{dis} steadily decreases, but their product M approaches 2.00×. Therefore, in the limit of the object going to the primary focal point (−5.00 cm), M goes to 2.00×.

An equation for the value of the angular magnification M when the object is at the primary focal point can be determined from Figure 17.4. For the object at the primary focal point, plane waves leave the magnifying lens and all the exiting rays are parallel. The nodal ray for the eye again subtends the angle w_m. However, the nodal ray for the eye is now parallel to the nodal ray for the magnifying lens, and hence the object O subtends an angle equal to w_m at the nodal point of the magnifying lens. Therefore,

$$\tan w_m = O/(-f_1)$$

The initial nodal angle w_e is given by

$$\tan w_e = O/(-u_e)$$

Then from Eq. 17.2,

$$M = (-u_e)/(-f_1)$$

The dioptric power P of the magnifying lens is related to f_1 by

$$P = -1/f_1$$

Therefore,

$$M = (-u_e)P$$

For all real objects, u_e is negative and

$$M = |u_e|P \qquad (17.10)$$

In Eq. 17.10, u_e must be in meters so that M is dimensionless. Equation 17.10 gives the angular magnification whenever the lens is used as a collimating magnifier (i.e., whenever plane waves leave the lens).

Note that Eq. 17.10 is independent of the distance d between the eye and the magnifying lens. This can be verified conceptually by noting that all the rays leaving the magnifying lens in Figure 17.4 are parallel and

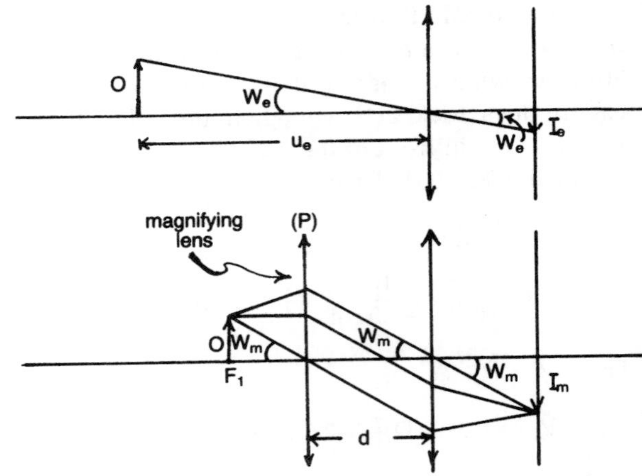

Figure 17.4 Unaided eye and eye aided by a collimating magnifier.

that no matter what the distance d is, the nodal ray incident on the eye subtends an angle equal to w_m. Consequently, the retinal image size I_m is also independent of the distance d.

EXAMPLE 17.6

Table 17.1 shows the angular magnification for a +20.00 D magnifying lens held 3 cm in front of the eye. The initial condition was that the person directly viewed the object 10 cm in front of his eye. According to Eq. 17.10, when the +20.00 D lens is used as a collimating magnifier,

$$M = (0.10\,\text{m})(+20.00\,\text{D}) = +2.00\times$$

The angular magnification of 2 agrees with the value arrived at by the limit procedure shown in Table 17.1.

EXAMPLE 17.7

In the above example, the person initially viewed the object 10 cm in front of his eye. Then the person used the +20.00 D lens as a collimating magnifier held 3 cm in front of his eye. The person increased his retinal image size by a factor of 2. What is the angular magnification relative to the initial 10 cm viewing distance when the person uses the +20.00 D lens as a collimating magnifier but holds the lens 18 cm in front of his eye?

Since for the collimating magnifier the person's retinal image and angular magnification are independent of the distance between the magnifying lens and the eye, M should again be +2×. Indeed, from Eq. 17.10,

$$M = (0.10\,\text{m})(+20.00\,\text{D}) \\ = +2.00\times$$

EXAMPLE 17.8
Marilyn Minnow has grown old, and has an uncorrected near point of 92 cm. Marilyn is trying to read the menu at a Hollywood restaurant. Finally, she pulls out a +32.00 D thin lens and uses it as a collimating magnifier. What is Marilyn's increase in retinal image size?

In this case, the best Marilyn can do without the magnifier is to hold the menu at her near point, and u_e is then 92 cm in magnitude. From Eq. 17.10,

$$M = (0.92\,\text{m})(+32.00\,\text{D}) \\ = 29.4\times$$

Note that the distance between the magnifying lens and the eye was not needed in the above example.

EXAMPLE 17.9
Elmer Towhead, an 8 year-old emmetrope, is dining at the table next to Marilyn's. Elmer's near point is 6.5 cm in front of his eye. Elmer sees Marilyn using the +32.00 D magnifying lens and wants to try it out. Will Elmer think it is as great as Marilyn does? Assume that Elmer uses the lens as a collimating magnifier.

Elmer achieves his largest retinal image without the magnifier by holding the menu at his near point. From Eq. 17.10, the increase in Elmer's retinal image size with the collimating magnifier is

$$M = (0.065\,\text{m})(+32.00\,\text{D}) \\ = 2.08\times$$

Elmer does get a 2.08 increase with the magnifying lens, but that is a factor of 14.2 less than Marilyn's 29.4×.

Clearly, their different near points are responsible for the different results. In fact, if Elmer held the menu at 92 cm (Marilyn's near point), and then brought the menu in to 6.5 cm, he would achieve an angular magnification due to the distance change of

$$M = 92\,\text{cm}/6.5\,\text{cm} = 14.2\times$$

which is exactly the difference between their angular magnifications.

17.6 THE CONVENTIONAL REFERENCE DISTANCE

As illustrated in Examples 17.8 and 17.9, different people get a different increase in retinal image size because of their different near points. This is important to keep in mind when prescribing magnifiers for a person with low vision.

However, to avoid confusion in the general public, it is desirable to label lenses with one magnification value so that a person can go to a store or a hobby shop and buy a specific magnifier (such as a 4× magnifier). To do this, a conventional, standard reference distance is needed.

The conventional standard reference distance is 25 cm. This distance is sometimes referred to as the *distance of most distinct vision*, although the latter title is meaningless. The 25 cm is a point that might be a typical near point for a group of people that includes both children, young adults, and some presbyopes. However, other people have variously argued that either 40 cm or 100 cm would be a better choice.

Since 25 cm is 1/4 meter, the angular magnification for a collimating magnifier of dioptric power P referenced to the standard distance is, from Eq. 17.10,

$$M = \frac{P}{4} \tag{17.11}$$

Consequently, a +20.00 D thin lens would be marked as a 5× magnifier, while the +32.00 D thin lens would be marked as an 8× magnifier.

Angular magnification was defined as the ratio of the magnified retinal image to an original unmagnified retinal image. The actual angular magnification matches the value given by Eq. 17.11 only when the initial direct viewing distance is 25 cm. When the initial direct viewing distance is not 25 cm, then the angular magnification achieved will not match the value given by Eq. 17.11.

EXAMPLE 17.10
Sylvia Frost, an emmetrope with a 5 D amplitude of accommodation, views a stamp held at her near point. Since she cannot see the fine detail, Sylvia buys a 6× thin magnifier at a hobby shop. What angular magnification does Sylvia achieve with the 6× magnifier relative to her near point?

From Eq. 17.11, the 6× thin magnifier is a +24.00 D lens. The default assumption is that Sylvia uses the lens as a collimating magnifier.

Sylvia's near point is 20 cm in front of her eye. Therefore,

$$M = (0.20\,\text{m})(+24.00\,\text{D}) = +4.8\times$$

Sylvia achieves an angular magnification of 4.8× relative to her near point. She does not achieve the full 6× because her near point is at 20 cm instead of the conventional 25 cm reference distance. In fact, if Sylvia moved the object from 20 cm to 25 cm and then used the 6× collimating magnifier, her total angular magnification would be the product of the angular magnification due to the distance change and the standard 6× of the magnifying lens. Specifically,

$$M = \frac{20\,\text{cm}}{25\,\text{cm}}(6\times)$$

or

$$M = (0.80)(6\times) = 4.8\times$$

which is the same value attained above.

EXAMPLE 17.11
Foster Grant has a near point 40 cm in front of his eye. Foster uses a collimating magnifier and achieves an angular magnification of 9× relative to his near point. What is the standard magnification rating of the lens?

From Eq. 17.10, the power of the lens is given by

$$\begin{aligned} P &= M/|u_e| \\ &= 9\times/0.40\,\text{m} = +22.50\,\text{D} \end{aligned}$$

From Eq. 17.11, the standard magnification is

$$\begin{aligned} M &= \frac{P}{4} \\ &= \frac{+22.50\,\text{D}}{4} = 5.6\times \end{aligned}$$

The lens would be marked as a 5.6× magnifier.

17.7 COLLIMATING MAGNIFIER: OBJECT TO EYE DISTANCE UNCHANGED

Equation 17.10 is the general equation for a thin lens collimating magnifier. Under a restricted condition, we can derive another equation for a collimating magnifier. The restricted condition is that the distance between the object and the eye is unchanged when the magnifier is put in place.

Notice that in Figure 17.4, the distance between the object and the eye changes when the magnifier is used. Figure 17.5 shows the restricted condition where the distance between the object and the eye is unchanged when the magnifier is used. In Figure 17.5a, the original viewing distance is u_e. The magnifier is placed so that the object is at the primary focal point of the lens. The distance between the lens and the eye is labeled d. From the restriction,

$$d = |u_e| - |f_1|$$

or

$$|u_e| = |f_1| + d$$

Then the general equation (Eq. 17.10) gives

$$M = [|f_1| + d]P$$

or

$$M = |f_1|P + dP$$

For a thin lens in air, the focal length and the dioptric power are reciprocally related so that

$$M = 1 + dP \qquad (17.12)$$

Equation 17.12 is the equation for a collimating magnifier *under the restricted condition* that the distance between the object and the eye is not changed when the magnifier is added. Equation 17.10 is the general

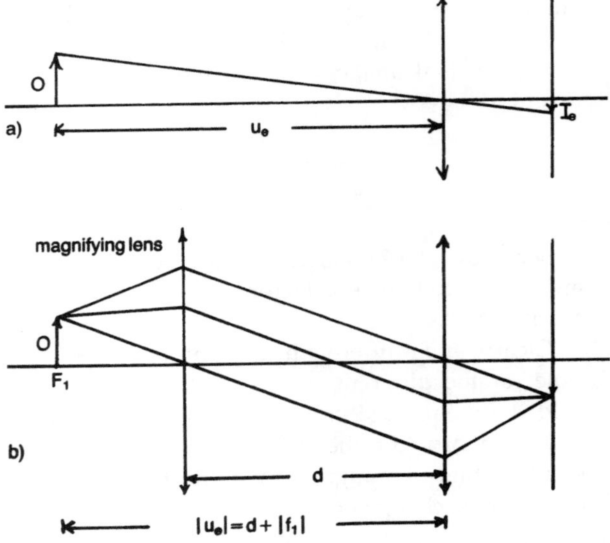

Figure 17.5 Special case where the distance between the object and the eye is unchanged between the initial and magnified viewing: a, unaided eye; b, eye viewing through a collimating magnifier.

equation. Historically, people have occasionally misused Eq. 17.12 in situations where it was not applicable.

EXAMPLE 17.12

Carmel Corn, an emmetrope with a neck cast, is viewing a stamp on a board in front of her. Carmel is unable to move her head or the board, but she is able to use a 4× magnifier to examine the fine detail on the stamp. Carmel places the 4× magnifier in front of her eye, notes that the image is blurred, and moves the magnifier towards the stamp until the image clears. At this point the magnifier is 30 cm from her eye. What angular magnification has Carmel achieved relative to her initial direct viewing?

When Carmel initially looked through the magnifier, the light leaving the magnifier was converging, which is why she saw a blurred image. The image clears when the light leaving the lens consists of plane waves, so Carmel is then using the lens as a collimating magnifier. From Eq. 17.11,

$$P = (4\,\times)4 = +16.00\,\text{D}$$

Because the restricted conditions apply in this case, we can use Eq. 17.12,

$$\begin{aligned} M &= 1 + dP \\ &= 1 + (0.30\,\text{m})(+16.00\,\text{D}) \\ &= 1 + 4.8 = 5.8\times \end{aligned}$$

EXAMPLE 17.13

Use the general equation (Eq. 17.10) to solve for the angular magnification in the previous example.

The general equation is

$$M = |u_e|P$$

where u_e is the original direct viewing distance. From the previous example the lens is a +16.00 D lens used as a collimating magnifier and held 30 cm from Carmel's eye. The focal length for a +16.00 D thin lens is 6.25 cm. Since Carmel is using the lens as a collimating magnifier and holding it 30 cm from her eye, the physical distance between the stamp and her eye is 36.25 cm. Under the conditions given, the 36.25 cm was Carmel's original viewing distance. Thus,

$$|u_e| = 36.25\,\text{cm} = 0.3625\,\text{m}$$

and Eq. 17.10 gives

$$\begin{aligned} M &= (0.3625\,\text{m})(+16.00\,\text{D}) \\ &= 5.8\times \end{aligned}$$

The general equation gives the same result as the restricted equation used in the previous example.

17.8 MAGNIFIERS AND MAXIMUM ACCOMMODATION

An emmetrope does not need to accommodate when looking through a collimating magnifier. However, the emmetrope might be able to achieve more magnification through a magnifier by accommodating. In this case, the light coming out of the magnifier is diverging, and Eq. 17.9 gives the angular magnification. Let us investigate the particular case in which an emmetrope uses the same amount of accommodation both initially and when viewing through the magnifier. Figure 17.6 shows the situation. The object is initially viewed at the distance u_e. When the magnifying lens is used, the object distance u_1 is adjusted until the virtual image that the emmetrope sees is at a distance u_m that is equal to u_e. From Eq. 17.9,

$$M = m_{\text{lens}} M_{\text{dis}}$$

but since $u_e = u_m$

$$M_{\text{dis}} = \frac{u_e}{u_m} = 1$$

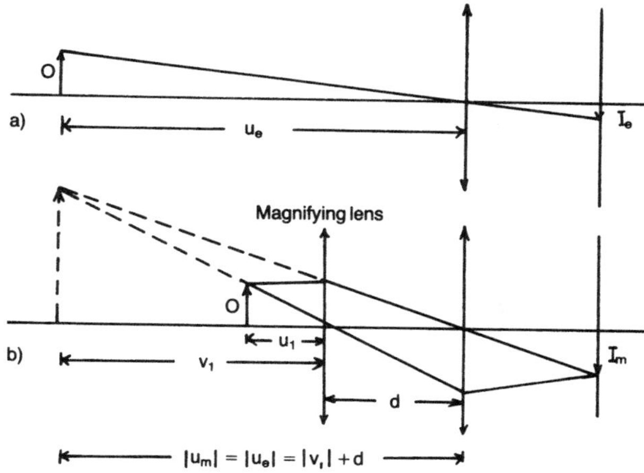

Figure 17.6 Special case where the ocular accommodative demand is unchanged between the initial and the magnified viewing: a, unaided eye; b, eye viewing through the magnifier.

Then for this case,

$$\begin{aligned} M &= m_{\text{lens}} \\ &= \frac{v_1}{u_1} = v_1 U_1 \\ &= v_1(V_1 - P) \\ &= 1 - v_1 P \\ &= 1 + |v_1| P \end{aligned}$$

From Figure 17.6b,

$$|u_e| = |v_1| + d$$

or

$$|v_1| = |u_e| - d$$

Then we can substitute the above equation into the last equation for M to obtain

$$M = 1 + (|u_e| - d)P \tag{17.13}$$

It is clear from Eq. 17.13 that the larger the distance d from the magnifying lens to the eye, the smaller the angular magnification M. When d is zero, Eq. 17.13 gives a maximum.

The d equal zero situation is not practical because it implies that the magnifying lens is pressed against (or in contact with) the eye. Nonetheless, let us assume d is zero and obtain the (mythical) maximum M:

$$M_{\max} = 1 + |u_e|P \tag{17.14}$$

Equation 17.14 is sometimes compared to Eq. 17.10, which was the magnification for a collimating magnifier. Note that for a finite u_e, the two equations describe different situations. Plane waves leave the collimating magnifier and an emmetrope does not have to accommodate. For the case of Eq. 17.14, the light leaving the magnifier is diverging, and the person needs to accommodate for the distance u_e. By using the accommodation, the person is able to add an additional one unit of magnification over what he or she could obtain while unaccommodated (assuming that d is zero).

EXAMPLE 17.14

Sylvia Frost, the emmetrope in Example 17.10, had an amplitude of accommodation of 5 D. When Sylvia used the +24.00 D lens as a collimating magnifier, the magnification rating was 6× but Sylvia's actual angular magnification was 4.8×. Relative to her near point, what is the maximum angular magnification that Sylvia can achieve?

The maximum angular magnification occurs when Sylvia accommodates maximally and when the distance d between the magnifier and the eye is zero. Equation 17.14 describes this case when u_e is equal to the near point distance (which is 20 cm for Sylvia), i.e.,

$$\begin{aligned} M_{\max} &= 1 + (0.20)(+24.00\text{ D}) \\ &= 1 + 4.8 = 5.8\times \end{aligned}$$

The maximum angular magnification is 5.8× compared to the 4.8× that Sylvia gets when she uses the lens as a collimating magnifier. Note that it is purely accidental that the 5.8× obtained for Sylvia is close to the 6× rating of the magnifier. For a different person (i.e., different set of numbers) these values may not be close.

Equation 17.14 gives the mythical maximum value of angular magnification available. Suppose this amount is referenced to the conventional 25 cm or 1/4 m viewing distance. Then $|u_e|$ in Eq. 17.14 equals 1/4 m and

$$M_{\max} = 1 + \frac{P}{4} \tag{17.15}$$

In conjunction with Eq. 17.15, the accommodative demand for an emmetrope is 4 D both when directly viewing the object and when viewing through the magnifier.

17.9 THE BADAL PRINCIPLE

The distance d between the magnifier and the eye does make a difference even though we set it equal to zero to obtain the mythical maximum. The d value tends to negate the value of u_e, and thus decrease M from the maximum value of Eq. 17.14. In fact, a large d can even make M smaller than the collimating magnifier value of Eq. 17.10.

This means that there is some d value for which the angular magnification is the same regardless of the accommodative demand. We can find this d value by equating Eqs. 17.10 and 17.13. Then,

$$1 + (|u_e| - d)P = |u_e|P$$

or

$$1 - dP = 0$$

and

$$d = 1/P = f_2$$

Thus, when d is equal to the secondary focal length of the magnifying lens, the angular magnification is independent of the vergence leaving the magnifying lens. This is called *Badal's Principle*.

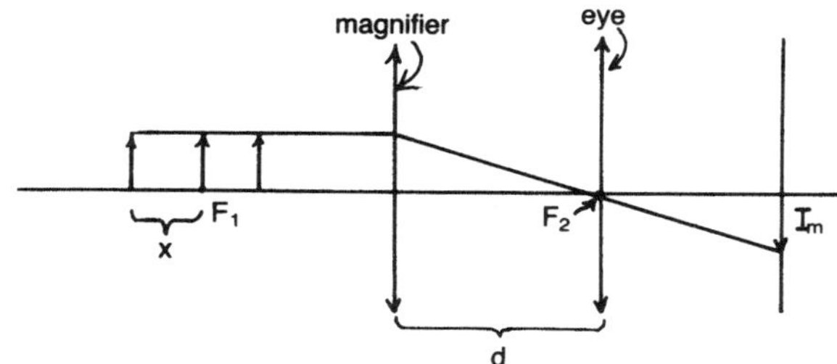

Figure 17.7 Badal Principle.

Figure 17.7 shows the optics of Badal's Principle. The lens representing the eye is placed at the secondary focal point of the magnifying lens. The figure shows three different object positions in front of the magnifier. The common incident ray parallel to the axis is common to all three objects, and the exiting ray passes through F_2 of the magnifier. Since F_2 of the magnifier coincides with the nodal point for the lens representing the eye, the ray proceeds straight through without bending and specifies the retinal image size I_m. Here as the object moves towards the magnifier, diverging light emerges from the magnifier, and the vergence incident on the eye changes. However if the eye accommodates correctly, the retinal image remains clear and its size does not change.

Badal's Principle supplies a way to measure accommodative responses independent of retinal image size changes. Badal's Principle is also used in some other ophthalmic instruments such as a lensmeter.

17.10 GENERAL EQUATION FOR A SIMPLE MAGNIFIER

Section 17.4 described an intuitive method for obtaining the angular magnification of a simple magnifier. We can derive an equation that replaces the intuitive method. The advantage of such an equation is that it conceptually ties much of the above discussion together. The disadvantage of the equation is that the optics involved are not as explicitly apparent as they were in the intuitive method.

The derivation starts with Equation 17.9,

$$M = m_{\text{lens}} M_{\text{dis}}$$

Figure 17.3 shows the situation. We can substitute the vergence equation for the lateral magnification and also the distances for the relative distance magnification to obtain

$$M = \left(\frac{U}{V}\right)\left(\frac{u_e}{u_m}\right)$$

In Figure 17.3, both u_m and v are negative, and so

$$M = \left(\frac{U}{V}\right)\left(\frac{u_e}{v - d}\right)$$

or

$$M = (u_e)\left(\frac{U}{1 - dV}\right)$$

For real objects, u_e is negative, and then

$$M = |u_e|\left(\frac{-U}{1 - dV}\right) \quad (17.16)$$

Equation 17.16 is a general equation for a thin lens used as a simple magnifier. In Eq. 17.16, U and V are the respective vergences of the wavefront incident on and leaving the lens, d is the distance between the lens and the eye, and u_e is the initial object distance (negative) for the unaided eye.

EXAMPLE 17.15

Use Eq. 17.16 to rework Example 17.5 involving Paula Bear.

From the data in Example 17.5, $u_e = -0.40$ m, $d = 0.04$ m, $U = -16.67$ D, and $V = -6.67$ D. Then Eq. 17.16 gives

$$M = |-0.40\,\text{m}|\frac{-(-16.67\,\text{D})}{1 - (0.04\,\text{m})(-6.67\,\text{D})}$$

or

$$M = (0.40\,\text{m})(13.16\,\text{D}) = 5.26\times$$

which is the same answer as that obtained in Example 17.5.

It is preferred to work this problem using the intuitive method as shown in Example 17.5. However, Eq. 17.16 does conceptually fit different aspects of simple magnifiers together. Specifically, Eq. 17.16 shows that, in general, the angular magnification depends on the initial observation distance u_e, the vergence U incident on the magnifying lens (which obviously depends on the object distance for the magnifier), the vergence V leaving the magnifying lens (where $V = P + U$), and the distance d between the magnifier and the eye.

There are, however, special circumstances, as previously discussed, in which the dependence on some of these variables drops out. For example, suppose the magnifier is used as a collimating magnifier. Then the object is placed at the primary focal point of the magnifier, and $U = -P$. Here plane waves leave the magnifier, so V is zero. Substitution into Equation 17.16 shows that it simplifies to Eq. 17.10,

$$M = |u_e|P \quad \text{for any } d$$

Alternatively, suppose that the object distance for the magnifier is free to vary, but that d is equal to the secondary focal length f_2 of the lens (Badal's Principle). Since $V = P + U$, Eq. 17.16 gives

$$M = |u_e|\left(\frac{-U}{1 - dP - dU}\right)$$

For $d = f_2$,

$$M = |u_e|\left(\frac{-U}{1 - f_2P - f_2U}\right)$$

Since $P = 1/f_2$,

$$M = |u_e|\left(\frac{-U}{-f_2U}\right) = \frac{|u_e|}{f_2}$$

or

$$M = |u_e|P \quad \text{for any } U$$

Here the angular magnification is independent of the vergence incident on the magnifier, and hence independent of the object distance u for the magnifier. The resulting angular magnification M is the same as that of a collimating magnifier.

17.11 THE COMPOUND MICROSCOPE

The compound microscope provides much higher magnifications than simple magnifiers. Compound microscopes first appeared in Holland in the early 1600s, possibly invented by the Dutchman Zacharias Janssen, 1588–1632. However, the full impact of the microscope did not develop until the work of the Dutchman Anothony van Leeuwenhoek (1632–1723). Starting in about 1673, Leeuwenhoek made microscopes that were superior to any others of that time. His first published microscopic report was on observations of the sting, mouth parts, and eye of the bee and the louse. He went on to make the first observations of microbes (bacteria and protozoa), and also made a series of important microscopic anatomical observations.

The simplest compound microscope consists of two thin lenses. The lens closest to the object is called the *objective lens,* and its function is to form a magnified real image inside the microscope (Figure 17.8). The lens closest to the eye is called the *ocular lens.* The ocular lens serves as a simple magnifier with the internal real image as its object. An unaccommodated emmetrope or corrected ametrope would focus the microscope so that plane waves leave the ocular lens.

The magnification of the microscope is expressed in terms of the increase in retinal image size achieved with the aid of the microscope. The comparison is with the retinal image size I_e of an object viewed directly at the standard reference distance of 25 cm. When looking through the microscope, one has a larger retinal image size I_m. Thus, the magnification of the microscope is

$$M = \frac{I_m}{I_e}$$

As before, the ratio of the retinal image sizes is equal to the ratio of the angles subtended at the nodal point of the eye. In Figure 17.4, w_e is the nodal angle in the initial viewing situation, while in Figure 17.8, w_m is the angle subtended at the nodal point of the eye by the rays leaving the microscope. Thus,

$$M = \frac{\tan w_m}{\tan w_e}$$

From Figure 17.4,

$$\tan w_e = O/u_e$$

For plane waves leaving the microscope, the internal image must be at the primary focal point of the ocular lens. Then from Figure 17.8,

$$\tan w_m = I_1/(f_1)_{oc}$$

Since

$$I_1 = m_{obj}O$$

where m_{obj} is the lateral magnification of the objective, the above three equations give

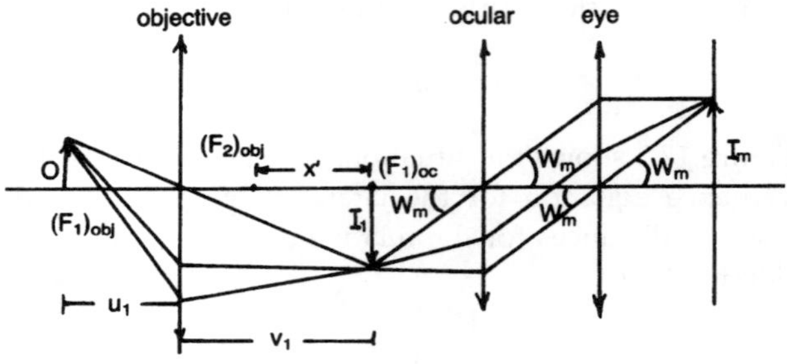

Figure 17.8 Compound microscope.

$$M = \frac{m_{obj} u_e}{f_1} = m_{obj}|u_e|P_{oc}$$

The 25 cm standard reference distance gives

$$M = m_{obj}\left(\frac{P_{oc}}{4}\right) \quad (17.17)$$

EXAMPLE 17.16

A compound microscope consists of a +50 D objective lens located 23.25 cm in front of a +80 D ocular lens. What is the magnification of the microscope when it is adjusted for plane waves leaving?

The most intuitive method to solve this problem is to reverse the light, in which case we consider plane waves incident on the ocular lens. Then we can follow the light back through the microscope and find the object position.

In the reversed system, $U_1 = 0$ and

$$V_1 = P_{oc} + U_1 = +80\,\text{D}$$

Then,

$$v_1 = +1.25\,\text{cm}$$
$$u_2 = -(23.25\,\text{cm} - 1.25\,\text{cm}) = -22.00\,\text{cm}$$
$$U_2 = -4.54\,\text{D}$$
$$V_2 = +45.45\,\text{D}$$

and

$$v_2 = +2.20\,\text{cm}$$

So in the forward direction, the object would be placed 2.2 cm in front of the objective lens (just 0.2 cm outside the primary focal point of the objective lens), and the internal image is formed 22.00 cm from the objective lens with a lateral magnification m of -10 (i.e., $22.0/-2.20$). From Eq. 17.17, the magnification of the microscope is

$$M = (-10)\left(\frac{+80\,\text{D}}{4}\right)$$
$$= (-10)(20\times) = -200\times$$

Relative to the standard reference distance, the magnification of the microscope is 200. The minus sign indicates that the microscope's image is inverted.

EXAMPLE 17.17

A microscope consists of a +30.00 D lens located 20 cm from the ocular lens. When focused for plane waves leaving, the object is 4.29 cm in front of the objective lens. What is the magnification of the microscope?

In this case, let us think in terms of the light traveling in the forward direction.

$$u_1 = -4.29\,\text{cm}$$
$$U_1 = -23.31\,\text{D}$$
$$V_1 = +30.00\,\text{D} + (-23.31\,\text{D}) = +6.69\,\text{D}$$
$$v_1 = +14.95\,\text{cm}$$
$$m = \frac{-23.31\,\text{D}}{+6.69\,\text{D}} = -3.48$$

The internal image is at the primary focal point of the ocular lens, so the focal length of the ocular lens must be

$$|f_1| = 20\,\text{cm} - 14.95\,\text{cm} = 5.05\,\text{cm}$$

Then,

$$P_{oc} = +19.80\,\text{D}$$

From Eq. 17.17, the magnification of the microscope is

$$M = (-3.48)\left(\frac{+19.80\,\text{D}}{4}\right) = -17.2\times$$

In the above examples, we obtained the lateral magnification of the objective lens from the image distance–object distance ratio or from the vergence ratio. Equation 9.8 was an alternative equation for the lateral magnification in terms of the extra-focal image distance x':

$$m = -\frac{x'}{f_2} = -x'P_{obj}$$

In the case of a microscope focused for plane waves leaving, the distance x' is the distance from the objective lens's secondary focal point to the internal image formed by the objective lens, which occurs at the ocular lens's primary focal point. The distance x' between these two focal points is called the *optical tube length* of the microscope (Figure 17.8). Note that the actual tube length is the distance from the objective lens to the ocular lens. When we substitute the above equation for m into Eq. 17.17, we obtain

$$M = \frac{-x'P_{obj}P_{oc}}{4} \quad (17.18)$$

Equation 17.18 is really just a disguised version of Eq. 17.17. Equation 17.18 has the advantage that the (angular) magnification of the microscope can be computed without the need to know the object distance for the objective lens.

In many microscopes the objective lens or lenses can be changed to increase the magnification. The design is typically such that the optical tube length x' remains the same when the objective lens is changed. 160 mm is a typical optical tube length. Equation 17.18 explicitly shows that the magnification increase is directly proportional to the increase in objective lens power.

EXAMPLE 17.18

A 100× compound microscope has an 18× ocular lens and a 160 mm optical tube length. Find the power of the objective lens, the distance from the objective lens to the ocular lens (the actual tube length) when the microscope is focused for plane waves leaving, and the distance from the objective lens to the object.

From Eq. 17.11,

$$P_{oc} = (18\times)(4) = +72.00\,\text{D}$$

Then from Eq. 17.18,

$$-100\times = -(0.160\,\text{m})P_{obj}(18\times)$$

and

$$P_{obj} = +34.722\,\text{D}$$

The distance between the two lenses equals the sum of the two focal lengths plus the optical tube length:

$$d = \frac{100\,\text{cm/m}}{+34.722\,\text{D}} + 16.0\,\text{cm} + \frac{100\,\text{cm/m}}{+72.00\,\text{D}} = 20.269\,\text{cm}$$

The image distance for the objective lens equals the secondary focal length of the objective plus the extrafocal image distance x'. Therefore,

$$v = +2.88\,\text{cm} + 16.0\,\text{cm} = 18.88\,\text{cm}$$

Then,

$$V = +5.297\,\text{D}$$

and from $V = P + U$,

$$U = +5.297\,\text{D} - 34.722\,\text{D} = -29.426\,\text{D}$$

or

$$u = -3.398\,\text{cm}$$

For plane waves leaving the microscope, the object must be 3.398 cm in front of the objective lens.

EXAMPLE 17.19

A 40× microscope has a +25.00 D objective lens. What is the magnification when the objective is switched to +93.75 D?

Here the ocular lens is unchanged, and the default assumption is that the optical tube length is also unchanged. Then we can use Eq. 17.18 to set up the ratio

$$\frac{M}{-40\times} = \frac{x'(+93.75\,\text{D})P_{oc}}{x'(+25.00\,\text{D})P_{oc}}$$

or

$$\frac{M}{-40\times} = \frac{+93.75\,\text{D}}{+25.00\,\text{D}}$$

which gives

$$M = -150\times$$

When an emmetrope or corrected ametrope uses a microscope, the focus condition for best visual comfort is to have plane waves leaving the microscope. However, the microscope can be focused for either converging or diverging light leaving. Equation 17.17 has the form that the angular magnification M of the microscope is equal to the lateral magnification m of the objective times the angular magnification of the ocular, or

$$M = (m_{lat})_{objective}(M_{ang})_{ocular} \tag{17.19}$$

Equation 17.19 is the general form for the magnification of a two-lens microscope even when the microscope is focused so that converging or diverging light is leaving (as opposed to plane waves). In the latter case, the appropriate equation for the angular magnification M_{ang} of the ocular lens is used. For example, if the person focuses the microscope for an accommodative demand of 4 D, then Eq. 17.15,

$$M_{ang} = 1 + \frac{P}{4}$$

would be the appropriate equation for the angular magnification of the ocular lens (instead of $M_{ang} = P/4$). Usually the dioptric power of the ocular lens is high and the resulting change in magnification is very small. In practical terms, this means that changing the focus of a high magnification microscope does not appreciably affect the magnification, so an emmetrope might as well focus for the comfortable situation of plane waves leaving.

17.12 EQUIVALENT POWER FORMULATION FOR MAGNIFICATION

The compound microscope consists of at least two lenses. The microscope, like any system of spherical lenses, has three dioptric power parameters: the neutralizing power P_n (also called the front vertex power), the back vertex power P_v, and the equivalent power P_e. In terms of the Gauss system, the compound microscope acts like a single lens with the equivalent power P_e.

In the Gauss system, the derivation for the magnification of the compound microscope (relative to the 25 cm standard reference distance) then proceeds exactly like that of Eq. 17.11 with P replaced by the equivalent power P_e. The result is

$$M = \frac{P_e}{4} \tag{17.20}$$

EXAMPLE 17.20

The compound microscope in Example 17.16 consisted of a +50.00 D lens located 23.25 cm in front of a +80.00 D lens. Find the magnification by using the equivalent power equation, and compare the results to those in Example 17.16.

For two separated lenses, Eq. 15.40 gives the equivalent power as

$$\begin{aligned} P_e &= P_1 + P_2 - \bar{d}P_1P_2 \\ &= +50.00\,\text{D} + 80.00\,\text{D} \\ &\quad - (0.2325\,\text{m})(+50.00\,\text{D})(+80.00\,\text{D}) \\ &= -800\,\text{D} \end{aligned}$$

From Eq. 17.20,

$$M = \frac{-800\,\text{D}}{4} = -200\times$$

The magnification of $-200\times$ agrees with Example 17.16. Note that here the negative equivalent dioptric power P_e relates directly to the inversion of the image.

Simple magnifiers are high plus lenses. In the real world, these lenses are thick. The reduced system corresponding to a thick lens consists of two thin lenses in air, respectively representing the front and back surfaces of the thick lens. Thus, the magnification theory of the thick lens exactly parallels that of the two-lens compound microscope. By interpreting the front surface as the objective and the back surface as the ocular, we can use Eq. 17.19 to find M. Alternatively, we can use the equivalent power of the thick lens and Eq.17.20.

EXAMPLE 17.21

A thick ($n = 1.50$) biconvex lens has front and back surface powers of +22.00 D and +16.00 D, respectively, and a central thickness of 33 mm. When this lens is used as a collimating magnifier, what is the magnification?

The default assumption is that the magnification requested is relative to the standard 25 cm reference distance. To use Eq. 17.19, we need to know where the object or the image for the front surface is. Since the thick lens is serving as a collimating magnifier, the object must be at the thick lens's primary focal point. We can find the primary focal point by reversing the light, in which case we consider plane waves incident on the back of the lens. For the reversed case,

$$U_1 = 0 \quad \text{and} \quad V_1 = +16.00\,\text{D}$$

The reduced thickness of the lens is 33 mm/1.50 or 22 mm. Then,

$$U_2 = +24.69\,\text{D} \quad V_2 = +46.69\,\text{D}$$

and

$$v_2 = +2.14\,\text{cm}$$

For light in the forward direction, the primary focal point of the lens is 2.14 cm in front of the +22.00 D surface. When the object is in the primary focal plane (light in the forward direction),

$$\begin{aligned} u_1 &= -2.14\,\text{cm} \\ U_1 &= -46.69\,\text{D} \\ V_1 &= -24.69\,\text{D} \\ U_2 &= -16.00\,\text{D} \end{aligned}$$

and

$$V_2 = 0$$

The lateral magnification for the +22.00 D surface, which serves as the objective, is

$$m = \frac{U_1}{V_1} = \frac{-46.69\,\text{D}}{-24.69\,\text{D}} = +1.89$$

The +16.00 D surface serves as the ocular, and from Eq. 17.19, the total magnification relative to the standard reference distance is

$$M = (+1.89)\left(\frac{+16.00\,\text{D}}{4}\right) = +7.56\times$$

The alternative formulation is to calculate the equivalent power of the thick lens and use Eq. 17.20. For the thick lens,

$$\begin{aligned} P_e &= P_1 + P_2 - \bar{d}P_1P_2 \\ &= +22.00\,\text{D} + 16.00\,\text{D} \\ &\quad - (0.022\,\text{m})(+22.00\,\text{D})(+16.00\,\text{D}) \\ &= +30.26\,\text{D} \end{aligned}$$

Then from Eq. 17.20,

$$M = \frac{+30.26\,\text{D}}{4} = +7.56\times$$

The two different methods give the same result.

EXAMPLE 17.22

This example considers a thick meniscus-convex lens ($n = 1.50$) used as a collimating magnifier. The lens has front and back surface powers of +22.00 D and −3.00 D, respectively, and a central thickness of 21 mm. What is the magnification?

Again, we could find the primary focal point by reversing the light and considering plane waves incident on the back of the lens, and then use Eq. 17.19. However here we'll just use Eq. 17.20. For the thick lens,

$$\begin{aligned} P_e &= P_1 + P_2 - \bar{d}P_1P_2 \\ &= +22.00\,\text{D} + (-3.00\,\text{D}) \\ &\quad - (0.014\,\text{m})(+22.00\,\text{D})(-3.00\,\text{D}) \\ &= +19.92\,\text{D} \end{aligned}$$

Then from Eq. 17.20,

$$M = \frac{+19.92\,\text{D}}{4} = +4.98\times$$

17.13 AFOCAL TELESCOPES

A slight modification of the compound microscope yields the telescope. We use a telescope to magnify a distant object, whereas the microscope was used to magnify a near object. *The direct viewing of the distant object without the aid of the telescope constitutes the initial situation.* Then the distant object is viewed through the telescope. The (angular) magnification of the telescope is the ratio of the retinal image size when the telescope is used to the retinal image size in the initial situation. When the telescope is afocal, it gives plane waves out for plane waves in.

Figure 17.9 shows a two-lens Keplerian or astronomical telescope. The Keplerian telescope has a converging objective lens and a converging ocular lens. The two lenses are separated by the reduced distance $\bar{d}$. (Johannes Kepler, 1571–1630, a contemporary of Tycho Brahe and Galileo Galilei, is the famous astronomer responsible for Kepler's Three Laws of Planetary Motion. Kepler also did research on basic optics and published an optics text entitled *Dioptrice*. He is responsible for the first telescopes that used converging ocular lenses.)

In the Keplerian telescope, the converging objective lens forms an inverted, real image inside the telescope. The ocular lens is then used as a simple magnifier to observe the internal image. In Figure 17.9, the incident rays belong to one bundle that originates at a distant off-axis image point. When the telescope is not present, the rays in the bundle subtend an angle w_e at the eye. When the telescope is present, the incident rays subtend the angle w_e at the objective lens of the telescope. The bundle of rays leaving the telescope is a parallel bundle subtending the angle w_m. The incident bundle of rays is traveling at a slight downward slope, indicating that the object point is above the axis. The emergent bundle of rays is traveling with an upward slope, indicating that the conjugate image point is below the axis. In other words, *the image seen through a Keplerian telescope is magnified and inverted.*

Assume that the observer looking directly at the distant object has a retinal image of size I_e, and that when the observer looks at the distant object through the telescope, the retinal image size is I_m. Then the (angular) magnification M is given by

$$M = \frac{I_m}{I_e} = \frac{\tan w_m}{\tan w_e}$$

Figure 17.9 Keplerian telescope.

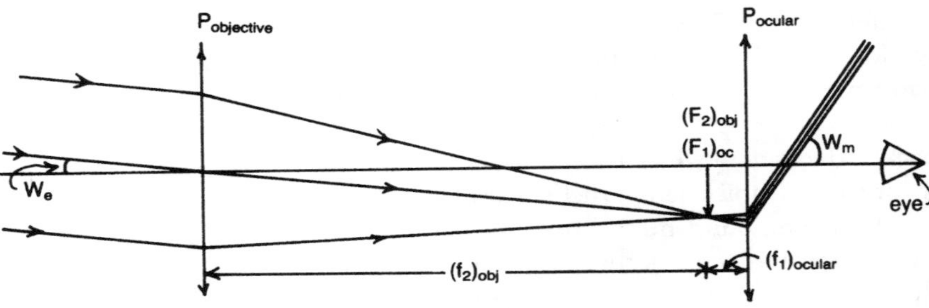

The internal image has a size I_1 (which is negative) and is formed at the secondary focal point of the objective lens. According to the sign convention for ray angles, the angle is positive when the ray slopes upward and negative when the ray slopes downward. The nodal ray for the objective lens shows that

$$\tan w_e = \frac{I_1}{(f_2)_{obj}} = I_1 P_{obj}$$

The nodal ray for the ocular lens shows that

$$\tan w_m = \frac{I_1}{(f_1)_{oc}} = -I_1 P_{oc}$$

The above equations give

$$M = -\frac{P_{oc}}{P_{obj}} \tag{17.21}$$

Also from Figure 17.9, the reduced length of the telescope is equal to the sum of the reduced secondary focal lengths of the ocular and objective lenses. In equation form,

$$\bar{d} = (\bar{f}_2)_{obj} + (\bar{f}_2)_{oc} \tag{17.22}$$

EXAMPLE 17.23

A Keplerian telescope has a +2.00 D objective lens and a +10.00 D ocular lens. What is the magnification and length of the telescope?

From Eq. 17.21,

$$M = -\left(\frac{+10.00\,\text{D}}{+2.00\,\text{D}}\right) = -5\times$$

The minus sign indicates that the image seen through the Keplerian telescope is inverted.

Air is between the two lenses, so the actual length of the telescope equals the reduced length, and Eq. 17.22 gives

$$d = \bar{d} = 50\,\text{cm} + 10\,\text{cm} = 60\,\text{cm}$$

Figure 17.10 shows an afocal Galilean (or Dutch) telescope. The Galilean telescope has a converging objective lens and a diverging ocular lens. It is unclear who first invented the telescope. Hans Lippershey (1587–1619) a Dutch spectacle maker made the first patent application for a telescope, and Lippershey's telescope had a diverging ocular lens. Soon after, word of the telescope's invention reached Galileo Galielei in Italy. Galileo built a number of telescopes and learned how to make higher magnification telescopes, all with diverging oculars. He used his telescopes to examine the moon, planets, and stars, and make his revolutionary astronomy discoveries.

For an afocal telescope, the incident light consists of plane waves. In a galilean telescope, the light leaving the objective lens is still converging when it hits the ocular lens. The virtual object for the ocular lens coincides with its primary focal point, so that the light leaving the ocular lens is again plane waves. In Figure 17.10, the incident ray bundle is sloping downward, indicating that the distant object point is above the axis. The emergent ray bundle again consists of parallel rays, and these rays are sloping downward at a larger angle than the incident rays. *Thus the image seen through the Galilean telescope is magnified and erect*. The equations for the galilean telescope are the same as those for the keplerian telescope.

EXAMPLE 17.24

A Galilean telescope consists of a +2.00 D objective lens and a –10.00 D ocular lens. Find the magnification and length of the telescope.

From Eq. 17.21,

$$M = -\left(\frac{-10.00\,\text{D}}{+2.00\,\text{D}}\right) = +5\times$$

Figure 17.10 Galilean telescope.

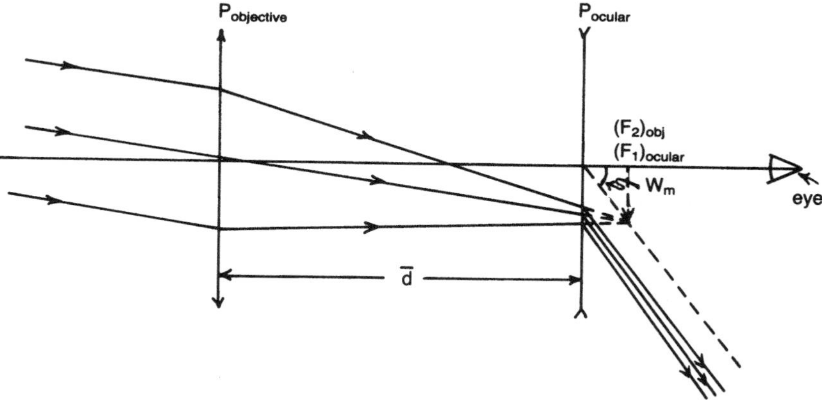

The magnification is positive, which is consistent with the fact that the image seen through the telescope is erect.

Again, air is between the two lenses, so the length is equal to the reduced length. Remember that the secondary focal length of the diverging lens is negative.

$$d = \bar{d} = 50.00\,\text{cm} + (-10.00\,\text{cm}) = 40\,\text{cm}$$

EXAMPLE 17.25

A solid glass ($n = 1.5$) rod 21 cm long is made into an afocal Galilean telescope. If the front surface of the rod has a +5 D surface power, what is the power of the back surface of the rod and what is the magnification of the telescope?

We could find the back-surface power by following incident plane waves through the telescope. The back surface has to have the correct power to give plane waves leaving the back. Alternatively, we can use Eq. 17.22,

$$\bar{d} = (\bar{f}_2)_{\text{obj}} + (\bar{f}_2)_{\text{oc}}$$

$$\frac{21\,\text{cm}}{1.5} = \frac{100}{+5.00\,\text{D}} + (\bar{f}_2)_{\text{oc}}$$

and it follows that

$$(\bar{f}_2)_{\text{oc}} = -6.00\,\text{cm} \quad \text{and} \quad P_{\text{oc}} = -16.67\,\text{D}$$

Then from Eq. 17.21,

$$M = -\left(\frac{-16.67\,\text{D}}{+5.00\,\text{D}}\right) = +3.33\times$$

The afocal telescope takes plane waves in and gives plane waves out. When one turns the telescope around, plane waves still leave when plane waves are incident, but now the telescope minifies instead of magnifies. The same equations (Eq. 17.21 and 17.22) still hold.

EXAMPLE 17.26

Amelia Airheart takes the telescope of Example 17.24 and looks through it backwards at a distant object. What magnification does Amelia achieve?

The telescope in Example 17.24 was a 5 Galilean telescope with a +2.00 D objective lens and a −10.00 D ocular lens. When Amelia looks through it backwards, the +2.00 D lens becomes the ocular and the −10.00 D lens becomes the objective.

Then from Eq. 17.21,

$$M = -\left(\frac{+2.00\,\text{D}}{-10.00\,\text{D}}\right) = \frac{1}{5}\times$$

Note that the 5× telescope minifies by a factor of 5 when used backwards.

Since an afocal telescope gives plane waves out for plane waves incident, the equivalent power P_e of the telescope is zero. Whenever the equivalent power is zero, the back vertex power and the neutralizing power are both zero.

17.14 ALTERNATE AFOCAL TELESCOPE EQUATIONS

The length of an afocal telescope and the dioptric powers of the two lenses are interrelated. In particular, for a two-lens telescope, only two of the three parameters are free parameters. It follows that we can derive alternate expressions for the afocal telescope magnification. One derivation method uses the system matrix for the telescope.

Consider the system matrix for a front vertex to back vertex multi-lens telescope. Let q and h be the incident ray parameters (i.e., q is the angle and h the perpendicular distance from the axis to the ray). For paraxial rays, the system matrix satisfies the equations,

$$\begin{pmatrix} q' \\ h' \end{pmatrix} = \begin{pmatrix} s_{11} & s_{12} \\ s_{21} & s_{22} \end{pmatrix} \begin{pmatrix} q \\ h \end{pmatrix}$$

where the determinant condition is

$$s_{11}s_{22} - s_{12}s_{21} = +1$$

For an afocal telescope,

$$s_{12} = -P_e = 0$$

and the determinant condition simplifies to

$$s_{22} = \frac{1}{s_{11}}$$

The paraxial magnification of the telescope is equal to the ratio of the angles subtended by the rays, or

$$M = \frac{q'}{q}$$

Since the matrix multiplications for q' give

$$q' = s_{11}q$$

it follows that

$$M = s_{11}$$

Then the simplification of the determinant condition gives

$$s_{22} = \frac{1}{M}$$

Therefore, the system matrix for a multi-lens afocal telescope is

$$\mathbf{S} = \begin{pmatrix} M & 0 \\ s_{21} & \frac{1}{M} \end{pmatrix} \tag{17.23}$$

The system matrix is the product of the individual refraction and translation matrices. For a two-lens afocal telescope,

$$\begin{aligned} \mathbf{S} &= \mathbf{R_{oc}TR_{obj}} \\ &= \begin{pmatrix} 1 & -P_{oc} \\ 0 & 1 \end{pmatrix}\begin{pmatrix} 1 & 0 \\ \bar{d} & 1 \end{pmatrix}\begin{pmatrix} 1 & -P_{obj} \\ 0 & 1 \end{pmatrix} \\ &= \begin{pmatrix} 1 & -P_{oc} \\ 0 & 1 \end{pmatrix}\begin{pmatrix} 1 & -P_{obj} \\ \bar{d} & 1-\bar{d}P \end{pmatrix} \end{aligned}$$

or

$$\mathbf{S} = \begin{pmatrix} 1-\bar{d}P_{oc} & 0 \\ \bar{d} & 1-\bar{d}P_{obj} \end{pmatrix} \tag{17.24}$$

Then from Eq. 17.23, it follows that

$$M = 1 - \bar{d}P_{oc} \tag{17.25}$$

or

$$M = \frac{1}{1-\bar{d}P_{obj}} \tag{17.26}$$

Equations 17.25 and 17.26 are alternate magnification equations for an afocal telescope. These two and Eq. 17.21 all give the same magnification values. Each of these equations contains two of the three variables present in a two lens afocal telescope. The spectacle magnification equations of the next chapter have the form of Eq. 17.26.

EXAMPLE 17.27

Use Eq. 17.26 to find the magnification of the telescope in Example 17.25. In Example 17.25, a solid glass ($n = 1.5$) rod 21 cm long was made into a Galilean telescope with a front surface power of +5.00 D. The reduced length of the rod is 14 cm.

From Eq. 17.26,

$$\begin{aligned} M &= \frac{1}{1-(0.14\,\text{m})(+5.00\,\text{D})} \\ &= \frac{1}{1-0.70} = +3.33\times \end{aligned}$$

which agrees with the answer found in Example 17.25.

EXAMPLE 17.28

A 12× Keplerian telescope has a length of 25 cm. What are the dioptric powers of the objective and ocular lenses?

The Keplerian telescope inverts, so

$$M = -12\times$$

From Eq. 17.26,

$$-12\times = \frac{1}{1-(0.25\,\text{m})P_{obj}}$$

Then,

$$\begin{aligned} \frac{1}{-12} &= 1-(0.25\,\text{m})P_{obj} \\ -0.0833 &= 1-(0.25\,\text{m})P_{obj} \\ P_{obj} &= +4.33\,\text{D} \end{aligned}$$

From Eq. 17.21,

$$\begin{aligned} P_{oc} &= -M\,P_{obj} = -(-12\times)(+4.33) \\ &= +52.00\,\text{D} \end{aligned}$$

We can verify the arithmetic by checking whether or not the dioptric powers give the correct length. From Eq. 17.22,

$$\begin{aligned} \bar{d} &= \frac{100}{+4.33\,\text{D}} + \frac{100}{+52.00\,\text{D}} \\ &= +23.08\,\text{cm} + 1.92\,\text{cm} = 25.00\,\text{cm} \end{aligned}$$

which is consistent. Note that it was crucial to use $-12\times$ as the magnification. When $+12\times$ is used, the lenses that make a Galilean telescope are found.

EXAMPLE 17.29

A 12× Galilean telescope has a length of 25 cm. What are the dioptric powers of the objective and ocular lenses?

For the Galilean telescope,

$$M = +12\times$$

From Eq. 17.26,

$$+12\times = \frac{1}{1-(0.25\,\text{m})P_{obj}}$$

Then,

$$\begin{aligned} \frac{1}{+12} &= 1-(0.25\,\text{m})P_{obj} \\ +0.0833 &= 1-(0.25\,\text{m})P_{obj} \\ P_{obj} &= +3.66\,\text{D} \end{aligned}$$

From Eq. 17.21,

$$P_{oc} = -M\,P_{obj} = -(+12\times)(+3.66)$$
$$= -44.00\,\text{D}$$

The Galilean telescope has a minus ocular lens as expected. We can further verify the arithmetic by checking whether or not the dioptric powers found give the correct length. From Eq. 17.22,

$$\bar{d} = \frac{100}{+3.66\,\text{D}} + \frac{100}{-44.00\,\text{D}}$$
$$= +27.27\,\text{cm} + (-2.27\,\text{cm}) = 25.00\,\text{cm}$$

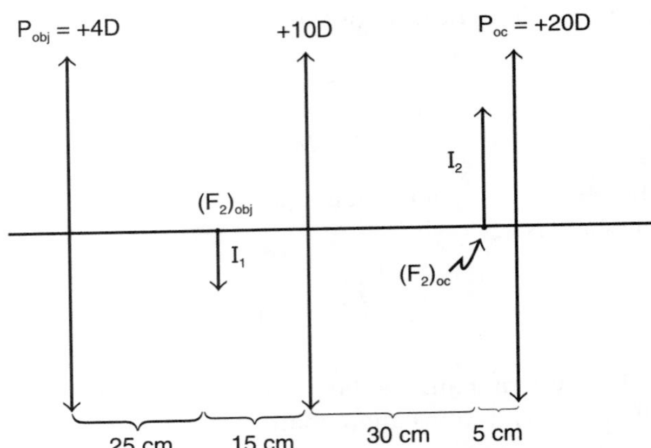

Figure 17.11 Keplerian telescope with a +10.00-D erecting lens that also magnifies. $M = +10\times$.

17.15 ERECTING SYSTEMS IN KEPLERIAN TELESCOPES

The inverted image of a Keplerian telescope is acceptable when looking at the stars. However for terrestrial use, one usually needs an erect image. A Galilean telescope gives an erect image, but a Keplerian telescope has a field of view advantage over a Galilean telescope (discussed in Chapter 19). Therefore, for terrestrial purposes one may want to use a Keplerian telescope with an erecting system, sometimes called a *terrestrial telescope*, rather than a Galilean telescope. The following example explores a thin lens erecting system in a keplerian telescope.

Consider a three lens afocal telescope consisting of a +4.00 D objective lens 40 cm in front of a +10.00 D lens, which in turn is 35 cm in front of a +20.00 D ocular lens. From Chapter 16, the system matrix for the three lens telescope is given by

$$\mathbf{S} = \mathbf{R}_3\mathbf{T}_2\mathbf{R}_2\mathbf{T}_1\mathbf{R}_1$$

Let $\mathbf{B}_i = \mathbf{T}_i\mathbf{R}_i$, where

$$\mathbf{B}_i = \begin{pmatrix} 1 & -P_i \\ \bar{d}_i & 1 - \bar{d}_i P_i \end{pmatrix}$$

Then,

$$\mathbf{S} = \mathbf{R}_3\mathbf{B}_2\mathbf{B}_1$$
$$= \begin{pmatrix} 1 & -20\,\text{D} \\ 0 & 1 \end{pmatrix}\begin{pmatrix} 1 & -10\,\text{D} \\ 0.35\,\text{m} & -2.5 \end{pmatrix}\begin{pmatrix} 1 & -4\,\text{D} \\ 0.40\,\text{m} & -0.60 \end{pmatrix}$$

or

$$\mathbf{S} = \begin{pmatrix} +10.0 & 0 \\ -0.65\,\text{m} & 0.10 \end{pmatrix}$$

The s_{12} element is zero, which confirms that the three-lens system is afocal. From Eq. 17.23, the magnification of this telescope is $+10.0\times$, so the image seen through the telescope is erect and 10 times larger than the object.

The system matrix approach gives the numbers, but does not supply much intuition about the optics. For the intuition, we will compare the three-lens telescope to a two-lens $5\times$ Keplerian telescope (i.e., $M = -5\times$) consisting of the +4.00 D objective lens and the +20.00 D ocular separated by 30.0 cm. Figure 17.11 shows the three-lens telescope. For a distant object, the +4.00 D objective lens forms an inverted real image, I_1, 25 cm to the right. I_1 serves as the object for the +10.00 D lens, so the object distance is −15 cm and the +10.00 D forms its image, I_2, 30 cm to the right. The lateral magnification of the +10.00 D lens is −2. I_2 is erect compared to the original distant object for the telescope and in the primary focal plane for the +20.00 D ocular lens. The ocular lens acts like a collimating magnifier. The total angular magnification M_t of the three-lens telescope is $+10\times$, which is equal to the product of the lateral magnification m_{erect} of the erecting lens times the angular magnification M of the two lens telescope consisting of the objective lens and the ocular lens, or

$$M_t = m_{erect}M \tag{17.27}$$

For this case,

$$M_t = (-2)(-5\times) = +10\times$$

When going from the two-lens $5\times$ telescope to the $10\times$ three-lens telescope, the length of the telescope increased from 30 cm to 75 cm. The increase in length is detrimental to the field of view. An erecting lens that merely flips the image without changing the magnification results in a (little) shorter three-lens telescope. In this case, the lateral magnification m_{erect} of the erecting lens would be −1. The object (I_1) for the erecting lens would be at its primary symmetry point ($u = 2f_1$), and the image for the erecting lens would be at its secondary symmetry point ($v = 2f_2$). Thus, when adding an erecting lens that flips the image without changing the magnification, the increase in telescope length is 4 times the focal length of the erecting lens.

Again let's start with the $M = -5\times$ Keplerian telescope of length 30 cm. When we use a +10.00 D erecting lens (secondary focal length of 10 cm) to flip the image without changing the magnitude of the magnification, the new telescope has a $+5\times$ magnification and a length of 70 cm (i.e., 30 cm + 40 cm). If a +20.00 D erecting lens is used to flip the image without changing the magnification, the length needs to be increased by 4 times 5 cm, or 20 cm.

Prism erecting systems (Section 11.15) have the advantage of being able to flip the image without increasing the length of the two-lens telescopes. Each tube of a common pair of binoculars consists of a Keplerian telescope with a Porro prism erecting system. The Amici roof prism is also sometimes used as an erecting prism in Keplerian telescopes.

17.16 VERGENCE AMPLIFICATION THROUGH AFOCAL TELESCOPES

When a person looks through an afocal telescope at a distant object, plane waves leave the telescope and are incident on the person's eye. When a person looks through an afocal telescope at a near object, the telescope amplifies the vergence of the exiting light. This usually results in a blurred image for the observer.

As an example, consider a $5\times$ Galilean telescope with a +4.00 D objective lens 20.0 cm in front of a −20.00 D ocular lens. When an emmetropic observer looks through this telescope at a distant lion, plane waves enter the telescope and magnified plane waves (traveling at a larger angle) leave the telescope and enter the emmetrope's eye. Now suppose the emmetrope looks through the telescope at a near object 25 cm from the objective lens. Here a vergence of −4.00 D is incident on the +4.00 D objective lens, plane waves travel across the interior of the telescope, and the wavefront emerging from the −20.00 D ocular lens has a vergence of −20.00 D. If the emmetrope's cornea is 1.0 cm behind the ocular lens, the vergence incident on it is −16.67 D which is greater than a typical emmetrope's amplitude of accommodation.

As a second example, consider a $5\times$ afocal Keplerian telescope consisting of a +4.00 D objective lens 30.0 cm in front of a +20.00 D ocular lens. Here for an object that is 25 cm from the +4.00 D objective lens, plane waves travel across the interior of the telescope, and a +20.00 D wavefront emerges from the back surface. In this case, the emmetrope is fogged.

In the general case of a near object in front of a telescope, the light waves crossing the interior of the telescope are not plane waves. Equation 16.35 is a general equation, in terms of the system matrix elements, that gives the vergence V_b of the light leaving the system's back vertex when the light incident on the system's front vertex has a vergence U_1:

$$V_b = \frac{P_e + s_{11}U_1}{s_{22} - s_{21}U_1}$$

When the system matrix elements from Eq. 17.23 for an afocal telescope of magnification M are substituted, the above equation becomes

$$V_b = \frac{M\,U_1}{(1/M) - s_{21}U_1}$$

or

$$V_b = \frac{M^2U_1}{1 - s_{21}MU_1} \tag{17.28}$$

Equation 17.28 is a vergence magnification equation that holds for any multi-lens afocal telescope. For a two-lens afocal telescope, s_{21} equals the reduced length $\bar{d}$ of the telescope.

The observer's accommodative demand equation is

$$A_o = U_{fp} - U_x$$

where U_x is the vergence incident on the cornea. For simplicity, neglect the vertex distance between the cornea and the ocular lens of the telescope. Then the vergence V_b of the light leaving the back of the telescope equals U_x, and

$$A_o = U_{fp} - V_b$$

For an emmetrope, U_{fp} is zero, and for a two-lens afocal telescope, we can combine the above equations to get

$$A_o = \frac{-M^2U_1}{1 - \bar{d}M\,U_1} \tag{17.29}$$

EXAMPLE 17.30

Ms. Computerina Bytes is a low vision patient with an emmetropic eye. As a distance low vision aid, Computerina uses a spectacle mounted afocal 5× Galilean telescope. A two-lens model of this telescope consists of a +32.00 D objective lens located 25.0 mm in front of a −160.00 D ocular lens. When Computerina looks through this telescope at an object 40 cm from the objective lens of the telescope, what is her accommodative demand? For simplicity, neglect the vertex distance between the ocular lens and her cornea.

Here $M = +5\times$ and $\bar{d} = d = 0.025\,\text{m}$, and $U = -2.50\,\text{D}$. Then Eq. 17.28 gives

$$A_o = \frac{-(5^2)(-2.50\,\text{D})}{1-(0.025\,\text{m})(5)(-2.50\,\text{D})} = \frac{62.50\,\text{D}}{1+0.313} = 47.60\,\text{D}$$

which clearly is way over any possible amplitude of accommodation for Computerina.

Hand held or spectacle mounted two-lens afocal telescopes used as low vision aids are fairly short telescopes, so $\bar{d}$, expressed in meters, is small. In this case, the right term in the denominator of Eq. 17.29 is small relative to 1, and the accommodative demand for an emmetrope looking through the afocal telescope is further approximated by

$$A_o \approx -M^2 U_1 \tag{17.30}$$

Equation 17.30 shows that for a short afocal telescope of magnification M, the telescope approximately amplifies the accommodative demand by a factor of M^2.

17.17 TELEMICROSCOPES

The vergence amplification problem discussed in the previous section can be avoided by placing a plus lens, called a reading cap, on the front of the telescope. In thin lens theory, the reading cap serves as a collimating magnifier. Thus, the diverging light from the object is incident on the reading cap, which converts the light into plane waves (Figure 17.12). The plane waves then pass through the telescope and are magnified in the normal manner. The total magnification is the product of the magnification of the reading cap and the magnification of the telescope.

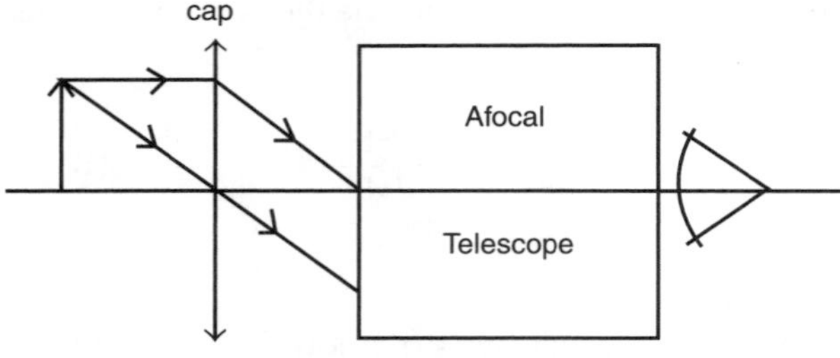

Figure 17.12 Afocal telescope with a reading cap. The cap would actually be against the objective lens.

$$M_{\text{tot}} = M_{\text{cap}} M_{\text{tel}} \tag{17.31}$$

Since we are again dealing with a near object, it is important to specify the initial conditions. Let's assume the conventional 25 cm reference distance. Then the magnification is the ratio of the observer's retinal image size that results from viewing the near object through the telescope with the reading cap to the retinal image size that the observer has when directly viewing the near object at 25 cm. Equation 17.31 then becomes

$$M_{\text{tot}} = \frac{P_{\text{cap}}}{4} M_{\text{tel}} \tag{17.32}$$

A Galilean or terrestrial telescope with the reading cap is actually a microscope that gives an erect image—a so-called *telemicroscope*. The microscope magnification equations in Section 17.12 are general equations that give the same M_{tot} as Eq. 17.32.

EXAMPLE 17.31a

A 3× telescopic low vision aid has a 24 mm length. The objective lens power is +27.78 D and the ocular lens power is −83.33 D. A +3.5 D reading cap is added to the telescope. What is the resulting magnification relative to the standard 25 cm initial viewing distance?

From Eq. 17.32,

$$M = \frac{+3.50\,\text{D}}{4}(3\times) = (0.875)(3\times) = 2.625\times$$

Note that the magnification of the cap is less than 1, or relative to the standard 25 cm reference distance the cap actually minifies.

EXAMPLE 17.31b

Treat the above telescope as a microscope and find the standardized magnification from the microscope equations.

The +3.50 D reading cap is placed against the +27.78 D objective. With the thin lens assumption, these two lenses act like a single new objective lens of power +31.28 D. The total system now looks like a microscope with a +31.28 D objective lens, a −83.33 D ocular lens, and a length of 24 mm. For correct focus, the object is placed at $100/(+3.50\,\text{D}) = 28.57\,\text{cm}$ from the reading cap. We can now use any of the microscope magnification equations to find the magnification relative to the standard near reference distance of 25 cm.

From Eq. 15.40, the equivalent power of a two lens system is

$$P_e = P_1 + P_2 - \bar{d}P_1P_2$$

So,

$$P_e = +31.28\,\text{D} + (-83.33\,\text{D}) - (0.024\,\text{m})(+31.28\,\text{D})(-83.33\,\text{D})$$

and

$$P_e = +10.50\,\text{D}$$

Then from Eq. 17.20,

$$M = \frac{P_e}{4} = \frac{+10.50\,\text{D}}{4} = 2.625\times$$

which is the same result as in part a.

Another way to focus a telescope for near (i.e. create a telemicroscope) is to adjust the length of the original afocal telescope. When a real object is brought in from optical infinity towards a telescope's objective lens, the real image of the objective lens moves back away from the lens. Thus we can increase the length of the telescope to keep this real image at the primary focal point of the objective lens.

Consider a 6× two lens afocal galilean telescope with a 5.0 cm length. The objective lens is +16.67 D and the ocular lens is −100.00 D. We want to adjust the length of the telescope so that an object that is 40 cm from the objective lens will result in plane waves leaving the ocular lens. Here for the objective lens,

$$u_1 = -40\,\text{cm} \quad \text{and} \quad U_1 = -2.50\,\text{D}$$

Then from $V = P + U$,

$$V_1 = +14.17\,\text{D} \quad \text{and} \quad v_1 = +7.06\,\text{cm}$$

To get plane waves leaving, this image must be at the primary focal point of the ocular lens. Since the ocular lens is −100.00 D, its primary focal point is virtual at 1 cm (or $f_1 = +1.0\,\text{cm}$). Thus the adjusted length of the telescope is 7.06 cm − 1.00 cm = 6.06 cm.

Since the telemicroscope is technically a microscope, the magnification can be found from any of the microscope equations. In particular, from Eq. 17.17,

$$M = m_{\text{obj}}\left(\frac{P_{\text{ocu}}}{4}\right) = \left(\frac{-2.50\,\text{D}}{+14.17\,\text{D}}\right)\left(\frac{-100\,\text{D}}{4}\right) = 4.41\times$$

Thus, relative to the 25 cm conventional reference distance, the adjusted telescope gives a 4.41× magnification. Alternatively, we could also find the magnification from the equivalent power of the adjusted telescope.

It is also possible to consider the adjusted telescope as a new afocal telescope with a reading cap. For the above telescope, consider the +16.67 D "old" objective lens as a combination of a +2.50 D reading cap and a +14.17 D "new" objective. The +14.17 D new objective located 6.06 cm in front of the −100 D ocular is an afocal telescope. For the magnification of the telemicroscope, Equation 17.32 gives

$$M = \left(\frac{2.50\,\text{D}}{4}\right)\left(\frac{-100\,\text{D}}{+14.17\,\text{D}}\right)$$

which is just a rearrangement of the numbers used in the previous paragraph, and again gives

$$M = 4.41\times$$

17.18 MAGNIFICATION TERMINOLOGY

Unfortunately, there is no standardized magnification terminology. Many optics authors use the name "apparent angular magnification" and contrast it with the name "actual angular magnification." Most of these authors define apparent angular magnification as the ratio of the magnified retinal image size relative to the unmagnified retinal image size when directly viewing the object at the standard 25 cm reference distance. They further define actual angular magnification as the ratio of the magnified retinal image size to the unmagnified retinal image size that exists when the magnification system is removed without changing the distance between the eye and the object.

A number of other optics authors use the phrase "magnifying power" in place of angular magnification. Most (but not all) of these authors define magnifying power as if it were apparent angular magnification. In some books, magnifying power is defined as actual angular magnification, but the equations used correspond to those for apparent angular magnification. As you might expect, some people get very confused by these terminology differences.

In this chapter, we avoided the use of the adjectives apparent and actual. Instead, we emphasized that angular magnification is a comparison of two different retinal image sizes. In particular, one needs to pay attention to exactly what unmagnified retinal image the magnified image is being compared to. For generality, the distance between the object and the eye is allowed to change when the magnification system is put in place. When the latter distance does remain constant, specialized equations such as Eq. 17.12 can be used. However, Eq. 17.12 cannot be used when the distance changes.

As noted in Section 1.1, models are used for economy and simplicity. In this chapter, a model based on retinal image size is used and the retinal image sizes are related to subtended angles. For simplicity, a thin lens and screen eye model is used. In Chapter 18, a more complicated eye model is used. The observer's eye can also be replaced with a camera, in which case the retina is replaced with a film or an electronic detector.

17.19 EQUATION SUMMARY

The following is a summary of the most important equations in this chapter.

Thin lens as a simple magnifier:

Not collimated $M = m_{\text{lens}} M_{\text{dis}}$ (17.9)

Collimated $M = |u_e| P$ (17.10)

Mythical maximum $M_{\max} = 1 + |u_e| P$ (17.14)

Compound Microscope or a thick lens:

$$M = m_{\text{obj}} \left(\frac{P_{\text{oc}}}{4} \right) \tag{17.17}$$

$$= \frac{-x' P_{\text{obj}} P_{\text{oc}}}{4} \tag{17.18}$$

where the optical tube length x' = actual tube length $- [(f_2)_{\text{obj}} + (f_2)_{\text{oc}}]$

$$M = \frac{P_e}{4} \tag{17.20}$$

Afocal Telescope:

$$M = -\frac{P_{\text{oc}}}{P_{\text{obj}}} \tag{17.21}$$

$$= 1 - \bar{d} P_{\text{oc}} \tag{17.25}$$

$$= \frac{1}{1 - \bar{d} P_{\text{obj}}} \tag{17.26}$$

where

$$\bar{d} = (\bar{f}_2)_{\text{obj}} + (\bar{f}_2)_{\text{oc}} \tag{17.22}$$

Reading Cap (telemicroscope):

$$M_{\text{tot}} = \frac{P_{\text{cap}}}{4} M_{\text{tel}} \tag{17.32}$$

PROBLEMS

1. Randy Vermin holds an object 50 cm from his cornea and then moves the object closer until it is 20 cm from his cornea. What gain in retinal image size does Randy obtain? What is the magnification name for this change?
2. Joe Brown holds a stamp 16 cm from his eye and views the stamp directly. He then picks up his +28.00 D magnifying lens, places the stamp at F_1 of the magnifying lens, and holds the magnifying lens 11 cm from his eye. What is the angular magnification in this situation?
3. What magnification will be marked on a +28.00 D magnifier in your local stamp collector's shop?
4. Suppose Joe Brown uses his left hand to hold a stamp 16 cm from his eye and then without moving either his left hand or his eye inserts his +28.00 D magnifying glass between the stamp and his eye so that the stamp is at the primary focal point of the magnifying glass. What is the magnification in this case?
5. Could Eq. 17.12 be used for problem no. 2? Could Eq. 17.12 be used for problem no. 4?
6. Emmy Trope directly views a stamp held 15 cm in front of her eye. Emmy then holds the stamp 3 cm in front of a +20.00 D lens. Her eye is 10 cm from the lens. How much must Emmy accommodate in order to see the magnified stamp? What is the magnification relative to the original 15 cm distance?
7. Barry Oilwater, an uncorrected 52 year-old emmetrope, uses a 4× magnifier to read the newspaper. What is the angular magnification when Barry first holds the paper at 40 cm and reads directly, and then holds the magnifying glass 20 cm from his eye and views the collimated light coming through the magnifier?
8. A compound microscope has a +50.00 D objective lens and a +40.00 D ocular lens. The microscope is adjusted so that the specimen is placed 2.25 cm from the objective lens of the microscope. What is the distance from the objective lens to the ocular lens? What is the magnification? What is the optical tube length of the microscope?
9. A Keplerian telescope has a +2.00 D objective lens and a +24.00 D ocular lens. What is the magnification and the length of this telescope?
10. What is the length and ocular lens dioptric power of a 10× Galilean telescope with an objective lens of +3.00 D?
11. A +8.00 D thin lens is used as an erecting lens in a 7× Keplerian telescope with an objective lens of +2.00 D. The length of the telescope without the

erecting lens is 57.14 cm. What is the length after the erecting lens is added?

12. A 4 cm thick biconvex glass ($n = 1.50$) lens has a +10.00 D front surface and a +6.00 D back surface. As a collimating magnifier, what is the angular magnification relative to the conventional 25 cm reference distance?

13. A 3× magnifying lens is held 5 cm in front of a 4× magnifying lens. An object is placed so that the light that travels through both lenses emerges collimated. What is the angular magnification for this system relative to the conventional 25 cm reference distance?

14. A 7× Galilean telescope has a +4.00 D objective lens, a −28.00 D ocular lens, and a length of 21.43 cm. The telescope is converted to a near magnification device by placing a 3× simple magnifier (a reading cap) against the front surface. What is the total magnification when plane waves emerge from the ocular lens (relative to the 25 cm conventional reference distance)?

CHAPTER 18

Spectacle Magnification and Relative Spectacle Magnification

18.1 THE APERTURE STOP AND THE ENTRANCE PUPIL

As discussed qualitatively in Chapter 6, an ametrope's retinal image size is dependent on whether the ametrope is corrected by a spectacle lens or a contact lens. This chapter considers these differences quantitatively. Spectacle magnification is the name given to the change that occurs in the retinal image size when a lens is placed in front of the eye. In spectacle magnification, one of the retinal images involved is usually blurred. The properties of a blurred image depend on both the lenses and the apertures in a system.

Apertures are placed in optical systems to control the amount of light passing through the system. The apertures also affect the field of view of the system (Chapter 19). Even when no apertures are present, the lenses or mirrors have finite sizes and act as apertures.

For an axial object point, one aperture or lens rim is most effective at limiting the amount of light that passes through the system. This particular aperture is called the *aperture stop* of the system. Note that a system may have many apertures or stops, but only one is called the aperture stop.

Figure 18.1a shows a two-lens system in which the 7first lens is the aperture stop, while Figure 18.1b shows a two-lens system in which the second lens is the aperture stop. The aperture stop is object distance dependent, and a system's aperture stop may switch when the object is moved. For example, Figures 18.1a and b might be the same system with a different object distance.

When the aperture stop is the first element in a system, then it is easy to specify the angular size ϕ of the bundle of incident rays that will get through the system (Figure 18.1a). When the aperture stop is not the first element in the system, then it is not as straightforward to specify the bundle size of the object space rays that will pass through the system.

For the system shown in Figure 18.1b, one of the easiest ways to find the angular bundle size of object space rays that pass through the system is to consider the second lens C as an object and trace rays from it backwards (left) through the first lens B, as shown in

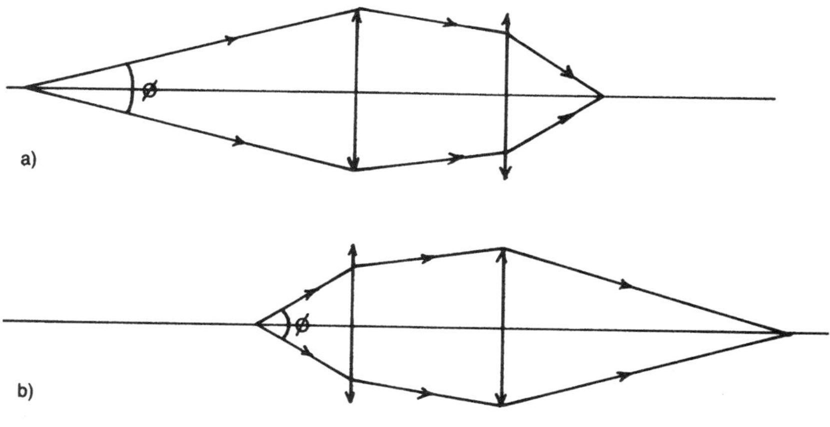

Figure 18.1 a, First lens is the aperture stop; b, second lens is the aperture stop.

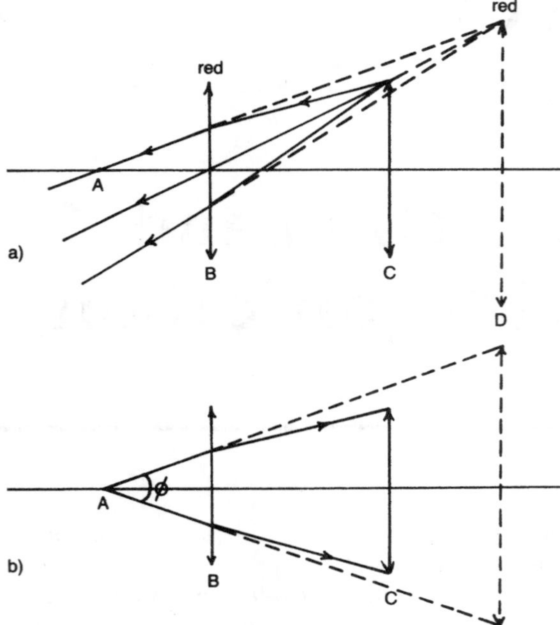

Figure 18.2 a, *D* is the image of *C* formed by lens *B*; b, the image *D* is the entrance pupil and the lens *C* is the aperture stop.

Figure 18.2a. The rays emerging backwards appear to be coming from the top of the virtual image *D* of the second lens formed by the first lens. One of the rays coming from the image point passes through the axial position *A*. Figure 18.2b shows the same system with the rays leaving an object point at the axial position *A* and traveling forward (right) through the first lens. By the principle of reversibility, the ray leaving the object point *A* pointing toward the top of the image *D* is bent by the first lens and passes through the top edge of the lens *C*. This ray is the top boundary ray for the bundle that gets through the system. Any rays aiming higher miss the second lens. A similar boundary ray exists on the bottom. Thus, when the lens *C* is the aperture stop, the bundle size ϕ of the object space rays that pass through the system is determined by the image *D*.

The image of the aperture stop formed by any lenses in front of it is called the entrance pupil. When there are no lenses in front of the aperture stop, the aperture stop itself is called the entrance pupil. Theoretically, when one looks from the axial object point toward the front of a system, all the possibilities for the entrance pupil are visible (either apertures, lens rims, or images of apertures and lens rims formed by the preceding lenses). *The entrance pupil itself is the candidate that subtends the smallest angle at the axial object point.* Because the entrance pupil subtends the smallest angle, it specifies the bundle size ϕ of the object space rays that ultimately pass through the system. Also, because the entrance pupil subtends the smallest angle, it appears smaller than the other candidates when viewed from the axial object point.

In Figure 18.2b, the image *D* is the entrance pupil. The bundle size ϕ of the object space rays that get through the system is specified by *D*. An observer at *A* looking toward the two lenses sees the first lens *B* and the image *D* of the second lens formed by the first lens. (Note that the observer cannot directly see the lens *C*.) The image *D* subtends a smaller angle at *A* than does the first lens *B*, so *D* (the entrance pupil) appears smaller to the observer than *B*.

Figure 18.3a shows a two-lens system with an iris diaphragm in the middle. The iris diaphragm may or may not be the aperture stop of the system. When the system is viewed from the axial object point *A*, the candidates for the entrance pupil are visible. As shown in Figure 18.3b, these candidates are the first lens *B*, the image *E* of the iris diaphragm formed by the first lens, and the image *G* of the second lens formed by the first lens. Of these candidates, the image *E* of the iris diaphragm formed by the first lens subtends the smallest angle and therefore is the entrance pupil (and would visually appear smallest from the position of the axial object point *A*). It follows that the aperture stop must be the iris diaphragm *C*.

In Figure 18.3c, the second lens *D* is smaller than in Figure 18.2c. The entrance pupil candidates are again the first lens *B*, the image *E* of the iris diaphragm formed by the first lens, and the image *G* of the second lens formed by the first lens. Of these candidates, the image *G* of the second lens formed by the first lens subtends the smallest angle, and therefore is the entrance pupil (and would visually appear smallest from the axial object point *A*). In this case, the second lens *D* is the aperture stop.

An equivalent air (reduced) system representation of the human eye is an example of a two-lens system together with an aperture. The cornea serves as the first lens and the crystalline lens serves as the second lens. The iris pupil serves as the aperture. Let us assume that the person is reading a book. If you place your eye at the book's position and look back at the reader's eye (Figure 18.4), you can see the cornea *B* and the image *E* of the iris pupil formed by the cornea. Of these two, the pupil's image *E* appears smaller. The remaining candidate for entrance pupil is the image *G* of the crystalline lens formed by the cornea, but this image subtends a larger angle than the pupil's image. Therefore the pupil's image *E* is the entrance pupil of the eye. You might think about this while closely observing someone else's eyes. Typically, the iris sits about 3.6 mm behind the cornea, and the image of the

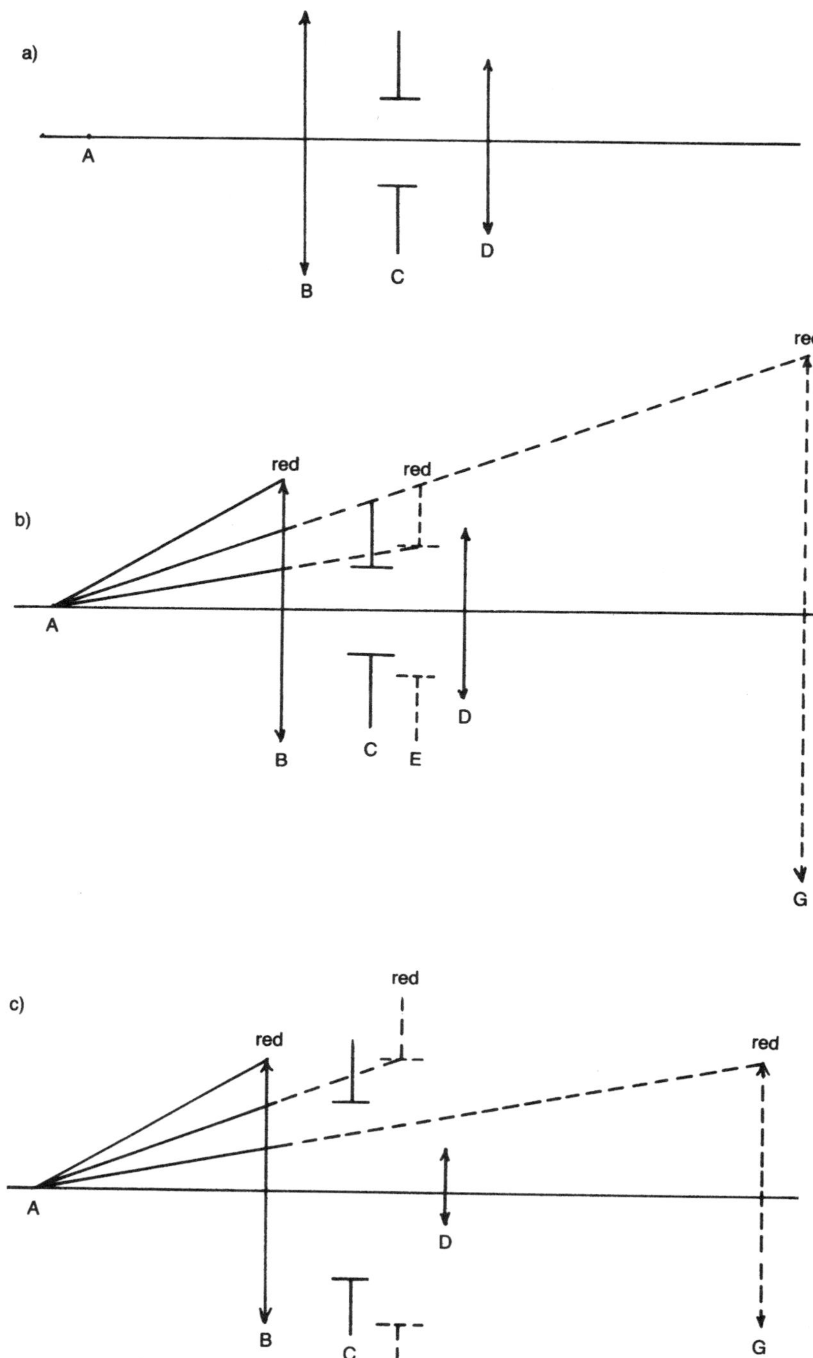

Figure 18.3 a, The system; b, the entrance pupil candidates are the lens *B*, the image *E* of the aperture *C*, and the image *G* of the lens *D*. Here the image *E* is the entrance pupil; c, entrance pupil candidates for changed sizes. Here the image *G* is the entrance pupil.

iris formed by the cornea is virtual and located about 3.0 mm behind the cornea (Example 7.18).

EXAMPLE 18.1

A +12.00 D lens is located 8 cm in front of a circular aperture with a 2 cm diameter. The lens itself has a circular shape and a diameter of 3 cm. An axial object point is 50 cm in front of the lens. Find the aperture stop of the system.

Remember to follow good problem-solving strategy and try to anticipate the answer before working out the solution. The general approach

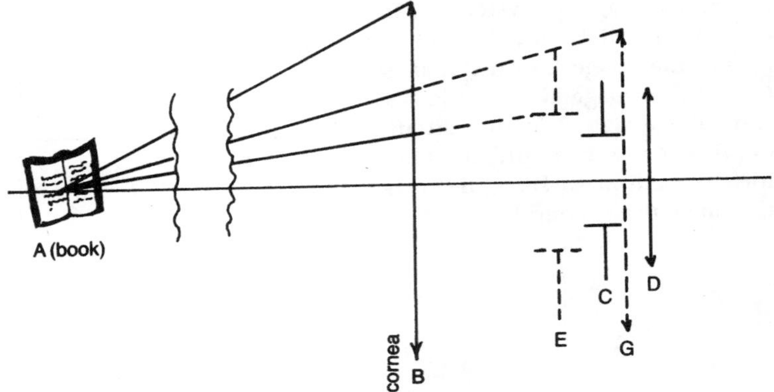

Figure 18.4 Entrance pupil representation for an eye. Lens *B* represents the cornea, aperture *C* represents the iris pupil, and lens *D* represents the crystalline lens. The entrance pupil candidates are the image *E* of the iris pupil (formed by the cornea), and the image *G* of the crystalline lens. *E* is the entrance pupil.

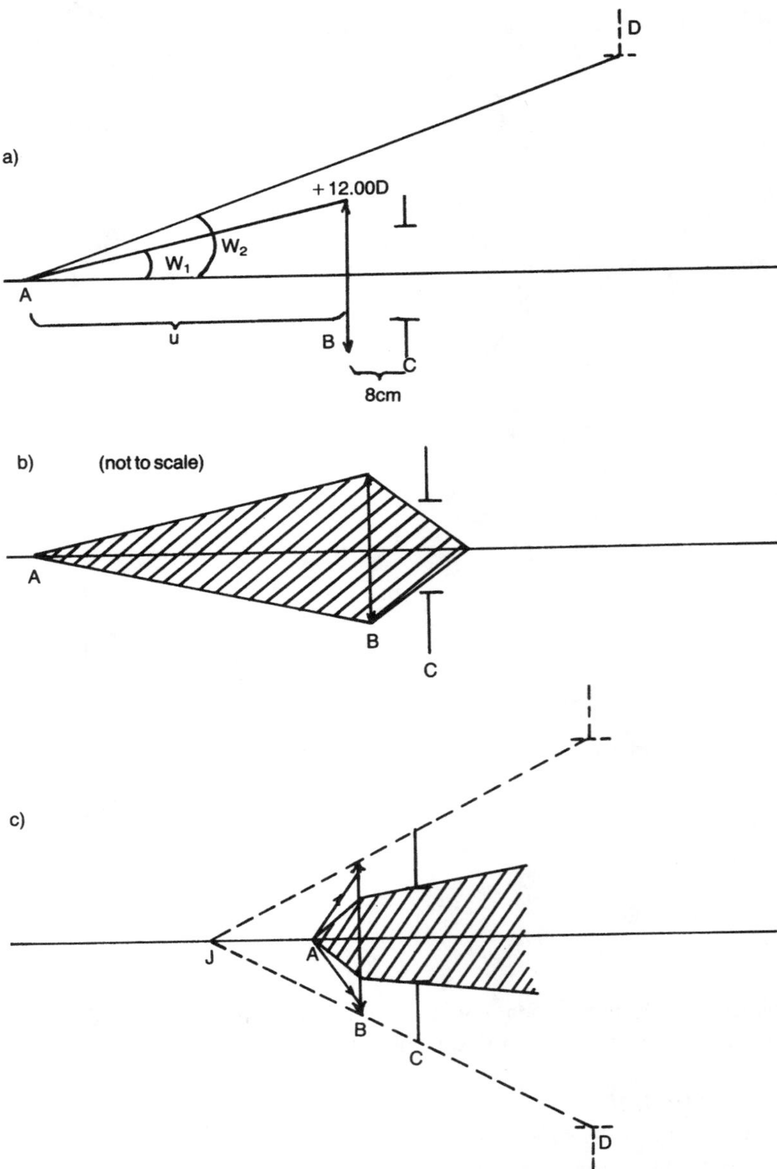

Figure 18.5 a, The entrance pupil candidates are the lens *B* and the image *D*. Here the lens *B* is the entrance pupil (and aperture stop); b, axial bundle size; c, for the closer object point *A*, the image *D* is the entrance pupil and the aperture *C* is the aperture stop. When the object point is at *J*, the lens *B* and the image *D* tie for the system's entrance pupil.

is to first find the entrance pupil. The entrance pupil is the candidate that subtends the smallest angle at the axial object point. The candidates are the +12.00 D lens (since it is directly visible from the axial object point) and the image *D* of the aperture formed by the +12.00 D lens (Figure 18.5a). Note that the aperture *C* is not directly visible from the object plane, but that the aperture's image *D* formed by the +12.00 D lens is directly visible from the object plane.

The top half of the lens subtends the angle w_1 at the axial object point *A* where,

$$\tan w_1 = \frac{1.5\,\text{cm}}{50\,\text{cm}} = 0.03$$

To find the image *D*, we take light coming from the aperture and image it through the +12.00 D lens. This light is traveling in the reversed direction (or left in Figure 18.5a). Thus,

$$u_r = -8\,\text{cm}$$
$$U_r = -12.5\,\text{D}$$
$$V_r = +12.00\,\text{D} + (-12.5\,\text{D}) = -0.5\,\text{D}$$
$$v_r = -200\,\text{cm}$$

The lateral magnification is

$$m = \frac{-12.5\,\text{D}}{-0.5\,\text{D}} = +25.0$$

Then the diameter of the image *D* is

$$(+25.0)(2\,\text{cm}) = 50\,\text{cm}$$

At the object point *A*, the top half of the image *D* subtends the angle w_2 where,

$$\tan w_2 = \frac{25\,\text{cm}}{(200 + 50)\,\text{cm}} = 0.10$$

Since both angles are acute (i.e., less than 90°), the angle with the smaller tangent is the smaller angle. In other words, since

$$\tan w_1 < \tan w_2$$

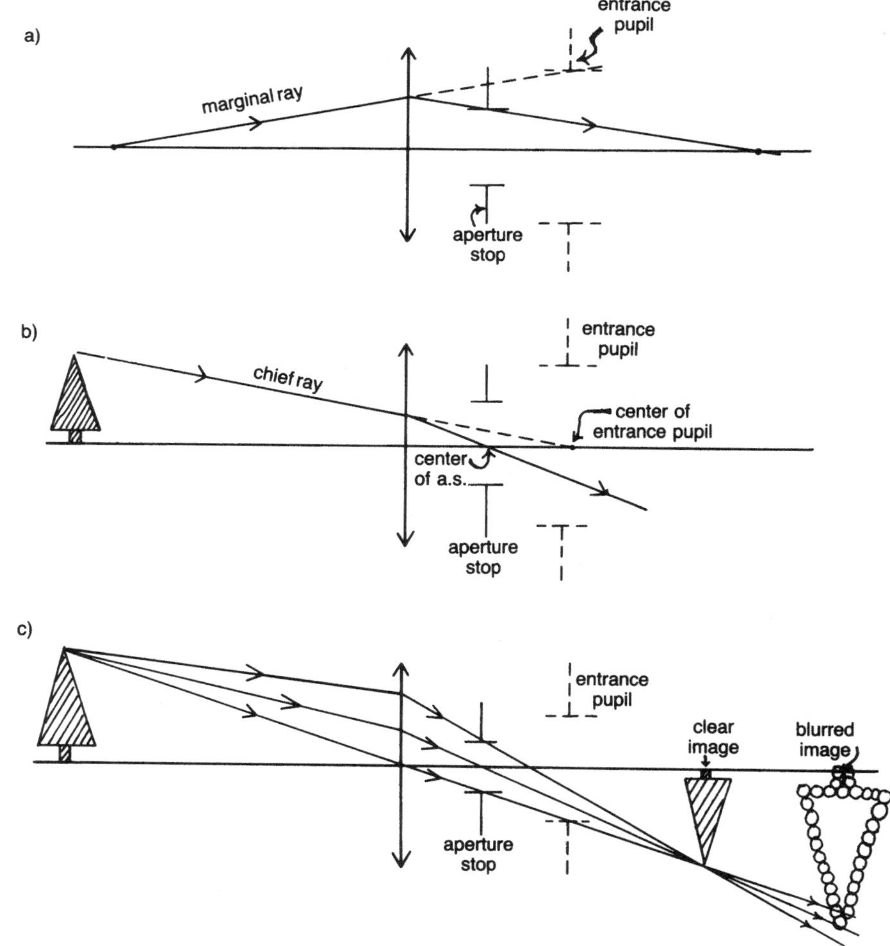

Figure 18.6 a, Marginal ray; b, chief ray; c, the chief ray determines a blurred image size.

it follows that

$$w_1 < w_2$$

and so the +12.00 D lens subtends the smaller angle at the object point A. Thus, the +12.00 D lens is the entrance pupil of the system. Since the +12.00 D lens is not an image, it is also the aperture stop of the system.

You may have initially expected that the circular aperture would be the aperture stop. However, the image conjugate to the axial object point A is only 10 cm behind the lens, and the entire converging axial bundle of image space rays gets through the aperture (Figure 18.5b). So the lens is the element that limits the amount of light from the axial object point.

EXAMPLE 18.2

For the same lens and aperture used in the preceding example, how close must the axial object point A be to the +12.00 D lens for the aperture to be the aperture stop?

Assume that the axial object point A is a distance u from the +12.00 D lens (Figure 18.5a). The top half of the lens then subtends the angle w_1 at A where,

$$\tan w_1 = \frac{1.5\,\text{cm}}{-u}$$

Note that u is negative, so minus u is positive. The image D of the aperture then subtends the angle w_2 at A where,

$$\tan w_2 = \frac{25\,\text{cm}}{200\,\text{cm} - u}$$

To find the turning point set,

$$\tan w_1 = \tan w_2$$

or

$$\frac{1.5}{u} = \frac{25}{200 - u}$$

Then,

$$300 - 1.5u = -25u$$

and

$$u = -12.77\,\text{cm}$$

The axial object point A would have to be closer than 12.77 cm to the lens for the aperture to be the aperture stop (Figure 18.5c). At 12.77 cm, the +12.00 D lens and the aperture tie for the aperture stop (the dashed line from J to D in Figure 18.5c). When the axial object point A is farther than 12.77 cm from the lens, the lens is the aperture stop.

The entrance pupil is conjugate to the aperture stop. Therefore, to get a ray to just pass through the edge of the aperture stop, one would aim the ray toward the edge of the entrance pupil as shown in Figure 18.6a. After refraction by any lenses in front of the aperture stop, the ray just passes the edge of the aperture stop. Such a ray is called a *marginal ray*.

Similarly, to get a ray to pass through the center of the aperture stop, one would aim the ray toward the center of the entrance pupil. After the refractions, this ray passes through the center of the aperture stop (Figure 18.6b). The ray from an object point that is incident on the system pointing toward the center of the entrance pupil is called the *chief ray*. After the appropriate refractions, the chief ray passes through the center of the aperture stop. For a paraxial bundle, the chief ray is the central ray of the bundle (Figure 18.6c) and takes on special significance when dealing with blurred image sizes.

18.2 THE EXIT PUPIL AND BLURRED IMAGE SIZES

The exit pupil is the image of the aperture stop formed by any lenses behind it. When there are no lenses behind the aperture stop, the aperture stop itself serves as the exit pupil (e.g., Figure 18.6c). Just as the entrance pupil specifies the bundle size of the object space rays, the exit pupil specifies the angular bundle size ϕ' of the image space rays.

In Figure 18.7a, the virtual image D is the image of the first lens B formed by the second lens C. The first lens B is the aperture stop, so the virtual image D is the exit pupil. The angular bundle size ϕ' of the image space rays is determined by the virtual image D. In Figure 18.7b, the first lens B is again the aperture stop. The real image D is the image of B formed by the second lens C. So the real image D is the exit pupil, and it determines the angular bundle size ϕ' of the image space rays.

In general, the candidates for exit pupil are the last lens, any aperture after the last lens, and the image of each lens and aperture formed by the lenses behind it. *At the axial image point, the exit pupil subtends the smallest angle of these candidates*. Theoretically, when viewed from the axial image position, the exit pupil appears to be the smallest of the candidates. (Note the analogous relations of image space properties and the

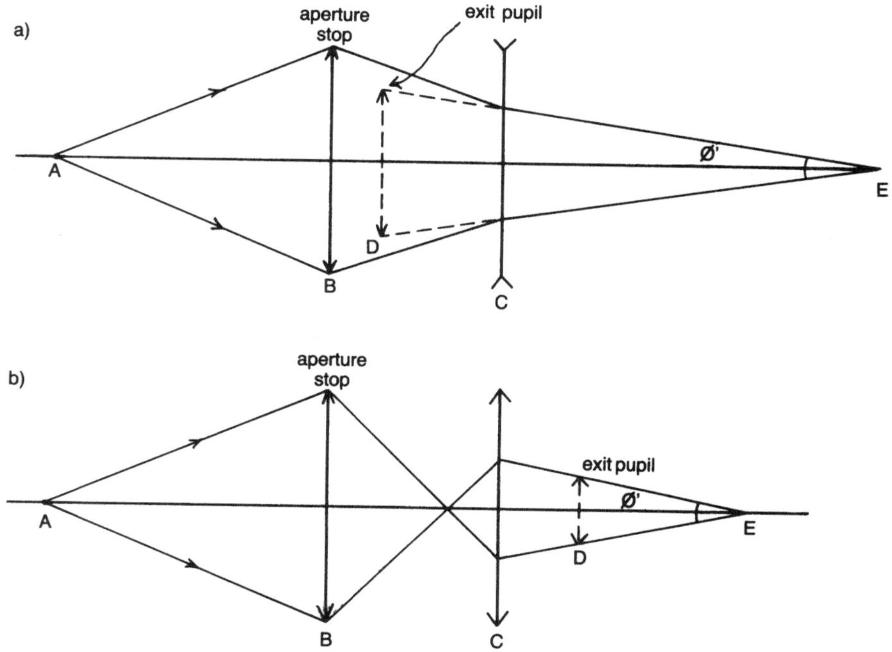

Figure 18.7 a, System with a virtual image as the exit pupil; b, system with a real image as the exit pupil.

exit pupil to the object space properties and the entrance pupil.)

The chief ray enters a system pointing toward the center of the entrance pupil, and after the appropriate refractions actually passes through the center of the aperture stop. The exit pupil is conjugate to the aperture stop, and so when the chief ray leaves the system, it appears to be coming from the center of the exit pupil. The chief ray is the center of any bundle of paraxial rays coming from an off-axis object point and in image space specifies the center of a blur circle formed by the bundle.

The system's entrance pupil is in object space, and the system's exit pupil is in image space. *For the entire system, the exit pupil is conjugate to the entrance pupil.* For example, if the entrance pupil happens to coincide with the primary principal plane H_1, the exit pupil is the same size as the entrance pupil ($m_t = +1$) and coincides with the secondary principal plane H_2.

Consider the human eye again (Figure 18.8). A tiny organism sitting on the retina and looking back toward the cornea would theoretically see the crystalline lens L, the image X of the iris pupil I formed by the crystalline lens, and the image of the cornea formed by the crystalline lens. Of these, the pupil's image X would appear smallest, so it is the exit pupil of the eye. When you hold a penlight at the primary focal point of your eye (about 1.67 cm in front of your

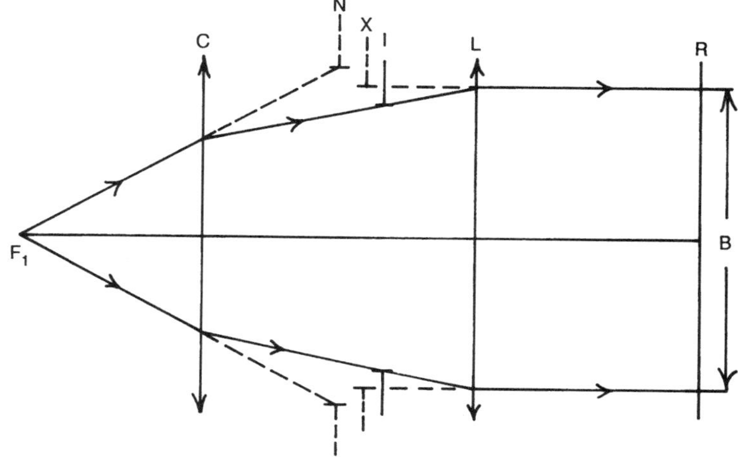

Figure 18.8 Schematic (not to scale) representation of the eye's cornea (*C*), crystalline lens (*L*), retina (*R*), primary focal point (*F*,), iris (*I*), entrance pupil (*N*), and exit pupil (*X*). The blur circle size (*B*) equals the exit pupil size.

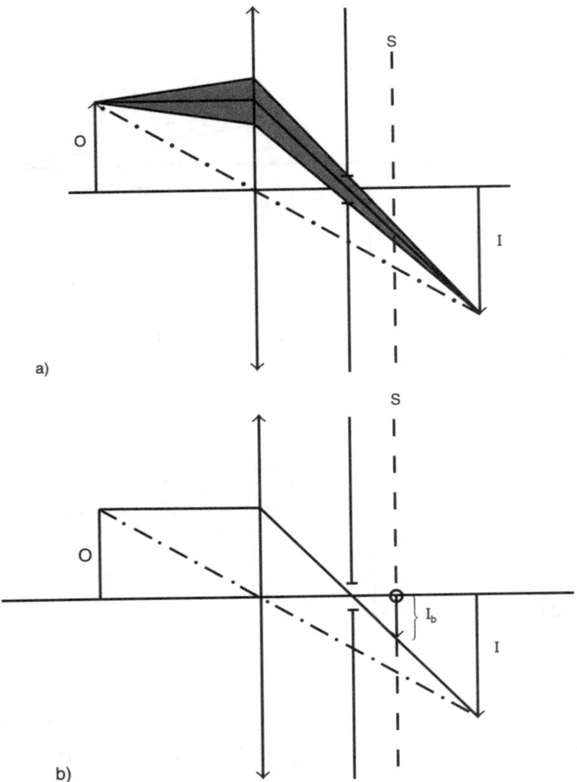

Figure 18.9 **A lens followed by an iris diaphragm, which is the aperture stop. *I* is the clear image conjugate to the object *O*: a, the bundle of rays that pass through the iris diaphragm. For a screen at *S*, this bundle forms a blur circle on the screen. The nodal ray (dot-dashed line) is blocked by the iris diaphragm; b, the chief ray, which passes through center of the aperture stop (the iris diaphragm), defines the blurred image size I_b on the screen *S*.**

cornea), the rays leaving the crystalline lens are parallel to the axis, and the resulting blur circle size *B* on the retina is equal to the size of the exit pupil *X*. Note that *X* is not equal to the actual size of the iris pupil *I*.

The system in Figure 18.9 consists of a lens followed by an iris diaphragm, which is the aperture stop. In this case, the iris diaphragm also serves as the system's exit pupil. The system has a real object *O* and a conjugate real image *I*. A blurred image is on the screen *S* that is in front of the clear image position. Figure 18.9a shows the bundle of rays from the top off-axis object point that passes through the system. This bundle forms a blur circle on the screen *S* and no light from the object point lies below this blur circle on the screen. In particular, the nodal ray (dot-dashed line) is blocked by the iris diaphragm and does not reach *S*. When we increase the diameter of the iris diaphragm, the blur circle size on screen *S* increases. When we decrease the diameter of the iris diaphragm, the blur circle size on the screen decreases.

The size of each individual blur circle is a measure of the amount of blur, but what is the measure of the size of the blurred image? It certainly is not the lens's nodal ray, which is blocked by the iris diaphragm and does not reach *S*. Neglecting diffraction, only the chief rays pass through a very small diaphragm (i.e., a pinhole). In this case, the pinhole effect gives a relatively clear image on screen *S*, and the top and bottom chief rays specify the size of the image (I_b in Figure 18.9b). Thus, *the paraxial convention is that blurred image sizes are specified by the chief rays.* These rays go to the center of the respective blur circles. So the blurred image size is taken to be from the center of the bounding blur circle on one side to the center of the bounding blur circle on the opposite side.

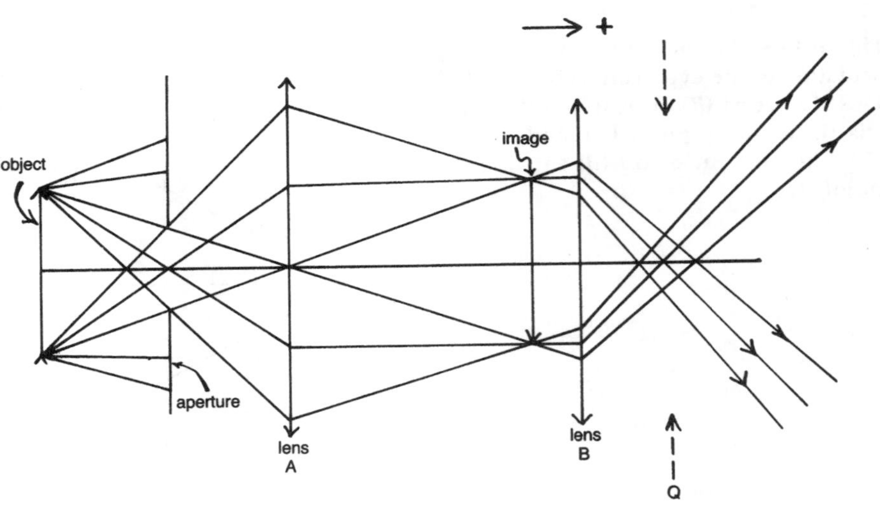

Figure 18.10 **The light from lens *B* to *Q* consists of a converging beam made up of diverging bundles. *Q* is the exit pupil.**

Figure 18.10 shows a two-lens system with an aperture in front of the lenses. The aperture is the aperture stop of the system. Two different pencils of rays are shown, from the top and bottom object points, respectively. Lens *A* forms a real image of the object. The real image serves as the object for lens *B*. The pencils leaving lens *B* are diverging, so lens *B* would have a virtual image (which is not shown, but which you can locate by tracing the exiting rays in each pencil backwards until they intersect). By following rays from the aperture to position *Q*, we see that the aperture is imaged by lenses *A* and *B* at *Q*. Since in this case, the aperture is the system's aperture stop, the aperture's image at *Q* is the system's exit pupil. (Note that the aperture's image is not conjugate to the arrow object.) When a screen is placed behind lens *B* and then moved back, the illumination on the screen appears to converge until position *Q* is reached and then diverges once *Q* is passed. Despite this convergence, no image of the system's object (the arrow) appears on the screen. The light between lens *B* and *Q* is an example of a converging beam made up of diverging bundles, the fourth logical possibility mentioned in Section 2.8.

18.3 THIN LENS SPECTACLE MAGNIFICATION

Figure 18.11a shows a reduced Gauss system representation of a possibly ametropic human eye viewing a distant object. The chief ray determines the size I_e of

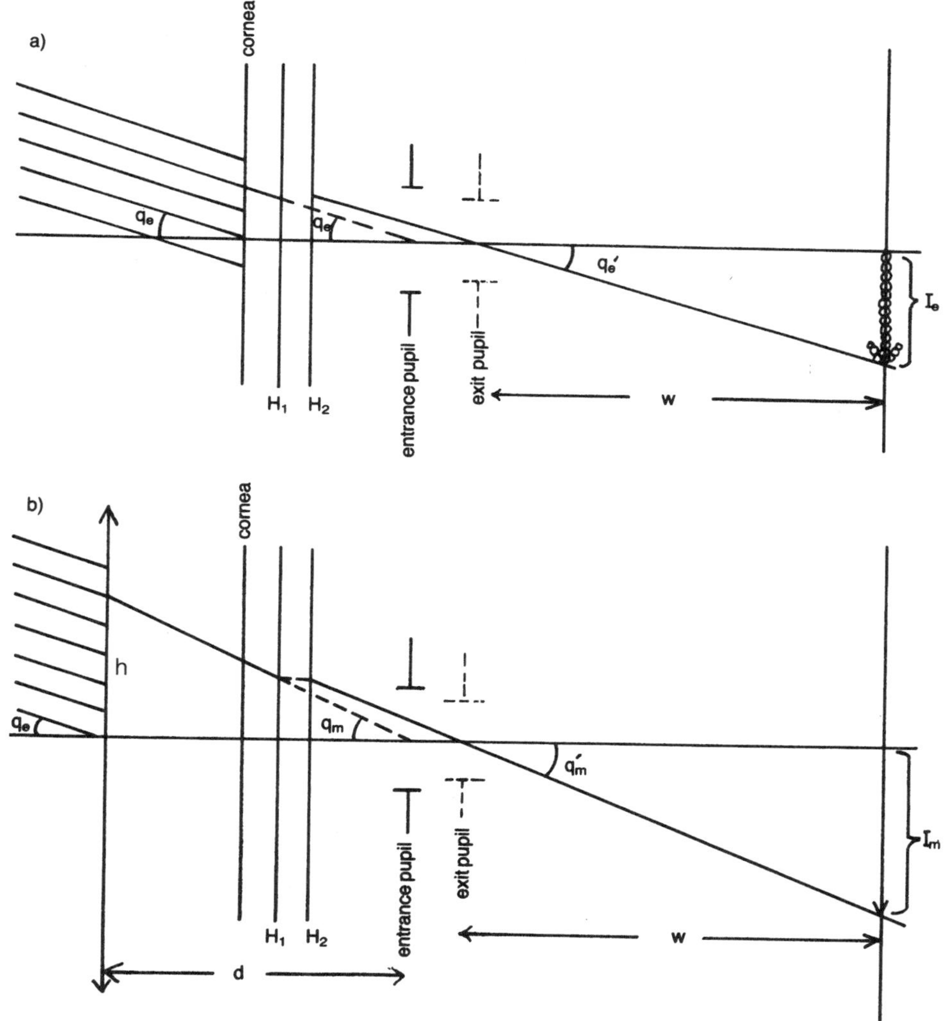

Figure 18.11 Spectacle magnification: a, blurred image size; b, spectacle corrected retinal image size.

the blurred image. *For a distant object, the spectacle magnification, M_{spec}, is defined as the ratio of the retinal image size when the person is wearing a spectacle lens to the retinal image size of the same eye when the person is not wearing a lens.*

Figure 18.11b shows the eye with a thin spectacle lens of power P located a distance d in front of the eye's entrance pupil. The resulting retinal image size is I_{m}. So

$$M_{\text{spec}} \equiv \frac{I_{\text{m}}}{I_{\text{e}}} \tag{18.1}$$

When the lens P is not the correction for the eye, then I_{m} is a blurred image. When the lens P is the correction for the eye, then I_{m} is a clear retinal image. In Figures 18.11a and b, the chief rays subtend respective angles q'_{e} and q'_{m} at the center of the exit pupils. The distance between the exit pupil and the retina is w. Thus, w times the tangent of the subtended angle equals to the image size. From Eq. 18.1, it follows that

$$M_{\text{spec}} = \frac{w \tan q'_{\text{m}}}{w \tan q'_{\text{e}}}$$

For paraxial rays, we can replace the tangent by the angle, and then

$$M_{\text{spec}} = \frac{q'_{\text{m}}}{q'_{\text{e}}}$$

The next paragraphs give a derivation of Eq. 14.3 for the spectacle magnification M_{spec}. In the derivation, we want to relate the above ratio of image space angles at the exit pupil to a ratio of object space angles at the entrance pupil. In Section 16.7, we saw that a front to back vertex system matrix could be expanded into an object–image matrix, or into any other convenient system matrix. Here it is convenient to use a system matrix that goes from the entrance pupil (in object space) to the exit pupil (in image space). Since for the whole system, the entrance pupil and exit pupil are conjugate to each other, the entrance to exit pupil system matrix has the general form of an object–image matrix, or

$$\mathbf{S}_{\text{en-ex}} = \begin{pmatrix} s_{11} & -P_{\text{e}} \\ 0 & s_{22} \end{pmatrix}$$

where P_{e} is the equivalent power of the system. The chief ray is defined in terms of the centers of the entrance and exit pupils. So in terms of the entrance pupil–exit pupil system matrix, the chief ray object space angles q_{m} and q_{e} are related to the respective image space angles by

$$\begin{pmatrix} q'_{\text{m}} \\ 0 \end{pmatrix} = \begin{pmatrix} s_{11} & -P_{\text{e}} \\ 0 & s_{22} \end{pmatrix} \begin{pmatrix} q_{\text{m}} \\ 0 \end{pmatrix}$$

and

$$\begin{pmatrix} q'_{\text{e}} \\ 0 \end{pmatrix} = \begin{pmatrix} s_{11} & -P_{\text{e}} \\ 0 & s_{22} \end{pmatrix} \begin{pmatrix} q_{\text{e}} \\ 0 \end{pmatrix}$$

From the matrix multiplications,

$$q'_{\text{m}} = s_{11} q_{\text{m}}$$

and

$$q'_{\text{e}} = s_{11} q_{\text{e}}$$

It follows that

$$M_{\text{spec}} = \frac{q'_{\text{m}}}{q'_{\text{e}}} = \frac{q_{\text{m}}}{q_{\text{e}}} \tag{18.2}$$

Equation 18.2 shows that in the reduced system the spectacle magnification is equal to the ratio of the object space angles subtended by the chief rays at the center of the eye's entrance pupil.

In Figure 18.11b, the ray angle at the center of the eye's entrance pupil is q_{m}. This particular ray was incident on the spectacle lens with an angle of q_{e} at a distance of h above the axis. From the refraction and translation matrices, the ray parameters of the ray incident on the lens are related to those at the entrance pupil plane by

$$\begin{aligned} \begin{pmatrix} q_{\text{m}} \\ 0 \end{pmatrix} &= \mathbf{TR} \begin{pmatrix} q_{\text{e}} \\ h \end{pmatrix} \\ &= \begin{pmatrix} 1 & 0 \\ d & 1 \end{pmatrix} \begin{pmatrix} 1 & -P \\ 0 & 1 \end{pmatrix} \begin{pmatrix} q_{\text{e}} \\ h \end{pmatrix} \\ &= \begin{pmatrix} 1 & -P \\ d & 1 - dP \end{pmatrix} \begin{pmatrix} q_{\text{e}} \\ h \end{pmatrix} \end{aligned}$$

The matrix multiplications give

$$\begin{pmatrix} q_{\text{m}} \\ 0 \end{pmatrix} = \begin{pmatrix} q_{\text{e}} - hP \\ dq_{\text{e}} + (1 - dP)h \end{pmatrix}$$

From the bottom equality,

$$h = \frac{-dq_{\text{e}}}{1 - dP}$$

Now substitute the above expression into the top matrix equality to find

$$\begin{aligned} q_{\text{m}} &= q_{\text{e}} + \frac{dPq_{\text{e}}}{1 - dP} \\ &= \frac{q_{\text{e}} - dPq_{\text{e}} + dPq_{\text{e}}}{1 - dP} \end{aligned}$$

or

$$q_{\text{m}} = \frac{q_{\text{e}}}{1 - dP}$$

Then from Eq. 18.2,

$$M_{spec} = \frac{1}{1 - dP} \quad (18.3)$$

Equation 18.3 is the spectacle magnification equation for a distant object and a thin spectacle lens of power P. The distance d is the distance from the spectacle lens to the entrance pupil of the eye.

For an emmetrope wearing a thin zero power (i.e., plano) spectacle lens (e.g., sunglasses) M_{spec} is equal to one. This means that the emmetrope's retinal image size is the same with or without the thin plano lenses.

Frequently, we talk about the percent gain G_{spec} when putting the spectacle lens on. Since for no change, M_{spec} is equal to one, the percent gain is defined as

$$G_{spec} = (M_{spec} - 1)100\% \quad (18.4)$$

EXAMPLE 18.3a

Veronica Vein's distance Rx is a +6.00 D (thin) spectacle lens at a 13 mm vertex distance. What is the difference between Veronica's uncorrected retinal image size and her retinal image when wearing the spectacle lens?

By definition, the difference is the spectacle magnification. The eye's entrance pupil is typically 3 mm behind the cornea (the default assumption), and then

$$d = 13\,\text{mm} + 3\,\text{mm} = 16\,\text{mm}$$

From Eq. 18.3,

$$M_{spec} = \frac{1}{1 - (0.016\,\text{m})(+6.00\,\text{D})} = \frac{1}{0.904} = 1.106$$

Veronica's retinal image size increases by a factor of 1.106 when she puts her spectacle lenses on. The percent gain is

$$G_{spec} = (1.106 - 1)100\% = +10.6\%$$

EXAMPLE 18.3b

What is Veronica's spectacle magnification when she switches to a thin contact correction?

Veronica's distance contact correction is +6.51 D. The contact sits on the cornea, so d is the 3 mm distance between the cornea and the entrance pupil. Here,

$$M_{spec} = \frac{1}{1 - (0.003)(+6.51\,\text{D})} = 1.020$$

and

$$G_{spec} = (1.020 - 1)100\% = 2.0\%$$

Veronica has almost an 11% gain in retinal image size with the spectacles versus a 2% gain with the contacts. In others words, Veronica's retinal image size with the spectacles is about 9% larger than with the contacts.

EXAMPLE 18.4a

Herman Turnip's distance Rx is a −4.00 D (thin) spectacle lens at a 12 mm vertex distance. What is the difference between Herman's uncorrected retinal image size and his retinal image when wearing the spectacle lens?

Again, the difference is the spectacle magnification. The eye's entrance pupil is typically 3 mm behind the cornea, and

$$d = 12\,\text{mm} + 3\,\text{mm} = 15\,\text{mm}$$

From Eq. 18.3,

$$M_{spec} = \frac{1}{1 - (0.015\,\text{m})(-4.00\,\text{D})} = \frac{1}{1.060} = 0.943$$

Herman's retinal image size decreases by a factor of 0.943 when he puts his spectacle lenses on. The percent gain is

$$G_{spec} = (0.943 - 1)100\% = -5.7\%\ \text{gain}$$

or

$$G_{spec} = +5.7\%\ \text{loss}$$

Note that a negative gain is equal to a positive loss.

EXAMPLE 18.4b

What is Herman's spectacle magnification when he switches to a thin contact correction?

Herman's distance contact correction is −3.82 D. The contact sits on the cornea, so d is the 3 mm distance between the cornea and the entrance pupil. Here,

$$M_{spec} = \frac{1}{1 - (0.003)(-3.81\,\text{D})} = 0.989$$

$$G_{spec} = (0.989 - 1)100\% = -1.13\%\ \text{gain}$$

or

$$G_{spec} = +1.13\%\ \text{loss}$$

Herman has about a 1% loss in retinal image size with the contacts versus about a 6% loss with the spectacles. In others words, Herman's retinal image size with the contacts is about 5% larger than with the spectacles. This is a noticeable difference, and is one of the advantages of a contact lens correction for a myope.

18.4 SPECTACLE MAGNIFICATION APPROXIMATION

For small x, an equation of the form

$$y = \frac{1}{1-x}$$

is approximated by the Taylor series expansion:

$$y \approx 1 + x + x^2 + x^3 + \ldots$$

The smaller x is, the less important are the higher order terms (e.g., when x is 0.1, x^2 is 0.01; and when x is 0.01, x^2 is 0.0001). Frequently, we can neglect the higher order terms, in which case

$$y \approx 1 + x$$

In the spectacle magnification equation (Eq. 18.3), d is in meters and dP is frequently much smaller than one. The approximation then yields

$$M_{spec} \approx 1 + dP \quad (18.5)$$

and from Eqs. 18.4 and 18.5,

$$G_{spec} \approx (dP)100\% \quad (18.6)$$

The approximation (Eq. 18.6) is most accurate for small values of G_{spec} and gets worse as G_{spec} increases.

The approximate equations clearly show the direct dependence of spectacle magnification on the power P of the lens and the distance d between the lens and the entrance pupil. For a plus lens, the percent gain increases with increasing power P of the lens (vertex distance fixed) or with increasing vertex distance (P fixed). Of course, for a clear retinal image the image of the lens must be at the far point of the eye. For a minus lens, the percent loss gets larger with a larger minus power (same vertex distance) or with increasing vertex distance (P fixed).

The (paraxially) exact spectacle magnification (Eq. 18.3) is not very different from 1, and sometimes people round it off to 1, in which case they have discarded all the percent gain information. When the approximation (Eq. 18.6) is used, the important information (the percent difference from 1) is directly available. In that sense, the use of the approximation (Eq. 18.6) sometimes actually improves the accuracy.

EXAMPLE 18.5

Rework Examples 18.4a and b using the approximate equation (Eq. 18.6).

In Example 18.4a, Herman wore a thin -4.00 D spectacle lens at a distance of 15 mm from the entrance pupil of the eye. From Eq. 18.6,

$$G_{spec} \approx (0.15)(-4.00\text{ D})100\% = -6.0\%$$

as opposed to the -5.7% exact answer.

In Example 18.4b, Herman wore a thin -3.82 D contact lens correction. The distance d is the 3 mm distance from the contact lens to the entrance pupil of the eye. From Eq. 18.6,

$$G_{spec} \approx (0.003\text{ m})(-3.82\text{ D})100\% = -1.15\%$$

as opposed to the -1.13% exact answer.

EXAMPLE 18.6

Rework Examples 18.3a and b using the approximate equation (Eq. 18.6).

In Example 18.3a, Veronica wore a thin $+6.00$ D spectacle lens at a distance of 16 mm from the entrance pupil of the eye. From Eq. 18.6,

$$G_{spec} \approx (0.016\text{ m})(+6.00\text{ D})100\% = +9.6\%$$

as opposed to the $+10.6\%$ exact answer.

In Example 18.3b, Veronica wore a thin $+6.51$ D contact lens correction. The distance d is the 3 mm distance from the contact lens to the entrance pupil of the eye. From Eq. 18.6,

$$G_{spec} \approx (0.003\text{ m})(+6.51\text{ D})100\% = +1.95\%$$

as opposed to the $+1.99\%$ exact answer.

Examples 18.3 through 18.6 illustrate a general principle already touched on in Chapter 6. For thin lens corrections, a hyperope has a larger retinal image size when corrected by spectacles (as opposed to a contact lens correction), while a myope has a larger retinal image when corrected by contacts as opposed to spectacles.

18.5 TELESCOPE CONCEPTS AND SPECTACLE MAGNIFICATION

The spectacle magnification equation (Eq. 18.3),

$$M_{spec} = \frac{1}{1-dP}$$

has the same form as the telescope magnification equation (Eq. 17.26). In the telescope magnification equation, P is the objective lens power and d is the length of the telescope.

For spectacle magnification of a corrective lens, we can think of the correcting lens as the objective lens of an afocal telescope. The spectacle or contact lens is neutralizing the refractive error as measured at the entrance pupil of the eye. So we can think of the ocular lens of the afocal telescope as the refractive error. The distance between the correcting lens and the entrance pupil is the length of the telescope.

A hyperope has a minus refractive error that is corrected by a plus lens. The correcting lens and the refractive error act like a Galilean telescope. The higher the refractive error (the ocular lens), the higher the correcting lens power (the objective lens), and the higher the magnification. For a fixed refractive error, the larger the vertex distance, the longer the length d of the telescope, and the higher the magnification.

A myope has a plus refractive error that is corrected by a minus lens. The correcting lens and the refractive error act like a reverse Galilean telescope (i.e., the person is looking backwards through the telescope). Therefore, the retinal image is minified. The higher the refractive error, the higher the correcting lens power, and the greater the minification. The larger the length d, the more the minification. The smaller the length d, the less the minification.

18.6 MAGNIFICATION PROPERTIES OF A THICK PLANO LENS

An ophthalmic lens typically has a converging front surface and a diverging back surface. An ophthalmic lens with an equivalent power of zero always has front vertex and back vertex powers of zero. In other words, the back surface just neutralizes the front surface, and the lens is an afocal system. Figure 18.12 shows several thick plano lenses, and the corresponding reduced systems. The reduced systems exactly match those of an afocal Galilean telescope.

For the thick plano lens, the spectacle magnification M is the ratio of the observer's retinal image size when viewing a distant object through the lens to the retinal image size of the person viewing the distant object directly. Since the thick plano lens acts like an afocal telescope, the spectacle magnification is just equal to the afocal telescope magnification given by Eq. 17.26;

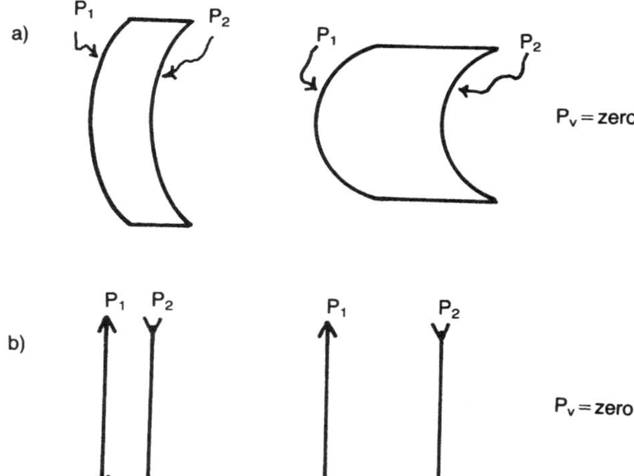

Figure 18.12 a, Afocal lenses; b, reduced systems.

$$M = \frac{1}{1 - \bar{d}P_{obj}}$$

where $\bar{d}$ is equal to the reduced center thickness c of the lens, and P_{obj} is the front surface power P_1. Since the plano lens has zero power, we say that the spectacle magnification is due to the shape of the lens. We can relabel the above equation as

$$M_{shape} = \frac{1}{1 - \bar{c}P_1} \tag{18.7}$$

The corresponding percent gain is

$$G_{shape} = (M_{shape} - 1)100\% \tag{18.8}$$

EXAMPLE 18.7a

Consider a thick CR-39 plastic ($n = 1.5$) lens with a zero equivalent power (i.e., a thick plano lens). The lens has a 9 mm central thickness and a front surface power of +10.00 D. What is the magnification of the lens?

The reduced central thickness is

$$\bar{c} = \frac{9\,\text{mm}}{1.5} = 6\,\text{mm}$$

From Eq. 18.7,

$$M_{shape} = \frac{1}{1 - (0.006\,\text{m})(+10.00\,\text{D})} = \frac{1}{1 - 0.060} = 1.064$$

From Eq. 18.8, the percent gain is

$$G_{shape} = (1.064 - 1)100\% = +6.4\%\text{ gain}$$

EXAMPLE 18.7b

Find the back surface power of the afocal lens and use it to verify the above magnification.

For plane waves incident on the front, $U_1 = 0$ and then $V_1 = +10.00\,\text{D}$. The reduced central thickness is 6 mm. From the downstream vergence equations, the vergence arriving at the back surface is $U_2 = +10.64\,\text{D}$. Since the lens is afocal, plane waves must leave the back surface, or $V_2 = 0$. Then the back surface power of the afocal lens is given by

$$P_2 = V_2 - U_2 = -10.64\,\text{D}$$

The front surface of the afocal lens serves as the objective lens of the telescope, and the back surface serves as the ocular lens. From Eq. 17.21, the magnification is

$$M = -\frac{P_{oc}}{P_{obj}}$$

$$= -\frac{-10.64\,\text{D}}{+10.00\,\text{D}} = 1.064$$

which agrees with the magnification found in Example 18.7a.

The small magnification approximations to Eqs. 18.7 and 18.9 are

$$M_{shape} \approx 1 + \bar{c}P_1 \tag{18.9}$$

and

$$G_{shape} \approx (\bar{c}P_1)100\% \tag{18.10}$$

where c is the actual central thickness and n is the index of refraction. For ophthalmic lenses, the central thickness c expressed in meters is small, and the shape factor approximations are frequently accurate.

Ophthalmic lenses typically have a converging front surface. For a converging front surface, Eq. 18.10 explicitly shows that the shape magnification increases with increasing front surface power. Ophthalmic lenses with a steeper front surface curvature (higher power) are said to be "bent" more. The higher the bend of the lens, the greater the shape magnification. The plano lens on the right in Figure 18.12a has a higher magnification than the plano lens on the left. For the same index, we can also increase the shape factor by increasing the center thickness c (since $\bar{c} = c/n$).

Both $\bar{c}$ and P_1 depend on the refractive index n. Therefore the effect of varying the refractive index without changing anything else is not necessarily obvious from Eq. 18.10. Lens clocks are calibrated for a 1.53 refractive index. Equation 7.35 related the true power of a spherical surface to the lens clock reading and for a front lens surface in air gives

$$P_1 = \frac{(n-1)}{0.53}P_{clock}$$

where n is refractive index of the lens. Then Eq. 18.10 can be written as

$$G_{shape} \approx \left(\frac{c}{n}\right)\frac{(n-1)}{0.53}P_{clock}100\%$$

or

$$G_{shape} \approx \left(1 - \frac{1}{n}\right)\frac{cP_{clock}}{0.53}100\% \tag{18.11}$$

Equation 18.11 shows that if the center thickness c is unchanged, and the front surface curvature, as measured by the lens clock is unchanged, then the shape factor increases with increasing refractive index.

EXAMPLE 18.8

A lens clock reads +6.00 D on the front surface of an afocal CR-39 hard resin ($n = 1.495$) with a 6.7 mm center thickness. This lens has a 2.5% gain shape factor. What is the percent gain shape factor for a $n = 1.71$ plastic lens with the same center thickness and the same front surface curvature (+6.00 D) as measured by a lens clock?

Here, only the index changes, so we expect a larger percent gain. From Eq. 18.11,

$$G_{shape} \approx \left(1 - \frac{1}{1.71}\right)\frac{(6.7 \times 10^{-3}\,\text{m})(+6.00\,\text{D})}{0.53}100\%$$

$$\approx (0.42)(7.55\%) = 3.1\%\ \text{gain}$$

Since G_{shape} is small, the above answer should be very accurate. You may use the exact equations (Eqs. 18.7 and 18.8) to check the results.

18.7 SHAPE AND POWER FACTORS

In the real world, all correcting lenses have thickness and shape. Ametropic correcting lenses also have a non-zero back vertex power P_v. Figure 18.13a shows a spectacle correction in front of an ametropic eye, while Figure 18.13b shows the reduced representation of the spectacle lens. P_1 and P_2 are the spectacle's respective front and back surface powers.

When plane waves are incident on the spectacle lens, the light is refracted by the front surface P_1, travels across the lens, is refracted by the back surface P_2, and exits the back surface with a vergence equal to the back vertex power P_v. The vergence U_2 incident on

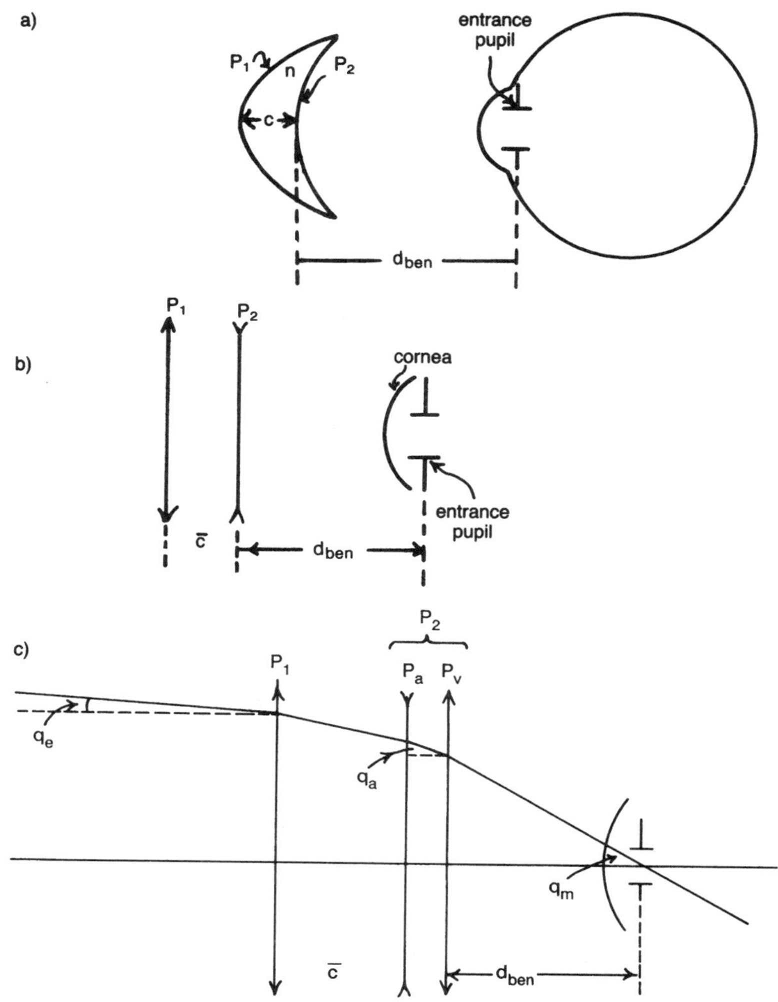

Figure 18.13 Spectacle magnification shape and power factors: a, actual parameters; b, reduced representation; c, P_2 represented as the sum of P_a and P_v, where P_a neutralizes P_1 and P_v is the back vertex power.

the back of the lens is given by the vergence effectivity relation:

$$U_2 = \frac{P_1}{1 - \bar{c}P_1}$$

From the standard $V = P + U$ equation.

$$P_v = P_2 + U_2$$

Then,

$$P_2 = P_v - U_2$$

or

$$P_2 = P_v + P_a \tag{18.12}$$

where,

$$P_a = -U_2 \tag{18.13}$$

It is easier to think in terms of the reduced system, in which the back surface is represented by a thin lens of power P_2. Equation 18.12 shows that we can consider the thin lens P_2 as the sum of thin lenses of respective powers, P_a and P_v (Figure 18.13c). As shown by Eq. 18.13, the lens P_a just neutralizes the vergence coming from the front surface power P_1. Therefore, P_1 and P_a are an afocal or telescopic system that has a magnification given by the shape factor, Eq. 18.7.

The remaining thin lens of power P_v acts like a thin lens correction, for which the spectacle magnification is given by Eq. 18.3. Since the latter contribution depends on the back vertex power, it is called the power factor. We can then relabel Eq. 18.3:

$$M_{power} = \frac{1}{1 - d_{ben}P_v} \tag{18.14}$$

where d_{ben} is the distance from the back vertex of the spectacle lens to the entrance pupil of the eye.

Figure 18.13c shows the ray angles for the reduced system. The incident rays subtend an angle q_e. The shape factor Galilean telescope then magnifies the ray angles, and the rays leaving P_a make an angle q_a where,

$$q_a = M_{shape} q_e$$

The lens P_v magnifies the ray angles so that at the entrance pupil the chief ray subtends an angle q_m, and

$$q_m = M_{power} q_a$$

The above two equations give

$$q_m = M_{power} M_{shape} q_e$$

Then from Eq. 18.2, the total spectacle magnification is the product of the power and shape factors, or

$$M_{tot} = M_{power} M_{shape} \tag{18.15}$$

The total percent gain is

$$G_{tot} = (M_{tot} - 1)100\% \tag{18.16}$$

EXAMPLE 18.9

George Wholecomb, an aphake, wears a +14.00 D CR-39 lens ($n = 1.495$) at a 10 mm vertex distance. The lens has a +17.00 D front surface and an 11 mm central thickness. What is George's total spectacle magnification?

The default assumption is that the eye's entrance pupil is 3 mm behind the cornea. Then,

$$d_{ben} = 10\,\text{mm} + 3\,\text{mm} = 13\,\text{mm}$$

The +14.00 D specified in the Rx is the back vertex power, so

$$M_{power} = \frac{1}{1 - (0.013\,\text{m})(+14.00\,\text{D})} = 1.222$$

The reduced central thickness is

$$\bar{c} = \frac{11\,\text{mm}}{1.495} = 7.36\,\text{mm}$$

and the shape factor is

$$M_{shape} = \frac{1}{1 - (0.00736\,\text{m})(+17.00\,\text{D})} = 1.143$$

From Eq. 18.15,

$$M_{tot} = (1.143)(1.222) = 1.397$$

or

$$G_{tot} = (1.397 - 1)100\% = +39.7\%\ \text{gain}$$

EXAMPLE 18.10

Victor Vegetable wears a −0.50 D ophthalmic crown ($n = 1.523$) lens at an 11 mm vertex distance. The front surface power of the lens is +7.00 D and the central thickness is 3 mm. What is the total spectacle magnification?

The default assumption gives

$$d_{ben} = 11\,\text{mm} + 3\,\text{mm} = 14\,\text{mm}$$

The −0.50 D specified in the Rx is the back vertex power, so

$$M_{power} = \frac{1}{1 - (0.014\,\text{m})(-0.50\,\text{D})} = 0.993$$

The reduced central thickness is

$$\bar{c} = \frac{3.3\,\text{mm}}{1.523} = 2.17\,\text{mm}$$

and the shape factor is

$$M_{shape} = \frac{1}{1 - (0.00217\,\text{m})(+7.00\,\text{D})} = 1.015$$

From Eq. 18.15,

$$M_{tot} = (1.015)(0.993) = 1.008$$

or

$$G_{tot} = (1.008 - 1)100\% = +0.8\%\ \text{gain}$$

We expect a myope to have a percent loss from the power factor, while the shape factor supplies a percent gain. Since Victor is such a low myope, the power factor was overidden by the shape factor.

18.8 SHAPE AND POWER FACTOR APPROXIMATIONS

When M_{shape} and M_{power} are each close to 1, we can make the small magnification approximations:

$$M_{shape} \approx 1 + \bar{c}P_1$$

and

$$M_{power} \approx 1 + d_{ben}P_v$$

The individual percent gain equations become

$$G_{shape} \approx \bar{c}P_1 100\%$$
$$G_{power} \approx d_{ben}P_v 100\%$$

From Eq. 18.15, the total spectacle magnification becomes

$$M_{tot} \approx (1 + d_{ben}P_v)(1 + \bar{c}P_1)$$

or

$$M_{tot} \approx 1 + d_{ben}P_v + \bar{c}P_1 + d_{ben}\bar{c}P_1P_v$$

The approximations depended on both $d_{ben}P_v$ and cP_1 being small. Therefore, the last term, which is the product of the two small terms, is negligible, and we can write the above equation as

$$M_{tot} \approx 1 + d_{ben}P_v + \bar{c}P_1$$

Then,

$$G_{tot} \approx (d_{ben}P_v + \bar{c}P_1)100\%$$

or

$$G_{tot} \approx G_{power} + G_{shape} \qquad (18.17)$$

Equation 18.17 shows that in the small magnification approximation the individual percent gains are additive. However, when the small magnification approximation is not applicable, the individual percent gains are not additive.

EXAMPLE 18.11

Dr. Michael Leaking wears a −3.00 D spectralite (plastic, $n = 1.54$) spectacle lens at a 12 mm vertex distance. The central thickness is 2.3 mm, and the front surface power is +4.00 D. What is the total spectacle magnification percent gain (loss)?

The shape factor should be small, and the approximation (Eq. 18.11) gives

$$G_{shape} \approx \frac{2.3 \times 10^{-3}}{1.54}(+4.00\,\text{D})100\%$$

$$\approx +0.60\%\ \text{gain}$$

The back vertex of the lens is a distance of 15 mm from the entrance pupil (i.e., 3 + 12). The power factor approximation gives

$$G_{power} \approx (15 \times 10^{-3})(-3.00\,\text{D})(100\%)$$

$$\approx -4.5\%\ \text{gain}$$

From Eq. 18.17,

$$G_{tot} \approx +0.60\% + (-4.5\%) \approx -3.9\%\ \text{gain}$$

or

$$G_{tot} \approx 3.9\%\ \text{loss}$$

18.9 COMPARISON OF DIFFERENT LENSES FOR THE SAME EYE

If the right retinal image differs in size from the left retinal image by a few percent (especially 5% or more), the human visual system has trouble fusing the two images. The problem of unequal retinal images is referred to as *aniseikonia* (*an* = not; *isos* = equal; *eikon* = image [Greek]). (The neural part of the human visual system can also be a source of *aniseikonia*.) The spectacle magnification shape and power factors are the tools for solving aniseikonic problems. The resulting lens is called an *iseikonic lens*.

Consider an eye with an uncorrected retinal image size I_e. Assume that one correcting lens results in a clear retinal image of size I_1 and that a second correcting lens results in a clear retinal image of size I_2. The comparison between the retinal image sizes of the same eye provided by the two lenses is quantified as the ratio I_2 to I_1:

$$M_{comp} = \frac{I_2}{I_1}$$

Then,

$$M_{comp} = \frac{I_2/I_e}{I_1/I_e} = \frac{M_2}{M_1}$$

or

$$M_{comp} = \frac{M_2}{M_1} \qquad (18.18)$$

where M_2 and M_1 are the respective total spectacle magifications for the two correcting lenses. The percent comparison between the spectacle magnifications for the two lenses is

$$G_{comp} = (M_{comp} - 1)100\% \qquad (18.19)$$

Equations 18.18 and 18.19 are the exact equations for the comparison. When the small magnification approximations are accurate, we can make a derivation similar to that of Eq. 18.17 to obtain

$$G_{comp} \approx G_2 - G_1 \qquad (18.20)$$

Within the accuracy of the small magnification approximation, the percent comparison between the two lenses is just the difference between the two individual percent gains.

EXAMPLE 18.12

Linda Swift-Spider wears a left −6.00 D CR-39 ($n = 1.498$) spectacle lens at a vertex distance of 11 mm. The lens has a 2.3 mm central thickness and a +2.00 D front surface. Linda has an aniseikonic problem. With her spectacle lens on, she still needs a 3% increase in her left retinal image. What spectacle lens at the same vertex distance will supply the extra 3% magnification?

Since the vertex distance is to remain fixed, the back vertex power must remain fixed. Therefore, the spectacle magnification power factor is fixed, and we have only the shape factor to work with. Since the shape factors are small, let us use the approximation (Eq. 18.17).

Linda's current lens has a percent gain given by

$$G_{\text{shape}} \approx \frac{2.3 \times 10^{-3}\,\text{m}}{1.498}(+2.00\,\text{D})(100\%)$$
$$\approx +0.31\%$$

From Eq. 18.20, Linda's new lens must then have a shape factor of 3.31%. Many lenses will work. Let us select a 1.60 index plastic lens ($n = 1.60$) with a +8.00 D front surface power. Then,

$$G_{\text{shape}} \approx 3.31\% \approx \frac{c}{1.60}(+8.00\,\text{D})100\%$$

and the solution for the center thickness c gives

$$c = 6.6 \times 10^{-3}\,\text{m} = 6.6\,\text{mm}$$

Note the iseikonic lens is thicker and bent more than the initial lens.

18.10 GAUSS FORMULATION FOR SPECTACLE MAGNIFICATION

As opposed to using the shape and power factors, we can make an alternate formulation of spectacle magnification in terms of the equivalent power and the principal planes. We can then treat the thick lens exactly like the thin lens.

Just as in Section 18.3, the spectacle magnification is defined as the ratio of the retinal image size with a lens in front of the eye to the retinal image size without the lens. Figure 18.14 shows the principal planes for a meniscus-convex correcting lens. The distant object subtends an angle q_e. The chief ray subtends an angle q_m at the eye's entrance pupil.

The derivation exactly parallels the derivation of the spectacle magnification equation for a thin lens (Eq. 18.3). The secondary principal plane H_2 is considered to be the image space surface of the equivalent lens of power P_e. This distance d_{Hen} is the distance from H_2 to the eye's entrance pupil. Then the total spectacle magnification for the thick lens is

$$M_{\text{tot}} = \frac{1}{1 - d_{\text{Hen}}P_e} \tag{18.21}$$

Equation 18.21 gives the same numerical results as the shape and power factor equations (Eqs. 18.7, 18.14, and 18.15). In fact, they can be directly derived from each other.

EXAMPLE 18.13

In Example 18.9, George Wholecomb wore a +14.00 D CR-39 ($n = 1.495$) lens at a 10 mm vertex distance. The lens had a +17.00 D front surface and an 11 mm central thickness. Use Eq. 18.21 to find the total spectacle magnification of the thick lens.

First, we need to find the equivalent power and the location of the secondary principal plane. The reduced center thickness $\bar{c}$ is 7.36 mm. To find the equivalent power we need to find the back surface power. The back vertex power of the lens is +14.00 D. So for plane waves incident on the front, the vergence V_2 leaving the back surface is +14.00 D. Then $U_1 = 0$, $V_1 = +17.00$ D, and the downstream vergence equations give $U_2 = +19.43$ D. Since V_2 must equal +14.00 D,

$$P_2 = V_2 - U_2 = +14.00\,\text{D} - 19.43\,\text{D} = -5.43\,\text{D}$$

From Eq. 15.40, the equivalent power is then given by

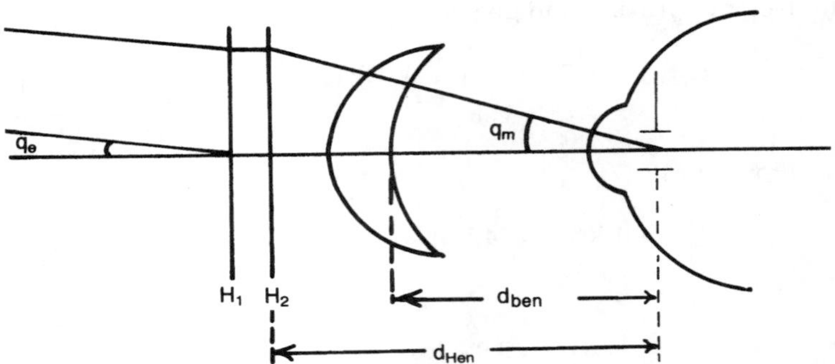

Figure 18.14 Spectacle magnification in terms of principal planes.

$$P_e = P_1 + P_2 - \bar{c}P_1P_2 = +12.25\,\text{D}$$

Equation 15.10 gives the secondary principal plane location from the back surface as

$$L_2H_2 = f_b - f_2 = \frac{1}{P_v} - \frac{1}{P_e}$$
$$= +71.42\,\text{mm} - 81.63\,\text{mm} = -10.21\,\text{mm}$$

Then,

$$d_{\text{Hen}} = 10.21\,\text{mm} + 10\,\text{mm} + 3\,\text{mm} = 23.21\,\text{mm}$$

From Eq. 18.21,

$$M_{\text{tot}} = \frac{1}{1 - (0.02321\,\text{m})(+12.25\,\text{D})} = 1.397$$

which agrees with the shape and power factor answer obtained in Example 18.9.

When a plus spectacle lens is bent more, the spectacle magnification increases. We explained this previously by noting that the shape factor increases as the lens is bent. How can the increase be explained in the Gaussian formulation?

Figure 18.15 shows a series of plus lenses with the same back vertex power. The principal planes are symmetrically located inside the equiconvex lens. For the convex-plano lens, the primary principal plane has moved forward to the front surface (which is the only surface with a non-zero dioptric power), and the secondary principal plane has also moved forward toward the front surface. For the meniscus-convex lens, the principal planes continue to move forward, and when the lens is bent enough, both of the principal planes are in front of the lens. The fact that H_2 is moving forward away from the spectacle's secondary focal point (and away from the entrance pupil of the eye) explains the increase in magnification. (This same general principle applies to a telephoto lens.)

Figure 18.16 shows a series of minus lenses with the same back vertex power. The principal planes are symmetrically located inside the equiconcave lens. For the planoconcave lens, the secondary principal plane has moved to the back surface and the primary principal plane has also moved backwards. For the meniscus-concave lens, the principal planes continue to move backwards; and when the lens is bent enough, both of the principal planes are in back of the lens. The fact that H_2 is again moving away from the minus spectacle's (virtual) secondary focal point explains the increase in magnification.

It is important to note that the power factor equation (Eq. 18.14) contains the back vertex power P_v and the distance d_{ben} from the back vertex of the lens to the entrance pupil. As indicated in Eq. 18.15, the power factor must be multiplied by the shape factor to obtain the total spectacle magnification. On the other hand, the Gauss equation (Eq. 18.21) contains the equivalent power and the distance d_{Hen} from the secondary principal plane to the entrance pupil. The shape and power information is encoded in the equivalent power and in the principal plane location.

In a clinical situation, the spectacle lens's equivalent power and the location of the secondary principal plane are not routinely known, although they can be calculated. For a spectacle lens of a given material, we know the refractive index. The back vertex power, front surface power (or lens clock reading), and central thickness are all routinely known in a clinical

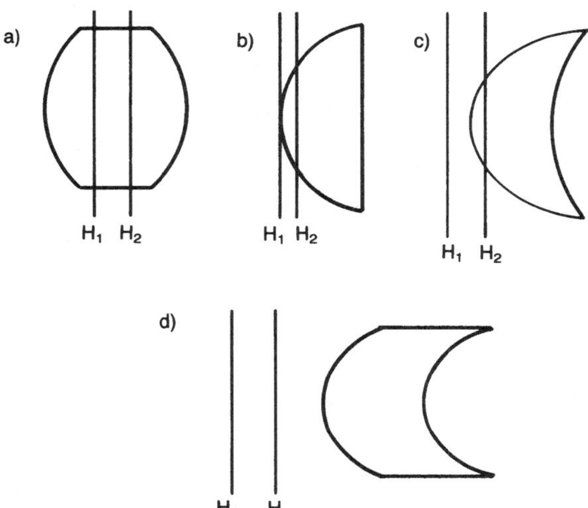

Figure 18.15 Principal planes as plus lens is bent.

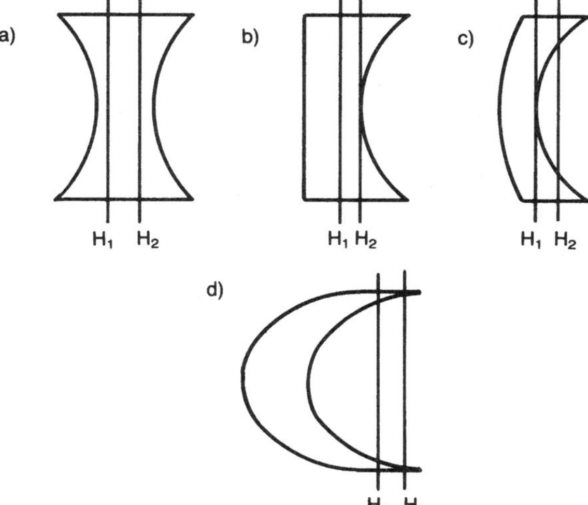

Figure 18.16 Principal planes as minus lens is bent.

situation. Hence clinically, the shape and power factor approach to spectacle magnification is easier to use than Gauss system approach.

18.11 TELESCOPES FOR AMETROPES

Consider an afocal telescope. For incident plane waves, plane waves leave the telescope. Suppose an uncorrected ametrope wants to use the telescope. The ametrope can adjust the length of the telescope so that the vergence leaving the telescope corrects the refractive error.

EXAMPLE 18.14

Juan Rodriguez has a +7.00 D thin spectacle correction at a 12 mm vertex distance. Juan has a focusable keplerian telescope with a +20.83 D objective lens and a +83.33 D ocular lens. When set as an afocal telescope the length is 60.0 mm (i.e., sum of the secondary focal lengths) and the magnification is −4×. Juan wants to take his spectacle off and use the focusable telescope to view a distant object. Assume that the telescope's ocular lens sits 12 mm from the eye. What new length will provide a clear image for Juan, and how much larger is Juan's retinal image when using the focussed telescope as compared to just using his spectacle correction?

There are several ways to figure the answer. A particularly quick way is to take the +83.33 D ocular lens and consider it as the sum of a +76.33 D lens and a +7.00 D lens. The +7.00 D supplies the correction for Juan, and the +76.33 D must work together with the +20.83 D objective lens as a new afocal telescope. From afocal telescope theory, the new reduced length is the sum of the secondary focal lengths (Eq. 17.22), or

$$\frac{1000}{20.83\,\text{D}} + \frac{1000}{76.33\,\text{D}} = 61.1\,\text{mm}$$

So Juan focuses the telescope by changing the length from 60.0 mm to 61.1 mm. The new magnification of the afocal portion of the telescope is

$$M = -\frac{P_{\text{oc}}}{P_{\text{obj}}}$$

$$= -\frac{76.33\,\text{D}}{+20.83\,\text{D}} = -3.66\times$$

The minus sign indicates the image seen through the telescope appears inverted (unless an erecting system is present in the telescope). With the focussed telescope, Juan's retinal image is 3.66 times larger than when just using the +7.00 D spectacle correction.

EXAMPLE 18.15

Racquel Mulch has a −4.00 D spectacle correction at an 11 mm vertex distance. To see a distant object, Mulch takes an afocal 5× Galilean telescope with a +2.00 D objective lens, a −10.00 D ocular lens, and a 40 cm length, and adjusts it so that the vergence leaving the telescope is −4.00 D. What is the new length of the adjusted telescope, and how much larger is Mulch's retinal image when using the adjusted telescope versus when just wearing her spectacle correction?

As in the previous example, an easy way to work this is to consider the −10.00 D ocular lens as the sum of a −6.00 D lens and a −4.00 D lens. The −4.00 D supplies the correction for Mulch. The −6.00 D lens must work together with +2.00 D objective lens as a new afocal telescope. From afocal telescope theory, the new reduced length is the sum of the secondary focal lengths, or

$$\frac{100}{+2.00\,\text{D}} + \frac{100}{-6.00\,\text{D}} = 33.33\,\text{cm}$$

So when Mulch focuses the telescope by changing the length from 40.0 cm to 33.33 cm. The new magnification of the afocal portion of the telescope is

$$M = -\frac{P_{\text{oc}}}{P_{\text{obj}}}$$

$$= -\frac{-6.00\,\text{D}}{+2.00\,\text{D}} = 3.00\times$$

With the focussed telescope, Mulch's retinal image is 3 times larger than when just using the −4.00 D spectacle correction.

In Example 18.14, Juan had to lengthen the Keplerian telescope and lost angular magnification when adjusting the telescope to correct his hyperopia. However a myope would have to shorten the Keplerian telescope and would gain angular magnification when adjusting the telescope to correct his myopia.

In Example 18.15, Mulch had to shorten the Galilean telescope and lost angular magnification when adjusting the telescope to correct her myopia. However a hyperope would have to lengthen the Galilean telescope and would gain angular magnification when adjusting the telescope to correct her hyperopia.

18.12 RELATIVE SPECTACLE MAGNIFICATION

Spectacle magnification dealt with a comparison of the "corrected" retinal image size to the uncorrected retinal image size *for the same eye*. For the optical analysis of *aniseikonia*, we want to compare the retinal image size of a person's left eye to the retinal image size of their right eye. Here, two different eyes are involved. Organizationally, it is easier to establish a standard eye and then compare the retinal image size of each eye (right and left) to the retinal image size of the standard eye. (This is analogous to establishing a standard length, such as a meter or a foot, and then comparing distances to the standard.) The conventional standard eye is a +60.00 D emmetropic eye.

For a distant object, relative spectacle magnification (RSM) is the ratio of the retinal image size I_a in the corrected ametropic eye to the retinal image size I_s in the standard emmetropic eye, or

$$\text{RSM} \equiv \frac{I_a}{I_s} \tag{18.22}$$

In order to understand RSM, it is helpful to first compare the uncorrected (blurred) retinal image size for the ametropic eye to the clear image of the standard emmetropic eye. Recall that there are two special cases of ametropia, axial and refractive. An axial ametropic eye has the same equivalent power as the standard emmetrope but differs in axial length. A refractive ametropic eye has the same axial length as a standard emmetrope but differs in equivalent power. In general, an ametropic eye may have both an axial and a refractive component of the ametropia.

Figure 18.17a shows the chief ray for a refractive hyperope, a refractive myope, and the standard emmetrope. The standard emmetrope's clear retinal image size is I_s. The retinal images for the ametropes are blurred and the chief ray specifies their size. For refractive ametropia, the blurred ametropic retinal image sizes are all equal to I_s. The correcting lenses clear the retinal images and change their size. From the spectacle magnification equation (Eq. 18.3), we know that a thin myopic correction decreases the retinal image size and a thin hyperopic correction increases the retinal image size.

Figure 18.17b shows the chief ray for an uncorrected axial hyperope, an uncorrected axial myope, and the standard emmetrope. The chief ray specifies the blurred image sizes for the ametropes. The clear

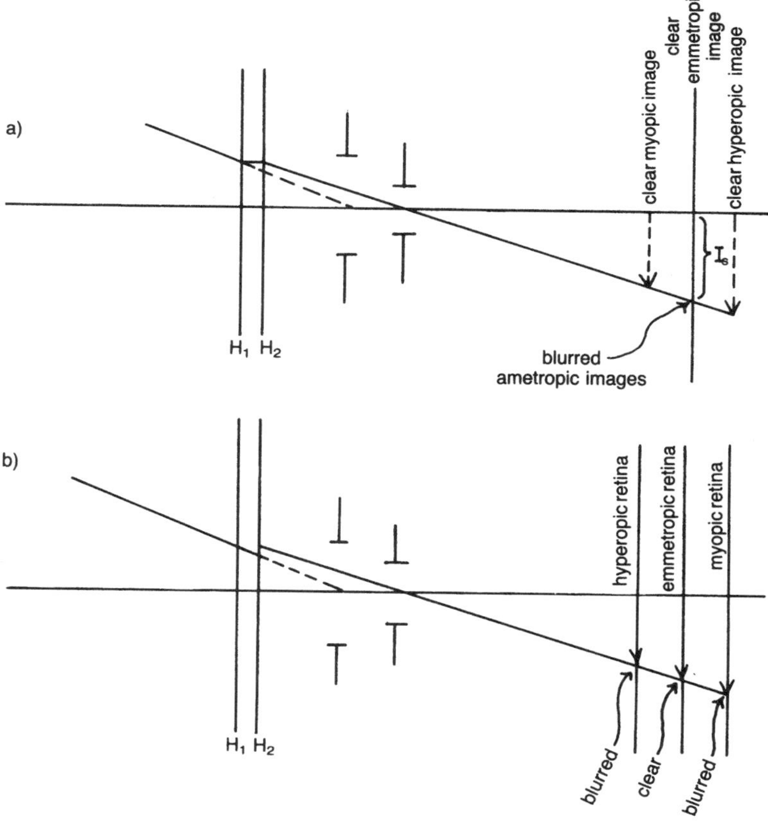

Figure 18.17 Ametrope versus emmetropic retinal image sizes: a, refractive ametropes; b, axial ametropes.

retinal image size for the +60.00 D standard emmetrope is I_s. The uncorrected retinal image size for the axial myope is larger than I_s, which in turn is larger than the retinal image size for the axial hyperope. From the spectacle magnification relations, we know that a thin correcting lens decreases a myope's retinal image size. However, the fact that the retinal image size for the uncorrected axial myope is larger than I_s raises the possibility that the retinal image size for the corrected axial myope might still be larger than I_s. Similarly, the fact that the retinal image size for the uncorrected hyperope is smaller than I_s raises the possibility that the retinal image size for the corrected axial hyperope might still be smaller than I_s even though the spectacle magnification gives a percent gain.

The spectacle magnification shape factor, M_{shape}, influences the RSM in the same way that it influences spectacle magnification. In other words, we can calculate the RSM for a thin correcting lens, and then simply multiple by the result by M_{shape} to get the RSM for a thick correcting lens. In this section, we will consider only thin correcting lenses.

Remember that the image sizes in a reduced system are the same as those in an actual system, and that the nodal points in a reduced system are located at the principal planes. Figure 18.18a is a reduced system representation for a hyperopic eye with a thin correcting lens. The principal planes for the uncorrected eye are dashed, while the principal planes for the corrected eye system (correcting lens and eye) are solid. The correction (power P_v) is at a distance of d_{bH} in

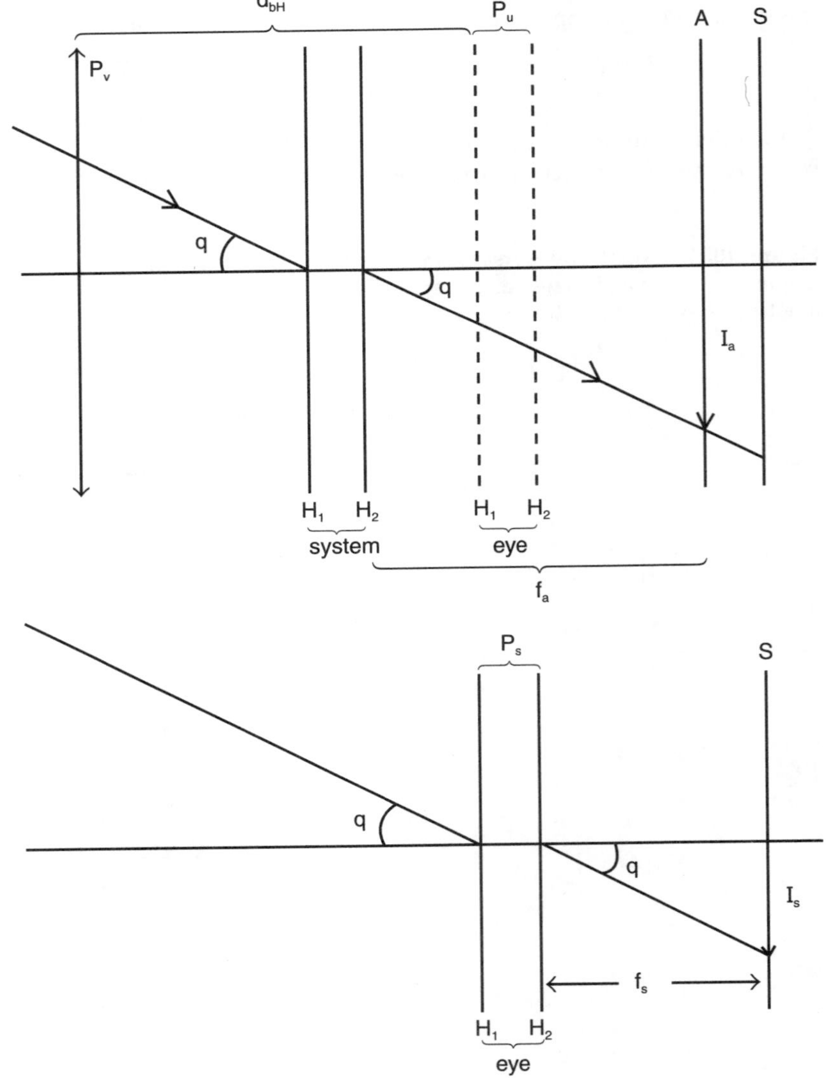

Figure 18.18 **Reduced system representation for a corrected hyperopic eye: a, the principal planes for the eye are dashed. The principal planes for the corrected eye system (correcting lens plus the eye) are solid. The nodal ray for the system subtends the angle *q* and specifies the clear retinal image size I_a; b, nodal ray for the standard emmetrope. For the same subtended angle *q*, the clear retinal image size is I_s.**

front of the primary principal plane H_1 (dashed) of the uncorrected eye. The position S would be the retinal location for a refractive hyperope. Position A is the retinal position for this hyperope, so there is both a refractive and an axial component to the hyperopia. The principal planes for the corrected eye system (i.e., correcting lens plus the eye) are solid. The ray shown is the nodal ray for the corrected eye system. The distant object subtends the angle q at the corrected eye system's primary principal plane H_1 (solid). The nodal ray leaving the corrected system's H_2 (solid) subtends the same angle q and specifies the clear retinal image I_a at the retinal position A. The distance from the system's H_2 (solid) to the retinal position A equals the corrected system's (reduced) secondary equivalent focal length f_a. Figure 18.18b is the reduced system diagram for the standard emmetropic eye, which has a retinal image I_s for the same object (i.e., same subtended angle q). The distance from the standard emmetrope's secondary principal plane to the emmetrope's retinal position S is the (reduced) secondary focal length f_s, of the standard emmetropic eye.

Let P_s be the +60.00 D equivalent power of the standard emmetropic eye. Let P_u be the equivalent power of the uncorrected ametropic eye. Assume a thin correcting lens of power P_v located at a distance d_{bH} from the uncorrected eye's primary principal plane. The Gauss theory equation (Eq. 15.40) gives the equivalent power P_a for the correction together with the ametropic eye (i.e., the corrected eye system) as

$$P_a = P_v + P_u - d_{bH} P_v P_u$$

From the nodal ray for the total system (Figure 18.18a), the retinal image size I_a is given by

$$I_a = f_a \tan q$$

where f_a is the secondary equivalent focal length for the corrected eye system. For the standard emmetropic eye viewing the same object (Figure 18.18b),

$$I_s = f_s \tan q$$

where $f_s = 1000/60\,\text{D} = 16.67\,\text{mm}$.

We can substitute the above two focal length equations into Eq. 18.22 to obtain

$$\text{RSM} = \frac{f_a}{f_s}$$

or

$$\text{RSM} = \frac{P_s}{P_a} \tag{18.23}$$

since each secondary focal length equals the reciprocal of the corresponding equivalent dioptric power. Equation 18.23 shows that RSM equals the ratio of the equivalent dioptric power for the standard eye to that of the corrected ametropic eye system.

EXAMPLE 18.16

For simplicity, represent Nick Name's left eye by a +56.00 D thin lens in air located 19.84 mm in front of a screen representing the retina. Nick's eye has both an axial and a refractive component to the refractive error, and the thin lens correction at a 12 mm vertex distance is −6.00 D. (You should be able to verify that with Chapter 6 methods.) What is the RSM for Nick Name's left eye?

What is our expectation before working the problem? The spectacle magnification for a −6.00 D thin correction would be a percent loss. However, Nick Name's eye is longer than that of the standard emmetrope, so Nick's uncorrected retinal image size is larger than that of a standard emmetrope. Therefore it's possible that the RSM is a percent gain.

The equivalent power of Nick's corrected eye system is

$$P_a = -6.00\,\text{D} + 56.00\,\text{D} - (12.0 \times 10^{-3}\,\text{m})(-6.00\,\text{D})(+56.00\,\text{D})$$

or

$$P_a = +54.03\,\text{D}$$

From Eq. 18.23,

$$\text{RSM} = \frac{+60.00\,\text{D}}{+54.03\,\text{D}} = 1.110$$

So Nick's corrected retinal image for his left eye is 11.0% larger than that of the standard emmetropic eye.

In the special cases of axial or refractive ametropia, there are equations that are easier to work with than Eq. 18.23. To start the derivation of the special equations, set the equivalent power P_u of the uncorrected ametropic eye equal to $P_s + P_w$, where P_s is +60.00 D. (In the previous numerical example, P_w would equal −4.00 D.) The thin lens correction (power P_v) is a distance d_{bH} from the primary principal plane for the uncorrected eye. Then from Gauss theory, the equivalent power P_a for the corrected eye system is

$$P_a = P_v + (P_s + P_w) - d_{bH} P_v (P_s + P_w)$$

We can substitute this equation into Eq. 18.23 to get

$$\text{RSM} = \frac{P_s}{P_v + (P_s + P_w) - d_{bH} P_v (P_s + P_w)} \tag{18.24}$$

Rearrangement in the denominator gives

$$\mathrm{RSM} = \frac{P_s}{(P_v + P_w - d_{bH}P_vP_w) + P_s(1 - d_{bH}P_v)} \qquad (18.25)$$

In the special case of a refractive ametrope, the correcting lens exactly neutralizes P_w . In other words, the equivalent power of a system consisting of thin lenses with respective dioptric powers P_v and P_w separated by d_{bH} equals zero. This means that the first term in the denominator vanishes, and the above equation simplifies to

$$\mathrm{RSM_r} = \frac{1}{1 - d_{bH}P_v} \qquad (18.26)$$

where RSM is subscripted with an r to represent the special case of a refractive ametrope. Equation 18.26 has the same form as the spectacle magnification Eq. 18.3 except that now the distance is from the thin correcting lens to the eye's primary principal plane H_1. Therefore for refractive ametropes, the RSM results are analogous to the spectacle magnification. Specifically, a refractive hyperope has a larger retinal image size than the standard emmetrope (analogous to a percent gain), and a refractive myope has a smaller retinal image size than the standard emmetrope (analogous to a percent loss). The percent gain (or loss) is larger in magnitude for a longer vertex distance and vice versa.

For an axial ametrope, the equivalent power P_u of the uncorrected ametropic eye equals the equivalent power P_s of the standard emmetropic eye. Therefore the power P_w in Eqs. 18.24 and 18.25 is zero. Then Eq. 18.25 becomes

$$\mathrm{RSM_a} = \frac{P_s}{P_v + P_s(1 - d_{bH}P_v)}$$

where RSM is subscripted with an a for the special case of an axial ametropic eye. Given that the secondary equivalent focal length f_s equals the reciprocal of P_s or 16.67 mm, we can divide both the numerator and the denominator by P_s and group like terms to obtain

$$\mathrm{RSM_a} = \frac{1}{1 - (d_{bH} - 0.01667\,\mathrm{m})P_v} \qquad (18.27)$$

where d_{bH} is in meters. Alternatively if d_{bH} is expressed in mm, we can write

$$\mathrm{RSM_a} = \frac{1}{1 - \left(\frac{d_{bH} - 16.67\,\mathrm{mm}}{1000\,\mathrm{mm/m}}\right)P_v} \qquad (18.28)$$

Equation 18.27 for an axial ametrope is different than Eq. 18.26 for a refractive ametrope. For thin correcting lenses, Eq. 18.26 shows that for refractive myopes $I_a < I_s$, while for refractive hyperopes $I_a > I_s$. However for axial ametropes, the situation also depends on whether d_{bH} is longer or shorter than the primary equivalent focal length 16.67 mm.

When the thin correcting lens for an axial ametrope is placed at the primary focal point of the eye, d_{bH} equals 16.67 mm, and then Eq. 18.28 becomes

$$\mathrm{RSM_a} = 1$$

This particular phenomenon is known as Knapp's law. The corresponding ray diagram is shown in Figure 18.19. The nodal ray for the thin correcting lens is also the ray that passes through the primary focal point of the eye, so the image space ray in the eye is parallel to the axis, and I_a is equal to I_s for both the axial myope and hyperope.

For either the axial or the refractive case, the percent gain G of the corrected retinal image I_a relative to the standard emmetropic image I_s is

$$G = (\mathrm{RSM} - 1)100\% \qquad (18.28')$$

Figure 18.19 Knapp's law.

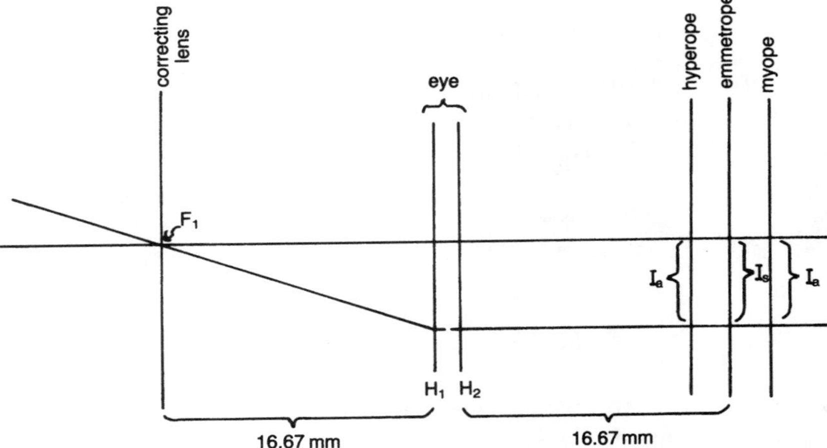

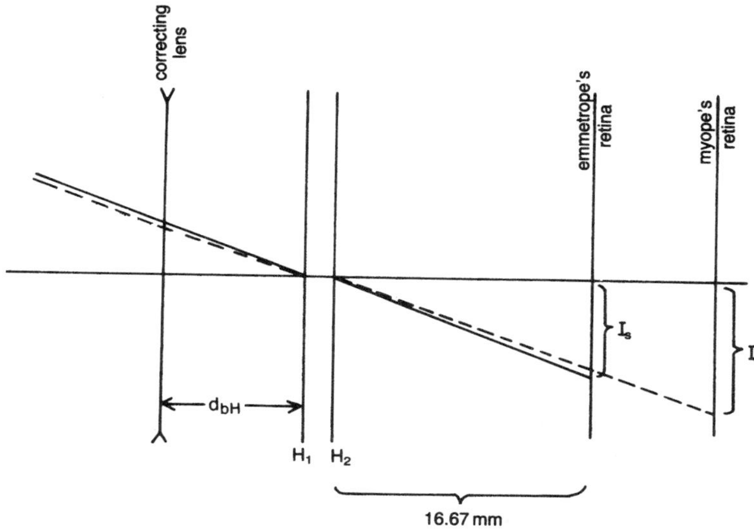

Figure 18.20 Superposition of standard emmetropic eye and corrected axial myope.

EXAMPLE 18.18

A myopic axial ametrope needs a −10.00 D thin spectacle correction at a distance of 13 mm from H_1 of the eye. What is the RSM?

From Eq. 18.27,

$$\text{RSM}_a = \frac{1}{\left[1 - \frac{(13\,\text{mm} - 16.67\,\text{mm})}{1000\,\text{mm/m}}(-10.00\,\text{D})\right]}$$
$$= \frac{1}{1 - 0.0367} = 1.038$$

The percent gain is

$$G = (1.038 - 1)100\% = 3.8\%$$

In this case, since the axial myopic eye is longer than the standard emmetropic eye, the corrected myope has a 3.8% larger retinal image than the standard emmetrope. Figure 18.20 shows a superposition of the reduced emmetropic eye and the corrected reduced ametropic eye. The solid ray is the nodal ray for the emmetrope, and the dashed nodal ray is for the myopic eye. The two rays come in parallel to each other. The dashed ray is bent up by the minus spectacle lens, so at the primary nodal point of the eye it subtends a smaller angle than the solid ray. However, since the axial myope has a longer eye, I_a turns out to be larger than I_s.

EXAMPLE 18.19

A refractive myope needs a −10.00 D correction at a distance of 13 mm from the primary principal plane of the eye. What is the RSM?

From Eq. 18.26,

$$\text{RSM}_r = \frac{1}{1 - (0.013\,\text{m})(-10.00\,\text{D})}$$
$$= \frac{1}{1 + 0.130} = 0.885$$

The percent gain is

$$G = (0.885 - 1)100\%$$
$$= -11.5\%\ \text{gain} = +11.5\%\ \text{loss}$$

While the axial myope in the previous example had a percent gain relative to the standard emmetrope, the refractive myope here has a large percent loss.

EXAMPLE 18.20

What is the RSM for the axial myope in Example 18.18 when wearing a (thin) contact correction?

From Gullstrand's #1 schematic eye, the primary principal plane sits 1.348 mm behind the cornea. From the vergence effectivity relations, the correction at the cornea is −8.96 D. From Eq. 18.27,

$$\text{RSM}_a = \frac{1}{\left[1 - \frac{(1.348\,\text{mm} - 16.67\,\text{mm})}{1000\,\text{mm/m}}(-8.96\,\text{D})\right]}$$
$$= \frac{1}{1 - 0.137} = 1.159$$

The percent gain is

$$G = (1.159 - 1)100\%$$
$$= +15.9\%\ \text{gain}$$

The contact corrected axial myope has a large percent gain.

Table 18.1 Retinal Image Sizes Relative to the Standard Emmetrope

	Uncorrected	*Spectacle Lens Correction at F_1 of the Eye*	*Contact Lens Correction*
Axial myope	Larger	Same	Larger
Axial hyperope	Smaller	Same	Smaller
Refractive hyperope	Same	Larger	About the same
Refractive myope	Same	Smaller	About the same

EXAMPLE 18.21

What is the RSM for the refractive myope of Example 18.19 when wearing a (thin) contact lens correction?

Again, the primary principal plane is 1.348 mm behind the cornea, and the power of the correction at the cornea is −8.96 D. From Eq. 18.25,

$$\text{RSM}_r = \frac{1}{1 - (0.001348\,\text{m})(-8.96\,\text{D})}$$
$$= \frac{1}{1 + 0.0121} = 0.988$$

The percent gain is

$$G = (0.988 - 1)100\%$$
$$= -1.2\%\ \text{gain} = +1.2\%\ \text{loss}$$

The contact corrected refractive myope has only a small percent loss relative to the standard emmetrope, while the spectacle corrected refractive myope has a larger percent loss.

Table 18.1 summarizes the comparisons of retinal image sizes relative to the standard emmetropic retinal image size I_s. Small percent differences are labeled as about the same. The myopic information corresponds to the above four examples.

Aniseikonia is usually associated with *anisometropia* (which is the condition of significantly different refractive errors in the right eye versus the left eye). When one eye is myopic and the other eye is hyperopic, the anisometropia is called antimetropia. From spectacle magnification relations, one might initially think that the retinal image size in a spectacle corrected myopic eye would be smaller than the retinal image size in a spectacle corrected hyeropic eye, but the RSM relations show this may not be true especially if the refractive errors are due to axial causes.

Clinically, one should keep in mind that the refractive error may not be just axial or just refractive but might be mixed. Also, the correcting lenses are thick. As mentioned earlier in this section, the RSM equations are modified for a thick correcting lens by simply multiplying the appropriate RSM equation by the shape factor, Eq. 18.7, of the thick lens.

18.13 PRISM EFFECTIVITY AND DYNAMIC MAGNIFICATION

Section 12.8 considered prism effectivity for thin lenses. For a distant object and no prescribed prism in the lens ($Z = 0$), Eq. 12.10 reduces to

$$Z_e = \frac{Z_c}{1 - c_{rot}P_v}$$

where P_v is the power of the thin lens, Z_c is the location of the object point in prism-diopters as measured at the lens plane, and Z_e is how much the eye has to rotate (in prism-diopters) from the straight-ahead direction to image the object point on the fovea. Examples presented in Section 12.8 show that plus lenses tend to increase the prism effectivity and minus lenses tend to decrease the prism effectivity. Some authors refer to this as an angular magnification effect (with names such as rotational magnification or dynamic magnification) instead of prism effectivity. In the dynamic magnification terminology, we can write the above equation as

$$Z_e = \text{DYM}_p Z_c$$

where,

$$\text{DYM}_p = \frac{1}{1 - c_{rot}P_v}$$

and DYM_p stands for the dynamic magnification power factor of the lens. When the lens is thin, P_v is the back vertex power of the lens, and c_{rot} is the distance from the lens's back vertex to the center of rotation of the eye.

For a real lens with shape, a distant object, and no prescribed prism in the lens, it is easy to show that the total dynamic magnification (or total prism effectivity) is the product of the dynamic magnification power factor times the shape factor of the lens.

$$\mathrm{DYM_{tot}} = \mathrm{DYM_p} M_{\mathrm{shape}}$$

where,

$$Z_e = \mathrm{DYM_{tot}} Z_c$$

Note that in this situation, the shape factor acts like an afocal telescope in front of a thin lens with a power equal to the back vertex power of the thick lens. For the thick lens, c_{rot} is the distance from the back vertex of the lens to the center of rotation of the eye, and P_v is the back vertex power of the lens. Thus the shape factor can influence prism effectivity or dynamic magnification, just as it influences the total spectacle magnification or the total RSM.

As mentioned in Section 12.8, substantially different spectacle lens powers for the right eye versus the left eye (i.e., anisometropia), frequently results in double vision when the person reads through the lower portion of the lens (i.e, there are significantly different Z_e values for the right and left eyes). The usual remedy for this is to use slab-off prism or reverse slab prism in the lower portion of one of the lenses. Remole has argued that using the shape factor to produce a corrected dynamic magnification eliminates the need for slab-off or reverse slab prism (*Optom Vis Sci* 1999; 76:783–95).

18.14 MERIDIONAL TELESCOPES

In spherocylindrical optical systems, the different powers in the different principal meridians cause different magnifications in those meridians. In a general thick obliquely crossed spherocylindrical lens system, the principal meridians of the magnification will differ from the principal meridians of the dioptric power. However, here we consider only some simpler cases where the principal meridians of the magnification are aligned with the principal meridians of the dioptric power.

A $+2.00 \times 180$ lens has a power of +2.00 D in the vertical meridian and zero power in the horizontal meridian. For a distant centered point source, the +2.00 D of power in the vertical meridian forms a real centered horizontal line image at 50 cm behind the lens. For a second point source located some distance vertically above the first point source, the 2.00 D of power in the vertical meridian forms a second horizontal line image at 50 cm behind the lens, and the second horizontal line image is vertically below the

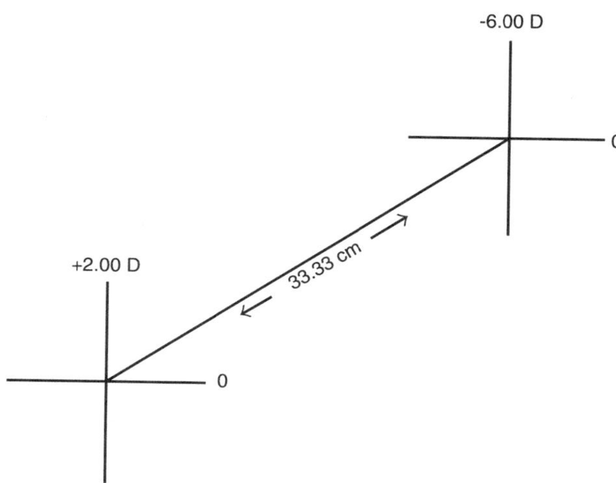

Figure 18.21 Power crosses for the objective and ocular lenses of a 3× axis 180 meridional telescope, which magnifies 3× in the vertical meridian and 1× (no change) in the horizontal meridian.

first horizontal line image. Here, magnification relates to the vertical distance between the two horizontal line images (i.e., for a higher plus cylinder dioptric power, the horizontal line images are formed closer to the lens and are vertically closer together, so the magnification is smaller in magnitude. For a lower power, the horizontal line images are formed farther from the lens and are vertically farther apart, so the magnification is larger in magnitude). Thus power in a vertical principal meridian is responsible for horizontal lines and is also responsible for vertical magnification, which relates to how far vertically apart the horizontal lines are. We can rotate the lens clockwise, in which case the line images and magnification effects rotate with the lens.

Recall that a 3× afocal Galilean telescope with a 33.33 cm length, a +2.00 D spherical objective lens, and a −6.00 D spherical ocular lens magnifies by 3× in all meridians. Now consider an afocal meridional telescope consisting of a $+2.00 \times 180$ objective lens 33.33 cm in front of a -6.00×180 ocular lens. Figure 18.21 shows the respective power crosses for the two lenses. When plane waves are incident on the objective, plane waves leave the ocular, and all meridians will be seen clearly through the meridional telescope. The zero power in the horizontal meridians provides neither a magnification nor a minification (Figure 18.22a). The respective vertical power meridians of the objective lens and the ocular lens work together to supply 3× magnification in the vertical meridian (Figure 18.22b). Thus a magnification "cross" for this meridional telescope is

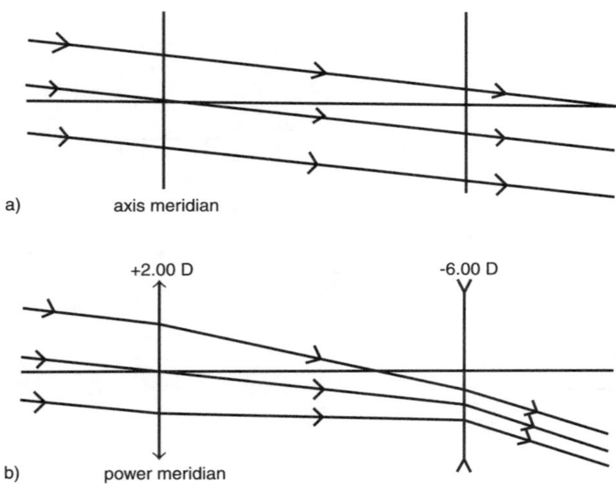

Figure 18.22 Principal meridian ray diagrams for a meridional telescope: a, the axis meridian (horizontal for the 3× axis 180 telescope in Figure 18.21); b, the power meridian (vertical for the 3× axis 180 telescope in Figure 18.21).

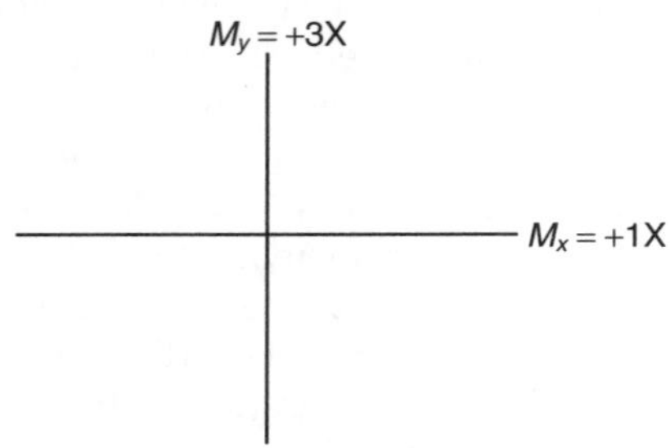

Consequently, a square with horizontal and vertical sides viewed through the meridional telescope would appear to be a rectangle that is three times longer vertically than horizontally (Figure 18.23). Similarly a circle would appear to be a vertically oriented ellipse, and a person would appear taller and thinner.

In terms of the internal optics of the meridional afocal telescope, the magnification differences occur as follows. The $+2.00 \times 180$ objective lens by itself forms a converging cylindrical wavefront for each point source in the object. Each of the cylindrical wavefronts would form a horizontal line image at 50 cm if the waves were allowed to propagate that far. When the converging cylindrical wavefronts hit the -6.00×180 ocular lens (at 33.33 cm from the objective lens), the ocular lens changes each cylindrical wavefront back into a plane wave, and increases the vertical angular separation of the wavefronts. The increase in the vertical angular separation of the two wavefronts (i.e., of the two different bundles) gives the 3× vertical magnification. There is no power in the

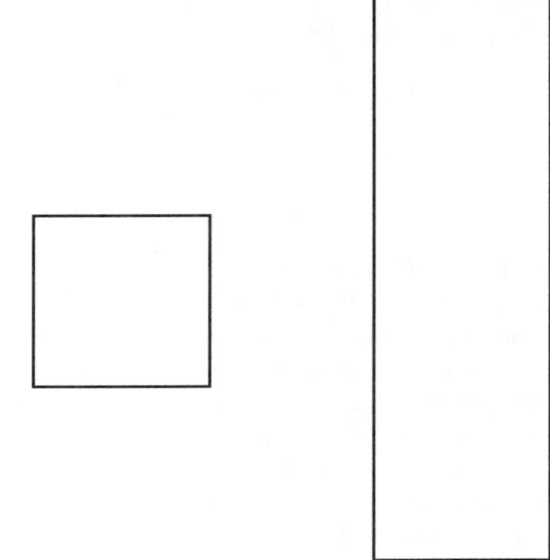

Figure 18.23 A square object (left) appears as a rectangle that is longer vertically (right) when viewed through the 3× axis 180 meridional telescope.

horizontal meridians, so the horizontal angular separation is unchanged, or the horizontal "magnification" is 1×.

Now consider an afocal meridional telescope with a $+2.00 \times 90$ objective lens and a -6.00×90 ocular lens. Here the power meridians are horizontal and 3× magnification occurs in the horizontal meridian, while the no magnification (i.e., $M = 1$) occurs in the vertical meridian. Through this telescope, a square with horizontal and vertical sides appears to be a rectangle that is three times longer horizontally than vertically (Figure 18.24). Similarly, a circle would appear to be a horizontally oriented ellipse, and a person would appear to short and wide.

Note that in Figure 18.24, the object square with horizontal and vertical sides has diagonal bars in it, where each diagonal bar makes an angle of 45° with the horizontal. Through the above meridional telescope, the square appears as a horizontally elongated

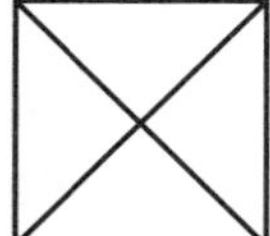
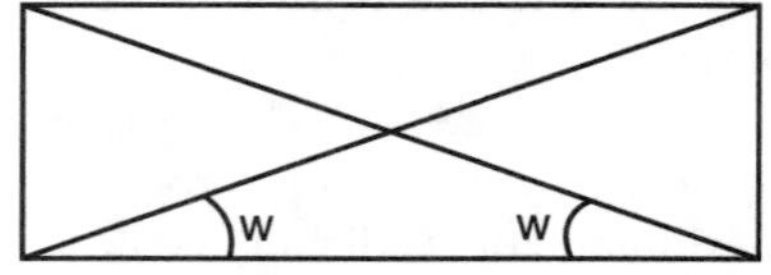

Figure 18.24 A square object (left) appears as a rectangle that is longer horizontally when viewed through a 3× axis 90 meridional telescope. The diagonals in the object are not lined up with the principal meridians. The image space diagonals appear to have rotated in opposite directions (scissors effect) and now make an angle w of 18.4° with the horizontal.

rectangle that still has horizontal and vertical sides. However, the diagonal bars are rotationally deviated and no longer make an angle of 45° with the horizontal. For a unit square object, the apparent rectangle has a three unit horizontal side together with a one unit vertical side. From the inverse tangent of 1/3, the apparent diagonals each make an angle w of 18.4° with the horizontal. Relative to the diagonals in the object, the apparent diagonals are rotated around the center in opposite directions (i.e., the scissors effect). Qualitatively, this is the same rotational deviation given by the prism properties of the $+2.00 \times 90$ objective lens for lines that are not aligned with the principal meridians (Section 12.4).

Consider a 1.5× afocal telescope with a $+4.00 \times 45$ objective lens located 8.333 cm in front of -6.00×45 ocular lens. The power meridian of each lens is the 135 meridian, and so the 1.5× magnification is in the 135 meridian. Figure 18.25 shows a distant clock as viewed through this telescope. Remember that this is the ocular view, and the 2:30 to 8:30 line is the 135 meridian. The 2:30 to 8:30 line is magnified 1.5 times, while the 10:30 to 4:30 line is unmagnified.

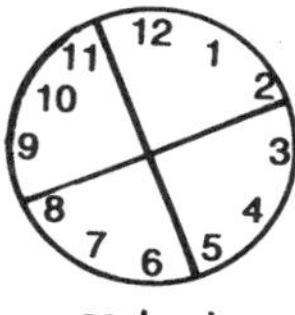

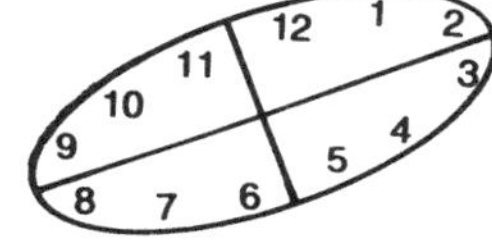

Figure 18.25 Ocular view of the oblique distortion of a clock dial seen through a meridional telescope that magnifies 1.5 times in the 135 meridian (i.e., a 1.5× axis 45 telescope).

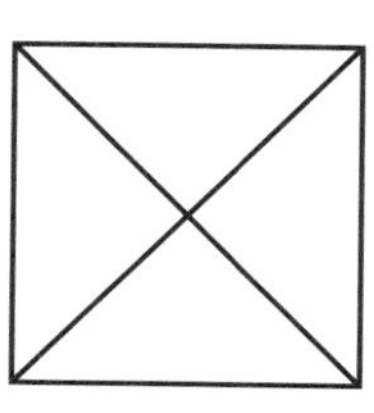

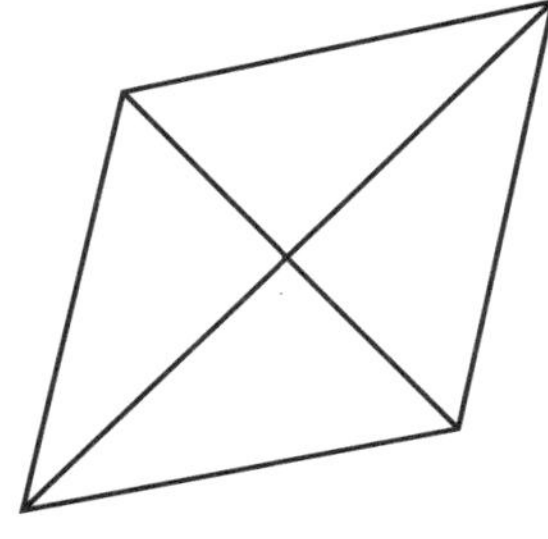

Figure 18.26 Ocular view of the oblique distortion of a square object (top) through the meridional telescope that magnifies 1.5 time in the 135 meridian. Here the diagonals are aligned with the principal meridians of the telescope lenses and are not rotated. The horizontal and vertical sides of the object square are not aligned with the principal meridians and in image space appear to have rotated in opposite directions (the scissors effect). The apparent image is a parallelogram.

Figure 18.26 shows the ocular view of how a square with horizontal and vertical sides would appear through the above 1.5× meridional telescope that magnifies in the 135 meridian. Since the diagonal bars are aligned with the principal meridians, they are not rotationally deviated. However, the horizontal and vertical sides of the object square are not aligned with the principal meridians, and the sides appear to have undergone a scissors movement. The object square now appears to be a parallelogram in which the sides are no longer horizontal and vertical.

18.15 POWER FACTOR IN SPHEROCYLINDRICAL CORRECTIONS

In a thick spherocylindrical correction with a spherical front surface, the total spectacle magnification in each principal meridian is the product of the shape factor and the power factor. Here we treat the lenses as thin, so in effect we are only considering the power factor part.

A thin spherocylindrical spectacle lens corrects the astigmatic refractive error. Thus, the spectacle lens together with the refractive error constitutes an afocal system. We can apply the power factor equation (i.e., Eq. 18.14),

$$M_{\text{power}} = \frac{1}{1 - d_{\text{ben}} P_{\text{v}}}$$

to each principal meridian to obtain the spectacle magnification in that meridian. The distance d_{ben} is the distance from the lens to the entrance pupil. Technically, the entrance pupil position may be slightly different for each principal meridian. However, it is usually a good approximation to assume that the entrance pupil is 3 mm behind the cornea regardless of the principal meridian powers.

Flo has a $+8.00 \times 180$ thin spectacle correction at a 12 mm vertex distance (so $d_{\text{ben}} = 15$ mm). Here the power meridian is vertical and the axis meridian is horizontal. The spectacle magnification power factor gives $M_{\text{spec}} = 1.136$ (or a 13.6% gain) in the vertical meridian, while $M_{\text{spec}} = 1.000$ (or a zero percent gain) for the horizontal meridian (since $P_{\text{v}} = 0$). When Flo looks at a square with horizontal and vertical sides, her retinal image will be a rectangle that is 13.6% longer vertically than horizontally. (Note that by transposition a $+8.00 \times 180$ correction is equivalent to a $+8.00 \bigcirc -8.00 \times 90$ correction.)

Cal has a -5.00×90 thin spectacle correction at an 11 mm vertex distance distance (so $d_{\text{ben}} = 14$ mm). Here the spectacle magnification power factor gives a 6.5% loss in the horizontal meridian and a zero percent loss in the vertical meridian. When Cal looks through this correction at a square with horizontal and vertical sides, Cal's retinal image will be a rectangle that is 6.5% shorter vertically than horizontally.

Pooch has a $+2.00 \bigcirc -6.00 \times 180$ thin spectacle correction at a 12 mm vertex distance. The power in the vertical meridian is -4.00 D and the power in the horizontal meridian is $+2.00$ D. Here the spectacle magnification power factor gives a 5.7% loss in the vertical meridian and a 3.1% gain in the horizontal meridian. When Pooch looks through this correction at a square with horizontal and vertical sides, Pooch's retinal image will be a rectangle that is approximately 8.8% longer horizontally than vertically (i.e., 3.1%–(–5.7%) = 8.8%).

There are cells the visual cortex area of the brain that fire when the person views a horizontal line, and different cells in the visual cortex that fire when the person views a vertical line. When spectacle corrected astigmats with horizontal and vertical principal meridians (such as Flo, Cal, and Pooch) look at a square with horizontal and vertical sides, their retina image is a a rectangle with horizontal and vertical sides. Here, since the sides are still horizontal and vertical, the same visual cortex cells still fire, and the person perceptually adapts to the small percentage horizontal–vertical magnification differences. Once adapted, these people perceive a square, even though their retinal image is actually a horizontal or a vertical rectangle.

However because of the oblique magnification differences that occur in a spectacle corrected high oblique astigmat, horizontal and vertical lines in the object are not imaged as horizontal and vertical lines on the retina. (This oblique distortion has the same nature as that in Figure 18.26 but is considerably smaller). Here, the various visual cortex cells responsible for either the horizontal lines or the vertical lines do not fire, and consequently the human visual system tends not to perceptually adapt to this situation.

Consider Pete, a high oblique astigmat, with a $-1.00 \bigcirc -7.00 \times 45$ thin spectacle correction at a 10 mm vertex distance. The power in the 45 meridian is -1.00 D and the power in the 135 meridian is -8.00 D. The spectacle magnification power factor gives a 1.3% loss in the 45 meridian and a 9.4% loss in the 135 meridian. When Pete looks through his correction at a square with horizontal and vertical sides, Pete's retinal image will be a parallelogram in which the sides are no longer horizontal and vertical.

Note that there is no blur in Pete's corrected image, but nevertheless due to the oblique distortion Pete may not adapt to the spectacle correction. In this case, reducing the magnitude of the spectacle's cylinder power and/or rotating the cylinder axis towards horizontal or vertical can minimize the oblique distortion. Either of these two methods leaves some astigmatic blur. The clinical result is that oblique astigmats tolerate the blur better than the distortions due to the different oblique magnifications. On the other hand, a rigid contact lens correction, instead of the spectacle correction, minimizes the spectacle magnification percent gains or losses and thus minimizes (or eliminates) the oblique distortions, while at the same time maintaining the clarity of the retinal image.

18.16 SUMMARY OF IMPORTANT EQUATIONS

Thin Lens Spectacle Magnification

$$M_{\text{spec}} = \frac{1}{1 - dP} \tag{18.3}$$

Thick Lens Spectacle Magnification

$$M_{\text{tot}} = M_{\text{shape}}\, M_{\text{power}} \tag{18.15}$$

$$M_{\text{shape}} = \frac{1}{1 - \bar{c}P_1} \tag{18.7}$$

$$M_{\text{power}} = \frac{1}{1 - d_{\text{ben}}P_{\text{v}}} \tag{18.14}$$

Alternatively,

$$M_{\text{tot}} = \frac{1}{1 - d_{\text{Hen}}P_{\text{e}}} \tag{18.21}$$

Special cases of RSM power factors

$$\text{RSM}_{\text{r}} = \frac{1}{1 - d_{\text{bH}}P_{\text{v}}} \tag{18.25$'$}$$

$$\text{RSM}_{\text{a}} = \frac{1}{1 - (d_{\text{bH}} - 0.01667\,\text{m})P_{\text{v}}} \tag{18.27}$$

Percent Gain

$$G = (M - 1)100\%$$

Generic Small Magnification Approximations

$$M = \frac{1}{1 - b} \approx 1 + b$$

and

$$G \approx b100\%$$

where b is small and its exact form depends on the particular magnification (spectacle, relative spectacle, dynamic). For small magnifications, the percent gains are additive.

PROBLEMS

1. A +5.00 D lens of diameter 4 cm is located 8 cm in front of an aperture of diameter 2 cm. What is the entrance pupil for a real object located 40 cm from the lens?
2. A +9.00 D lens of diameter 4 cm is located 10 cm in front of an aperture of diameter 2 cm. What is the entrance pupil for a real object located 50 cm from the lens?
3. A +6.50 D lens is located 10 cm in front of a −3.50 D lens. A small aperture is located midway between the lenses. For a distant object, the aperture is the aperture stop. Find the entrance pupil and the exit pupil.
4. A 9× Keplerian telescope has a +4.00 D objective lens located 27.78 cm in front of a +36.00 D ocular lens. If the objective lens is the aperture stop, find the entrance pupil and the exit pupil.
5. An eye has a +44.00 D cornea located 3.7 mm in front of a 3 mm pupil. Assume the cornea and aqueous humor both have a 1.336 refractive index. Locate the entrance pupil and give its size.
6. A hyperope has a +5.75 D spectacle correction worn at a 10 mm vertex distance. What is the spectacle magnification in terms of the percent gain or loss? (Assume the entrance pupil is 3 mm behind the cornea.)
7. A myope has a −7.25 D spectacle correction worn at a 12 mm vertex distance. What is the spectacle magnification in terms of the percent gain or loss? (Assume the entrance pupil is 3 mm behind the cornea.)
8. An afocal lens ($n = 1.50$) has a +12.00 D front surface, a 5 mm central thickness, and a −12.50 D back surface. Verify that the equivalent and back vertex powers are zero. Find the shape factor of the spectacle magnification for this lens. Report it as a percent gain or loss.
9. Mary Proudfoot needs a −5.00 D spectacle lens at a 10 mm vertex distance. The lens ($n = 1.58$) used has a +4.00 D front surface power and a 4 mm central thickness. Give the shape factor, power factor, and total spectacle magnification. (Assume the entrance pupil is 3 mm behind the cornea.)
10. Antonio Termite wears a +6.00 D spectacle correction ($n = 1.53$) with a +12.50 D front surface power and an 8.0 mm central thickness. For a 10 mm vertex distance, give the shape factor, power factor, and total spectacle magnification. (Assume the entrance pupil is 3 mm behind the cornea.)
11. Rowena Meadowbrook has a −5.00 D spectacle correction ($n = 1.523$) for her left eye. The vertex distance is 10 mm, the front surface power is +2.00 D, and the central thickness is 2.3 mm. Due to an *aniseikonia* problem, Rowena needs an increase of 3% in her spectacle magnification for this lens. Specify a lens fit at the same vertex distance that could provide the additional 3% gain. You may use the small magnification approximations.
12. Sam Fox is an axial hyperope with a +8.00 D spectacle correction worn at a 10 mm vertex distance. Sam's entrance pupil is 3 mm behind his cornea, and his primary principal plane is 1.34 mm behind the cornea. What is the RSM? Compare this result to that of a refractive hyperope with the same correction.
13. Millie Yuppie is an axial myope with a −9.00 D spectacle correction at a 10 mm vertex distance. Millie's entrance pupil is 3 mm behind her cornea, and her primary principal plane is 1.44 mm behind her cornea. What is the RSM? Compare this result to that of a refractive myope with the same correction.
14. Consider a thin lens and screen model for an emmetrope eye. The entrance pupil and the principal planes are both located at the thin lens representing the eye. For a distant object the retinal image is clear without any lenses in front of the eye. Suppose a −2.00 D lens is placed 14 mm in front of the lens representing the eye. By accommodation, the retinal image would again be clear. How much larger or smaller (percent gain or percent loss) is the retinal image for the accommodated state versus the retinal image for the unaccommodated state. (Hint: You could consider the accommodation as a refractive error and the −2.00 D lens as the correction.) This example gives an indication of retinal image size changes when a patient is over-minused.
15. A meridional telescope consists of a +2.00 × 90 objective lens located 40.00 cm in front of a −10.00 × 90 ocular lens. List the magnification in the horizontal and vertical meridians. Describe how a distant square would appear through the telescope.
16. An afocal telescope has a 20 cm length, and a +4.00 ◯ −1.00 × 90 objective lens. What is the magnification of the telescope in each meridian? What are the parameters of the ocular lens?
17. Ryan O'Coughin has a +10.00 ◯ −4.00 × 90 spectacle correction at a 12 mm vertex distance. What is the spectacle magnification (percent loss or percent gain) in each principal meridian? When spectacle corrected, Ryan looks at a distance square. Is Ryan's retinal image a square, a rectangle longer vertically than horizontally, or a rectangle that is longer horizontally than vertically. (Assume the entrance pupil is 3 mm behind the cornea.)
18. Mary Spack wears a −7.50 ◯ −6.00 × 180 spectacle correction at a 13 mm vertex distance. What is the spectacle magnification percent gain or loss in each principal meridian? Is Mary's retinal image of a distant square a rectangle? If so, which side is larger? (Assume Mary's entrance pupil is 3 mm behind his cornea.)
19. A distant square has horizontal and vertical sides. Cheri Tree views the square through her +2.00 ◯ −5.00 × 135 spectacle lens. Cheri's vertex distance is 12 mm, and the entrance pupil is 3 mm behind the cornea. Give the spectacle magnification percent loss or percent gain in each principal meridian. Is Cheri's retinal image a square, a rectangle, or a parallelogram? (Hint: Consider the magnification for the diagonals of the square.)

CHAPTER 19

Stops and Related Effects

19.1 FIELD OF VIEW—TWO COMPONENT SYSTEMS

The field of view of an optical system is the extent of the object plane that is imaged by the system. For example, stand on one side of a room and look out a window on the opposite side. The amount of the outside world that you can see through the window is your field of view (maybe two cars where one is parked to the left of the other). A smaller window would give you a smaller field of view (maybe one car), and a larger window would give you a larger field of view (maybe three cars). For a fixed window size, you can increase your field of view by walking towards the window. Specifically, if your field is two cars when you are on the opposite side of the room from the window, your field might be three cars when you are in the middle of the room, and your field continues to increase as you walk still closer to the window. Once you stick your head through the (open) window, it no longer limits your field of view. Thus both the size of the window and your distance from the window play a role in limiting the field of view.

An optical system needs at least two separated components to limit the field of view. The window and your eye constitute the two components in the previous paragraph. For two component systems, one of the components is the system's aperture stop (defined in Section 18.1). The other component is called the field stop. The *field stop* works in conjunction with the aperture stop to limit the system's field of view.

The entrance and exit pupils are the object and image space images of the aperture stop. Similarly, the entrance and exit ports are the object and image space images of the field stop. In principle, the entrance port is the image of the field stop as seen from the object plane. More formally, *the entrance port is the image of the field stop formed by any lenses in front of it.* When there are no lenses in front of the field stop, then the field stop itself is (in principle) visible from the object plane, and so the field stop also serves as the entrance port.

In principle, the exit port is the image of the field stop as seen from the image plane. More formally, *the exit port is the image of the field stop formed by any lenses behind it.* When there are no lenses behind the field stop, it is (in principle) visible from the image plane, and here the field stop also serves as the exit port. (Some authors use the terms entrance and exit window instead of entrance and exit port.)

Figure 19.1 shows an iris diaphragm I located some distance in front of a thin lens P. (An ideal iris diaphragm has a circular aperture that can be varied in diameter.) The iris diaphragm is set at a semidiameter that is larger than the semidiameter of the lens. (As in Chapter 18, we use the word semidiameter instead of radius to avoid confusion with the radius of curvature.) For a distant object, the lens (rim) is the aperture stop, and therefore the iris diaphragm I must be the field stop. Since neither has a lens in front of it, the lens P also serves as the entrance pupil and the iris diaphragm I also serves as the entrance port.

In Figure 19.1a, the rays (shown as dashed) incident parallel to the axis come from the distant axial object point A and after passing through the lens form the conjugate image point A'. In the paraxial region, there are object points on either side of the point A for which the same amount of light (luminous flux) passes through the system. The object point B is the farthest point above A for which this occurs. The incident rays (shown as solid) from the distant point B are parallel to each but make an angle with the optical axis. After passing through the lens, these rays form the conjugate image point B'. The top bounding ray for this bundle is the ray that grazes the top edge of the entrance port (the iris diaphragm I) and is incident at the top edge of the entrance pupil (the lens P). For both image points A' and B', the entire entrance pupil (the lens) is filled with light. Therefore when the

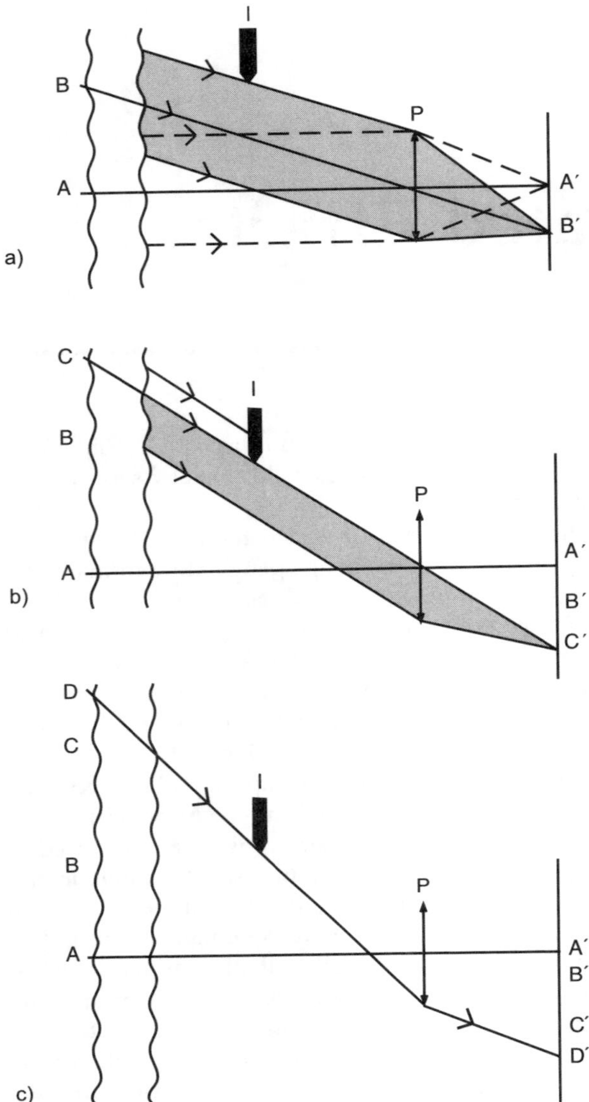

Figure 19.1 For a distant object, an iris diaphragm *I* is in front of a lens *P*. *I* is the field stop (and entrance port) and *P* is the aperture stop (and entrance pupil). The vertical wavy lines represent a large distance: a, the light from object point *B* fills the entire lens; b, the light from object point *C* fills half the entrance pupil *P*; c, only one ray from object point *D* gets through to the image plane.

paraxial object points *A* and *B* have the same luminance, the image points *A′* and *B′* have the same illuminance. This same illuminance also occurs for the image points between *A′* and *B′* (i.e., for object points between *A* and *B*). However for object points that are higher than *B*, the illuminance at the image plane decreases since the iris diaphragm *I* now blocks some of the rays (Figure 19.1b). The set of object points that range from *B* to *A* together with the symmetric set below the optical axis constitutes the *field of uniform illumination*.

Figure 19.1b shows off-axis rays that come from a distant object point *C* that is above point *B*. After passing through the lens, these rays form the conjugate image point *C′*, which is below *B′*. The top bounding ray in the bundle from *C* is the ray that grazes the top edge of the entrance port (the iris diaphragm *I*) and goes to the center of the entrance pupil (the lens *P*). Recall that the chief ray is the incident ray that points towards the center of the entrance pupil, so the top bounding ray here is the chief ray for the bundle from object point *C*. In the cross sectional view of Figure 19.1b, the rays that pass through the entrance pupil (the lens *P*) only fill up half of it. In that sense, the illuminance at *C′* is only half of the cross sectional illuminance of the image points *A′* and *B′*. So for image points below *B′*, the illuminance start to decrease and is down to the 50% level at *C′*. The set of object points from *C* to *A* above the optical axis together with the symmetric set below the axis constitutes the *field of at least one-half illumination* (or the field of at least 50% illumination).

For object points that are higher than *C*, even less light gets through the system. Figure 19.1c shows an incident ray coming from a distant object point *D* that grazes the top of the entrance port (the iris diaphragm *I*) and after passing through the bottom edge of the entrance pupil (the lens *P*) goes to the conjugate image point *D′*. Out of all the rays leaving the point *D*, this ray is the only ray that gets through the system. Any rays above this ray miss the top of the entrance port (are blocked by the iris diaphragm) and any rays below this ray miss the bottom edge of the entrance pupil (do not go through the lens). The object point *D* is the highest object point for which any light gets through the system. For object points between *D* and *A*, more than one ray gets through the system. The set of object points from *D* to the axial point *A* together with the symmetric set below the optical axis constitutes the *total field of view*.

Figure 19.2 shows the illuminance behavior across the image plane. The illuminance is uniform (constant) from *A′* to *B′*, then starts decreasing and is at one-half of the maximum at *C′*, and then falls to zero for points outside of *D′*. The plot is symmetric for image points above the optical axis, in which case the conjugate object points are below the optical axis. The fall-off in illumination for points away from the optical axis is referred as *vignetting*.

The uniform field, the field of at least one-half illumination, and the total field of view are the most frequently used fields to specify the field of view.

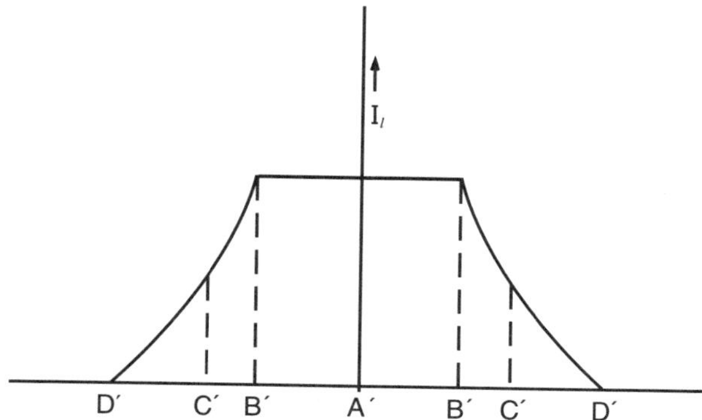

Figure 19.2 The illuminance fall-off in the image plane of the system in Figure 19.1.

However, when needed, other fields can be specified (e.g., the field of at least 70% illumination, etc.).

A criticism of the total field of view is that it may be too liberal for some situations. If only one ray gets through the system, the conjugate image point D' may be below the threshold of the system to detect and as such is not useful. On the other hand, a criticism of the uniform field of view is that it may be too conservative. The bounding image point C' for the field of at least one-half illumination is not in the uniform field, but may be a perfectly useful image point even though its illuminance is decreased relative to that of the image points in the uniform field. The field of at least one-half illumination is the compromise choice for the *conventional field of view*, and the words "field of view" without any other identification refer to the field of at least one-half illumination.

The following exercise is a way to visualize how vignetting occurs. Stand about 2 m from a window and look centrally through it at a somewhat distant neighboring building. Pick out a centrally located distant window that is completely visible through your window (or use some other object to imagine a window). Assume that one of your eyes in glowing (like in an imaginary movie), and think of your glowing eye as the object point for the system that consists of the two windows. (If you like, you can imagine a Fresnel plus lens that fills the neighboring window and forms a real image of your glowing eye on a screen inside the neighboring house.) The amount of light from your centrally located glowing eye that gets through this two-window system is limited by the size of the neighboring window. So the neighboring window is the system's aperture stop, and your window is the system's field stop. Now move to your left until the left edge of the neighboring window appears to be lined up with the left edge of your window. At this position, you can still see the entire neighboring window through your window, hence the light from your glowing eye can still fill up all of the neighboring window. This position is the limit of the field of uniform illumination for your glowing eye. When you move farther to the left, you can no longer see all of the neighboring window and thus the light from your glowing eye can no longer fill up all of the neighboring window. Continue to move left until you can see exactly half of the neighboring window. This is the limit of the field of at least one-half illumination for your glowing eye, since now the light from it can fill up only half of the neighboring window. Now move still further to the left until the only part of the neighboring window that you can see is a sliver sandwiched between the left edge of your window and the right edge of the neighboring window. Light from your glowing eye can now only get through this sliver, and your glowing eye is at the limit of the total field of view for the two-window system. When you move still further to the left, you can no longer see the neighboring window and so no light from your glowing eye can get through the two-window system.

For all but relatively near objects, it is convenient to specify the field of view in angular terms. Figure 19.3a shows an entrance port G with a semidiameter a located a distance d_p in front of an entrance pupil E with a semidiameter b. The line that passes through the top edge of the entrance port and the top edge of the entrance pupil specifies the bounding ray for the field of uniform illumination. This bounding ray makes an angle of $F_u/2$ with the axis, where F_u is the total angular size of the field of uniform illumination. An easy way to find an equation for F_u is to start at the top edge of the entrance pupil and draw a line parallel to the optical axis (shown as dashed in Figure 19.3a). The angle α between this line and the bounding ray is equal to $F_u/2$. At each position, the new horizontal line is a vertical distance b above the optical axis. Dropping a vertical line from the top edge of the entrance port to the dashed horizontal line forms a right triangle containing α. In the right triangle, the side opposite to α has a length that is equal to a minus b, and the adjacent side has the length d_p between the entrance port and the entrance pupil. It follows that

$$\tan\left(\frac{F_u}{2}\right) = \frac{a-b}{d_p} \tag{19.1}$$

Figure 19.3b shows the bounding ray for the field of at least one-half illumination. This ray grazes the top edge of the entrance port G and goes to the center of the entrance pupil E. The bounding ray makes an angle $F_h/2$ with the optical axis, where F_h is the angular expression for the field of at least one-half

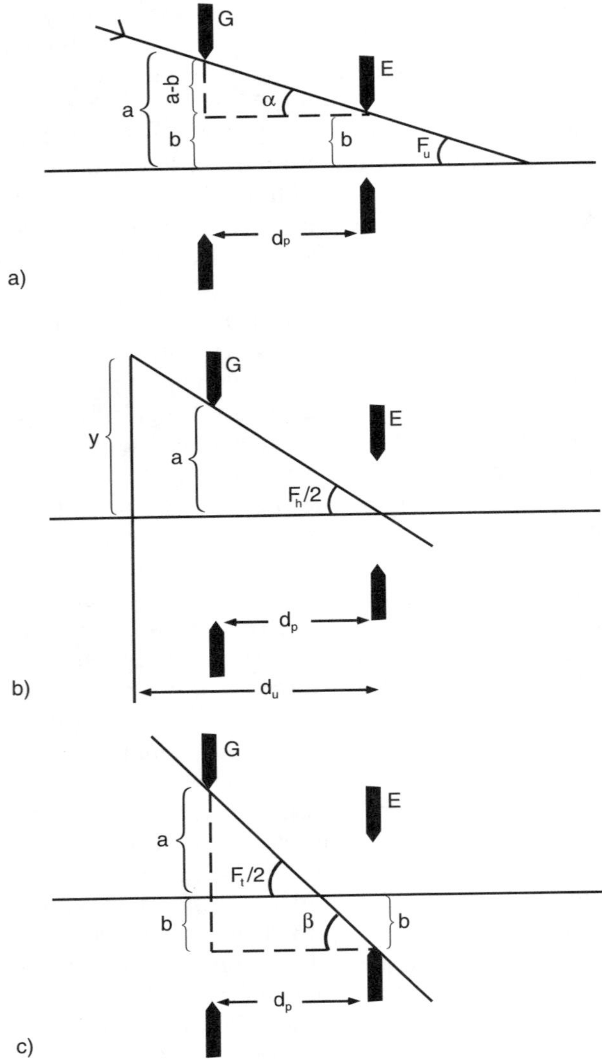

Figure 19.3 An entrance port G with semidiameter b located a distance d_p in front of an entrance pupil E with semidiameter a: a, bounding ray for the field of uniform illumination; b, bounding ray for the field of at least one-half illumination. The object plane is a distance d_u from E, and the bounding object point C is located a distance y above the axis; c, bounding ray for the total field of view.

illumination (i.e., the conventional field of view). When a vertical line is dropped from the top edge of the entrance port to the optical axis, it follows from the right triangle that

$$\tan\left(\frac{F_h}{2}\right) = \frac{a}{d_p} \tag{19.2}$$

Figure 19.3c shows the bounding ray for the total field of view. This ray lies grazes the top edge of the entrance port G and goes to the bottom edge of the entrance pupil E. The bounding ray makes an angle of $F_t/2$ with the optical axis. An easy way to find the equation for $F_t/2$ is to start at the bottom edge of the entrance pupil and draw a line (shown as dashed) parallel to the optical axis. At any position, this line is a vertical distance B below the optical axis. The angle β that this line makes with the bounding ray is equal to $F_h/2$. Dropping a vertical line (shown as dashed) from the top edge of the entrance port to this line forms a right triangle that contains the angle β, and it follows that

$$\tan\left(\frac{F_t}{2}\right) = \frac{a+b}{d_p} \tag{19.3}$$

Equations 19.1 and 19.3 show that F_u and F_t depend on the entrance port semidiameter a, the entrance pupil semidiameter b, and the distance d_p between the entrance port and the entrance pupil. In particular, the total field of view F_t increases as semidiameter b of the entrance pupil increases. Equation 19.2 shows that F_h depends only on the entrance port semidiameter a and the distance d_p. In particular, F_h does not depend on the semidiameter b of the entrance pupil.

EXAMPLE 19.1

Assume that the lens in Figure 19.1 is a +8.00 D lens with a 20 mm diameter, and that the iris diaphragm has a 26 mm diameter and is located 22 cm in front of the lens. Find F_u, F_h, and F_t.

Here $a = 26\,\text{mm}/2 = 13\,\text{mm}$, and $b = 20\,\text{mm}/2 = 10\,\text{mm}$. The distance d_p is 220 mm. From Eq. 19.1,

$$\tan\left(\frac{F_u}{2}\right) = \frac{13\,\text{mm} - 10\,\text{mm}}{220\,\text{mm}} = 0.0136$$

The inverse tangent then gives

$$\frac{F_u}{2} = 0.78^\circ \quad \text{and so} \quad F_u = 1.56^\circ$$

From Eq. 19.2,

$$\tan\left(\frac{F_h}{2}\right) = \frac{13\,\text{mm}}{220\,\text{mm}} = 0.0591$$

The inverse tangent gives

$$\frac{F_h}{2} = 3.38^\circ \quad \text{and so} \quad F_h = 6.76^\circ$$

From Eq. 19.3,

$$\tan\left(\frac{F_t}{2}\right) = \frac{13\,\text{mm} + 10\,\text{mm}}{220\,\text{mm}} = 0.1045$$

The inverse tangent gives

$$\frac{F_t}{2} = 5.97^\circ \quad \text{and so} \quad F_t = 11.94^\circ$$

The three angular fields in the above example have quite different values. Equations 19.1 through 19.3 show that when the entrance port is much larger than the entrance pupil (i.e., $a >> b$), the three fields have values that are very close together. In such cases, the illuminance drops abruptly at the F_u boundary.

The field of view can also be expressed as a linear distance in the object plane. In Figure 19.3b, the object plane is a distance d_u from the entrance pupil, and the top half of the object field (linear size y) subtends the angle $F_h/2$. It follows that

$$\tan\left(\frac{F_h}{2}\right) = \frac{y}{|d_u|} \tag{19.4}$$

In Example 19.1, $F_h/2$ was 3.38°. So for at $d_u = 1000$ m, y is given by

$$y = |d_u| \tan\left(\frac{F_h}{2}\right)$$
$$= (1000\,\text{m}) \tan(3.38^\circ) = 59.1\,\text{m}$$

The top to bottom linear extent of the field is $2y = 118.2$ m. Similarly, for a system with an object at

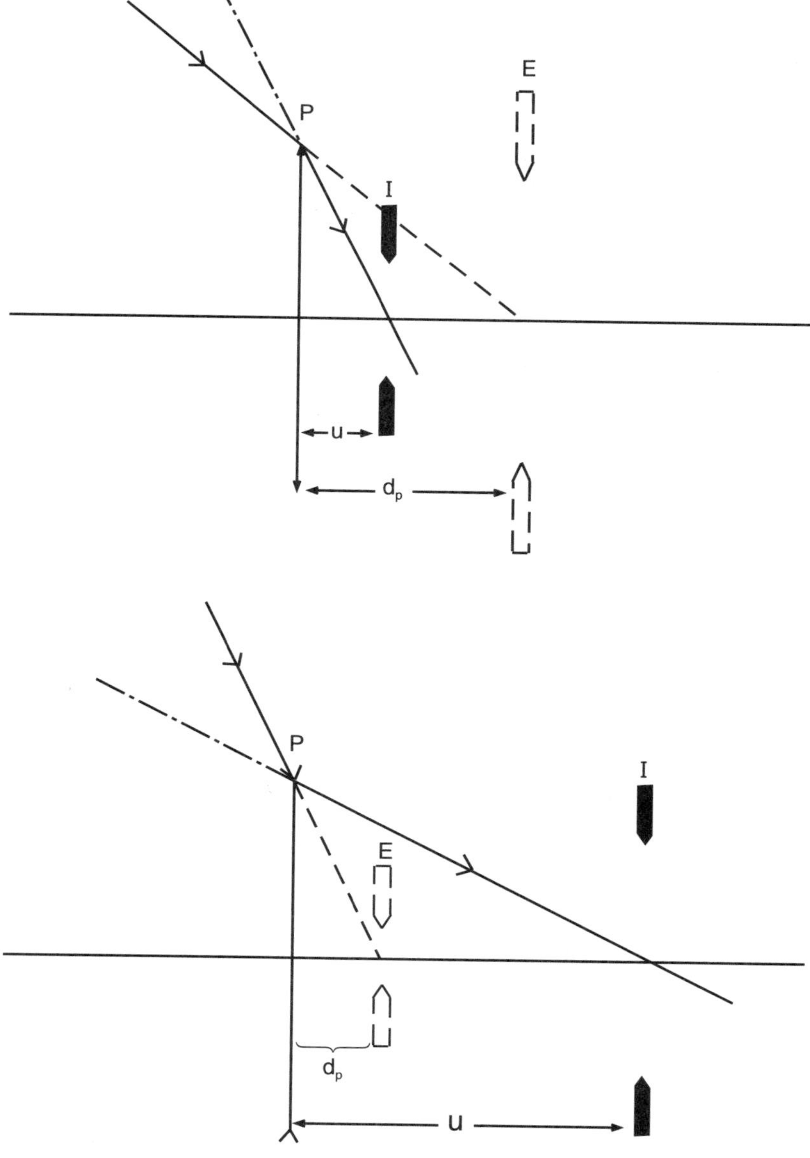

Figure 19.4 A lens P (which is the field stop and entrance port) in front of an iris diaphragm I, where I is the aperture stop. The entrance pupil E is the virtual image of I by the lens. (I could also be an aperture that simulates the entrance pupil of a human eye looking through the lens P.) a, the lens is plus, and the image E is larger and farther from the lens than I; b, the lens is minus, and the image E is closer to the lens and smaller than I.

40 cm and the same F_h, the top to bottom linear field ($2y$) is 4.72 cm. For near objects, the field of view angles are sometimes confusing, and so the linear field of view is especially useful in those cases.

Figure 19.4a shows a thin lens P in front of a smaller iris diaphragm I that is the system's aperture stop. Then by default the lens P must be the field stop. Since the lens is visible from the object plane, it also serves as the entrance port. The aperture stop I is closer to the lens than the focal length of the lens, so it's virtual image E formed by the lens P is the system's entrance pupil. The distance between P and E is d_p. The incident ray that points toward the top edge of the entrance port (the lens P) and the center of the entrance pupil E is the bounding ray for the field of at least one-half illumination. The lens bends this ray so that in image space it physically passes through the center of the aperture stop I.

When the arrows on this ray are reversed, they indicate that for light traveling to the left, an object point at the center of the aperture stop is conjugate to the virtual image point at the center of the entrance pupil. This is consistent with the fact that an observer at the system's object plane sees the image E and not the actual iris diaphragm I.

EXAMPLE 19.2a

Nanook, an uncorrected hyperope, holds a +3.00 D trial lens (diameter 36 mm) 20 cm in front of her eye's entrance pupil (diameter 4 mm) and looks through it to clearly see some distant skyscrapers. When Nanook keeps her eye fixed on the distant axial object point, what is her field of view? (The fixed eye is referred to as a "static" eye. An eye that is allowed to rotate, in order to look around, is a "dynamic" eye.)

The field of view without any other descriptors refers to F_h. We can simulate Nanook's field of view by the two component system shown in Figure 19.4a. Let an aperture I of size 4 mm simulate the entrance pupil of Nanook's eye. The +3.00 D trial lens P is located 20 cm in front of I. In general, either the aperture or the lens rim could be the system's aperture stop. To determine this, we first need to look at the system's entrance pupil candidates.

The entrance pupil candidates are the lens (rim) with a 36 mm diameter, and the image E of the aperture formed by the +3.00 D lens. We find this image as follows. For light traveling to the left: $u = -20.0$ cm, $U = -5.00$ D, $V = -2.00$ D, and $v = -50.0$ cm. The lateral magnification m equals +2.5 (from $m = U/V$), so the image diameter is 10 mm (i.e., +2.5 times 4 mm).

Normally, the entrance pupil candidate that subtends the smallest angle at the axial object point is the entrance pupil. However, *in the limit of a distant object, the smallest entrance pupil candidate is the entrance pupil*. So here the image E, with its 10 mm diameter, is the system's entrance pupil. This makes the aperture I (simulating the entrance pupil of Nanook's eye) the aperture stop, and the +3.00 D lens (P) the field stop. The +3.00 D lens also serves as the entrance port, and its semidiameter a is 18 mm. Note the difference between the entrance pupil of Nanook's eye, simulated by I, and the system's entrance pupil, which is the image E.

The magnitude of the image distance v is the distance d_p, and from Eq. 19.2,

$$\tan\left(\frac{F_h}{2}\right) = \frac{1.8\ \text{cm}}{50\ \text{cm}} = 0.0360$$

The inverse tangent gives

$$\frac{F_h}{2} = 2.06^\circ \quad \text{and so} \quad F_h = 4.12^\circ$$

EXAMPLE 19.2b

Nanook has enough accommodation that she can take the trial lens out of the metal lens rim, and look through the empty lens rim (diameter 36 mm) held 20 cm in front of her entrance pupil to clearly see the distant skyscrapers. What is her (static eye) field of view through the lens rim?

In this situation, the aperture I simulating the entrance pupil of Nanook's eye is also the system's entrance pupil. The empty lens rim serves as both the field stop and the entrance port (so a is still 18 mm), and d_p is now the 20 cm distance between the lens rim and I. The dot-dashed extension of the straight line from the center of I through the lens rim is the boundary for F_h. From Eq. 19.2,

$$\tan\left(\frac{F_h}{2}\right) = \frac{1.8\ \text{cm}}{20\ \text{cm}} = 0.0900$$

The inverse tangent gives

$$\frac{F_h}{2} = 5.14^\circ \quad \text{and so} \quad F_h = 10.28^\circ$$

EXAMPLE 19.2c

What is the spectacle magnification M_p for the +3.00 D thin lens held 20 cm in front of Nanook's entrance pupil, and how does M_p relate to the field of view change in parts a and b?

From Eq. 18.14,

$$M_p = \frac{1}{1 - d_{ben}P_v} = \frac{1}{1 - 0.20\,\text{m}(+3.00\,\text{D})} = \frac{1}{0.40} = 2.50$$

The spectacle magnification shows that Nanook's retinal image is 2.50 times larger when she looks through the +3.00 D as opposed to looking through the empty lens rim, while parts *a* and *b*, show that the +3.00 D lens shrinks Nanook's field of view by a factor of 2.50 (i.e., 10.28°/4.12°). In effect, when Nanook has a larger retinal image, she has a decreased field of view (or can image less of the object space on the same sized retina). (Note that this example is a two-component example with a distant object. For more complicated systems, there is not necessarily such a direct relationship between angular magnification and field of view.)

In general, a hyperope has a larger retinal image size when spectacle corrected than when contact corrected. Similar to the preceding example, this results in a smaller field of view for the hyperope when spectacle corrected as opposed to the field of view when contact corrected. The smaller field of view is a major complaint for spectacle corrected high hyperopes or aphakes.

EXAMPLE 19.3a

Admiral Rich Destiny, an emmetrope, sits at his desk and looks at some distant warships through a porthole of diameter 20 cm. If the entrance pupil of Rich Destiny's eye is 300 cm from the porthole, what is the field of view for the static eye?

Here we can simulate the situation with a two component system by representing the entrance pupil of Destiny's eye by an aperture placed 300 cm from the porthole. The aperture serves both as the system's aperture stop and entrance pupil, while the porthole serves both as the system's field stop and entrance port.

From Eq. 19.2,

$$\tan\left(\frac{F_h}{2}\right) = \frac{10\,\text{cm}}{300\,\text{cm}} = 0.0333$$

and

$$F_h = 3.81°$$

EXAMPLE 19.3b

A −2.00 D Fresnel lens (20 cm diameter) is now mounted in the porthole. What is Rich Destiny's new field of view for (static eye) while he is sitting at the same desk?

The ray diagram in Figure 19.4b shows that the minus lens increases the field of view. In this case, the porthole remains the system's field stop and entrance port. The aperture *I* simulating Rich Destiny's eye is the system's aperture stop, and the system's entrance pupil *E* is the virtual image *E* of the aperture *I* formed by the −2.00 D Fresnel lens. For the image location (light traveling left) $u = -300$ cm, $U = -0.33$ D, $V = -2.33$ D, and $v = -42.86$ cm. The entrance pupil *E* is virtual and 42.86 cm behind the porthole. The porthole (semidiameter $a = 10$ cm) is still the field stop and entrance port. From Eq. 19.2,

$$\tan\left(\frac{F_h}{2}\right) = \frac{10\,\text{cm}}{42.86\,\text{mm}} = 0.2333$$

and

$$F_h = 26.3°$$

This angle is somewhat outside the paraxial zone. For an "idealized" paraxial (or first order) comparison purposes with the spectacle magnification, one should use the small angle approximation to the tangent. Here the small angle approximation gives 26.7° for F_h.

EXAMPLE 19.3c

What is the spectacle magnification M_p for the −3.00 D Fresnel lens that is 300 cm in front of Destiny's entrance pupil, and how does M_p relate to the field of view change in parts a and b?

The spectacle magnification (Eq. 18.14) for a −2.00 D lens located 300 cm in front of the person is

$$M_p = \frac{1}{1 - d_{ben}P_v} = \frac{1}{1 - 3.0\,\text{m}(-2.00\,\text{D})} = \frac{1}{7.0} = 0.143$$

The −2.00 D Fresnel lens decreases Destiny's retinal image by a factor of 7, and at the same time it increases his field of view by a factor of 7 (i.e., from parts a and b, 26.7°/3.8°).

The above example shows how a diverging (minus) lens increases the field of view. Large diameter minus Fresnel lenses are sometimes used on the backs of vans or motor-homes to increase the field of view of the driver while backing up.

Similarly, convex (diverging) mirrors are frequently used to increase the field of view. One common example is the security mirrors in stores. Another common example is the side mirror on the passenger side of a car. This side mirror is usually a diverging mirror that forms a smaller, erect, virtual image, and the smaller image results in a larger field of view. A driver glancing in the center rear view plane mirror (lateral magnification +1, so the image size equals the object size) may make a judgement as to how close the following car is based on the image size seen in the mirror. The same driver glancing at the passenger side mirror is looking at the smaller virtual image, and may therefore judge a following car to be farther away than it actually is. Because of this, a warning decal stating "Objects in the mirror are closer than they appear" is often on the side mirror.

EXAMPLE 19.4

Cola Swig looks through a +20.50 D thin lens (diameter 30 mm) at a real object that is 200 cm in front of the lens. Cola holds the lens so that the entrance pupil of her eye is 50 cm from the lens. What is Cola's field of view through the lens, and how does it compare to Cola's field through the empty lens rim at the same position?

As before, Cola's eye can be simulated by an aperture placed at the entrance pupil of her eye. Assume that this aperture is small enough to be the system's aperture stop.

For the empty lens rim case, the lens rim is the system's field stop and entrance port, while the simulating aperture is the system's aperture stop and entrance pupil. Then in Eq. 19.2, $a = 1.5\,\text{cm}$, $d_p = 50\,\text{cm}$. So

$$\tan\left(\frac{F_h}{2}\right) = \frac{1.5\,\text{cm}}{50\,\text{cm}} = 0.030$$

and F_h is 3.44°

For the +20.50 D lens case: the lens is the field stop and the entrance port, and the image of the simulating aperture by the +20.50 D lens is the entrance pupil. Here for light going left, $u = -50.0\,\text{cm}$, $U = -2.00\,\text{D}$, $V = +18.50\,\text{D}$, and $v = +5.41\,\text{cm}$. Then in Eq. 19.2, $a = 1.5\,\text{cm}$, $d_p = 5.41\,\text{cm}$. So

$$\tan\left(\frac{F_h}{2}\right) = \frac{1.5\,\text{cm}}{5.41\,\text{cm}} = 0.28$$

and F_h is 31.0°

Note that for the object at $u = -200\,\text{cm}$ (light going right), the +20.50 D lens forms a conjugate real, image (inverted and much smaller) at $v = +5\,\text{cm}$ behind it with a lateral magnification m of -0.025 (i.e., v/u). Cola is actually looking at this small real image as an aerial image, and this results in her much larger field of view with the lens (compared to without the lens). (This example is similar to how an indirect ophthalmoscope, Section 19.8, provides a larger field of view.)

For a unique field stop, Eqs. 19.1 through 19.3 give the angular expressions for the *object space field of view*. In Figure 19.1, the image points B', C', and D' were limits to the linear field of view as expressed in image space. Equations for angular *image space field of view* have the same structure as Eqs. 19.1 through 19.3. The difference is that in the image space equations, the exit port appears instead of the entrance port, the exit pupil appears instead of the entrance pupil, and the distance is between the exit port and the exit pupil.

19.2 FIELD OF VIEW OF A THIN COLLIMATING MAGNIFIER

Consider the linear field of a plus thin lens used as a collimating magnifier. Figure 19.5 shows a two component simulation. In the simulation, the aperture I represents the entrance pupil of the observer's eye and is the system's aperture stop. The magnifier P is the system's field stop (and entrance port). In Figure 19.5,

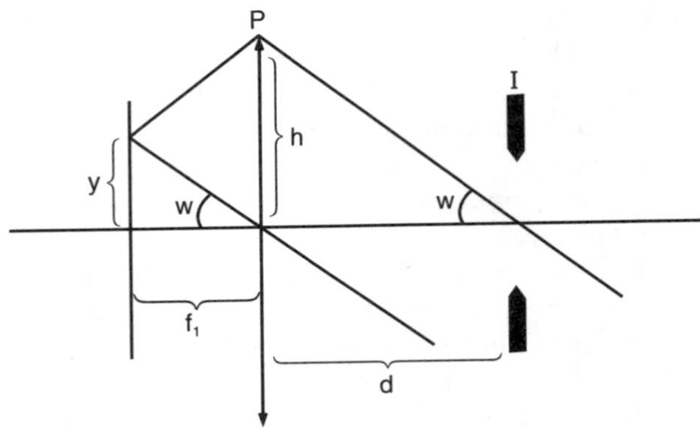

Figure 19.5 A collimating magnifier P (semidiameter h) at a distance d in front of an iris diaphragm I that is simulating the entrance pupil of an observer's eye. The object plane is a distance f_1 from the lens. The lens semidiameter is h, and the distance y is the top half of the linear field of view in object space.

the top object point in the linear field is a distance y above the optical axis, the magnifier's semidiameter is h, and the aperture simulating the observer's eye is a distance d from the magnifier. Since the object is in the primary focal plane of the magnifier ($u = f_1$), all of the rays leaving the magnifier are parallel to the nodal ray, and all subtend an angle of magnitude w at the optical axis. We could go ahead and find the system's entrance pupil (which is to the left of the object plane) and then use Eq. 19.2 to find the angular field. However, the linear field is more useful in this case and is easy to find by using the tangents of the angles w.

In the image space of the magnifier, the bounding ray for the field of at least one half illumination extends from the top of the magnifier to the center of the aperture I, and subtends the angle w there. From the triangle involving this ray,

$$|\tan w| = h/d$$

For the object point at y, the nodal ray subtends the angle w at the optical center of the lens. From the triangle involving this ray,

$$|\tan w| = y/(-f_1) = y/f_2$$

We can equate the right hand sides of these two equations to obtain

$$y = \frac{f_2 h}{d} \qquad (19.5)$$

or

$$y = \frac{h}{dP} \qquad (19.6)$$

where $P = 1/f_2$ is the dioptric power of the magnifier. The whole linear field of view is $2y$, and $2h$ is the diameter of the lens, so it follows that

$$\text{linear field of view} = \frac{\text{lens diameter}}{dP} \qquad (19.7)$$

This equation shows that the linear field of the magnifier depends directly on the size of the lens, inversely on the distance d between the eye and the magnifier, and inversely on the dioptric power P of the magnifier. Since for a collimating magnifier, $M = |u_e|P$, the linear field also depends inversely on the angular magnification M. In particular, when the power is doubled to increase the magnification, the field of view is cut in half.

EXAMPLE 19.5

Judge Judi Lee-Gall uses a +28.00 D thin lens as a collimating magnifier. The lens has a 36 mm diameter and Judge Judi holds it 15 cm from the entrance pupil of her eye. What is the conventional angular magnification and the total linear field of view?

From $M = P/4$, the magnification is 7.0×. From Eq. 19.7,

$$\text{linear field of view} = \frac{3.6\,\text{cm}}{15\,\text{cm}(+28.00\,\text{D})} = 8.57 \times 10^{-3}\,\text{m} = 8.57\,\text{mm}$$

Note that Judge Judi can substantially increase her field of view by moving her eye closer to the magnifier.

19.3 MULTI-COMPONENT SYSTEMS

In optical systems where there are more than two components, one component serves as the aperture stop, but there are still several possibilities for the field stop. *In general, the field stop is the aperture or lens rim that together with the aperture stop is most effective at limiting the field of view.* One complication though is that a system, such as that in Figure 19.6, may not have a unique field stop.

Figure 19.6 shows two iris diaphragms, A and B in front of a lens P. For distant objects, the lens P is the system's aperture stop and entrance pupil. Ray #1, which grazes the top edge of A and goes to the top edge of P, is the top bounding ray for the field of uniform illumination (F_u). So the iris diaphragm A serves as the entrance port in this situation. (Since A is not an image, it is also the system's field stop in this situation.)

If A is also the entrance port for the field of at least one-half illumination (F_h), the top bounding ray would lie along line #2, which grazes the top edge of A and goes to the center of P. However, an incident ray along line #2 would be blocked by iris diaphragm B. Therefore, for F_h, iris diaphragm B serves as the entrance port, and the top bounding ray grazes the top edge of B and goes to the center of P (ray #3). Note that as a function of increasing subtended angles of the off-axis object points, there is an angle at which the entrance port switches from A to B. (In this case since A and B are not images, this means that there is an angle at which the field stop switches from A to B.)

Figure 19.7 shows a plot of the image plane illuminance for a case with a field stop switch. The illuminance is constant from A' to B', and then starts to fall off at B'. At the position C' that corresponds to the field stop switch, the fall off in illuminance abruptly

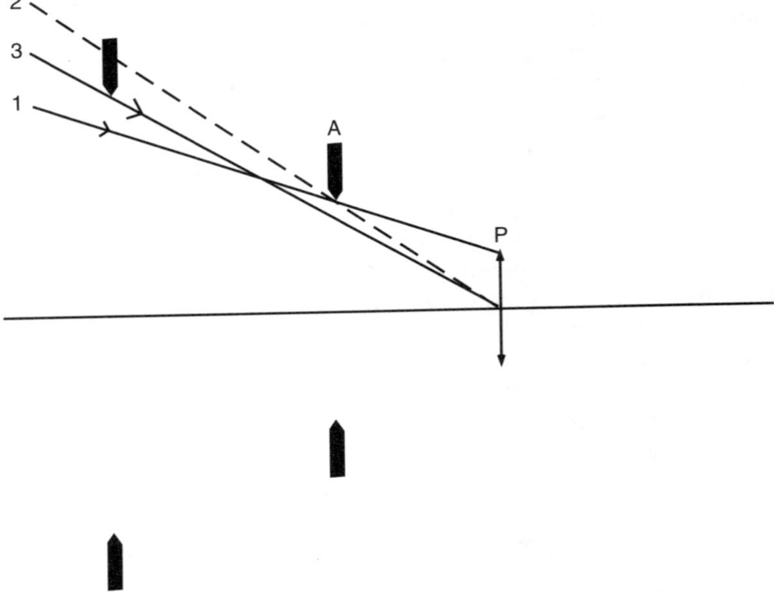

Figure 19.6 Two diaphragms, *B* and *A*, in front of a lens *P*, which is the aperture stop. Ray 1 is the bounding ray for the uniform field of view, while ray 3 is the bounding ray for the field of at least one-half illumination.

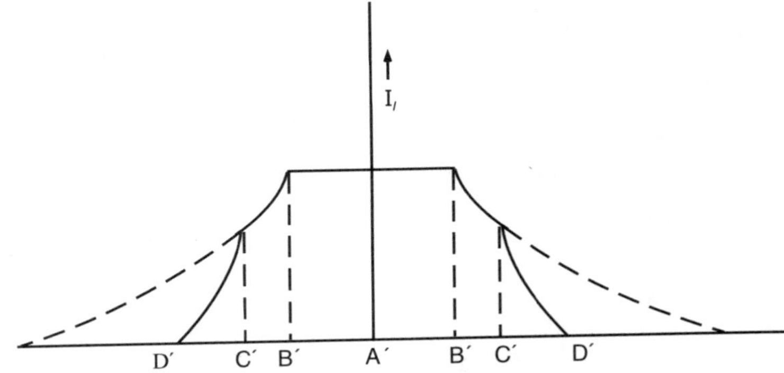

Figure 19.7 The fall-off in illuminance in the image plane for the system in Figure 19.6.

increases. The dashed line shows the "no switch" fall-off in illuminance that would occur if iris diaphragm *B* was not present.

Consider a general case in which there is a different entrance port for each of the fields F_u, F_h, and F_t. (Ray tracing is one way to determine this.) Let a_u be the semidiameter of the entrance port for F_u, and d_u be its location from the entrance pupil. Let a_h be the semidiameter of the entrance port for F_h, and d_h be its location from the entrance pupil. Let a_t be semidiameter of the entrance port for the total field of view, and d_t be its location from the entrance pupil. Then Eqs. 19.1 through 19.3 switch to

$$\tan\left(\frac{F_u}{2}\right) = \frac{a_u - b}{d_u} \quad (19.8)$$

$$\tan\left(\frac{F_h}{2}\right) = \frac{a_h}{d_h} \quad (19.9)$$

and

$$\tan\left(\frac{F_t}{2}\right) = \frac{a_t + b}{d_t} \quad (19.10)$$

When there is a unique entrance port and a unique field stop for the system, then the same *a* and *d* values can be used, and Eqs. 19.8 through 19.10 respectively reduce to Eqs. 19.1 through 19.3.

Figure 19.8a shows a two lens system that has vignetting. Each lens is a +10.00 D equal diameter lens, and the lenses are separated by 40 cm. The object (top point *O*) is 20 cm in front of the first lens, and has a size equal to that of the first lens. An internal real image (bottom point I_1), inverted and the same size as the object, is formed 20 cm behind the first lens (i.e., this is the symmetry point situation: $u = -2f_1$, $v = 2f_2$, and $m = -1$). The internal real image is the object for the second lens, and it forms a real image (top point I_2)

Figure 19.8 a, A two lens system with vignetting. O is the top object point that bounds the total field of view. I_1 is the conjugate internal image point, and I_2 is the final image point. Note that only one ray gets through the system from O. A is the image of lens 2 by lens 1, and can be considered the entrance port. H is the bounding object point for the field of at least one-half illumination; b, the field lens L_F eliminates the vignetting. O is now the bounding point for the field of uniform illumination. Note that now all the rays that get through L_1 also get through L_2.

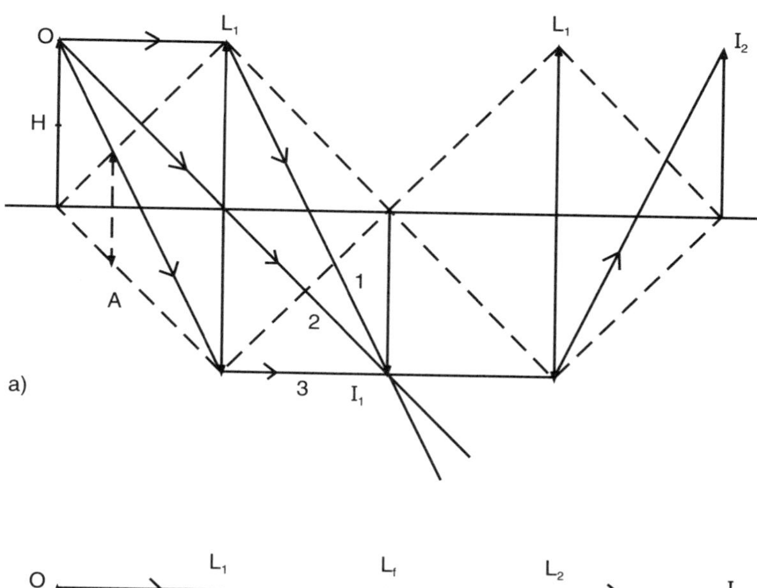

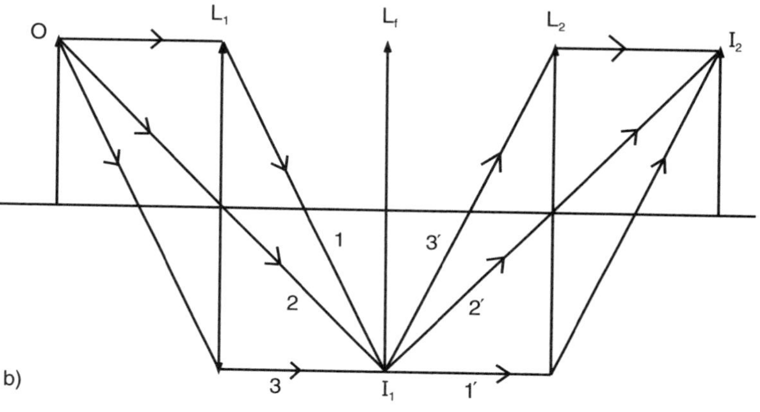

20 cm behind it. The final image I_2 is erect and the same size as the original object O.

The dashed rays from the axial object point show that the two lenses tie for the system's aperture stop. In this case, we can pick either one as the aperture stop and the other acts as the field stop. When we pick the first lens as the aperture stop, then it also serves as the entrance pupil. The second lens is then the field stop, and its inverted image A by the first lens is the entrance port. Since the dashed rays from the axial object point pass through the edges of the second lens (after passing through the edges of the first lens), the incident dashed rays also pass through the edges of the entrance port A (principle of conjugacy). These rays are therefore the bounding rays for the field of uniform illumination, and only the axial object point is in the field of uniform illumination. In other words, for non-axial object points, the illumination starts falling off immediately. A ray (not shown) that passes through the top edge of the entrance port A and goes to the center of the entrance pupil (lens 1) is the bounding ray for the top part of the field of at least one-half illumination, and the corresponding object point is H.

The bounding ray for the top part of the total field of view is the solid ray from the top object point O that passes through the top edge of the entrance port and goes to the bottom edge of the lens. This ray (labeled as 3) comes out of the first lens parallel to the axis, goes through the internal real image position, is incident on the bottom edge of the second lens, and then goes to the top point I_2 on the final image. Any rays leaving point O below ray 3 miss the first lens, and any rays leaving point O above ray 3 miss the entrance port, and hence the field stop (the second lens). In particular, the rays labeled 1 and 2 both miss the second lens.

The vignetting in this case can be minimized or eliminated by placing a plus thin lens, called a *field lens*, at the internal real image position. The optimum field lens images the second lens at the position of the first lens (Figure 19.8b). (This field lens would also be a +10.00 D lens.) The image of the second lens by the field lens is inverted, so that the bottom edge of the second lens is imaged at the top edge of the first lens. For the light passing through the system from the object point O, the internal real image I_1 is the object for the field lens. For the field lens, u is zero, v is zero, m is $+1$, and the field lens has no effect on the location or size of the final image I_2. Note that the base up prism in the bottom section of the field lens bends ray 1, which is coming from the top of the first lens, up so that it travels parallel to the axis (ray now labeled 1′) and passes through the bottom edge of the second lens. Similarly ray 2, which is coming from the optical center of the first lens, is bent up by the field lens (ray now labeled 2′) and travels through the optical center of the second lens. Ray 3, which is traveling parallel to the axis from the bottom edge of the first lens, is bent up by the field lens (ray now labeled 3′) and travels to the top edge of the second lens. For the light leaving the top object point O, the rays that fill the entire first lens (the entrance pupil) now all get through the second lens (and in fact fill the second lens). In that sense, the illumination at the image point I_2 is the same as the illumination at the axial image point!

The prism base directions of the plus field lens all point towards the optical center, so the same effect occurs in all meridians. Hence the entire object bounded by O on the top and a symmetric point on the bottom is in the field of uniform illumination. Object points beyond O are outside the field of view, so there is a sharp field cutoff at O.

The field lens eliminated the vignetting in this system. Another way of phrasing this is that the field lens increased the field of uniform illumination (bounding point now O), and also increased the field of at least one-half illumination (from object point H to O). In the three lens system, the first and the third lenses are still tied for the aperture stop, but the field lens is now the field stop. Since the field lens is at the internal real image position, it is conjugate to the object for the first lens, and conjugate to the final image for the second lens. Therefore, the system's entrance port is at the object position and the exit port is at the final image position.

An internal real image is conjugate to a system's final image. Therefore when the field lens is at an internal real image position, any dust or scratches on it are also imaged at the final image plane. Therefore in practice, the field lens is usually displaced a little away from the internal real image position.

There is another way to minimize or eliminate vignetting, but it does not increase the field of view. This way is simply to place an appropriately sized stop at or near the final image position, or at or near an internal real image position. The size of the stop is such that it blocks the light from all field points outside the

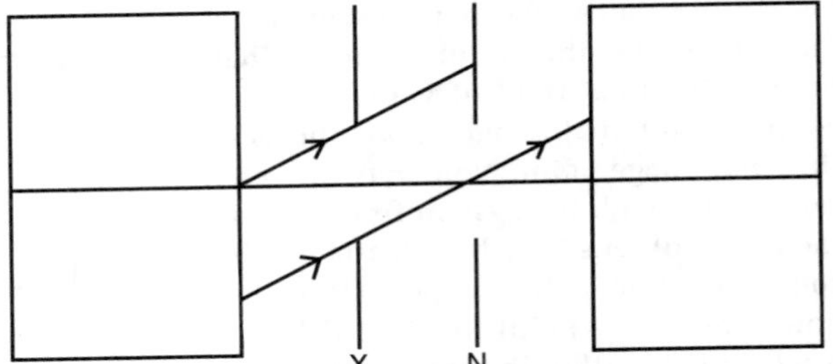

Figure 19.9 ***X*** **is the exit pupil of the first system and** ***N*** **is the entrance pupil of the second system. Vignetting occurs between the two systems even though** ***N*** **is the same size as** ***X*****.**

field of uniform illumination. This provides a sharp cut-off of the field of view at the boundary of the field of uniform illumination.

An optical system in general may consist of several sub-systems that are being used together. Figure 19.9 shows two sub-systems in which the entrance pupil N of the second sub-system is the same size as the exit pupil X of the first sub-system. However since N is some distance behind X, not all of the light that goes through X gets through N, and there is vignetting between the two systems. We can maximize the amount of the light that gets through both systems by placing N at the same place as X. This is called *pupil matching*.

In general, there is an inverse type relationship between field of view and magnification. The solid curve in Figure 19.10 represents the decreasing field

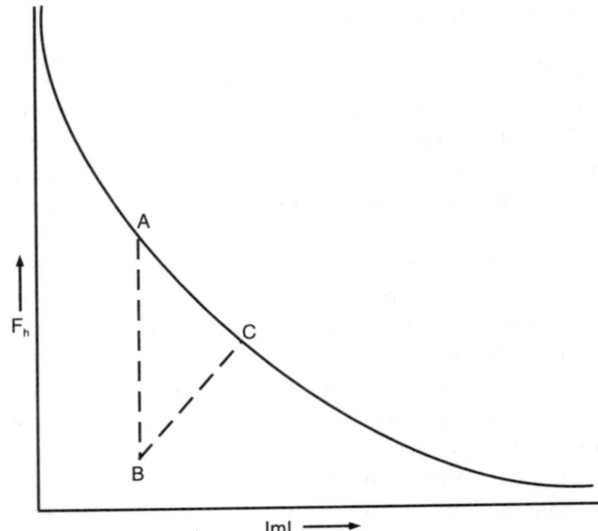

Figure 19.10 Relationships between the angular field of view F_h **and the magnification** m**.**

of view F_h with increasing magnification m for maximally efficient systems (e.g., A to C). However if only the central part of the field is of interest, one can always put a new aperture in a system that decreases the field of view without changing the magnification (e.g., A to B). When one starts with a reduced field system, one can increase both the field of view and the magnification until the boundary for maximally efficient systems is reached (e.g., B to C).

19.4 TELESCOPE ENTRANCE AND EXIT PUPILS

Two lens Keplerian telescopes have a plus objective lens (power P_{obj}) and a plus ocular lens (power P_{oc}). The apparent image seen through the Keplerian telescope is magnified and inverted. Figure 19.11a shows rays parallel to the axis incident on a Keplerian telescope. The emerging ray bundle has a smaller diameter than the incident ray bundle, and the objective lens is the telescope's aperture stop. The exit pupil X is the image of the objective by the ocular lens, and here X is a real image located behind the ocular lens. The size of the exit pupil determines the size of the bundle of rays leaving the telescope.

Figure 19.11b shows the top and bottom bounding rays for the telescope's field of at least one-half illumination (object space angular size F_h). The rays from the top object point are solid and the rays from the bottom object point are dashed. Between the ocular lens and the exit pupil X, the beam leaving the telescope is a converging beam made up of parallel bundles. The beam is smallest at X, and changes to a diverging beam after X. The exit pupil of the Keplerian telescope has been referred to as the *Ramsden circle.* It's contemporary generic name is the *eye ring*. The optimum position for an observer with a static eye is to place the entrance pupil of their eye at the Ramsden circle (i.e., pupil matching). The distance that the Ramsden

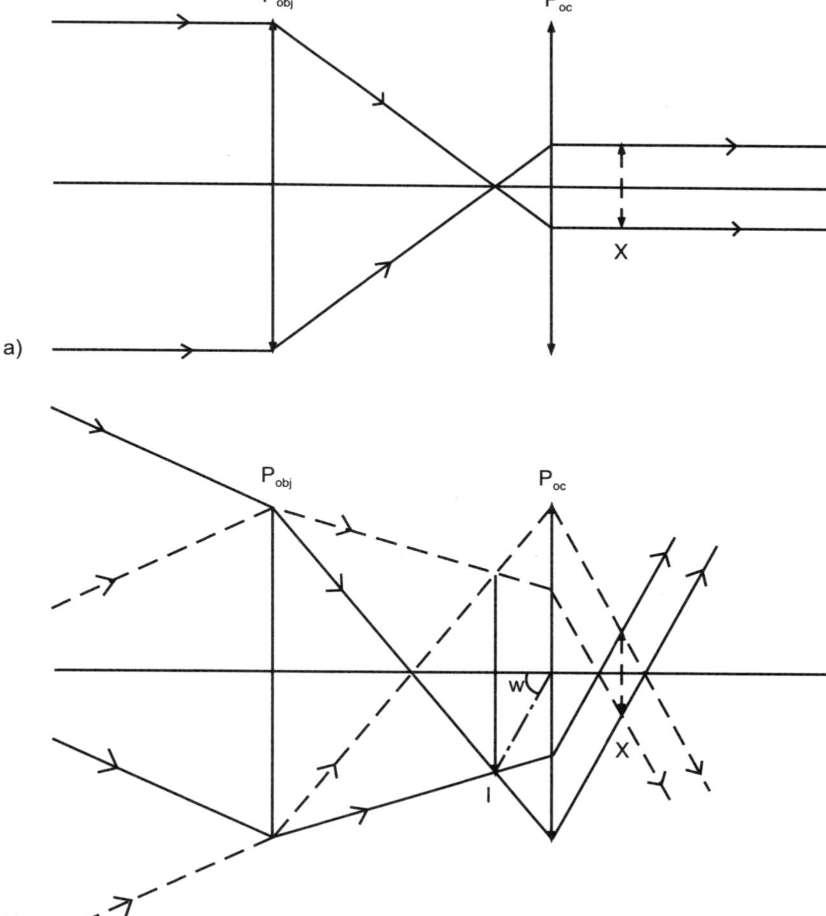

Figure 19.11 **a, Rays from an axial object point passing through a Keplerian telescope where P_{obj} is the objective lens and P_{oc} is the ocular lens. The exit pupil or Ramsden circle, located at X, is the image of the objective lens by the ocular lens; b, bounding rays for the field of uniform illumination (solid from the top object point, dashed from the bottom object point). I is the internal real image. Between the ocular lens and X, there is a converging beam made up of bundles of plane waves.**

circle is behind the ocular lens is called the *eye relief*. The exit pupil size and the eye relief are important parts of the design of a Keplerian telescope.

Consider a two lens Keplerian telescope with length d and angular magnification M (where M is negative, since the apparent image is inverted). Then the Ramsden circle location (position X in Figure 19.12a) is a distance of $d/|M|$ behind the ocular lens, and its size is smaller than the objective lens size by a factor of $|M|$. To prove this, take the objective lens as the object and image it by the ocular lens. Here the light is traveling right, and

$$\begin{aligned} u &= -d \\ V &= P_{oc} + U \\ &= P_{oc} + \left(\frac{1}{-d}\right) \\ &= \frac{-dP_{oc} + 1}{-d} \end{aligned}$$

and

$$v = \frac{-d}{1 - dP_{oc}}$$

From Eq. 17.25, $M = 1 - dP_{oc}$, so

$$v = \frac{d}{-M} \tag{19.11}$$

Since M is negative, Eq. 19.11 can be written as

$$v = d/|M|$$

The lateral magnification m is given by $m = v/u$, and substitution from above shows that

$$m = \frac{1}{M} \tag{19.12}$$

The lateral magnification m equals the image size I divided by the object size O, and it follows that

$$|M| = \frac{\text{objective lens diameter}}{\text{Ramsden circle diameter}} \tag{19.13}$$

Since the Ramsden circle is a real image, it is visible on a screen. When one shines light backwards through the telescope, the Ramsden circle appears as a sharp circle (i.e., focussed image) filled with light, and its

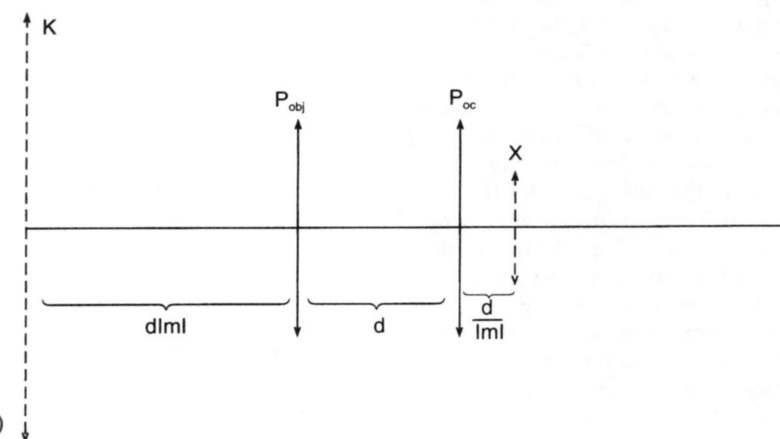

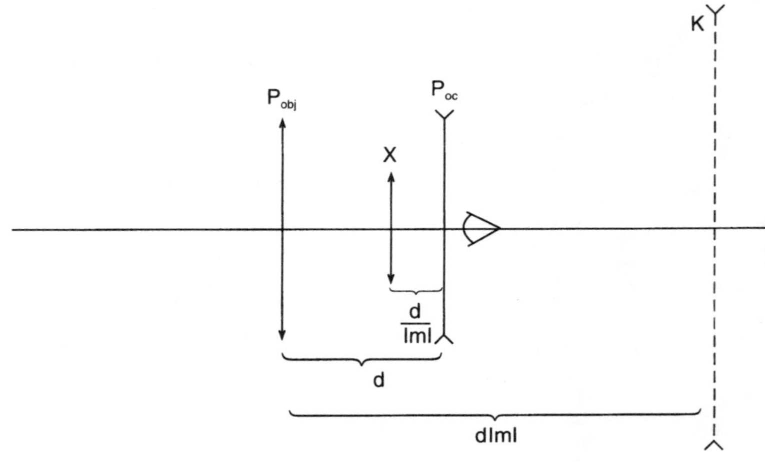

Figure 19.12 Two lens telescopes of magnification M and length d. The image of the objective lens by the ocular is X, and the image of the ocular lens by the objective is K: a, for a Keplerian telescope, the images X and K are both real; b, for a Galilean telescope, the images X and K are both virtual.

diameter is measurable. The objective lens diameter is also measurable, and then Eq. 19.13 gives the magnitude of the telescope's angular magnification M. (Equation 19.13 is also good for a multi-lens afocal telescope.)

For the two lens Keplerian telescope, we can show in a similar manner that the image of the ocular lens by the objective is a real image (K in Figure 19.12a) located at a distance equal to d times $|M|$ in front of the objective lens, and that K is $|M|$ times larger than the ocular lens. That is, for light traveling left in Figure 19.12a,

$$v = -dM \tag{19.14}$$

and

$$m = M \tag{19.15}$$

EXAMPLE 19.6a

A 4× Keplerian telescope consists of a +2.50 D objective lens and a +10.00 D ocular lens. The two lenses are 50 cm apart and each has a 36 mm diameter. What is the location and size of the Ramsden circle?

In Figure 19.12a, light is traveling right, and $M = -4\times$. For the location v, Eq. 19.11 gives

$$v = \frac{50\,\text{cm}}{4} = +12.5\,\text{cm}$$

In other words, the eye relief is 12.5 cm. For the size, Eq. 19.13 gives

$$\text{Ramsden circle diameter} = \frac{36\,\text{mm}}{4} = 9\,\text{mm}$$

EXAMPLE 19.6b

For the same Keplerian telescope, where is the image of the ocular by the objective and what is its size?

Here light is traveling to the left in Figure 19.12a, and Eq. 19.14 gives

$$v = -(50\,\text{cm})(-4\times) = 200\,\text{cm}$$

It follows from Eq. 19.15 that

$$I = M(\text{ocular lens size})$$

or

$$I = (-4)(36\,\text{mm}) = -144\,\text{mm}$$

Figure 19.12b shows an afocal Galilean telescope. Here M is positive, since the apparent image seen through the telescope is erect. For the Galilean telescope, the image X of the objective lens by the ocular lens is a smaller, virtual image that is located inside the telescope. The derivation of Eqs. 19.11 and 19.12 is good for any afocal telescope, so it applies to the Galilean telescope as well as the Keplerian telescope. Thus the virtual image is located at a distance of $-d/M$ from the ocular lens, and the virtual image is M times smaller than the objective lens. Similarly from Eqs. 19.14 and 19.15 for the two lens Galilean telescope, the image K of the ocular lens by the objective lens is virtual, is located a distance of d times M away from the objective lens, and is M times larger than ocular lens.

EXAMPLE 19.7a

A 4× Galilean telescope consists of a +1.50 D objective lens and a −6.00 D ocular lens. The two lenses are 50 cm apart and each has a 36 mm diameter. What is the location and size of the exit pupil?

In Figure 19.12b, light is traveling right and $M = +4\times$. For the location v, Eq. 19.11 gives

$$v = \frac{50\,\text{cm}}{-4} = -12.5\,\text{cm}$$

It follows from Eq. 19.13 that

$$\text{virtual image size} = \frac{36\,\text{mm}}{4} = 9\,\text{mm}$$

EXAMPLE 19.7b

For the same Galilean telescope, where is the image of the ocular by the objective and what is its size?

Light is traveling left in this case, and the image is virtual. Equation 19.14 gives

$$v = -(50\,\text{cm})(+4\times) = -200\,\text{cm}$$

It follows from Eq. 19.15 that the image size I is

$$\begin{aligned} I &= M(\text{ocular lens size}) \\ &= (+4)(36\,\text{mm}) = +144\,\text{mm} \end{aligned}$$

The location of the exit pupil plays an important role in the field of view that an observer has when using a telescope. Somewhat simplistically, the exit pupil of the telescope acts like a keyhole. The observer can maximize the field of view by placing the entrance pupil of their eye as close as possible to the exit pupil. For the Keplerian telescope, the exit pupil (the Ramsden circle) is a real image behind the ocular lens and the observer can place their entrance pupil at this position (pupil matching). For the Galilean telescope, the exit pupil is a virtual image inside the telescope and the observer cannot obtain pupil matching. The best the observer can do is to get their eye as close as possible to the ocular lens.

In the examples above, the two lenses in the telescope were of equal size. However for object points near the axis, Figure 19.11a shows that much of the ocular lens does not have light passing through it, and the same effect occurs for Galilean telescopes. Because of this, and because of the image quality concerns (see aberrations in the next chapter), the ocular lenses are usually smaller in size than the objective lenses.

19.5 GALILEAN TELESCOPE FIELD OF VIEW

When an observer makes a two lens Galilean telescope with trial lenses and looks through it at a distant object, it appears that their field of view is limited by the objective lens. In other words, the objective lens is the field stop for the telescope–eye system. Furthermore the observer's field of view decreases as the observer backs away from the telescope. The largest field of view is obtained when the observer has their eye as close as possible to the ocular lens (i.e., as close as possible to the internal virtual image at X in Figure 19.12b). In general, the telescope's exit pupil size may be larger, equal to, or smaller than the observer's entrance pupil size. For field of view purposes, the essential general principles are the same regardless of the size relationship. Therefore in the following discussion, we assume for simplicity that the observer's entrance pupil size is less than the telescope's exit pupil size.

For field of view purposes, we can (as before) simulate the observer's static eye by an aperture placed at the entrance pupil location of the observer's eye. The entrance pupil of the eye is typically about 3 mm behind the cornea and cannot be made coincident with the ocular lens. However for further simplification, we assume that the simulating aperture can be placed directly against the ocular lens. The latter assumption slightly over-estimates the field of view, so we'll refer to it as the "mythical" maximum field of view. With these assumptions, the simulating aperture is the aperture stop of the telescope–eye system. Since the simulating aperture is coincident with the ocular lens, the ocular lens cannot be the field stop. This leaves the objective lens as the field stop of the telescope–eye system, and since it is not an image it also serves as the entrance port. Let h_{obj} be the semidiameter of the objective lens.

The entrance pupil of the telescope–eye system is then the image of the simulating aperture formed by the lenses in front of it. Since this aperture is against the ocular lens, u equals zero, v equals zero, and the lateral magnification m equals +1. In other words, the ocular lens has no imaging effect in this situation. Then the image (the entrance pupil) of the simulating aperture by the objective lens occurs at the same position (K in Figure 19.12b) as the image of the ocular lens by the objective. From the previous section, this is a virtual image located a distance of $d|M|$ behind the objective lens, where d is the distance between the lenses. So in Eq. 19.2, $a = h_{obj}$ and $d_p = dM$, or for the Galilean telescope

$$\tan\left(\frac{F_h}{2}\right) = \frac{h_{obj}}{dM} \tag{19.16}$$

For the assumptions made in this section, Eq. 19.16 shows that for the Galilean telescope, $\tan(F_h/2)$ depends directly on the semidiameter of the objective lens, inversely on the distance d between the objective and ocular lenses, and inversely on the magnification.

EXAMPLE 19.8

For the 4× Galilean telescope in the previous example, what is the (mythical) maximum field view of the telescope–eye system?

The semidiameter h_{obj} of the entrance port (the objective lens) is 1.8 cm, the telescope length d is 50 cm, and M is +4. From Eq. 19.16,

$$\tan\frac{F_h}{2} = \frac{1.8\,\text{cm}}{(50\,\text{cm})(+4)} = 9.00 \times 10^{-3}$$

and

$$F_h = 1.03^\circ$$

Consider a series of Galilean telescopes of increasing (angular) magnification M, where each telescope has the same length and the same lens diameters. Equation 19.16 shows that the field of view decreases directly with increasing M. For example, when M is doubled, the field of view is cut in half.

19.6 KEPLERIAN TELESCOPE FIELD OF VIEW

When an observer makes a two lens Keplerian telescope with trial lenses and looks through it at a distant object, the field of view changes as the person backs away from the telescope's ocular lens. When the eye is as close as possible to the ocular lens, it appears that the objective lens is limiting the field of view (just as in a Galilean telescope), but now as the person slowly backs their eye away from the ocular lens, the field of view starts to *increase*. At a certain position of the eye, the field stop appears to shift from the objective lens to the ocular lens. Then as the person continues to slowly back away from the telescope, the field of view may appear not to change for a bit, but soon starts to decrease (while the ocular lens still appears to be the field stop or the exit port). Finally, as the person continues to back away, there is a position where the exit port appears to shift from the ocular lens to the Ramsden circle, and after that the field of view decreases even more rapidly as the person backs up.

Again let's simulate the observer's static eye by an aperture placed at the entrance pupil location of the observer's eye, and again for simplicity assume that the simulating aperture is smaller in size than the telescope's exit pupil (the Ramsden circle). With these assumptions, the simulating aperture is the aperture stop of the telescope–eye system. One can derive equations for the field of view as a function of the distance between the eye and the ocular lens, however we're primarily interested in the largest field, which usually occurs the observer's entrance pupil is at the Ramsden circle (X in Figure 19.12a).

For light going to the right, the Ramsden circle is the image conjugate to the objective lens. Therefore for light going left, the simulating aperture at the Ramsden circle is imaged at the objective lens position (principle of reversibility), and the objective lens has no further imaging effect on it (u equals zero, v equals zero, m equals $+1$). So when the simulating aperture at the Ramsden circle is the aperture stop of the telescope–eye system, the system's entrance pupil is formed at the objective lens position. (In effect the observer's eye is imaged at the objective lens.) This means that the objective lens cannot be the field stop, and so the ocular lens must be the field stop (in agreement with the two lens observations). The image of the ocular lens by the objective lens is then the entrance port of the telescope–eye system (K in Figure 19.12a). For a distance d between the objective lens and the ocular lens, Eq. 19.14 shows that the entrance port is located a distance of d times $|M|$ in front of the objective lens (which is the entrance pupil location), and so d_p in Eq. 19.2 equals $d|M|$. From Eq. 19.15, the entrance port is $|M|$ times larger than the ocular lens (semidiameter h_{oc}), so the entrance port semidiameter a equals $|M|h_{oc}$, and Eq. 19.2 gives

$$\tan\left(\frac{F_h}{2}\right) = \frac{|M|h_{oc}}{d|M|}$$

or

$$\tan\left(\frac{F_h}{2}\right) = \frac{h_{oc}}{d} \qquad (19.17)$$

For the assumptions made in this section, Eq. 19.17 shows that the tangent of the $F_h/2$ for the keplerian telescope depends directly on the ocular lens semidiameter h_{oc}, and inversely on the distance d between the ocular lens and the objective lens. For equal magnification galilean and keplerian telescopes with the same length and the same lens diameters, Eqs. 19.16 and 19.17 show that the maximum field of the galilean is M times smaller than the maximum field of the keplerian.

EXAMPLE 19.9

For the 4× Keplerian telescope in Example 19.6, what is the maximum field view of the telescope-eye system?

The semidiameter h_{oc} of the ocular lens is 1.8 cm, d is 50 cm, and M is -4. From Eq. 19.17,

$$\tan\frac{F_h}{2} = \frac{1.8\,\text{cm}}{50\,\text{cm}} = 3.60 \times 10^{-2}$$

and

$$F_h = 4.12^\circ$$

(Since the keplerian telescope provides angular magnification, the angular field of at least on half illumination, F'_h as measured in image space is 4 times 4.12°, or 16.48°.)

The 4× Keplerian telescope in the above example has a 4.12° maximum field of view. When the person moves their eye significantly forward or backward away from the Ramsden circle, the field of view decreases. This 4× Keplerian telescope had the same length and the same lens diameters as the 4× Galilean telescope in Example 19.8. The maximum field of the Galilean was 1.03°, which was obtained for the simulating aperture placed against the ocular lens. It turns out that when the simulating aperture is placed against the ocular lens of the Keplerian telescope, its field is also 1.03°.

Equation 19.17 shows no dependence on M for the field of view of the Keplerian telescope provided that the ocular lens size and the length of the telescope are unchanged. Hence for a series of Keplerian telescopes of the same length and same lens diameters, one can increase the magnification without changing the field of view. However a different effect eventually places a limit on this series. For the higher magnifications, the image space rays emerge from the telescope at large angles (i.e., outside the paraxial range). Here the optical aberrations (discussed in the next chapter) will decrease image quality (maybe even to the extent that there is no image). It turns out that there is a maximum image space angle beyond which image quality is no longer acceptable. (For expensive multi-lens systems, this angle is about ±30° from the optical axis. It is smaller for simpler, less expensive systems.) The internal real image of the Keplerian telescope is in the primary focal plane of the ocular lens, and the angle of a bundle of light emerging from the telescope is parallel to the nodal ray for the ocular lens. For an internal image of size I, the rays from the bottom point make a nodal angle w at the ocular lens (Figure 19.11b) where,

$$\tan w = -I/f_1 = IP_{oc}$$

For a fixed I, the image quality restriction on the magnitude of the angle w, places a restriction on the magnitude of the power P_{oc} of the ocular lens. In other words, to maintain good image quality there is a maximum P_{oc}, or a minimum secondary focal length for the ocular lens. Since $M = -P_{oc}/P_{obj}$, once the maximum P_{oc} is reached, the only way to further increase the magnification of the telescope is to decrease the power of the objective lens P_{obj}. A smaller P_{obj} has a longer secondary focal length, so the length d of the telescope increases, and then Eq. 19.17 shows that the field of view then decreases. We can explicitly show this as follows:

$$M = -\frac{P_{oc}}{P_{obj}} = -\frac{(f_2)_{obj}}{(f_2)_{oc}}$$

so

$$(f_2)_{obj} = |M|(f_2)_{oc}$$

Since

$$d = (f_2)_{obj} + (f_2)_{oc}$$

it follows that

$$d = (|M| + 1)(f_2)_{oc}$$

Substitution into Eq. 19.17 results in

$$\tan\left(\frac{F_h}{2}\right) = \frac{h_{oc}}{(|M| + 1)(f_2)_{oc}} \qquad (19.18)$$

In Eq. 19.18, it is explicitly clear that for a fixed (minimum) secondary focal length of the ocular lens, the field of view decreases with increasing magnification $|M|$.

The Galilean telescope does not have an internal real image, but the Keplerian telescope does. A reticle is a series of lines, circles, or markers imprinted on a transparent piece of glass. When a reticle is placed at the internal real image position of the Keplerian telescope, the image of the distance object and the image of the reticle will be superposed. The reticle marks are used for sighting or measurements.

Another advantage of the internal real image of the Keplerian telescope is that a field lens (Section 19.3) can be placed there to increase the field of view (Figure 19.13). When added to a two lens Keplerian telescope, a plus field lens does not change the size of the Ramsden circle (i.e., the image of the objective lens by the lenses behind it), but it does move the image towards the ocular lens (X to X'). In other words, the field lens shortens the eye relief. The addition of the field lens at the internal real image position does not change the size of the image of the ocular lens by the lenses in front of it, but it does moves that image closer to the objective lens (K to K'). (In multi-element systems, ray traces are frequently needed to determine the vignetting effects in the system. In practice, there is an optimum power for a field lens.)

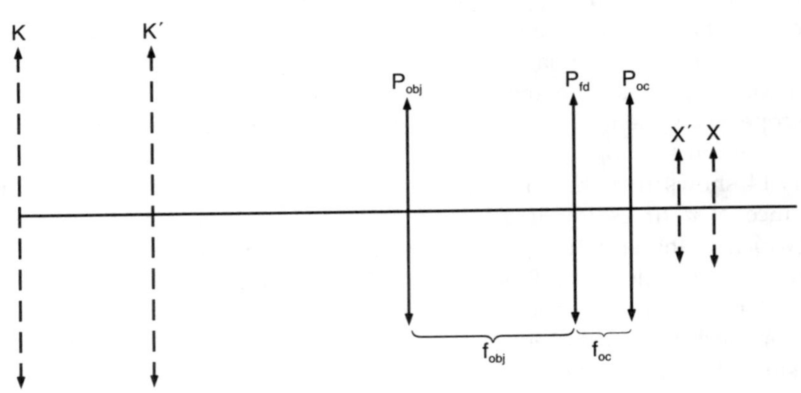

Figure 19.13 A field lens P_{fd} added at the internal real image of a Keplerian telescope. Here f_{obj} is the focal length of the objective lens and f_{oc} is the focal length of the ocular lens. When the field lens is added, the exit pupil moves from X to X' without a size change, and the entrance port moves from K to K' without a size change.

EXAMPLE 19.10a

A +2.50 D field lens is added to the 4× Keplerian telescope of Example 19.14. (There the telescope had a 50 cm length, a +2.50 D objective lens, a +10.00 D ocular lens, lens diameters of 36 mm, and a 4.12° F_h. The ocular lens was the field stop and the entrance pupil location was at the objective lens.) For a static eye at the Ramsden circle, what is the new entrance port location and the new field of view?

The field lens is at the internal real image position, which is 40 cm behind the objective lens and 10 cm in front of the ocular lens. To find the new entrance port, we take the ocular lens as the object and find its image formed by the field lens and the objective lens. Here light is traveling to the left, and

$$u_1 = -10\,\text{cm}$$
$$U_1 = -10.00\,\text{D}$$
$$V_1 = +2.50\,\text{D} + (-10.00\,\text{D}) = -7.50\,\text{D}$$
$$v_1 = -13.333\,\text{cm}$$
$$u_2 = -13.333\,\text{cm} - 40\,\text{cm} = -53.333\,\text{cm}$$
$$U_2 = -1.875\,\text{D}$$
$$V_2 = +2.50\,\text{D} + (-1.875\,\text{D}) = +0.625\,\text{D}$$

and

$$v_2 = +160\,\text{cm}$$

Also $m_1 = U_1/V_1$ and $m_2 = U_2/V_2$, and $m_t = m_1 m_2$. So

$$m_t = (+1.333)(-3.00) = -4.00$$

and the diameter of the entrance port is 144 mm (i.e., |−4| times 36 mm), which is the same size that the entrance port had without a field lens. Since the objective lens is the entrance pupil, d_p is 160 cm, and Eq. 19.2 gives

$$\tan\left(\frac{F_h}{2}\right) = \frac{7.2\,\text{cm}}{160\,\text{cm}} = 0.045$$

and

$$F_h = 5.15°$$

Note that in this case, the field lens provides a 25% increase in the field of view over the 4× Keplerian without the field lens.

EXAMPLE 19.10b

What is the eye relief for the 4× Keplerian telescope with the field lens?

To find the eye relief, we need to image the objective lenses by the lens behind it (i.e., the field lens and the ocular lens). Here light is traveling to the right, $U_1 = -2.50\,\text{D}$, $V_1 = 0.00\,\text{D}$, $U_2 = 0.00\,\text{D}$, $V_2 = +10.00\,\text{D}$, and $v_2 = +10.00$ cm. The eye relief without the field lens was 12.5 cm, so the +2.50 D field lens shortened the eye relief to 10 cm.

19.7 TERRESTRIAL TELESCOPES

Because of the field of view advantage of the Keplerian telescope over the Galilean telescope, it is desirable to use a Keplerian with an internal erecting system for terrestrial uses. Figure 19.14 shows a Keplerian telescope with a thin lens erecting system that does not change the angular magnification M of the telescope. The erecting lens (secondary focal length f_{er}) is placed

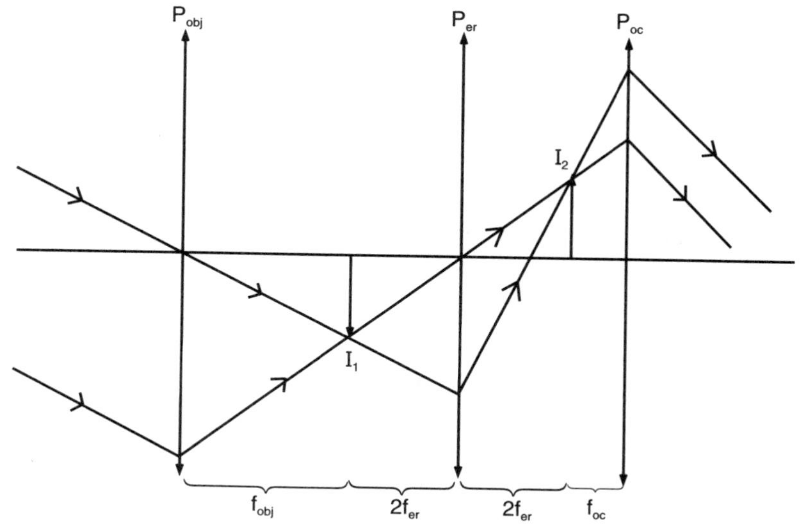

Figure 19.14 An erecting lens P_{er} of focal length f_{er}, added to a Keplerian telescope. I_1 is the image formed by the objective lens and I_2 is the flipped image formed by the erecting lens.

so that it is $2f_{er}$ behind the objective lens's secondary focal point and is $2f_{er}$ in front of the primary focal point of the ocular lens. For a distant object, the objective lens forms a real image I_1 at its secondary focal point. The image I_1 serves as the object for the erecting lens, and the erecting lens forms its image I_2 at primary focal point of the ocular lens. The lateral magnification for the erecting lens is -1 (symmetry point case), so I_2 is flipped relative to I_1 without a size change. Since the internal image I_2 is at the primary focal point for the ocular lens, plane waves leave the ocular lens. The length of the two lens telescope was equal to the sum of the focal lengths of the objective lens and the ocular lens (i.e., $f_{obj} + f_{oc}$). In order to put the erecting lens into the Keplerian telescope, it length has to be increased by 4 times the secondary focal length f_{er} of the erecting lens (i.e., new length $= f_{obj} + 2f_{er} + 2f_{er} + f_{oc}$).

Consider a two lens Keplerian telescope with angular magnification M. Erecting lenses can also be added that increase the magnification of the telescope. Here the length increase is greater than $4\,f_{er}$, and the resultant angular magnification M_r of the telescope is the product of M and the lateral magnification m_{er} of the erecting lens, i.e.,

$$M_r = Mm_{er} \tag{19.19}$$

A rifle scope is a Keplerian telescope (with a long eye relief) that contains an erecting lens, and a reticle for sighting assistance.

There are prism-erecting systems that flip the image without changing the length of the telescope. One system uses the pair of Porro prisms discussed in Chapter 11. Common binoculars consist of Keplerian telescopes with Porro prism erecting systems. The beam coming out of the Porro prisms is laterally inset from the incoming beam. A prism that flips the image without an inset is the Amici Roof prism. The tolerances are the roof prisms are very exacting, and the optical quality of the roof prism systems may be poorer than the optical quality of the Porro prism systems.

Binoculars (and other terrestrial telescopes) are usually marked with numbers like 8×40. The first number is the angular magnification ($8\times$) and the second number is the diameter of the objective lens in mm. Telescopes with larger diameter objectives lenses gather more light from the object than telescopes with smaller diameter objectives. It follows from Eq. 19.13 that the Ramsden circle diameter is 5 mm (i.e, 40 mm/8), which is a typical size.

For brightness considerations, it is desirable to have a large objective lens, and to have a Ramsden circle equal to or larger than the entrance pupil of the observer's eye. Binoculars designed for low light levels may have 7 mm or 8 mm diameter Ramsden circles. Rifle scopes have Ramsden circles that range from 5 mm to 10 mm, which make them easier to sight through. Surveying instruments are designed more for accuracy and usually have smaller Ramsden circles (e.g., 1.0–1.5 mm).

The eye relief is also important. Usually telescopes are designed so that a person gets their maximum field of view when the entrance pupil of their eye is about 15 mm from the ocular lens of the telescope. A shorter eye relief results in the observer's eye lashes making contact with the ocular lens. A longer eye relief is needed for spectacle lens wearers. A longer eye relief is also needed for special uses, such as a rifle scope.

Despite the field restrictions, short spectacle mounted Galilean telescope do have some advantages over the short spectacle mounted Keplerian telescopes for low vision patients. As with any spectacle frame, bumps, wear, and oily skin can cause the frames to change position relative to the eye. In a Keplerian telescope which has its exit pupil at the entrance pupil of the eye, such a bump may cause the exit pupil to no longer be coincident with the eye's entrance pupil, in which case the person cannot see through the telescope (a pupil mis-match). On the other hand, since the exit pupil (virtual image) of a Galilean telescope is in front of the observer's entrance pupil, the Galilean telescope is not as sensitive to frame position changes, and the observer can more easily sight through it even when the frame position shifts. Consequently, a low vision patient may find the spectacle mounted Galilean telescope easier to use than the spectacle mounted Keplerian, even though the Keplerian gives a larger field of view.

19.8 DIRECT AND INDIRECT OPHTHALMOSCOPES

The ocular fundus is the concave interior of the eye consisting of the retina, choroid, optic disc, and blood vessels. The optic disk is about 1.5 mm in diameter, and the fundus itself is about 25 disc diameters (DD) across. The major blood vessels are only 0.1–0.2 mm in diameter. Examination of the fundus by looking through the patient's cornea and crystalline lens is an important part of an ocular health assessment.

Figure 19.15a represents a patient's eye P and an examiner's eye E. Some of the light from the light source S enters the patient's eye and illuminates region B on the patient's fundus. The fundus then acts as a secondary source, and the light rays (solid)

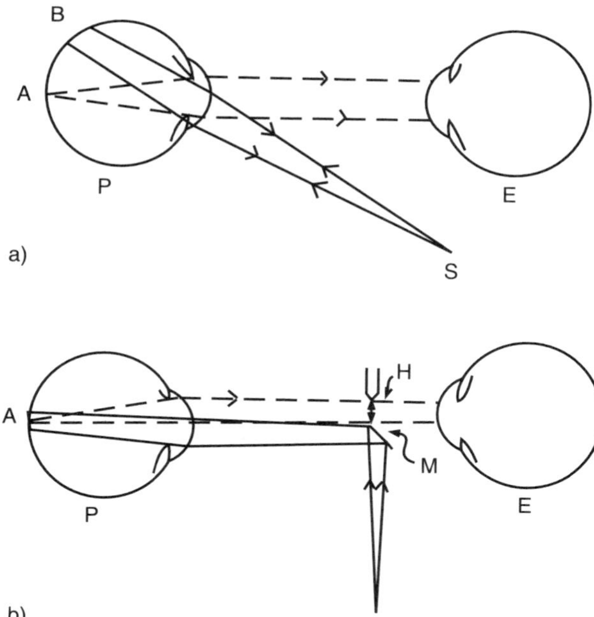

Figure 19.15 a, Light from source *S* illuminates area *B* of a patient's fundus and the light leaving the fundus as a secondary source is refracted back towards (solid rays). To the examiner *E*, the patient's pupil looks black and area *B* is not visible. If area *A* of the patient's fundus was illuminated, then the light coming out of the patient's eye is refracted towards the examiner's eye and the examiner can now see the patient's fundus (dashed rays); b, schematic of a direct ophthalmoscope. *M* is a mirror (or prism). *H* is the ophthalmoscope sighthole, which may have a lens or filter in it.

coming back out of the patient's eye are refracted back towards the source *S*, and not towards the examiner's eye. Thus, to the examiner, the patient's pupil looks black, and the examiner cannot see the fundus. However if region *A* on the patient's fundus was illuminated, then the examiner could see it, since the rays (dashed) from region *A* would be refracted by the patient's eye and travel to the examiner's eye. For this to occur, the light source *S* (or its image) must be close to the visual axis of the examiner. In such a case, when the examiner focuses on the patient's pupil it appears to have a red glow (the red reflex) due to the light that comes from the blood-filled choroid acting as a secondary source in region *A*. Similarly, a photograph of a person taken by a camera may show the red reflex if the flash is close to the camera's optical axis.

An ophthalmoscope is an instrument that enables an examiner to clearly see the patient's fundus by looking through the cornea and crystalline lens of the patient's eye. There are two basic types of ophthalmoscopes—direct and indirect. Figure 19.15b is a schematic representation of the essentials of a *direct ophthalmoscope*. The examiner *E* looks at the patient's eye *P* through a sighthole *H* in the ophthalmoscope. The direct ophthalmoscope has a series of lenses and/or filters that can be rotated into the sighthole to assist the examiner to clearly see fundus detail. The mirror *M* (or a prism) reflects light from source *S* so that it is traveling close to the examiner's visual axis when it is incident on the patient's eye and illuminates region *A* of the patient's fundus. For the fundus as a secondary source, some of the light coming back out of the patient's eye is refracted back towards the sighthole *H* and the examiner's eye. For an emmetropic patient, this light consists of plane waves, and no lens needs to be in the ophthalmoscope sighthole for an emmetropic examiner. For uncorrected ametropic patients and/or an uncorrected ametropic examiner, a lens needs to be rotated into the sighthole in order for the examiner to see a clear image of the patient's fundus.

With the direct ophthalmoscope, the patient's crystalline lens and cornea function as a high plus magnifier, and the examiner sees an erect, magnified virtual image of the patient's fundus, but with a small field of view. Optical irregularities or opacities in the patient's eye may degrade the quality of the apparent image seen with the direct ophthalmoscope.

Since the light source or its image must be close to the examiner's line of sight, a potential problem in ophthalmoscopy is that the reflected images (reflexes) from the patient's cornea and crystalline lens can obscure parts of the patient's fundus. Allvar Gullstrand was the first to explain the principles of "reflexless ophthalmoscopy." Here, the light incident on the patient's eye must pass through one part of the patient's pupil (bottom part in Figure 19.15b), while the light coming back out of the patient's eye and going to the examiner's eye must pass through a different part of the patient's pupil (top part).

When the patient is an emmetrope, the patient's cornea and crystalline lens function as a collimating magnifier. For +60.00 D emmetropic eye, the angular magnification (relative to the standard reference distance) provided by the patient's eye is $P/4$, or 15×. This means that the examiner's retinal image with the direct ophthalmoscope is 15 times larger than it would be if the examiner looked directly at an excised fundus held 25 cm in front of his or her cornea. The 15× magnification helps the examiner to see fundus detail in small areas. An emmetropic patient with a +56.00 D eye would result in 14× magnification, etc.

Equation 19.7 gives the linear field of view for a collimating magnifier. This equation would apply to the direct ophthalmoscopy situation if the incident light beam illuminated a substantial area of the patient's fundus. However, a direct ophthalmoscope typically illuminates a fundus area that is only about 1 disc diameter in size. Hence, it is usually the illuminating system, and not the viewing system that limits the field of view.

The light coming back out of the eye of an ametrope is either converging (for a myope) or diverging (for a hyperope). For these cases, an unaccommodated emmetropic examiner needs to rotate a lens into the ophthalmoscope sighthole to change the light into plane waves. The lens needed is the patient's correction as measured at a vertex distance that corresponds to the sighthole position. The direct ophthalmoscope lenses are a finite series of spherical lenses, so in practice the lens only approximates the Sp Eq of the patient's correction.

The angular magnification achieved with a direct ophthalmoscope varies with the patient's refractive error and the correcting lens in the sighthole. The patient's eye and the separated correcting lens constitute a system that has an equivalent power P_e. Relative to the standard reference distance, the angular magnification for this system is $P_e/4$. For two lenses of power P_1 and P_2 separated by the distance d, Eq. 15.40 gives

$$P_e = P_1 + P_2 - dP_2P_1$$

In a thin lens eye model, the equivalent power depends on both the power of the eye (P_1), the correcting lens power (P_2), and the vertex distance d. When the ametropia is purely refractive relative to a standard emmetrope, the decreased power of the hyperope's eye results in a smaller magnification and the increased power of a myope's eye results in a larger magnification. When the ametropia is purely axial and the sighthole is at the primary focal point of the patient's eye (16.67 mm), the magnification is the same as that for a standard emmetrope (reminiscent of Knapp's Law in spectacle magnification). In the general case, the resultant magnification relative to the standard emmetrope varies depending on how much of the ametropia is refractive versus axial, and how far the direct ophthalmoscope is away from the eye.

EXAMPLE 19.11a

A thin lens and screen (fundus) model for a standard emmetropic eye consists of a +60.00 D lens located 16.67 mm in front of the screen. For a refractive hyperope (thin lens model) with a virtual far point that is 10.00 cm far point from the cornea, what magnification is obtained with a direct ophthalmoscope held 16.67 mm from the cornea?

Since the ametropia is refractive, the lens–screen separation is still 16.67 mm, so the power of the eye must be +50.00 D. The calculated correction at 16.67 mm is +8.57 D. (For purposes of this calculation, we'll use the +8.57 D as opposed to the approximate value.) Then the equivalent power of the eye and correction is given by

$$P_e = +50.00\,\text{D} + 8.57\,\text{D} - (16.67 \times 10^{-3}\,\text{m})(+50.00\,\text{D})(+8.57\,\text{D})$$

and

$$P_e = +51.43\,\text{D}$$

So $M = P_e/4 = 12.9\times$. This is less than the $15\times$ obtained for the +60.00 D emmetrope.

EXAMPLE 19.11b

For an axial hyperope (thin lens model) with a virtual far point that is 10.00 cm from the cornea, what magnification is obtained with a direct ophthalmoscope held 16.67 mm from the cornea

Since the ametropia is axial, the power of the eye (thin lens model) is still +60.00 D, and the lens–screen (fundus) separation must be 14.29 mm. The calculated correction at 16.67 mm is again +8.57 D. The equivalent power of the eye and correction is given by

$$P_e = +60.00\,\text{D} + 8.57\,\text{D} - (16.67 \times 10^{-3}\,\text{m})(+60.00\,\text{D})(+8.57\,\text{D}) = +60.00\,\text{D}$$

So $M = P_e/4 = 15.0\times$ (which is the same as the +60.00 D emmetrope). Note that for a shorter distance between the ophthalmoscope and the axial hyperopic eye, the equivalent power exceeds +60.00 D, and the magnification is larger than $15\times$.

EXAMPLE 19.11c

Consider a 10.00 D ocular hyperope with an eye represented by a +55.00 D thin lens located 15.38 mm in front of a screen (fundus). Here the ametropia has both an axial and a refractive component. The far point of this eye is still virtual and 10.00 cm from the cornea, and the correction at 16.67 mm is still +8.57 D. What magnification is obtained with a direct ophthalmoscope held 16.67 mm from this eye?

The equivalent power of the eye and correction is given by

$$P_e = +55.00\,\text{D} + 8.57\,\text{D} - (16.67 \times 10^{-3}\,\text{m})(+55.00\,\text{D})(+8.57\,\text{D})$$
$$= +55.71\,\text{D}$$

So $M = P_e/4 = 13.9\times$ (which, as might be expected, is between the purely refractive and purely axial results of parts a and b).

When the (unaccommodated) examiner also has an uncorrected refractive error, the lens that needs to be in the ophthalmoscope is the sum of the patient's correction and the examiner's correction both as measured at the plane of the sighthole. Consider an uncorrected hyperopic patient who needs a +4.00 D correction at the sighthole. Suppose the examiner is an uncorrected myope who needs a −1.00 D correction at the sighthole. Then the sum specifies that a +3.00 D lens needs to be in the ophthalmoscope sighthole. One can confirm this as follows. The light leaving the hyperopic patient's eye is diverging and has a −4.00 D vergence when it hits the +3.00 D lens. From $V = P + U$, the light leaving the +3.00 D lens has a −1.00 D vergence, which is the vergence required to correct the myopic examiner.

With an *indirect ophthalmoscope*, a high plus lens called a condenser lens is used to form a real, inverted aerial image of the patient's fundus, and the examiner views the aerial image from a distance of 33–35 cm (13–14 in). The aerial image is inverted in all meridians, so not only is the up and down orientation reversed, but the left and right orientation is also reversed. Relative to the virtual image seen in direct ophthalmoscopy, the optical irregularities and/or opacities in the patient's eye have a smaller effect on the quality of the real, aerial image, and it has been described as "incredibly brilliant." Also relative to the direct ophthalmoscope, the indirect ophthalmoscope provides less angular magnification but a much larger field of view. The brilliance of the apparent image and the larger field of view make it possible for the examiner to see subtle changes in the fundus that can be early indications of disease.

There are both monocular and binocular indirect ophthalmoscopes. With the monocular scope, the examiner uses one eye to look at the aerial image; while with the binocular indirect ophthalmoscope, the examiner uses both eyes to view the aerial image. In a binocular indirect ophthalmoscope, the examiner wears a head-mounted set that contains the light source and the optics for the illumination beam, along with an optical unit that splits the light from the patient's eye and redirects it so that it enters both eyes of the examiner. This results in a stereoscopic view of the inverted aerial image of the patient's fundus. For an adequate field of view, the patient's pupil is usually dilated for indirect ophthalmoscopy.

The condenser lens is hand-held by the examiner about a focal length away from the patient's eye. In order to maximize the field of view, the condenser lens performs two other functions besides forming the aerial image. For the light incident on the patient's eye, the condenser lens forms a small image of the ophthalmoscope's light source in the patient's pupil. The second function of the condenser lens is to image the patient's pupil at the pupil of the examiner (i.e., pupil matching). The condenser lens can meet both of these functions when the ophthalmoscope's light source and the examiner's pupil are the same distance from the patient's pupil. For reflex free viewing the light source must be imaged in one part of the patient's pupil (e.g., the top part), while the examiner's pupils are imaged in the opposite part (e.g., the bottom part).

An emmetropic examiner who looks directly at the aerial image from 33 to 35 cm away must accommodate to have a clear retinal image. An emmetropic examiner who is presbyopic can view the aerial image through a plus spectacle lens (essentially an "add") that changes the diverging light from the aerial image into plane waves, which then enter the examiner's eye. In binocular indirect ophthalmoscopy, examiners who are not presbyopic also often use an add that helps with fusion for stereopsis.

Hand-held condenser lenses range from about +14.00 D to +40.00 D. A slit lamp can be modified to work as a more complicated indirect ophthalmoscope, and those condenser lenses can range as high as +90.00 D. The higher powered condenser lenses have shorter focal lengths and form smaller aerial images. Therefore, the angular magnification decreases as the condenser lens power increases. The smaller aerial images result in a larger field of view, so the field of view increases as the condenser lens power increases.

Figure 19.16 shows a simplified model (not to scale) for the viewing optics of indirect ophthalmoscopy when both the patient and the examiner are unaccommodated emmetropes. Even though this is a simplified model, it gives numbers that are quite close to the actual values. We use thin lens and screen models to represent both the patient's eye (lens P) and the examiner's eye (lens E). The pupil of each eye is assumed to be at the thin lens representing that eye and determines the effective size of the lenses. Lens C represents the condenser lens and lens A represents the add. The vertex distance between the add and the examiner's cornea does not significantly change the numbers, so for simplicity lens A is placed against the front of lens E. The rays (solid) leaving point H on the patient's fundus are converged by lenses P and

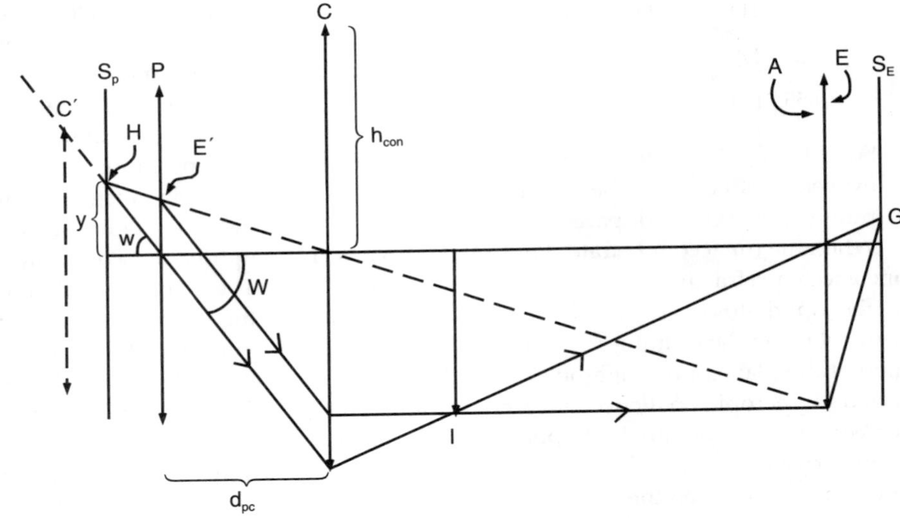

Figure 19.16 Diagram (not to scale) of the viewing system optics of an indirect ophthalmoscope. The thin lens P and screen S_p represent the patient's eye, the thin lens E and screen S_E represent the examiner's eye, C is the condenser lens (semi-diameter h_{con}), A is the add, I is the aerial image of the patient's fundus, and C' is the entrance port (i.e., the image of the condenser lens C by P). The distance between P and C is d_{PC}. For simplicity, the vertex distance between A and E is neglected. Lens C images the bottom of lens E at the point E' on P. The fundus point H, which subtends the angle w at P, is the field of view boundary point on the patient's fundus and is a linear distance y above the optical axis.

C to form the conjugate image point I on the aerial image. The light diverging from I is then incident on the lenses A and E, and they form the image point G on the examiner's retina.

The condenser lens C also images the examiner's pupil (which is assumed to be at E) in the patient's pupil at P. So the center of P is conjugate to the center of E. The bottom point on E is conjugate to the image point E' at P, where the nodal ray (dashed) through C determines the location of E'. Note that the image E' of the examiner's pupil is smaller than the patient's pupil (lens P). (While this is not shown, a nodal ray from the bottom edge of lens P through the center of lens C would show that the image of the patient's pupil at lens E is larger than the examiner's pupil.)

For the patient's fundus as the object, the image of the examiner's pupil (top point E') is the viewing system's entrance pupil, and thus the examiner's pupil at E is the system's aperture stop. Lens P cannot be the field stop since the entrance pupil E' is coincident with it. In reality, the add (lens A) cannot be the field stop since it is much larger than the examiner's entrance pupil. (So for simplicity in the figure, the add lens A is represented as the same size as E.) This leaves the condenser lens C as the system's field stop (which is typical in real world indirect ophthalmoscopy with a dilated patient pupil).

The object point H on the patient's fundus is the boundary for the field of at least one half illumination. The chief ray (solid) from H goes through the center of lens P (which is coincident with the center of the entrance pupil) to the bottom edge of the condenser lens C (the system's field stop), then through the aerial image point I to the center of the examiner's eye E (the aperture stop), and on to the image point G on the examiner's fundus. The marginal ray from H goes through point E' (the top edge of the entrance pupil), comes out of the patient's eye parallel to the chief ray (i.e., plane waves), travels to the condenser lens C, is converged by C, passes straight through the aerial image point I (located at the intersection of the two solid rays), goes to the bottom edge of lens E, and then goes to the G. Only the bottom half of lens E, the system's aperture stop, is filled with light.

Assume that lens P representing the patient's eye is +60.00 D, lens C is a +14.00 D condenser lens with a 50 mm diameter, lens A is a +3.00 D add, lens E representing the examiner's eye is also +60.00 D, and that the examiner is viewing the aerial image point I from a 33.33 cm distance. For each eye, the distance from the lens representing the eye to the screen representing the fundus of that eye is 16.67 mm. For the patient's fundus as an object (e.g., point H), plane waves leave the emmetropic patient's eye, and the condenser lens C forms the aerial image point I at its focal length, or 7.14 cm to the right of C. Then the lens C is a total of 40.47 cm from lens E (i.e., 33.33 cm + 7.14 cm), and the examiner needs to hold the condenser lens 8.67 cm from lens P in order to image the examiner's pupil at the patient's pupil, and vice versa (i.e., for light going left from lens E, $u = -40.47\,\text{cm}$, $U = -2.47\,\text{D}$, $V = +14.00\,\text{D} + U = +11.53\,\text{D}$, and $v = +8.67\,\text{cm}$).

Since the aerial image is at the primary focal point of the add, the light leaving the add (lens A) consists of plane waves, which are immediately incident on the examiner's eye (lens E). Therefore, for the examiner's eye, the patient's eye (lens P), the condenser lens C, and the add (lens A) together act like a collimating magnifier with the patient's fundus as the object. Relative to the standard reference distance, the angular magnification M is $P_e/4$, where P_e is the equivalent power of the three lens system. An easy way to find the equivalent power for a three lens system is to compute the system matrix. Here,

$$\mathbf{S} = \mathbf{R}_3\mathbf{T}_2\mathbf{R}_2\mathbf{T}_1\mathbf{R}_1$$

where lens 1 is P, lens 2 is C, and lens 3 is A. When the **T** and **R** matrices are combined into the matrix **B**,

$$\mathbf{S} = \mathbf{R}_3\mathbf{B}_2\mathbf{B}_1$$

where,

$$\mathbf{B}_i = \begin{pmatrix} 1 & -P_i \\ d_i & 1 - d_iP_i \end{pmatrix}$$

The matrix multiplications in this case give

$$\mathbf{S} = \begin{pmatrix} -0.214 & +12.86\,\text{D} \\ 0.00 & -4.676 \end{pmatrix}$$

The equivalent power P_e is $-12.86\,\text{D}$, and $M = -12.86\,\text{D}/4 = -3.21\times$. The minus sign indicates that the image seen by the examiner is inverted. The zero in the second row-first column element confirms that in this model the patient's pupil is imaged at the examiner's pupil (i.e., **S** is an object–image matrix). The -4.67 in the second row-second column element is the lateral magnification and it shows that the image of the patient's pupil is inverted and 4.67 times larger than the examiner's pupil. So by reversibility, the image of the examiner's pupil at the patient's pupil is 4.67 times smaller than the patient's pupil (i.e., the lateral magnification is -0.214, which is the first row-first column element).

The entrance port is the real image C' of the condenser lens C (the field stop) by the patient's eye (lens P). The bounding ray for the field of at least one-half illumination lies on the line extending from the top edge of the entrance port C' through the center of the entrance pupil (at P). In Figure 19.16, this line passes through the fundus point H, intersects the bottom edge of lens C, and subtends the angle w at the center of lens P. Here $w = F_h/2$, where F_h is the angular field of at least one-half illumination. We could calculate the entrance port size and location and use Eq. 19.2 to find the tangent of $F_h/2$. However since the bounding ray is the nodal ray that goes straight through lens P, the subtended angle w on the right side of the lens P also equals $F_h/2$. Then from the triangle involving this ray, lens C, and the optical axis,

$$\tan\left(\frac{F_h}{2}\right) = \frac{h_{con}}{d_{PC}} \tag{19.20}$$

where h_{con} is the semidiameter of the condenser lens C and d_{PC} is the distance between the patient's eye (lens P) and C. Then,

$$\tan\left(\frac{F_h}{2}\right) = \frac{2.5\,\text{cm}}{8.67\,\text{cm}} = 0.29$$

On the patient's fundus, the distance y from the optical axis to the point H is the top half of the linear field of view. From the triangle involving the nodal ray to point H, the distance y, and the optical axis,

$$\tan\left(\frac{F_h}{2}\right) = \frac{y}{16.67\,\text{cm}} = 0.29$$

which gives $y = 4.8\,\text{mm}$. The whole linear field (top and bottom parts) across the patient's fundus is $2y$ or 9.6 mm, which is about 6.4 disc diameters.

The angular magnification of a microscope equals $P_e/4$. The angular magnification of a microscope also equals the lateral magnification of the objective lens times the angular magnification of the ocular. We can treat the system S (lens P to lens A) as a microscope with lenses P and C together acting as the objective, and lens A acting as the ocular. For lenses P and C, the lateral magnification is the ratio of the aerial image size to the fundus size. For the case, where plane waves are traveling between the two lenses, we can use the subtended nodal angles to show that this lateral magnification m is given by

$$m = -\frac{P}{C}$$

where P is the power of the patient's eye and C is the power of the condenser. Let A be the power of the add (lens A). The angular magnification of the add is then $M = A/4$. So the total angular magnification M_t with the indirect ophthalmoscope is

$$M_t = mM$$

or

$$M_t = \left(-\frac{P}{C}\right)\left(\frac{A}{4}\right) \tag{19.21}$$

For the +14.00 D condenser,

$$M_t = \left(-\frac{+60.00\,\text{D}}{+14.00\,\text{D}}\right)\left(\frac{+3.00\,\text{D}}{4}\right)$$
$$= (-4.29)(0.75\,\text{D}) = -3.21\times$$

which is the same value that the system matrix method gave.

When the examiner switches to a +20.00 D condenser lens C with a 47 mm diameter, the aerial image is 5.0 cm behind C. In this case, the condenser lens must be 5.75 cm from the patient's eye (lens P) in order to achieve pupil matching. Then Eq. 19.21 gives

$$M_t = \left(-\frac{60.00\,\text{D}}{+20.00\,\text{D}}\right)\left(\frac{+3.00\,\text{D}}{4}\right)$$

and

$$M_t = (-3.00)(.75) = -2.25\times$$

From Eq. 19.20, the field of view is

$$\tan\left(\frac{F_h}{2}\right) = \frac{2.35\,\text{cm}}{5.75\,\text{cm}} = 0.41$$

We can then find the linear field of view on the patient's fundus from

$$\tan\left(\frac{F_h}{2}\right) = \frac{y}{16.67\,\text{mm}} = 0.41$$

which give $y = 6.8$ mm, or $2y = 13.6$ mm. The whole field here is about 9.1 DD

The direct ophthalmoscope gave a 15.0× angular magnification and a 1.0 DD field of view. The indirect ophthalmoscope with the +14.00 D condenser lens gave a −3.21× angular magnification and a 6.4 DD field of view. The indirect ophthalmoscope with the +20.00 D condenser lens gave a −2.25× angular magnification and a 9.1 DD field of view. Still higher powered condenser lenses give smaller aerial images, and therefore less magnification and a larger field of view.

Suppose a lesion results in a 1 mm elevation on a patient's fundus. The axial magnification specifies the height of the elevation in the aerial image. From Section 9.10, the axial magnification for object points that have only a small axial separation equals square of the lateral magnification. For the patient's eye and the +14.00 D condenser lens, the lateral magnification ratio between the aerial image and the patient's fundus was −4.29, so the axial magnification is $(4.29)^2$ or 18.4. This indicates that the elevation is significantly magnified in the stereoscopic view of the aerial image.

The magnification and field of view in indirect ophthalmoscopy are not particularly sensitive to low and moderate amounts of uncorrected ametropia in the patient. The examiner compensates for the uncorrected refractive error by simply shifting the position of the condenser lens slightly.

19.9 DYNAMIC OR FOVEAL FIELD OF VIEW

The previous field of view discussions were for static optical systems including a static eye. However, the human visual system's resolution of detail comes from the foveal area of the retina only. When our head is fixed, we see detail by turning our eyes to look at directly at the object. During the turn, the eye rotates around its center of rotation in order to image the object on the fovea. This results in a foveal field of view, sometimes called a dynamic field of view, that is different than the static field of view. For a rotated eye, the ray incident on the eye that defines the dynamic field of view is a ray that points toward the eye's center of rotation (C in Figure 19.17a). This same ray appeared in the prism effectivity calculations in Chapters 11 and 12. The location of the eye's center of rotation varies from person to person. The average location is about 13.5 mm behind the cornea.

Figure 19.17a shows a lens in front of an eye. The dynamic field of view is defined in object space by the bounding ray incident on the edge of the lens. This ray is pointing towards C', which is the image of the eye's center of rotation C by the lens, and makes an angle of $F_d/2$ with the axis, where F_d is the angular expression for the dynamic field of view.

In Figure 19.17b, the dashed ray incident on the edge of the lens is the bounding ray for the static field of view (i.e., the field of at least one-half illumination). After passing through the lens, the dashed ray passes through the center of the static eye's entrance pupil E. The solid ray is the boundary for the dynamic field of view. After passing through the lens, the solid ray passes through the eye's center of rotation C. The two rays show that for a plus lens, the dynamic field is less than the static field.

EXAMPLE 19.12

A patient has a +16.00 D thin lens correction (diameter 40 mm) at a 12 mm vertex distance. The patient's entrance pupil is 3 mm behind the cornea, and the center of rotation of the patient's eye is 13.5 mm behind the cornea. What is the static and dynamic field of view?

The lens is the field stop, and its semidiameter is 20 mm. For the static field, first find the image of the eye's entrance pupil by the lens.

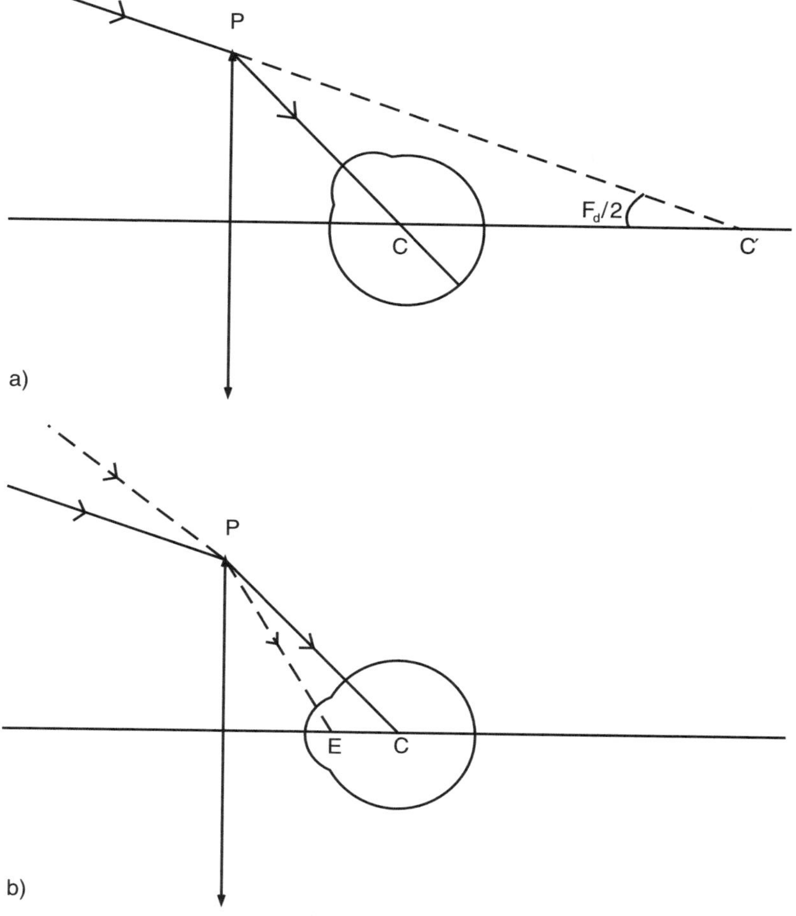

Figure 19.17 a, Bounding ray for the dynamic (or foveal) field of view. C' is the image of the eye's center of rotation C by the lens P. The bounding ray incident on P points towards C' and makes an angle of $F_d/2$ with the axis. The ray leaving P points towards C; b, the static field of view (defined by the dashed rays) is larger than the dynamic field of view (solid rays). The dashed ray leaving P points towards E, which is the eye's entrance pupil.

Here $u = -(12+3)\,\text{mm} = -15\,\text{mm}$, $U = -66.67\,\text{D}$, $V = P + U = -50.67\,\text{D}$, and $v = -19.74\,\text{mm}$. This image is the system's entrance pupil. Then Eq. 19.2 gives

$$\tan\frac{F_h}{2} = \frac{20\,\text{mm}}{19.74\,\text{mm}} = 1.01$$

and the static field is $F_h = 90.6°$.

For the dynamic field, first find the image of the eye's center of rotation. Here $u = -(12+13.5)\,\text{mm} = -25.5\,\text{mm}$, $U = -39.22\,\text{D}$, $V = P + U = -23.22\,\text{D}$, and $v = -43.07\,\text{mm}$. Then from the triangle in Figure 19.17a,

$$\tan\frac{F_d}{2} = \frac{20\,\text{mm}}{43.07\,\text{mm}} = 0.46$$

and the dynamic field is $F_d = 49.8°$.

(The numbers calculated here illustrate the differences between the static and dynamic fields of view. However the calculated angles are not paraxial angles, and a +16.00 D lens would not be a thin lens. Therefore aberration effects, discussed in Chapter 20, as well as the lens shape factor, Eq. 18.7, would need to be considered in a real world situation.)

The previous example shows that for high plus lenses, the dynamic field is significantly smaller than the static field. For ametropes, such as aphakes, with high plus spectacle corrections, this results in the so-called "jack-in-the-box" effect. Consider a spectacle corrected aphake viewing a centrally located white object (the white is for clarity of presentation and is not crucial). While fixating on the white object, the aphake may become aware of a different object, perhaps red, at the edge of their static field of view. When the aphake turns their eye (while keeping their head fixed) to look at the red object, it vanishes since it is not in the dynamic field. Then when the aphake turns their eye back (keeping the head fixed) to fixate on the white object, the red object again appears at the edge of the static field. When the aphake turns the eye back to view the red object, it again vanishes. Thus, the peripheral (red) object appears and disappears like a jack-in-the box.

19.10 FILM EXPOSURE AND THE *F*-NUMBER

The *exposure* is the amount of luminous flux (light energy) delivered to a film. On a simple level, the exposure E equals the illuminance I_l, on the film times the time t that the film is exposed, or

$$E = I_l t \tag{19.22}$$

Equation 19.22 is known as the *reciprocity law*, since it says we can obtain the same exposure with a high illuminance and a short exposure time or with a low illuminance and a long exposure time. (This law works well over the linear region of the film response but breaks down at the extremes.)

Obviously, the illuminance on the film plane depends on the amount of light let into the system, which in turn depends on the area of the entrance pupil. The area of the entrance pupil is proportional to the square of the diameter d_m of the entrance pupil, so

$$I_l \propto d_m^2$$

For a fixed entrance pupil, the illuminance on the film plane varies inversely with the image area. In other words, for a small image, the illuminance is higher (the energy is more concentrated); while for a large image the illuminance is smaller (i.e., the energy is spread out more). The image area is directly proportional to the square of the image size I. (i.e., the area of an image of a square with both sides of length I is I^2, while the image of a circle of diameter I is $\pi I^2/4$). The image size I equals the image distance v times the tangent of the nodal angle. Therefore, the image area is directly proportional to the square of v, and then

$$I_l \propto \frac{1}{v^2} \tag{19.23}$$

From the above two equations

$$I_l \propto \frac{d_m^2}{v^2} \tag{19.24}$$

Ordinary cameras usually have a high enough dioptric power and deal with objects that are far enough away that the image distance v is approximately equal to the secondary equivalent focal length f, so

$$I_l \propto \frac{d_m^2}{f^2} \tag{19.25}$$

The ratio of the reduced secondary equivalent focal length to the entrance pupil diameter is called the *f*-number:

$$f\text{-number} = \frac{f}{d_m} \tag{19.26}$$

Equations 19.25 and 19.26 together show that the illuminance is inversely proportional to the *f*-number squared, or

$$I_l \propto \frac{1}{f\text{-number}^2} \tag{19.27}$$

The *f*-number is conventionally preceded by the symbols, $f/$. For example, an *f*-number of 11 is written as $f/11$, an *f*-number of 5.6 is written as $f/5.6$. Many cameras have the *f*-number settings marked on them. The larger the aperture, the smaller the *f*-number. Fast camera systems (i.e., short exposure times) have small *f*-numbers (e.g., $f/1.8, f/2.8$). The smaller the aperture, the larger the *f*-number. Slow camera systems (longer exposure times) have larger *f*-numbers (e.g., $f/11$, $f/16$). Instamatics and older single lens cameras are $f/11$ systems. The better the image quality of the camera lens system, the wider the aperture can be, and so the smaller the minimum *f*-number. Camera lens systems rated $f/1.8$ are now common.

For a fixed exposure E, the reciprocity law, Eq. 19.22, gives the exposure time t:

$$t = \frac{E}{I_l}$$

Then substitution of Eq. 19.27 gives

$$t \propto E(f\text{-number})^2$$

For the same exposure E in a camera or system, it follows that the exposure times are directly proportional to the *f*-number squared, or

$$\frac{t_2}{t_1} = \frac{(f\text{-number})_2^2}{(f\text{-number})_1^2} \tag{19.28}$$

Suppose that for $f/2$, the exposure time t_1 is 1 unit. Then the *f*-number setting that doubles t for the same E is

$$\frac{2}{1} = \frac{(f\text{-number})_2^2}{2^2}$$

or

$$(f\text{-number})_2^2 = 8$$

and

$$(f\text{-number})_2 = 2.8$$

This is written as $f/2.8$. Similarly, the *f*-number that doubles the exposure time again (i.e., $t = 4$) is $f/4$. For the same exposure, Table 19.1 completely shows how the exposure time t varies with the *f*-number.

Table 19.1 Exposure Time versus *f*-number for the same Exposure

t	*f-number*
1	2
2	2.8
4	4
8	5.6
16	8
32	11.3
64	16
128	22.6

The *f*-number settings on a camera are called the *f*-stop settings. On a modern camera, there may also be some half or third stop settings. A typical real sequence is $f/1.8$, $f/2.8$, $f/4$, $f/5.6$, $f/8$, $f/11$, $f/16$, and $f/22$. Diffraction effects due to the small aperture start to become noticeable at $f/22$.

EXAMPLE 19.13

A 35 mm camera (the 35 mm is the film width), has a 55 mm focal length lens ($P = +18.18$ D). What is the entrance pupil size for *f*-numbers of $f/1.8$, $f/11$, and $f/22$?

From Eq. 19.26, the entrance pupil diameter for $f/1.8$ is

$$d_{\mathrm{m}} = \frac{f}{f\text{-number}} = \frac{55\,\mathrm{mm}}{1.8} = 30.6\,\mathrm{mm}$$

Similarly, $f/11$ gives 5 mm and $f/22$ gives 2.5 mm.

EXAMPLE 19.14

Consider a thin lens and screen model for a +60.00 D human eye. For a 3 mm entrance pupil, what is the *f*-number of the eye?

The focal length is 16.67 mm, and Eq. 19.26 gives

$$f\text{-number} = \frac{16.67\,\mathrm{mm}}{3\,\mathrm{mm}} = 5.6$$

So $f/5.6$ is the rating for this eye. (The human eye functions from about $f/2$ when dark adapted to $f/8$ in high illuminations.)

The *f*-number system enables one to change lens systems on a camera, and yet still use the same type of film. No matter what lens system is being used, if it is set for $f/8$, then the exposure time is the same. Thus, for the same distant object, a +10.00 D lens with a +12.5 mm entrance pupil diameter has the same exposure time as a +20.00 D lens with a 6.25 mm opening. For illumination purposes, we simply describe both lenses as $f/8$.

In *macrophotography* or photography of very near objects, the image distance v differs significantly from the focal length f. Here there is an effective *f*-number, or *f*-effective, defined as

$$f\text{-effective} = \frac{v}{d_{\mathrm{m}}} \qquad (19.29)$$

Then from Eq. 19.24,

$$I_{\mathrm{I}} \propto \frac{1}{(f\text{-effective})^2}$$

The lateral magnification m is negative for a real image conjugate to a real object. From $V = P + U$, and $m = U/V$, it follows that $v = (1 - m)f$, where f is the secondary focal length. For such a case, when we substitute this relation and Eq. 19.26 into Eq. 19.29, we obtain

$$f\text{-effective} = (1 + |m|)f\text{-number} \qquad (19.30)$$

For a fairly distant object, m is small, and *f*-effective is approximately equal to the *f*-number. As the object gets nearer, m gets larger, and *f*-effective begins to differ from the *f*-number. For example, for $m = -0.5$, *f*-effective is 1.5 times the *f*-number.

EXAMPLE 19.15

For a near object, a bellows added to a camera extends the lens away from the film plane until the image size is equal to the object size. The camera lens has regular *f*-number settings for distance marked on it. Which of the distance settings should be used when the lighting conditions and film speed require an $f/8$ setting for the near object?

Here f-effective $= 8$. Both the object and the image are real, so $m = -1$ (the symmetry point case). Then Eq. 19.30 gives

$$f\text{-number} = f\text{-effective}/2 = 8/2 = 4$$

So $f/4$ is the setting. Relative to the image for a distant object, this makes sense because the image for the near object is larger than the image for a distant object. Therefore for the same amount of light incident on the camera lens, the illuminance on the film will be less for the near object, and the compensation is to open the aperture up from $f/8$ to $f/4$. (Actually, macrophotography may have more complications than this, but for these you are referred to the photographic literature.)

19.11 COSINE TO THE FOURTH LAW

For the lens P, Figure 19.18a shows the nodal ray from a non-paraxial (off-axis) object point that subtends the angle ϕ. Since this is a one component system, it has no field stop. Nevertheless, there is an illuminance fall-off in the image plane as a function of the subtended ϕ for the non-paraxial object points. This illuminance fall-off has a cosine to the fourth power dependence. There are three different factors that contribute to the fourth power fall-off.

The first factor is the actual (peripheral) image distance along the light wave. The center part of the light wave from the object point follows the nodal ray (subtended angle ϕ) through the lens, and the peripheral image distance v_{per} from the nodal point to the non-paraxial image point is longer than the paraxial image distance v_{par} along the axis. From the triangle involving the nodal ray, and the image point,

$$v_{per} = \frac{v_{par}}{\cos\phi}$$

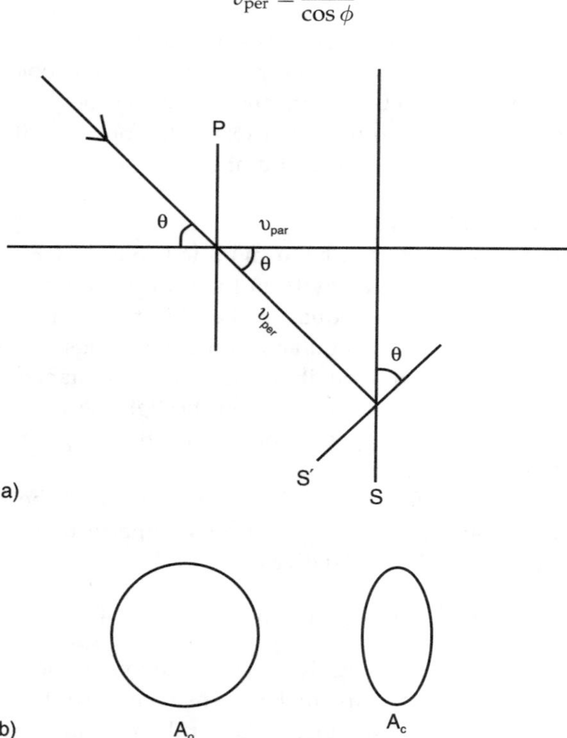

Figure 19.18 a, A non-paraxial nodal ray subtends the angle ϕ with the optical axis of the lens P. S' (dashed) is an image screen normal to the nodal ray. The (vertical) screen S is the image screen normal to the optical axis; b, A_o is the cross-sectional area of a circular shaped lens as viewed from the optical axis. A_c is the cross-sectional area of a rotated lens (or the cross-sectional area as viewed from a non-paraxial object point).

From Eq. 19.24, the illuminance at the peripheral image point is proportional to the reciprocal of the image distance squared, which results in

$$I_I \propto \frac{1}{(v_{per})^2} = \frac{\cos^2\phi}{(v_{par})^2}$$

The second factor is the cross-sectional area of the lens for the non-paraxial object point. When you view a circularly shaped lens normal to the surface, you see the full circular area A_o of the lens. However when you view the lens at an angle ϕ to the optical axis, you see a cross-sectional area A_c that is smaller than A_o (Figure 19.18b). The vertical size of the lens is the same in the two views, but for the off-axis view the horizontal cross sectional size decreases by a factor of cos ϕ with the result that $A_c = A_o \cos\phi$. If your eye was an off-axis glowing object point, then less light would get through the smaller cross sectional area than would get through from an object point on the optical axis. The illuminance in the image plane is proportional to the cross-sectional area A_c of the lens that is presented to the incoming light wave. When this is combined with the above equation,

$$I_I \propto \frac{A_c\cos^2\phi}{(v_{par})^2} \propto \frac{A_o\cos^3\phi}{(v_{par})^2}$$

The third factor is that the incident angle of the non-paraxial light illuminating the image screen S differs significantly from normal incidence. In 19.18a, the tilted screen S' (dashed) is normal to the incident light traveling along the nodal ray. Assume that this results in a circular illumination patch on S'. Then for the non-tilted (vertical) screen S, the light along the nodal ray is incident at an angle ϕ relative to the screen's normal, and this results in an elongated elliptical illumination patch on the screen. The area of the elliptical patch is larger than the circular patch by

$$\text{elliptical patch} = \frac{\text{circular patch}}{\cos\phi}$$

(Note that this is exactly the opposite of the cross sectional argument for the lens area.) Since illuminance is the luminous flux per unit area, the reciprocal of the above equation places the cos ϕ in the numerator of the proportionality for the illuminance, or

$$I_I \propto \frac{A_o\cos^3\phi\cos\phi}{(v_{par})^2} \propto \cos^4\phi \tag{19.31}$$

For $\phi = 1°$, $\cos^4\phi = 1.00$. For $\phi = 5°$, $\cos^4\phi = 0.98$. For $\phi = 10°$, $\cos^4\phi = 0.94$. For $\phi = 20°$, $\cos^4\phi = 0.78$. For $\phi = 30°$, $\cos^4\phi = 0.56$. These numbers show that the cosine to the fourth fall-off is fairly negligible in the paraxial region, but grows rapidly for angles outside the paraxial zone. For light outside the paraxial zone incident on multi-component systems, the cosine to the fourth illuminance fall-off needs to be considered along with the field of view considerations.

19.12 DEPTH OF FIELD

Figure 19.19 shows a fixed image screen at a distance v behind a thin lens of power P. The conjugate object point distance is u. Normally, there is a range of object distances (u_d for distal to u_p for proximal) for which the image on the screen does not have any detectable blur. (For u_d the rays are dashed, and the image distance is v_d. For u_p the rays are solid, and the image distance is v_p.) The object range, u_d to u_p, is called the *linear depth of field*.

The diameter of the lens is d_m, and the maximum tolerable blur circle diameter is b. (In other words, blur circles of diameter up to b do not result in detectable blur.) The depth of field clearly depends on b. From the similar triangles in Figure 19.19,

$$\frac{v_d}{d_m} = \frac{v - v_d}{b}$$

Then,

$$\frac{b}{d_m} = \frac{v - v_d}{v_d}$$

or

$$\frac{b}{d_m v} = \frac{1}{v_d} - \frac{1}{v}$$

and

$$\frac{b}{d_m} V = V_d - V$$

where V_d and V are the corresponding dioptric values. Now

$$V_d = P + U_d$$

and

$$V = P + U$$

where $U = 1/u$ and $U_d = 1/u_d$. By subtraction,

$$V_d - V = U_d - U$$

Thus, the distal part of the depth of field expressed dioptrically is:

$$U_d - U = \frac{b}{d_m} V$$

Similarly, we can show that the proximal part of the depth of field is

$$U - U_p = \frac{b}{d_m} V$$

Therefore, as expressed dioptrically, the distal part of the depth of field equals the proximal part. Let δ stand for each part, or

$$\delta = \pm \frac{b}{d_m} V = \pm \frac{b}{d_m v} \qquad (19.32)$$

δ is the dioptric expression for the depth of field. (The total dioptric depth is sometimes expressed as 2δ.)

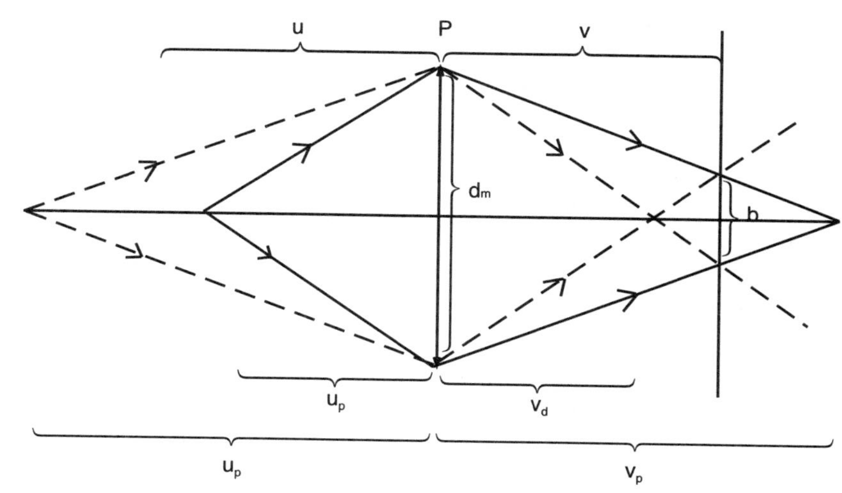

Figure 19.19 Depth of field for a lens P (diameter d_m) with a maximum tolerable blur circle diameter b. The image screen is a distance v behind the lens, and the conjugate object distance is u. The distal limit (dashed rays) is u_d, and the conjugate image distance is v_d. The proximal limit (solid rays) is u_p, and the conjugate image distance is v_p.

Equation 19.32 shows that for a tolerable blur circle size b and a fixed vergence V (i.e., a fixed image distance v), we can increase the depth of field by decreasing the aperture diameter d_m. This is consistent with the pinhole effect.

EXAMPLE 19.16

A +7.00 D lens has a 36 mm diameter and an image screen is precisely conjugate to an object at 50 cm. When the tolerable blur circle diameter is 1 mm, what is the dioptric and linear depth of field?

For the object at 50 cm, $U = -2.00\,\text{D}$ and $V = +5.00\,\text{D}$. Then from Eq. 19.32,

$$\delta = \pm \frac{1.0\,\text{mm}}{(36\,\text{mm})} 5.00\,\text{D} = \pm 0.14\,\text{D}$$

The dioptric depth of field is ±0.14 D. The dioptric range is

$$-2.00\,\text{D} + 0.14\,\text{D} = -1.86\,\text{D}$$

to

$$-2.00\,\text{D} - 0.14\,\text{D} = -2.14\,\text{D}$$

The linear depth of field ranges from

$$\frac{100}{-1.86\,\text{D}} = -53.8\,\text{cm}$$

to

$$\frac{100}{-2.14\,\text{D}} = -46.7\,\text{cm}$$

Note that relative to the 50 cm object point, the linear depth extends out farther on the distal side (3.8 cm) than it does on the proximal side (3.3 cm). The exact focus is dioptrically halfway between the distal limit and the proximal limit, but for larger values of δ is not linearly halfway between. (This is similar to the calculation the circle of least confusion location in astigmatism.)

EXAMPLE 19.17

An iris diaphragm with a 9 mm aperture diameter is placed against a +10.00 D lens. With this aperture, the linear depth of field is 43.3–33.9 cm. What is the dioptric depth of field and what is the tolerable blur circle size?

Here,

$$U_p = \frac{100}{-33.9\,\text{cm}} = -2.95\,\text{D}$$
$$U_d = \frac{100}{-43.3\,\text{cm}} = -2.31\,\text{D}$$

Then the dioptric midpoint, $(U_p + U_d)/2$, is −2.63 D, and 38.0 cm (i.e., 100/−2.63 D) is the precise focus for the system. The dioptric depth of field is half of the total depth, or $\delta = \pm 0.32\,\text{D}$. For an object at the precise focus, $V = P + (-2.63\,\text{D}) = +7.37\,\text{D}$. From Eq. 19.32,

$$\pm 0.32\,\text{D} = \pm \frac{b}{9\,\text{mm}} 7.37\,\text{D}$$

which gives $b = 0.39\,\text{mm}$.

EXAMPLE 19.18

Consider a +60.00 D lens–screen model for the human eye. The typical diameter of a cone in the fovea of the human eye is 3 μm (microns). Assume that the eye cannot detect blur until the blur circles are at least the size of these cones. For distant objects, what is the dioptric depth of field of the eye when the pupil diameter is 3 mm?

For distant objects, $U = 0$, and $V = P$. From Eq. 19.32,

$$\delta = \frac{3 \times 10^{-6}\,\text{m}}{3 \times 10^{-3}\,\text{m}} (+60.00\,\text{D})$$

and

$$\delta = \pm 0.06\,\text{D}$$

So the depth of field is ±0.06 D. The typical ±0.25 D clinical depth of field of a human eye corresponds to blur circles of diameter 12.5 μm.

For distant objects, there is a direct relationship between the dioptric depth of field δ_d and the *f*-number. Here, V is approximately equal to P. We can multiply both the numerator and the denominator of Eq. 19.32 by the secondary focal length f to obtain

$$\delta_d = \pm \frac{bf}{d_m f} P$$

Then from Eq. 19.26 and the fact that the dioptric power equals the reciprocal of the focal length,

$$\delta_d = \pm b(f\text{-number})P^2 \tag{19.33}$$

Thus, for distant objects, the dioptric depth of field is directly proportional to the *f*-number, and we can set up the ratio:

$$\frac{\delta_2}{\delta_1} = \frac{(f\text{-number})_2}{(f\text{-number})_1} \tag{19.34}$$

Consider a camera set for $f/8$ with a ±0.36 D depth of field. Equation 19.34 shows that when set at $f/2$, this camera will have a ±0.09 D depth of field.

The power squared dependence in Eq.19.33 shows that higher powered systems (shorter focal lengths) have a larger dioptric depth of field. Newborn infants typically have about +2.75 D of hyperopia, and an accommodation system that is not yet well developed. A typical equivalent dioptric power for newborn human infants is +89.6 D. Thus, compared to the +60.00 D of an adult eye, the infant eye has a larger depth of field, which helps the infant while the accommodation system is developing.

When a camera with a ±0.167 D depth of field is precisely focused for optical infinity ($U = 0$ D), the dioptric proximal limit of the field is at $U = -0.167$ D, or the linear proximal limit is a real object point at $u = -6$ m. The dioptric distal limit is at $U = +0.167$ D, or the linear distal limit is a virtual object point at $u = +6$ m. That is, the linear depth of field extends from a real object point at −6 m through optical infinity to a virtual object point at +6 m (recall the distorted circle representations in Chapter 6). Here half of the depth of field covers virtual object points. To maximize the depth of field for real object points, the camera's focus needs to be at the real object distance closer than optical infinity that puts the distal limit at optical infinity.

The *hyperfocal distance* is the distance at which a camera (or system) is focused so that the distal limit of the depth of field is at optical infinity. Actually, the image distance v differs slightly from f when the system is focused for the hyperfocal distance. However, if we neglect this small difference, then the hyperfocal distance u_h equals the reciprocal of the dioptric depth of field δ_d, or

$$|u_h| = \left|\frac{1}{\delta_d}\right| \qquad (19.35)$$

When the system is focused for the hyperfocal distance, the dioptric range is $\delta_d \pm \delta_d$, so the distal limit is 0 D (i.e., optical infinity), and the proximal limit is $2\delta_d$ (i.e., at half of the hyperfocal distance).

EXAMPLE 19.19

An eye has a depth of field of ±0.25 D. What is the depth of field for the eye when focused on optical infinity? What is the depth of field for the eye when focused on the hyperfocal distance?

For the eye focused on optical infinity, the dioptric range is 0 ± 0.25 D, which is +0.25 D to −0.25 D. For real objects, the depth is from 0 to −0.25 D, and the linear depth is from optical infinity to 4 m.

From Eq. 19.35, the hyperfocal distance u_h is 1/0.25 D or 4 m. For the eye focused on the 4 m hyperfocal distance, the dioptric range is −0.25 D ± 0.25 D, which is 0 D to −0.5 D. The linear range is from infinity to 2 m.

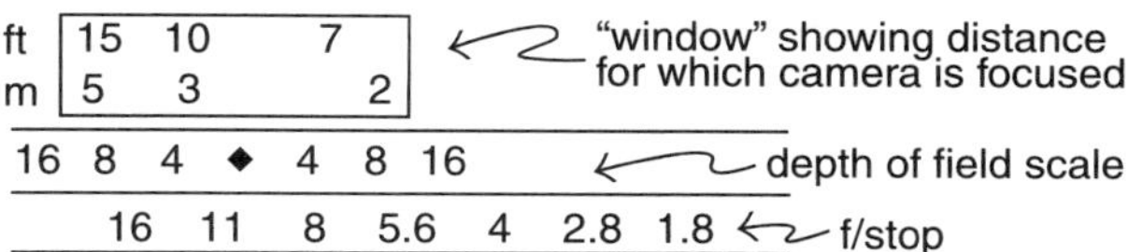

Figure 19.20 Depth of field scale as a function of *f*-stop.

Many good cameras have a depth of field scale marked one of the rings around the lens. To set the depth (assuming one is not limited by the film speed), one could proceed as follows: first focus the camera with a wide aperture (e.g., $f/1.8$), then set the f-number to give the desired depth, and finally set the correct exposure time. Figure 19.20 shows the settings for a camera that is focused for 2.8 m (above the diamond) and set at $f/11$ (below the diamond). To estimate the depth of field, look out on the depth scale to where 11 would be (between 8 and 16), and then go directly up to the distance ring. From the distance ring, the depth of field ranges from 5 m to 1.8 m. For the same focus with a $f/4$ setting, the depth would range from 3.5 m to 2.4 m.

Since for real objects and real images, $v = (1 + |m|)f$, where m is the lateral magnification, Eq. 19.32 becomes

$$\delta = \pm\frac{b}{d_m(1 + |m|)f}$$

and it follows that

$$\delta = \frac{\delta_d}{(1 + |m|)} \qquad (19.36)$$

In macrophotography with $m = -1$ (symmetry point situation), Eq. 19.36 shows that the dioptric depth of field δ is 1/2 of the distal depth of field δ_d. This means that optical system focussing must be more precise for the near objects.

When humans look from far to near, the eyes converge, accommodate, and the pupil constricts. This is the so-called *near triad*. The constriction of the pupil helps with the depth of field for near objects. As an object is moved from far to near, the eye's retinal image increases in size, and the tolerable blur circle size may also increase. This also helps the depth of field of near objects.

A *telecentric stop* is an aperture stop that is located at a focal point of an optical system. In a telecentric system, either the entrance pupil or the exit pupil is located at optical infinity. Telecentric stops are widely

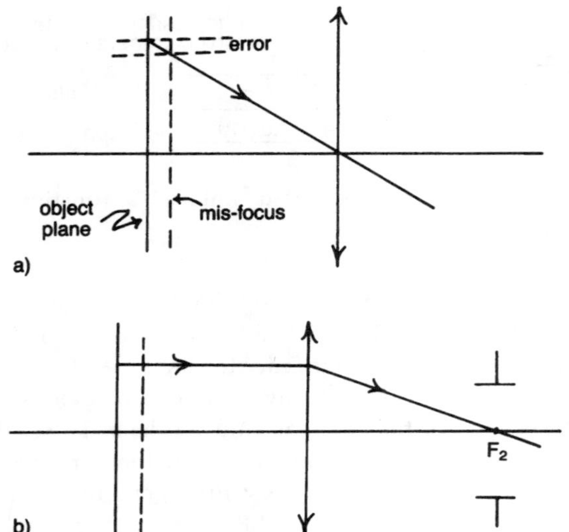

Figure 19.21 a, Size error; b, telecentric system to eliminate the error.

used in measurement systems. The telecentric stop minimizes the measurement error made by a slight defocus of the system. (A slight defocus can occur because of the depth of focus.) In Figure 19.21a, the stop is at the lens. The chief ray is then the nodal ray for the lens, and the place where it intersects the scale is the reading, which has some error in it. In Figure 19.21b, the aperture stop is at the secondary focal point of the lens. The incident chief ray is now parallel to the axis and, hence, gives no error if slightly defocused. Aperture stops can also be placed at the primary focal point (telecentric in object space).

19.13 DEPTH OF FOCUS

Given a tolerable blur circle size and a fixed object distance u, there is a range of image distances over which a screen can be moved before any blur is detected. This range is the *depth of focus*.

Just as for the depth of field, we can set up similar triangles and work out equations for the depth of focus. In general, this results in equations that are different from the depth of field equations. However, for a single thin lens with distant objects and small dioptric depths, the dioptric depth of focus equals the dioptric depth of field δ_d to a good approximation (e.g., depth of field = depth of focus = ±0.25 D).

EXAMPLE 19.20

Consider a +20.00 D lens with a ±0.2 D depth of field. For distant objects, what is the linear depth of focus?

When the depth of focus is approximately equal to the depth of field, the dioptric range for the depth of focus is +19.8 to +20.2 D. The linear range is then,

$$\frac{1000}{19.8\,\text{D}} = 50.5\,\text{mm}$$

to

$$\frac{1000}{20.2\,\text{D}} = 49.5\,\text{mm}$$

This means that the camera film has to be flat within a tolerance of plus or minus 0.5 mm, and is the reason cameras have pressure plates to flatten the film.

PROBLEMS

1. A window of width 100 cm is located 4 m in front of the pinhole of a pinhole camera. For a distant object (assuming the film size is not a limiting factor), what is the angular field of view of the camera?
2. A +7.00 D lens is located 6 cm in front of a −2.00 D lens. Each lens has a 30.0 mm diameter. For a real object 50 cm in front of the first lens, find the entrance pupil, entrance port, and the angular fields of view F_u, F_h, and F_t. Also what is the linear field for the field of at least one-half illumination?
3. Archie Meedes is looking through a round paper tube at a distant object. The tube has a 40 mm diameter, and is 30.0 cm long.

   a. Find Archie's field of view through the tube assuming that his eye's entrance pupil is located at the back end of the tube.
   b. When Archie holds at a −3.00 D lens (diameter 4.0 cm) at the objective end of the tube, what is his field of view?
   c. What is the ratio of the field of view in part b to the field in part a, and how does this ratio relate to the spectacle magnification for the −3.00 D lens?
   d. Archie Meedes is an uncorrected hyperope and can hold a +2.00 D lens at the end of the tube and still see distant objects clearly when looking through the tube. What is Archie's angular field of view through the tube under these circumstances?
   e. What is the ratio of the field of view in part d to the field in part a, and how does this ratio relate to the spectacle magnification for the +2.00 D lens?
   f. Finally, Archie Meedes holds a +20.00 D lens at the objective end of the tube and views the aerial image formed by the +20.00 D lens. What is Archie's field of view under these circumstances?

4. Ms. Octa Hedron has a 6.25× magnifier with a 50 mm diameter. When Octa uses this lens as a collimating magnifier held 8 cm from the entrance pupil of her eye, what is the linear field of view? Can Octa increase her field of view with this lens? If yes, how? If no, why not? Would a higher powered collimating magnifier with the same diameter and held at the same position give a larger or a smaller field of view?
5. An 8.5× Galilean telescope has a +2.368 D objective lens with a 40 mm diameter, a −20.132 D ocular lens with a 20 mm diameter, and a 37.255 cm length. The observer's entrance pupil has a diameter of 5 mm. Find the angular field of view assuming the observer's entrance pupil can be placed at the ocular lens of the telescope. Also specify the telescope's exit pupil location. Why can't a field lens be added to a Galilean telescope?
6. An 8.5× Keplerian telescope has a +3.000 D objective lens with a 40 mm diameter, a +25.500 D ocular lens with a 20 mm diameter, and the length of the telescope is 37.255 cm. The observer's entrance pupil has a diameter of 5 mm.

   a. Specify the entrance pupil, entrance port, and the angular field of view.
   b. Also specify the exit pupil location.
   c. The 8.5× Keplerian of this problem has the same lens diameters and length as the 8.5× Galilean of the previous problem. Which has the larger field of view, or are the fields equal in size?

7. A +4.00 D field lens is now added to the 8.5× Keplerian telescope of the previous problem. Assume that the ocular lens remains the field stop. What is the new entrance port location? What is the new angular field of view? What is the percent increase in the field of view? Also specify the new exit pupil location.
8. A pair of binoculars has a +4.00 D $f/5.6$ objective lens and a 6 mm diameter Ramsden circle. What is the angular magnification of the binoculars?
9. An $f/11$ lens has a 4.6 mm diameter. What is the diameter of an $f/2.8$ lens of the same power?
10. If the correct exposure time is 1/120 second for an $f/5.6$ setting, what is the exposure time for an $f/16$ setting?
11. In dim light, a human entrance pupil opens up to an 8 mm diameter. For a +60.00 D eye, what is the *f*-number?
12. An optical system focused for 40 cm has a depth of field that ranges from 33.33 cm to 50.00 cm. What is the dioptric depth of field? If the lens in the system is +12.00 D with a 36 mm size, what is the tolerable blur circle size?
13. For a distant object, a +16.00 D $f/16$ lens has a ±1.00 D depth of field. What is the depth of field for the +16.00 D lens with an $f/1.8$ setting?
14. A camera has a 5 m hyperfocal distance. For real objects, what is the camera's linear depth of field when focused for optical infinity? When focussed for the hyperfocal distance?
15. For a refractive myope with a far point that is 23.53 cm from the cornea, what magnification is obtained with a direct ophthalmoscope held 16.67 mm from the cornea?
16. What lens needs to be in a direct ophthalmoscope in order for an uncorrected 2.00 D myopic examiner to clearly see the fundus of an uncorrected 5.00 D patient. Assume that neither is accommodating and that the specified corrections are at the plane of the sighthole.
17. In indirect ophthalmoscopy, an examiner with +2.75 D of accommodation uses a +18.00 D condenser lens (diameter 52 mm) to examine the fundus of a +60.00 D emmetrope. Use a thin lens and screen model of the patient's eye and of the examiner's eye to answer the following questions.

   a. How far is the aerial image from the condenser lens?
   b. How far must the examiner hold the condenser lens from her eye?
   c. How far must the examiner hold the condenser lens from the patient's cornea (thin lens model) in order to make the pupils conjugate?
   d. What is the linear field of view, and how many DD does it correspond to?
   e. What is the angular magnification for this situation?
   f. Would a higher powered condenser lens give more or less magnification? Would a higher powered condenser lens give a larger or a smaller field of view?

CHAPTER 20

Aberrations

20.1 DETRIMENTS TO IMAGE QUALITY

In a good quality image, both the gross and the fine detail are sharp and clear. In a poor quality image, the fine detail is blurred out, even though the gross detail may still be resolvable. For example, we may be able to identify a person (gross detail) in a blurred photograph, but we might not be able to see the wrinkles by their eyes (fine detail). The use of a magnifying system to examine the blurred photograph only magnifies the blur, and confirms the fact that the fine detail is degraded or lost.

Besides a misfocus (blur), another source of image degradation is stray light caused by extraneous light sources, reflections, or by scatter in the system. Sources of scatter include scratches, dirt, or inhomogenities in the media. For example, a cataract in the crystalline lens degrades the retinal image by scattering light.

Even for properly focused systems free of stray light, there are optical sources of image degradation. These sources are referred to as the aberrations. The aberrations can be divided into chromatic aberration (CA) and the so-called monochromatic aberrations.

Chromatic aberration is due to the fact that the refractive index of a material varies slightly with the wavelength. Thus, the refracting (dioptric) power of the material varies slightly with the wavelength, and consequently, a single lens does not focus all wavelengths at precisely the same position.

The theoretical reason for the monochromatic aberrations of spherical systems is that the paraxial equations, including $V = P + U$, break down as the light paths leave the thread-like paraxial region. Consequently, the nonparaxial light paths give wavefronts that are not quite spherical. This means that perfect point images are no longer formed, and extended images are degraded in quality. Besides degradation, image distortion may occur for nonparaxial paths.

Diffraction is the ability of waves to bend around corners. Even if all the aberrations are controlled, the ability of an optical system to image fine detail is still limited by diffraction. Diffraction is discussed in Chapter 22.

20.2 DISPERSION AND CHROMATIC ABERRATION

When white light is incident on a thick prism, the light is dispersed into a rainbowlike spectrum (Figure 20.1a). The physical reason for the dispersion is that the refractive index of the material is slightly different for each wavelength of light.

Figure 20.1b shows the index of refraction of ophthalmic crown glass as a function of the incident

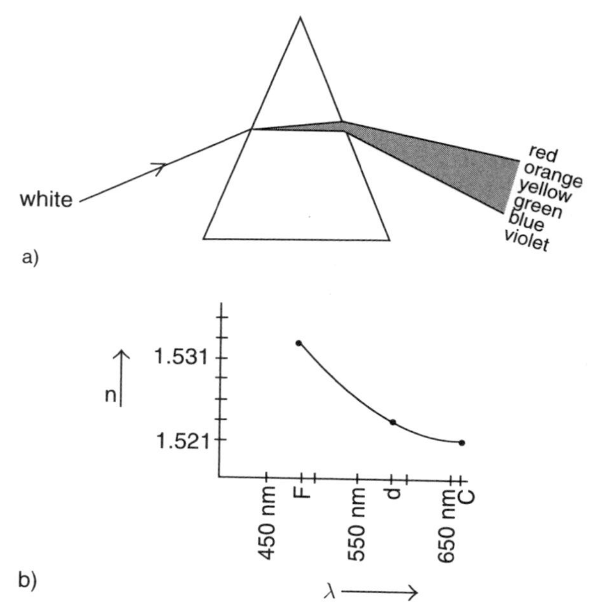

Figure 20.1 a, Dispersion by a thick prism; b, refractive index versus incident wavelength.

wavelength. One way to obtain such data is to use an ophthalmic crown prism and measure the minimum deviation angle for each incident wavelength. Then we can use the minimum deviation equation (Eq. 11.7) to solve for the index of refraction for each wavelength.

As shown in Figure 20.1a, the shorter wavelengths (violets and blues) are bent more than the longer wavelengths (reds). This occurs because the refractive index is greater for the shorter wavelengths (Figure 20.1b). Thus, the violet and blue wavelengths have a larger refractive index than the reds. The human eye is not as sensitive to violet as it is to blue, so frequently in dealing with CA, we label the short wavelength zone as blue.

For a thin prism of refractive index n in air, Eq. 11.9 gave

$$d = (n - 1)A \tag{20.1}$$

where d is the deviation angle and A is the apex angle. It is obvious from the equation that the higher indices give the larger deviations. Figure 20.2 shows a white light bulb located in front of a BD prism. The prism forms a virtual image that appears to be deviated toward the apex. Since the prism bends the shorter wavelengths down the most, a blue blur fringe appears on the top of the white virtual image. Similarly, a red blur fringe appears on the bottom of the white virtual image. These colored fringes are CA due to the dispersion.

While dispersion is the cause of CA, it is also the cause of considerable aesthetic joy. For example, dispersion is the cause of the colors of a rainbow. Figure 20.3 shows the ray path for light that makes the primary rainbow. The ray enters the raindrop near its edge, is reflected once inside the raindrop, and then exits the drop. The dispersion occurs at the two refractions (entering and exiting). The color that appears on top of the primary rainbow is found by extending the outgoing rays back toward the virtual image position. This shows that red appears on top of the primary rainbow. Similarly, the "fire" (play of colors) in a diamond is due to dispersion. The dispersion occurs at the refractions when the light enters and exits the diamond.

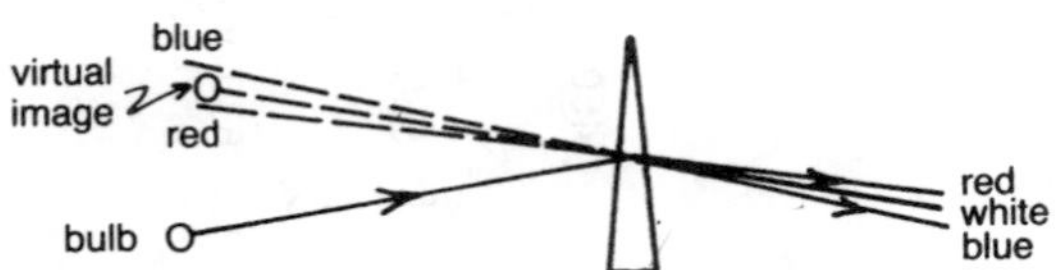

Figure 20.2 Chromatic blur due to a prism.

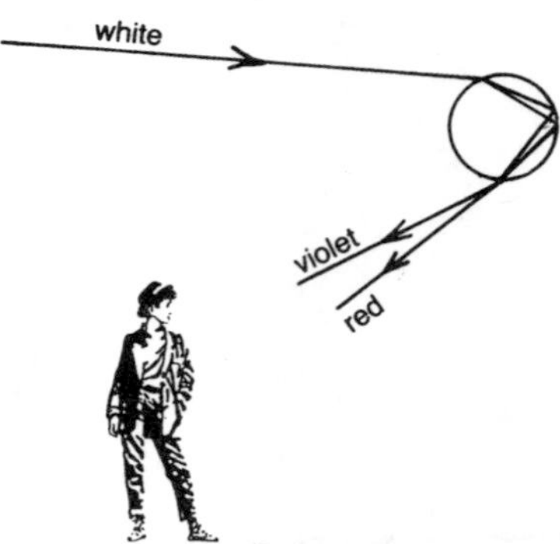

Figure 20.3 Rainbow rays.

20.3 LONGITUDINAL AND LATERAL CHROMATIC ABERRATION

Consider a convex lens with red and blue wavelengths incident from a distant axial point source. The convex lens is thickest at the optical center. We can crudely represent the convex lens as two prisms base to base (Figure 20.4a). Since the prisms deviate blue light the most, we see that the blue point image is formed before the red point image. For the lens, the linear separation of the blue and red point images is a longitudinal (or axial) manifestation of chromatic aberration. Experimentally, this corresponds to moving the image screen between the clear image positions.

If we place an image screen at the position of the red image, then a blue blur circle (Figure 20.4b) surrounds the red point image. The blur circle is a lateral (or transverse) manifestation of CA. Similarly, when the image screen is placed at the position of the blue image, a red blur circle surrounds the blue point image.

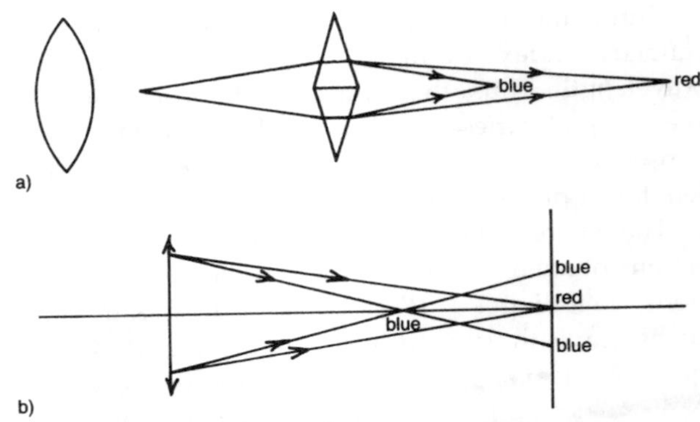

Figure 20.4 a, Base to base prisms provide intuition on the origin of longitudinal CA for a plus lens; b, longitudinal and lateral CA.

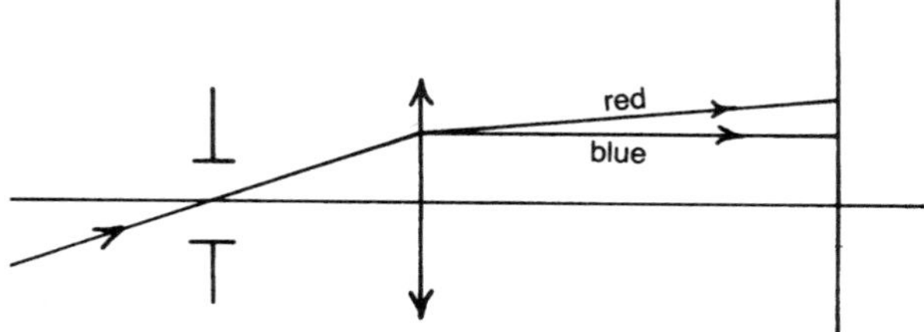

Figure 20.5 Chief ray and size manifestation of lateral CA.

Figure 20.5 shows the chief ray for an off-axis object in front of a system consisting of a separated aperture and lens. Due to the longitudinal CA, either the red or the blue image will be slightly blurred. When the aperture is small enough, the depth of focus may be large enough that the blur is not noticeable. However, the chief ray also specifies the size of the blurred image. Consequently, on the screen, the blue image is smaller in size than the red image. The image size difference is also a lateral manifestation of CA, and may be noticeable even when the blur is not. This lateral manifestation is sometimes referred to as a *chromatic difference in magnification*.

The human visual system is more sensitive to lateral manifestations of CA than it is to longitudinal manifestations. A system that has a zero (or minimal) longitudinal CA may have a noticeable lateral CA. We can design systems that have minimal lateral CA by leaving some longitudinal CA.

Systems that consist of only front surface mirrors are free of CA. This is because CA depends on the refractive index, while the basic law of reflection states that the angle of reflection equals the angle of incidence independent of the refractive indices. Thus, the image formation by a front surface mirror does not depend on the refractive index.

20.4 STANDARD WAVELENGTHS AND ABBE NUMBER

In order to quantify the discussion of CA for refraction, we need to use specific (vacuum) wavelengths. Sodium was the source historically used as the standard for specifying the index of refraction. Sodium gives a very strong orangish-yellow "doublet line" emission at an average (vacuum) wavelength of 589.29 nm. In lower precision instrumentation, the sodium doublet line effectively functions as a monochromatic line. However the sodium doublet line actually consists of two slightly different wavelengths, one at 589.59 and the other at 588.95 nm, with 589.29 nm as the average of the two. During the last third of the twentieth century, the precision of modern laser systems developed to the point that the sodium doublet was no longer acceptable as the wavelength standard.

An attempt in the 1990s to universally adopt a new standard wavelength was not successful. The United States chose to use the monochromatic helium d "singlet line" with a 587.56 nm wavelength, since the helium d wavelength is quite close to the old sodium standard. Europe and Asia chose to use the monochromatic mercury e "singlet line" with a 546.07 nm wavelength, since it is closer to the middle of the visible spectrum.

The indices of refraction for the two standard wavelengths are $n_d = 1.523$ and $n_e = 1.525$ for ophthalmic crown glass, $n_d = 1.498$ and $n_e = 1.500$ for CR-39 hard resin plastic, and $n_d = 1.586$ and $n_e = 1.590$ for polycarbonate. There is a clinically significant difference in higher dioptric or higher prism powers measured using the two different indices. So until a universal standard is adopted, it is important that those who buy and use optical lens and instruments are keenly aware of which index was used to calibrate the equipment.

This book uses the helium d wavelength for the standard index of refraction. This corresponds to using the helium d wavelength as the source to measure the refracting powers of lenses or prisms. For example, a +4.00 D lens means that the lens is +4.00 D specifically for helium d light. Similarly, a 6^{Δ} prism means the prism is 6^{Δ} specifically for helium d light.

A hydrogen gas discharge tube emits only a few visible wavelengths (singlet lines) across the visible spectrum. Two of the hydrogen wavelengths are used, together with the standard helium d wavelength, to quantify CA. These are the hydrogen C line at 656.28 nm (red), and the hydrogen F line at 486.13 nm (aqua blue). The refractive indices of ophthalmic crown glass for these wavelengths are $n_F = 1.530$, $n_d = 1.523$, and $n_C = 1.521$.

The refracting power for a single spherical air–glass interface of radius r for each of the three conventional wavelengths is

$$P_d = \frac{n_d - 1}{r}$$

$$P_F = \frac{n_F - 1}{r}$$

and

$$P_C = \frac{n_C - 1}{r}$$

Of these, P_d is the conventional geometric optics dioptric power. The dioptric CA is defined as

$$CA = P_F - P_C \tag{20.2}$$

It follows from the above four equations that

$$CA = P_d\left(\frac{n_F - n_C}{n_d - 1}\right)$$

The term on the right is a characteristic of the material only, and is called the *dispersive power*. Its reciprocal,

$$v_d = \frac{n_d - 1}{n_F - n_C} \tag{20.3}$$

is more commonly used and is variously called the *refractive efficiency, the constringence, or the Abbe number.* Then,

$$CA = \frac{P_d}{v_d} \tag{20.4}$$

A six number code is used to classify transparent materials. The first three numbers are the three digits behind the decimal in n_d, and the second three digits equal the Abbe number v_d times 10. For ophthalmic crown glass, $n_d = 1.523$, $v_d = 58.6$, and the code is then 523–586. The codes for some common transparent materials are presented in Table 20.1.

For transparent lens materials, the Abbe number v_d ranges from about 20 to 90. Equations 20.4 shows that the higher Abbe values are better in that they give lower chromatic aberration. For example: The CA for a +16.00 D ophthalmic crown surface is

$$CA = \frac{+16.00\,D}{58.6} = +0.27\,D$$

while for polycarbonate, the Abbe number is 30.0 and the CA for a +16.00 D polycarbonate surface is

$$CA = \frac{+16.00\,D}{30.0} = +0.53\,D$$

Table 20.1 Refractive Parameters for Some Transparent Materials

Material	*Code*
Water	334–556
Alcohol	363–606
CR-39 hard resin plastic	498–580
Ophthalmic crown glass	523–586
Spectralite (plastic)	537–470
Polycarbonate	586–300
MR-6 plastic	597–360
Dense barium crown glass	617–549
MR-7 plastic	660–320
Highlite glass	701–310

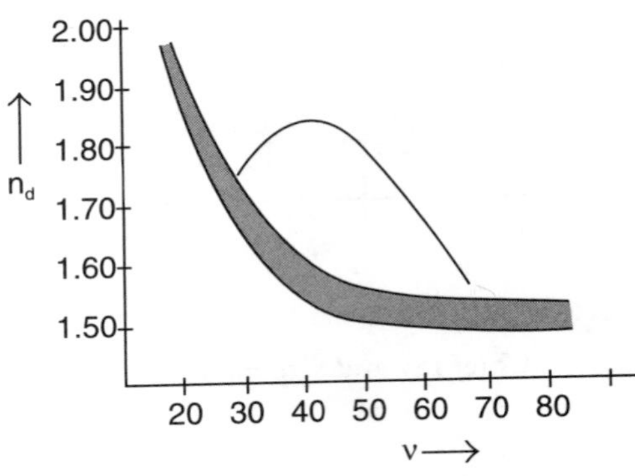

Figure 20.6 Refractive index versus refractive efficiency for various types of glass.

Figure 20.6 is a plot the index of refraction versus the Abbe number for various types of glass and plastic. The majority of types are in the shaded area. The tendency is for higher index materials to have lower Abbe numbers. However, as a result of considerable research, there are some modern glass materials that have a high index with an improved Abbe value. On the plot, these glasses fall between the bowed curve and the shaded area.

A +60 D spherical refracting interface between air and water (334–556) is a fairly accurate simple model for the CA of the human eye. From Eq. 20.4, this model gives

$$CA = \frac{+60\,D}{55.6} = +1.08\,D$$

with blue focusing before red (like Figure 20.4b). Experimental measurements of the CA of the eye agree well with the +1.08 D of CA predicted by this simple model. (This simple model deviates from actual measurements at the short wavelength end of the spectrum.) In view of the ±0.25 D clinical significance level, the amount of CA in the eye is surprising.

Due to the CA of the eye, a person corrected for the orangish-yellow helium d light would be myopic for blue light, slightly myopic for green light, and slightly hyperopic for red light. The CA of the eye is the basis for the red-green test (or duochrome test) commonly used in clinical refraction. The CA of the eye differs from the simple SSRI water model at the lower (blue) wavelengths. This difference is due to the CA of the crystalline lens.

For a thin lens, the total CA is the sum of that for each surface, or

$$CA_{lens} = \frac{P_1}{v} + \frac{P_2}{v}$$

where P_1 and P_2 are the front and back surface powers. (Here we assume that the Abbe number v

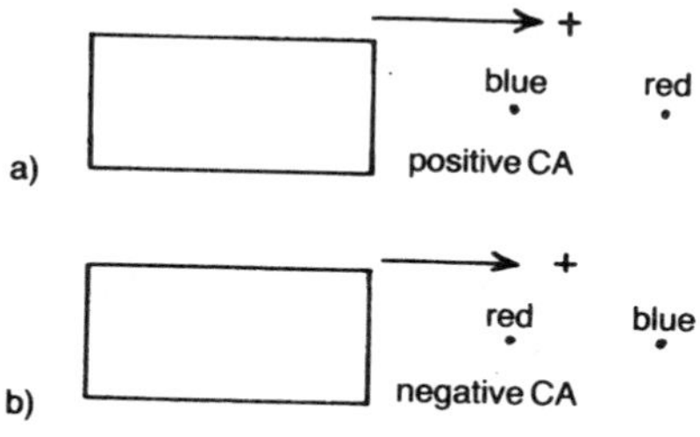

Figure 20.7 Longitudinal CA for a system: a, positive; b, negative.

means v_d.) Since the thin lens power is the sum of the surface powers it follows that

$$\mathrm{CA}_{\mathrm{lens}} = \frac{P_{\mathrm{lens}}}{v} \tag{20.5}$$

A plus lens converges the blue more than the red, while a minus lens diverges the blue more than the red. Thus, a minus lens tends to correct the CA of a plus lens. For converging systems that consist of both plus and minus lens, the resulting CA is called positive when the F (blue) image is formed closer to the system than the C (red) image (Figure 20.7a), and negative when the C image is formed closer than the F image (Figure 20.7b). The longitudinal CA is zero when the F and C images are focused in the same place.

20.5 THE ACHROMATIC DOUBLET

Since some materials have different Abbe numbers, it is possible to combine a positive lens and a negative lens of different materials into an achromatic doublet (Figure 20.8a). In the thin lens design of an achromatic doublet, the total dioptric power of the doublet is the sum

$$P_t = P_1 + P_2 \tag{20.6}$$

where P_1 and P_2 are the dioptric powers of the individual lenses. Similarly, the total CA is the sum

$$\mathrm{CA}_t = \mathrm{CA}_1 + \mathrm{CA}_2$$

or

$$\mathrm{CA}_t = \frac{P_1}{v_1} + \frac{P_2}{v_2} \tag{20.7}$$

where v_1 and v_2 are the respective Abbe numbers for the different lens materials. CA_t is zero for an achromatic doublet. Once the materials are specified, we can solve Eqs. 20.6 and 20.7 for the unknown powers P_1 and P_2 of the components.

EXAMPLE 20.1
Design a +10.00 D achromatic doublet using ophthalmic crown glass (523–586) and dense flint glass (617–366).

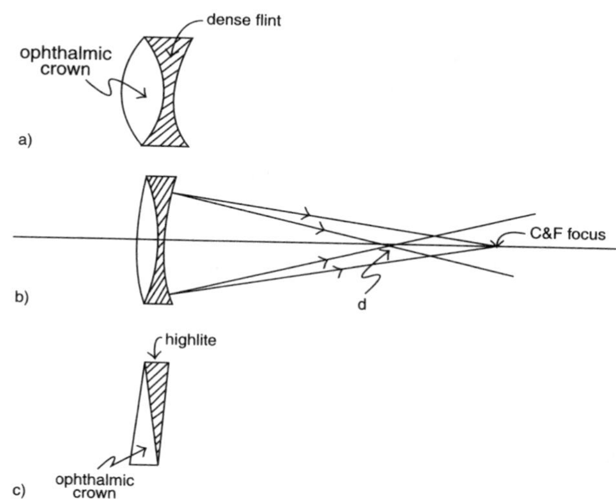

Figure 20.8 a, Achromatic doublet; b, exaggeration of focus differences; c, achromatic prism.

From the condition for zero CA,

$$0 = \frac{P_1}{58.6} + \frac{P_2}{36.6}$$

Then,

$$P_1 = -\frac{58.6}{36.6} P_2 = -1.60 P_2$$

The power condition is

$$+10.00\,\mathrm{D} = P_1 + P_2$$

Substitution for P_1 gives

$$\begin{aligned} +10.00\,\mathrm{D} &= -1.60 P_2 + P_2 \\ &= -0.60 P_2 \end{aligned}$$

or

$$P_2 = -16.64\,\mathrm{D}$$

Then,

$$P_1 = -1.60 P_2 = +26.64\,\mathrm{D}$$

So a +10.00 D doublet lens made of a +26.64 D ophthalmic crown component and a −16.64 D flint glass component has zero CA (Figure 20.8a). We can check the arithmetic in the above example by noting that the sum of +26.64 D and −16.64 D is +10.00 D, and by noting that

$$\begin{aligned} \mathrm{CA}_t &= \frac{+26.64\,\mathrm{D}}{58.6} + \frac{-16.64\,\mathrm{D}}{36.6} \\ &= +0.46\,\mathrm{D} + (-0.46\,\mathrm{D}) = 0 \end{aligned}$$

Note that in the achromatic doublet, the material with the higher power (in magnitude) has to also have the higher Abbe number, while the material with the lower power (in magnitude) has to have the lower Abbe number.

In the achromatic doublet, the zero CA condition specifies that the dioptric powers are equal for the hydrogen C (red) and F (blue) wavelengths. That does not mean that the dioptric power for helium d light is equal to the dioptric power for the C and F wavelengths. The achromatic doublet focuses the C and F light at the same position, but does not necessarily focus d light there (Figure 20.8b shows an exaggerated view). The remaining CA (which is small) is referred to as the *secondary spectrum*.

One way to focus three wavelengths at one position is to use a triplet lens (three components with three different materials). The equations involved consist of three equations in three unknowns. The resulting lens is called an *apochromatic* lens. Actually, a triplet lens that does better than focusing three wavelengths in one position can be designed by considering the exact form of the index of refraction as a function of wavelength. Such lenses are referred to as *superachromats*.

20.6 ACHROMATIC PRISMS

Equation 20.1 gives the deviation for a thin prism of index n and apex angle A. The prism-diopter rating is given by

$$Z = 100 \tan d \tag{20.8}$$

When d in radians is small,

$$Z \approx 100\, d$$

and then

$$Z \approx 100\,(n-1)A$$

The standard prism-diopter value specified in terms of the helium d wavelength is

$$Z_d \approx 100\,(n_d - 1)A \tag{20.9}$$

We can write similar expressions for the prism-diopter ratings for hydrogen C (red) and F (blue) light. Then the (lateral) CA of the prism (in prism-diopters) is defined by

$$CA = Z_F - Z_C \tag{20.10}$$

It follows that

$$CA = \frac{Z_d}{v_d} \tag{20.11}$$

where v_d is the Abbe number of the material. The CA of two thin prisms in contact is then

$$CA_t = \frac{Z_1}{v_1} + \frac{Z_2}{v_2} \tag{20.12}$$

We can use Eq. 20.12 and prism additivity to design achromatic prisms just as we design achromatic lenses.

EXAMPLE 20.2

Design a 6^Δ BD achromatic prism using ophthalmic crown (523–586) and highlite (701–310) glass.

The zero CA condition is

$$0 = \frac{Z_1}{58.6} + \frac{Z_2}{31.0}$$

or

$$Z_1 = -\frac{58.6}{31.0} Z_2 = -1.89 Z_2$$

The power condition is

$$-6^\Delta = Z_1 + Z_2$$

where the minus sign comes from the required BD. We can substitute for Z_1 to obtain

$$\begin{aligned} -6^\Delta &= -1.89 Z_2 + Z_2 \\ &= -0.89 Z_2 \end{aligned}$$

or

$$Z_2 = +6.74^\Delta$$

The plus sign means the prism is BU. Then,

$$Z_1 = -1.89 Z_2 = -12.74^\Delta$$

So a 12.74^Δ BD ophthalmic crown prism combined with a 6.74^Δ BU highlite prism constitutes a 6^Δ BD achromatic doublet (Figure 20.8c). We can check the arithmetic by first noting that 12.74^Δ BD combined with 6.74^Δ BU is indeed equivalent to a 6^Δ BD. Second, the CA for this doublet is

$$\begin{aligned} CA_Z &= \frac{-12.74^\Delta}{58.6} + \frac{6.74^\Delta}{31.0} \\ &= -0.22^\Delta + 0.22^\Delta = 0 \end{aligned}$$

20.7 THICK LENSES AND CHROMATIC ABERRATION

Achromatic doublets of high dioptric power are actually thick lenses. A thick lens system that has zero longitudinal CA might still have some lateral CA. The reason is that the Gaussian principal planes for

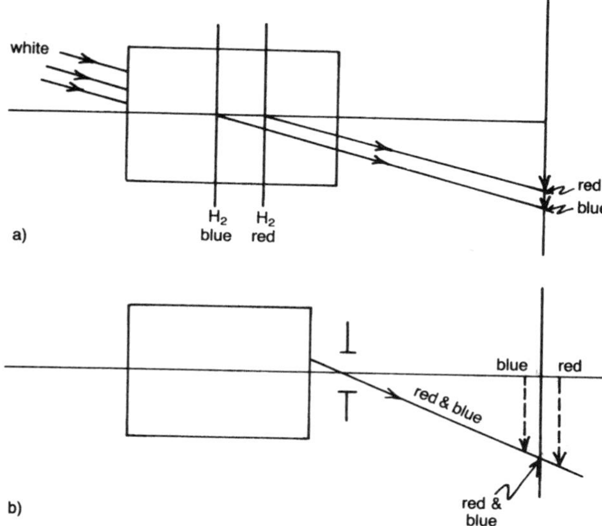

Figure 20.9 a, System with lateral CA even though longitudinal CA is zero; b, system with minimized lateral CA.

the hydrogen C light (red) can occur at positions different from the principal planes for the hydrogen F light (blue). Figure 20.9a shows the secondary principal planes and the image space nodal rays for this situation. The image screen has clear red and blue images (zero longitudinal CA), but the image sizes are different.

Figure 20.9b shows a system in which the lateral CA is minimized by leaving some longitudinal CA. The blue image is focused slightly in front of the screen position, while the red image is focused slightly behind the screen position. The system is designed so that the red and blue chief rays coincide. Therefore, at the screen position, the red and blue image sizes (as specified by the chief rays) are equal.

20.8 SEPARATED LENSES OF THE SAME MATERIAL

High magnification telescopes and microscopes are not possible unless special care is taken to control the aberrations. In the ocular lens, it is much more important to control the lateral CA as opposed to the longitudinal CA. This can be done with two separated lenses of the same material by minimizing the equivalent power with respect to variations in the refractive index. Since the magnification depends on the equivalent power, this procedure minimizes the variations in image size (lateral CA) rather than variations in image location (longitudinal CA). (For comparison purposes, you might think of minimizing longitudinal CA by minimizing the appropriate vertex power as opposed to the equivalent power.)

The standard calculus procedure for finding an extreme (maximum or minimum) is to set the derivative equal to zero. For a SSRI,

$$P = (n-1)/r = (n-1)R$$

where R is the curvature. Then the derivative with respect to the index is

$$\frac{dP}{dn} = \frac{d}{dn}(n-1)R = R$$

This can be rewritten as

$$\frac{dP}{dn} = R\frac{(n-1)}{(n-1)} = \frac{P}{(n-1)} \tag{20.13}$$

For a thin lens of power P_t it follows that

$$\frac{dP_t}{dn} = \frac{P_t}{(n-1)} \tag{20.14}$$

The equivalent power for two thin lenses in air separated by a distance t is

$$P_e = P_1 + P_2 - tP_1P_2$$

Then the derivative is

$$\frac{dP_e}{dn} = \frac{dP_1}{dn} + \frac{dP_2}{dn} - t\frac{d(P_1P_2)}{dn}$$

The chain rule for differentiation gives

$$\frac{dP_e}{dn} = \frac{dP_1}{dn} + \frac{dP_2}{dn} - t\frac{dP_1}{dn}P_2 - tP_1\frac{dP_2}{dn}$$

or

$$\frac{dP_e}{dn} = \frac{P}{(n-1)} + \frac{P_2}{(n-1)} - \frac{tP_1P_2}{(n-1)} - \frac{tP_1P_2}{(n-1)}$$

The condition for the minimum is

$$\frac{dP_e}{dn} = 0$$

and this occurs when

$$2tP_1P_2 = P_1 + P_2$$

We can solve for t to obtain

$$t = \frac{1}{2}\left(\frac{1}{P_1} + \frac{1}{P_2}\right)$$

The reciprocal of the power is the secondary focal length of the lens, so

$$t = \frac{1}{2}[(f_2)_1 + (f_2)_2] \tag{20.15}$$

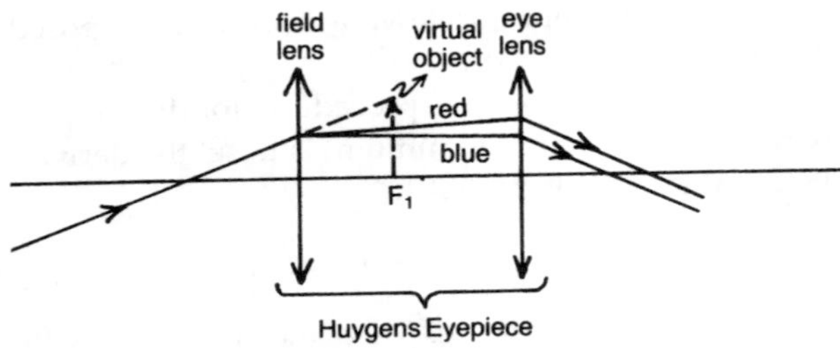

Figure 20.10 Huygens eyepiece.

Equation 20.15 says that for the two lenses, the lateral CA is minimized when the separation t equals one half the sum of the secondary focal lengths.

The Huygens eyepiece is a classic design that meets the above criterion. The Huygens eyepiece incorporates a field lens together with an ocular lens (Figure 20.10), and the power of the ocular lens is twice that of the field lens.

EXAMPLE 20.3

A Huygens eyepiece consists of a +20.00 D ophthalmic crown field lens and a +40.00 D ophthalmic crown ocular lens. What is the separation between the lenses, and the magnification of the eyepiece?

The separation is equal to one half of the sum of the secondary focal lengths or

$$t = \frac{1}{2}(50.0\,\text{mm} + 25.0\,\text{mm}) = 37.5\,\text{mm}$$

The magnification of the eyepiece (for plane waves leaving) is equal to the equivalent power divided by 4. Here,

$$P_e = (+20.00\,\text{D}) + (40.00\,\text{D}) - [(0.0375\,\text{m})(+20.00\,\text{D})(+40.00\,\text{D})]$$
$$= +30.00\,\text{D}$$

Therefore,

$$M = P_e/4 = 7.5\times$$

The neutralizing power P_n of this Hugygen's eyepiece is −60.00 D, so the front focal point is virtual and at +16.67 mm behind the first (field) lens. Hence, the Huygens eyepiece is positioned such that the light converging from the objective lens would form its image 16.67 mm behind the first lens.

We can get an intuitive feel for how the Huygens eyepiece works by following the rays in Figure 20.10. The blue ray bends more than the red ray at the first lens (the field lens). So when the blue ray leaving the first lens is parallel to the optical axis, the red ray is traveling slightly upward between the lenses. Hence, the red ray strikes the second lens at a point farther from its optical center than the blue ray. Prentice's rule for the second lens gives

$$Z = -Ph$$

The dioptric power P is smaller for the red than for the blue. However, this is offset by the larger h value for the red ray. The net effect, for the correct lens separation, is for the red and blue rays to come out parallel to each other, which gives zero lateral CA.

20.9 THE MONOCHROMATIC WAVEFRONT ABERRATION

Consider a centered spherical system consisting of uniform media and illuminated by monochromatic light. In Chapter 7, we derived the vergence equation, $V = P + U$, with the help of the sagittal approximation. While the vergence equation works well in the threadlike paraxial region, the light that passes through nonparaxial parts of the system does not behave as predicted by the paraxial equations.

The box in Figure 20.11a represents a centered spherical system with incident monochromatic light from an axial point source. The dashed curve represents the spherical wavefront predicted by the paraxial equations. This spherical wavefront is also the wavefront required to give a perfect point image (neglecting diffraction). The solid curve represents the actual wavefront leaving the system. In the paraxial region, there is essentially no difference between the predicted and the actual wavefront. However, as a function of the distance from the axis, the actual wavefront differs more and more from the spherical curve. In general, the deviation of the actual wavefront from the perfect sphere is referred to as the *wavefront aberration*. For an axial point source, the wavefront aberration has only one component, which is called spherical aberration.

We can also describe spherical aberration in terms of rays. The rays in Figure 20.11b correspond to the actual wavefront in Figure 20.11a. The paraxial rays focus at the desired image point, but each set of nonparaxial (or peripheral) rays focus progressively farther from the paraxial image point. These peripheral rays cause a circular illumination patch to occur around the paraxial image point. For an extended object, these peripheral rays cause image degradation (or loss of contrast).

Fast optical systems are those with short exposure times. One way to make systems faster is to increase the aperture size. As the aperture size increases, part

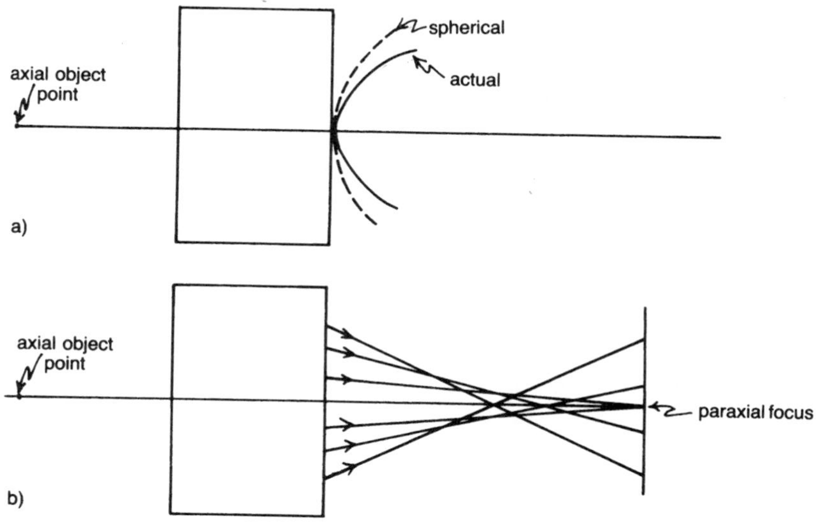

Figure 20.11 Spherical aberration: a, wavefront; b, rays.

of the light path becomes nonparaxial. Consequently, unless corrected, fast systems have an inherent image degradation problem due to spherical aberration.

For a non-paraxial off-axis object point, the actual wavefront leaving the system also differs from the spherical wavefront required for a perfect image. For the off-axis case, the symmetry that occurs for the axial case is broken, and the actual exiting wavefront may even contain a toricity factor (e.g., the wavefront shape might be toric, ellipsoid, hyperboloid, or some other awful shape). Thus, for off-axis point sources, the wavefront aberration has spherical aberration plus additional components.

Systems that have a wide field of view deal with light that makes a large angle with the axis. Thus, these systems are nonparaxial, and unless corrected have an inherent image degradation problem due to the wavefront aberration. Precision fast or wide-field optical systems give an actual exiting wavefront that is closer to a sphere than that of other systems. Consequently, precision systems have a better image quality.

It is important to note that the design of precision systems is object-distance dependent. A system that is designed to minimize the wavefront aberration for an object at optical infinity may have significant wavefront aberration for a near object, and vice versa.

20.10 THE SEIDEL OR THIRD ORDER ABERRATIONS

For an arbitrary system, there are no closed form algebraic equations that describe the exact actual wavefront. Therefore, how can we predict what an optical system will do? In other words, how are precision optical systems designed?

One tool is to numerically determine the exact actual wavefront for a given system. We can do this by calculating exact ray traces through the system and then using the rays to reconstruct the wavefront. An exact ray trace involves the use of Snell's law,

$$n_1 \sin \theta_i = n_2 \sin \theta_r \tag{20.16}$$

at each refracting surface. The exact ray trace is contrasted to a paraxial ray trace that involves the small angle approximation,

$$n_1 \theta_i \approx n_2 \theta_r \tag{20.17}$$

However, the use of numerical calculations without any theory is analogous to looking for a needle in a haystack. The theory provides a guide for where to look. In the absence of exact equations, we can improve the theory with better approximations. For small angles (expressed in radians), the sine function is approximated by

$$\sin \theta \sim \theta - \frac{\theta^3}{3!} + \frac{\theta^5}{5!} - \frac{\theta^7}{7!} + \cdots \tag{20.18}$$

We could start with the paraxial version of Snell's law and derive the vergence equation $V = P + U$. The next higher order approximation keeps the third order terms for the sine function. Then Snell's law becomes

$$n_1\left(\theta_i - \frac{\theta_i^3}{3!}\right) = n_2\left(\theta_r - \frac{\theta_r^3}{3!}\right) \tag{20.19}$$

When we use the third order terms, we find that the difference between the actual wavefront and the perfect sphere can be described by the sum of five terms. While these terms are all interrelated, we tend to think of them as five separate aberrations, each of which contributes to the wavefront aberration. The five terms are called *spherical aberration, coma, radial astigmatism, curvature of field, and distortion*. Of these, spherical aberration is present for both on-axis and off-axis object points. The other four are present only for off-axis object points.

The five aberrations that result from the third order terms were first described by Ludwig von Seidel in the 1850s, and so they are sometimes referred to as the Seidel aberrations. They are also referred to as the primary aberrations, the third order aberrations, or as the aberrations of form – since they depend on the exact form (biconvex, equiconvex, meniscus-convex) of the lens. After Seidel, there were a number of other scientists who further improved our understanding of the aberrations and their correction.

We could proceed further with the approximations and keep the fifth order term. This would generate another set of aberrations, the fifth order aberrations. For ray angles less than 35°, the fifth order aberrations are usually an order of magnitude smaller than the third order aberrations. Here, we discuss only the third order or Seidel aberrations.

For systems with spherical surfaces, the five Seidel aberrations are interrelated. This complicates lens design work because the design that minimizes one of the five frequently makes one or more of the others worse.

20.11 SPHERICAL ABERRATION

For a centered spherical system, spherical aberration is the only Seidel aberration that occurs for both on-axis and off-axis object points. Figure 20.12 shows spherical aberration for a distant axial monochromatic point source located in front of a convex SSRI. After refraction, the paraxial rays intersect at the on-axis paraxial image position. The peripheral rays obey the exact form of Snell's law, and they intersect at a point closer to the interface than the paraxial focus.

Note that Figures 20.11 and 20.12 are both symmetric about the optical axis. Consider a centered circle of semidiameter h on the SSRI. For an axial object point, all of the incident rays that hit this circle go to the same focus along the axis. The larger the circle, the farther the focus is from the paraxial focus. The deviation of the rays from the paraxial focus varies like the square of h. This means that when the aperture size is doubled, the longitudinal spherical aberration for the outer rays quadruples.

Both surfaces of a lens contribute to the spherical aberration of the lens. For plus thin lenses, the peripheral rays focus closer to the interface than the paraxial rays (as in Figure 20.11b). The longitudinal manifestation of spherical aberration is the difference between the image location for the peripheral rays versus the image location for the paraxial rays. For a screen at the paraxial image position, the lateral manifestation of spherical aberration is the circular illumination patch due to the peripheral rays.

Consider an extended object in front of a thin biconvex lens next to an aperture. When the aperture is small, only the paraxial region is exposed, and a good quality image is formed. As the aperture is opened up, the stray light coming from the peripheral rays degrades the paraxial image. For a large aperture setting, we can actually obtain a better image by moving the screen forward from the paraxial image position to a position that would correspond to a circle of least confusion due to the spherical aberration. In fact, while spherical aberration degrades the image quality, it may actually increase the depth of focus of the resulting image. When we use an annular aperture that lets through only a narrow region of peripheral rays (i.e., blocks the paraxial rays), then the image screen must be moved even further forward to the image position for the peripheral rays. The quality of the "peripheral" image is poorer than that of the paraxial image.

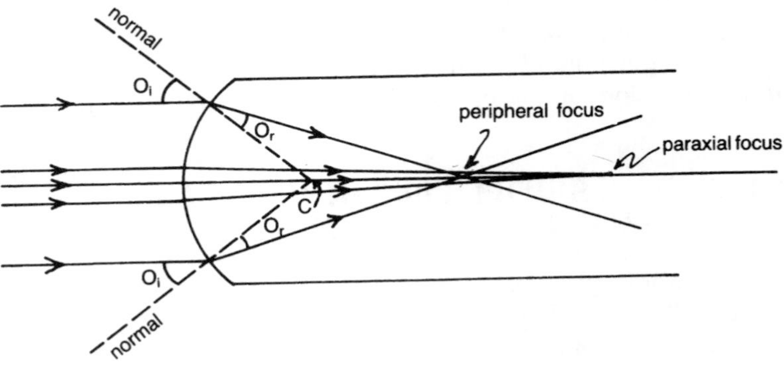

Figure 20.12 Spherical aberration for a convex SSRI.

Spherical aberration is sensitive to the exact shape or form of a lens. This is understandable in terms of Prentice's rule and thick prism theory. Consider the meniscus-convex lens in Figure 20.13a. The concave side of the lens is facing the incident direction. We can think of the peripheral section of the lens as a thick prism (large apex angle). The incident ray makes an angle on the apex side of the normal to the first surface. This results in a prism deviation that is close to maximum (Section 11.3). Now what happens when we turn the lens around so that the convex side faces the incident direction? Then the incident ray makes an angle on the base side of the normal to the first surface (Figure 20.13b), and the resulting prism deviation is close to minimum. The spherical aberration for the convex side forward (minimum deviation) is less than the spherical aberration for the same lens with the concave side forward (maximum deviation). Thus, the same meniscus lens when turned around gives differing amounts of spherical aberration.

For light traveling right, Figure 20.14 shows a plot of longitudinal spherical aberration as a function of lens form for a fixed aperture size and a distant object. The worst spherical aberration occurs for the meniscus-convex lens with the concave side forward. The spherical aberration never goes to zero, but there is a form (biconvex with the front side curved more than the back), that gives the minimum spherical aberration.

The third order aberrations are dependent on the object distance. The biconvex form minimizes spherical aberration for a distant object point, but when the object and image are equidistant from the lens (the symmetry point case, object at $2f_1$ and image at $2f_2$), it is an equiconvex lens that minimizes the spherical aberration.

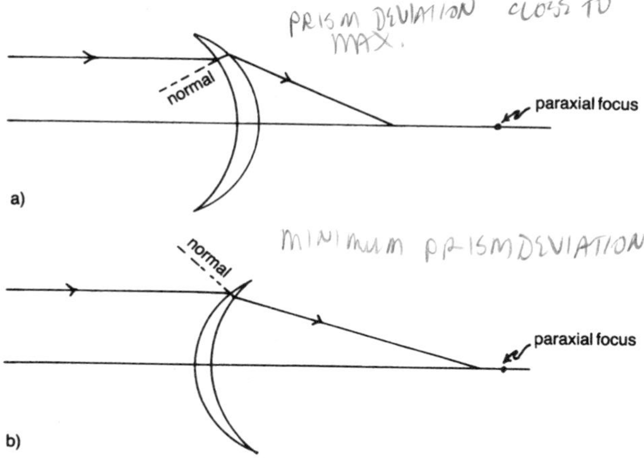

Figure 20.13 Shape dependence of spherical aberration: a, light incident on concave side of a lens; b, light incident on the convex side of the same lens.

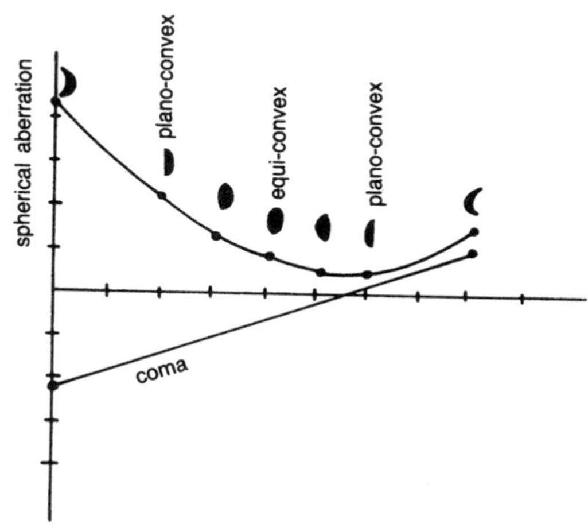

Figure 20.14 Spherical aberration and coma as a function of lens shape.

Another method to minimize (or eliminate) spherical aberration is to use aspheric surfaces. Given an axial set of conjugate points, there is some surface for which every ray leaving the object point passes after refraction through the image point. These surfaces are referred to as *Cartesian ovals*. They are usually not spherical. Instead they tend to flatten out away from the axis (Figure 20.15), and might be elliptical, parabolic, hyperbolic, or a higher order aspheric surface. (It is interesting to note that the human cornea flattens out away from the axis.) For a spherical surface, we can then think of spherical aberration as occurring because the surface is not the proper Cartesian oval for that object distance.

In a system consisting of plus and minus lenses, the peripheral rays are diverged too much by the minus lenses and converged too much by the plus lenses. Therefore, the spherical aberration from the minus lenses works to correct the spherical aberration from the plus lenses. For a system that forms a real image, the spherical aberration is called positive (or undercorrected) when the peripheral rays focus closer to the back vertex than the paraxial rays, and negative (or overcorrected) when peripheral rays focus farther

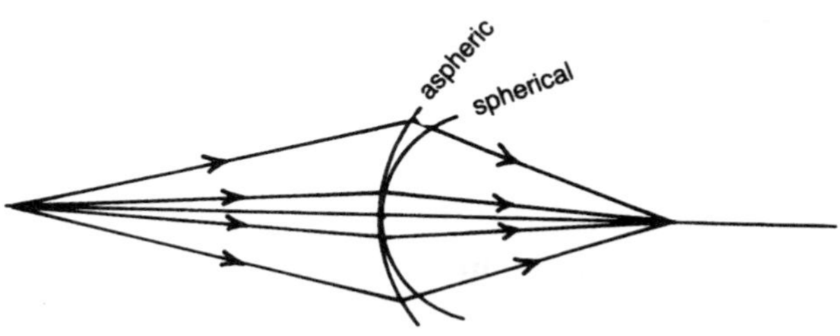

Figure 20.15 Aspheric refracting interface to correct spherical aberration.

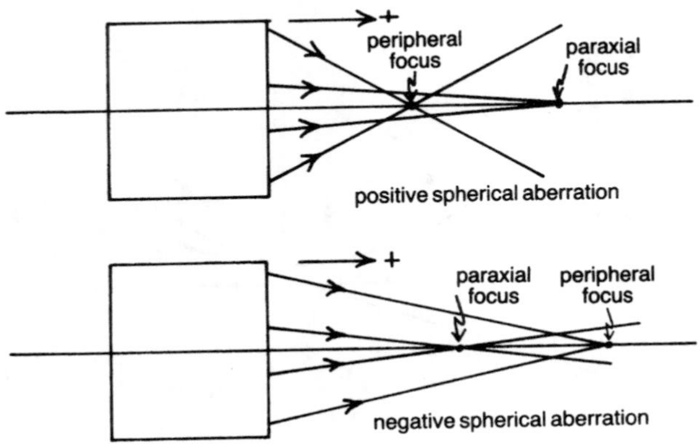

Figure 20.16 Positive versus negative spherical aberration.

from the back vertex than the paraxial rays (Figure 20.16). The spherical aberration is corrected (zero) when the peripheral rays focus in the same place as the paraxial rays.

Figure 20.17 shows a plot of longitudinal spherical aberration as a function of aperture semidiameter h for a single lens compared to that for a doublet lens of the same back vertex power. The doublet lens consists of a positive component of one material and a negative component of a different material. The horizontal displacement of the doublet curve has been multiplied by 10 in order to make it visible. The performance of the doublet is far superior to that of the single lens. Below h values of 14 mm, the doublet undercorrects the spherical aberration, and then overcorrects it for h values greater than 14 mm. By adjusting the thicknesses and surface curves, doublets can be designed to control both spherical and CA.

Clearly, spherical aberration can be corrected by keeping the apertures small. However, this does not work for fast or wide field systems. Then lens form, doublets, systems of separated lenses, or aspheric surfaces need to be used to control spherical aberration for a given object distance.

20.12 COMA

For an on-axis monochromatic point source in front of a centered spherical system, a screen placed at the paraxial image position shows if there is any spherical aberration or not (previous section). For an off-axis monochromatic point source, there may also be one or more of the other Seidel aberrations.

When the point source is moved off-axis, the illumination pattern on the screen at the paraxial image position frequently changes to a comet shaped pattern with a head and a tail (Figure 20.18). This is the Seidel aberration called *coma*. Coma is particularly detrimental to image quality because the comet shaped illumination pattern is not circular but instead the tail flares out in a definite direction.

We can develop some understanding about how coma occurs with the aid of Figure. 20.19. Figure 20.19 shows a SSRI between media of index n_1 and n_2 together with an aperture stop E in front of the SSRI. (In this case, the aperture stop E also serves as the system's entrance pupil.) The center of curvature of the SSRI is at C, and the optical axis for the system is the horizontal line that passes through the center of E and then through C. For a monochromatic axial object point at A, the conjugate paraxial image point is A'.

The monochromatic off-axis object point at O is vertically below the optical axis, and so the side view in Figure 20.19 is a cross sectional view of the vertical meridian. A ray that leaves O and points towards the SSRI center of curvature C is a nodal ray and does not bend when it passes through the interface. When all

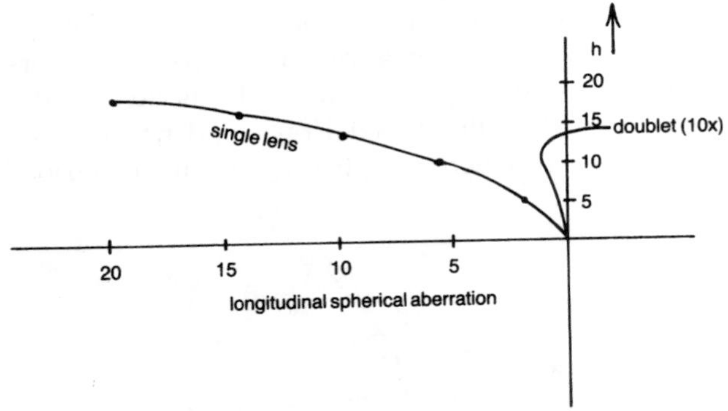

Figure 20.17 Longitudinal spherical aberration as a function of distance from the optical center for a single lens and for a doublet lens. The doublet lens values are multiplied by 10 in order to make them visible on this scale.

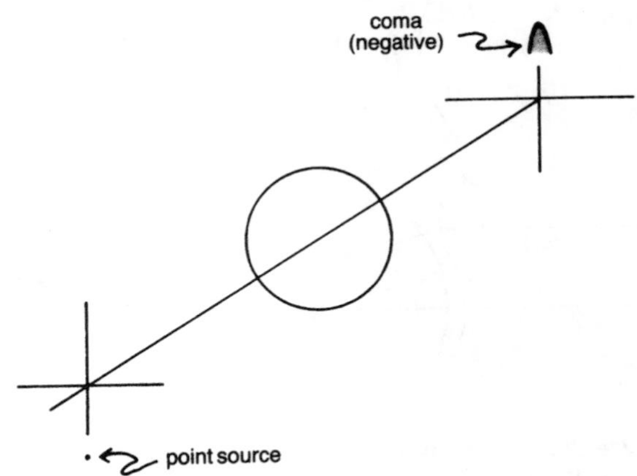

Figure 20.18 Coma for an off axis point source.

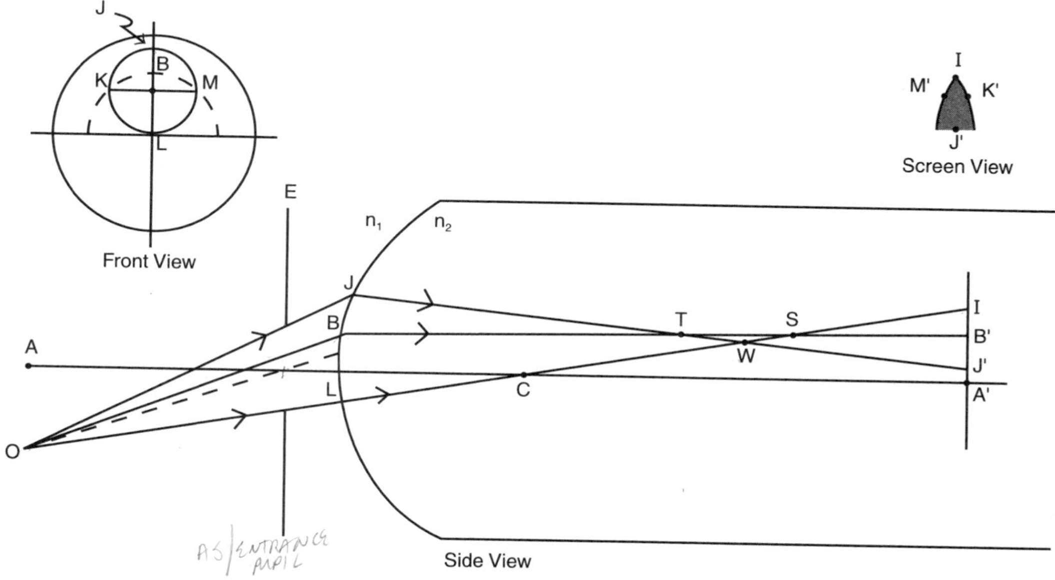

Figure 20.19 Side view of a single spherical refracting interface between media of index n_1 and n_2 with an aperture stop E in front of it. The upper left inset shows the front view from the object point O. The upper right inset is the screen view that shows the coma illumination pattern.

aberrations are neglected, the paraxial image point is at point I, which is where the nodal ray intersects the paraxial image plane. In Figure 20.19, the nodal ray from O just happens to graze the bottom edge of the aperture E.

Temporarily assume that the aperture E is not present. Since the straight line O to I passes through C, it is a symmetry line. Therefore, for a cone of incident rays from O hitting the SSRI in a circle of fixed semidiameter h centered on the point L, the image space rays all go to a common point on the line O to I. From the spherical aberration discussions, we know that increasing the semidiameter h results in the common point moving along the symmetry line away from point I toward the SSRI. When the aperture E is present in front of the SSRI, it blocks part of the cone of rays, but the rest still go to the common point.

Coma and radial astigmatism are usually analyzed in terms of the tangential and sagittal planes. *For a given off-axis object point, the tangential plane is the plane that contains the chief ray together with the system's optical axis.* In Figure 20.19, the chief ray (dashed line) leaves O and passes through the center of the aperture stop E, while the optical axis lies along the line from A to A'. Thus the vertical meridian shown in Figure 20.19 is the tangential plane for the point O. The bottom bounding ray, incident on the SSRI at point L, is in the tangential plane, as is the top boundary ray incident at point J, as well as the ray incident at point B.

For an off-axis object point, the sagittal plane is the plane that contains the chief ray and is perpendicular to the tangential plane. For the side view in Figure 20.19, the sagittal plane is the plane that contains the chief ray (dashed line) and is perpendicular to the plane of the figure.

The upper left inset shows a front view as seen from the object point O, which is just outside the paraxial zone. The outer circle represents the boundary of the SSRI that would be seen from O in the absence of the aperture E. The inner solid circle represents the surface of the SSRI that is seen from O when looking through the aperture E. The bottom-bounding ray hits the SSRI at point L, which is on the bottom of the inner circle, and the top bounding ray hits the SSRI at point J, which is on the top of the inner circle. All the rays hitting the SSRI on the vertical line between J and L lie in the tangential plane (including the ray that hits at point B).

As in spherical aberration, the non-paraxial ray that hits the SSRI at J will be bent too much (as computed by the exact form of Snell's Law), and so it intersects the symmetry line (O to I) at point W, which is in front of the paraxial image point I. This ray continues on and intersects the paraxial image plane at point J'. The ray that hits the SSRI at B is closer to being paraxial, so it intersects the symmetry line at point S, which is between W and I, and then intersects the paraxial image plane at B', which is between I and J'.

The chief ray from O hits the SSRI at the center of the inner circle (i.e., at the intersection of the vertical line and horizontal line in the front view). Since the sagittal plane contains the chief ray and is perpendicular to the tangential plane, it intersects the SSRI along the horizontal line from K to M. Thus a fan of rays that leave O and hit the SSRI along the line from K to M lie in the sagittal plane. (In the side view, point K is below the plane of the figure and point M is above the plane of the figure.)

In the front view, the dashed circle represents a circle perpendicular to and centered on the symmetry line (O to I). The semidiameter of the circle is such that points K and M lie on the circle. Point B, in the tangential meridian, also lies on this circle. The fact that the line O to I is a symmetry line dictates that all the incident rays that hit the SSRI along this dashed circle intersect the symmetry line at the same point. Since the ray through point B intersects the symmetry line at S, this means that the sagittal rays through points K and M also intersect the symmetry line at point S. The rays from K and M then diverge from S and are spreading out horizontally when they hit the paraxial image plane. However the horizontal (or left-right) spread is not as large as the vertical spread. The upper right inset shows the screen view of the resultant illumination (coma) pattern in the image plane. The head of the coma pattern is at point I and its tail flares downward away from I. The point J' is centered at the end of the tail. The ray from point K hits at K', and the ray from point M hits at M'.

In a lens (or a series of lenses) with an off-axis object point O, each surface has a different symmetry line, and the contribution to the final coma varies from surface to surface. Some surfaces contribute coma with a tail flaring one way, while other surfaces contribute coma with a tail flaring the opposite way. When the coma tail is closer to the optical axis than the head, as in Figures 20.18 and 20.19, the coma is labeled negative. Positive coma has its head closer to the axis than the tail. Coma can be corrected (made zero) by the right combination of positive and negative coma.

For a single spherical lens, we can use the thick prism characteristics in the peripheral sections of the lens to predict which way the coma tail will flare near the paraxial focus. In particular, rays that undergo minimum deviation (or close to it) go to the head of the coma pattern, while rays that undergo maximum deviation (or close to it) go to the tail end of the coma pattern.

Figure 20.20a shows a meniscus convex lens, with the convex side facing the object plane, and an image screen at the paraxial image position. Let's approximate the top and bottom sections of the lens by thick prisms. Two rays from a distant off-axis point are incident on the lens. The ray that is incident on the top "prism" is incident at an angle that is close to grazing incidence, and so this ray undergoes a deviation that is close to the maximum. This ray is bent too much and goes to the tail of the coma pattern. The ray that is incident on the bottom "prism" is at an angle that is closer to the symmetric case of minimum deviation, and this ray goes to the head of the coma pattern. This results in the tail of the coma pattern being closer to the axis than the head (negative coma).

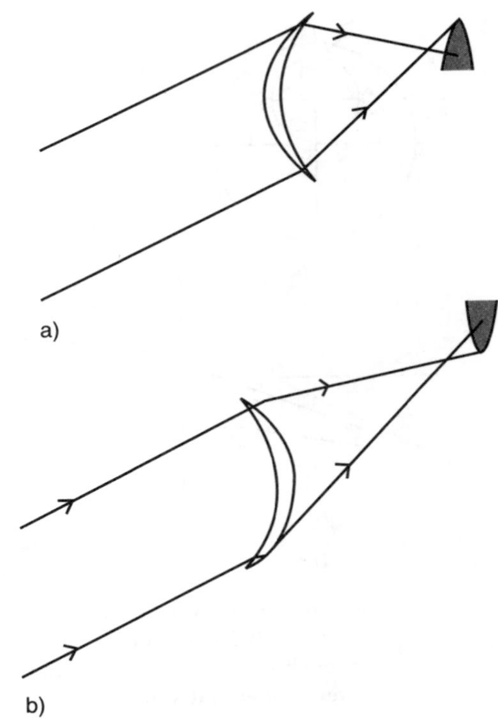

Figure 20.20 Meniscus lenses showing a reversal of the coma direction. The top and bottom edges of the lenses can be considered as thick prisms. When the prismatic deviation is closest to minimum, the rays go to the head of the coma illumination pattern. When the prismatic deviation is closest to maximum, the ray goes to the tail of the coma pattern.

When the same lens is turned around (Figure 20.20b), the coma flares the other way. Here the ray incident on the bottom "prism" is coming in on the apex side of the normal, which results in a deviation close to maximum. This ray is bent too much and goes to the tail of the coma pattern. The ray incident on the top "prism" is closer to the symmetric angle that gives minimum deviation and goes to the head of the coma pattern. The result is that the tail of the coma pattern is farther from the axis than the head (positive coma).

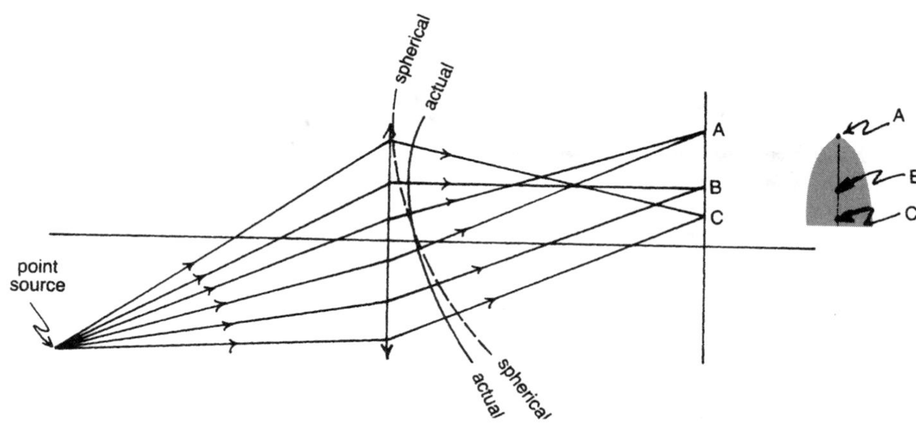

Figure 20.21 Wavefront, rays, and illumination patch for coma.

Clearly coma is strongly dependent on lens form. In fact, the thick prism argument suggests that there is a lens form that would give zero coma. For a distant object, Figure 20.14 showed a plot of coma (together with spherical aberration) as a function of lens form. The form of the lens that gives zero coma is close to the form that gives minimum spherical aberration.

Figure 20.21 shows the tangential meridian of a lens that has only coma and no other Seidel aberrations. Here the rays through the middle of the lens go to point *A*, which is at the head of the coma pattern. The rays through a zone further out go to point *B*, which is roughly in the middle of the coma tail, and the rays near the edge go to point *C* which is near the bottom of the tail. In other words, the image size as defined by points *A*, *B*, and *C* varies with the zone semidiameter *h*. Thus in the tangential meridian, coma can be defined as the variation of lateral magnification with the distance *h*.

Figure 20.21 also shows how the actual wavefront for coma differs from the perfect spherical wavefront in the tangential meridian. Here the top part of the actual wavefront is curved too much relative to the spherical wavefront, while the bottom is not curved enough. In the sagittal meridian (not shown), the actual wavefront for coma matches the perfect spherical wavefront.

Like spherical aberration, coma depends on the square of the aperture size. When the aperture is stopped down, the coma flare is eliminated. Spherical aberration is independent of the location of the aperture stop. When spherical aberration is corrected, then coma is also independent of the aperture stop location. However, when both spherical aberration and coma are present, coma is dependent on the location of the aperture stop in the system. Some aperture stop locations result in positive coma, some in negative coma, and one eliminates coma leaving only the spherical aberration.

Spherical aberration and coma are the two monochromatic aberrations most important to control in the design of high magnification microscopes. The *aplanatic points* of a system are conjugate object and image points that are free of both spherical aberration and coma. Aplanatic points satisfy an equation called the *Abbe sine condition* (after Ernst Abbe, 1840–1905), which is widely used by lens designers.

For a SSRI, the aplanatic object point is in the higher index medium. In microbiology, the oil immersion microscope objective for high magnification uses the aplanatic point for a spherical surface. The first lens in the objective has a plano front surface and a spherical back surface. The oil drop has the same refractive index as the first lens in the microscope objective. When the oil drop is placed on the microscope slide and the microscope is focussed, the plano surface makes contact with the index matched oil, which results in no refraction at that surface. In this case, the object is effectively in the higher index medium at the aplanatic point for the second (spherical) surface.

20.13 RADIAL ASTIGMATISM

For an on-axis object point in front of a centered spherical system with wide apertures, spherical aberration showed that the exiting wavefront is no longer perfectly spherical. For an off-axis peripheral object point, coma showed that the exiting wavefront is asymmetric (i.e., it has one shape in the tangential meridian and a different shape in the sagittal meridian). Another effect of the asymmetry is that the exiting wavefront has a toric-type component that results in the Seidel aberration called *radial astigmatism* (RA). Radial astigmatism is sometimes referred to as *marginal* or *oblique astigmatism*.

For an off-axis point source, RA results in a centered spherical system producing a conoid of Sturm complete (for moderate to small size apertures) with two perpendicular line images—one associated with the tangential meridian and one associated with the sagittal meridian. For larger apertures, the tangential "line" image appears to have a slight curvature to it, while the sagittal line image remains straight.

Figure 20.19 also shows the origins of the RA (although it is intermixed with the coma). As discussed in the previous section, the vertical meridian shown in the side view is the tangential meridian. Suppose the bottom half of the aperture E is now covered. The rays between J and B in the tangential meridian (vertical) still pass through the aperture, and these rays converge to point T. Similarly the rays in the sagittal meridian (horizontal) between K and M still pass through the aperture, and these rays converge to point S. Thus the rays passing through the top half of the aperture give a conoid of Sturm with line images at S and T. The line image at S (from the horizontal sagittal meridian) is a vertical line image that extends vertically down to the ray that goes from J to J'. The line image at T is a horizontal line, which is perpendicular to the plane of the side view. (The rays from K to K' and M to M' would pass through the ends of the horizontal line image at T.)

For the convex SSRI, the tangential image T occurs in front of the sagittal image S (as in Figure 20.19). For a non-paraxial situation, this means that the tangential meridian of the SSRI has an *effective power* that is greater than that of the sagittal meridian.

Radial astigmatism is negligible in the paraxial zone, but like the other aberrations increases in magnitude as the object point gets farther off-axis. Figure 20.22 shows a thin lens and a nodal ray from an off-axis object point that subtends an angle ϕ at the optical axis. For this object point, the position of the tangential image is where this ray intersects the (solid) curved surface marked T. The sagittal image position occurs where the ray intersects the curved surface marked S. For different values of ϕ, the resulting image positions trace out the curved tangential (T) and sagittal (S) image surfaces. In the paraxial region, the T and S surfaces coincide and are indistinguishable from the paraxial image position. Outside of the paraxial image position, the tangential image occurs in front of the sagittal image, and the tangential image surface is curved more than the sagittal image surface. We can rotate this figure about the optical axis to trace out the entire three-dimensional tangential image surface and the entire sagittal image surface. (The dashed line represents the rim of the 3 D tangential image surface.)

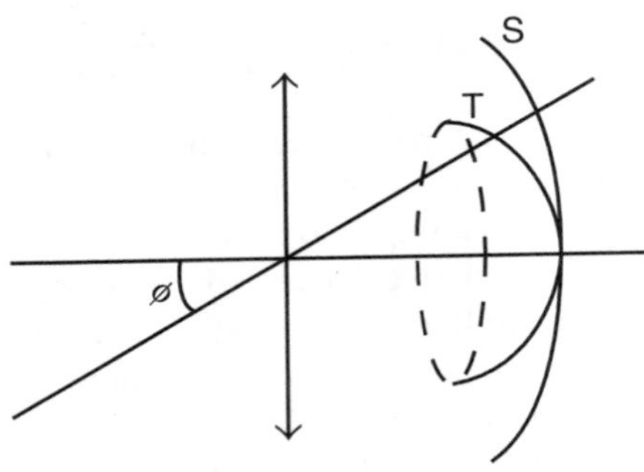

Figure 20.22 The teacup and saucer diagram for radial astigmatism. The tangential image surface is the teacup, while the sagittal image surface is the saucer. For a distant object point that subtends the angle ϕ, the tangential focus occurs closer to the lens than the sagittal focus.

One way to remember these surfaces is to think of a vertical optical axis with the light traveling downward. Then, the three dimensional tangential image surface resembles a teacup, and the sagittal image surface resembles the saucer under the teacup. Thus, it is sometimes referred to as the *teacup and saucer diagram*.

An important factor in RA (and in coma) is that the tangential and sagittal planes vary with the meridional location of the object point. Figure 20.23a shows front views of four off-axis object points that are respectively above, below, left, and right of the optical axis. For the object point vertically below the optical axis (just as in Figure 20.19), the tangential meridian of the lens is vertical and the sagittal meridian is horizontal. For a small enough aperture, the vertical tangential meridian forms a horizontal line image (on the top in the tangential image plane), while the horizontal sagittal meridian forms a vertical line image (on the top in the sagittal image plane). The tangential and sagittal meridians have the same orientation for the top object point, in which case the line images are now on the bottom in the image planes.

For the object point that is horizontally to the left of the optical axis in Figure 20.23a, the chief ray and the optical axis lie in a horizontal plane, which is then the tangential plane for this object point. The sagittal plane contains the chief ray and is perpendicular to the tangential plane. So the sagittal plane intersects the lens along the vertical meridian. The horizontal tangential meridian of the lens forms a vertical line image and the vertical sagittal meridian of the lens forms a horizontal line image (both on the right in the image planes). The tangential and sagittal meridians have the same orientation for the object point that is horizontally to the right of the optical axis, in which case the line images are on the left. Note that the sagittal line images all point toward the optical axis. In other words, the sagittal line images for a spherical lens are all radial lines pointing toward the optical axis.

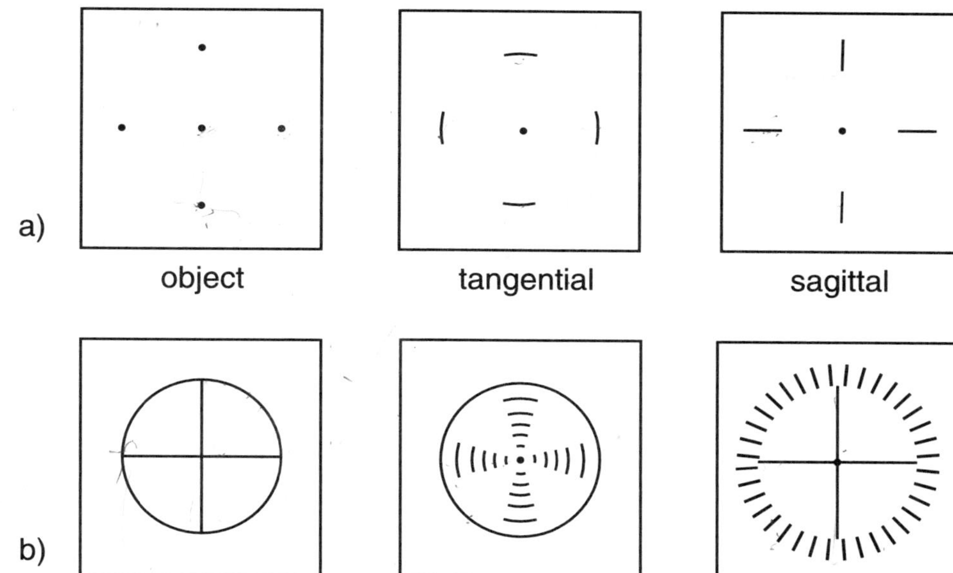

Figure 20.23 **Object and the respective images on the tangential and sagittal image surfaces: a, the object consists of 4 point sources symmetrically located about the optical axis, which passes through the center; b, the object is a large spoked wheel target.**

If the object point is rotated in a circle around the optical axis, the tangential and sagittal planes rotate with the object point. In particular, an oblique object point gives oblique tangential and sagittal planes. Figure 20.23b shows a large spoked wheel target centered on the optical axis of a plus spherical lens. On the sagittal image surface, the spokes of the wheel are imaged clearly, since each point on a spoke results in a sagittal line image that points towards the optical axis. The circular rim of the wheel is blurred on the sagittal image surface, since each point on the rim is imaged as a short radial line.

The tangential line images are perpendicular to the radial sagittal line images (Figure 20.23b). On the tangential image surface, this results in a clear rim of the wheel while the spokes are blurred. The blur of the spokes gets progressively worse away from the optical center, since the RA gets worse for object points that are further off-axis (i.e., the tangential line images get longer). For small enough aperture sizes, individual tangential line images looks straight, but for larger aperture sizes the tangential "line" images appear curved (to match the image plane curvature of the wheel's rim.)

Normally we don't deal with large targets like the spoked wheel, but rather we deal with smaller targets in a specific off-axis location. For example, given a small cross located vertically above the axis, the tangential meridian of the lens is vertical and the sagittal meridian of the lens is horizontal. Thus the image at the tangential focus would have a clear horizontal line and a blurred vertical line (since each point on the vertical line is imaged as a horizontal line). Similarly, the image at the sagittal focus would have a clear vertical line and a blurred horizontal line.

Coddington derived a set of equations for dealing with RA. Consider a narrow bundle of light from an off-axis point source that passes through the center of a thin lens of index n and power P. (This case is classically referred to as *oblique central refraction*.) When the distant point source subtends an angle ϕ with the optical axis of the lens, the result of RA is a differential increase in the magnitude of the effective refracting powers E_t and E_s in the tangential and sagittal meridians respectively. To third order, Coddington's equations can be written as

$$E_t = PT_c \tag{20.20}$$

and

$$E_s = PS_c \tag{20.21}$$

where T_c is the tangential RA change factor given by

$$T_c = \frac{2n + \sin^2 \phi}{2n \cos^2 \phi} \tag{20.22}$$

and S_c is the sagittal RA change factor given by

$$S_c = 1 + \frac{\sin^2 \phi}{2n} \tag{20.23}$$

Note that the RA change factors depend only on the lens's refractive index n and the subtended off-axis angle ϕ.

When $n = 1.5$, $2n = 3$. Then for a point source that is 20° off-axis, Eq. 20.22 gives

Table 20.2 Radial Astigmatism Change Factors for $n = 1.5$

ϕ	T_c	S_c	H_c
1°	1.000	1.000	1.000
5°	1.010	1.003	1.006
10°	1.041	1.010	1.026
15°	1.096	1.022	1.059
20°	1.177	1.039	1.108
25°	1.290	1.060	1.175
30°	1.444	1.083	1.264

$$T_c = \frac{3 + \sin^2 20°}{3\cos^2 20°}$$

or

$$T_c = \frac{3.117}{2.649} = 1.177$$

while Eq. 12.23 gives

$$S_c = 1 + \frac{\sin^2 20°}{3} = 1.039$$

For $n = 1.5$, Table 20.2 gives the results of the change factors T_c and S_c for various values of the off-axis subtended angle ϕ. Note that for 1°, T_c and S_c both equal 1.000 to 3 digits. This is clearly in the paraxial region. As ϕ increases, the sagittal change factor S_c increases slowly, while the tangential change factor T_c increases much faster.

It will also sometimes be convenient to use a RA change factor H_c that is halfway between T_c and S_c. I.e.,

$$H_c = \frac{T_c + S_c}{2} \tag{20.24}$$

For 20°, the above values give $H_c = 1.108$. H_c values are also shown in Table 20.2.

Radial astigmatism, in diopters, is the difference between the effective tangential and sagittal powers, or

$$\text{RA} = E_t - E_s \tag{20.25}$$

We can calculate the RA directly from Eq. 20.25. However we can also use Eq. 20.20 through 20.25 to derive the following common approximation to Eq. 20.25:

$$\text{RA} \approx P\tan^2\phi \tag{20.26}$$

As third order equations, Eqs. 20.20 through 20.25 are accurate out to angles of about 30 to 35° (and perhaps some beyond depending on the precision needed).

Consider a distant point source that is 20° vertically below the axis of a +15.00 D spherical lens. Here the tangential meridian is vertical and the sagittal meridian is horizontal. From Eq. 20.20 and Table 20.2, the effective power in the vertical meridian is

$$E_t = (+15.00\,\text{D})(1.177) = +17.66\,\text{D}$$

while from Eq. 20.21 and Table 20.2, the effective power in the horizontal meridian is

$$E_s = (+15.00\,\text{D})(1.039) = +15.59\,\text{D}$$

From Eq. 20.25,

$$\text{RA} = +17.66\,\text{D} - (+15.59\,\text{D}) = +2.07\,\text{D}$$

The approximation, Eq. 20.26, gives

$$\text{RA} \approx +15.00\,\text{D}\tan^2 20° = +1.99\,\text{D}$$

The effective powers can be put on a power cross:

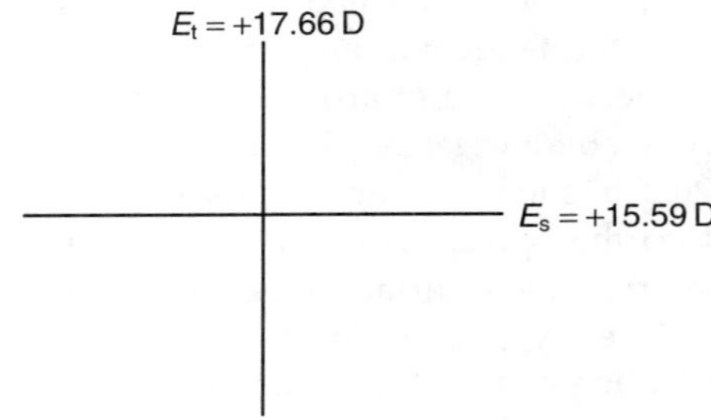

From the power cross, we can write down effective spherocylindrical lens parameters $S_e \bigcirc C_e \times \theta_e$ that the spherical lens has for the object point that is 20° vertically below the optical axis. As a sphere-plus cylinder combination, the effective parameters are $+15.59 \bigcirc +2.07 \times 180$, while as a sphere-minus cylinder combination, the effective parameters are $+17.66 \bigcirc -2.07 \times 90$.

EXAMPLE 20.4

Figure 1.3 shows that the fovea is displaced horizontally on the temporal side from the eye's optical axis. A representative value is that the fovea of the human eye is about 5.2° horizontally away from the optical axis. Consider a +60.00 D thin lens ($n = 1.333$) and screen model of the human eye. For foveal imaging, the light passes through the lens at an angle of $\phi = 5.2°$. Taking RA into account, what are the effective parameters of the eye based on this model?

The chief ray (here the nodal ray) and the optical axis lie in the horizontal plane, and so it is the tangential plane. The sagittal plane inter-

sects the +60.00 D lens along the vertical meridian, which is then the sagittal meridian.
From Eqs. 20.22 and 20.23

$$T_c = \frac{2.666 + \sin^2 5.2^\circ}{2.666 \cos^2 5.2^\circ} = 1.011$$

and

$$S_c = 1 + \frac{\sin^2 5.2^\circ}{2.666} = 1.003$$

Then Eqs. 20.20 and 20.21 give

$$E_t = (+60.00\,\text{D})(1.011) = +60.66\,\text{D}$$
$$E_s = (+60.00\,\text{D})(1.003) = +60.18\,\text{D}$$

From Eq. 20.25,

$$\text{RA} = +60.66\,\text{D} - (+60.18\,\text{D}) = +0.48\,\text{D}$$

The approximation, Eq. 20.26, gives

$$\text{RA} \approx +60.00\,\text{D} \tan^2 5.2^\circ = +0.50\,\text{D}$$

The effective powers can be put on a power cross:

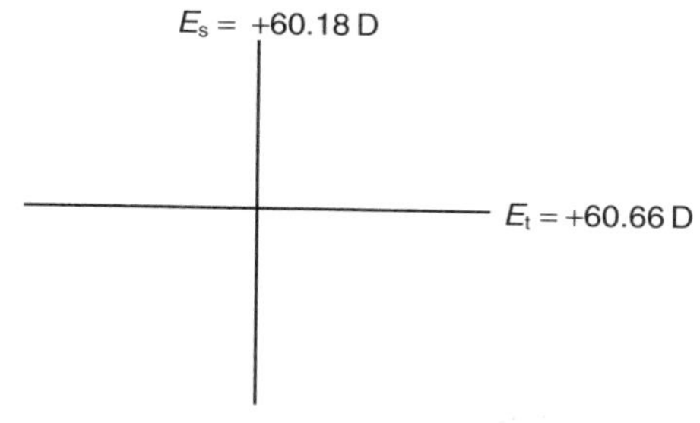

From the power cross, the effective spherocylindrical lens parameters $S_e \bigcirc C_e \times \theta_e$ are $+60.18 \bigcirc +0.48 \times 90$.

In this model, the +60.00 D lens was spherical, but the eye still has about 0.50 D of against-the-rule astigmatism. (The clinically rounded astigmatic correction is −0.50 × 90.) This is called internal *astigmatism* since it is not due to a toric front surface of the cornea (which is external). Indeed Javal's Rule from keratometry and refraction data is that the human eye has on the average has a half diopter of against the rule internal astigmatism. This model suggests that the average internal astigmatism is due to RA from the off-axis fovea location.

When ϕ is not tremendously large, the most noticeable effect of RA may be the power gain in both the sagittal and tangential meridians (as opposed to the RA difference). For a distant off-axis object point, the power gain is best represented by the dioptric location of the circle of least confusion (which dioptrically halfway between the tangential and sagittal powers). From basic astigmatism theory, the dioptric location

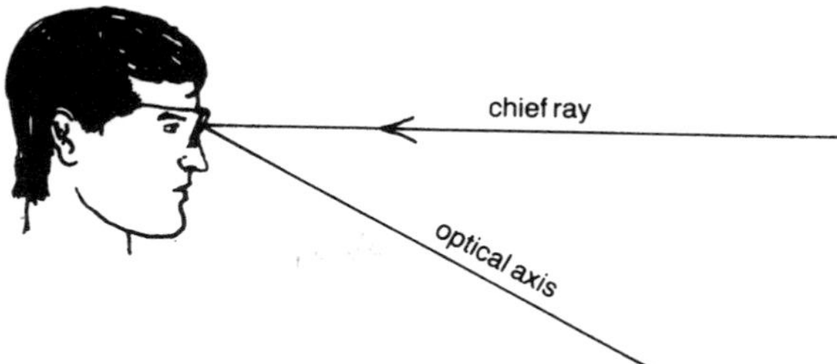

Figure 20.24 Effective power gain by tilted lenses.

of the circle of least confusion is also called the spherical equivalent (Sp Eq). So the effective spherical equivalent $(\text{Sp Eq})_e$ is given by

$$(\text{Sp Eq})_e = \frac{E_t + E_s}{2} \tag{20.27}$$

which from Eqs. 20.20 through 20.24 is equivalent to

$$(\text{Sp Eq})_e = PH_c \tag{20.28}$$

H_c was 1.108 for 20°, so Eq. 20.28 gives +16.62 D as the $(\text{Sp Eq})_e$ for the +15.00 D spherical lens. We could also get +16.62 D directly from Eq. 20.27, or from $(\text{Sp Eq})_e = S_e + (C_e/2)$.

People (especially myopes and hyperopic presbyopes) who need a slightly stronger spectacle correction frequently notice that when they tilt their spectacles, as in Figure 20.24, they can see better. They have "discovered" the power gain due to RA.

EXAMPLE 20.5

Professor Walter Nutty wears a spherical correction of −5.75 D. Its been a while since his last refraction, and he is having trouble seeing a distant straight-ahead object. Nutty discovers that if he tilts his spectacles 25° about a horizontal meridian (Figure 20.24) and looks through the center of the tilted lens (oblique central refraction), he can see the distant object better. What are the effective spherocylindrical lens parameters and the $(\text{Sp Eq})_e$ of the tilted lens?

In this case, the tangential plane, defined by the chief ray and the optical axis, is the vertical meridian. The change factors for 25° are given in Table 20.2. Then from Eq. 20.20 through 20.24,

$$E_t = -5.75\,\text{D}(1.290) = -7.42\,\text{D}$$

while

$$E_s = -5.75\,\text{D}(1.060) = -6.10\,\text{D}$$

Since the tangential meridian is vertical and the sagittal is horizontal, we can write the effective

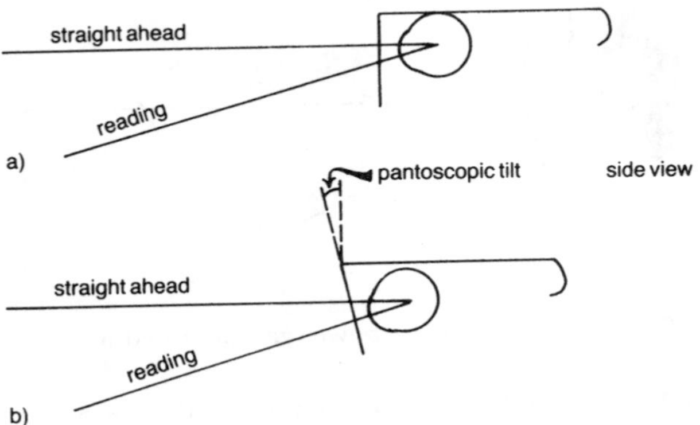

Figure 20.25 Lines of sight for distance and reading: a, no tilt; b, pantoscopic tilt.

powers on a power cross, and then get the −5.75 D spherical lens's effective spherocylindrical parameters, which are $-6.10 \bigcirc -1.32 \times 180$.

The $(\text{Sp Eq})_e$ of the tilted lens is −6.76 D (from either Eq. 20.27 or 20.28). Nutty's spherical lens was −5.75 D, so in terms of Sp Eq, he got an effective increase of −1.01 D of minus power by tilting his lens.

People typically look straight ahead at a distant object, and drop their line of sight when reading (Figure 20.25a). For a spectacle lens with no tilt, this results in the presence of RA while reading. However, spectacle frames usually have a pantoscopic tilt as shown in Figure 20.25b. The pantoscopic tilt is equivalent to a rotation around a horizontal meridian. Besides a cosmetic improvement, the pantoscopic tilt minimizes the RA while reading (at the expense of leaving a little radial astigmatism at distance). The typical pantoscopic tilt is about 7.5°.

Some spectacle frames also have a face-form tilt, which is equivalent to rotating the lens around a vertical meridian (Figure 20.26). As a result of the tilts, strong prescriptions may behave differently in the spectacle frame than during the visual exam when the tilts are not present.

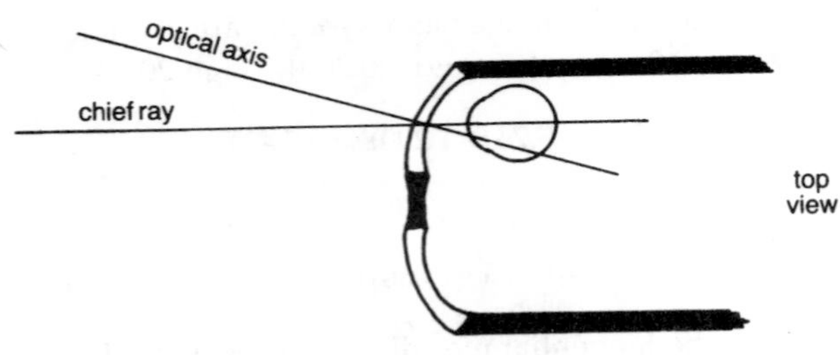

Figure 20.26 Face form tilt.

When a *plus* spherical lens is tilted through the angle ϕ around a meridian M and the effective spherocylindrical parameters $S_e \bigcirc C_e \times \theta_e$ are expressed in *plus cylinder* form, then S_e is the effective sagittal power E_s and θ_e is the meridian M around which the tilt occurred. When a *plus* spherical lens is tilted through the angle ϕ around a meridian M and the effective spherocylindrical parameters $S_e \bigcirc C_e \times \theta_e$ are expressed in *minus cylinder* form, then S_e is the effective tangential power E_t and θ_e is perpendicular to the meridian M around which the tilt occurred. Similarly, when a *minus* spherical lens is tilted through the angle ϕ around a meridian M and the effective spherocylindrical parameters $S_e \bigcirc C_e \times \theta_e$ are expressed in *minus cylinder* form, then again S_e is the sagittal power E_s and θ_e is the meridian M around which the tilt occurred. We can use the standard transposition relations to go back and forth between the plus and minus cylinder expressions.

Consider an on-axis point source in front of a plus lens–aperture combination, and assume negligible spherical aberration. When the lens is rotated, both coma and radial astigmatism are present. Thus, at each line image position, a coma flare is detectable. By decreasing the aperture size, the coma flare can be eliminated without changing the position of the line images. In other words, the interval of Sturm caused by radial astigmatism is unchanged when the aperture is made smaller. (This contrasts with the behavior of longitudinal spherical aberration.) If we continue to decrease the aperture size, we run into the pinhole effect. Here the length of the line images decreases, and, consequently, the blur due to RA decreases.

For oblique central refraction, RA is not very sensitive to the form of the lens. However, RA through a peripheral part of the lens, as shown in Figure 20.27a, is dependent on the form of the lens. Figure 20.27b shows a plot of the form of a spherical thin lens that gives zero radial astigmatism for one off-axis angle. The plot is for front surface power versus back vertex power. The curves turn out to be elliptical and are referred to as the *Tscherning ellipses*. (Tscherning derived the third order equations that first gave this ellipses.) The inside (smaller) ellipse is for a distant object, while the outside (larger) ellipse is for a near object.

For a distant object, lens forms that give zero RA exist for back vertex powers ranging from about −22 D to +8 D. For most back vertex powers, there are two forms that work: a steep form (top of the ellipse) and a shallower form (bottom of the ellipse). The shallower form is the starting point for the design of *corrected curve* spectacle lenses. Note that when near objects are taken into account, the designs are flatter than for

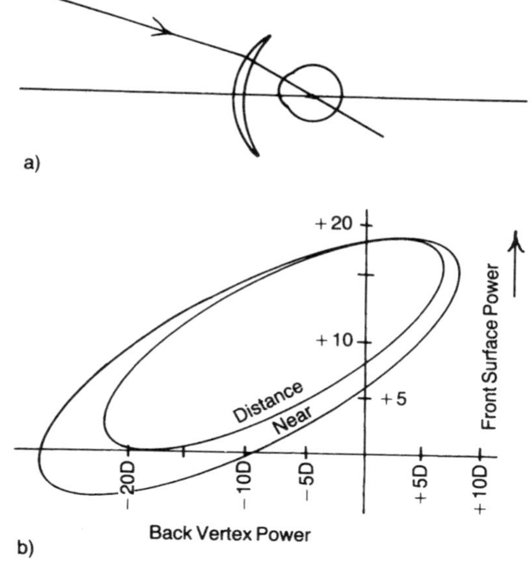

Figure 20.27 a, Radial astigmatism through peripheral portion of the lens; b, Tscherning ellipses for distance and near.

distant objects only. Also note that for high plus lenses (high hyperopes or aphakes), there is no spherical lens that gives zero RA. However there are aspheric lenses that give zero RA for one angle for high plus lenses. Typically the aspheric lenses for zero RA have flatter front surfaces than the spherical lenses.

In systems with plus and minus lenses, the RA from the minus lens acts to correct the RA from the plus lenses. Therefore besides lens form, we can use doublets and systems of separated plus and minus lenses to control RA.

20.14 CURVATURE OF FIELD

When the previous Seidel aberrations are corrected, then an off-axis monochromatic point source would give a perfect point image (neglecting diffraction). However, for a specified object plane, the conjugate image points for the non-paraxial off-axis object points lie on a curved surface rather than a flat plane. This is the Seidel aberration called curvature of field. In the presence of curvature of field, an extended image on a flat screen gets progressively blurred as a function of distance from the optical axis.

We can get an intuitive feeling for curvature of field, in the absence of RA, by considering a convex single spherical refracting interface between air and glass ($n_2 = 1.50$). Figure 20.28 shows three different narrow pencils of rays coming from the distant object. In each pencil, the central ray points toward the interface's center of curvature C and so does not bend. Consider the pencil traveling straight ahead. The rays are refracted and form an image at the secondary focal point, which is a distance of f_2 from the SSRI or a distance of $f_2 - r$ from the center of curvature C.

The interface has exactly the same geometry for the other two pencils. The central ray in each pencil passes straight through without bending, and the other rays converge on the central ray to form a real point image at a distance equal to $f_2 - r$ from the center of curvature C. Since the central rays in each pencil pass through C, the surface specified by all the image points is a sphere of radius $f_2 - r$ centered on C.

The Petzval surface is the image surface conjugate to a flat object. For the distant object, the curvature K of the Petzval surface is the reciprocal of the distance $f_2 - r$. For a SSRI, the sum of the primary and secondary focal points equaled the radius of curvature r, so $f_2 - r = -f_1$. Since the dioptric power P equals $-1/f_1$, it follows that $K = P/n_1$. Then dividing both sides by n_2 gives

$$\frac{K}{n_2} = \frac{P}{n_2 n_1}$$

For a lens, the light starts in the object space medium of index n_1, passes through (is refracted by) the first

Figure 20.28 Curvature of field for a convex single refracting interface.

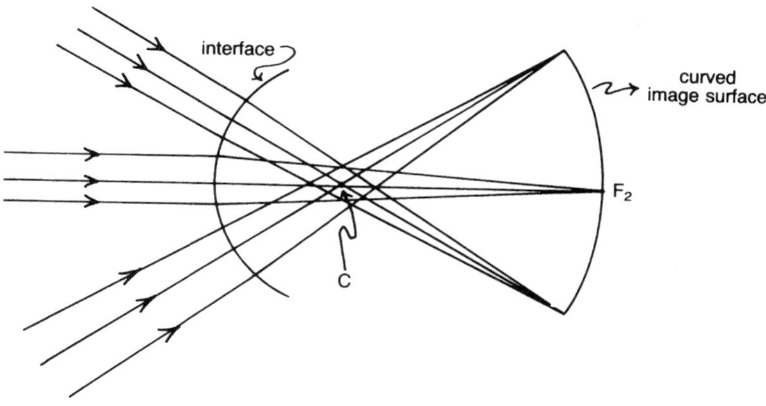

surface of power P_1, goes through the lens medium n_2, and then passes through the second surface of power P_2, and enters the image space medium of index n_3. Petzval showed that in the absence of RA, the final image surface curvature K_3 for the lens is given by

$$\frac{K_3}{n_3} = \frac{K_1}{n_1} + \frac{K_2}{n_2}$$

or

$$\frac{K_3}{n_3} = \frac{P_1}{n_2 n_1} + \frac{P_2}{n_3 n_2} \quad (20.29)$$

Petzval also showed that this sum can be further extended for multiple surfaces.

For a thin lens in air, $n_1 = n_3 = 1$, and Eq. 20.29 reduces to

$$K_3 = \frac{P_t}{n_2} \quad (20.30)$$

where P_t is the thin lens power (i.e., $P_1 + P_2$). Equation 20.30 shows that to third order, the curvature of field depends only on the lens power and index, and not on the shape. The higher the power P of the lens, the greater the Petzval curvature.

For a distant object, the curvature K of the image surface for a series of separated thin lenses in air is given by

$$K = \sum_j \frac{P_j}{n_j} \quad (20.31)$$

Equation 20.31 is called the Petzval equation (after Josef Petzval, 1807–1891, who first discovered it). Positive lenses introduce an inward curvature in the field (concave relative to the back vertex of the system), and minus lenses introduce an outward curvature in the field. The image surface is flat when K equals zero (the Petzval condition). Petzval used this condition to design by far the best portrait lens system of his time.

It is interesting to note that for a plus system, a minus lens introduced very close to the image plane makes a full contribution to the Petzval condition for a flatter field, and yet makes very little contribution to the other aberrations. Another point of interest is that two separated lenses of the same material, one with a power of $+P$ and the other with a power $-P$, give a flat field ($K = 0$). For example, a +10.00 D ophthalmic crown lens 5 cm in front of a −10.00 D ophthalmic crown lens has a flat field, a +5.00 D equivalent power, and a +10.00 D back vertex power.

Curvature of field and RA are intimately related, although we can have one without the other. In the absence of RA, the best image surface is called the Petzval surface. In the presence of RA and curvature of field, the tangential image plane and the sagittal image plane are both curved. (The curvature of the tangential and sagittal image planes was already implicit in the RA equations of the last section.) There is a mathematical relation that says the tangential image surface is always farther from the Petzval surface than the sagittal image plane. However, when RA is present, the best image surface is specified by the circles of least confusion in the conoids and not by the Petzval surface.

Figure 20.29a shows the image surfaces for a distant object in front of an equiconvex lens. The tangential image surface is curved more than the sagittal image surface (teacup and saucer). From the mathematical

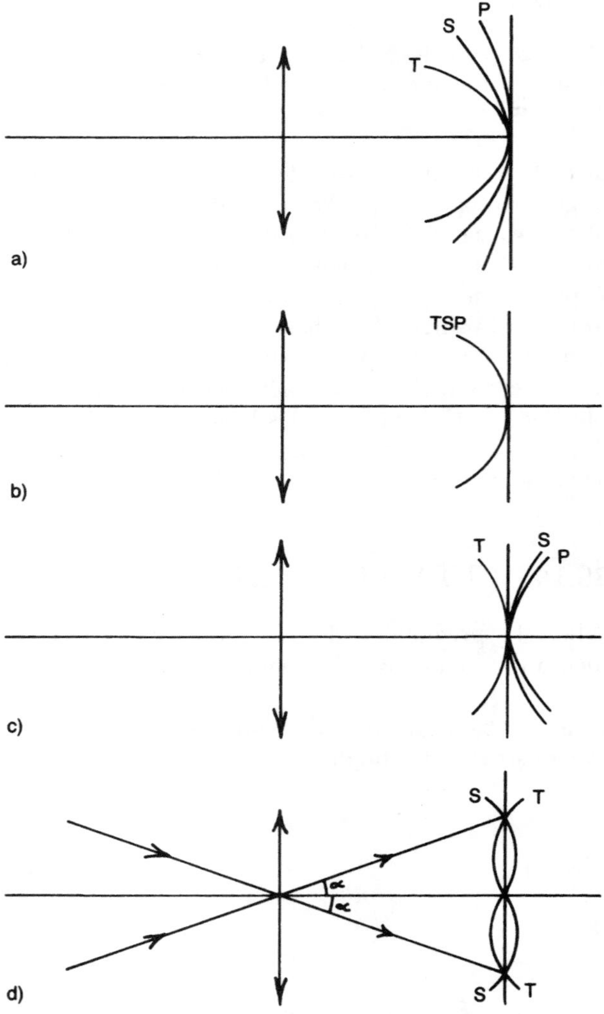

Figure 20.29 Tangential, sagittal, and Petzval surfaces: a, equiconvex lens; b, zero RA; c, zero curvature of field; d, anastigmat projector system.

relationship, the Petzval surface is then the "plate" under the teacup and saucer.

For zero RA, the T, S, and P surfaces all coincide (Figure 20.29b). We say that such a system is corrected for RA but not for curvature of field. In the presence of RA, we say that curvature of field is corrected when the surface specified by the circles of least confusion is flat (Figure 20.29c).

Figure 20.29d shows the tangential and sagittal image surfaces for an anastigmat projector system. The anastigmat has a flat field and zero RA at one off-axis angle α. The RA between α and the axis is minimal; however, beyond α it quickly gets worse.

Radial astigmatism and curvature of field are the two most important aberrations to control in the design of corrected curve spectacle lenses. (The third most important is lateral CA.) When curvature of field is taken into consideration as well as RA, the lenses tend to be flatter than those given by the Tscherning ellipse.

20.15 DISTORTION

Distortion is the last Seidel aberration. Distortion differs from the other aberrations in that it does not cause any blur or loss of resolution. Distortion is due to the fact that the lateral magnification for off-axis points depends on the exact image and object distances along the chief rays. Distortion has the result that any straight line in the object plane is imaged as a straight line only when the object line passes through the optical axis. All other lines are curved (Figure 20.30).

For a grid target in front of a spherical lens, there are two types of distortion: pincushion (in which the image "lines" are convex relative to the axial point) and barrel (in which the image "lines" are concave relative to the axial point). Pincushion distortion results when the peripheral lateral magnification is greater (in magnitude) than the paraxial lateral magnification. Barrel distortion results when the peripheral lateral magnification is less than the paraxial lateral magnification.

In general, distortion depends on lens form and is quite sensitive to the aperture location. Figure 20.31a shows an object in front of a thin plus lens with an aperture at the secondary focal point (a telecentric stop). The chief ray for the peripheral object point is incident parallel to the axis. Thus, the object distance for the chief ray equals the paraxial object distance. The image distance for the chief ray is the diagonal distance g, which is greater than the paraxial image distance v. The lateral magnification m_{per} for the off-axis point is equal to g/u, and

$$|m_{per}| = \left|\frac{g}{u}\right| > \left|\frac{v}{u}\right| = |m_{par}|$$

where m_{par} is the paraxial lateral magnification. Since the peripheral magnification is greater than the paraxial magnification, the outer part of the image is magnified more, resulting in pincushion distortion.

The same argument can be repeated for a stop located in front of the lens at the primary focal point (Figure 20.31b). In that case, the chief ray emerges parallel to the axis, and the peripheral image distance is equal to the paraxial image distance. The diagonal object distance for the chief ray is greater in magnitude

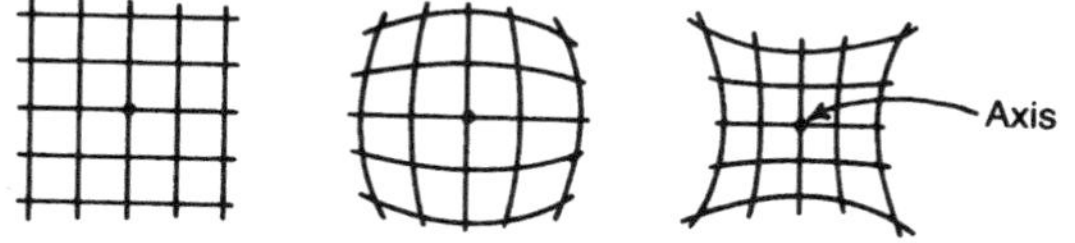

Figure 20.30 Barrel and pincushion distortion for a grid object.

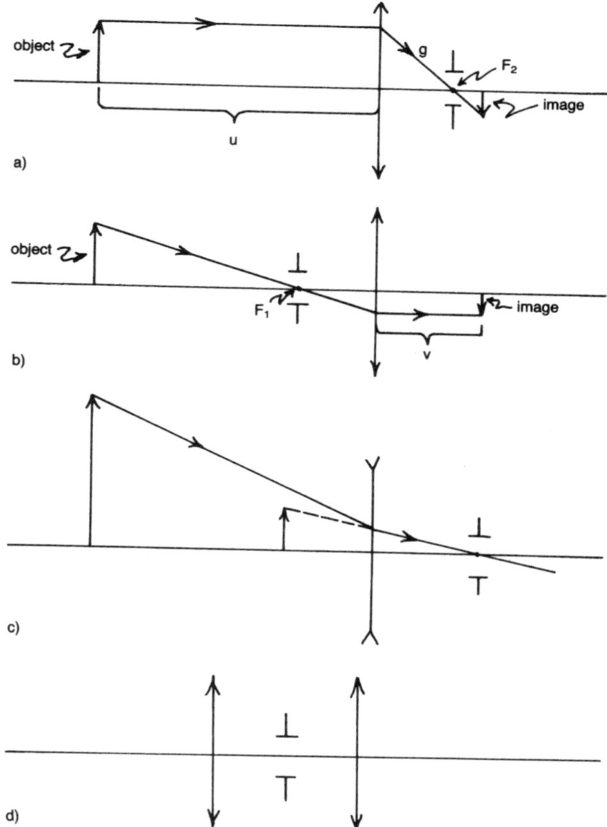

Figure 20.31 a, Chief ray for pincushion distortion; b, chief ray for barrel distortion; c, chief ray for aperture simulating observer's entrance pupil; d, orthoscopic system.

than the paraxial object distance, so the peripheral lateral magnification is less than the paraxial lateral magnification, resulting in barrel distortion. When the thin lens is by itself (no other aperture), there is no distortion. Similarly, a pinhole by itself forms a distortion-free image, and, consequently, pinhole cameras with long exposure times are sometimes used for wide field photography of stationary objects such as buildings or landscapes.

When we view an object through a lens, our own pupil acts as the aperture stop of the system. An object viewed through a minus lens shows barrel distortion. In Figure 20.31c, the aperture behind the lens simulates the pupil of the observer's eye. Here both the peripheral image and object distances are greater in magnitude than the corresponding paraxial distances. However, the object distance difference is greater than the image distance difference, so the peripheral lateral magnification is less than the paraxial magnification, and the result is barrel distortion.

One way to correct distortion is to design a symmetric system so that the barrel distortion introduced by one part of the system is counteracted by the pincushion distortion from the other part. A simple example is the *orthoscopic lens* system in which an aperture is located midway between two lenses of the same power (Figure 20.31d).

Distortion in asymmetric systems can be minimized by making the system satisfy a geometric tangent condition. Distortion can also be minimized with aspheric lenses. However, the wider the field of a lens, the harder it is to correct for distortion. Photographs taken with the very wide field "fish eye" lenses have barrel distortion.

20.16 LENS DESIGN

Lens design is a complicated process since the design that improves one of the aberrations frequently makes another worse. For large angles, fifth and larger order aberrations also come into play. As an example, let us briefly consider how camera lens design has progressed.

Figure 20.32a shows a simple meniscus lens design developed by Wollaston about 1812. Wollaston did not have a coherent theory to guide him. Instead, he tried different lenses and different forms until he empirically found one that worked well. Around 1840, Chevalier replaced Wollaston's meniscus lens with an achromatic doublet. Chevalier's lens could be used at about $f/16$. Petzval's portrait lens, also about 1840, was the first designed lens. It could be used at $f/3.5$ provided the field of view was not large (Figure 20.32b).

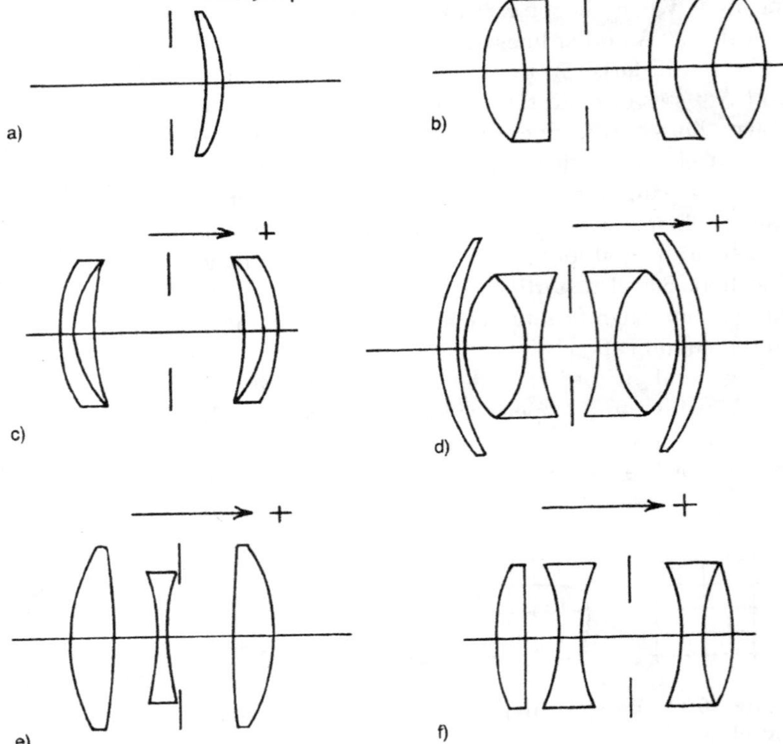

Figure 20.32 Examples of camera lens system design: a, Wollaston; b, Petzval portrait lens; c, Rapid rectilinear; d, Zeiss planar; e. Cooke triplet; f, Zeiss Tessar.

As mentioned, a symmetric lens system is free of distortion. In fact, a perfectly symmetrical lens system is also free of lateral CA and free of coma for one zone. In 1866, Dallmeyer developed a symmetric system called the rapid rectilinear lens, which could be used at $f/8$ with a field as wide as 50° (Figure 20.32c). A number of modern systems, such as the Zeiss planar, are symmetric systems operating as fast as $f/1.4$ (Figure 20.32d).

According to third order theory, a designer has to control eight variables: the system power, the five Seidel aberrations, and longitudinal and lateral CA. Hence, a good lens system has to have at least eight free variables in the design. The Cooke triplet lens, first designed by Taylor in 1893, is an elegant design that uses just eight variables (Figure 20.32e). These include the three lens materials, the form of each lens, and the two spacings between the lenses. The original Cooke triplet could operate at $f/4$. Modern variations of the Cooke triplet, such as the Zeiss Tessar, can operate as fast as $f/1.9$ (Figure 20.32f).

In the 1930s lens design work got a major boost from the introduction of antireflecting coatings. The antireflecting coatings enabled people to use more air-spaced lenses without having to worry about internal reflections. The development of new high index glass types has enabled people to achieve the same quality systems with fewer lenses, e.g., a Tessar style versus a Planar style. Finally the use of aspheric surfaces, particularly on plastic lenses, can also reduce the number of surfaces needed.

20.17 OBLIQUE CENTRAL REFRACTION FOR SPHEROCYLINDRICAL LENSES WITH HORIZONTAL AND VERTICAL PRINCIPAL MERIDIANS

The previous sections applied to systems of spherical lenses. Ophthalmic optics is complicated by the use of spherocylindrical lenses with toric surfaces to correct astigmatism in the human eye. Such spherocylindrical lenses have all the previous aberrations plus some additional asymmetric aberrations that are not present in spherical systems.

As mentioned, the two most important aberrations to control in spectacle lens design are RA and curvature of field. The oblique central refraction equations are easily modified for a spherocylindrical lens tilted (or effectively tilted) around a principal meridian. The actual spherocylindrical power in the sagittal meridian is used to compute the effective sagittal power E_s, while the actual spherocylindrical power in the tangential meridian is used to compute the effective tangential power E_t.

EXAMPLE 20.6

A +14.00 ⊂ −6.00 × 90 lens ($n = 1.5$) has a 10° pantoscopic tilt. What are the effective spherocylindrical parameters for viewing an object straight-ahead?

Here the tangential meridian is vertical and the sagittal meridian is horizontal. The power cross for the lens is

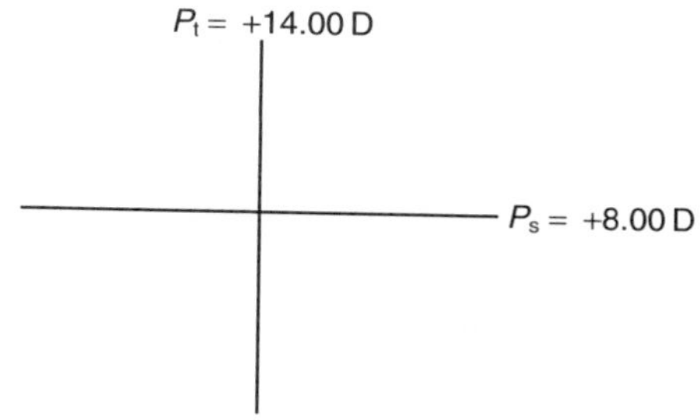

From Eq. 20.20 (modified for the tangential meridian),

$$E_t = P_t T_c$$

We can either calculate T_c from Eq. 20.22 (or use Table 20.2) to obtain

$$E_t = +14.00\,\text{D}\ (1.041) = +14.57\,\text{D}$$

From Eq. 20.21 (modified for the sagittal meridian),

$$E_s = P_s S_c$$

Then,

$$E_s = +8.00\,\text{D}\ (1.010) = +8.08\,\text{D}$$

The effective power cross is

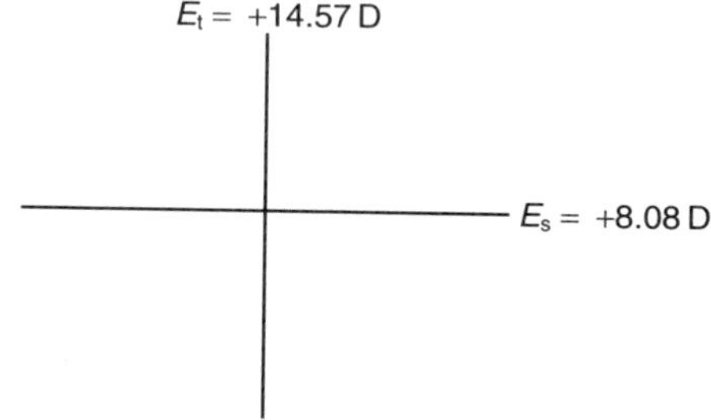

The effective spherocylindrical parameters of the +14.00 ⊂ −6.00 × 90 lens are +14.57 ⊂ −6.49 × 90.

Some people feel that their vision is not as good through sports safety lenses as through their regular lenses, and they are often told that nothing can be done to help this. However the poorer optics may be due to a sports frame with a considerable faceform tilt. If so, there are a variety of solutions. One is contact lenses and a plano sports safety frame. A second is a sports safety frame with less tilt. A third is to keep the same frame with the large amount of tilt, and order lenses that compensate for the tilt. In the latter case, the effective parameters of the compensated lens match the person's Rx.

EXAMPLE 20.7

Dr. Carol Bright-Gem has an Rx of $-7.00 \bigcirc -2.00 \times 90$. Carol wants these lenses in a sports frame with an 18° faceform tilt. What compensated lens will give effective parameters that match Bright-Gem's Rx? Assume that Carol is looking at a distant straight-ahead object through the center of her lenses (oblique central refraction).

From Eqs. 20.22 and 20.23, the RA change factors are

$$T_c = \frac{3 + \sin^2 18°}{3\cos^2 18°} = 1.141$$

and

$$S_c = 1 + \frac{\sin^2 18°}{3} = 1.032$$

In the faceform tilt situation, the tangential meridian is horizontal and the sagittal meridian is vertical. Here the effective parameters of the compensated lens must match the $-7.00 \bigcirc -2.00 \times 90$ Rx, or

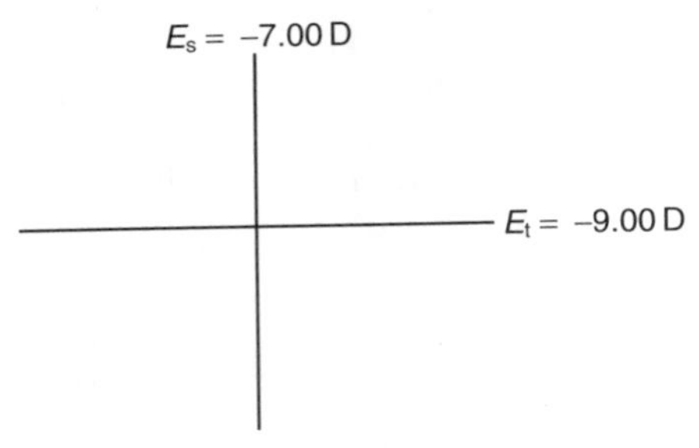

From Eq. 20.20, the compensated lens needs a power P_t in the tangential meridian, where

$$P_t = E_t/T_c$$

or

$$P_t = -9.00\,\mathrm{D}/1.141 = -7.89\,\mathrm{D}$$

From Eq. 20.21, the compensated lens needs a power P_s in the sagittal meridian, where

$$P_s = E_s/S_c$$

or

$$P_s = -7.00\,\mathrm{D}/1.032 = -6.78\,\mathrm{D}$$

The power cross for the compensated lens is

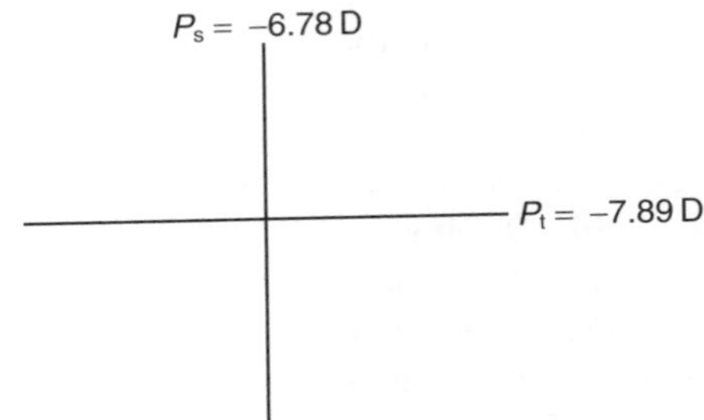

From the power cross, the spherocylindrical parameters of the compensated lens are $-6.78 \bigcirc -1.10 \times 90$. When placed in the frame with the 18° faceform tilt, the $-6.78 \bigcirc -1.10 \times 90$ lens has effective parameters of $-7.00 \bigcirc -2.00 \times 90$, which match Bright-Gem's Rx and give her good vision. (When rounded to clinically significant values, the compensated lens is a $-6.75 \bigcirc -1.00 \times 90$.)

20.18 OBLIQUE CENTRAL REFRACTION IN SPHEROCYLINDRICAL LENSES WITH OBLIQUE PRINCIPAL MERIDIANS

Given a spherocylindrical lens with parameters $S \bigcirc C \times \theta$, when a tilt or effective tilt is around a principal meridian, the effective spherocylindrical parameters $S_e \bigcirc C_e \times \theta_e$ have the same meridional orientation. In other words, $\theta_e = \theta$. However when a tilt or effective tilt is around a non-principal (or off-axis) meridian, then the effective spherocylindrical parameters $S_e \bigcirc C_e \times \theta_e$ may have a different meridional orientation. In other words, θ_e may differ from θ. In particular, θ_e may differ considerably from θ when $|S|$ is large compared to $|C|$. When $|C|$ is large compared to $|S|$, θ_e will be close to θ.

For the spherocylindrical lens with parameters $S \bigcirc C \times \theta$, we can use the dioptric power matrix to easily find the effective dioptric power matrix. For the spherocylindrical lens, Eq. 13.23 gives the dioptric power matrix

$$\mathbf{P} = \begin{pmatrix} P_x & P_t \\ P_t & P_y \end{pmatrix}$$

while Eqs. 13.25 through 13.27 give

$$P_x = S + C\sin^2\theta$$
$$P_y = S + C\cos^2\theta$$

and

$$P_t = -C\sin\theta\cos\theta$$

For a faceform tilt situation, the tangential meridian is horizontal and the sagittal meridian is vertical. Then the effective dioptric power matrix in a faceform tilt situation (tangential meridian is horizontal, sagittal meridian is vertical) is

$$\mathbf{E} = \begin{pmatrix} P_xT_c & P_tH_c \\ P_tH_c & P_yS_c \end{pmatrix} \qquad (20.32)$$

Note that the horizontal component and vertical components (the x–y components) change as expected. The change factor for the torsional component P_t is H_c.

In a compensated lens situation, the effective dioptric power matrix **E** is equal to the dioptric power matrix of the Rx, and then the compensated lens dioptric power matrix **P** is given by

$$\mathbf{P} = \begin{pmatrix} E_x/T_c & E_t/H_c \\ E_t/H_c & E_y/S_c \end{pmatrix} \qquad (20.33)$$

EXAMPLE 20.8a

Mark Whiskers has an Rx of $+8.00 \bigcirc -1.50 \times 130$. When this lens is put into a frame with a 20° faceform tilt, what are the effective parameters of the lens?

From Eqs. 13.23 through 13.27,

$$\mathbf{P} = \begin{pmatrix} +7.120\,\text{D} & -0.739\,\text{D} \\ -0.739\,\text{D} & +7.380\,\text{D} \end{pmatrix}$$

Then from Eq. 20.32 and Table 20.2

$$\mathbf{E} = \begin{pmatrix} (+7.120\,\text{D})(1.177) & (-0.739\,\text{D}(1.108) \\ (-0.739\,\text{D})(1.108) & (+7.380\,\text{D})(1.039) \end{pmatrix} = \begin{pmatrix} +8.380\,\text{D} & -0.818\,\text{D} \\ -0.818\,\text{D} & +7.668\,\text{D} \end{pmatrix}$$

Then from Eqs. 13.41 through 13.44, the effective spherocylindrical parameters of the $+8.00 \bigcirc -1.50 \times 130$ lens are $+8.92 \bigcirc -1.79 \times 146.8$. Note that the effective cylinder axis is different from the cylinder axis of the lens.

EXAMPLE 20.8b

What compensated lens can be ordered for Mark (so that the effective parameters of the tilted lens match the Rx)?

From Eq. 20.33,

$$\mathbf{P} = \begin{pmatrix} +7.120\,\text{D}/1.177 & -0.739\,\text{D}/1.108 \\ -0.739\,\text{D}/1.108 & +7.380\,\text{D}/1.039 \end{pmatrix} = \begin{pmatrix} +6.049\,\text{D} & -0.667\,\text{D} \\ -0.667\,\text{D} & +7.103\,\text{D} \end{pmatrix}$$

Then from Eqs. 13.41 through 13.44, the compensated lens parameters are $+7.43 \bigcirc -1.70 \times 115.8$. When placed in the frame with the 20° faceform tilt, this lens gives effective parameters of $+8.00 \bigcirc -1.50 \times 130$, which match Mark's Rx. (When rounded to clinical accuracy, the compensated lens is $+7.50 \bigcirc -1.75 \times 116$.)

In pantoscopic tilt (or tilt of a lens around a horizontal meridian), the tangential meridian is vertical and the sagittal meridian is horizontal. For a lens with a dioptric power matrix **P**, the effective dioptric power matrix is then

$$\mathbf{E} = \begin{pmatrix} P_xS_c & P_tH_c \\ P_tH_c & P_yT_c \end{pmatrix} \qquad (20.34)$$

Similarly, a compensated lens matrix is

$$\mathbf{P} = \begin{pmatrix} E_x/S_c & E_t/H_c \\ E_t/H_c & E_y/T_c \end{pmatrix} \qquad (20.35)$$

EXAMPLE 20.9

When a $+5.00 \times 45$ cylindrical lens is rotated 25° around a horizontal axis, what are the effective parameters of the lens?

From Eqs. 13.23 through 13.27,

$$\mathbf{P} = \begin{pmatrix} +2.500\,\text{D} & -2.500\,\text{D} \\ -2.500\,\text{D} & +2.500\,\text{D} \end{pmatrix}$$

Then from Eq. 20.34,

$$\mathbf{E} = \begin{pmatrix} (+2.500\,\text{D})(1.060) & (-2.500\,\text{D})(1.175) \\ (-2.500\,\text{D})(1.175) & (+2.500\,\text{D})(1.290) \end{pmatrix} = \begin{pmatrix} +2.650\,\text{D} & -2.938\,\text{D} \\ -2.938\,\text{D} & +3.225\,\text{D} \end{pmatrix}$$

Then from Eqs. 13.41 through 13.44, the effective spherocylindrical parameters of the $+5.00 \times 45$ lens are $-0.01 \bigcirc +5.90 \times 42.2$, or approximately $+6.00 \times 42$.

EXAMPLE 20.10

When a $-2.50 \bigcirc +5.00 \times 45$ spherocylindrical lens (a JCC) is rotated 25° around a horizontal axis, what are the effective parameters of the lens?

From Eqs. 13.23 through 13.27,

$$\mathbf{P} = \begin{pmatrix} 0 & -2.500\,\text{D} \\ -2.500\,\text{D} & 0 \end{pmatrix}$$

Then from Eq. 20.35,

$$\mathbf{E} = \begin{pmatrix} (0)(1.060) & (-2.500\,\text{D})(1.175) \\ (-2.500\,\text{D})(1.175) & (0)(1.290) \end{pmatrix} = \begin{pmatrix} 0 & -2.938\,\text{D} \\ -2.938\,\text{D} & 0 \end{pmatrix}$$

From Eqs. 13.41 through 13.44, the effective spherocylindrical parameters of the $-2.50 \bigcirc +5.00 \times 45$ lens are $-2.94 \bigcirc +5.88 \times 45$.

For an oblique cylinder axis θ, the effective cylinder axis θ_e normally differs from θ. The lens in this example is an exception because of the zero P_x and P_y dioptric power curvital components.

20.19 MIRRORS

Front surface mirrors are free of CA. However, front surface mirrors do suffer from the monochromatic aberrations of form, including the Seidel aberrations. The first clue to this occurred in Chapter 14 where we used the paraxial approximation to derive the power equations of a mirror. Of the Seidel aberrations for a mirror, distortion is particularly easy to observe in a convex mirror (such as those used for wide fields of view in stores).

The Cartesian oval was the surface that for a conjugate object and image point gives no spherical aberration. For a mirror, the Cartesian ovals are the second order conic surfaces (ellipses, parabolas, and hyberbolas). For an ellipse, the conjugate points that are free of spherical aberration occur at the two focii of the ellipse (both near points). For a parabola, the conjugate points free of spherical aberration are optical infinity and the focus of the parabola. A practical application of this is the use of parabolic mirrors in automobile headlights, or the use of parabolic mirrors in searchlights.

20.20 TAYLOR AND ZERNIKE CLASSIFICATIONS

There are other methods, in addition to the Seidel method, of classifying the monochormatic aberrations. One of these utilizes a Taylor Series expansion, while another utilizes an expansion in terms of Zernike Polynomials. These methods are inter-related in that if one has a complete aberration classification in one of the methods, then one can convert that classification to any of the other methods.

As a function of the rectangular coordinates x and y, let $W(x, y)$ be the difference between the actual wavefront and the perfect spherical wavefront. The Taylor method expands $W(x, y)$ into a power series expansion

$$\begin{aligned} W(x, y) = W_1 + W_2x + W_3y + W_4x^2 + W_5xy + W_6y^2 \\ + W_7x^3 + W_8x^2y + W_9xy^2 + W_{10}y^3 \\ + W_{11}x^4 + W_{12}x^3y + W_{13}xy^3 + W_{14}y^4 \\ + \text{higher order terms} \end{aligned}.$$

The above Taylor series is general and can therefore be used to describe aberrations for spherocylindrical systems as well as spherical systems. In the Taylor series, W_1 is called the piston term and is set to zero whenever there is no aberration at the center of the wavefront. The W_2 and W_3 terms are prismatic errors, and the W_4, W_5, and W_6 terms are the common spherocylindrical defocus terms. The W_7 through W_{10} terms are "coma-like" aberrations, while the W_{11} through W_{14} terms are "spherical aberration-like" terms, etc. When the Taylor series is expressed in polar coordinates, $W(\rho, \theta)$, and applied to spherical systems only, then the primary Seidel aberrations each appear as a separate term in the series.

The Zernike series is an expansion of $W(\rho, \theta)$ in a series of polynomials that are orthogonal over a unit circle. An advantage of the Zernike series is that each Zernike term is orthogonal to the other terms. (Recall that when two vectors are perpendicular to each other, they are said to be orthogonal. In other words, when vector **A** is orthogonal to vector **B**, vector **A** has no component along vector **B**. The orthogonality of the Zernike series is similar.) Another advantage of the Zernike series is that the effects of diffraction (Chapter 22) can be incorporated into the aberration theory.

A reference to the interrelations of the different ocular aberration series is: Atchison DA, Scott DH Cox MJ. Mathematical Treatment of Ocular Aberrations: a User's Guide. OSA TOPS 2000; 35: 110–130.

PROBLEMS

1. What is the CA for a +7.00 D ophthalmic crown (523–586) lens? Compare this to the CA for a +7.00 D polycarbonate (580–300) lens.
2. What is the CA for a −6.00 D CR-39 (495–580) lens? Compare this to the CA for a −6.00 D MR6 plastic (597–360) lens.

3. When a human eye is emmetropic for helium d light (orangish yellow), is it myopic or hyperopic for blue light (F line)? For red light (C line)?
4. Design a +7.00 D achromatic doublet using ophthalmic crown glass (523–586) and highlite glass (701–310).
5. Design a 5^{Δ} BU achromatic prism using ophthalmic crown (523–586) and dense flint glass (617–366).
6. For oblique central refraction: what are the effective spherocylindrical parameters for a +7.00 D lens with a 12° pantoscopic tilt and an object point straight ahead? In terms of a Sp Eq, did the lens gain or lose power? What compensated spherocylindrical lens with a 12° pantoscopic tilt would have an effective power of +7.00 D?
7. For oblique central refraction: what are the effective spherocylindrical parameters or a +9.00 D lens that is rotated 15° around a vertical axis with an object point that is straight ahead? In terms of a Sp Eq, did the lens gain or lose power? What compensated spherocylindrical lens with a 15° tilt around a vertical axis would have an effective power of +9.00 D?
8. A −8.00 ⊂ −4.00 × 180 lens has a 20° faceform tilt. For oblique central refraction, what are the effective spherocylindrical parameters for viewing an object straight ahead? What compensated lens would have an effective power of −8.00 ⊂ −4.00 × 180?
9. Babe Ruff has an Rx of −6.00 ⊂ −1.00 × 35. For oblique central refraction, what compensated lens with a 20° faceform tilt would have an effective power that matches Babe's Rx?

CHAPTER 21

Waves and Superposition

21.1 INTRODUCTION

In the eighteenth century, people thought that electricity, magnetism, and light were independent physical entities, but in 1820, Hans Christian Oersted discovered that an electrical current induces a magnetic field. (Specifically, an electrical current causes a compass needle to turn.) In 1830, Michael Faraday added to the relationship by discovering that a changing magnetic field induces an electric field. Today we know that electricity and magnetism are different manifestations of the same basic force called the electromagnetic force.

Faraday also made another curious discovery. He found out that a magnetic field rotates the polarization plane of a light beam that is propagating in a medium. This was the first apparent connection between light and the electromagnetic force. Subsequently, in 1886 James Clerk Maxwell summarized the then known electromagnetic phenomena in four equations. With great physical intuition, Maxwell decided that a term was missing in one of the equations. After introducing the missing term, he derived the fact that accelerating electrically charged particles should radiate energy, and this energy propagates through space according to wave equations. Furthermore, the calculated propagation speed of the electromagnetic waves turned out to be the speed of light. So Maxwell proposed that electromagnetic radiation exists and that light is part of the electromagnetic radiation spectrum.

A few years later, Henrich Hertz generated the first man-made electromagnetic waves. Hertz's waves were in the region of the electromagnetic spectrum that we now call radio waves. Today we are familiar with many other parts of the electromagnetic spectrum. From long to short wavelengths some of these are: radio waves, television waves, radar waves, microwaves, infrared radiation, visible light, ultraviolet radiation, X-rays, and gamma rays.

21.2 BASIC WAVE PROPERTIES

In order to discuss the wave properties of light, let us first review some elementary wave concepts. In general, a wave is a disturbance or change that propagates through the available space or medium. Three characteristics of low energy wave motion are: energy is transmitted, the medium is not transmitted, and an oscillation with a return to equilibrium is involved.

In a high energy wave propagation, the return to equilibrium does not necessarily occur. For example, tapping on your desk with your finger generates low energy sound waves traveling through the desk. Igniting a stick of dynamite on the desk initially sends very high energy sound waves (i.e., shock waves) through the desk. On about the third shock wave through, the material begins to tear apart, and there is no longer a return to equilibrium. In regards to light, typical everyday light waves are low energy waves. High energy light waves can be generated by modern lasers.

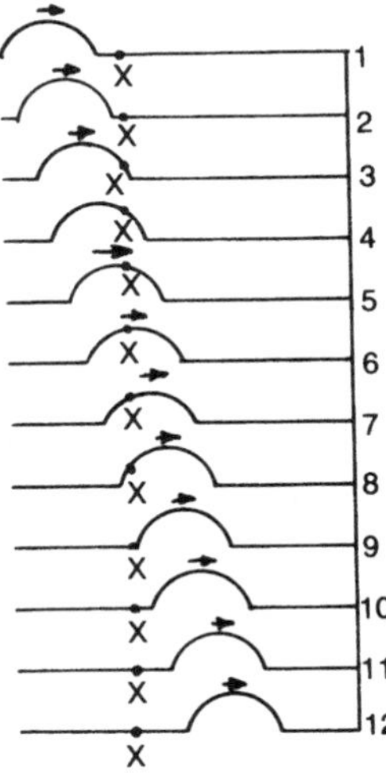

Figure 21.1 Transverse pulse traveling down a rope.

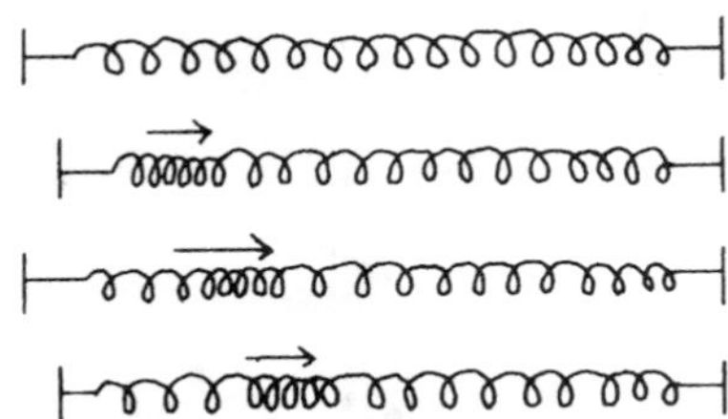

Figure 21.2 Longitudinal waves in a slinky.

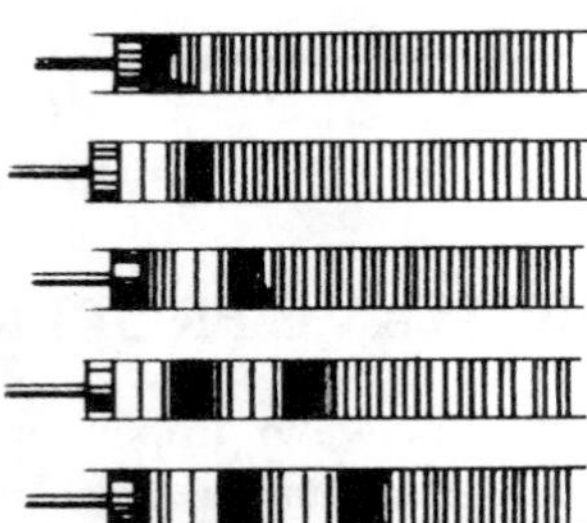

Figure 21.3 Longitudinal sound waves.

For an example of the three characteristics of low energy wave motion, consider a pulse propagating down a rope (Figure 21.1). Point *X* on the rope, which for conceptual purposes can be marked with red dye, is at the equilibrium position in nos. 1 and 2. When the pulse reaches point *X*, that part of the rope gains energy and moves up (nos. 3 through 5). As the pulse moves on, point *X* loses energy and returns to the equilibrium position (nos. 5 through 9). Eventually, point *X* is back in its original position (nos. 10 through 12).

We refer to the pulse as a transverse wave. A transverse wave is one in which the oscillation is perpendicular to the direction of propagation. The pulse oscillation was vertical (up and down), while the propagation direction was horizontal (to the right).

Another type of wave is a longitudinal wave in which the direction of oscillation is in the same plane as the direction of propagation. Figure 21.2 shows a stretched slinky. When the slinky is pushed in (right) and then pulled back (left), a longitudinal pulse propagates to the right along the slinky. A point on the slinky would first be at equilibrium, then oscillate right and left as the pulse passes through.

Sound waves are longitudinal waves. Figure 21.3 shows a sound wave in air generated in a tube. A piston generates a compression pulse traveling right. The compression is followed by a rarefaction (a less dense region). The rarefaction is then followed by another compression. A stationary air molecule oscillates left and right as each pulse passes through.

When a stone is dropped into a pond, a series of ripples or transverse water waves move outward on the surface (Figure 21.4). Each water molecule vibrates up and down as the ripples pass through. Light waves are transverse waves similar to the ripples except that

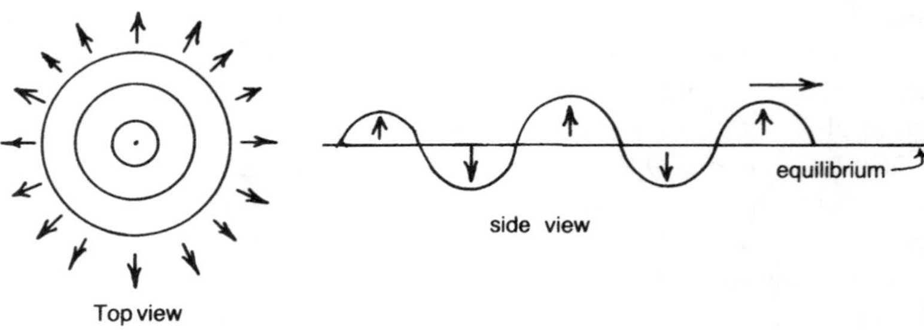

Figure 21.4 Top and side views of transverse waves generated by a point source.

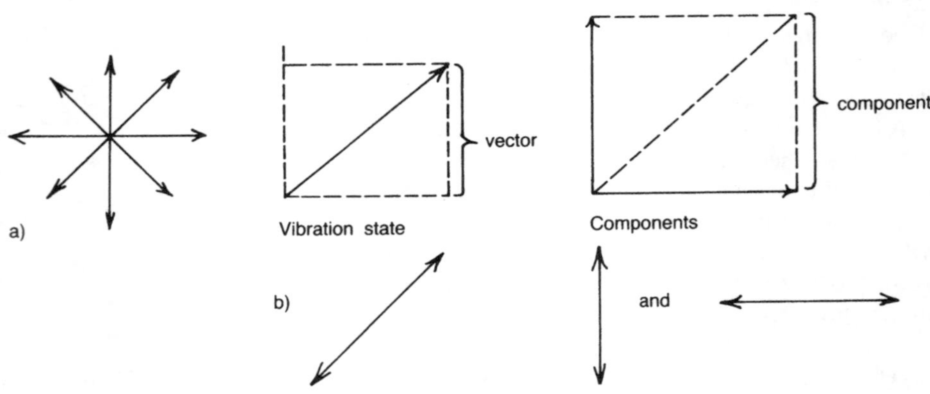

Figure 21.5 a, Some polarization states for transverse waves propagating perpendicular to the plane of the paper; b, resolution of polarized light into perpendicular components.

they propagate in three dimensions (whereas the ripples only propagate along the two-dimensional surface of the water).

Each double-headed arrow in Figure 21.5a represents a possible vibration state for a three-dimensional transverse wave that is propagating perpendicular to the plane of the paper. One vibration state is vertical, one is horizontal, and two are oblique. We can resolve a vibration state into two perpendicular components just as we can resolve a vector into two perpendicular components. Figure 21.5b shows the horizontal and vertical components of an oblique vibration state. The phenomenon of separating a transverse wave into components is called *polarization*. Light waves are transverse waves and can be polarized. Sound waves are longitudinal waves and cannot be polarized.

21.3 HARMONIC WAVES

When a pulse is regularly repeated, a periodic wave is formed. Figure 21.6a shows some periodic waveforms.

A *harmonic wave* is a periodic wave that can be mathematically described by a single sine function:

$$y = A \sin p \tag{21.1}$$

where y is the displacement, A is the *amplitude* or maximum displacement, and p is called the *phase*. For a harmonic wave, Figure 21.6b shows a plot of the displacement y as a function of the phase p.

A harmonic wave results when the restoring force (the force that causes the return to equilibrium) is a linear function of the displacement y, i.e.,

$$F = ky$$

where F is the restoring force and k is the proportionality constant. In low energy situations, many restoring forces satisfy this condition. Therefore, harmonic waves are ubiquitous.

In dealing with harmonic waves, it is frequently convenient to talk about the crests or the troughs. However, we can use the phase p to pick out any point on the wave that we wish to discuss. From Eq. 21.1, the phase of a crest is 90°, i.e.,

$$y = A \sin 90° = +A$$

(In radians, the phase of the crest is $\pi/2$.) The sine of 270° is −1. Therefore,

$$y = A \sin 270° = -A$$

and we see that 270° is the phase of a trough. The phase difference between a crest and a trough is 180° (i.e., 270°−90°).

Each of the other parts of the wave has a specific phase value. For example, consider a wave with an amplitude of 4 units. At a phase of 30° the displacement is:

$$y = 4 \sin 30° = 4(+0.5) = +2$$

Zero displacement occurs when the phase is 0°, 180°, or 360°. The phase difference between a zero and the nearest crest or trough is 90°.

A *wavefront* is a curve on a wave connecting points of equal phase. It is easy to think of the crests (phase 90°) as wavefronts (Figure 21.4). However, we could connect all points on the wave with phases of 63° (or any other value), and use these curves as the wavefronts.

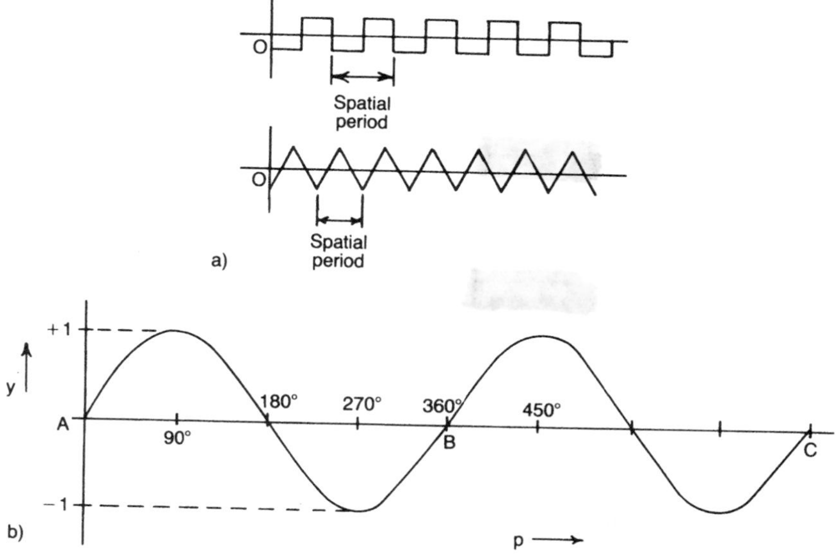

Figure 21.6 a, Periodic nonharmonic waves; b, harmonic wave.

For a periodic wave, the spatial period is the length of each repeating cycle. The spatial period of a harmonic wave is called a wavelength, and is represented by the greek letter λ (lambda). In Figure 21.6b, the distance between A and B equals the wavelength, as does the distance between B and C. Similarly, the distance between two adjacent crests equals the wavelength. In fact, the distance between any two points that have a 360° phase difference equals one wavelength. So one wavelength corresponds to a phase difference of 360°. Half of a wavelength corresponds to a phase difference of 180°, etc.

For conceptual simplicity, let us consider a water wave or ripple propagating to the right. As the wave moves right, each water molecule on the surface vibrates up and down. Figure 21.7 shows a double exposure picture of the wave. The solid curve indicates the wave at time t_1, while the dashed curve indicates the wave at the later time t_2. The water molecule at A rises during the time $t_2 - t_1$, while the water molecule at B falls.

If the double exposure is taken at times t_1 and t_2, in-between which the wave traveled one wavelength, the resulting side view is identical to that of the initial wave. During this time, each water molecule makes one complete up–down cycle or vibration. The time required for a complete vibration is called the (temporal) *period* T of the wave. The number of cycles per unit time is called the (temporal) *frequency* f of the wave, and

$$f = 1/T \tag{21.2}$$

For example, a harmonic water wave with a period of 1/4 second (s), has a frequency of 4 cycles/s.

Since the distance the wave moves during a period T is just one wavelength, we have the following relation:

$$\text{distance} = (\text{speed})(\text{time})$$

or

$$\lambda = vT$$

We can solve for the speed v, and substitute from Eq. 21.2 to obtain

$$\lambda f = v \tag{21.3}$$

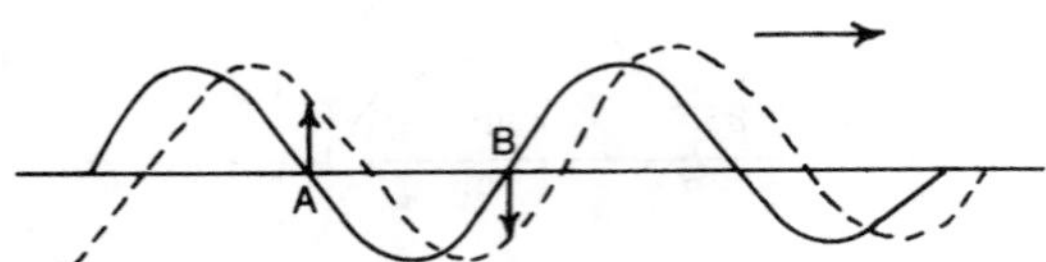

Figure 21.7 Double exposure of a harmonic wave moving right.

Equation 21.3 is a very important relation between the wavelength, frequency, and speed of a wave. In particular, for a fixed speed, Eq. 21.3 says that the wavelength and frequency are inversely related.

EXAMPLE 21.1

A harmonic wave is traveling 10 cm/s and has a temporal frequency of 4 cycles/s. What is the wavelength? From Eq. 21.3,

$$\lambda = (10\,\text{cm/s})/(4\,\text{cycles/s}) = 2.5\,\text{cm/cycle}$$

Usually we just write

$$\lambda = 2.5\,\text{cm}$$

21.4 INTENSITY

The *intensity* I of a wave is the energy carried or delivered by the wave per unit area per unit time, i.e., for a small area and a small time.

$$I = (\text{energy delivered})/[(\text{area})(\text{time})] \tag{21.4}$$

The intensity I of a harmonic wave is proportional to the square of the wave's amplitude:

$$I \propto A^2 \tag{21.5}$$

Equation 21.5 follows from basic physics. Consider a water wave. A water molecule on the surface vibrates up and down as the wave comes through. The kinetic energy that the wave delivers to the water molecule equals $1/2\,\text{m}(v_{\text{vib}})^2$ where m is the molecule's mass and v_{vib} is the vibration velocity. The vibration velocity equals the derivative of the displacement y with respect to the time t, or

$$v_{\text{vib}} = dy/dt$$

From Eq. 21.1,

$$\begin{aligned} v_{\text{vib}} &= d(A \sin p)/dt \\ &= Ad(\sin p)/dt \\ &= A \cos p \end{aligned}$$

Since the kinetic energy is proportional to the square of the vibration velocity, the kinetic energy delivered to the molecule is proportional to $(A \cos p)^2$.

The potential energy of a particle displaced a distance y by a wave is proportional to $1/2\,ky^2$ where k is the proportionality constant in the restoring force. For an incident harmonic wave, the potential energy is then proportional to $(A \sin p)^2$.

The total energy delivered to the molecule is the sum of the kinetic energy plus the potential energy. Then,

$$I \propto (A\cos p)^2 + (A\sin p)^2$$
$$\propto A^2(\cos^2 p + \sin^2 p)$$

Since $\cos^2 p + \sin^2 p = 1$, it follows that

$$I \propto A^2$$

For our purposes, we can choose the units to make the proportionality constant equal to 1. Then,

$$I = A^2$$

It is the intensity of a sound wave that is the stimulus for perceived loudness, and it is the intensity of a light wave that is the stimulus for perceived brightness. Frequently, only relative intensities are considered, in which case

$$I_{rel} = I_2/I_1 = (A_2)^2/(A_1)^2 \quad (21.6)$$

EXAMPLE 21.2

A water wave has an amplitude of 2, and a second water wave has an amplitude of 6. What is the relative intensity of the second wave to the first?

From Eq. 21.6,

$$I_{rel} = (6)^2/(2)^2 = 36/4 = 9$$

In general wave theory, the word intensity refers to the energy delivered by the wave per unit area and per unit time. By international convention, when dealing with electromagnetic waves, the word intensity is replaced by the word *irradiance*. From Eq. 21.5, the irradiance is proportional to the square of the amplitude of the electromagnetic wave. When the irradiance is evaluated according to its ability to produce a brightness response in a human observer, we refer to it as the *illuminance*.

21.5 FREQUENCY INVARIANCE AND WAVELENGTH CHANGES

The visible region of the electromagnetic spectrum is a narrow band centered on a vacuum wavelength of 550 nm. One nanometer (nm) equals 10^{-9} m. Another unit that has been used for wavelength is the angstrom (Å), which equals 10^{-10} m (or 0.1 nm).

As discussed in Section 1.7, light of a single wavelength typically stimulates a single color response. The color–wavelength relations given in Table 21.1 are repeated here.

Table 21.1 Color Response versus Vacuum Wavelength

Color Response	*Vacuum Wavelength (nm)*
Red	780–620
Orange	620–590
Yellow	590–560
Green	560–490
Blue	490–450
Indigo	450–430
Violet	430–380

For electromagnetic radiation, the unit for frequency is called the hertz (Hz). Visible light is a narrow part of the electromagnetic spectrum centered on a frequency of about 5.45×10^{14} Hz. The frequency is a very important parameter because it does not change when the light moves from one medium to the next. For example, Figure 21.8 shows a system with plane interfaces between air, water, and glass. The light incident in air has a frequency of 5.45×10^{14} Hz. When the light enters the water its frequency is unchanged, and similarly when the light enters the glass its frequency is unchanged.

The invariance property for the frequency does not hold for the wavelength. The velocity v for light in transparent materials is slower than it is in a vacuum, and

$$v = \frac{c}{n}$$

where n is the refractive index of the medium.

Now consider light of frequency f in a medium of index n. From Eq. 21.3,

$$f\lambda_m = v$$

where λ_m is the wavelength in the medium. Then,

$$f\lambda_m = \frac{c}{n}$$

and

$$\lambda_m = \frac{c}{fn}$$

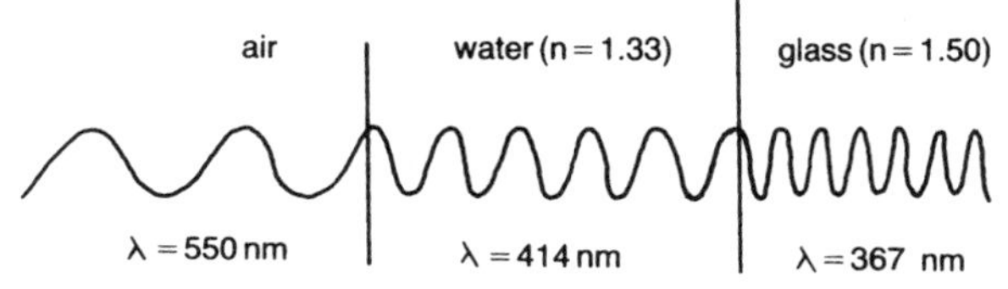

Figure 21.8 Wavelength changes as monochromatic light moves into different media.

The vacuum wavelength λ equals c/f. Therefore,

$$\lambda_m = \frac{\lambda}{n} \tag{21.7}$$

In Figure 21.8, the vacuum wavelength is 550 nm, the wavelength in water ($n = 1.33$) is 414 nm, and the wavelength in glass is 367 nm.

Since the wavelength changes whenever the light enters a different media, it would be better to identify monochromatic light by its frequency, which is invariant. However, in many physical optics experiments, it is the wavelength that is directly measured, and so we tend to identify light by its vacuum wavelength. (The index of refraction of air is about 1.0003, so normally we think of the wavelength in air as being equal to the vacuum wavelength. For precision work, the difference must be taken into account.)

Under normal circumstances, light of vacuum wavelength 633 nm incident on the eye produces a red response. The frequency of the light is

$$f = \frac{c}{\lambda} = \frac{3 \times 10^8\,\text{m/s}}{633 \times 10^{-9}\,\text{m}} = 4.74 \times 10^{14}\,\text{Hz}$$

The frequency remains the same as the light propagates through the cornea, the aqueous humor, the crystalline lens, the vitreous humor, and into the cones. The light is absorbed in the cones, and the resulting neural signal ultimately produces the red response. However, when the light is incident on the cones, the wavelength is not 633 nm. The wavelength has changed each time the light enters a new medium. In particular, the wavelength in the vitreous humor is

$$\lambda_m = \frac{633\,\text{nm}}{1.336} = 474\,\text{nm}$$

So for light of vacuum wavelength 633 nm incident on the eye, the wavelength in the vitreous humor is 474 nm. In each of the media, this light has a frequency of 4.74×10^{14} Hz. Thus, we could say that light of frequency 4.74×10^{14} Hz is the stimulus for the red response. It is more common to say that the incident light of (vacuum) wavelength 633 nm is the stimulus for the red response even though the wavelength in the vitreous is 474 nm.

EXAMPLE 21.3

Light of frequency 6.52×10^{14} Hz is incident on a human eye. What is the frequency and wavelength in the vitreous humor? What is the normal color response?

The frequency is invariant, so it remains 6.52×10^{14} Hz in all the media. The vacuum wavelength is

$$\lambda = \frac{c}{f} = \frac{3 \times 10^8\,\text{m/s}}{6.52 \times 10^{14}\,\text{Hz}} = 0.460 \times 10^{-6}\,\text{m}$$

or

$$\lambda = 460 \times 10^{-9}\,\text{m} = 460\,\text{nm}$$

From Table 21.1, the normal color response is blue. The wavelength in the vitreous humor is

$$\lambda_m = \frac{\lambda}{n} = \frac{460\,\text{nm}}{1.336} = 344\,\text{nm}$$

Remember that the wavelength–color tables are for vacuum wavelengths, not for wavelengths inside the eye.

21.6 SUPERPOSITION

The *superposition principle* states that when two or more low energy waves are superposed on the same space or medium, the waves travel independently through each other, and the resultant displacement at each position is the algebraic sum of the displacements due to each wave.

As an example, consider two pulses traveling in opposite directions down a rope. Figure 21.9a shows the resulting effect as a function of time. Initially, the pulses are traveling toward each other but are not superposed. In exposure no. 2, the waves are superposed, and the resultant displacement on the rope is the sum of the individual displacements. Exposure nos. 3 and 4 are similar. In exposure no. 5, the pulses have passed each other, and each continues on its way.

In Figure 21.9b, an upward and downward pulse are incident from opposite directions. In exposure nos. 2 through 5, the resultant displacement is the sum of

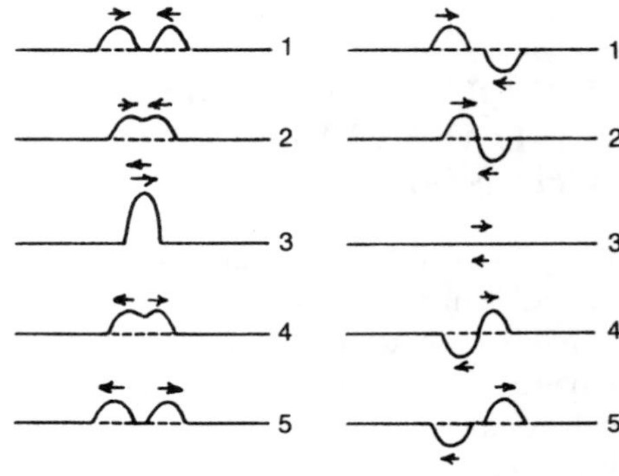

Figure 21.9 a, Superposition of two upward pulses; b, superposition of an upward pulse with a downward pulse.

the individual displacements due to each pulse. In exposure no. 3, one pulse has counteracted the other and there is no resultant displacement. However, at the time of exposure no. 3, the points on the rope still have a non-zero vertical velocity. In other words, for exposure no. 3 all the energy carried by the wave is kinetic, while in the other exposures some of it is kinetic and some potential. In exposure no. 6, the pulses have passed each other and each proceeds as if the other pulse had not been present.

When two harmonic waves of the same frequency propagate in the same direction, the resultant displacement is that of a harmonic wave of the same frequency, i.e.,

$$y_r = A_1 \sin p_1 + A_2 \sin p_2 = A_r \sin p_r$$

The two waves are said to be in phase if their crests line up ($p_1 = p_2$). In this case, the resultant amplitude equals the sum of the two component amplitudes (Figure 21.10a), i.e.,

$$y_r = A_1 \sin p_1 + A_2 \sin p_1$$
$$= (A_1 + A_2) \sin p_1$$

and so

$$A_r = (A_1 + A_2) \quad (21.8)$$

while $p_r = p_1$.

This is referred to as *constructive interference*. (Be careful of the word interference here. Nothing has interfered in a normal sense; the two waves have simply superposed.) When the component waves are in phase and have the same amplitude, the amplitude of the resultant wave is twice that of either component.

When the crest of one component lines up with the trough of the other component, the waves are 180° out of phase. In this case, the amplitudes subtract (Figure 21.10b), a situation referred to as *destructive interference*, i.e.,

$$y_r = A_1 \sin p_1 + A_2 \sin (p_1 + 180)$$

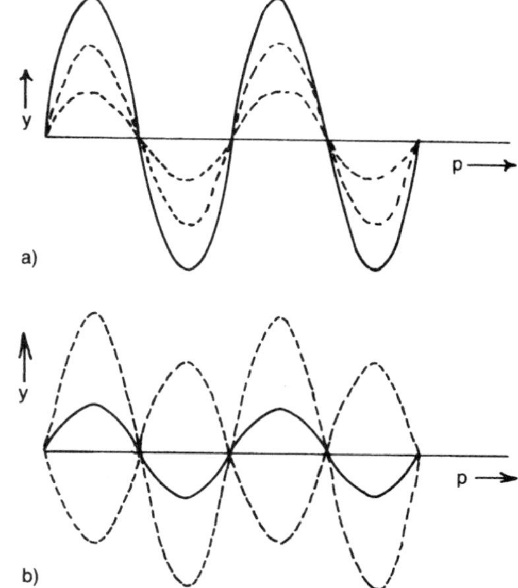

Figure 21.10 a, Constructive interference; b, destructive interference.

Since

$$\sin (p_1 + 180) = - \sin p_1$$

we have

$$y_r = A_1 \sin p_1 + A_2[(-1) \sin p_1]$$

or

$$y_r = (A_1 - A_2) \sin p_1$$

So

$$A_r = (A_1 - A_2) \quad (21.9)$$

while $p_r = p_1$.

For two equal amplitude waves that are 180° out of phase, the amplitude of the resultant wave is zero (complete destructive interference).

When two harmonic waves of different frequencies are superposed, the resultant waveform is periodic but not harmonic (Figure 21.11a). It turns out that

Figure 21.11 a, Superposition of harmonic waves of different frequency; b, beats from superposition of two harmonic waves of slightly different frequency.

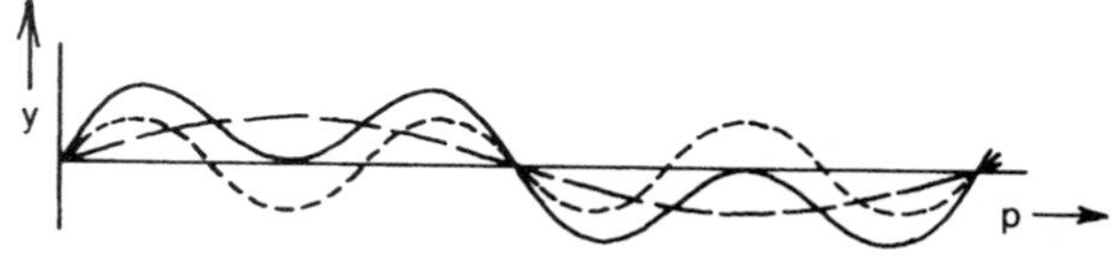

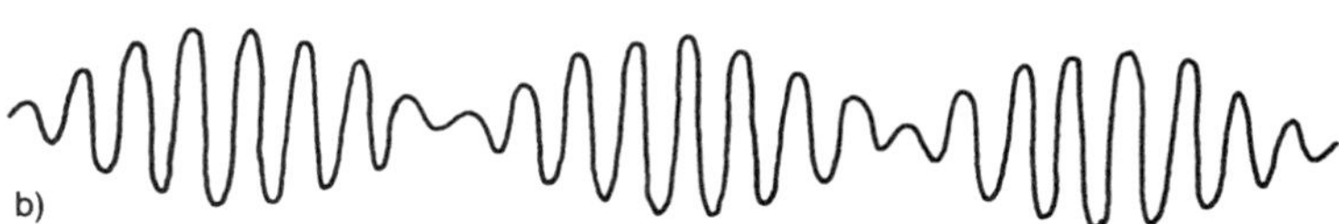

essentially any periodic waveform can be synthesized by adding together a series of harmonic waves of different frequencies (e.g., Fourier series in Chapter 25). In that sense, harmonic waves are a set of fundamental waves.

When we superpose two harmonic waves of slightly different frequencies, we get the waveform shown in Figure 21.11b. In those regions where the waves are pretty much in phase (crests lined up), we get a constructive interference effect. Since the waves are at a slightly different frequency, the two crests drift farther apart until we have a region where a crest and a trough tend to line up. Then we get a destructive interference effect. The result is the beat phenomenon, where it appears that the energy carried by the waves is clustered into groups or beats. Conceptually, the beat phenomenon begins to show that light can have both a wave-like and a particle-like character.

21.7 INTERFERENCE IN A RIPPLE TANK

Ripple tanks are great for developing physical intuition about wave motion. Consider two vibrators hooked together in a ripple tank. A circular wave travels out from each vibrator. According to the superposition principle, the waves travel independently through each other and the resultant displacement on the water's surface is the algebraic sum of the displacements from each wave. The circular curves in Figure 21.12 represent the crests of each wave. There are some positions where the two waves always arrive 180° out of phase (e.g., a trough from one always arrives at the same time as a crest from the other). Destructive interference occurs at those positions resulting in a node (i.e., no resultant vibration on the water surface). Curves connecting the nodal regions are actually hyperbolas with the point sources serving as the focal points of the hyperbolas. The hyperbolic nodal curves become straight lines at points far away from the two sources.

In between the destructive interference zones, there are regions where a wave from one source always arrives in phase with a wave from the other source, and constructive interference occurs. At points far away from the sources, the effect of the constructive interference is a resultant wave that travels outward in between the nodal curves.

Consider the waves incident on the plane G, which is distant from the two sources (Figure 21.12). The energy carried by the waves is proportional to the square of the amplitude. The curve in Figure 21.13 is a plot of the resultant intensity I as a function of the distance x across the plane G. Because of the interference, the energy carried by the waves (the intensity) is redistributed. At the constructive interference positions, the resultant amplitude is twice that of each component wave, so the energy available is actually 4 times that of each component wave. (Naively, this looks like $1 + 1 = 4$.) In effect, energy is removed from the destructive interference zones and placed in the constructive interference zones. Energy is conserved in the process, but it is redistributed.

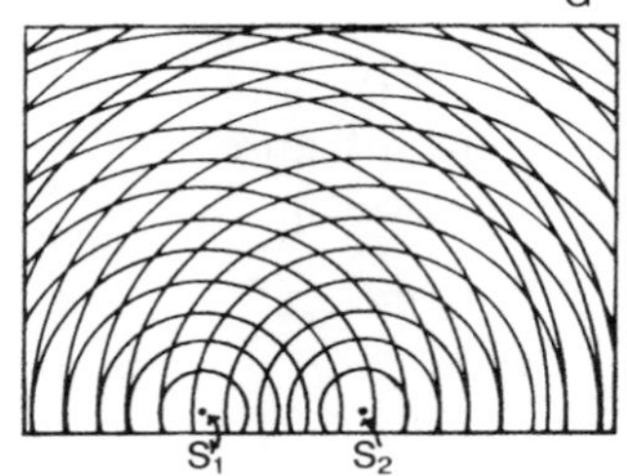

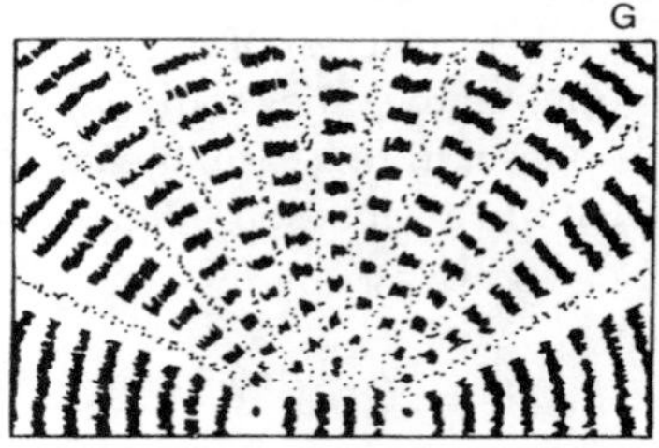

Figure 21.12 Top view of interference by two coherent waves.

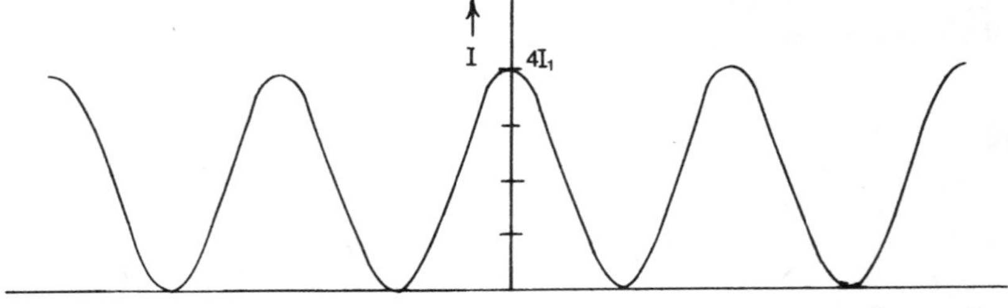

Figure 21.13 Intensity plot for interference of two coherent waves (each of intensity I_1).

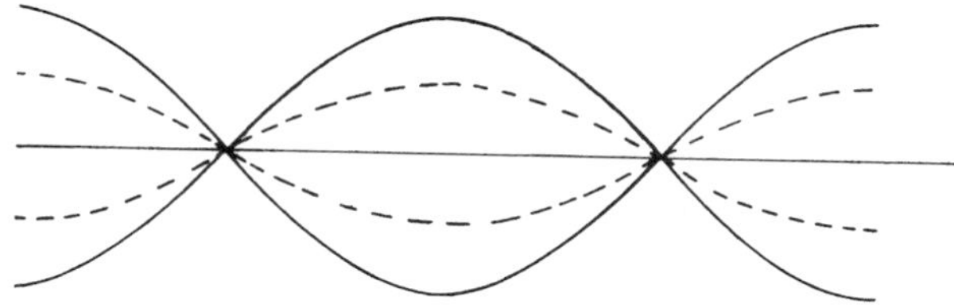

Figure 21.14 Time exposure of standing wave.

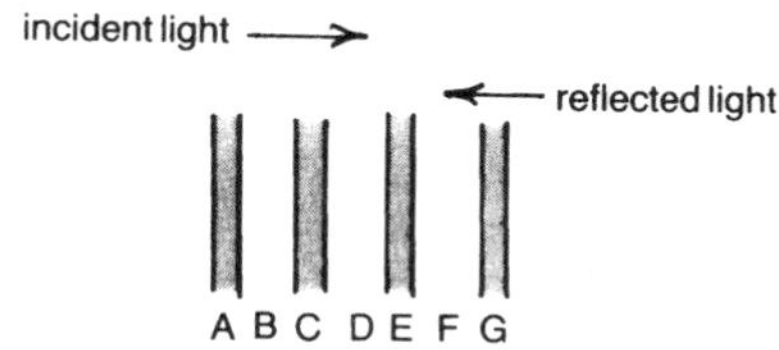

Figure 21.15 Standing wave exposure pattern.

21.8 STANDING WAVES

In the ripple tank, the region directly in between the two sources has two component waves propagating in opposite directions. The resultant superposition results in significant effects only when the distance between the two sources corresponds to an integer multiple of half the wavelength. Then a standing wave is formed by the superposition. The standing wave has stationary nodes that are separated by stationary vibration regions (the antinodes).

The stationary nodes are formed by destructive interference between the two component waves, i.e., when the two sources have the right separation (integer multiple of half wavelength), the two component waves are always 180° out of phase at the nodal positions. Constructive interference occurs at the antinode positions, so the amplitude of the standing wave is twice that of the components. Each curved line in Figure 21.14 shows the standing wave at a particular time. The envelope for the curved lines shows the standing wave motion over a time interval.

While energy is available to a detector at the antinodes, no energy is available at the nodes. Standing waves have been set up with visible light. The original experiment set standing waves up in a photographic film about 20 wavelengths thick. Exposure occurred in the antinode regions (*A*, *C*, *E*, and *G* in Figure 21.15), but there was no exposure at the nodes (*B*, *D*, and *F*). So the film had exposed layers separated by unexposed layers.

21.9 COHERENCE

Whenever two monochromatic light sources vibrate together, ripple tank-type interference patterns result. More precisely, the phase difference between the two sources must remain constant with time, i.e.,

$$(\text{Phase of } S_1) - (\text{Phase of } S_2) = k \quad \text{(at all times)}$$

Note that the phase of S_1 could abruptly jump, but if the phase of S_2 makes the same jump, then the condition is still satisfied. When the condition is satisfied, the sources and the resulting waves are said to be *mutually coherent*.

At the other extreme, suppose the phase difference between the two sources undergoes abrupt changes with time:

$$(\text{Phase of } S_1) - (\text{Phase of } S_2) = k_1 \quad (\text{from } 0 \text{ to } t_1)$$
$$(\text{Phase of } S_1) - (\text{Phase of } S_2) = k_2 \quad (\text{from } t_1 \text{ to } t_2)$$
$$(\text{Phase of } S_1) - (\text{Phase of } S_2) = k_3 \quad (\text{from } t_2 \text{ to} t_3)$$

etc. When the phase changes are completely random, then the sources and waves are said to be *mutually incoherent*. For incoherent waves, the energy delivered to a particular area changes with time. During one time period there may be destructive interference, while during another time period there may be constructive interference.

For two harmonic waves superposed together, the resultant displacement is the sum of the individual displacements

$$y_r = A_1 \sin p_1 + A_2 \sin p_2 = A_r \sin p_r$$

The resulting irradiance (intensity) I_r at a point is proportional to $(A_r)^2$. It follows from the above that

$$I_r = (A_1)^2 + (A_2)^2 + 2A_1A_2 \cos(p_1 - p_2) \qquad (21.10)$$

The first two terms on the right are just the irradiances that would be achieved by the respective waves individually. The third term is called the interference term.

To investigate the interference term, let us first consider the case of waves in phase. Then p_1 equals p_2 and the cosine is +1. Thus,

$$I_r = (A_1)^2 + (A_2)^2 + 2A_1A_2$$

or

$$I_r = (A_1 + A_2)^2 \qquad (21.11)$$

Since I_r equals the square of A_r, the above equation is just the typical constructive interference result that the amplitudes add. For the additional condition that $A_2 = A_1$

$$I_r = (2A_1)^2 = 4I_1$$

where I_r is the irradiance of each component wave by itself.

When there is a 180° phase difference, the cosine equals −1. Then,

$$I_r = (A_1)^2 + (A_2)^2 - 2A_1A_2$$

or

$$I_r = (A_1 - A_2)^2 \tag{21.12}$$

This is the typical destructive interference result in that the amplitudes subtract. When we have the additional condition that the amplitudes are equal, the resultant irradiance I_r is zero.

Suppose the waves are incoherent. Then the phase difference fluctuates as a function of time. The average irradiance delivered to a detector is

$$(I_r)_{avg} = (A_1)^2 + (A_2)^2 + 2A_1A_2[\cos(p_1 - p_2)]_{avg}$$

The cosine is sometimes positive (up to +1) and sometimes negative (down to −1). If the phase differences are random and the average is done over a long enough period of time, then the cosine term averages to zero (i.e., every plus value is ultimately canceled by a minus value). Then,

$$(I_r)_{avg} = (A_1)^2 + (A_2)^2$$

or

$$(I_r)_{avg} = I_1 + I_2 \tag{21.13}$$

Equation 21.13 says that for incoherent sources, the average irradiance distribution is just the sum of the irradiances of each individual source. This is our typical everyday experience since our common light sources are highly incoherent. Specifically, they usually change phase much faster than 10^{-8} s, and the human visual system cannot detect changes faster than about 1/20 s. (In other words, the human visual system averages over about a 1/20 s period.)

EXAMPLE 21.4

A wave has an irradiance of 25 units, and another wave has an irradiance of 9 units. (a) What is the resulting (average) irradiance when the waves are incoherent? (b) What is the resulting irradiance when the waves are coherent and 180° out of phase? (c) What is the resulting irradiance when the waves are coherent and in phase?

For (a), the irradiances add, and

$$(I_r)_{avg} = 25 + 9 = 34$$

For (b), the amplitudes subtract. The wave with irradiance 25 has an amplitude of 5, while the wave with irradiance 9 has an amplitude of 3. Then,

$$A_r = 5 - 3 = 2$$

and

$$I_r = (A_r)^2 = 2^2 = 4$$

For (c), the amplitudes add.

$$A_r = 5 + 3 = 8$$

and

$$I_r = (A_r)^2 = 8^2 = 64$$

Note that from common experience with incoherent sources, we expect a result of 34 units. At the constructive interference positions, we get 64 units. At the destructive interference positions, we get 4 units. Also the average of the irradiances at the constructive and destructive interference positions is $(64 + 4)/2 = 34$.

21.10 YOUNG'S DOUBLE-SLIT EXPERIMENT

In 1800, the predominant opinion of the scientific community was that light was not a wave. Certain known light properties could be explained by the wave theory, but these properties could also be explained by the nonwave theories. In 1801, Thomas Young conceived the following experiment. He wanted to demonstrate that light was a wave by generating interference effects similar to those in a ripple tank. Young wanted to use two pinholes to generate the interference effects, and he realized the need for mutual coherence of the light coming through the pinholes. He decided to run sunlight through a single pinhole and then have that light illuminate the double pinholes (Figure 21.16). Since the double pinholes were both illuminated by the light that went through the single pinhole, Young reasoned that whatever phase changes the light incident on the left pinhole underwent would equal the phase changes of the light incident on the right pinhole. Thus, the light coming through the double pinholes would be mutually coherent.

A modification of Young's original experiment was to use slits instead of pinholes. The slits maintain the needed coherence requirements while letting more light through. For monochromatic light, the result of the double-slit experiment is a series of bright and dark interference fringes exactly analogous to the ripple tank experiment. The dark fringes (unilluminated

Figure 21.16 Young's interference experiment.

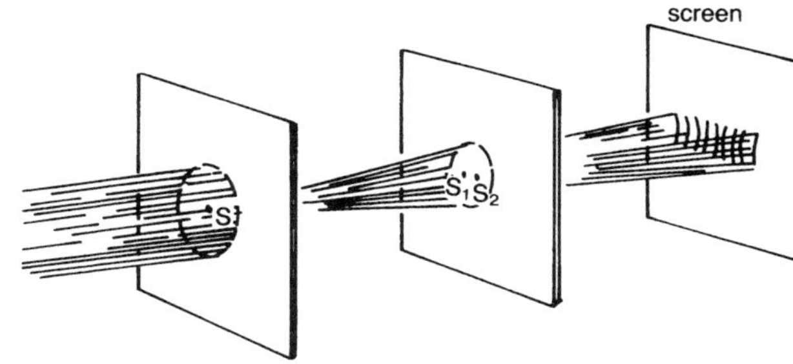

Figure 21.17 Geometry for double-slit interference pattern.

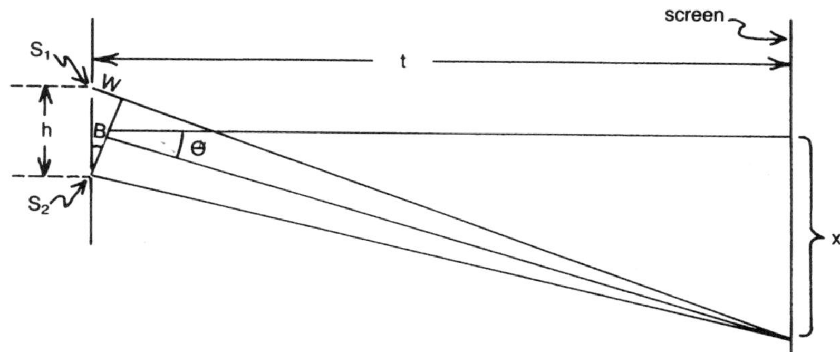

regions) correspond to the nodal regions of the ripple tank (destructive interference). The bright fringes were due to constructive interference.

Let us analyze Young's double-slit experiment for a screen far from the double slits. In Figure 21.17, h is the distance between the slits S_1 and S_2. The wave leaving S_1 has to travel a distance w farther than the wave leaving S_2. Since angles with perpendicular sides are equal, the angle B in the triangle involving w and h is equal to θ. Therefore,

$$\sin\theta = \sin B = w/h$$

At the constructive interference positions, the crest of one wave has to arrive at the same time as the crest of the other wave. For this to occur, the path difference w must be 0, λ, 2λ, 3λ, etc. The condition for the constructive interference maximums is:

$$w = m\lambda \quad \text{where } m = 0, 1, 2, \ldots$$

From the above two equations,

$$h\sin\theta = m\lambda \quad \text{where } m = 0, 1, 2, \ldots \tag{21.14}$$

The interference maximums are located at the angular locations given by Eq. 21.14. The central or zero order maximum results for $m = 0$. The maximums given by the other m values are called the mth order maximums, i.e., $m = 1$ gives the first order maximums, $m = 2$ gives the second order maximums, etc.

The screen is a distance t from the slits. Since we are dealing with a screen far away, we can use the small angle approximation to obtain

$$\theta \approx \sin\theta \approx \tan\theta = x/t \tag{21.15}$$

where x is the distance from the center of the screen. The linear location x of the mth order maximum is given by

$$hx/t = m\lambda$$

or

$$x = m\lambda t/h$$

In the small angle region, the maximums are equidistant from each other, and the fringe spacing s equals the distance x between the central and first order maximum ($m = 1$), or

$$s = \lambda t/h \tag{21.16}$$

Destructive interference gives a minimum or a dark fringe. Here the path difference must be a half integer multiple of λ, i.e.,

$$w = (m + 1/2)\lambda \quad \text{where } m = 0, 1, 2, \ldots$$

Then,

$$h\sin\theta = (m + 1/2)\lambda \quad \text{where } m = 0, 1, 2, \ldots \tag{21.17}$$

In the small angle region, the minimums occur halfway between each maximum.

For a fixed wavelength λ, the fringes are wider when the slits are closer together (small h). Wide fringes are easy to see. The fringes are narrow or finer when the slits are far apart (large h). Fine fringes are harder to see, and may lie below the resolution ability of the human eye.

For a fixed slit separation (fixed h), the fringes are wider for a longer wavelength λ. Hence, red fringes are spread out farther than blue fringes. Thus, for white light illumination, interference fringes are colored.

EXAMPLE 21.5a

Light of wavelength 600 nm (orange) is used to produce double-slit interference fringes. What is the angular and linear location of the second order maximum when the two slits are 0.5 mm apart and the screen is 7 m away?

The second order maximum is described by $m = 2$ in Eq. 22.14. Then,

$$\begin{aligned}\sin\theta &= 2\lambda/h \\ &= 2(600 \times 10^{-9}\,\text{m})/0.5 \times 10^{-3}\,\text{m} \\ &= 2.40 \times 10^{-3}\end{aligned}$$

From the small angle approximation, θ is 2.40×10^{-3} rad. Alternatively, θ is 0.14° or 8.25 min (i.e., there are 60 min per degree, so 0.14° = 8.25 min).

From Eq. 21.15,

$$\begin{aligned}x &= t\theta \\ &= (7\,\text{m})(2.40 \times 10^{-3}) \\ &= 16.8 \times 10^{-3}\,\text{m} = 16.8\,\text{mm}\end{aligned}$$

EXAMPLE 21.5b

For the same slits, what is the location of the second order maximum for light of 480 nm (blue) incident on the same slits?

Here,

$$\begin{aligned}\sin\theta &= 2(480 \times 10^{-9}\,\text{m})/0.5 \times 10^{-3}\,\text{m} \\ \sin\theta &= 1.92 \times 10^{-3}\end{aligned}$$

From the small angle approximation, θ is 1.92×10^{-3} rad (or 0.11°, which is 6.6 min).

From Eq. 21.15,

$$x = (7\,\text{m})(1.92 \times 10^{-3}) = 13.4\,\text{mm}$$

The second order blue maximum is not out as far as the second order orange maximum. This is consistent with the fact that the fringe spacing increases with increasing wavelength.

EXAMPLE 21.6

Monochromatic light is used to produce double-slit interference fringes with a spacing of 3 mm. The screen is 5 m from the slits and the slits are 0.83 mm apart. What is the wavelength?

From Eq. 21.16,

$$\begin{aligned}\lambda &= sh/t \\ &= (3 \times 10^{-3}\,\text{m})(0.83 \times 10^{-3})/(5.0\,\text{m}) \\ &= 0.498 \times 10^{-6}\,\text{m} \\ &= 498 \times 10^{-9}\,\text{m} = 498\,\text{nm}\end{aligned}$$

This wavelength is in the green region near the blue border, so it would actually appear as bluish-green.

21.11 PARTIAL COHERENCE AND FRINGE VISIBILITY

Assume that each slit by itself provides the same irradiance on the screen ($I_1 = I_2$). When the light coming through the slits is incoherent, there is no interference and the irradiance distribution on the screen in the small angle region is $2I_1$. When the light coming through the slits is coherent, interference fringes appear on the screen with a maximum of $4I_1$, and a minimum of zero (Figure 21.13).

Suppose each slit is illuminated with a mixture of 60% coherent and 40% incoherent light. When I_1 equals I_2, the coherent light contributes zero at the minimums and $4(0.6I_1)$ or $2.4I_1$ at the maximums. The incoherent light adds an irradiance of $0.4(2I_1) = 0.8I_1$ to every point on the screen. The net effect is that the maximums now have an irradiance of $2.4I_1 + 0.8I_1$ or $3.21I_1$, while the minimums now have an irradiance of $0.8I_1$. As compared to the 100% coherent case, the interference fringes are still there, but the visibility (contrast) is reduced (Figure 21.18).

The fringe visibility is defined as

$$\text{Visibility} = \frac{I_{max} - I_{min}}{I_{max} + I_{min}} \tag{21.18}$$

For 100% coherent light the fringe visibility equals 1.0, while for incoherent light the fringe visibility equals zero. For the 60–40 mixture, the fringe visibility is

$$\text{Visibility} = \frac{3.2I_1 - 0.8I_1}{3.2I_1 + 0.8I_1}$$

or

$$\text{Visibility} = \frac{2.4}{4.0} = 0.6$$

Note that the fringe visibility equals the percent of coherent light.

The above example shows that partially coherent waves can generate interference fringes, but the visibility or contrast of the fringes is reduced. The percent

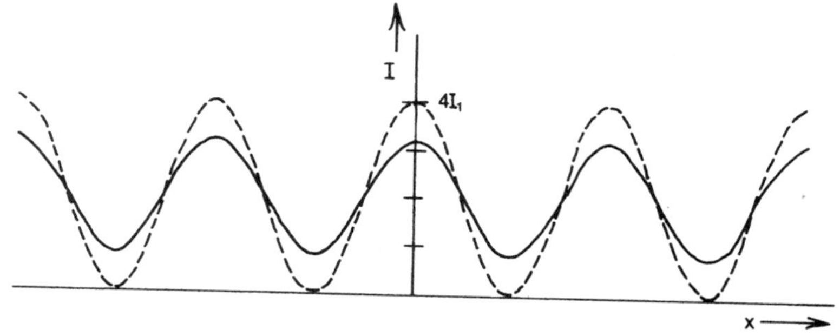

Figure 21.18 Reduction in fringe visibility due to partial coherence.

of coherent light is called the *degree of coherence*. The numerical argument can be repeated for any percentage. Thus, we have a general principle. The fringe visibility equals the degree of coherence of the light coming through the two slits.

One cause of partial coherence (or incoherence) is the finite emission time of atoms. An isolated atom emits light for 10^{-8} s at the most, and then needs to recycle before emitting again. In materials, interactions or collisions with neighboring atoms further shorten the emissions. (Hot solids can have emission times as short as 10^{-15} s.)

During a finite emission time, the atom emits a wave packet, which has a finite length (Figure 21.19). Now consider a pair of double slits illuminated by the atom. When the emission time is long enough, the waves that overlap after passing through the slits belong to the same wavepacket, are therefore mutually coherent, and give fringes that have a visibility equal to 1. For a shorter emission time, the wavepackets may only partially overlap, so that interference occurs only part of the time. This decreases fringe visibility (partial coherence). For still shorter emission times, the same wavepackets may not overlap at all. This results in no interference and zero fringe visibility (incoherence).

The *longitudinal coherence length* is essentially the length of the wavepacket emitted during a typical emission. In a tungsten filament (a hot solid) light bulb, the typical coherence length is only 3 or 4 wavelengths. For a low pressure gas discharge tube, the collisions are less frequent, and coherence lengths of 5,000 wavelengths (about 2 mm) can result. The laser (invented in 1960) is an incredible source in which the coherence length can be as long as 10^{11} wavelengths (about 50 km). The longer the longitudinal coherence length, the easier it is to produce visible interference fringes.

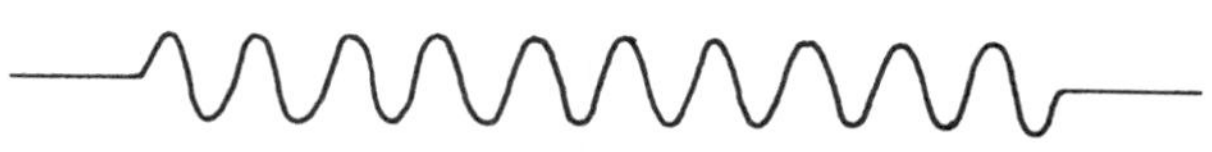

Figure 21.19 Finite length of a wavepacket (due to finite emission time).

For extended sources, there is also a lateral coherence effect. Consider a pair of double slits illuminated by two point sources that are close together. Suppose that each point source by itself produces interference fringes of good visibility. The resultant irradiance on the screen due to both point sources is the sum of the irradiances in the two interference patterns.

Because the point sources are angularly separated, the central maximums in the two interference patterns are not quite lined up. This means that the resultant irradiance pattern has fringes of slightly reduced visibility. If the two point sources are separated further, the visibility of the fringes in the resultant pattern decreases still further. The fringe visibility drops to zero when the two point sources are separated by an amount such that the maximum from one interference pattern lines up with the minimum from the other.

Now consider an extended source consisting of many points. Suppose the source has a small angular size θ_s and illuminates a pair of double slits. Then the light from each point source produces an interference pattern each slightly misaligned with the others. This results in a slightly decreased fringe visibility. As the angular size of the source gets larger, the different interference patterns are more and more misaligned, and the interference patterns tend to counteract each other, resulting in decreasing fringe visibility. For an angular source size θ_s and a slit separation h, the fringe visibility is negligibly small when

$$\theta_s \geq \lambda/h \tag{21.19}$$

Thus, interference fringes are visible when θ_s is much less than λ/h. Note that the required angular size depends on the slit separation h.

Why couldn't Thomas Young have directly illuminated his double slits with light from the sun, and observed interference fringes? The answer is that for Young's slit separation h, the sun's angular size θ_s was too large. Young solved this by running the sunlight through a pinhole before illuminating the double slits. The pinhole's angular size was sufficiently small to give visible interference fringes. Later, Emile Verdet made double slits close enough together ($h < 0.05$ mm) so that he obtained visible interference fringes with the slits illuminated directly with sunlight.

Verdet's experiment is startling because we normally think of the sun as an incoherent source. However, it is probably better to think of the sun as having a small degree of coherence that can be manifested under the right conditions. One way to specify those conditions is in terms of the h value that first gives zero visibility in Eq. 21.19. This h value is sometimes called the *lateral coherence length* l_w. From Eq. 21.19,

$$l_w = \lambda/\theta_s \tag{21.20}$$

where θ_s is the angular size of the source. (Remember that by moving extended sources far enough away, we can make them act like point sources, i.e., we increase l_w by decreasing θ_s.)

In astronomy, the angular size of red dwarf stars has been determined by measuring the lateral coherence length l_w of light from the star, and calculating θ_s. (Even more impressive, but outside the scope of this book are the second order coherence measurements, developed by Hanbury-Brown and Twiss, to determine the angular size of stars smaller than red dwarfs.)

In summary, *the longitudinal coherence length depends on the finite emission time of the atoms, while the lateral coherence length depends on the angular size of extended sources.*

21.12 ACUITY TESTING OF THE VISUAL PATHWAYS BY INTERFERENCE FRINGES

Since interference fringes are easy to form with lasers, we can use a laser to bypass the optics of the eye and test the integrity of the neural part of the human visual system (retina, optic nerve, brain). The method is to project two small spots of the coherent light in the patient's entrance pupil. The light then diverges from these spots and forms interference fringes on the retina. The orientation of the fringes can be changed by rotating the spots. Furthermore, the fringe spacing can be changed by moving the spots closer together or farther apart. We thus have the tools to ascertain which set of fringes the patient can resolve.

For example, suppose a person with a history of retinal disease has cataracts. The surgeon is unsure whether to do cataract surgery since the retina may not be functional. Furthermore, the cataracts obscure the retina, so it cannot be examined by normal means. To use the interference fringe method to check the visual pathways, all we need to do is find a small clear enough area in the crystalline lens to project the two spots of coherent light. Then we can vary the fringe orientation and spacing and get a subjective measure of the potential acuity after cataract surgery. Since the interference fringes do not depend on a clear image being in focus on the retina, the patient does not need to be corrected during this procedure. A positive result (good acuity) would indicate that the patient is a good candidate for surgery. A negative result is inconclusive, since we may not be sure that the interference fringes actually get to the retina.

21.13 OTHER METHODS FOR PRODUCING INTERFERENCE

Interference fringes similar to those from the double-slit experiment can be produced by a number of other methods. One way is to use a Fresnel biprism (Figure 21.20a). When the biprism is illuminated by a point source, it forms two virtual image points. In effect, the two virtual images function as the two point sources in Young's original interference experiment. The waves that go through the different parts of the biprism then overlap and produce the interference fringes. In the same manner, two slightly tilted mirrors can be used to generate interference fringes in the reflected light.

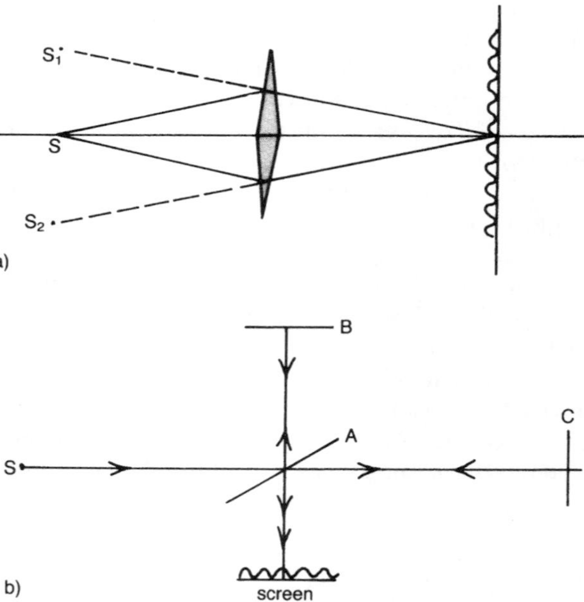

Figure 21.20 a, Interference fringes by Fresnel biprism; b, Michelson interferometer.

The Michelson interferometer is a famous device that uses interference fringes to make precision measurements (Figure 21.20b). Interference fringes are great for precision measurements since a variation of just a half a wavelength (about 280 nm) gives a clear shift in the interference fringes. The basic ingredients of a Michelson interferometer are a partially silvered mirror (A) together with two fully silvered mirrors (B and C). The light incident on A is split in two, and each part travels to a different mirror. The part that goes to B reflects, and travels back to A at which point partial transmission occurs with the transmitted part going to the screen. The part that goes to C reflects and travels back to A at which partial reflection occurs with the reflected part going to the screen. The two different paths introduce the phase differences that lead to the formation of the interference fringes on the screen.

Michelson used this interferometer to make precision measurements on the speed of light. In particular, he showed that the speed of light is independent of the relative motion of the source and the measurement system. In other words, an observer moving toward a light beam, and an observer moving away from a light beam will both measure the relative speed of the beam as C. This is one of the experimental foundations of the special theory of relativity. (In 1907 Albert Michelson became the first American to win the Nobel Prize in Physics.)

21.14 SPECKLES AND LASER REFRACTION

As mentioned, lasers are highly coherent sources. When a diverging laser beam illuminates a diffuse reflecting surface such as a wall, the illuminated region appears to have a series of small black spots in it (similar to a bunch of fly specks). This speckle pattern is due to interference of the diffusely reflected coherent light.

Figure 21.21 shows a highly magnified view of the diffusely reflecting surface. The waves arriving at position 3 have reflected from different positions on the surface, and thus have different path lengths. Depending on the path difference, either destructive interference (dark speckles) or constructive interference (bright speckles) can occur. Similar statements can be made about any other position, such as 1 or 2.

When an observer views the wall, the interference of the diffusely reflected light occurs at the retina, and thus the observer sees the speckles. (A camera records the speckles on film in the same manner.) Since the speckles are formed by interference, the observer sees the speckles even if the wall is blurred. In fact, we can consider the speckles on the retina to be conjugate to speckles in the eye's far point plane.

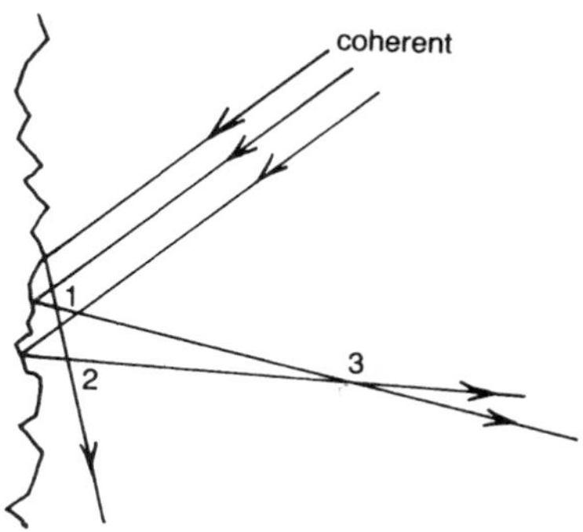

Figure 21.21 Speckle formation due to path length differences from diffuse reflection.

Consider a myope viewing a distant wall (Figure 21.22a), and assume that a dark speckle is formed by destructive interference in the myope's far point plane (position 1). The two waves travel independently through each other, continue on to the eye, and are recombined at the retina. The path lengths for each wave are the same between the far point plane (position 1) and the retina (position 1′) so the waves again destructively interfere at the retina. In effect, the dark

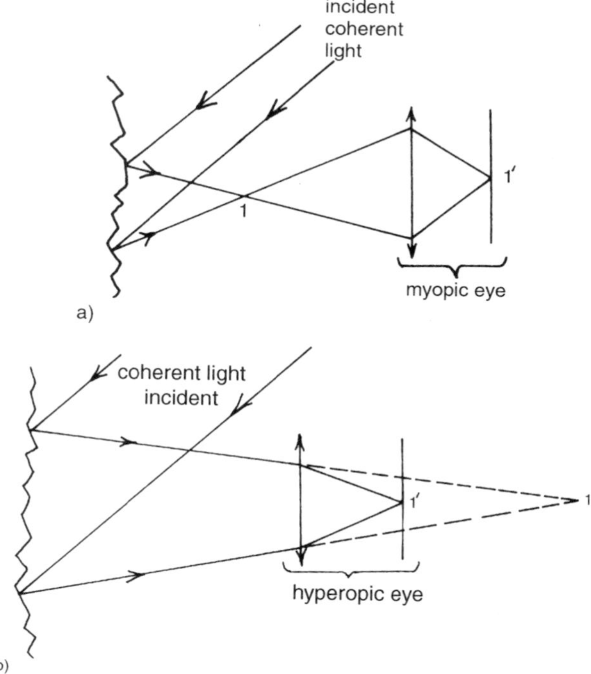

Figure 21.22 a, Speckle in myope's far point plane is conjugate to speckle on the retina; b, virtual speckle in hyperope's far point plane is conjugate to the speckle on the retina.

speckle at the retina (position 1′) is conjugate to the dark speckle in the far point plane (position 1).

Figure 21.22b shows an uncorrected, unaccommodated hyperope viewing the wall. Again, assume the diffusely reflected light going into the eye destructively interferes, giving a dark speckle at 1′. This speckle is conjugate to the speckle that would have been formed at position 1. In terms of geometric optics, the real speckle on the retina (1′) is conjugate to a virtual speckle at position 1.

Not only are the speckles present, but when an ametrope moves his or her head back and forth (or up and down), the speckles also appear to move. In fact, they appear to move in opposite directions for a myope as compared to a hyperope. The speckles do not appear to move for an emmetrope. It should be obvious then that the speckle movement can be used to determine the refractive error of the observer's eye. This is the basis for *laser refraction*.

Let us consider the motion for a myope, hyperope, and emmetrope (Figure 21.23). In each case, we will start with a dark speckle on the center of the retina. This speckle is conjugate to a speckle in the far point plane; then the eye moves up (dashed lines). For the myope, the speckle in the far point plane does not shift, but now the nodal ray (dashed) for the eye intercepts the retina at a position above the center. The nodal ray defines the new retinal speckle position, and it is shifted up relative to the retinal center. However, retinal images are inverted, so an upward shift on the retina is perceived as a downward motion. Hence the eye moved up (EM), the speckle on the retina shifted up (RM), and the perceived speckle motion is down (PM). Thus, the myope who moves his or her head perceives the speckles to move in the opposite direction.

For the hyperope, the solid line shows the rays for the speckle formed on the center of the retina. The dashed lines show the eye shifted up, in which case the incident top ray becomes the nodal ray for the shifted eye. The nodal ray (dashed) shows that the speckle position is now below the center of the retina. So the speckle moved down on the retina, which is perceived as an up motion. Here the speckle appears to move with the motion of the retina.

The bottom drawing is for the emmetropic eye. This time when the eye is shifted up so that the top ray becomes the nodal ray, the speckle remains on the

Figure 21.23 Speckle motion for myope, hyperope, and emmetrope.

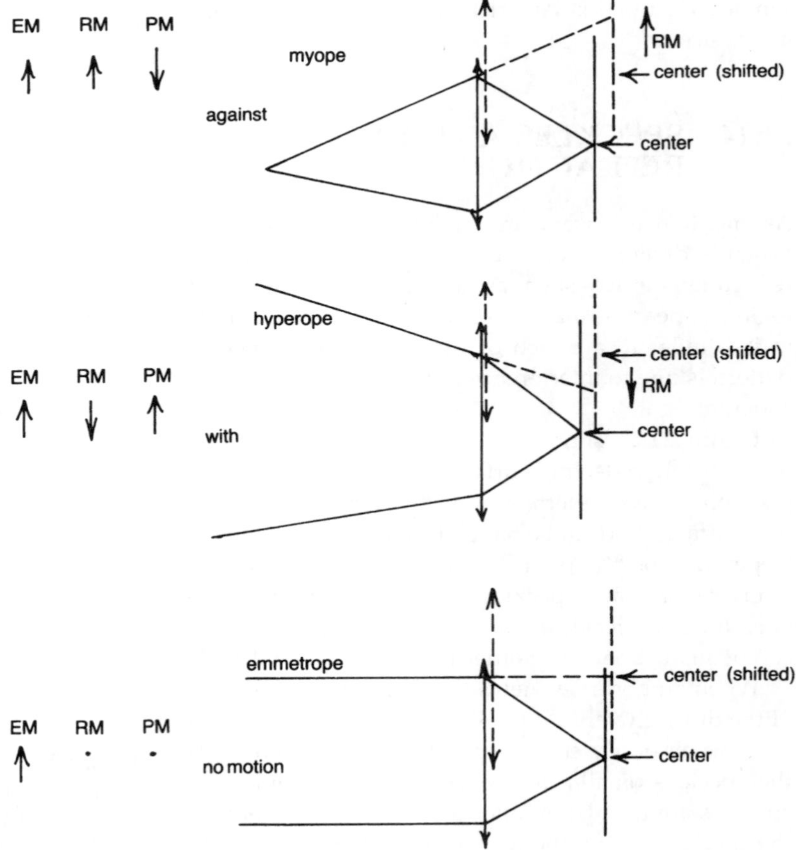

center of the retina, and no speckle motion is perceived.

So relative to a head movement, the myope perceives against motion, the hyperope perceives with motion, and the emmetrope perceives no motion. The higher the degree of ametropia, the faster the perceived motion. The lower the degree of ametropia, the slower the perceived motion.

Laser refraction is actually performed by illuminating a very slowly moving surface with laser light. Then the observer does not need to make a head movement to perceive the motions. A drum that rotates one revolution per hour works well. Under incoherent illumination, the drum appears stationary. Under coherent illumination, the drum still appears stationary, but now speckle motion is perceived by an ametrope. A corrected ametrope (or an emmetrope) sees no definite with or against motion, although the speckles may appear to boil around in a random fashion. (Note that a surface moving one direction while the patient's head is stationary is equivalent to the patient moving his or her head the opposite direction while the surface is stationary. Therefore an uncorrected myope perceives the speckles to move opposite to his or her head motion, or with the motion of a moving surface.)

Laser light is monochromatic, so the terms emmetropic, myopic, and hyperopic refer to the conditions for that wavelength. The low energy laser (1 mW) helium–neon laser puts out a coherent monochromatic beam with a 632.8-nm vacuum wavelength. Because of the eye's chromatic aberration, blue focuses before red. A person emmetropic for the middle of the visible spectrum is actually hyperopic for the helium–neon laser beam.

Optometers based on laser refraction have been very useful is studying the subjective accommodative response of the eye. A beam splitter is used so that the person can simultaneously view the object (the accommodative stimulus) and a slowly rotating drum. The laser light is flashed onto the drum for short periods of time. While the laser is on, the person sees the speckle pattern simultaneously with the accommodative stimulus. If the person sees no speckle motion, the subjective accommodative response equals the stimulus. If the person sees speckle motion, then the response leads or lags the stimulus. The speckles themselves do not act as an accommodative stimulus, after all, they are formed on the retina independent of the focus. These laser optometers have been a prime tool for testing the accommodative intermediate resting state hypothesis.

The speckle size is a function of the diffuseness of the surface and the size of the optical system's aperture stop. If the drum is rotating vertically, the speckle motion is vertical and power is checked in the vertical meridian of the eye. The axis of the drum can be rotated so that any other meridian can be checked, and hence laser refraction can be used as a meridional refraction technique. For an off-axis meridian of an astigmat, the torsional component of the dioptric power causes the speckle motion to appear in a meridian different from the meridian of rotation. This complicates the use of laser meridional refraction.

21.15 THIN FILM INTERFERENCE

Thin films of various materials create colorful interference fringes. These fringes are quite common because the films are thin enough so that even short wavepackets give the interference effects. Hence, the fringes show under illumination by sunlight or other common light sources. Some frequently observed examples are the color of oil slicks on wet roads and the colored fringes in soap bubbles. Two clean microscope slides that adhere together give the fringes because of trapped thin layers of air. Some chemical interactions produce thin film surface changes, which then result in colored interference fringes (e.g, the bottoms of some cooking pans, weathered glass). Some sea shells also show thin film interference colors because of their thin film shell structure.

Thin film interference is formed as a result of multiple reflection processes. This is a wave effect; however, we will use rays to simplify the figures. In Figure 21.24, the incident ray hits the thin film at point *A*. Part of the light is reflected (ray 1) and part is transmitted. The transmitted ray travels to point *B*, where part of it is transmitted (ray u) and part is reflected. The reflected part travels to point *C*, where part of it is transmitted (ray 2) and part reflected. The part reflected travels to point *D* where again part is transmitted (ray v) and part reflected. The process continues on resulting in the reflected waves 1 to 5 and the transmitted waves u through y.

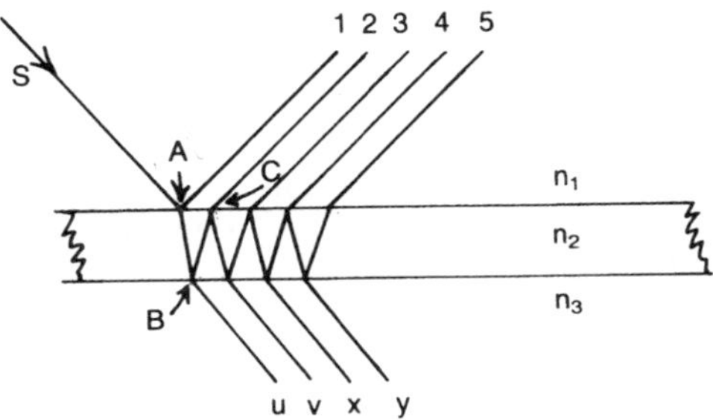

Figure 21.24 Multiple reflections responsible for thin film interference.

For a thin film, the coherence length of ordinary light is long enough so that all the overlapping multiple reflected waves give interference effects. For a complete analysis, all the multiple reflected waves need to be taken into account, but for our purposes we will consider only the largest amplitude waves—namely, 1, 2, u, and v.

If waves 1 and 2 are out of phase, then destructive interference occurs in the reflected light. When this happens, waves u and v are in phase resulting in constructive interference in the transmitted light. As before, energy is conserved in the process, but it is redistributed from the reflected light to the transmitted light.

By adjusting the thickness of the thin film, we could make the destructive interference occur between waves u and v, in which case the constructive interference occurs between waves 1 and 2. Again energy is conserved. The energy that is removed from the transmitted light is channeled into the reflected light.

21.16 PHASE CHANGES AT REFLECTION

For thin films, one obvious source of the phase differences is the over and back path differences across the film. A second source is phase changes at the reflections. To gain some intuition about phase changes at a reflection, let us consider a pulse propagating along a rope (Figure 21.25). The rope consists of a lightweight section (thin line) connected to a heavyweight section (thick line). Some reflection occurs when the pulse moves from one section to the other. When the crest is initially in the heavy section, the reflected pulse is also a crest (no phase change). However, when the crest is initially in the lightweight section, the reflected pulse is a trough (a 180° phase change on reflection).

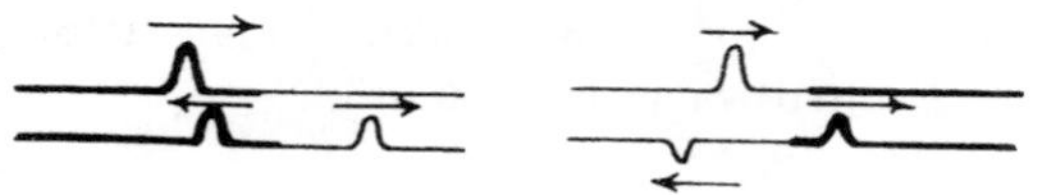

Figure 21.25 Relation of reflected pulse phase to incident pulse phase.

G.G. Stokes (1819–1903) used the principle of optical reversibility to prove that light waves must exhibit reflected phase changes analogous to the rope pulses. Consider an interface between two dielectric media of refractive indices n_1 and n_2. In Figure 21.26a, the incident ray represents a wave of amplitude A incident on the interface. The amplitude of the reflected wave is $r_{12}A$. The amplitude of the transmitted light is $t_{12}A$.

In the optically reversed situation, two waves are incident on the interface (Figure 21.26b). The wave $r_{12}A$ is partially reflected, $r_{12}(r_{12}A)$, and partially transmitted, $t_{12}(r_{12}A)$. The wave $t_{12}A$ is partially reflected, $r_{21}(t_{12}A)$ and partially transmitted, $t_{21}(t_{12}A)$. According to the reversibility principle, the reversed situation must give us back the original wave of amplitude A traveling in the opposite direction. Hence, the two waves traveling to the bottom left in medium n_2 must cancel each other out (destructive interference). In terms of amplitudes,

$$r_{12}t_{12}A + t_{12}r_{21}A = 0$$

and it follows that

$$r_{12} = -r_{21}$$

The minus sign indicates that the two reflections differ by a phase change of 180°. For dielectrics in situations not involving total internal reflection, Maxwell's equations show that when the light is initially in the optically less dense (lower n) medium, the reflected light has a 180° phase change, whereas when the light is in the optically more dense medium (higher n), the reflected light does not have a phase change. For example, light in air that reflects at an air–glass interface undergoes a 180° phase change (Figure 21.27), while light in the glass that reflects at a glass–air interface does not change its phase.

For completeness, consider the light traveling up and to the left in the reversed situation. According to the principle of reversibility,

$$t_{12}t_{21}A + r_{12}r_{12}A = A$$

or

$$t_{12}t_{21} + (r_{12})^2 = 1$$

Figure 21.26 a, Reflection and refraction of incident light; b, reflection and refraction of reversed light.

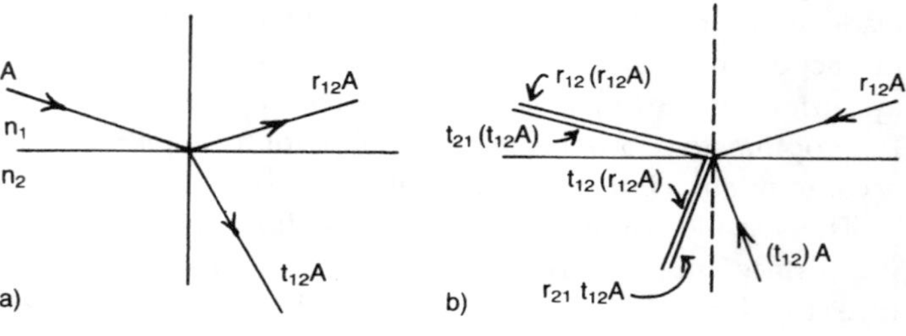

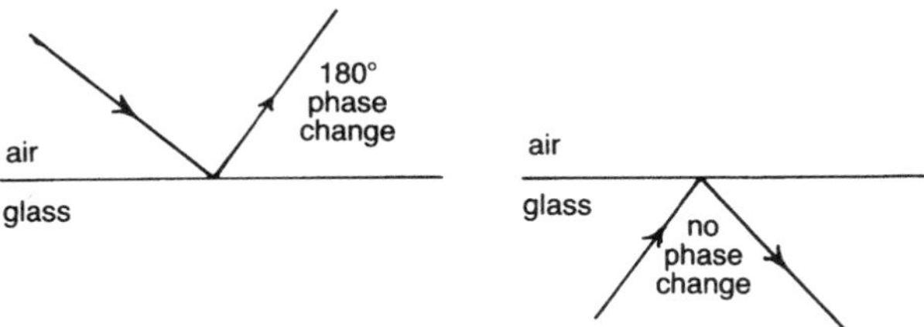

Figure 21.27 Phase behavior at reflection.

There are no phase changes with transmission so t_{12} equals t_{21}. Then,

$$(t_{12})^2 + (r_{12})^2 = 1$$

Let

$$T = (t_{12})^2 \quad \text{and} \quad R = (r_{12})^2$$

Then

$$T + R = 1$$

and we see that T and R are the geometric optics transmission and reflection factors (no absorption). For near normal incidence, Fresnel's law of reflection gave

$$R = \frac{(n_2 - n_1)^2}{(n_2 + n_1)^2}(100\%)$$

21.17 SOAP FILMS

Consider monochromatic light incident on a soap film of thickness t in air (Figure 21.24). Here n_1 and n_3 equal 1, while n_2 is approximately 1.33. At the first reflection (point A), the reflected light changes phase by 180°. The transmitted wave travels to B. A percentage of the wave reflects at B and travels back to C where part is transmitted (wave 2). For almost normal incidence, wave 2 has traveled over and back or a distance of $2t$ farther than wave 1. Suppose

$$2t = m\lambda_{tf} \quad \text{where} \quad m = 0, 1, 2, \ldots$$

and λ_{tf} is the wavelength in the thin film. Then the path difference does not introduce a phase difference between waves 1 and 2. However, wave 1 had a 180° phase change at its reflection whereas wave 2 did not. Thus, wave 1 is 180° out of phase with wave 2, and they will destructively interfere.

What about the transmitted light? At C the light reflects with no phase change and travels back to D, where part of it is transmitted (wave v). The only source of phase differences between waves u and v is that wave v traveled $2t$ (over and back) farther than wave u. Then for the thickness condition above, waves u and v are in phase and constructively interfere.

Because of the interference, there is a minimum or dark fringe in the reflected light, while there is a maximum or bright fringe in the transmitted light. More energy is transmitted and less is reflected.

Since

$$\lambda_{tf} = \frac{\lambda}{n_2}$$

the condition for a minimum in the reflected light becomes

$$2t = m(\lambda/n_2) \quad \text{where } m = 0, 1, 2, \ldots$$

where λ is the vacuum wavelength.

For $m = 1$, the reflected light has a dark fringe for

$$2t = \lambda/n_2$$

For $m = 0$, the condition for a dark fringe in the reflected light is

$$2t = 0$$

If there is no film, we obviously do not expect any reflected light, and the above condition agrees with that. However, as the film thickness goes to zero, the mechanism by which the reflection goes to zero is interesting. The air–film reflection gives a 180° phase change, while the interior film–air reflection does not give a phase change. If the thickness is negligible, then these two reflected waves (1 and 2) overlap and destructively interfere. Gravitational forces cause a soap film to thin with time. As t goes to zero, the reflected light turns black even before the film breaks, thus confirming the above analysis.

By a similar analysis, constructive interference in the reflected light (and hence destructive interference in the transmitted light) occurs when

$$2t = \left(m + \frac{1}{2}\right)\frac{\lambda}{n_2} \quad m = 0, 1, 2, \ldots$$

EXAMPLE 21.7a

Monochromatic light of 656 nm (red) is incident on a soap film. What is the smallest non-zero thickness that will give a dark fringe in the reflected light?

Here $m = 1$, and

$$2t = \lambda/n_2$$

or

$$t = \frac{656\,\text{nm}}{2(1.33)} = 246.6\,\text{nm}$$

EXAMPLE 21.7b

When white light is incident on the above film, what color will the reflected light tend to have?

The thickness of 246.6 nm gives a maximum or bright fringe in the reflected light for a wavelength given by

$$2(246.6\,\text{nm}) = \left(m + \frac{1}{2}\right)\frac{\lambda}{1.33}$$

or

$$4(246.6\,\text{nm})(1.33) = (2\,\text{m} + 1)\lambda$$

For

$$m = 0 \quad \lambda = 1311.9\,\text{nm}$$
$$m = 1 \quad \lambda = 437.3\,\text{nm}$$
$$m = 2 \quad \lambda = 262.4\,\text{nm}$$

Of these wavelengths, 437.3 nm is in the visible range (indigo or violet). Therefore, a thickness of 246.6 nm gives destructive interference in the reflected light for 656 nm (red) and constructive interference in the reflected light for 437.3 nm. There are other wavelengths around 437.3 nm (especially the blues) that will also tend to have a constructive interference effect. Hence in white light, the reflected fringe shifts from the violet toward a blue.

Normally in soap bubbles, the film thickness varies from position to position on the surface, and also varies with time. For incident white light, the resulting thin film colored interference fringes drift around with time. If you watch the top of a soap bubble, these interference fringes turn black or disappear just prior to the bubble breaking.

21.18 ANTIREFLECTION COATINGS

In lens systems, the amount of light lost by reflection rapidly increases with the number of lenses. For example, if 4% is reflected at each surface, the transmission factor T is 0.96 per surface. Consider a system consisting of five separated lenses in air. There are ten surfaces, and the resultant transmission of the primary wave is $(0.96)^{10}$ or 0.66. The primary transmitted wave is down to 66% even though only 4% is being reflected at each surface. Furthermore multiple reflections can generate ghost images or glare (haziness) that degrade the final image quality of the system.

In the 1930s, vacuum technology advanced to the point where a material could be vaporized in a vacuum chamber and deposited in very thin films on a lens surface. This made possible the design of uniform thickness antireflecting thin films. These thin films reduced the percent reflection by destructive interference and at the same time increased the percent transmission by constructive interference. The first antireflection (AR) thin film coatings were for glass lenses, but near the end of the twentieth century good quality AR coatings were also developed for plastic lenses.

Antireflection thin films work similar to soap bubbles except that the index sequence is now different. In Figure 21.28, n_3, n_2, and n_1 are the refractive indices of the glass, thin film, and initial medium, respectively. In order for a single layer AR thin film to work with maximum efficiency, we need the percent reflectance R_{12} at the n_1–n_2 interface to equal the percent reflectance R_{23} at the n_2–n_3 interface. For normal incidence, Fresnel's law of reflection (Chapter 14) gives

$$R_{12} = \frac{(n_2 - n_1)^2}{(n_2 + n_1)^2}100\%$$

$$R_{23} = \frac{(n_3 - n_2)^2}{(n_3 + n_2)^2}100\%$$

The ideal single layer thin film has an index n_2 that makes R_{12} equal to R_{23}. We can set the above two expressions equal to each other, cross multiply, and solve for n_2 to obtain

$$n_2 = \sqrt{n_1 n_3} \tag{21.21}$$

This is the refractive index for an ideal single layer AR thin film. For example, consider ophthalmic crown glass ($n = 1.523$) in air ($n = 1.000$), the ideal refractive index is $\sqrt{1.523}$, or 1.234.

Practical thin films do not necessarily have the ideal index. A thin film of magnesium fluoride ($n = 1.38$) is widely used as an AR coating for glass lenses. Some of the practical reasons are good adhesion and relatively good stability over time.

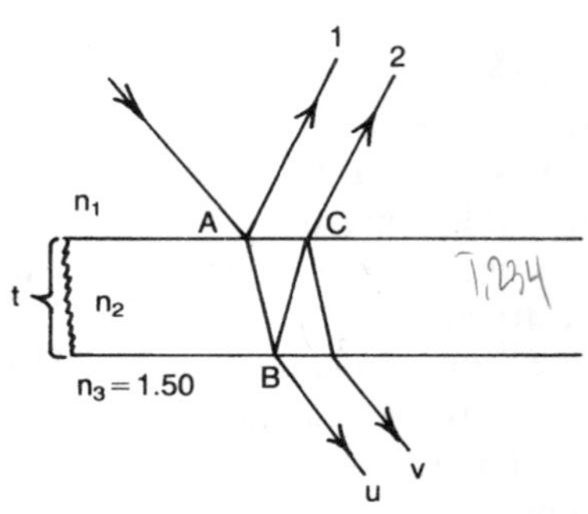

Figure 21.28 Antireflection thin film.

The thickness condition for an AR thin film is different from that of a soap film in air because of different phase changes at the reflections. In Figure 21.28, there is a 180° phase change for the light reflected at position *A*. There is also a phase change for the light reflected at position *B*. Therefore, the only phase difference between waves 1 and 2 is due to the over and back ($2t$) distance that wave 2 traveled. For destructive interference between 1 and 2, we then need

$$2t = (m + 1/2)\lambda_{tf} \quad m = 0, 1, 2, \ldots$$

For $m = 0$,

$$2t = \lambda_{tf}/2$$

or

$$t = \lambda_{tf}/4$$

The minimum thickness of an antireflecting thin film on glass is a quarter of the wavelength in the thin film (λ_{tf}). Since

$$\lambda_{tf} = \frac{\lambda}{n_2}$$

we have

$$t = \frac{\lambda}{4n_2} \tag{21.22}$$

or

$$tn_2 = \frac{\lambda}{4}$$

The product of the thickness and the refractive index, tn_2, is called the *optical thickness*. Thus, we can say that the reflected light has a minimum when the optical thickness is a quarter wavelength.

EXAMPLE 21.8

A MgFl ($n = 1.38$) AR coating is placed on a glass lens. What is the minimum thickness of the film for incident light of wavelength 552 nm?

From Eq. 21.22,

$$t = \frac{552\,\text{nm}}{4(1.38)} = 100\,\text{nm}$$

Figure 21.29 gives the reflectance as a function of incident wavelength for uncoated glass, a single layer AR coating, and multiple layer AR coatings. The single layer coating is not ideal, so the minimum is not zero. The performance is improved by using layered thin films consisting of quarter wavelength thick stacks of different thin film materials. Zinc sulfide ($n = 2.32$) is one of the materials used with MgFl to achieve the layered results for glass lenses. Typically

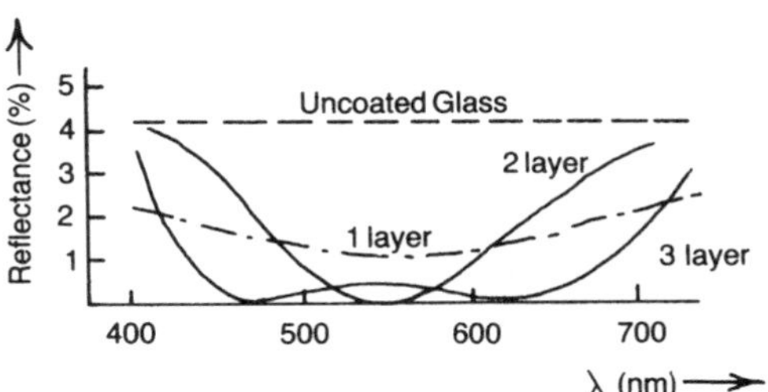

Figure 21.29 Reflectance as a function of incident wavelength for uncoated and various layer antireflection films.

the high index thin film is deposited first on the glass lens followed by the low index thin film. Multilayered thin films also increase the range of incident angles over which the coating will be antireflective.

When the coating is antireflecting for the middle of the visible spectrum, some reflection occurs at both the red and violet ends of the spectrum. This gives the lens a purplish appearance similar to that of a ripe plum. (Such a lens is sometimes referred to as a bloomed lens.) Multi-layer AR thin films can be designed to essentially eliminate all visible reflection, or can be tailored to leave a residual reflection with a particular desired color.

The thin film thickness that gives destructive interference in the reflected light gives constructive interference in the transmitted light. In Figure 21.28, consider the wave traveling from position *A* to *B*. At *B*, part is transmitted (wave u) and part is reflected with a 180° phase change. The reflected light travels back to position *C*, and part is reflected without a phase change. The light then travels back across the film, and part is transmitted at point *D* (wave v). Wave v differs from u by a 180° phase change due to the reflection at *B* and by the phase difference due to the over and back distance ($2t$). The condition for destructive interference in the reflected light was

$$2t = (m + 1/2)\lambda_{tf} \quad m = 0, 1, 2, \ldots$$

The above condition gives a 180° phase difference due to the path difference. This 180° phase difference adds to the 180° phase difference due to the reflection at *B*. The result is a 360° phase difference, which means that the two waves (u and v) are in phase and constructively interfere. The energy that is not reflected (because of the destructive interference) is transmitted (because of the constructive interference).

Thus, an AR coated lens has an increased transmission over an uncoated lens. This is important to remember since at a quick glance an AR coated lens can look like a lens with a light absorbing tint. However, the lens with the absorption tint decreases transmission, whereas the AR coated lens increases transmission. This can make a difference in low illumination conditions such as night driving.

In studies, patients who wear AR coated spectacle lenses report that they see detail more crisply and that the environment appears brighter. The higher the refractive index of an uncoated lens, the higher the reflection at each surface (i.e., Fresnel's law of reflection). Therefore, the higher the refractive index of the lens, the larger the benefits of an AR coating. Antireflection coatings also provide a cosmetic benefit in that reflections from the spectacle lens that interfere with eye contact or appearance of the person are cut down by the AR coatings. It turns out that eliminating all of the reflection by a multilayer AR coating is not cosmetically desirable because it gives the lens a dark or dirty appearance (sometimes called a "dead" gray). Therefore AR spectacle lens coatings are designed with a cosmetically pleasing residual reflection (or residual "color"). Bluish-green is a frequently used residual color, although blues and golds are also used. Some patients prefer specific residual colors.

The shift from glass to plastic for spectacle lenses created challenges for the AR coating industry. Plastic lenses sometimes softened and warped under the temperatures required for evaporation coating. The resulting AR coats sometimes cracked, crazed, and peeled off the plastic lenses. Recent advances in the AR coating industry have solved many of these problems. Different materials (e.g., silicon, zirconium, and titanium oxides) are used for coating plastic lenses. Ion beams are used to optimize the lens surface for coatings, and to improve the thin film by packing it with heavy ions (ion assisted deposition). A buffer coat is also used to improve adhesion and reduce cracking and crazing of the AR multilayers.

A historical disadvantage of AR coatings is that they attracted dirt and oils, exaggerated the dirty appearance of the lens, and were hard to clean. Near the end of the twentieth century, the best AR multilayer coatings were covered with an easy-to-clean hydrophobic topcoat that helps repel dirt and oils.

Just as thin films can be antireflecting, we can design layers of thin films that give constructive interference in the reflected light. Such thin film stacks can give a much higher percent reflection than silvered surfaces.

Thin film stacks can also be designed to do specific tasks with different parts of the electromagnetic spectrum or with different parts of the visible spectrum. For example, there are thin film stacks that reflect infrared while transmitting visible light (a so-called *hot mirror*). Similarly, there are thin film stacks that reflect visible light while transmitting infrared (a so-called *cold mirror*). These types of films are important in that high intensity filament or arc sources radiate much more energy in the infrared than in the visible light region. In higher intensity situations, the infrared radiation can generate damaging heat levels.

21.19 INTERFERENCE FILTERS

Interference filters work on thin film interference principles. They are designed to transmit a very narrow band of visible light (by constructive interference) while reflecting all other wavelengths.

An interference filter consists of a thin film sandwiched between highly reflecting surfaces. The higher the reflectance of the surfaces, the narrower the wavelength band of transmitted light. Figure 21.30 compares the transmission of a narrow band interference filter to that of an absorption filter. The absorption filter is a broad band filter that also absorbs much of the desired light. The interference filter is a high transmittance narrow band filter. An absorption filter heats up under high illumination conditions, whereas an interference filter tends to stay cool, since it is reflecting the unwanted light instead of absorbing it.

Consider an interference filter that transmits a wavelength λ. The thickness of the film that gives constructive interference between the multiply-reflected transmitted waves is exactly the correct thickness for a standing wave of that light to be formed in the film (between the highly reflecting surfaces). In the ideal situation, this is the only wavelength for which there is a large buildup of energy inside the thin film, and consequently, the only wavelength that is transmitted. Increasing the reflectance of the surfaces helps to finely tune the allowed standing wave, and consequently, the transmission band narrows. When an interference filter is tilted, the effective thickness changes and the transmitted wavelength decreases.

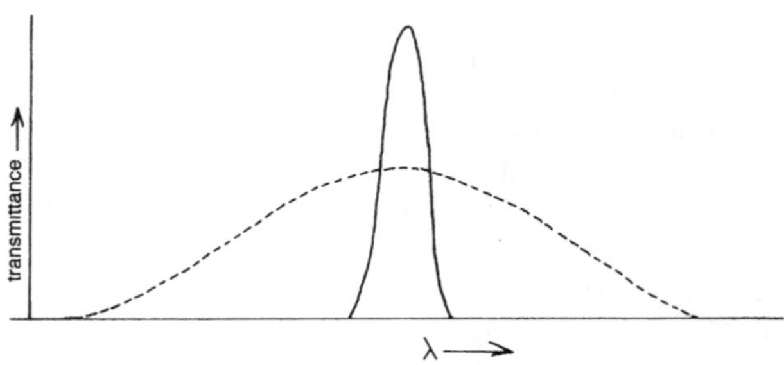

Figure 21.30 Transmittance for interference filter versus absorption filter.

(The decrease may seem counterintuitive, but a complete geometric analysis shows that it is correct.)

Precision interference filters are made with multi-thin film layers between the reflecting surfaces. The Fabry–Perot interferometer is a precision interferometer that works much like an interference filter.

21.20 NEWTON'S RINGS

Thin air layers can also generate thin film interference. One example is the thin film interference fringes visible when two clean microscope slides adhere together trapping some air between them. In optics, such thin film interference is used to test the precision of surfaces to within a fraction of a wavelength of the light. The simplest set-up for spherical surfaces generates circular interference fringes called Newton's rings (after Newton who experimentally discovered them even though he did not believe the wave theory).

In Figure 21.31, the light in the glass incident on A is partially transmitted and partially reflected (without a phase change). The light in air incident on B is partially reflected with a 180° phase change. Since the reflections introduce a 180° phase difference, waves 1 and 2 will be out of phase if the path difference between them is

$$2t = m\lambda \quad m = 0, 1, 2, \ldots$$

where λ is the wavelength in the air gap. There are then circular dark fringes in the reflected light for thicknesses corresponding to air gap thicknesses t, which corresponds to integer multiples of a half wavelength. Bright fringes occur between the dark fringes.

Note that a dark fringe occurs for $t = 0$, or for the contact point. This is not surprising since we do not expect reflection from an ophthalmic crown–ophthalmic crown interface. Actually, we already get destructive interference for a non-zero air gap provided the gap thickness is considerably smaller than a quarter wavelength.

Surface flaws that change t by a quarter wavelength (or $2t$ by a half wavelength) shift a dark fringe to a bright fringe and are thus clearly visible by inspection of Newton's rings. Similarly, thin film interference methods are used to calibrate precision manufacturing equipment.

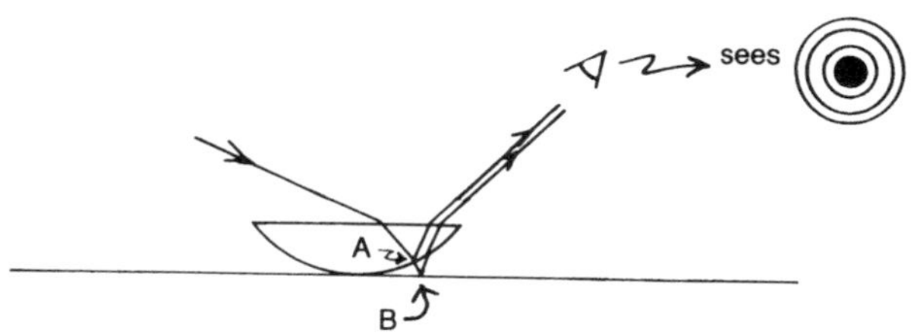

Figure 21.31 Newton's rings.

PROBLEMS

1. A light wave has a frequency of 5.00×10^{14} Hz. What is the vacuum wavelength in nm? What is the color classification of this light? When this light enters glass ($n = 1.50$), what is the frequency and wavelength? Does the color classification change? Why or why not?
2. A harmonic wave has an amplitude of 3 units. A second harmonic wave has an amplitude of 12 units. What is the relative intensity of the second wave to the first?
3. Light in the vitreous humor has a 406 nm wavelength. What is the normal color classification for this light?
4. A harmonic wave of amplitude 5 units is superposed with a harmonic wave of amplitude 7 units. What is the resultant intensity when the waves are incoherent? When the waves are coherent and in phase? When the waves are coherent and 180° out of phase?
5. Sodium D light has a 589.3 nm vacuum wavelength. When this light passes through two narrow slits 0.1 mm apart, what is the interference fringe spacing on a screen 300 cm from the slits? Same question for the slits 0.5 mm apart.
6. Light from an arc source passes through an interference filter and is incident on two narrow slits 0.06 cm apart. The interference pattern is formed on a screen 250 cm away. The interference fringe spacing on the screen is 2.28 mm. What is the wavelength of the light?
7. For a given wavelength, does the lateral coherence length of a source increase or decrease with increasing source size?
8. When light of wavelength 489 nm is incident on soap film ($n = 1.33$) in air, what is the smallest thickness that gives a maximum in the reflected light?
9. What is the ideal index and thickness for an antireflecting thin film on a high index glass ($n = 1.68$) lens in air. Assume the incident wavelength is 560 nm.
10. A 90 nm thick MgFl ($n = 1.38$) antireflecting thin film is placed on a glass lens with a 1.523 index. What is the incident wavelength for the thin antireflecting film?
11. A helium–neon laser beam (wavelength 632.8 nm) is incident on double slits of separation 0.8 mm. On a screen located 6 m from the slits, how far is the third order maximum from the center of the interference pattern?

CHAPTER 22

Diffraction

22.1 THE HUYGENS–FRESNEL PRINCIPLE

We are very familiar with the ability of sound waves to travel around corners. You may have even noticed the ability of water waves to propagate around obstacles. The ability of a wave to propagate around corners is called diffraction. The importance of diffraction depends on the size of the obstacle or aperture relative to the size of the wavelength. Music and speech wavelengths range from 1.7 cm to 17 m. A door (an aperture) is perhaps a meter across, so that for the long wavelengths, the sound waves bend easily around the doorway. Diffraction is less evident for the short wavelengths.

The wavelengths of visible light are so short (10^{-7} m) that at first glance it appears no bending occurs (i.e., the law of rectilinear propagation). However, careful observations show that visible light waves do diffract. For example, look at a distant street light at night and squint. The light appears to streak out from the light bulb, i.e., it has bent around the "corners" formed by your eyelids. Alternatively, stand in a dark room and look at a distant light bulb in another room. Now move until the doorway blocks half of the distant light bulb. Due to diffraction around the doorway, the light appears to streak out into the umbra region of the dark room.

There are several approaches to explaining diffraction. The most intuitive approach is based on a principle first put forth by Christian Huygens (1629–1695, inventor of the pendulum clock). Huygens' principle states:

> All points on a wavefront can be considered as point sources for the production of spherical secondary wavelets, and at any later time the new wavefront position is the envelope (or surface of tangency) to these secondary wavelets.

Huygens' principle can be used to derive the geometric optics laws of reflection and refraction (see Section 22.18).

Figure 22.1a shows Huygens' principle applied to plane waves. The points *A*, *B*, *C*, and *D* each serve as a point source for a secondary spherical wavelet. After a time *t*, each of the secondary wavelets has propagated downstream. The new position of the wavefront is specified by the envelope (or surface of tangency) of the secondary wavelets. This envelope is a straight line indicating that the new wave is still a plane wave (i.e., flat).

Figure 22.1b shows plane waves incident on a straight-edged obstacle. High above the obstacle, the envelope is still flat indicating rectilinear propagation. In the lower region, the obstacle blocks some of the secondary wavelets. In the region behind the obstacle, the secondary wavelets from points above the obstacle give an envelope that is curved similar to that of a sphere. This curved envelope indicates that some light bends around the obstacle and propagates into the geometric optics umbra region. This is the diffracted light. Since the amount of diffracted light (the luminous flux) is small, any background light may mask it. However, with a dark background, it is easy to observe.

For a screen some distance behind the obstacle, the dashed curve in Figure 22.1c indicates the expected irradiance predicted by geometric optics when diffraction is ignored. The "dark" zone behind the obstacle is to the right of where the dashed line drops to zero. The solid curve in Figure 22.1c is the actual irradiance on the screen. The actual curve shows some diffracted light in the zone behind the obstacle. While the fall-off in the diffracted light behind the obstacle is smooth, the irradiance in the illuminated region at a height above the obstacle shows a ripple-like variation. Augustin Fresnel (1788–1827) expanded Huygens' principle to explain the ripple effect. A

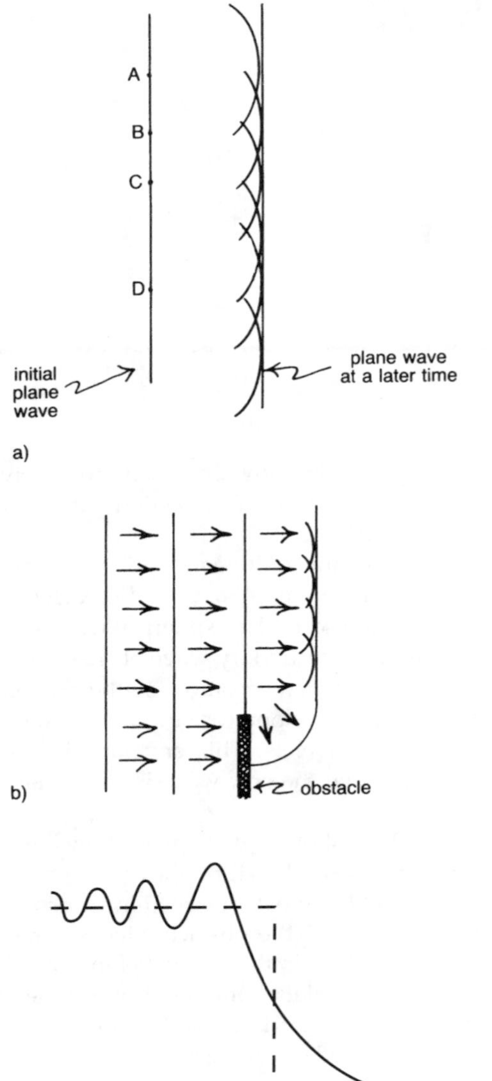

Figure 22.1 Huygens principle: a, plane waves; b, diffraction; c, rippled irradiance in the diffraction pattern.

simplified statement of Fresnel's addition to Huygens' principle is:

> For light in the same bundle (i.e., waves from the same point source) the secondary wavelets undergo mutual interference.

So the Huygens' principle explanation is that the ripple effect in the diffraction pattern is due to the constructive and destructive interference of the secondary wavelets.

22.2 SINGLE-SLIT DIFFRACTION

Consider monochromatic plane waves (wavelength λ) incident on a single slit of width d. Figure 22.2a shows a cross-sectional view in the plane perpendicular to the slit length. When the aperture is large, the waves going through the middle remain plane waves (little or no diffraction). When the aperture is very small, only one secondary wavelet comes through, and the resulting cross-sectional shape of the envelope is the circular shape of that wavelet. The circular shape indicates a large amount of diffraction (lateral spreading) of the light.

In Figure 22.2a, the slit has a size such that several secondary wavelets pass through the slit. At the distant screen, these secondary wavelets superpose giving a rippled irradiance distribution, which is referred to as the single-slit diffraction pattern (Figure 22.2b). The irradiance in the pattern has a central maximum at P_0, and then falls to zero (the first minimum). Past the first minimum, the irradiance rises to a relatively small second maximum before again dropping to zero (the second minimum). The rippling continues with each maximum having less magnitude than the previous maximum.

According to Huygens' principle, each point on the screen receives secondary wavelets from each point on

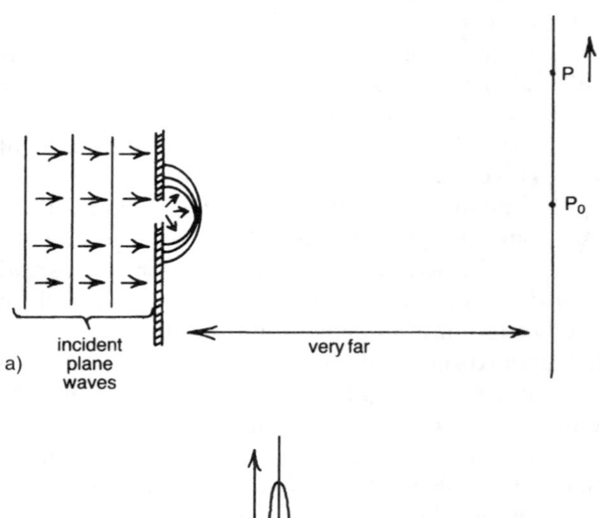

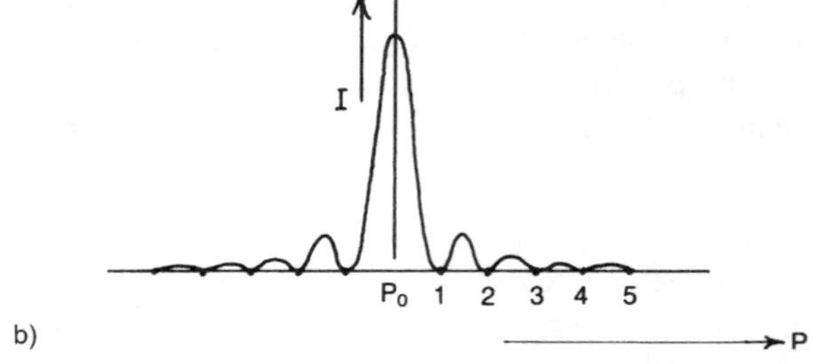

Figure 22.2 a, Single-slit diffraction; b, irradiance in single-slit diffraction pattern.

the wavefront in the slit. The resultant displacement is the sum of the displacements of the secondary wavelets. In the limit of a distant screen, the central point becomes equidistant from each point on the slit's cross section so that all the secondary wavelets arrive in phase, and the resulting constructive interference gives the large central maximum I_0. The other points on the screen are not equidistant from each point on the slit; therefore, the secondary wavelets arriving at these points are not all in phase, so the resultant displacement is smaller than that of the central maximum.

Figure 22.3 shows a view of the geometry for the irradiance at the point P on the distant screen (where P subtends an angle θ with the axis). For a distant screen the points on the line AC are equidistant from P. Therefore, the relative phase distribution of the wave along AC is identical to the relative phase distribution of the wavelets arriving at P. Figure 22.4a shows the relative phase distribution along the line AC for the angle θ that gives the first minimum. The first minimum occurs because each upward displacement along AC is matched by a downward displacement of equal magnitude. When these wavelets are superposed, the upward and downward displacements cancel each other and give a zero resultant displacement.

The distribution shown in Figure 22.4a cuts across one complete spatial period of the wave. Consequently, the length of the line segment BC in Figure 22.3 must equal one wavelength, and the first minimum in a single-slit diffraction pattern occurs at

$$BC = \lambda$$

From the triangle ABC,

$$AB \sin\theta = \lambda$$

or

$$d \sin\theta = \lambda \tag{22.1}$$

For angles greater than the first minimum, there is no longer complete destructive interference, and the resulting irradiance increases for awhile. Figure 22.4b shows the distribution along the line BC that results in the first maximum away from the center (at approximately $BC = 3/2\lambda$). Here the downward lobe cancels one of the upward lobes. The first maximum is then due to the remaining upward lobe. Due to the cancellations, the resultant displacement at the first maximum is significantly smaller in magnitude than the central maximum.

Figure 22.4c shows the distribution along the line AC that occurs when BC equals 2λ. Here the two downward lobes cancel the two upward lobes, and the resultant displacement on the distant screen is again zero. This is the second minimum location, and the angular location is given by

$$d \sin\theta = 2\lambda$$

In general, the minimum locations are given by

$$d \sin\theta = m\lambda \quad \text{where} \quad m = 1, 2, 3, \ldots \tag{22.2}$$

The secondary maximums occur approximately halfway between the local minimums.

Note that Eq. 22.2 is an equation for the minimums in a single slit diffraction pattern. The structure of the equation is easy to confuse with Eq. 21.14, which is the equation for the maximums in the double-slit interference pattern. Be careful not to confuse the two situations.

Figure 22.3 Geometry of single-slit diffraction.

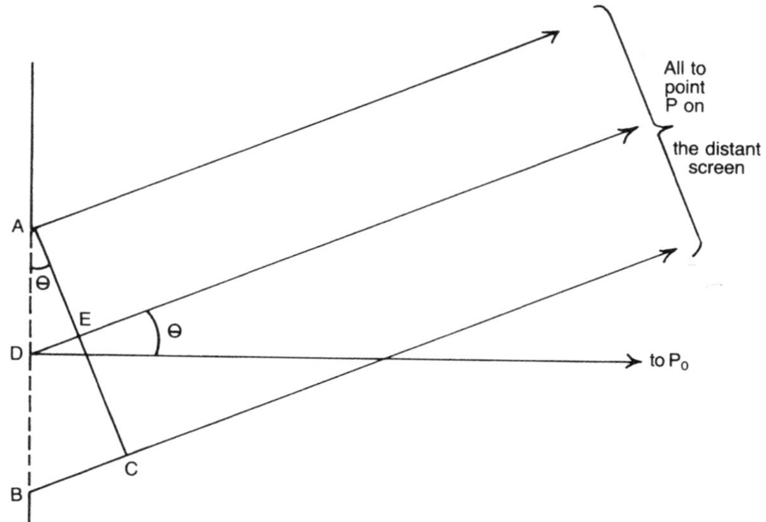

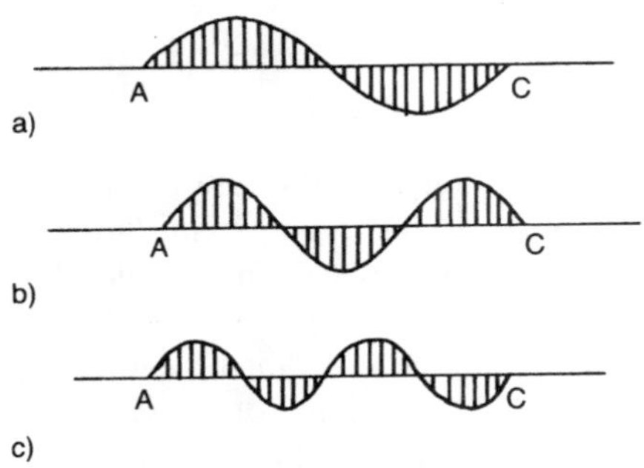

Figure 22.4 Wave displacement (phase distribution) along the line *AC* of the previous figure: a, first minimum; b, next maximum; c, second minimum.

Since most of the irradiance occurs inside the first minimum, we can use Eq. 22.1 to learn about single-slit diffraction. Consider a slit with width d equal to 10 times the wavelength λ. Then from Eq. 22.1,

$$10\lambda \sin\theta = \lambda$$

or

$$\sin\theta = 0.10$$

and

$$\theta = 5.7^\circ$$

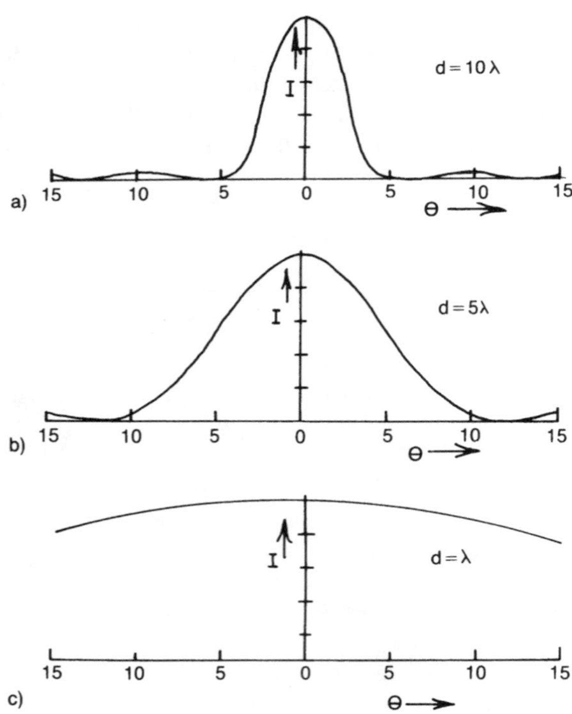

Figure 22.5 Single-slit diffraction irradiances as the slit width varies.

Most of the irradiance is spread out between the center maximum and the 5.7° angular location for the first minimum.

Suppose the slit width is halved (becomes 5 λ). Then the first minimum location is given by

$$5\lambda \sin\theta = \lambda$$

or

$$\theta = 11.5^\circ$$

Decreasing the aperture size from 10λ to 5λ caused the diffraction pattern to spread out about twice as far.

An aperture with a width d equal to one wavelength λ causes the first minimum to fall at 90°. Consequently, no ripples are formed, and a monotonic fall-off in the irradiance occurs. The three cases discussed are shown in Figure 22.5.

EXAMPLE 22.1a

A slit of width 0.5 mm is illuminated with 633 nm red light from a helium–neon laser. What angular location gives the first minimum in the single-slit diffraction pattern on a distant screen? On a screen 10 m from the slit, what is the linear distance between the central maximum and the first minimum?

From Eq. 22.1,

$$(0.5 \times 10^{-3}\,\text{m}) \sin\theta = 633 \times 10^{-9}\,\text{m}$$

or

$$\sin\theta = \frac{6.33 \times 10^{-7}}{5 \times 10^{-4}} = 1.27 \times 10^{-3}$$

From the small angle approximation,

$$\theta = 1.27 \times 10^{-3}\,\text{rad}$$

Alternatively, either from the inverse sine or from the fact that there are 57.30°/rad,

$$\theta = 7.25 \times 10^{-2}\text{degrees},$$

or

$$\theta = 4.35'$$

since there are 60′ per degree.

Here the amount of diffraction is quite small. For a screen 10 m from the slit, the linear location of the first minimum away from the central maximum is

$$y = (10\,\text{m}) \tan\theta$$

From the small angle approximation,

$$y = (10\,\text{m})\theta = (10\,\text{m})(1.27 \times 10^{-3}\,\text{rad})$$
$$= 1.27 \times 10^{-2}\,\text{m} = 1.27\,\text{cm}$$

For a given slit width, the spread in the pattern depends directly on the wavelength λ. In fact for small angles, the spread θ is directly proportional to the wavelength. Hence long wavelengths (the reds) are diffracted or spread more than the short wavelengths (blue or violets).

EXAMPLE 22.1b
For the same slit width, where is the first minimum for 486 nm (blue) light?
From Eq. 22.1,

$$(0.5 \times 10^{-3}\,\text{m}) \sin\theta = 486 \times 10^{-9}\,\text{m}$$
$$\sin\theta = 9.72 \times 10^{-4}$$
$$\theta = 5.57 \times 10^{-2}\,\text{degrees}$$
$$= 3.34'$$

As specified by the location for the first minimum, the blue light is diffracted about 23% less than the red light.

When white light illuminates a single slit, each wavelength is diffracted independently. The result is an irradiance distribution with a white center surrounded by colored fringes. The outer part of the pattern tends to be reddish since the long wavelengths (red) are diffracted the most. You can easily observe a white light single-slit diffraction pattern by looking through the tines of a dinner fork at a match or candle. The room illumination should be dim or dark. Twist the dinner fork about its handle so that the cross-sectional area between the tines decreases. As soon as the cross-sectional area is small enough, the diffraction pattern will be evident. (This is a potential conversation topic for a candle light dinner.)

22.3 DIFFRACTION BY A SQUARE APERTURE

When a single slit is vertical, the waves are diffracted horizontally (Figure 22.6a). When the slit is horizontal, the waves are diffracted vertically (Figure 22.6b).

When a vertical slit is placed against a horizontal slit of the same width, the combination forms a square aperture. To determine the diffraction pattern for the crossed slits (or square aperture), we can first consider the horizontally diffracted waves leaving the vertical slit. Each of the horizontally diffracted waves is associated with one of the maximums in the diffraction pattern for the vertical slit, and the wave amplitude decreases rapidly for the higher order maximums. Each of the horizontally diffracted waves then passes through the horizontal slit and is diffracted vertically. The result is a series of vertical diffraction patterns centered on each of the horizontal maximums (Figure 22.6c).

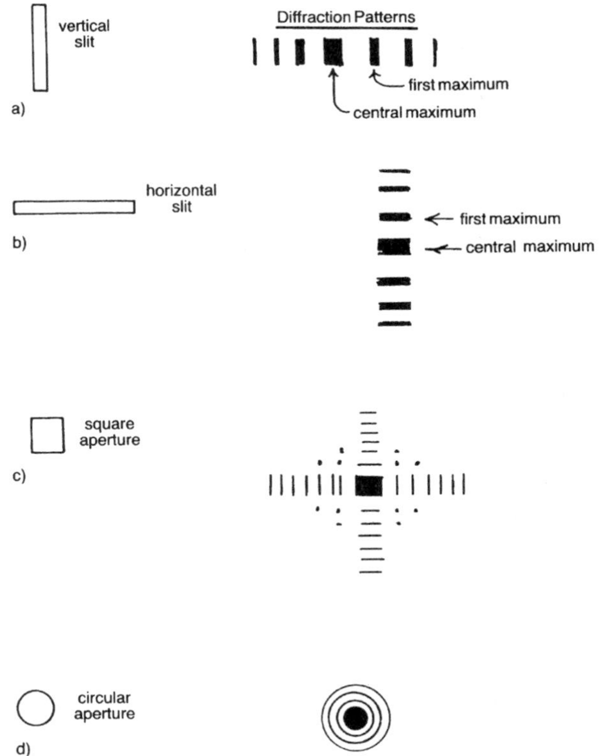

Figure 22.6 Apertures and resulting diffraction patterns: a, vertical slit; b, horizontal slit; c, square aperture; d, circular aperture.

The total pattern for the crossed slits or square aperture is dominated by the maximums along the horizontal and vertical axes. The other local maximums are much fainter due to the amplitude fall-off with increasing order of the diffracted waves.

22.4 DIFFRACTION BY A CIRCULAR APERTURE

When a circular aperture is illuminated by a monochromatic plane wave, the waves are diffracted equally in all directions. The resulting diffraction pattern has a central maximum surrounded by a first minimum, and then by a series of progressively fainter rings (Figure 22.6d). The bright center bounded by the first minimum is known as Airy's disk. (Sir George Airy, 1801–1892, is credited with being the first person to use spherocylindrical lenses to correct astigmatism, and is well known for the Airy integral that occurs in the mathematical theory of the rainbow.) The boundary for Airy's disk is given by the first minimum, which has an angular location of

$$d \sin \theta = 1.22\lambda \tag{22.3}$$

As compared to Eq. 22.1, Eq. 22.3 contains the weird 1.22 number. Perhaps we shouldn't be too surprised at this, because we are already familiar with the weird number π that appears in the equation for the area of a circle. The 1.22 comes from the first zero of the J_1 Bessel function. For those not familiar with Bessel functions, a more intuitive explanation is given in the next section.

Diffraction by a circular aperture behaves as we would expect from single-slit considerations. The smaller the aperture, the larger the diffraction (i.e., Airy's disk is larger as shown by a larger θ in Eq. 22.3). The larger the wavelength the larger the diffraction, so again red is diffracted more than blue.

EXAMPLE 22.2

Plane waves of 500 nm are incident on a circular aperture of diameter 0.4 mm. What is the angular location of the first minimum in the diffraction pattern? What is the diameter of Airy's disk on a screen 6 m behind the aperture?

From Eq. 22.3,

$$(0.4 \times 10^{-3}\,\text{m}) \sin \theta = 1.22(500 \times 10^{-9}\,\text{m})$$
$$= 610 \times 10^{-9}\,\text{m}$$
$$\sin \theta = 1.53 \times 10^{-3}$$

From the small angle approximation,

$$\theta = 1.53 \times 10^{-3}\,\text{rad}$$

Alternatively,

$$\theta = 8.77 \times 10^{-2}\text{degrees} = 5.2'$$

On the screen 6 m away, the linear location x of the first minimum is

$$x = (6\,\text{m}) \tan \theta$$

From the small angle approximation,

$$x = (6\,\text{m})(1.53 \times 10^{-3}\,\text{rad})$$

or

$$x = 9.2 \times 10^{-3}\,\text{m} = 9.2\,\text{mm}$$

The value x is the radius of Airy's disk, so the diameter is 18.4 mm.

You can observe a white light circular diffraction pattern by making a small pinhole in a sheet of aluminum foil. Then stand in a dark or dim room, and look through the pinhole at a small source (e.g., match, candle, a distant light bulb).

22.5 CHANGING FROM A SQUARE TO A CIRCULAR APERTURE

This section provides some intuition about the factor of 1.22 that appears in the Eq. 22.3. The method used is to consider the change in the diffraction patterns as the aperture is smoothly changed from a square aperture of width d to a circular aperture of diameter d.

The series of apertures in Figure 22.7 shows a smooth change from a square aperture to a circular aperture. The n values listed correspond to aperture boundaries specified by

$$[x^n + y^n]^{1/n} = 1$$

The square aperture is the limit for large n values ($n \to \infty$). The circular aperture is given by $n = 2$. As n is decreased to 2, the aperture smoothly changes to circular.

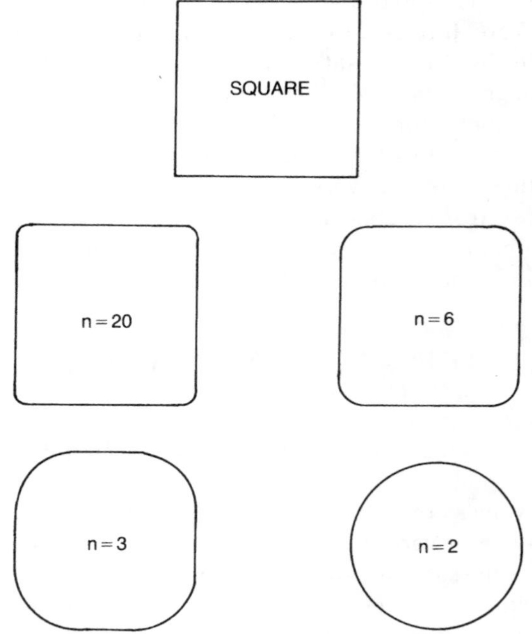

Figure 22.7 Smooth change of a square aperture to a circular aperture.

As the smooth aperture change is made, the corresponding diffraction pattern smoothly changes from that of a square aperture to that of a circular aperture. Figure 22.8 shows the topographical representation of the irradiance distributions in the corresponding diffraction patterns. In each case the solid lines are the minimums, the dots are the local maximums, and the dashed lines are the irradiance values at 50% of the local maximum.

All of the diffraction patterns are dominated by the large central maximum. The minimums in the diffraction pattern for the square aperture are intersecting horizontal and vertical lines, while the minimums in the diffraction pattern for the circular aperture are circles.

We are particularly interested in the first minimum surrounding the central maximum. Because of the intersecting horizontal and vertical lines, the first minimum is not well defined for the square aperture.

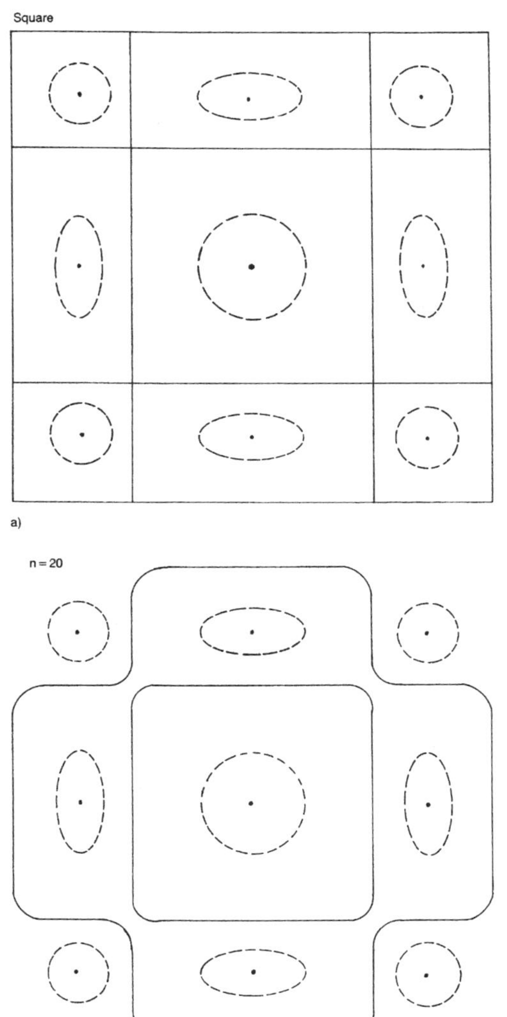

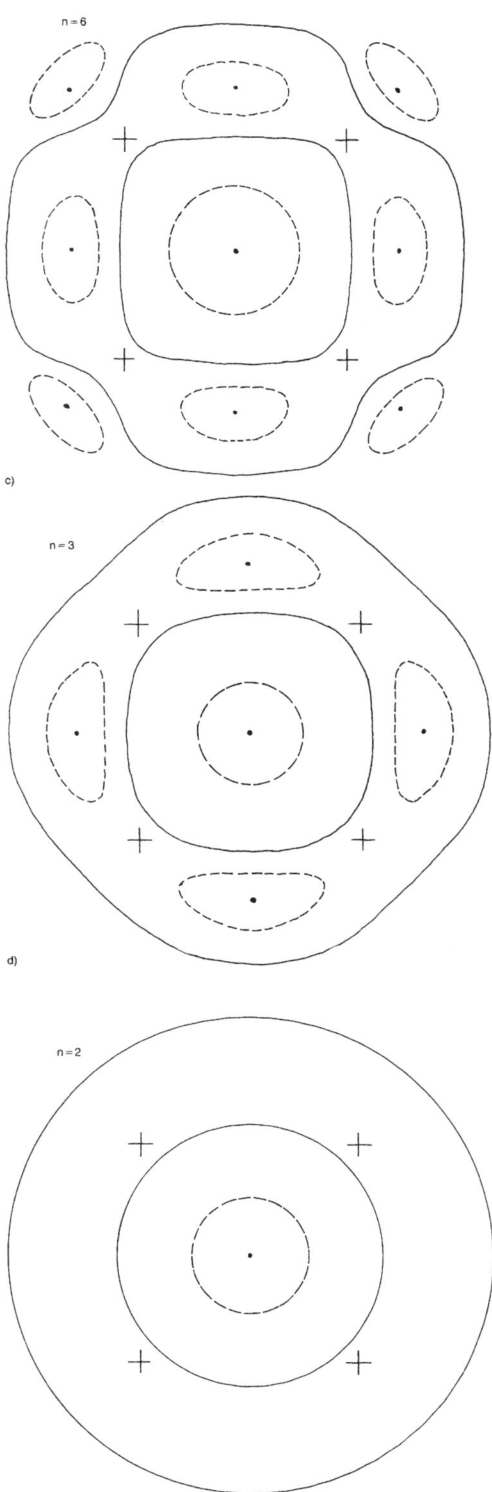

Figure 22.8 Diffraction patterns corresponding to the apertures of Figure 22.7. The four crosses in c, d, and e mark the positions of the horizontal and vertical minimum intersection points in the square aperture diffraction pattern.

The $n = 20$ aperture is basically square except that the corners have been rounded in. A comparison of Figures 22.8a and b shows that the corresponding diffraction patterns are also quite similar. The major change is that while the square pattern had intersecting horizontal and vertical minimums, the $n = 20$ pattern has minimums that do not quite intersect. In particular, there is a clearly defined first minimum that surrounds the central maximum.

It is now easy to visualize how the pattern will change as the apertures are changed from $n = 20$ to $n = 2$. The diffraction pattern will circularize. In particular, each minimum curve will circularize. To follow how this occurs, the four intersection points closest to the central maximum in the square pattern are marked on the $n = 6$ through the $n = 2$ patterns. It is clear from these marks that the first minimum is circularizing by moving in toward the central maximum along the diagonals. On the other hand, the first minimum is moving out along the horizontal and vertical axes (see especially the $n = 3$ to $n = 2$ step). In fact, the total inward movement along the diagonal is approximately equal to the total outward movement along the axes. In other words, the first minimum for the circular aperture lies approximately halfway between the diagonal and axial locations of the first minimum for the square aperture.

In the diffraction pattern for the square aperture, the angular location for the first minimum along either the horizontal or vertical axis (x_0 and y_0 in Figure 22.9) is given by Eq. 22.1. In the small angle approximation, the angular location is λ/d. From the Pythagorean theorem, the distance to the first diagonal minimum q_0 is given by $\sqrt{2}\lambda d$.

Since the first minimum for the circular aperture lies approximately halfway between the axial and diagonal locations, we have

$$(1 + \sqrt{2})/2 \sim 1.21$$

A more exact treatment shows that the 1.21 value is actually 1.22.

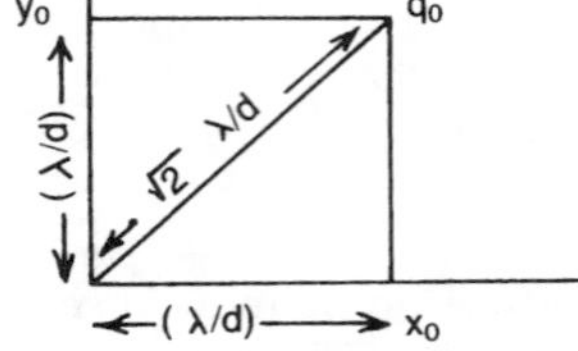

Figure 22.9 Geometry for the diagonal location of the first minimum in the square aperture diffraction pattern.

Here we gained some intuition about the 1.22 that appears in Eq. 22.3 for the first minimum in the circular aperture diffraction pattern. The method was to consider the change in the diffraction patterns as the aperture is smoothly changed from square to circular. The result was that the first minimum moves approximately equal distances in along the diagonals and out along the axes. This consideration alone gives us a factor of 1.21, which is within 1% of the exact 1.22 value.

22.6 FRAUNHOFER VERSUS FRESNEL DIFFRACTION

In each of the obstacles and apertures discussed above, plane waves were incident and the diffraction pattern was viewed on a distant screen (Figure 22.10a). In these cases, we can consider the diffracted waves as plane waves (Figure 22.10b), and we refer to the diffraction as *far field*. Far field diffraction is also known as *Fraunhofer diffraction*. (Joseph von Fraunhofer, 1787–1826, was a major figure in optics and a pioneer in the development of diffraction gratings and their application to the study of optical spectra.)

When the waves incident on the aperture are converging or diverging, or when the distance from the aperture to the observation screen is small, the diffraction is referred to as *near field* or *Fresnel diffraction*. In this case, the curvature of the diffracted waves is important (Figure 22.11a).

One of the differences between Fresnel and Fraunhofer diffraction is that the Fresnel patterns can change significantly as the distance from the aperture is varied. On the other hand, the Fraunhofer patterns are not sensitive to distance changes, and thus, we can

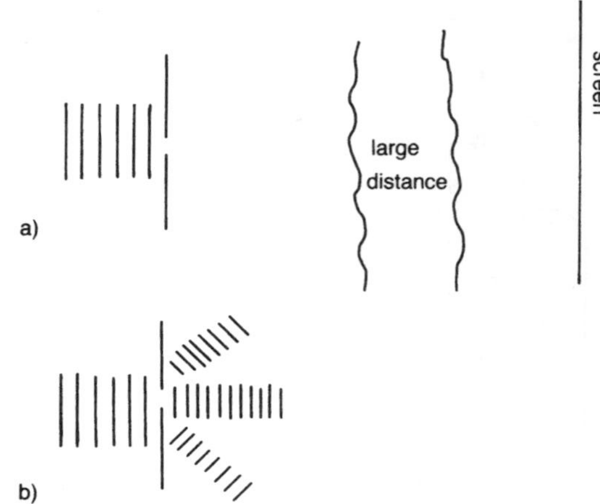

Figure 22.10 a, Geometry for Fraunhofer or far field diffraction; b, plane wave representation for Fraunhofer diffraction.

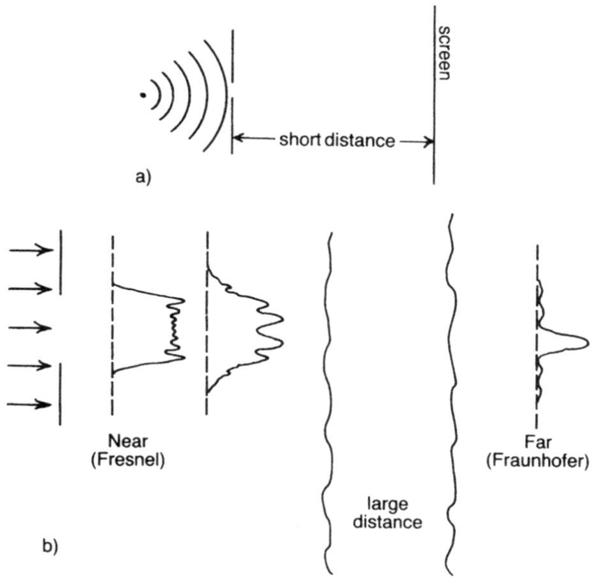

Figure 22.11 a, Geometry for Fresnel or near field diffraction; b, variation of diffraction patterns.

express the Fraunhofer pattern by its angular location as long as the screen is in the far field zone.

Figure 22.11b shows cross sections of a circular aperture with incident plane waves. Immediately behind the aperture, the illumination is exactly as predicted by the law of rectilinear propagation (geometric optics). As the screen is moved away from the aperture, we enter the Fresnel or near field zone. Here the illuminance on the screen starts deviating from that predicted by geometric optics and we start getting the diffraction ripple effects. These ripples give illumination in umbra zones together with decreased illumination in the unobstructed zones. The ripples change character as we move through the Fresnel zone, finally blending into those of the Fraunhofer or far field diffraction zone. Once into the Fraunhofer zone, the ripples no longer change character but maintain the same angular relationship.

Fresnel diffraction can result in some counterintuitive behavior of light. The famous Poisson spot is an example. In 1818, Fresnel had presented his mathematical work on near field diffraction to a committee in Paris. One of the committee members was the very adept mathematician Simeon Poisson. Poisson studied Fresnel's work, and then pointed out that if the work was correct, there should be a maximum (a bright spot) directly in the middle of the umbra region at a specific distance in the near zone behind a circular obstacle. Poisson felt that this prediction was ridiculous and that Fresnel's work was wrong. On hearing Poisson's comments, one of the other committee members, Dominic Arago, set up the experiment and found that the bright spot does exist.

Some people perceive dark floaters in their eyes. These floaters are naively described as shadows cast on the retina by debris, such as blood cells, floating in the vitreous humor. However, these floaters are not geometric optics shadows but rather Fresnel diffraction patterns formed by the debris. (A good way to observe floaters is to look at a uniformly illuminated blank field such as a gray sky.)

Figure 22.12a shows a way to observe Fraunhofer diffraction in situations where space is limited. A lens collimates the light from a near point source. The collimated light (plane waves) passes through the diffracting aperture. The diffracted waves are also plano but have an angular deviation. A second lens is then used to bring the diffracted plane waves to a focus. The Fraunhofer diffraction pattern appears in the image plane of the second lens.

The two lenses and aperture can be combined into one lens with a finite aperture size (Figure 22.12b), in which case the Fraunhofer diffraction pattern appears in place of the geometric optics point image. The geometric optics assumption is that the lens apertures are large and the diffraction spread is small enough that the result is effectively a point image. However, if the lens aperture is small, or if we are interested in very fine detail, then the difference between a point image and the Fraunhofer diffraction pattern becomes important.

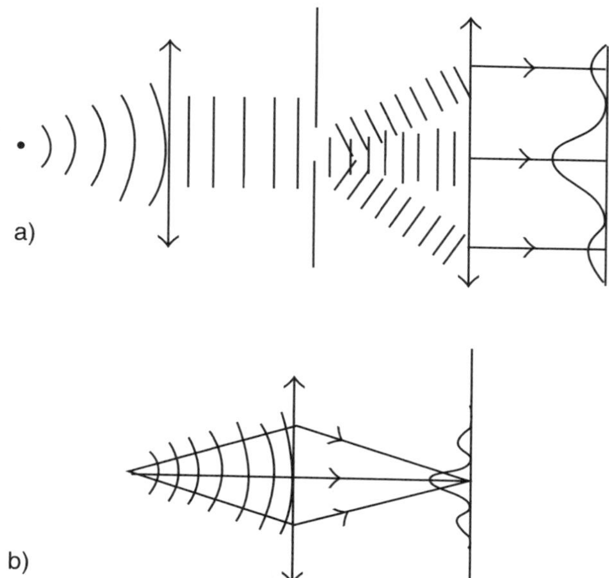

Figure 22.12 a, System to observe Fraunhofer diffraction in a small area; b, Fraunhofer diffraction pattern at the image point.

For a point object, blur due to a misfocus or a refractive error, aberrations, scatter, or diffraction can all spread out the light from a perfect point image. In general, the spread in the light intensity (or illuminance) is referred to as a *point spread function*. When there is no misfocus, no abberations, and no scatter, then there is still a non-zero point spread function due to diffraction.

22.7 DIFFRACTION LIMIT ON RESOLUTION

In the previous section, we saw that an image point is actually a Fraunhofer diffraction pattern. In other words, when the light waves pass through the lens, they suffer some diffraction effects (usually small). Thus, a perfect optical system (correct focus, all aberrations corrected) still does not form a perfect point image. Instead the light is spread out some due to the diffraction. This means that diffraction places a limit on the ability of the system to form good quality images. In other words, diffraction places a limit on the ability of the system to transmit perfect information about the object. Optical systems that are "perfect" (correct focus, aberrations sufficiently corrected) are referred to as *diffraction limited* systems.

The ability of an optical system to resolve two points is one example of the detrimental (or limiting) effects of diffraction. Figure 22.13a shows two point sources (A and B) in front of a lens with a circular aperture. The point sources subtend an angle θ at the nodal point of the lens, and so the geometric image points A' and B' also subtend the angle θ at the nodal point.

Because of the circular aperture, each image point is actually an Airy's disk with its surrounding rings. Airy's disk contains 84% of the intensity, while the rings contain the remaining 16%. For simplicity we will neglect the surrounding rings and just consider Airy's disk.

When the aperture is large, there is little diffraction and Airy's disk is small. In this case, the two illumination patterns are very close to points, and it is easy to tell from the image plane that two points existed in object space. As the aperture size is decreased, the

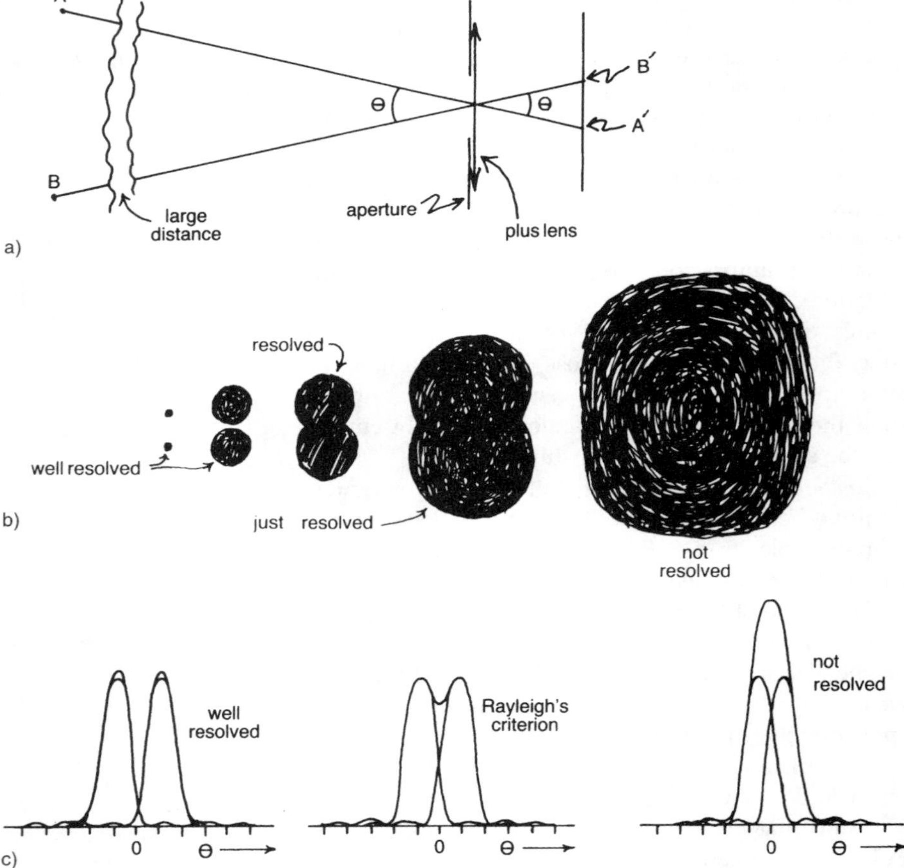

Figure 22.13 Two point resolution: a, geometry; b, diffraction patterns; c, irradiance distributions.

diffraction increases. Now there is a sizable Airy's disk centered on each image point (A' and B'). Initially, A' and B' are far enough apart that the two Airy's disks do not overlap. Hence we can still tell from the image plane that there were two point sources in object space (i.e., we can still resolve the two points).

When the aperture is decreased still further, the diffraction increases and Airy's disks get larger and begin to overlap (Figure 22.13b). An experienced observer looking at the image plane can still tell that there are two point sources in object space. As the process continues (aperture size decreases, diffraction increases), the Airy's disks eventually overlap until they look like one large diffraction pattern. Here even experienced observers (as well as automated photodetection systems) can no longer tell that there were two points in object space. In this case, we say the two points are not resolvable.

There are several criteria for the resolution limit. Rayleigh's criterion is one that is widely used because of its simplicity. (John William Strutt, the Baron Rayleigh, 1824–1919, was very active in optical research.) *Rayleigh's criterion* states that the two point resolution limit occurs when the first minimum (the boundary of Airy's disk) of one diffraction pattern coincides with the center maximum of the other diffraction pattern. When the patterns overlap more than this, the points are not resolvable. When the patterns overlap less than this, the points are resolvable.

Equation 22.3 gives the angular location for the first minimum in the diffraction pattern for a circular aperture. For the resolution limit, the angles are small, and then Rayleigh's criterion states that the just resolvable angle $\theta_{\min}$ is

$$\theta_{\min} = \frac{1.22\lambda}{d} \qquad (22.4)$$

where d is the diameter of the circular aperture (or of the lens rim). Then for two points subtending an angle θ at the lens, there is resolution when $\theta \geq \theta_{\min}$ and no resolution for $\theta < \theta_{\min}$. Figure 22.13c shows intensity plots for an unresolved, just resolved (Rayleigh limit), and resolved situation.

In diffraction-limited systems, the larger apertures give the best resolution. Note, however, that large aperture systems are usually limited by aberrations as opposed to diffraction. The smaller apertures help with the aberrations but make diffraction worse.

EXAMPLE 22.3

Two dots are on a chart 6 m from a pinhole camera with a diameter of 0.5 mm. For light of wavelength 550 nm (the middle of the visible spectrum), how close can the two dots be and still be resolved according to Rayleigh's criterion?

From Eq. 22.4,

$$\theta_{\min} = 1.22(550 \times 10^{-9}\,\text{m})/(0.5 \times 10^{-3}\,\text{m})$$
$$= 1.34 \times 10^{-3}\,\text{rad}$$

From the rays in Figure 22.13a, the separation of the two points is

$$y = (6\,\text{m}) \tan \theta_{\min}$$

From the small angle approximation,

$$y = (6\,\text{m})\theta_{\min}$$
$$= (6\,\text{m})(1.34 \times 10^{-3})$$
$$= 8.04 \times 10^{-3}\,\text{m} = 8.04\,\text{mm}$$

EXAMPLE 22.4

A +5.00 D thin lens has an overall diameter of 3.2 cm. What angular separation gives the resolution limit for two distant point objects emitting light of wavelength 589 nm? Also, how many wavelengths apart are the two image points when just resolvable?

From Eq. 22.4,

$$\theta_{\min} = 1.22(589 \times 10^{-9}\,\text{m})/(3.2 \times 10^{-2}\,\text{m})$$
$$= 2.25 \times 10^{-5}\,\text{rad}$$

From the rays, the separation of the two image points is

$$y = (f_2) \tan \theta_{\min}$$

The secondary focal length f_2 is 20 cm or 0.20 m. Then from the small angle approximation,

$$y = (0.20\,\text{m})\theta_{\min}$$
$$= (0.20\,\text{m})(2.25 \times 10^{-5})$$
$$= 4.50 \times 10^{-6}\,\text{m}$$

The number of wavelengths is $4.50 \times 10^{-6}\,\text{m}/589 \times 10^{-9}\,\text{m}$, or 7.6 wavelengths.

In complicated optical systems, the aperture stop provides the maximum amount of diffraction. The image space effects of this diffraction are figured by using the exit pupil. The object space effects are figured by using the entrance pupil. For a telescope, the object space angle for two point resolution is then easy to find.

EXAMPLE 22.5

A 7× Keplerian telescope has a +2.00 D $f/12.5$ objective lens. What is the angular resolution limit of the telescope for 486 nm light?

The objective lens is the entrance pupil of the telescope. The *f*-number is the focal length divided by the diameter of the lens, so the objective lens diameter is 50 cm/12.5, or 4 cm. Then Eq. 22.4 gives

$$\begin{aligned}\theta_{\min} &= 1.22(486 \times 10^{-9}\,\text{m})/(4 \times 10^{-2}\,\text{m}) \\ &= 1.48 \times 10^{-5}\,\text{rad}\end{aligned}$$

(or 3.06 s).

For a microscope, we want to know the minimum distance s between two resolvable points in the object plane. From Rayleigh's criterion, we can show that the minimum distance s between two resolvable incoherent point sources is given by

$$s = \frac{1.22\lambda}{2\ n \sin i} \tag{22.5}$$

where λ is the vacuum wavelength, $2i$ is the angle subtended by the objective lens at the object plane, and n is the object space index (normally air, but can be oil as in the oil-immersion objective). The term (n sin i) is called the *numerical aperture*, and is printed on microscope objectives together with the relative magnification. Typical microscope objectives have numerical apertures ranging from 0.16 up to 1.25. In special cases, the numerical aperture may get as high as 1.5.

EXAMPLE 22.6

A diffraction-limited 50× microscope objective has a numerical aperture of 1.22. For 600 nm incoherent illuminance, how close can two points be and still be resolved by the microscope?

In this case,

$$s = \frac{1.22(600\,\text{nm})}{2(1.22)} = 300\,\text{nm}$$

In diffraction-limited systems, the resolution ability clearly depends on the wavelength. Long wavelengths (reds) are diffracted the most, while short wavelengths (blues and violets) are diffracted the least. Therefore, resolution is better for the short wavelengths. This is the reason why the ultraviolet microscope has better resolution than the visible light microscope.

Electrons are quantum particles as opposed to electromagnetic radiation. However, all quantum particles propagate according to wave equations and so suffer from diffraction. The electron's wavelength is much less than that of visible light. Thus, the electron microscope has considerably less diffraction and gives resolution that is orders of magnitude better than the ultraviolet or visible light microscopes.

22.8 DIFFRACTION AND ACUITY

At large pupil sizes, the human eye does not form a perfect point image due to aberrations. However, at smaller pupil sizes (2.4 mm) or less, the human eye appears to be a diffraction-limited system. We can use a simple thin lens and screen model of the human eye to investigate the effects of diffraction on visual acuity.

The most familiar acuity system is Snellen acuity (20/20, 20/40, 20/60, etc.). When expressed as a decimal, Snellen acuity is equal to the reciprocal of the minimum resolvable angular detail expressed in minutes, for example, 20/40 = 0.5, which has a reciprocal of 2. Therefore, the smallest letters that a person with 20/40 acuity can resolve have detail that subtends an angle of 2′. The 20/20 letters have detail that subtends an angle of 1′, and 20/60 letters have detail that subtends an angle of 3′.

Snellen acuity is considerably more complicated than two point resolution. Nevertheless, we can gain intuition by using Rayleigh's criterion to estimate Snellen acuity. Consider a thin lens and screen model of the human eye with a 3 mm pupil size. According to Rayleigh's criterion, what is the expected visual acuity for the middle of the visible spectrum (555 nm)?

From Eq. 22.4, the smallest resolvable angle is

$$\begin{aligned}\theta_{\min} &= 1.22(555 \times 10^{-9}\,\text{m})/(3 \times 10^{-3}\,\text{m}) \\ &= 2.26 \times 10^{-4}\,\text{rad}\end{aligned}$$

We can convert to minutes by multiplying by 57.30°/rad and then by 60′/degree, which gives

$$\theta_{\min} = 0.78'$$

Then,

$$1/0.78' = 1.29 = \text{Snellen acuity}$$

or

$$1.29 = 20/x$$

and

$$x = 20/1.29 = 15.5$$

So the predicted Snellen acuity is essentially 20/15, which is about what we would expect.

The pinhole is used clinically to see if poor acuity is due to optical causes (blur) or pathological causes (e.g., senile macular degeneration). If the poor acuity is due to blur (misfocus), then the pinhole effect minimizes the blur and increases the acuity. If the poor acuity is not due to optical blur, then in theory the pinhole gives no improvement in acuity. In reality, the pinhole test works better for some conditions than it does for others.

What happens when an emmetrope with good acuity looks through a pinhole? Here the pinhole introduces diffraction, and the person's acuity may actually decrease through the pinhole. Again, we can use a thin lens and screen model to predict the acuity through a pinhole.

EXAMPLE 22.7

Based on Rayleigh's criterion, what is the expected visual acuity through a pinhole with a 1.5 mm diameter?

Let us use the middle of the visible spectrum or the wavelength (555 nm). From Eq. 22.4, the smallest resolvable angle is

$$\theta_{\min} = 1.22(555 \times 10^{-9}\text{ m})/(1.5 \times 10^{-3}\text{ m}) = 4.51 \times 10^{-4}\text{ rad}$$

We can convert to minutes by multiplying by 57.30°/rad and then by 60′/degree, which gives

$$\theta_{\min} = 1.55'$$

Then,

$$1/1.55' = 0.64 = \text{Snellen acuity}$$

or

$$0.64 = 20/x$$

and

$$x = 31.0$$

So in this case, the expected visual acuity through the pinhole is about 20/30.

According to this example, a person with 20/20 acuity would lose acuity when looking through the 1.5 mm pinhole. A person with about 20/30 acuity would show no change when looking through the pinhole. A person with 20/250 acuity due to optical blur would gain acuity (something between 20/250 and 20/30) when using the pinhole.

Raleigh's criterion is a simple rule of thumb for the diffraction limited two point resolution limit. It works very well for resolution of stars. For extended objects that are more complicated than two points, many optical systems do somewhat better than Raleigh's criterion. In fact, for small aperture sizes the human eye tends to do better than Raleigh's criterion. (Further discussion of imaging limits for extended objects occurs in Chapter 25 under modulation transfer functions.)

22.9 DIFFRACTION HALOS

Consider a random array of many small circular apertures. If this array is illuminated by plane waves from a white point source, each aperture will generate an Airy type diffraction pattern. When the apertures are small and close together, the diffraction patterns are large and overlap. The overlapping diffraction patterns produce a readily visible halo—namely, a central white disk surrounded by circular colored rings (red outermost, blue or violet innermost).

Similar halos occur when the diffraction is due to a random array of circular obstacles. The obstacles do not even have to be opaque. Suspended water ($n = 1.33$) droplets in air ($n = 1.00$) can give diffraction halos. When observed through a light cloud cover around the sun or moon, these diffraction halos are referred to as coronas. The diffraction halos are easy to distinguish from ice crystal halos. Ice crystal halos are due to refraction and dispersion by the ice crystals; they have red on the inside of the rings, whereas diffraction halos have red on the outside of the rings.

The sometimes brilliant halos seen through fogged up car windows are diffraction halos. You can easily see such halos by breathing on the side of a clear glass, and then looking through the fogged area at a small source (e.g., match, penlight, or distant bulb).

When the cornea swells (becomes edematous), small droplets of fluid form randomly between the stromal fibers. These random droplets produce a diffraction halo that the person sees when looking at lights. Such halos are one of the warning signs of high ocular pressures produced by uncontrolled glaucoma. These halos can also be produced by epithelial damage due to poorly fitting contact lenses.

22.10 APODIZED CIRCULAR APERTURE

Sections 22.4, 22.7, and 22.8 considered diffraction by a clear circular aperture. The resulting Fraunhofer diffraction pattern consisted of Airy's disk and its surrounding rings.

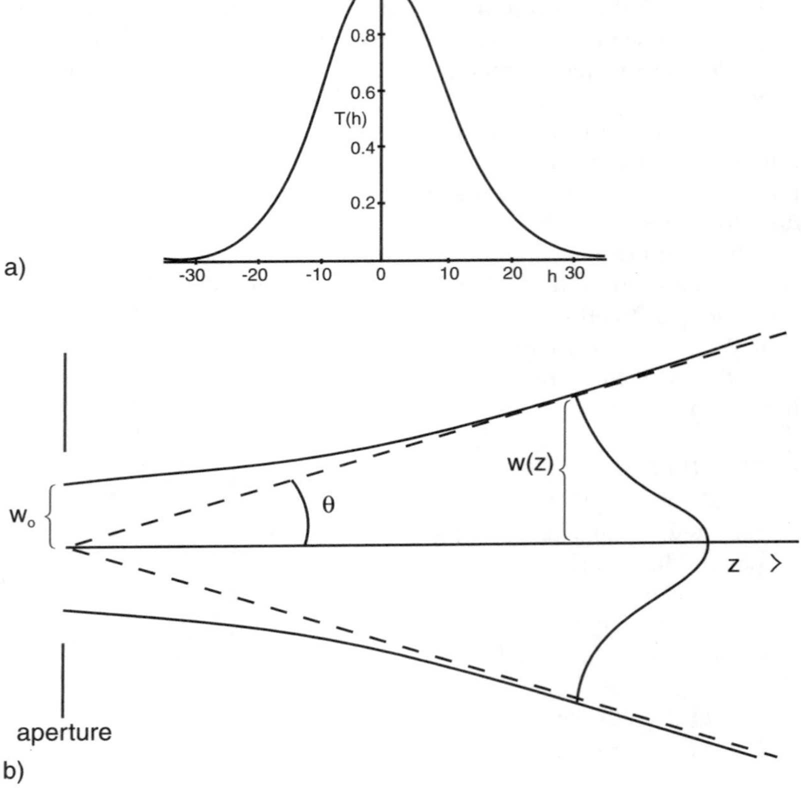

Figure 22.14 a, Gaussian intensity transmission function of a gradient filter placed over a circular aperture; b, side view of the Gaussian diffracted wave. The solid curves are hyperbolic and represent the Gaussian semidiameter parameter $w(z)$ as a function of the distance z from the aperture. Each asymptote forms the angle θ with the axis.

Let the z-axis be a line that is perpendicular to the circular aperture and passes through its center. Now consider plane waves traveling along the z-axis incident on a circular aperture with a centered circularly symmetric gradient filter placed over it. Let $z = 0$ be the location of the filtered aperture, and let $T(h)$ be the intensity transmission function of the filter as a function of the radial distance h away from the z-axis. For example, when the filter has a value of $T(h) = 0.25$ for a particular h, then the filter transmits 25% of the intensity at that position.

Since the intensity is proportional to the square of the amplitude, the wave amplitude transmission function $t(h)$ equals $\sqrt{T(h)}$. For the wave leaving the filtered aperture, the amplitude of the various secondary spherical wavelets varies like $t(h)$. In the use of the Huygens–Fresnel principle, we need to take this amplitude variation into account when adding the secondary wavelets together to get the resultant diffracted wave.

There could be many different transmission functions. A rather special situation occurs when the gradient filter has the Gaussian transmission function

$$T(h) = e^{-2h^2/w_o^2} \tag{22.6}$$

where the semidiameter of the circular aperture is significantly larger than the distance w_o. A Gaussian gradient filter of this type has $T(0) = 1$, so the transmission is 100% at the center. Similarly $T(w_o) = e^{-2} = (2.718)^{-2} = 0.135$, so that the transmission has dropped to 13.5% at a distance of $h = w_o$ from the center. In Eq. 22.6, h and w_o must be in the same units (e.g., both μm, or both mm, etc.). Figure 22.14a shows a plot of the intensity transmission function $T(h)$ for $w_o = 20\,\mu m$.

For a Gaussian filter, the amplitude transmission function becomes

$$t(h) = \sqrt{T(h)} = e^{-h^2/w_o^2} \tag{22.7}$$

For plane waves incident on the Gaussian filtered aperture, the diffracted wave (given by the Huygens–Fresnel principle) at a distance z along the axis has an amplitude distribution $A(h)$ that is also Gaussian with

$$A(h) \propto e^{-h^2/w^2(z)} \tag{22.8}$$

where,

$$w(z) = w_o\sqrt{1 + \left(\frac{\lambda z}{\pi w_o^2}\right)^2} \tag{22.9}$$

It follows from Eq. 22.8 that the amplitude distribution is a maximum on the axis ($h = 0$), and falls to $1/e$ of its maximum value at the perpendicular distance $h = w(z)$ from the axis. It is convenient to use the value $w(z)$ as a representative measure of the semidiameter width of the diffracted wave. For a fixed wavelength λ, the plot of $w(z)$ versus z in Figure 22.14b (solid curves) shows the spread of the wave as it leaves the aperture. At the aperture ($z = 0$), Eq. 22.9 shows that $w(z) = w_o$. As the wave propagates down the z axis, it spreads out (diffracts) according to Eq. 22.9.

By squaring both sides of Eq. 22.9, it is easy to show that $w(z)$ plotted as a function of z is hyperbolic. For distances far away from the aperture, the hyperbolas are asymptotic to straight lines that make an angle θ with the axis. For a large distance z, the small angle approximation for the tangent results in

$$\theta = \tan\theta = \frac{w(z)}{z}$$

When z is large in Eq. 22.9, the 1 under the square root is insignificant and can be dropped. Then taking the square root and substituting the result into the above equations leads to

$$\theta = \frac{\lambda}{\pi w_o} \qquad (22.10)$$

The parameter w_o directly relates to the effective size of the filtered aperture. When w_o is small, the diffracted angle θ is large (as we would expect), and vice versa. Equation 22.10 also shows that the diffracted angle θ depends directly on the wavelength (which is also what we would expect).

In a plane perpendicular to the optical axis at a distance z from the aperture with the Gaussian filter, the diffracted amplitude distribution results in a Gaussian intensity distribution given by

$$I(h) \propto [A(h)]^2 \propto e^{-2h^2/w^2(z)}$$

The intensity is a maximum on the axis ($h = 0$), drops to $1/e^2$ of its maximum value at $h = w(z)$, and then continues to smoothly fall off. In other words, there are no rings in the diffraction pattern from the Gaussian filter, only a smooth illumination fall-off. For a clear circular aperture, Airy's disk contains 84% of the intensity (light) in the diffraction pattern. In the Gaussian diffraction pattern, 86% of the intensity is inside the circle described by $h = w(z)$.

EXAMPLE 22.8

For 633 nm plane waves incident on a clear circular aperture with a 60 µm diameter (i.e., 30 µm semidiameter), Eq. 22.3 gives 0.74° as the angular boundary of Airy's disk, and on a screen 6 m from the aperture the semidiameter of Airy's disk is then 7.72 cm. When a Gaussian transmittance function with a 20-µm semidiameter size parameter w_o (Figure 22.14a) is placed over this aperture, what is the shape and size of the diffraction pattern on a screen 6 m from the aperture. Also, what is the diffraction angle θ?

Here $w_o = 20$ µm, and the intensity distribution in the diffraction pattern is Gaussian with a size parameter $w(z)$ at a distance z from the filtered aperture. For $z = 6$ m, Eq. 22.9 gives

$$w(z) = (20 \times 10^{-6}\,\text{m})\left[1 + \left(\frac{(633 \times 10^{-9}\,\text{m})6\,\text{m}}{\pi(20 \times 10^{-6}\,\text{m})^2}\right)^2\right]^{1/2}$$
$$= (20 \times 10^{-6}\,\text{m})[9.13 \times 10^6]^{1/2}$$
$$= (6.04 \times 10^{-2}\,\text{m}) = 6.04\,\text{cm}$$

The semidiameter parameter $w(z)$ of the Gaussian diffraction pattern is 6.04 cm. That is, 86% of the intensity is within a circle with a 6.04-cm semidiameter (or a circle with a 12.08 cm diameter).

From Eq. 22.10,

$$\theta = \frac{633 \times 10^{-9}\,\text{m}}{\pi(20 \times 10^{-6}\,\text{m})}$$

or

$$\theta = 1.01 \times 10^{-2}\,\text{rad} = 0.58°$$

The above example shows that on a screen 6 m from the aperture, the Gaussian filter concentrated 86% of the intensity into a circle of semidiameter 6.04 cm, while the semidiameter of Airy's disk, which encloses 84% of the intensity, for the clear aperture was 7.72 cm. Thus the Gaussian filter gives less diffraction spread than the clear aperture. (However the Gaussian filtered aperture transmits less than half of the light intensity transmitted by the clear circular aperture.)

Since the diffraction pattern from the Gaussian filtered aperture is smaller than that of the clear circular aperture, the resolution limit may be better with the filtered aperture (assuming enough incident light). The process of using a filtered aperture to suppress or remove the rings around the central maximum and concentrate the light more into the center of the diffraction pattern is referred to as *apodization* (''a'' = no, ''pod'' = feet, so "no feet" or by analogy "no rings").

It turns out that many diffraction limited lasers emit a coherent Gaussian shaped beam. As discussed in Section 24.8, the equations in this section also apply to the propagation of the Gaussian laser beams.

22.11 DIFFRACTION GRATINGS

Interference is clearly present in the phenomenon of diffraction. In fact, the distinction between the two is sometimes murky. We did not worry about diffraction in our initial discussion of the double-slit experiment because the width of each slit was so small that the first diffraction minimums were very far out (Figure 22.15a). When the slit width is larger, the diffraction minimums are closer to the central maximum. Figure 22.15b shows the right half of a single-slit diffraction pattern for this case. For this slit width, the double-slit interference maximums are modulated by the single-slit diffraction pattern (Figure 22.15c, where the two patterns are superposed). The double-slit separation is the same for Figures 22.15a and c; only the slit width is different. Note that the single-slit minimums can actually wipe out some of the double-slit maximums (the "missing" orders).

Let us keep each slit width very narrow, and consider the effect of adding more slits. Initially we have the double-slit pattern in which all the interference maximums have essentially the same irradiance (Figure 22.16a). What changes occur in the pattern when a third slit (at the same spacing) is added?

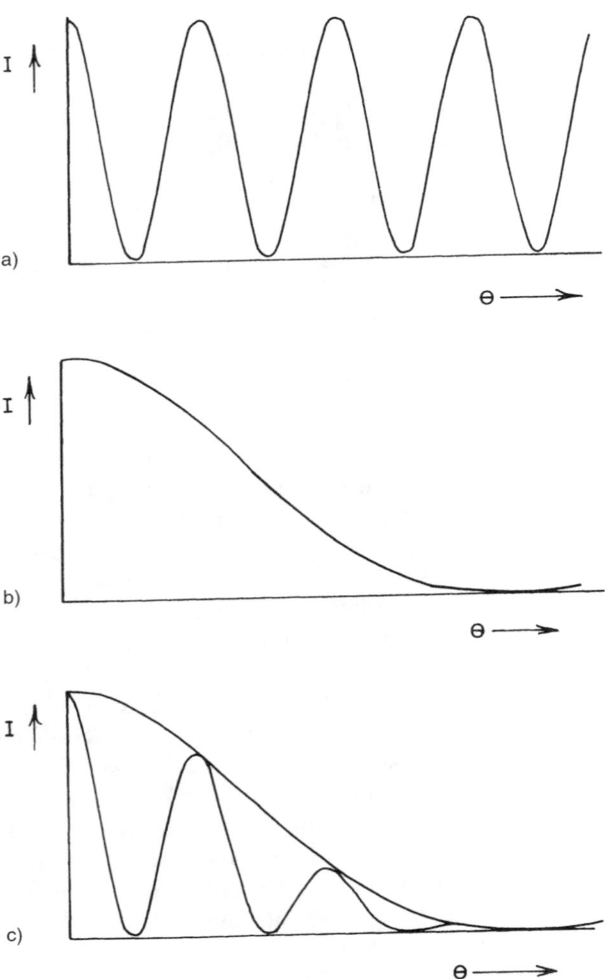

Figure 22.15 a, Double-slit interference pattern for narrow widths; b, single-slit diffraction pattern for wider slit; c, double-slit interference pattern for wider slits.

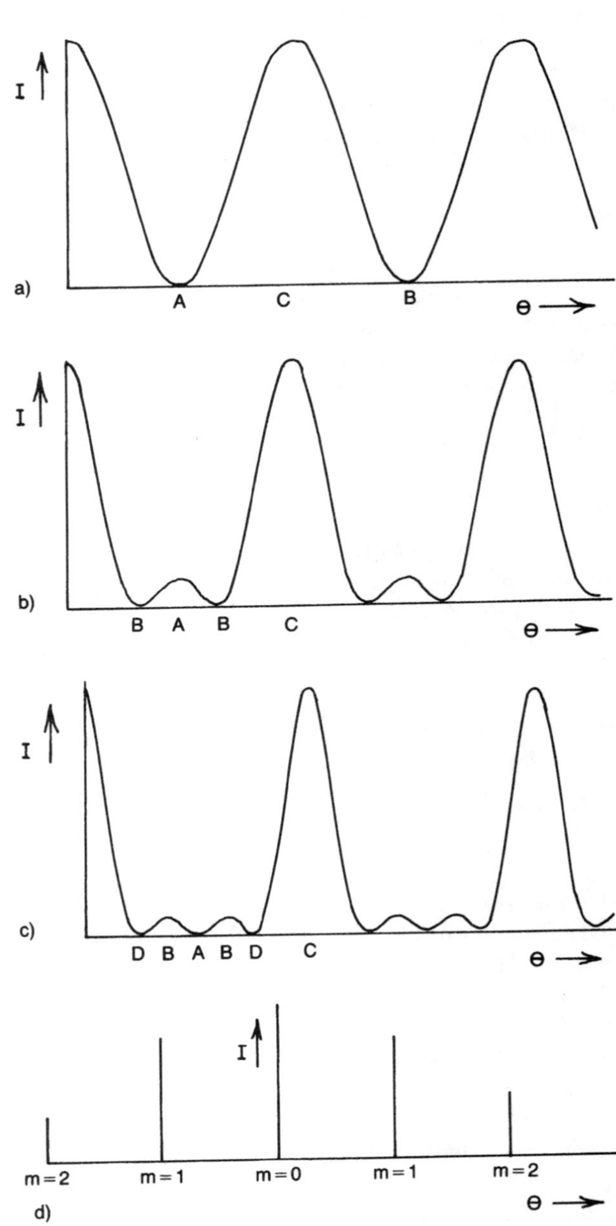

Figure 22.16 Interference patterns for the same slit spacing: a, two slits; b, three slits; c, four slits; d, many slits (a diffraction grating).

The minimums will certainly be affected. For the double-slit case, the minimums result when the two waves destructively interfere. Consider a double-slit minimum at position A. With three slits, three waves are incident on A. Two of these waves still destructively interfere, leaving the third wave to produce some irradiance at A. On either side of A, there are positions B where the resultant displacement of the three waves is zero (the three waves give destructive interference). At the double-slit maximum positions C, the two waves arrive in phase. When the third slit is added (at the same spacing), it produces a third wave that arrives in phase with the other two. Therefore, the maximum positions remain at C. The net effect is that the main maximums still occur at the same positions, but now there is a little bump in the irradiance between each main maximum (the relative irradiance distribution is shown in Figure 22.16b).

Suppose we now go to four slits (at the same spacing). The fourth wave will arrive in phase at C, so the location of the major maximums is unchanged. However, the minimums are again affected. The three-slit minimums occurred at B where the three incoming waves resulted in complete destructive interference. At B, the fourth wave now gives some irradiance. On either side of B, there are positions D where the superposition of the four waves gives a zero resultant displacement (destructive interference).

Consider position A, which is halfway between the major maximums. For the three slits, A was the center of the little bump; while for two slits, A was a minimum. For four slits, A is again a minimum because each pair of two waves gives destructive interference (i.e., the four waves pair off two by two). For four slits, the result is two little bumps between each major maximum (Figure 22.16c).

Because of the little bumps, the irradiance spread around each major maximum gets narrower as the number of slits increases, i.e., in the two-slit case, the irradiance falls off slowly around a major maximum, while in the four-slit case, the irradiance falls off much quicker.

In general, j equally spaced slits produce major maximums at the same angular θ positions as the double-slit maximums:

$$h \sin \theta = m\lambda \quad m = 0, 1, 2, 3, \ldots \tag{22.11}$$

where h is the distance between slits. As j is increased, each major maximum becomes narrower and narrower. Between each major maximum are $j-2$ little bumps in the irradiance. However, the maximum irradiance in each little bump gets smaller and smaller as j increases. For a very large number of slits, the irradiance of the little bumps becomes negligible, and all the light is channeled into very narrow major maximums. A diffraction grating consists of many slits with a very small slit separation. Figure 22.16d shows the zero, first, and second order maximums for monochromatic light incident on a diffraction grating. As in Figure 22.16c, the irradiance at each of the maximums is modulated by the single slit diffraction pattern.

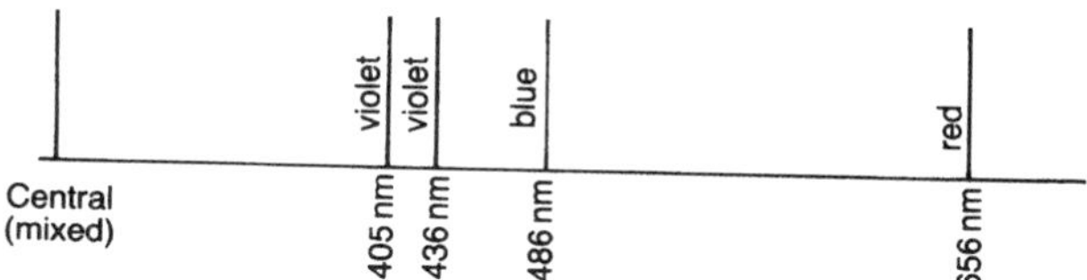

Figure 22.17 Line spectra from a hydrogen gas discharge tube showing the central and the first order maximums that are right of center.

For the zero order maximum, there is no angular separation of incident wavefronts. However, for the first and higher order maximums ($m \geq 1$), the maximum locations are wavelength-dependent. In particular the longer wavelength maximums are out farther than the shorter wavelength maximums. Since the maximums are very narrow, diffraction gratings become a fantastic tool for analyzing the spectrum of wavelengths present in a source.

A low pressure hydrogen gas discharge tube emits only certain specific wavelengths. A diffraction grating can be used to resolve the wavelengths emitted. Figure 22.17 shows the central and first order visible maximums that are to the right of the center. Besides the F (486 nm) and C wavelengths (656 nm), hydrogen also emits two violet wavelengths in the visible spectrum.

For double slits, the irradiance of the interference maximums depended on the relationship between the slit separation and the coherence of the incident light. The coherence must be high for the larger slit separations. For smaller slit separations, the coherence can be lower. For a diffraction grating (many slits), the slit separation is automatically very small, so that the coherence requirements are not particularly high. Hence, the maximums from the diffraction grating can be seen with ordinary extended light sources. Perhaps that is why it is called a diffraction grating as opposed to an interference grating.

One way to make a diffraction grating is use a diamond point to edge (or rule) the slits on a piece of glass. The slits can also be made with a prism shape, which then channels the light away from the central maximum into one or more higher order maximums. These gratings are called *blazed gratings*. The slits can also be made in a reflective material, and these work as diffraction gratings in reflected light.

22.12 SIMPLE OBSERVATIONS

You can easily observe diffraction grating effects. At night, look through a window or door screen at a distant car, street, or porch light. The screen acts like a pair of perpendicularly crossed diffraction gratings, and the light appears to streak out in a cross-shaped pattern. (Recall the discussion of diffraction by a square aperture.) The spacing of the screen may not be fine enough to resolve the colors in the source's spectrum. You can do even better by looking through a pair of sheer curtains at the same light. The threads in the curtains are closer together than those of the screen.

Many feathers are natural diffraction gratings and give very nice spectrums. The fine track spacings on compact disks (CDs) act as a diffraction grating and give diffraction grating colors (spectra) in the reflected light.

Panty hose give brilliant diffraction halos due to the randomly occurring orientation of the threads. (These act like many different crossed diffraction gratings.) Silk gives similar results. (In fact, the colors produced by silk were the motivation for David Rittenhouse's invention of the first diffraction grating in 1785. Later, in 1816 Joseph Fraunhofer independently invented the diffraction grating and made it famous with a series of spectral experiments.)

In the crystalline lens of the human eye, radial lens fibers form a randomly oriented diffraction grating known as Rabl's laminae on the periphery of the lens. In a normal eye, Rabl's laminae give a dim halo called the physiologic halo. Note this halo is different from the pathologic halos due to corneal swelling. You can see the physiologic halo by looking at a bright relatively small source at night. You might stand on a sidewalk, and use the lights of a car coming down the street. (When viewing through a stenopeic slit, only part of the physiologic halo is visible, whereas all of a pathologic halo from the cornea is visible.) The radial diffraction grating properties of the crystalline lens also give the radial streaks that people see when looking at a star or other bright small light source. These streaks are referred to as the ciliary corona.

22.13 IRIDESCENCE IN NATURE

Diffraction grating effects are surprisingly common in nature. The iridescent green on the neck of a male mallard duck is due to the diffraction grating effect of the feathers. Similar natural diffraction gratings give the iridescent blue wings of the Morpho butterflies, and even the beautiful colors of the eye of the peacock's feathers. The metallic-like sheen from a number of beetles is due to the diffraction grating structure of their shells. The metallic green reflection from a cat's eye at night is due to a layered structure in the cat's retina (a reflection grating).

Diffraction gratings give maximums at specific angles that depend on the wavelengths. Therefore, a clue to diffraction grating colors in nature are the saturation of the colors (i.e., fairly monochromatic) and a dependence of the observed color with viewing angle.

The gemstone opal is another example of a natural diffraction grating. Opal actually has a series of randomly oriented gratings. The fire or play of color in the opal comes from the diffraction grating maximums. Shells containing layers of calcium carbonate also give a diffraction grating effect. Examples are pearls and mother-of-pearl. The silvery pearl-like appearance of some fish scales (e.g., the belly scales of herring) come from plate-like crystals that lie in the scale and produce a diffraction grating effect.

22.14 SINUSOIDAL AMPLITUDE GRATING

The diffraction grating discussed in Section 22.11 is sometimes called a *square wave grating* with a spacing of h between each slit (or there are $f = 1/h$ slits per unit length). Let $T(x)$ be the transmission function for the intensity. Then $t(x) = \sqrt{T(x)}$ is the decimal expression for the transmission of the amplitude of the wave. The opaque bars of the square wave grating block all of the light, so $t(x) = 0$, and all of the light is transmitted at each opening, so $t(x) = 1$. The dashed lines in Figure 22.18a shows a plot of $t(x)$ for the square wave grating. The diffraction pattern for the square wave grating consists of the central maximum plus a pair of first order maximums ($m = 1$ in Eq. 22.5), a pair of second order maximums ($m = 2$), etc. Figure 22.18b shows the angular dependence of the zero to third order maximums.

There are gratings that have a variation in the transmission function across the grating. One such grating is the so-called *sinusoidal amplitude grating* in which the transmission is described by

$$t(x) = \left[\frac{1}{2} + \frac{1}{2}\cos(2\pi f x)\right] \tag{22.12}$$

where f is the cycles per unit length (i.e., $h = 1/f$ is the length between cycles). The solid curve in Figure 22.18a shows $t(x)$ for the sinusoidal grating. For monochromatic plane waves from a distant point source incident on the grating, the secondary wavelets

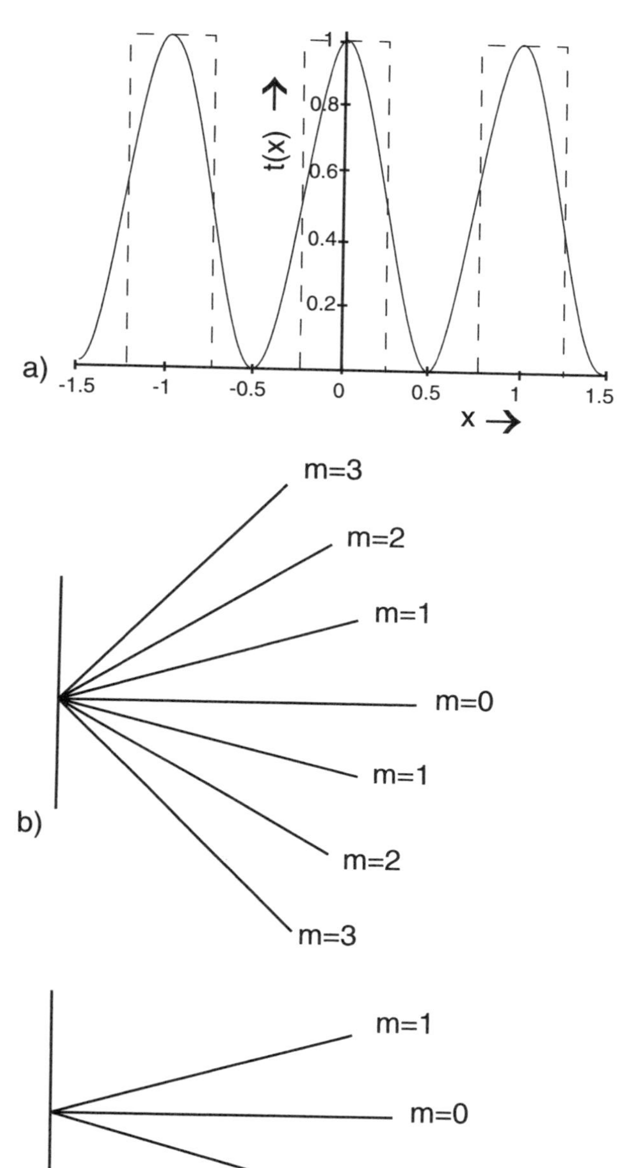

Figure 22.18 a, The dashed lines are the amplitude transmission function for a square wave diffraction grating. The solid curve is for a sinusoidal amplitude transmission function; b, side view of a square wave grating, which results in zero ($m=0$), first ($m=1$), and second ($m=2$), and higher order diffracted waves; c, side view of a sinusoidal grating, which results in only zero ($m=0$) and first order ($m=1$) diffracted waves.

leaving the sinusoidal amplitude grating have different amplitudes due to $t(x)$. When these secondary wavelets superpose to give the diffraction pattern, it consists only of the central maximum and one pair of first maximums on either side of the central maximum, where the angular location of the first order maximums is given by

$$h \sin\theta = \lambda$$

Unlike the square wave diffraction grating, there are no higher order maximums (Figure 22.18c).

22.15 ZONE PLATES

Consider monochromatic plane waves incident on a diffraction grating made of circular "slits." Because of the circular symmetry, the diffracted waves also have circular symmetry, and are either diffracted inward or diffracted outward. The most startling phenomenon is that a sequence of zones can be found for which the inward diffracted waves are spherical in nature. Such a grating is called a *zone plate* (Figure 22.19). The inward spherical diffracted waves from a zone plate can form a "point" image. In other words, the diffraction maximum for a zone plate is the "point" image. If we can form a point image by diffraction, we can also form an extended image by diffraction. In that sense a zone plate functions like a lens.

Fresnel zone plates were the earliest zone plates made. The transmission across a Fresnel zone plate changes abruptly from 0% to 100% at the zone boundaries (like a square wave grating). For a monochromatic plane wave incident on a Fresnel zone plate, the center order diffracted light goes straight through the zone plate. Then the first order inward diffracted light gives a point image (diffraction maximum) at a distance f_2 from the grating (Figure 22.20). The second order diffracted light is diffracted inward at a larger angle, and it gives a point image (diffraction maximum) at a distance of $f_2/2$ from the grating. Similarly the third order inward diffracted light gives a maximum at $f_2/3$, etc.

Figure 22.21 shows a side view of a zone plate with an object point at A, which is a distance u from the zone plate. The goal is for the zone plate to form a conjugate point "image" at B, which is a distance v from the zone plate. Consider the light that travels through the zone plate at point C, which is a perpendicular distance h_m from the axis. In object space, this

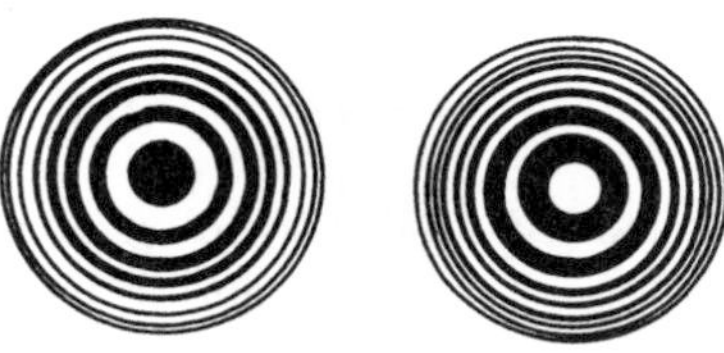

Figure 22.19 Fresnel zone plates.

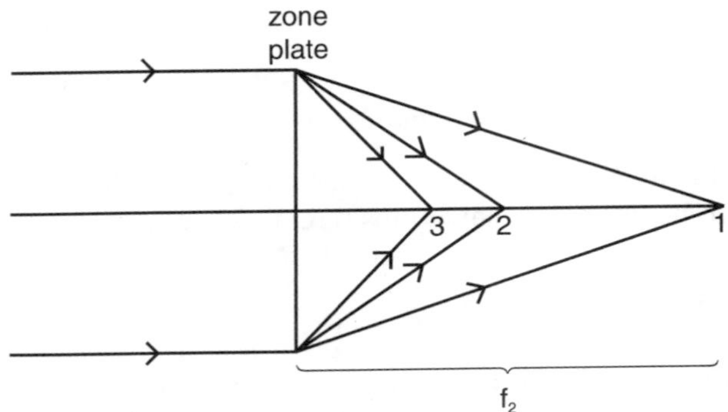

Figure 22.20 Side view of the inward diffracted orders for a Fresnel zone plate. Only the end rays of the diffracted waves are shown. The first order ($m = 1$) diffracted wave forms a maximum (point image) at position 1. The second and third order diffracted waves form respective maximums at positions 2 and 3.

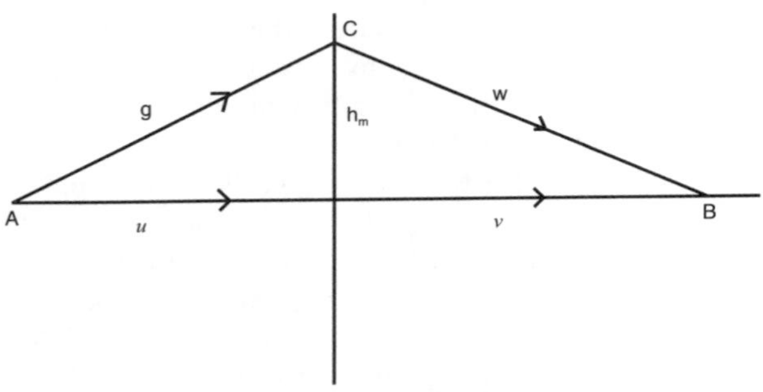

Figure 22.21 Geometry for the Fresnel zones of semidiameter h_m.

wave travels from point A to point C along the diagonal of length g. In "image space," we are considering the part of a secondary spherical wavelet (Huygens' Principle) that travels from point C to point B along the diagonal of length w.

The light wave that travels from A to B through point C has a path length that is equal to the sum of the diagonal distances g and w. The light wave that travels along the axis from point A to point B has a path length equal to the sum $|u| + |v|$. At B, these two waves will be in phase or out of phase with each other depending on the difference in path lengths. Specifically for

$$g + w - (|u| + |v|) = m\frac{\lambda}{2} \quad m = 1, 2, 3, \ldots$$

the diagonal wave will be 180° out of phase with the axial wave for $m = 1, 3, 5$, etc, and in phase with the axial wave for $m = 2, 4, 6, \ldots$ etc. The in phase waves result in constructive interference at B, while the 180° out of phase waves result in destructive interference at B.

When no zone plate is present, there is no particular build-up of light at B because of the mixture of constructive and destructive interference. The idea of the zone plate is to block the waves that contribute the destructive interference by circular opaque rings with the appropriate semidiameters. Then all of the waves arriving at B contribute constructive interference, and we expect a build-up in the light intensity at B (i.e., a diffraction maximum).

We can find an (approximate) equation for the required zone plate semidiameters h_m as follows. From the Pythagorean theorem,

$$g = \sqrt{|u|^2 + |h_m|^2}$$

Then,

$$g = |u|\sqrt{1 + \frac{|h_m|^2}{|u|^2}}$$

In Chapter 7, we used the sagittal approximation to derive the vergence equation $V = P + U$. Here, h_m is usually much smaller than $|u|$, and we can again use the sagittal approximation to obtain

$$g \approx |u|\left(1 + \frac{|h_m|^2}{2|u|^2}\right)$$

Similarly,

$$w = \sqrt{|v|^2 + |h_m|^2}$$

and

$$w \approx |v|\left(1 + \frac{|h_m|^2}{2|v|^2}\right)$$

When we substitute the approximations into the path difference equation, we get

$$|u|\left(1 + \frac{|h_m|^2}{2|u|^2}\right) + |v|\left(1 + \frac{|h_m|^2}{2|v|^2}\right) - (|u| + |v|) = m\frac{\lambda}{2}$$

which results in

$$\frac{h_m^2}{2}\left(\frac{1}{|u|} + \frac{1}{|v|}\right) = m\frac{\lambda}{2}$$

In terms of vergences, this becomes,

$$\frac{h_m^2}{2}(-U + V) = m\frac{\lambda}{2}$$

or

$$h_m^2 P = m\lambda \tag{22.13}$$

where P is the "dioptric power" of the zone plate. Since (in air) the secondary "focal length" f_2 equals the reciprocal of P, it follows that

$$h_m = \sqrt{m\lambda f_2} \tag{22.14}$$

When the zones for $m = 1, 3, 5, \ldots$ are blocked, the resulting zone plate acts like a lens with a focal length f_2 and a dioptric power P. The spacing of the zones gets closer as m gets larger. The zones of 100% transmission are $m = 2, 4, 6$, etc. zones. (Note, some authors number the zones by a full wavelength change instead of a half wavelength change, and then refer to constructive and destructive interference "half" zones.)

EXAMPLE 22.9
For a +2.00 D power (standard Helium d wavelength of 587.56 nm), what are the radii of the first four dark rings in a Fresnel zone plate with a bright center?

Here we need $m = 1, 3, 5$, and 7 respectively. For $m = 1$, Eq. 22.14 gives

$$h_m = \sqrt{(587.56 \times 10^{-9}\,\text{m})(0.50\,\text{m})}$$
$$= 5.4 \times 10^{-4}\,\text{m} = 0.54\,\text{mm}$$

Similarly, $m = 3, 5$, and 7 give radii of 0.94 mm, 1.21 mm, and 1.43 mm respectively.

One could also make a Fresnel zone plate by blocking the center zone and $m = 2, 4, 6$, etc. zones. The waves coming through the odd integers are all phased shifted by the same amount and so are in phase with each other, and will all constructively interfere at B.

Dennis Gabor, the inventor of holography, pointed out a zone plate modification in which only the zero and first order diffracted waves are present. In Gabor's modification, the circular zones change transmission according to a sinusoidal amplitude variation (such as discussed in the previous section). For collimated plane waves incident on Gabor's zone plate, there is a central order diffracted wave, a first order outgoing (diverging) diffracted wave, and a first order inward (converging) diffracted wave. The inward diffracted wave forms a real image point at a focal distance $+f_2$, while the outward diffracted wave forms a virtual image point (at a focal distance $-f_2$). There are no higher order foci in the Gabor zone plate.

Since diffraction depends directly on the wavelength, a zone plate illuminated by white light has considerable CA. In particular, longer wavelengths

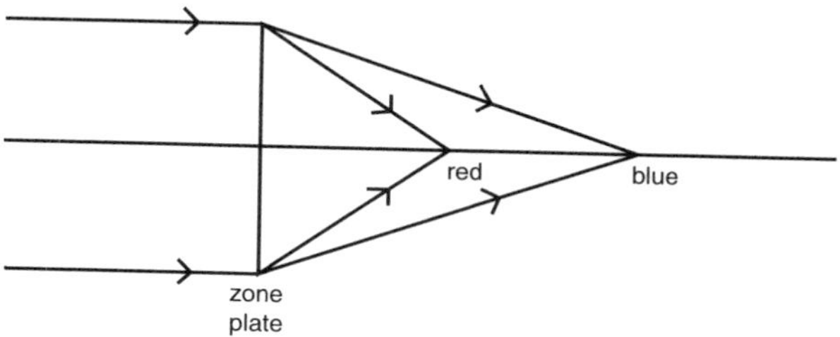

Figure 22.22 For a zone plate, long wavelengths (red) are diffracted inward at a larger angle than short wavelengths (blue).

are diffracted inward at a larger angle than the shorter wavelengths, so the longer wavelengths have shorter focal lengths (Figure 22.22). This is the opposite of the CA of a single plus lens.

We can work out an effective Abbe value for a zone plate as follows. From Eq. 22.14, the zone plate radii are the same for a constant q equal to λf_2. For the same order, it follows that

$$P = \frac{1}{f_2} = \frac{\lambda}{q}$$

or

$$P = k\lambda$$

where $k = 1/q$. We can subscript P and λ for each wavelength: helium d, $\lambda_d = 587.56$ nm; hydrogen C, $\lambda_C = 656.28$ nm; and hydrogen F, $\lambda_F = 486.17$ nm. Then the CA of the zone plate is

$$\begin{aligned}\text{CA} &= P_F - P_C \\ &= k\lambda_F - k\lambda_C \\ &= k\lambda_d\left(\frac{\lambda_F - \lambda_C}{\lambda_d}\right)\end{aligned}$$

or

$$\text{CA} = \frac{P_d}{v}$$

where,

$$v = \frac{\lambda_d}{\lambda_F - \lambda_C} = -3.45$$

For comparison, typical Abbe values for a refractive (glass or plastic) lens range from +90 to +20. Relative to a lens, the −3.45 Abbe value confirms that the zone plate has the opposite CA and that the CA is much larger in magnitude.

A Fresnel zone plate can be made by printing the appropriate dark circular stripes on white paper, and then photographically reducing it to give the proper

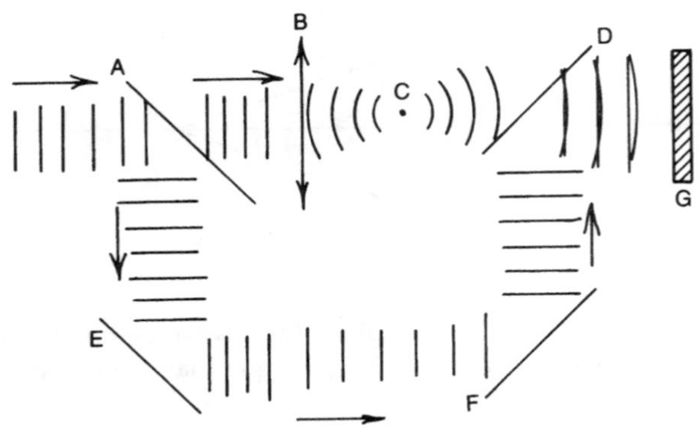

Figure 22.23 Optical method to make a Gabor zone plate by film exposure to an interference pattern.

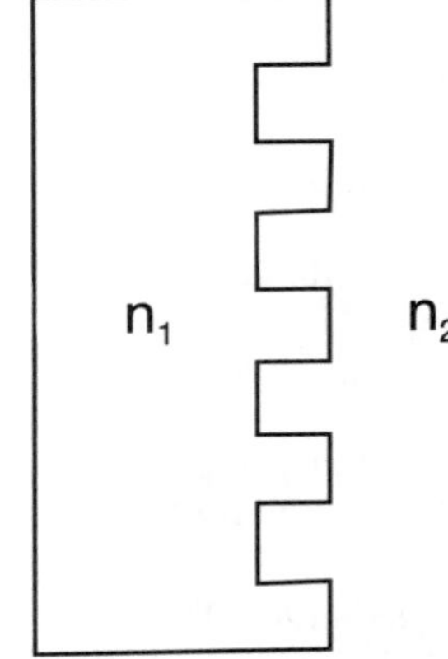

Figure 22.24 Side view of phase plate grooves (square wave design).

scale in the zone plate. It is more complicated to print a Gabor zone plate. However, a Gabor zone plate can also be made optically by recording a set of circular interference fringes on appropriate film. The invention of the laser made the optical method easy to use.

Figure 22.23 schematically represents the optical method to make a Gabor zone plate. Mirrors *A* and *D* are partially reflecting and partially transmitting. Mirrors *E* and *F* are plane reflectors. An expanded laser beam is split in two by *A*. One part of the beam is converged by lens *B* to form a point image at *C* (actually a small Airy's disk and ring pattern). The diverging spherical waves from the point *C* are then superposed with the plane waves from the other part of the beam. Because of the phase differences, a set of circular interference fringes are formed by the superposition. When the appropriate film *G* is placed at the superposition position, the interference fringes are recorded on the film. The circular interference fringes on the developed film have the required spacing and sinusoidal amplitude transmission of a Gabor zone plate. The process of optically making a Gabor zone plate, and then using it to form an image is better known as *holography* (Section 22.17).

Fresnel and Gabor zone plates work by blocking the light waves that would contribute destructive interference at the diffraction maximum (or image point). This image is dimmer because of the blocked light. Suppose that instead of blocking these waves, they are phased shifted by 180°. Then the phase shifted waves would be in phase with the axial wave, and would contribute to the constructive interference with the result that the diffraction maximum (or image point) is brighter. This is the idea of a *phase plate.*

There are various ways to introduce the required 180° phase shift in a phase plate. One way is to make very small (microscopic) grooves of a depth d in a material of index n_1 (Figure 22.24). The grooves might be filled with air ($n_2 = 1$), or might be filled with a different material of index n_2 where $n_2 \neq n_1$. The depth of the grooves is designed to introduce the required 180° (half wavelength) phase shift in zones 1, 3, 5, etc. The (fractional) number of wavelengths in each material equals the thickness d divided by the wavelength of the light in that material (λ/n). A relative 180° phase shift will occur in the light emerging from the different materials when the difference in the (fractional) number of wavelengths equals $\pm 1/2$, or

$$\frac{d}{\lambda/n_1} - \frac{d}{\lambda/n_2} = \pm\frac{1}{2}$$

Then,

$$n_1 d - n_2 d = \pm\frac{\lambda}{2} \tag{22.15}$$

A thickness of material multiplied by the index of refraction of that material is called the *optical path length.* Another way of stating Eq. 22.15 is to say that the grooves introduce a half wavelength difference in the optical path lengths. The groove depth equals one wavelength when $n_1 = 1.50$ and $n_2 = 1.00$. For indices that are closer together, the required depth d is larger. (For example, when $n_1 = 1.43$ and $n_2 = 1.33$, the groove depth is 5λ.)

Just as with blazed gratings, the efficiency of a phase plate at concentrating the light into one or more desired maximums can be improved by appropriately shaping the grooves (i.e., we could let the dashed lines in Figure 22.18a represent square wave grooves, while the solid curve represents shaped grooves). The appropriately shaped grooves are referred to as kinoforms. A zone plate with kinoform shaped grooves is referred to as a *diffractive lens.* The same idea can be optically achieved in a zone plate, as opposed to a phase plate, and these zone plates are sometimes called *holographic lenses*.

In the closing years of the twentieth century, the use of small diffractive lenses in monochromatic laser optical systems grew rapidly. Diffractive lenses also have a place in white light systems where the CA is balanced by a combination of regular (refractive) lenses and diffractive lenses. A single refractive lens with a phase plate imbedded on one of its surfaces is referred to as a *hybrid lens*.

22.16 OPHTHALMIC DIFFRACTIVE LENSES

In spectacle lenses for a presbyope, there is an area on the lens with the distance vision dioptric power and another area (usually in the bottom portion of the lens) that has the near vision dioptric power. The wearer moves his eyes to look through either the distance or the near portion. However, a contact lens rides on the cornea and moves with the eye. Therefore for a bifocal contact lens, some of the light goes through the distance portion of the lens and some goes through the near portion, and both of these light waves are incident on the retina simultaneously. This simultaneous incidence acts to reduce the contrast in the images on the retina.

There are a number of bifocal contact lens designs, some that are rotationally symmetric and some that are not. Figure 22.25a shows a front view of a concentric design with the center zone having the near power and the outer zone having the distance power. Such a design is sensitive to pupil size fluctuations. Among the available designs is a diffractive bifocal contact lens (Figure 22.25b shows a front view). The diffractive bifocal contact lens is really a hybrid lens, since it is a regular (refractive) contact lens with a grooved (kinoform) phase plate on its back surface. The depth of the groves is microscopic. The refractive surfaces of the contact lens provide the distance vision power (the zero order light), and the phase plate provides the near vision power (the first order diffracted light). On the eye, the grooves fill with tear fluid, and the path difference between the tear fluid and the lens material introduces the appropriate phase shift.

Since all parts of the diffractive bifocal contact lens are contributing to both the distance and the near powers, the performance of the lens is relatively independent of pupil size fluctuations. However centration of the lens seems to be important in patient satisfaction. As with other bifocal contact lenses, there is a clinical protocol for determining the potential success of the diffractive bifocal contact lens on a patient.

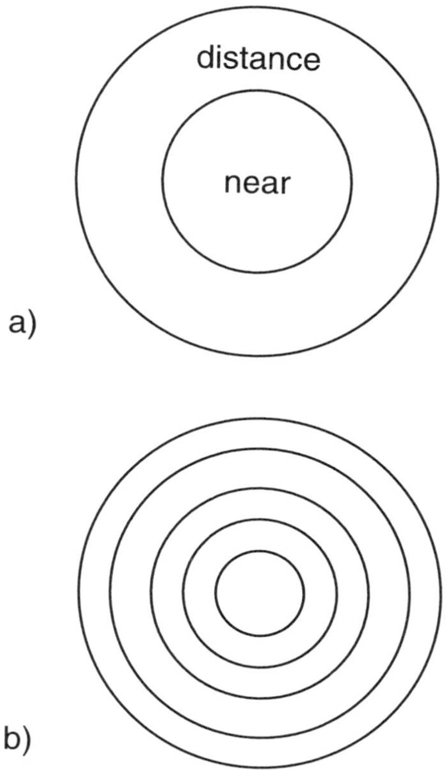

Figure 22.25 a, Front view of concentric bifocal contact lens design; b, front view of diffractive bifocal contact lens design. The distance power comes from refraction of the zero order wave by the lens shape (meniscus convex or concave). The near power comes from diffraction of the first order wave by the phase plate grooves. Note that each area of the lens contributes to both the distance and the near powers.

There are also diffractive lenses in use for Intraocular lens (IOL) implants. These lenses are implanted in the eye when a cataractous crystalline lens is removed. A single vision IOL does not provide any change in focus, so that eye is completely presbyopic. A bifocal IOL, such as a diffractive IOL, provides two powers, as does the diffractive bifocal contact lens. The two focii do reduce contrast in the retinal image. In laser refractive surgery, laser produced diffractive lenses grooves on the cornea have been proposed as a way to make the cornea into a bifocal lens.

22.17 HOLOGRAPHY

In a general sense, a hologram is a very complicated diffraction grating (or zone plate) that when properly illuminated results in diffracted waves (maximums) that forms real and/or virtual images. The diffracted waves are actually reconstructions of the waves that would come from real objects. Once these waves are reconstructed, an observer viewing them sees the objects in three dimensions. Another startling property of the hologram is that each small section of it contains all the information needed to reconstruct the whole scene. In other words, when a hologram is cut in half and one of the halves is properly illuminated, the diffracted wave from that half still forms the whole image. The Greek word for whole is *holos*, thus the name *hologram*.

Holography was invented by Dennis Gabor in 1947 as a method to improve electron microscopy. Visible light holograms did not become practical until after the invention of the laser in 1960. In 1971, Gabor was awarded the Nobel prize in physics for his discovery of holography.

A Gabor zone plate is essentially a hologram of a point source. Suppose we want to make a hologram of two point sources separated both laterally and longitudinally. We could do this by separating the initial laser beam into three parts (*A*, *B*, and *C*). We converge *A* to form one of the points, and *B* to form the other. Then *C* is used to form two sets of circular interference fringes, one from the superposition with *A*, and one from the superposition with *B* (Figure 22.26a). The two sets of circular fringes are recorded by direct exposure of the film (Figure 22.26b). (Cross modulation between the two sets of fringes can limit quality of the hologram).

When the hologram is properly reilluminated, it generates first order diffracted waves that propagate inward and outward. The two first order waves that are diffracted outward are spherical. One has *A* as its

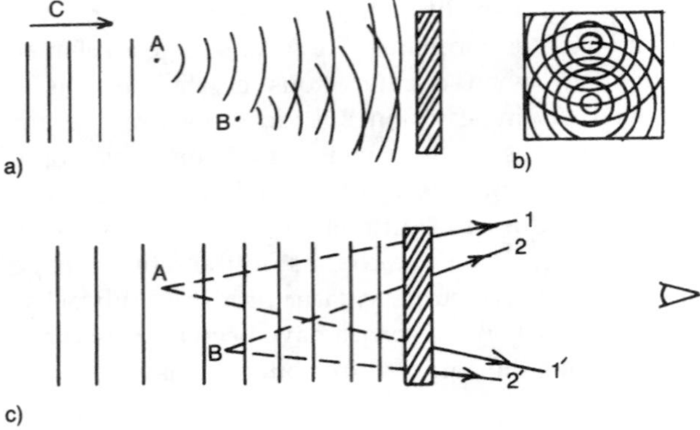

Figure 22.26 a, Method to make a hologram of two point sources; b, schematic representation of interference fringes on the holographic film; c, generation of virtual image points by diffracted waves from the hologram.

center of curvature, and the other has *B* as its center of curvature. The zero order wave is plane and associated with the wave *C*. In Figure 22.26c, rays 1 and 1′ represent the spherical diffracted wave that has *A* as its center of curvature (virtual image), while rays 2 and 2′ represent the spherical diffracted wave that has *B* as its center of curvature. An observer looking at the diffracted waves sees the two virtual image points spatially separated both longitudinally and laterally. (The zero order wave *C* provides the background illumination.)

Consider a real three dimensional object, such as a small box in front of a cat. When viewed from an angle the cat is visible behind the box. When viewed from straight ahead (axially), the cat is hidden by the box. This relative shift in position of the objects is referred to as parallax, and is a monocular depth perception cue.

Figure 22.27a shows a top view of the set-up to make a hologram of the cat box scene. The cat is represented by the circle *C* and the box by the square *D*. The hologram film is *F*. Mirrors *B* and *E* are plane mirrors, and mirror *A* is partially reflecting and partially transmitting. An expanded laser beam is split at *A*. The transmitted part of the laser beam is reflected at *B*, and illuminates the cat box scene *C* and *D*. The diffusely reflected light is incident on the film *F*. (The rays represent the diffusely reflected light from two of the points in the cat box scene.) The part the laser beam reflected at *A* is called the reference beam. It remains plane, is reflected at *E*, and is then incident on the film *F*. At the film plane the reference beam and the diffusely reflected light superpose and result in a complicated interference pattern that is recorded on the film *F*. The developed slide is the hologram. If we examine the slide through a phase contrast microscope, we see only the fringes of the recorded interference pattern.

When the hologram is properly illuminated by light incident at the same angle as the reference beam, it forms two diffracted waves (the first order maximums), together with the zero order or central maximum. One of the first order maximums is converging (and forms a real image), while the other is diverging (and is associated with a virtual image).

Let us consider the diffracted waves associated with the virtual image. These diffracted waves are a reconstruction of the waves that would have come from the object. Therefore, the observer sees a conjugate virtual image in three dimensions just as if the objects were there. For example, by viewing the hologram from a side angle near ray 2′, the cat is behind the box and therefore not visible. By viewing the hologram from the normal (between rays 2 and 1′) we can

Figure 22.27 a, Set-up to make a hologram; b, set-up to view the hologram's image.

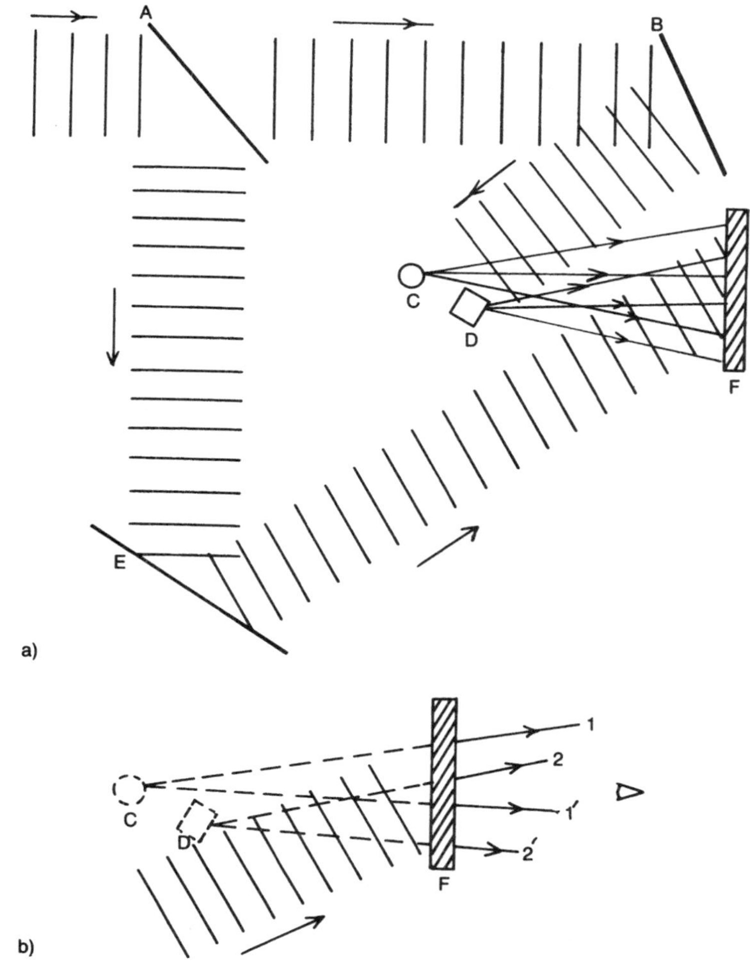

see the cat behind the box. (In Figure 22.27b, rays 1 and 1′ correspond to the diffracted spherical wave that has a center of curvature at a point on the cat, while rays 2 and 2′ correspond to the diffracted spherical wave that has a center of curvature at a point on the box.)

Let us contrast a hologram with a normal photographic slide made with a camera. The information recorded in a normal photograph relates only to the amplitude distribution of the waves. The information (interference pattern) recorded on the hologram relates to both the amplitude and the phase distribution of the waves. In technical terms, it is the ability of the hologram to record phase information, as well as amplitude information, that distinguishes it from the camera's photographic slide.

When the hologram is made, each small part of the film receives diffusely reflected light from each point on the object. Hence, each small part of the hologram contains the whole information. Imagine viewing the hologram through a circular aperture. The whole three-dimensional image is still present, although the angular view is restricted. A small enough aperture introduces its own diffraction, and this diffraction introduces blur into the hologram's image. Thus, if the aperture is made smaller and smaller (or equivalently a hologram is cut smaller and smaller), we lose the holographic image, not by cutting off parts of it, but rather the whole image eventually blurs out.

The geometry of making a hologram can be varied to emphasize either the real or the virtual image. The angle of the diffracted waves from a hologram depends directly on the wavelength of the source. Therefore, holograms tend to have CA problems. Holograms also tend to have image quality problems when illuminated by extended sources. "Second generation" holograms remedy many of these problems. One method of minimizing both the extended source and CA problem is to limit the depth of the hologram's image to a fraction of the viewing distance.

The rainbow hologram, invented by Stephen Benton in 1969, is an example of second generation holography. The rainbow hologram's image can be viewed with ordinary room illumination. This is achieved by sacrificing vertical parallax (which does not change the three-dimensionality much, since it is mostly horizontal parallax that we use as a depth cue). When scanning horizontally, the person sees the three dimensional image (horizontal parallax). When scanning vertical, the person does not perceive vertical parallax, but instead sees the same angular view in different colors (hence the name rainbow, although that is not very accurate scientifically). The different colors are due to the wavelength dependence of the diffraction in the vertical direction.

The initial rainbow holograms were actually the second hologram of a two hologram process. First a typical hologram is made of the scene (e.g., the cat and box). This is referred to as the master hologram. Then a laser beam is split into a reference beam and an illuminating beam. The illuminating beam passes through a horizontal slit and then through the master hologram and is incident on a film. The reference beam is also incident on the film, so that an interference pattern is recorded (a hologram of a hologram—or a copy hologram). The developed film is the rainbow hologram.

When the rainbow hologram is reilluminated, the light diffracted by it shows the three-dimensional scene (cat and box) as viewed through the slit. (You can think of the rainbow hologram as forming an image of the slit, so even when it is illuminated by an extended source, the diffracted light passes through the slit's image.) At the primary viewing angle, typical room illumination gives a good quality black and white image. At higher and lower angles, the diffracted waves give the image in a series of different colors. (There are now specialized one-step processes for making rainbow holograms.)

The holograms discussed above are transmission holograms. Reflection holograms can also be made. Reflection-type rainbow holograms are now fairly common (i.e., on stamps, stickers, magazine covers, telephone cards, jewelry items, and on credit cards and some currencies to hinder counterfeiting). In each case the three-dimensional images are visible under ordinary room illumination.

Holograms are also used in supermarket checkout lines to help the electro-optical system read the bars and stripes of the universal product code (UPC). Typically, laser light is passed through a rotating disk of 21 wedge shaped holograms, each of which deflects the beam in a different way. At least one of the beam deflections will reach and be diffusely reflected from the UPC onto a photodetector, which electronically reads the signal and feeds it to a computer. The computer has the product's name, size, and price stored in memory. It gives the price, prints the receipt, and updates the store's inventory. (All that for a can of beans!)

22.18 SNELL'S LAW FROM HUYGENS' PRINCIPLE

This chapter used Huygens' principal of wave propagation and focused on diffraction. Huygens' principle can also be used to derive the geometric optics laws of reflection and refraction (Snell's Law). Here we focus on refraction.

Figure 22.28 shows plane waves in air (index n_1) incident at an angle on a flat glass surface (index n_2). The plane wave in air at time t_1 contains the points A, B, and C. This plane wave makes the angle θ_i with the glass surface. According to Huygens' principle, secondary spherical wavelets from points B and C reach points E and F respectively at time t_2. The envelope for the new wavefront passes through points E and F, and gives another plane wave in air that also makes an angle θ_i with the surface. However, point A is on the glass surface. The secondary spherical wavelet leaving point A at time t_1 is in the glass, and during the time interval $\Delta t = t_2 - t_1$ it travels a shorter distance than the secondary wavelets in air. At t_2, the wavelet from point A reaches point D. For the new wavefront in the glass, the envelope lies on the straight line that passes through D and E. The result is a plane wave in the glass that makes an angle θ_r with the surface. The secondary wavelets leaving points D, E, and F respectively reach points G, H, and I at time t_3, giving another plane wave in the glass that also makes an angle θ_r with the surface. The sequence (times t_1, t_2, and t_3) shows the refraction of the plane waves at the air–glass interface.

We can obtain Snell's Law as follows. First note that a ray is perpendicular to the wavefront, and that the normal is perpendicular to the surface. Therefore when the plane wave makes an angle of θ_i with the surface, the corresponding ray makes an angle of θ_i with the normal (since angles with sides perpendicular to each other are equal). A similar argument holds for θ_r and rays in the glass. Now from the triangle ABE,

$$\sin\theta_i = \frac{BE}{AE}$$

and from triangle ADE

$$\sin\theta_r = \frac{AD}{AE}$$

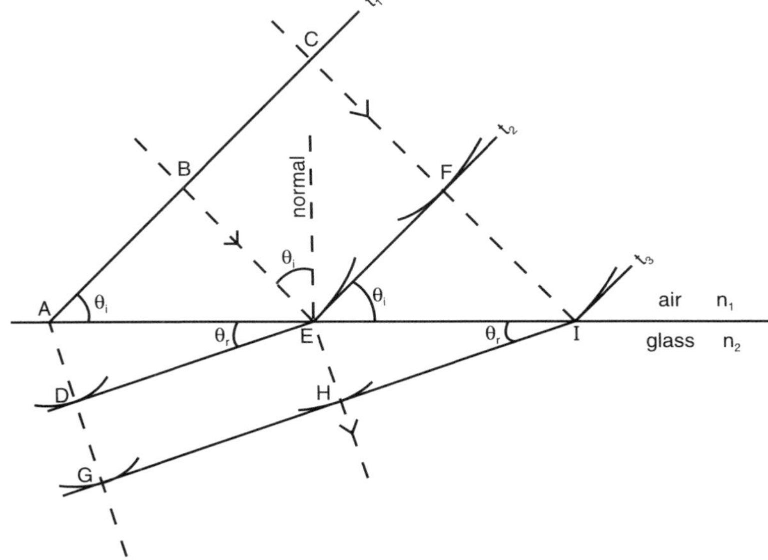

Figure 22.28 Huygens Principle construction to derive Snell's Law.

It follows that

$$\frac{\sin\theta_i}{BE} = \frac{\sin\theta_r}{AD}$$

The length BE equals the velocity v_1 of the light in the air times the time Δt, while the length AD equals the velocity v_2 of the light in the glass times the time Δt. Since $v_1 = c/n_1$ and $v_2 = c/n_2$, we can substitute to obtain

$$\frac{\sin\theta_i}{(c/n_1)\Delta t} = \frac{\sin\theta_r}{(c/n_2)\Delta t}$$

This simplifies to

$$n_1 \sin\theta_i = n_2 \sin\theta_r$$

which is Snell's Law (or the Snell–Descartes Law) first introduced in Chapter 1.

PROBLEMS

1. A single slit has a width of 0.03 mm. For incident light of wavelength 520 nm, what is the angular location of the first minimum in the single-slit diffraction pattern? What is the angular location of the first minimum for 620 nm incident light?
2. A circular pinhole has a 0.1 mm diameter. What is the angular location of the first minimum in the diffraction pattern when the incident light has a 565 nm wavelength? What is the size of Airy's disk on a screen located 400 cm behind the pinhole? Same questions for incident light of 465 nm wavelength.
3. Two dots are on a chart 4 m from a pinhole camera with a 0.2 mm diameter. For light of wavelength 550 nm, what is the minimum distance between the two dots that gives resolution according to Rayleigh's criterion?
4. For a distant object plane, what angular separation in minutes gives the two-point resolution limit for a +20.00 D lens set at $f/5.6$? Use a 570 nm wavelength.
5. Based on Rayleigh's criterion alone, what is the expected acuity for a human eye with a 3 mm pupil and an incident wavelength of 600 nm? (Use a thin lens and screen model.) Based on Rayleigh's criterion alone, what is the expected acuity for looking through a pinhole of diameter 1.5 mm?
6. When a diffraction grating has 5,000 lines per cm, what is the angular location of the second order maximum for incident light with a 543 nm wavelength? Same question for light of wavelength 533 nm.
7. A filtered small circular aperture has a Gaussian transmission function with a 0.1 mm semidiameter size parameter. For monochromatic light of wavelength 565 nm incident from a distant point source, what is the semidiameter size parameter of the beam on a screen 400 cm behind the aperture? How does the beam size on the screen compare to Airy's disk size in problem #2 above?

CHAPTER 23

Scattering, Absorption, Dispersion, and Polarization

23.1 DIPOLE RADIATION

A dipole consists of equal amounts of positive and negative electrically charged particles separated by a distance *s*. The dipole is electrically neutral, but will emit electromagnetic waves of frequency *f* when the charges periodically oscillate toward and away from each other with frequency *f*.

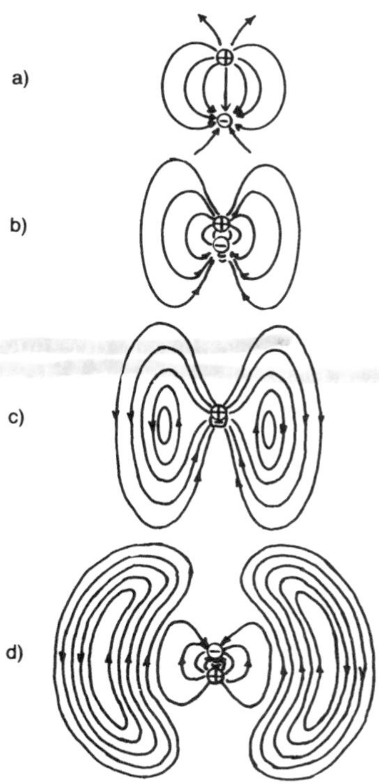

Figure 23.1 Sequence of electric field curves for an oscillating dipole.

Figure 23.1 shows a sequence of electric field curves for an oscillating dipole with a vertical axis. As the charges move toward each other, the electric field curves form closed loops. Once the charges pass each other, the closed loops propagate away from the dipole and represent the radiated electromagnetic wave. Note that no radiation propagates out directly along the dipole axis.

Atoms or molecules consist of equal numbers of negatively charged electrons and positively charged protons. The atoms and molecules are thus electrically neutral. When electromagnetic waves are incident on the atoms or molecules, the electrons are driven to oscillate in a direction opposite to the protons. Hence, the incident radiation sets up a dipole oscillation in the atoms or molecules. The dipole oscillation causes a re-radiation of an electromagnetic wave of the same wavelength as the incident wave. The re-radiated light propagates out in the allowed directions, and is a major component of scattered light.

23.2 INCOHERENT SCATTERING

Section 1.10 pointed out that scattering is due to inhomogeneities in a medium. For convenience, let us refer to the inhomogeneities as particles. (The particles might be molecules, water droplets, ice crystals, aerosol pollutants, fat globules, etc.) Scattering depends on the size of the particles, the distance between particles, and the strength of the interaction between the light and the particles. The strength of the interaction depends on the refractive index and the absorption strength of the particles.

In this section, we will assume that the incident light is white and that the particles are far enough

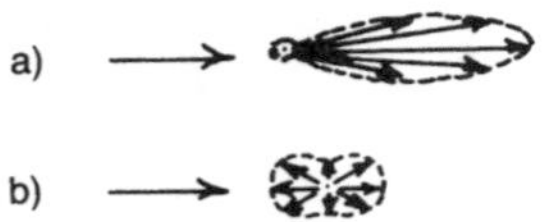

Figure 23.2 a, Scattering by a large particle; b, scattering by a small particle.

apart so that the light scattered by different particles is incoherent. The total effect of the scattering is then obtained by adding the intensities of the light scattered from each particle. (The incoherent scattering condition is met when the spacing between the particles is much greater than the coherence length of the light.)

For elementary discussion purposes, it is convenient to divide the dependence of incoherent scattering on particle size into three categories. The three categories respectively consist of particles much larger than the wavelength of light, particles about the size of the wavelength of light, and particles much smaller than the wavelength of light. In reality, there is a gradual transition between these three regions.

When transparent particles (i.e., weak absorbers) are much larger than the wavelength of light, the geometric optics processes of reflection and refraction are the dominant causes of the scattering. The scattering from large transparent particles is strongly peaked in the forward direction, and tends to be wavelength-independent (Figure 23.2a). Common examples are single scattering from fog and clouds. (The rainbow can be considered as scattering from raindrops, and it is an exception to the wavelength independence.)

When transparent particles are about the size of a wavelength, wave effects inside the particle can occur (e.g., diffraction, standing waves or resonances). These interior wave effects result in scattering that is spread out much more in direction, is wavelength dependent, and is very sensitive to the particle size. The halos seen through a fogged-up car window is a common example.

When transparent particles are much smaller than the size of a wavelength (e.g., less than a tenth of the wavelength) then dipole re-radiation is the prime contributor to the scattered light. Here the scattered light is fairly isotropic in direction (Figure 23.2b), and the intensity is much stronger for short wavelengths than for long wavelengths, which results in a bluish appearance of the scattered light.

The large and small particle extremes of incoherent scattering are easily observed on partly cloudy days. The white of the clouds is due to scattering by the large transparent water droplets or ice crystals. The blue of the sky is due to Rayleigh scattering by the small transparent air molecules. Since both are made up of transparent particles, there is no "white" in the clouds, nor "blue" in the sky.

Gustave Mie (1868–1957) gave a general mathematical formulation of scattering. For small particles, Mie's equations give Rayleigh scattering. For large particles, Mie's equations give the wavelength-independent scattering of the geometric optics limit. With the aid of computers, Mie's equations can be numerically solved for any other region (e.g., particle size about the size of the wavelength).

Mie's theory applies to particles that absorb as well as scatter. In fact, Mie developed his theory to explain the colors of colloidal gold solutions in water. Gold particles of diameter 40 nm form a solution that appears red in the transmitted light. (This effect is also used to make ruby red glass). Here the effect is primarily due to absorption of blue and green by the gold, while the scattered light is weak and yellow-green in color. Gold particles of diameter 140 nm form a solution that appears blue in the transmitted light. Here the absorption is weaker, the scattering is stronger than the absorption, and the scattered light is red.

In a similar manner, oil droplets in the atmosphere from large forest fires have, on rare occasions, resulted in a bluish appearing sun and moon. (This has been verified by spectroscopy measurements.) It is conjectured that this is the origin of the phrase *once in a blue moon.*

23.3 RAYLEIGH SCATTERING

John Tyndall, a contemporary of Lord Rayleigh, was the first person to experimentally confirm that the scattered intensity from small transparent particles is larger for the short wavelengths (violets and blues) than for the longer wavelengths. Rayleigh showed that theoretically the scattering dependence of the intensity depends directly on the fourth power of the frequency. Since frequency and wavelength vary inversely, this means that the intensity dependence of the scattering varies inversely with the fourth power of the wavelength. Rayleigh also pointed out that molecular scattering would follow the fourth power dependence, and hence the blue color of the sky was due to scattering by the air molecules.

Where does the $1/\lambda^4$ dependence come from? Rayleigh gave the following dimensional argument. First, it is obvious that the amplitude of the scattered wave is directly proportional to the amplitude of the incident wave. Second, Rayleigh pointed out that the amplitude of the scattered wave is also directly proportional to the volume of the scattering particle.

(Volume has dimensions of length cubed.) Third, he assumed that the scattered wavefront is spherical. The energy carried by a small part of the spherical wavefront is inversely proportional to the surface area of the sphere. (The surface area of a sphere is 4π times the radius squared.) Since the amplitude of a wave is proportional to the square root of the energy carried, it follows that the amplitude of the spherical scattered wave is inversely proportional to the radius of the wavefront.

The ratio of the amplitude of the scattered wave to that of the incident wave is dimensionless. Since the amplitude of the scattered wave is directly proportional to the volume of the particle (length cubed), and inversely proportional to the radius of the wavefront (length), there is still an unaccounted factor in the denominator that varies as a length squared. The only other length in this situation is the wavelength of the light, and so the scattered amplitude must be inversely proportional to the square of the wavelength. Hence, the scattered intensity (irradiance) is inversely proportional to the fourth power of the wavelength, or

$$I_{scat} \propto \frac{1}{\lambda^4} \tag{23.1}$$

A considerably more detailed mathematical analysis shows that the $1/\lambda^4$ dependence is characteristic of dipole radiation under the conditions that the dipole size is much smaller than the wavelength of the light.

Consider the relative Rayleigh scattering intensity I_{rel} for hydrogen F light (blue) compared to hydrogen C light (red). Here,

$$I_{rel} = I_2/I_1$$

where I_2 is for the F light and I_1 for the C light. We would expect that I_{rel} is greater than 1, since the scattered intensity of blue light is greater than the scattered intensity of red light. From Eq. 23.1,

$$I_{rel} = \frac{1/\lambda_2^4}{1/\lambda_1^4}$$

which simplifies to

$$I_{rel} = \left(\frac{\lambda_1}{\lambda_2}\right)^4 \tag{23.2}$$

The F wavelength (λ_2) is 486 nm, and the C wavelength (λ_1) is 656 nm, so

$$I_{rel} = (656\,\text{nm}/486\,\text{nm})^4 = 3.3.$$

Thus, for Raleigh scattering, the intensity of the scattered blue F light is 3.3 times greater than that of the scattered red C light. Even more impressive is the fact that the intensity of 400 nm scattered light is 7.2 times greater than that of 656 nm light.

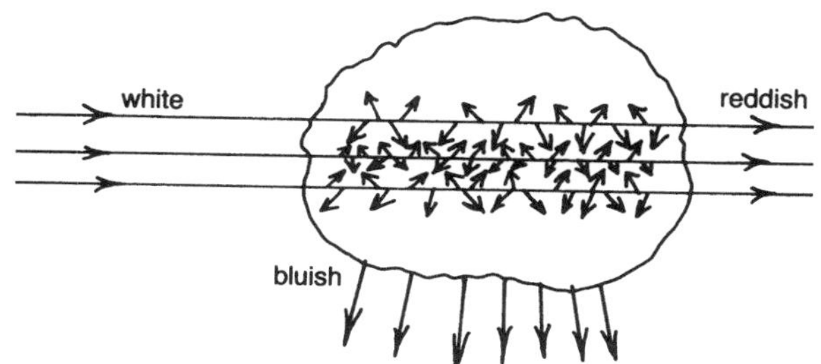

Figure 23.3 Rayleigh scattering.

The smoke coming from the end of a cigarette has a bluish appearance (especially when viewed against a dark background). The blue component is due to Rayleigh scattering by the small smoke particles. However, the smoke that is exhaled by the smoker appears white. The exhaled smoke particles are coated with water, and are much larger than a wavelength. This gives the wavelength-independent scattering of the large particle (geometric optics) scattering.

In Rayleigh scattering, the transmitted light and the scattered light have a complementary appearance (Figure 23.3). Sunrises and sunsets appear orange or red since the light reaching the observer's eye has traveled a long path through the atmosphere, and has lost more blues than reds (Figure 1.6). The red color of a sunset is enhanced by the presence of small dust particles in the lower atmosphere. (You can simulate atmospheric scattering by placing a few drops of milk in a clear glass of water, and then illuminating the glass with a penlight. The transmitted light will have a definite orangish appearance, while the scattered light has a faint bluish appearance.)

23.4 MULTIPLE INCOHERENT SCATTERING

When there are just a few scattering particles per unit volume, the dominant scattering process is single scattering. Suppose you want to see the path of a collimated light beam by looking from the side (i.e., perpendicular to the beam path). If there is no scattering, you cannot see the beam path, since no light is coming to your eye. If there is a suitable amount of single scattering, the beam path is well defined by the scattered light that reaches your eye. Now suppose there are so many scattering particles per unit volume that multiple scattering occurs. Then when looking at the scattering medium, you see a glow coming from an area that is considerably larger than the incident beam path. For example, light might first scatter up (or

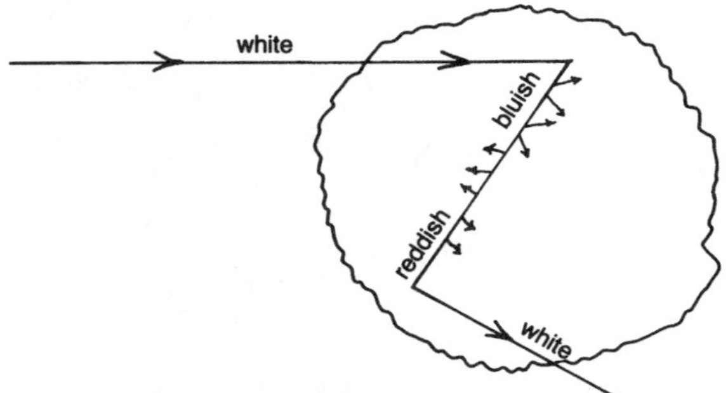

Figure 23.4 Multiple scattering.

down), travel outside the incident beam's path, and then scatter again back toward your eye. (You can experimentally observe the two extremes of single scattering and multiple scattering by starting with a collimated beam going through clean water in an aquarium tank or other suitable container. For single scattering, add a few drops of milk to the tank. Then keep adding milk until you get multiple scattering.)

Multiple scattering rapidly decreases any wavelength dependence regardless of the size of the particles. Figure 23.4 shows a double scattering path for small particles. The light initially scattered appears bluish (i.e., more blues than reds). However, this light loses blues faster than it loses reds as it travels through the scattering medium. So the light incident on the second scattering center is loaded with reds. When the second scattering occurs, the relatively deficient blues scatter more than the relatively abundant reds. Hence, the scattered light returns toward a balance of the blues and reds, and thus appears white. The more times the light is scattered, the less the wavelength dependence of the scattered intensity.

Let I_o be the intensity of the light incident on the scattering medium. Let $I_f(d)$ be the intensity of the light that ends up traveling forward at the far end of a scattering medium of thickness d. Then we can define the *transmission coefficient* T as

$$T = \frac{I_f(d)}{I_o}$$

Let $I_b(0)$ be the intensity of light that ends up traveling backward at the front surface of the scattering medium. Then the *albedo* R is defined as

$$R = \frac{I_b(0)}{I_o}$$

The albedo R acts like a reflection coefficient, although the light traveling backwards is due to multiple scattering from the medium as opposed to a reflection at the surface.

One of the parameters involved in a quantitative analysis of scattering is the *scattering coefficient* β, where $1/\beta$ has units of length and is the average distance between scattering events. On the average, there is a small distance between scattering events when β is large, and there is a large distance between scattering events when β is small. Another parameter involved is the *asymmetry parameter* g defined as the cosine of the mean scattering angle. For mostly forward scattering, the scattering angle is small and g (the cosine) is close to +1. For isotropic scattering, the mean scattering angle is 90°, so g is 0. For backward scattering, the scattering angle is 180° and g is −1. (The asymmetry parameter g is about 0.85 for cloud droplets and about 0.93 for snow.)

In general, the mathematical theory of multiple scattering is quite complicated. However, we can get some intuitive understanding by considering the results of a simple "two-stream" model given by Craig Bohren. Consider a large scattering medium bounded by parallel planes normal to the incident light. Let d be the thickness of the medium. In the two-stream model, the light can scatter only forward or backward. So light traveling in the forward direction may go straight without scattering, may be scattered forward, or may be scattered backward. Light that is going backward (because it's been scattered at least once) may go straight backward without scattering, may scatter in the backward direction, or may scatter back into the forward direction. The asymmetry parameter g is related to the different probabilities for forward and backward scattering. Let's further assume that the light that gets through the scattering medium does not return to it (either because there is nothing else to scatter it, or because a successive media absorbs it). Here the two-stream theory gives the following simple equations for the albedo R and the transmission coefficient T:

$$R = \frac{\tau}{2+\tau} \tag{23.3}$$

and

$$T = \frac{2}{2+\tau} \tag{23.4}$$

where

$$\tau = (1-g)\beta d \tag{23.5}$$

This scattering medium has no absorption, and therefore energy conservation requires that $T + R = 1$. Note that if T is small, then R must be large and vice versa. Therefore, a thick layer of clouds that appear relatively dark when viewed from below (T close to zero), will appear quite bright when viewed from above (R close to 1). (You can also observe this by looking away from the sun and noting the brightness of a thick cloud floating in the sky.)

The parameter τ is called the *scaled optical thickness*. It depends on the asymmetry parameter g, the scattering coefficient β, and the physical thickness d. Therefore, different scattering media with the same value for τ will appear the same, even though the values for g, β, and d differ among the media. In other words, there are different scattering media that can give the same multiple scattering appearance.

When $g = 1$ (forward scattering only), Eqs. 23.3 through 23.5 give $\tau = 0$, $R = 0$, and $T = 1$. Note however, when $g = -1$ (backward scattering only), $\tau = 2\beta d$, and $R = \beta d/(1 + \beta d)$, which in general is not 1. When $g = 0$, $\tau = \beta d$, and forward and backward scattering are equally probable (i.e., this is isotropic scattering in the two-stream model).

When the scaled optical thickness τ is very large, Eqs. 23.3 through 23.5 give $R \approx 1$ and $T \approx 0$. In this case, the scattering material is said to be *optically thick*. One meter of snow is optically thick. Storm clouds during the day may cause it to get relatively dark for daytime, but some light is still transmitted (T is small but not zero).

When $\tau = 1$, Eqs. 23.3 and 23.4 give $R = 1/3$ and $T = 2/3$. When $\tau = 0.1$, $R = 0.048$ and $T = 0.952$. When τ is small, we can approximate Eq. 23.4 by

$$T \approx 1 - (\tau/2) \tag{23.6}$$

For $\tau = 0.1$, the approximation term gives 0.950.

Let's contrast multiple scattering with single backward scattering ($g = -1$). When the average distance between scattering particles is $1/\beta$, the number of particles in a scattering medium with a small thickness Δz is $\Delta z/(1/\beta) = \beta \Delta z$. For single backward scattering, the amount of light lost to the forward direction is directly proportional to the number of particles and to the incident intensity. Then,

$$I(z + \Delta z) = I(z) - \beta \Delta z\, I(z)$$

or

$$\frac{I(z + \Delta z) - I(z)}{\Delta z} = -\beta I(z)$$

In the limit of Δz going to zero, this becomes the differential equation

$$\frac{dI}{dz} = -\beta I$$

and the solution is

$$I = I_o e^{-\beta z} \tag{23.7}$$

Thus, single backward scattering gives an exponential fall-off in intensity as the light moves through the scattering medium. For single backward scattering in a scattering medium of thickness d, Eq. 23.5 gives $\tau = 2\beta d$. Then Eq. 23.7 can be substituted into 23.4 to give

$$T = e^{-(\beta d)} = e^{-(\tau/2)} \tag{23.8}$$

For small τ values, this exponential is also approximated by Eq. 23.6. I.e., for $\tau = 0.1$, the exponential in Eq. 23.8 is 0.951, while Eq. 23.6 gave 0.950. So the two-stream multiple scattering equations automatically give the single scattering results for a small τ. Now consider a case where $\tau = 2$. Here the single scattering equation (23.8) gives $T = e^{-1} = 0.37$, while the multiple scattering equation (Eq. 23.4) gives $T = 0.50$. In other words, the multiple scattering medium transmits more light than the single scattering medium. This is because in multiple scattering, some of the light that is initially scattered backwards is re-scattered back into the forward direction.

By differentiating Eq. 23.3 with respect to the wavelength, we also see mathematically that multiple scattering is wavelength independent in spite of the wavelength dependence of the single scattering particles. That is, from Eq. 23.3, the derivative is

$$\frac{dR}{d\lambda} = \frac{2}{(2 + \tau)^2} \frac{d\tau}{d\lambda}$$

The term $dR/d\lambda$ is the wavelength dependence of the albedo of the multiple scattered light, while the term $d\tau/d\lambda$ gives the wavelength dependence of the scattering by the individual particles. Note that we can have a significant $d\tau/d\lambda$ term, as in small particle scattering, and yet for a large τ, $dR/d\lambda$ is still small. Hence, for a thick enough multiple scattering medium, there is little or no wavelength dependence even if the individual scattering particles do have a wavelength dependence. For example, the sky appears bluer closer to the zenith (thinner amount of air and therefore single scattering), than it does near the horizon (much thicker amount of air and therefore multiple scattering). Pollutants or dust in the lower atmosphere may enhance the whitish appearance of the sky near the horizon.

We can extend this argument to particles that absorb (are colored) as well as those that scatter. Consider three different glasses that are respectively clear, blue, and red. When each of these is hammered into a pile of small enough grains to give a significant amount of multiple scattering, they all appear white in the scattered light.

Small grains of sugar and salt are colorless by themselves, but larger amounts of sugar and salt appear white because of multiple scattering. Foam consists of tiny thin film bubbles of the material, and appears white due to multiple scattering. White oil-based paint is made by a suspension of small transparent particles in a film of oil, and the white appearance is due to multiple scattering. (The old toxic lead based paints used lead carbonate as the particles. Newer nontoxic paints use titanium dioxide as the particles.) Many colored paints are suspensions of absorbing particles, and the appearance of the color is due to a combination of scattering and absorption.

Multiple scattering greatly enhances absorption, since the light path in a multiple scattering medium can be very long (imagine a path where the light has scattered 37 times). Snow and ice, like water, weakly absorb in the red. The light emerging after multiple scattering in snow (a "snow hole") or ice may be a beautiful blue due to the long light path in the weakly absorbing scattering medium.

23.5 COHERENT SCATTERING

When the particles are much closer together than the coherence length of the light, constructive and destructive interference occurs between the waves scattered from different particles. Even for ordinary sources (the sun, light bulbs, etc.) coherent scattering occurs when the particles are much closer together than the wavelength of the light.

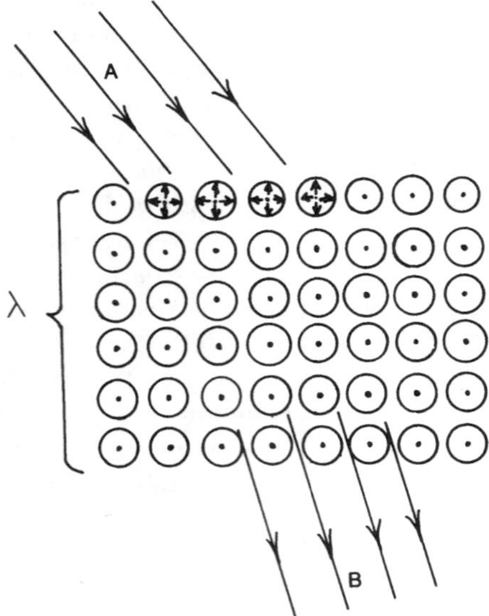

Figure 23.5 Coherent Scattering.

Coherent scattering is involved with the transmission of light through transparent materials that are inhomogeneous on a microscopic level. Figure 23.5 shows light (represented by the rays A) in a vacuum incident on a regular array of transparent particles in which the spacing is much less than the wavelength of the light. Each particle acts as a source for the coherent scattered waves.

The scattered waves propagate outward and overlap. The material acts similar to a diffraction grating in that for most directions the resultant superposition of the many coherent scattered waves is destructive interference. However, two directions give constructive interference (analogous to the maximums from a diffraction grating). One of the constructive interference directions is parallel to the incident light (a forward scattered component). This component is 180° out of phase with the unscattered part of the incident wave, and destructively interferes with it. This interference wipes out the unscattered portion of the incident wave, a very commonsense result since we usually do not think of the incident wave as existing in the material. (The mathematical proof of this is known as the Ewald–Oseen extinction theorem.) The other constructive interference direction is that given by Snell's law, and the resultant scattered wave in this direction is the refracted wave.

This constructive interference in the scattered wave gives a refracted wave that is phase-shifted relative to the incident wave. Each successive scatterer contributes an additional component to the phase shift, thus making it appear that the light travels through the medium at a speed v that is different from c. We refer to the ratio c/v as the refractive index n of the medium. In principle, we can derive the refractive index n from the scattering properties in the medium. (Of course, it is far easier just to use Snell's law to determine it.) Since Rayleigh scattering is wavelength dependent, we might now expect that the refractive index also has some wavelength dependence.

Deep in the material, there is no reflected component because of the destructive interference of the scattered waves in the direction of the reflected light. However, within a half wavelength of the surface, there are fewer scattering centers with the result that complete destructive interference does not occur in the reflected direction. In fact, the reflected light comes from the scattering roughly within a half wavelength zone of the surface. For a transparent material, blue light scatters more than red light. On the other hand, the half wavelength zone for red is larger than that for blue. The result is that the amount of light reflected from a transparent material is wavelength-independent.

23.6 INTRAOCULAR LIGHT SCATTER

The corneal stroma consists of collagen fibrils that are approximately 25 nm in diameter and have an interfibril spacing of 60 nm. These dimensions are much less than the wavelength of visible light, so coherent scattering theory applies to the transparent cornea. Some residual scattering occurs (about 10%) since the destructive interference is not complete. This scattered (or diffusely reflected) light enables us to examine the structure of the cornea with a slit lamp.

The corneal endothelium pumps excess water out of the cornea into the aqueous humor. In cases of endothelial trauma, the pumping action decreases and "lakes" of water begin to form between the stromal fibers. Once these lakes approach a size of 1/2 the wavelength, the efficiency of the destructive interference in the scattered light declines. This results in increased scattering, in which case the cornea starts to lose its transparency and takes on a greyish appearance. Scar tissue on the cornea may appear a bright white due to multiple scattering.

In the scleral area, the collagen fibers are much larger, and the spacing is about a wavelength. Here there is little or no coherent scattering, and the sclera appears whitish due to large particle incoherent scattering. In cases of scleral thinning, the fibers get smaller and the sclera takes on a bluish appearance due to single Rayleigh-type scattering. (In fact, if you look carefully, you will see that most normal scleras have a slight bluish appearance due to some single scattering.)

Another difference between the sclera and the cornea is that the collagen fibers in the human cornea are laid down in parallel bundles, while those in the sclera are laid down in a random order. However, this regularity does not seem to be crucial to transparency. In 1967 Goldman and Benedek observed that the very thick Bowman's zone of a shark cornea has a completely random arrangement of collagen fibers and yet still meets the coherent scattering conditions for transparency.

The crystalline lens is not as transparent as the cornea. The lens has a slight yellow pigment to it, and also scatters more light. In cataract formation, the protein in the crystalline lens clumps together, fluid pools form, and this causes additional scattering. Thus, a cataract degrades vision by scattering light. As the cataract grows, the amount of scatter increases. Eventually, in order to restore useful vision, the cataractous crystalline lens must be surgically removed.

The vitreous is a composite of a 1% hyaluronic acid solution interspersed with collagen fibers approximately 10 nm in diameter. These fibers are much smaller than the corneal fibers and the vitreous scatters only 0.1% of the incident light. With age, vitreous collagen fibers can coalesce, fluid pockets form, and localized scattering develops. In this case the patient reports seeing floating specks and threads. (In some cases, the floaters may resemble Fresnel diffraction patterns.)

The healthy retina scatters about as much light as the cornea. However, when the blood supply is interrupted, the retinal integrity is damaged, and edema fluid starts collecting in the nerve fiber layer. This increases the retinal light scattering, and that area turns milky gray (clinically referred to as cotton wool spots).

23.7 SCATTERING AND SELECTIVE ABSORPTION

In the animal world, Rayleigh scattering and selective absorption often combine to give a Tyndall blue color. The basic mechanism is for the scattering particles to appear in front of a layer of dark melanin pigment. The scattering particles might be collagen fibers, air vesicles, protein, keratin, or guanine crystals. The blue in the feathers of a blue jay is caused by scattering from air vesicles. Tyndall blues include those on baboons, on a turkey's neck, and on many reptiles including chameleons. One can distinguish between iridescent blues due to diffraction and interference effects (e.g., the Morpho butterly) from Tyndall blues (scattering) by the fact that interference colors change rapidly with viewing angle, and are immediately altered by immersion in a fluid; whereas Tyndall blues are independent of viewing angle and do not change color rapidly upon immersion.

Iris color is due to the scattering–selective absorption combination. The human iris is backed by a heavily pigmented epithelial layer. The apparent iris color depends on the amount of pigment that lies in the layers anterior to the epithelial layer. When the layers in front have little pigment, the eyes are blue. The bluish appearance is due to Rayleigh scattering from the fine gossamer stromal fibers in the anterior layers. When the anterior layers have more pigment, the pigment contributes a yellow component. This yellow coupled with the scattered blue gives green eyes. Still more pigment in the anterior layers results in brown eyes. Albino eyes have no pigment. Here the reddish light diffusely reflected (scattered) from the blood in the iris capillaries coupled with the scattered blue from the stromal fibers gives a pinkish appearance.

23.8 RESONANCE RADIATION

In the previous section, we considered scattering from transparent structures in the presence of a selective absorber. Here we want to consider "scattering" from the absorbers themselves.

First we need to further consider how the atomic electrons respond to the incident radiation. The atomic electrons are bound to the nucleus by attractive electromagnetic forces. For our present purposes, let us conceptually represent the electromagnetic binding force by a spring. In this model, we consider the electrons to have certain natural vibration frequencies (i.e., the natural vibration frequencies of the spring). These natural vibration frequencies are called the resonance frequencies of the atom.

When an electromagnetic wave is incident on the atom, it drives the electron into a dipole vibration that has the same frequency as that of the incident radiation. When the incident frequency is far from the resonance frequency f_o, the dipole vibration is small (Figure 23.6). However, when the incident frequency f matches the resonance frequency f_o, the vibration is greatly amplified.

We can intuitively understand the amplification as follows. When the incident radiation is at f_o, each push that it gives the atomic electron matches the electron's natural vibration direction (just like correctly pushing a swing). Hence the resulting vibration becomes very large. On the other hand, when the incident frequency is very different from f_o, the resulting vibration is small, because the resonance amplification does not occur. (This is analogous to trying to push a swing at the wrong times.)

The magnitude of the electron's vibration is limited by the damping factor q. The damping factor depends on those things that drain off energy from the electron. These include re-radiation, loss of energy through atomic collisions (heat), or chemical changes. From the differential equations for a damped oscillator, the square of the electron's vibration amplitude is proportional to

$$\frac{1}{(f_o^2 - f^2)^2 + (qf)^2}$$

For a medium that is not too dense (few atomic collisions), the damping factor q is small. Then when f is far from f_o, the first term in the denominator is large and the vibration amplitude is small. However, when f equals f_o, the first term in the denominator vanishes, and only the small second term remains. Here the vibration amplitude is very large (i.e., the resonance amplification).

For a material, we would expect the absorption strength k to somehow depend on the electron's vibration amplitude. We would also expect that k would depend on the density δ of the material. For materials that are not too dense (e.g., a gas), we can use some simplifying approximations together with the electron's vibration amplitude to derive the following expression for the absorption strength k:

$$k = \frac{-\delta E g f}{(f_o^2 - f^2)^2 + (qf)^2} \quad (23.9)$$

where E is a parameter that depends on the atomic electron's mass and charge. Note that the denominator is the same as that of the square of the electron's vibration amplitude.

Figure 23.7 is a plot of the absorption strength as a function of the incident frequency f. For a small q, the absorption strength k forms a deep, narrow "hole" centered on f_o. For a larger q, the hole is shallower.

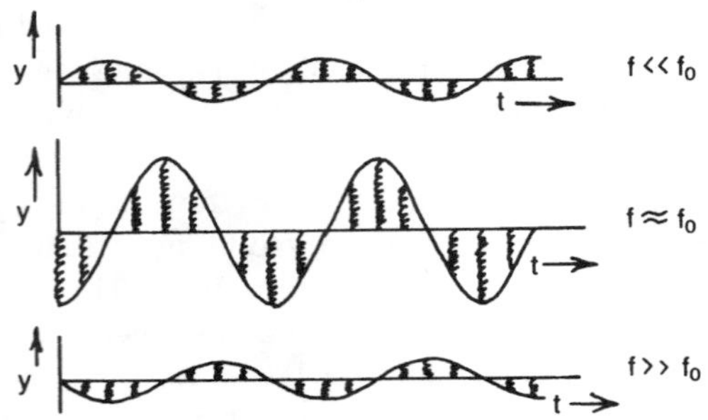

Figure 23.6 Vibration response of an atomic electron with a resonance frequency f_o illuminated by light of frequency f.

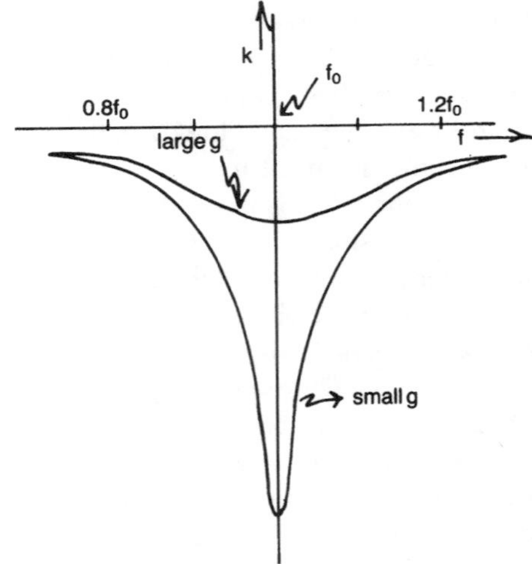

Figure 23.7 Absorption strength k for two different damping factors.

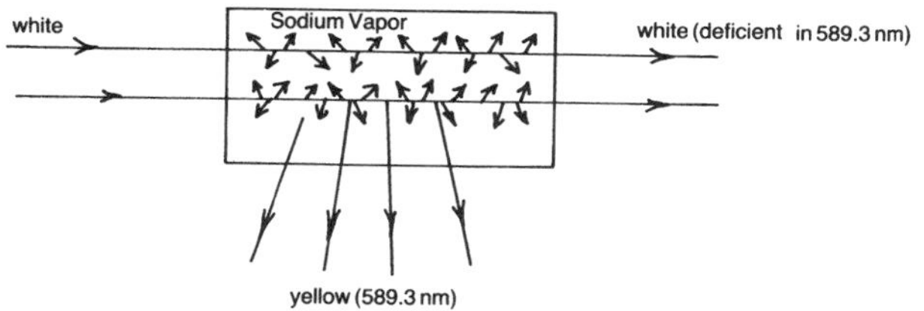

Figure 23.8 Resonance radiation (or resonance scattering).

Now we are ready to consider resonance radiation. Consider white light incident on a sodium vapor. Sodium has a strong resonance (small g) at the sodium D wavelength of 589.3 nm. (Actually, there are two overlapping resonances—at 589.0 nm and 589.6 nm with 589.3 nm as the average of the overlapping resonances.) For transparent particles (no resonances in the visible spectrum), we would expect Rayleigh scattering from the vapor. However, the sodium atoms have an amplified vibration response to 589.3 nm, and hence re-radiate very strongly at that wavelength. Consequently, the yellow re-radiated light of the sodium doublet overwhelms the expected Rayleigh scattering (Figure 23.8). The re-radiation of the light at the resonance frequency of the atom is referred to as *resonance radiation* or sometimes as *resonance scattering*. As a consequence, the transmitted light is deficient in the sodium yellow wavelengths.

A good diffraction grating shows that sunlight is missing some very specific wavelengths including the sodium D wavelength. The hot core of the sun emits these wavelengths, but the "cooler" vapors in the sun's outer atmosphere undergo resonance scattering. Hence, the transmitted light that is incident on earth is deficient in the resonance wavelengths of the elements in the vapor.

23.9 DISPERSION

In Section 23.5, we saw that a refracted wave is actually made by a coherent scattering process. The refracted wave appears to travel through the medium at a speed of c/n, where n is the refractive index of the medium. The refractive index is a function of the frequency (or wavelength) of the incident light. The fact that the different frequencies of electromagnetic radiation travel through a material at different speeds is called dispersion. Dispersion is responsible for chromatic aberration.

The higher the refractive index, the slower a wave propagates through a medium. We would intuitively expect that the refractive index would depend on the density δ of the medium. Since a coherent scattering process makes the refracted wave, we might also intuitively expect that it would depend on the vibration response of the electrons in the medium. Again, for a material that is not too dense (e.g., a gas), we can make some simplifying approximations, and derive that

$$n = 1 + \frac{\delta E(f_o^2 - f^2)}{(f_o^2 - f^2)^2 + (qf)^2} \tag{23.10}$$

Note that the denominator of the second term is the same as that of the square of the electron's vibration amplitude. In fact, it is the same as the denominator for the absorption strength k.

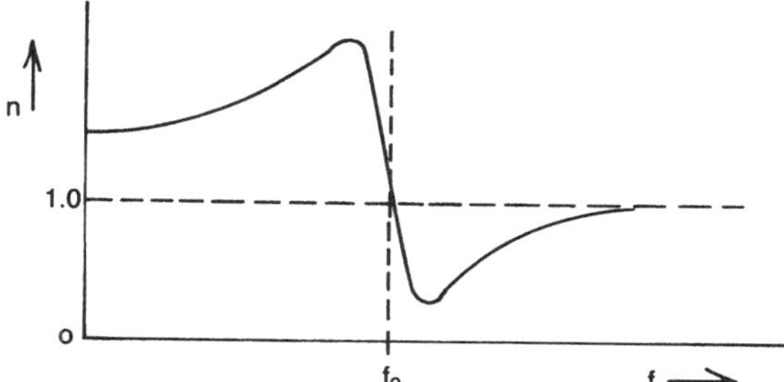

Figure 23.9 Dispersion curve for a single resonance.

Figure 23.9 shows a plot of the refractive index n versus the incident frequency f for a small non-zero damping factor q. For f well below the resonance frequency f_o, the refractive index increases slowly with increasing f. This slow increase is characteristic of transparent materials and is referred to as *normal dispersion*. As f approaches the resonance, the refractive index starts to increase much faster. For a zero damping factor, the refractive index n would go to infinity at the resonance frequency f_o. However, the non-zero damping factor prohibits the refractive index from going to infinity. Instead, the damping factor causes the refractive index curve to turn down and equal 1 at f_o. Above the resonance, n decreases some more and then starts to increase again. As f goes to infinity, the refractive index increases to 1. The behavior of the refractive index near and above f_o is referred to as *anomalous dispersion*. (The meaning of $n < 1$ is discussed in the next section).

Even though the above equations are derived under a low density approximation, they actually work well for many optical materials. For a material with multiple resonances, the resonance term in Eq. 23.10 is replaced by the sum of the terms for each resonance:

$$n = 1 + \sum_{i=1}^{m} \frac{\delta E(f_i^2 - f^2)}{(f_i^2 - f^2) + (qf)^2} \tag{23.11}$$

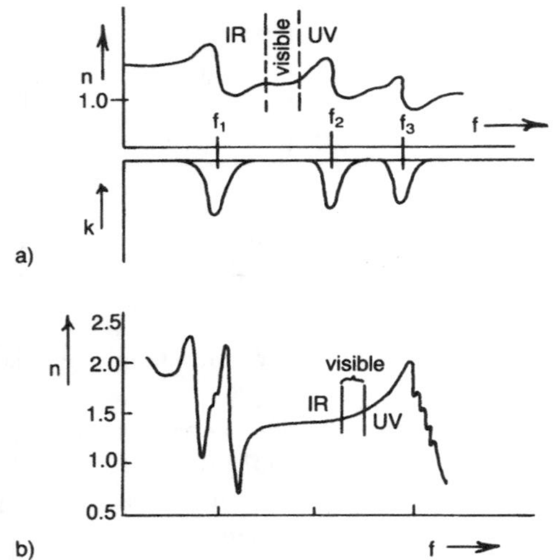

Figure 23.10 a, Dispersion and absorption curves for a material with three resonances; b, dispersion curve for crown glass.

where m is the number of resonances and f_i is the ith resonance frequency. Figure 23.10a shows plots of the index of refraction and the absorption strength curve for a hypothetical material with three resonances. Figure 23.10b shows the actual refractive index (dispersion curve) for clear crown glass. The glass has several strong resonances well below the visible region. The closest resonance to the visible region is the resonance in the ultraviolet. The resonance in the ultraviolet means that normal glass becomes opaque in the ultraviolet. The dispersion in the visible region is due to the nearness of the resonance in the ultraviolet. If that resonance had been further away, the dispersion would be smaller in the visible region.

One way to achieve a higher index glass is to pick a chemical composition that results in the ultraviolet resonance being closer to the visible region. These high index glasses tend to absorb some blue (hence, the transmitted light is slightly yellowish). The high index glasses also tend to have more dispersion than the lower index glasses. Barium crown glass is an exception in the sense that it has low dispersion for a high index glass.

It is clear from the Eqs. 23.9 through 23.11 that both absorption and dispersion are tied to the magnitude of the electron's vibration response to the incoming radiation. In that sense, both the absorption behavior and the dispersion behavior are determined by the resonances of a material. The relationship is so strong that the refractive index n and the absorption strength k can be combined into a complex index of refraction η where

$$\eta = n + ik$$

and $i = \sqrt{-1}$. This leads to a modification of Frensel's Law of reflection from an interface between air ($\eta_1 = n_1 = 1$) and an absorbing medium ($\eta_2 = n_2 + ik$). Now the decimal reflection coefficient R is given by

$$R = \frac{(n_2 - 1)^2 + k^2}{(n_2 + 1)^2 + k^2} \tag{23.12}$$

When k is zero (no absorption, a transparent material), Eq. 23.12 is equivalent to Eq. 14.2. However, when k is non-zero, then it contributes to the reflection coefficient R. In particular, R approaches 1 for a very strong absorption strength k. In other words, a very strong absorber (such as a metal) is also a very strong reflector.

EXAMPLE 23.1

A transparent glass with an 1.50 index reflects 4.0% of the incident light (i..e., $R = 0.04$). How much light is reflected by an absorbing glass with $\eta = 1.50 + i3.00$?

Here 3.00 is the absorption strength k. From Eq. 23.12,

$$R = \frac{(1.50 - 1)^2 + 3^2}{(1.50 + 1)^2 + 3^2} = \frac{9.25}{15.25} = 0.61$$

So the absorbing glass reflects 61% of the incident light.

23.10 GROUP VERSUS PHASE VELOCITY

The speed v, where $v = c/n$, is the speed at which a point of fixed phase propagates in a harmonic wave of frequency f. For example, a crest is a fixed phase of 90°. When two harmonic waves of slightly different frequencies are superposed, the result is the beat phenomenon (Section 21.6). In a vacuum, both harmonic waves travel with speed c, and so the beat also travels with speed c.

However, in a dispersive medium, the two harmonic waves travel at different phase velocities. Therefore, the crests of the two waves will not stay lined up, and the beat is going to propagate at a different speed than either component. Usually the beat velocity is slower than that of either component, and is called the group velocity u. The group velocity u is related to the phase velocity v by

$$u = v - (\text{dispersive term})$$

or

$$u = \frac{c}{n} - (\text{dispersive term})$$

In a vacuum, the dispersive term is zero, and n equals 1, so $u = v = c$. When n is less than 1 (anomalous dispersion), the dispersive term is large enough so that u stays less than c.

Light sources have a finite emission time; consequently, wavepackets have a finite length (Figure 21.19). Similar to beats, we can consider the wavepackets to be made up of a superposition of a number of harmonic waves each of slightly different frequency. In a vacuum all the harmonic components, and consequently the packet itself, move with the speed c. In a dispersive medium, each harmonic component moves with a different speed. This has two effects: (1) the packet spreads out as it moves through the medium; (2) the packet moves slower than the phase velocity of the harmonic components (exactly analogous to the beat behavior except that more than two components are involved).

The theory of relativity says that energy (information) cannot propagate faster than the vacuum speed c of light. The packets convey the energy (or the information), and the relativity limit says that the packet or group velocity must be less than c. For anomalous dispersion where $n < 1$, the group velocity is still less than c because of the dispersive term. (Michelson was the first to actually measure a difference between a phase and a group velocity. He found that when the phase velocity for CS_2 is $c/1.64$, the group velocity is $c/1.76$.)

23.11 POLARIZATION FUNDAMENTALS

Electromagnetic waves are transverse and can therefore be polarized. For electromagnetic waves propagating perpendicular to the plane of the paper, the double-headed arrows in Figure 23.11 show the vibration plane of the electrical field component for three different polarization states: vertical, horizontal, and diagonal.

A dipole with a vertical axis produces vertically polarized light. However, in our natural environment,

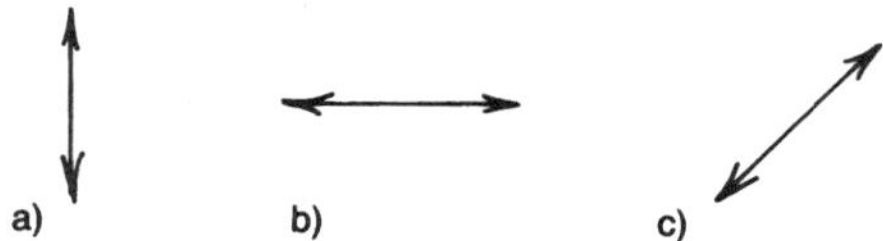

Figure 23.11 Vibration meridians for polarized light: a, vertical; b, horizontal; c, oblique.

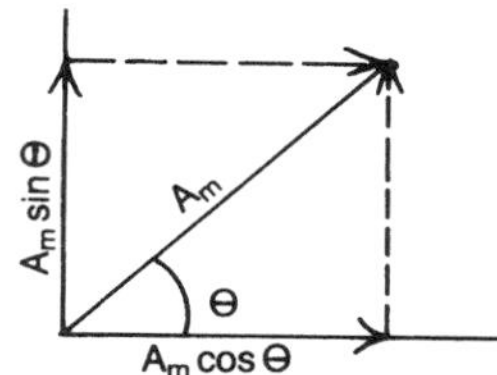

Figure 23.12 Resolution into perpendicular polarization components.

light is incident from many atomic and molecular dipoles with differing orientations. In addition, the same atomic dipole radiates for at most 10^{-8} s, and then may change orientation before radiating again. Hence, the light in our normal environment is a completely random mixture of waves vibrating in all planes. Such light is called unpolarized. In unpolarized light, there is a randomly fluctuating phase relationship between the waves vibrating in different planes. Partially polarized light can be made by mixing polarized and unpolarized light.

The arrow in Figure 23.12 represents the amplitude A_m of a wave that is plane-polarized at an angle θ with the horizontal. The irradiance (intensity) I_m of the wave is proportional to $(A_m)^2$. Like a vector, the polarized light can be resolved into perpendicular components. From Figure 23.12, the horizontal component has an amplitude of $A_m \cos\theta$, while the vertical component has an amplitude of $A_m \sin\theta$. The oscillations of the horizontal and vertical components are correlated in that both reach their maximums at the same time, both reach their minimums at the same time, etc. The irradiance I_x of the horizontal component varies like the square of its amplitude:

$$I_x = (A_m \cos\theta)^2$$

Then,

$$I_x = I_m \cos^2\theta \tag{23.13}$$

A similar equation for the vertical component contains the square of the sine function. Eq. 23.13 is known as the law of Malus, named after Etienne Malus (1775–1812), who discovered polarization of light in 1808.

The superposition of two perpendicularly polarized waves never gives destructive interference. After all, a vertical displacement cannot cancel a horizontal displacement. For complete destructive and constructive interference to occur, the light that is superposed must be identically polarized.

In Young's double-slit experiment, the incident light was unpolarized. This unpolarized light consisted of equal amounts of uncorrelated horizontal and vertical polarization components. The interference fringes were produced by the right slit horizontal components interfering with the left slit horizontal components, and similarly the vertical components interfering with each other. This can be checked using polarization filters, such as polaroids, over the slits. When the filters both transmit only vertically polarized light, the interference fringes still have a visibility of 1. Fringe visibility of 1 also occurs when both filters transmit only horizontally polarized light. However, when one filter transmits vertically polarized light and the other transmits horizontally polarized light, no interference fringes occur (i.e., zero visibility). Thus, for two waves to be mutually coherent, the waves must have the same polarization state together with a correlated phase relation.

Partial coherence (fringe visibility less than 1) can occur for polarization states that are neither aligned nor perpendicular. Here, the horizontal components of one beam interfere with the horizontal components of the other beam, and similarly for the vertical components. Suppose the diagonally polarized light in Figure 23.12 is superposed with horizontally polarized light. When the two beams have a fixed phase relation, the horizontal components give constructive and destructive interference. The vertical component of the diagonally polarized light has nothing to interfere with, so it provides the uniform background that decreases the visibility of the interference fringes.

23.12 POLAROID

In a dielectric material, the electrons are bound to the atoms and/or the molecules. In a metal, the conduction electrons are free to move throughout the metal. Because the conduction electrons are free to move, they respond very strongly to incident light, which is why metals are such fantastically strong absorbers of light.

When light is incident normally on a thin metal disk, the vertically polarized component drives the electrons to vibrate vertically, while the horizontally polarized component drives the electrons to vibrate horizontally. Suppose the metal disk is replaced by a grid of very fine vertical metal wires. The conduction electrons are free to run up and down the metal wires, and so they still strongly absorb light that is plane-polarized vertically. However, the horizontal movement of the conduction electrons is restricted. When the wire diameters are small relative to the wavelength of the light, the restriction prevents the absorption of the horizontal component, and it is transmitted (Figure 23.13). (In other words, the vertical grid "looks" like a solid metal disk to the vertically polarized light, and "looks" transparent to the horizontally polarized light.)

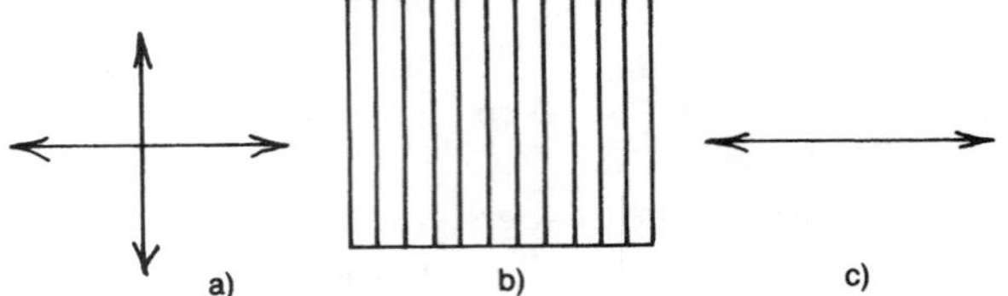

Figure 23.13 a, Unpolarized light-components are not correlated; b, wire grid polarizer; c, transmitted component.

A standard oven rack would serve as a wire grid polarizer for microwaves. A wire grid polarizer has been constructed for infrared (2,160 wires/mm). While no wire grid polarizer has been constructed for visible light, polaroid works on the same principle.

J-sheet polaroid was invented in 1928 by Edwin Land, then a 19-year-old undergraduate student at Harvard. Besides polarizing, J-sheet scattered light and thus had a hazy appearance. In 1938, Land invented the widely used H-sheet polaroid. The process consists of heating a sheet of clear polyvinyl alcohol, and stretching it in one direction. During the stretching, the sheet's long hydrocarbon molecules become aligned. The sheet is then dipped in an ink solution rich with iodine. The iodine impregnates the plastic and attaches to the straight long chained molecules effectively forming a chain of its own. The iodine's conduction electrons can move along the iodine chains as if they were long thin wires.

The absorption axis of the polaroid is aligned with the iodine chains. The transmission axis of the polaroid is perpendicular to the iodine chains. Thus, when the iodine chains are vertical, the transmission axis is horizontal. (Warning: many elementary books have simplified picket fence models that give the impression that the chains are aligned with the transmission axis.)

When two perfect polaroids are perpendicularly crossed (e.g., one with a horizontal absorption axis and one with a vertical absorption axis), no light is transmitted. The second polaroid is frequently referred to as the *analyzer* since it is analyzing the plane polarization properties of the light incident on it. H-sheet starts to lose its effectiveness for the shorter visible wavelengths (the violets), so when two H-sheet polaroids are crossed, a little violet is transmitted. For the most part, we will neglect the violet leakage.

When unpolarized light is incident on an ideal polaroid, the transmitted light consists of the 50% that is vibrating in the plane of the polaroid's transmission axis. Such an ideal polaroid is referred to as HN-50. In reality, there are surface reflections (about 4%) at each surface. So we would be down to a 42% transmission for unpolarized light (HN-42). In real polaroids, some absorption also occurs. The widely used types of H-sheet polaroid are HN-38, HN-32, and HN-22.

For plane-polarized light incident on an ideal polaroid (HN-50), the irradiance of the light transmitted varies like the law of Malus (Eq. 23.13), provided θ is the angle between the polarization plane of the incident light and the transmission axis of the polaroid. When the polarization plane is aligned with the transmission axis of an ideal polaroid ($\theta = 0$), 100% of the light is transmitted. When the polarization plane is parallel to the absorption axis, it is perpendicular to the transmission axis. Here, θ equals 90°, and no transmission occurs.

EXAMPLE 23.2
Vertically polarized light is incident on an ideal polaroid with an absorption axis rotated 35°, from the vertical. What percent of the light is transmitted?

The transmission axis is perpendicular to the absorption axis, or 55° from the vertical (Figure 23.14). Before calculating, you should ask whether you expect the percent transmission to be high (greater than 50%) or low (less than 50%). Since the absorption axis is closer to the polarization plane, we should expect a low transmission.

For the ideal polaroid (HN-50), we neglect the surface reflections. From Eq. 23.13,

$$I = I_m \cos^2 (55°)$$
$$= I_m(0.57)^2 = I_m(0.33)$$

So for this case, 33% of the incident light (i.e., I_m) is transmitted (in agreement with the expectations).

EXAMPLE 23.3
Unpolarized light is incident on a two polaroid system. The second polaroid has a transmission axis rotated 25° relative to the first. Neglecting surface reflections, what is the percent of the original incident light that is transmitted through both polaroids?

We will assume the polaroids are ideal (HN-50). Then the first polaroid transmits 50%. We should expect a high transmission for the second polaroid since the incident polarization plane is fairly close to the transmission axis. Equation 23.13 gives the transmission of the second as:

$$I = I_m \cos^2 (25°)$$
$$= I_m(0.82)$$

The total transmission is the product, (0.50) (0.82), or 41%.

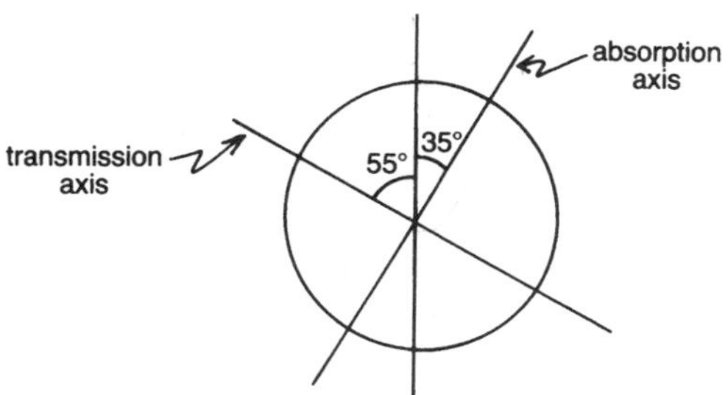

Figure 23.14 Polaroid with an absorption axis 35° from the vertical.

23.13 POLARIZATION PLANE ROTATION BY POLAROIDS

An ideal system with two crossed polaroids transmits no light. A remarkable property of polaroids is that when a third polaroid is placed between the two crossed polaroids, transmission can occur. This transmission is due to rotation of the polarization plane by the middle polaroid.

EXAMPLE 23.4
Consider a three polaroid system in which the first polaroid has a vertical transmission axis and the last polaroid has a horizontal transmission axis. Assume that the transmission axis of the middle polaroid makes an angle of 30° with the vertical. For incident unpolarized light, what percent of the original light is transmitted through the system?

We will assume HN-50 (ideal) polaroids, so the first polaroid transmits 50% of the light, and that light is polarized vertically. We can find the transmission of the second polaroid from the law of Malus, (Eq. 23.13),

$$I = I_m \cos^2 (30°)$$
$$= I_m(0.75)$$

This light is polarized at an angle of 30° with the vertical, or 60° with the horizontal. So the transmission for the last polaroid is

$$I = I_m \cos^2 (60°)$$
$$= I_m(0.25)$$

The total transmission for the three polaroid system is then

$$(0.50)(0.75)(0.25) = 0.094$$

or 9.4% of the incident light.

Thus, when all three polaroids are present, 9.4% of the incident light is transmitted. When the middle polaroid is removed, leaving only the two crossed polaroids, no light is transmitted. The 9.4% transmission occurs because the middle polaroid acts to rotate the plane of the polarized light. When the first and last polaroid are perpendicularly crossed, the maximum transmission for incident unpolarized light through a three polaroid system occurs when the middle polaroid has a transmission axis at 45° to that of the first polaroid (see the problems).

23.14 POLARIZATION BY REFLECTION

Light can be partially or completely polarized by specular reflection from dielectrics. Anyone who has looked through polaroid sunglasses at the sun's reflection from water has probably noticed this effect. It is only necessary to tilt the head from side to side, thus tilting the polaroids, to observe the intensity changes in the reflected light that is transmitted through the polaroids.

We can use Figure 23.15 to help understand why the reflected light may be partially or completely polarized. Unpolarized light in the medium of refractive index n_1 is incident on the flat surface of the medium with refractive index n_2. Figure 23.15 shows the case where the angle between the refracted ray and the reflected ray is 90°. The incident unpolarized light can be resolved into two perpendicular components: one oscillating perpendicular to the paper (represented by the dots) and the other oscillating in the plane shown by the double-headed arrows.

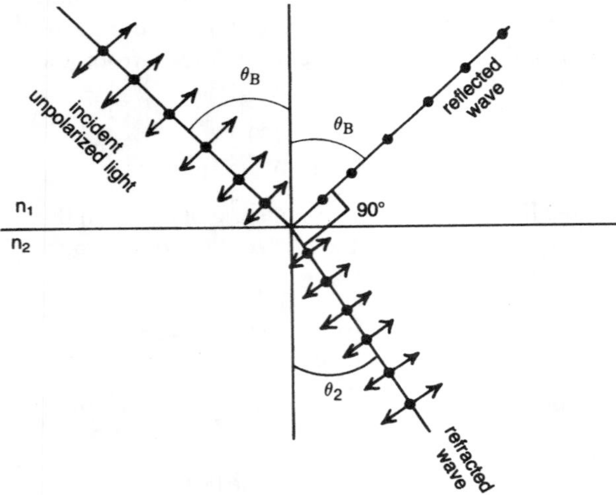

Figure 23.15 Geometry for polarization by reflection.

The light represented by the dots sets up dipole vibrations in the surface zone of the second medium. The axis of these dipoles is perpendicular to the plane of the paper, and so the dipoles re-radiate maximally in that plane. From a coherent scattering viewpoint, both the reflected and refracted waves are then generated by constructive interference of the re-radiated waves.

The light represented by the double-headed arrows sets up dipole vibrations that are in the same plane as the arrows. The axes of these dipoles are parallel to the direction of the reflected light. Since dipoles do not radiate along their axes, no light is re-radiated in the reflected direction. Hence, no reflection occurs for this component of the incident light.

Thus, when the reflected direction is perpendicular to the refracted direction, the light that is specularly reflected is plane-polarized in the plane of the surface. The incident angle at which this occurs is referred to as Brewster's angle. We can derive an equation for Brewster's angle by starting with Snell's Law

$$n_1 \sin \theta_B = n_2 \sin \theta_2$$

Because the angle of reflection equals the angle of incidence, and because of the 90° angle between the reflected and the refracted rays, we have

$$180° = \theta_B + 90° + \theta_2$$

or

$$\theta_2 = 90° - \theta_B$$

Then,

$$n_1 \sin \theta_B = n_2 \sin (90° - \theta_B)$$

Since $\cos \theta = \sin (90° - \theta)$, Snell's law becomes

$$n_1 \sin \theta_B = n_2 \cos \theta_B$$

and it follows that

$$\tan \theta_B = \frac{n_2}{n_1} \tag{23.14}$$

Equation 23.14 is referred to as Brewster's law after Sir David Brewster who discovered it empirically. (Brewster also invented the kaleidoscope). Equation 23.14 specifies that for dielectrics Brewster's angle depends only on the ratio of the refractive indices of the two materials. In particular, for a material of index n_2 in air ($n_1 = 1$), Brewster's angle can be used to determine the refractive index of the material.

EXAMPLE 23.5
Unpolarized light in air is incident on ophthalmic crown glass ($n = 1.523$). At what incident angle is the reflected light completely polarized?

From Eq. 23.14,

$$\tan \theta_B = 1.523/1$$

or

$$\theta_B = 56.7^\circ$$

Similarly, Brewster's angle for an air–water ($n = 1.333$) surface is 53.1°.

The above discussion shows that when unpolarized light is incident at Brewster's angle on a horizontal dielectric plane (e.g., glass or water), the light specularly reflected is plane-polarized horizontally. When vertically polarized light is incident at Brewster's angle on a horizontal dielectric plane, no light is specularly reflected.

Polaroid sunglasses with a vertical transmission axis do not transmit the horizontally polarized light reflected at Brewster's angle from flat horizontal surfaces. Such sunglasses reduce the glare that arises from specular reflection from water and from roads. These sunglasses do not reduce glare arising from reflections from a vertical surface, such as office building windows.

While specular reflection tends to polarize light, diffuse reflection does not. In fact, polarized light that is diffusely reflected is depolarized.

23.15 POLARIZATION BY SCATTERING

Scattered light can become either completely or partially polarized for essentially the same reasons that apply to specularly reflected light. Figure 23.16 shows unpolarized light incident on a scattering center. The dots represent the component vibrating perpendicular to the plane of the paper. This light sets up a dipole vibration in the scattering center, and the dipole re-radiates maximally in the plane of the paper (including points *A*, *B*, and *C*). The vertical double-headed arrows represent the other polarization component of the incident light. This component sets up a dipole vibration with a vertical axis. Since dipoles do not radiate along their axes, no re-radiation occurs in the vertical direction (point *B*). Thus, the scattered light reaching point *B* is plane-polarized perpendicular to the plane of the paper. At other points (e.g., *A* and *C*), the scattered light is partially polarized.

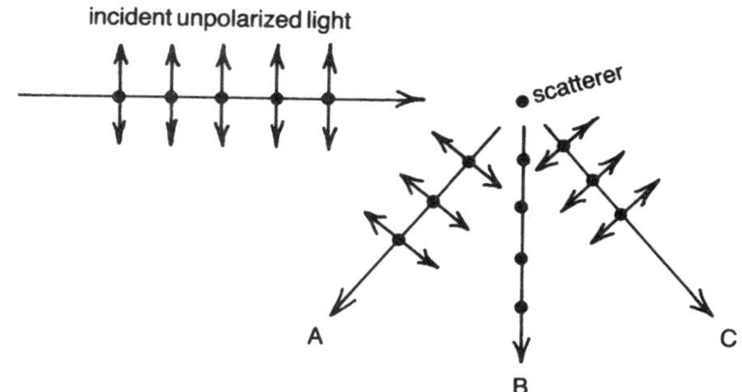

Figure 23.16 Geometry for polarization by scattering.

As a consequence, skylight at 90° to the sun is polarized. As the angle varies from 90°, the polarization decreases. The polarization of skylight is noticeable when wearing polaroid sunglasses. (Bee's eyes have built-in polarization detectors, and they appear to use the polarization information in their dance that tells other bees where to look for honey sources.)

Multiple scattered light is depolarized. Thus, while the blue sky tends to be polarized, the white clouds are not.

23.16 BIREFRINGENCE

When one views objects through a properly oriented, transparent, polished calcite crystal, the image is doubled (Figure 23.17). This phenomenon is known as birefringence, or double refraction. The light associated with each image is plane-polarized perpendicular to that of the other.

The underlying reason for the appearance of the double images is that the calcite crystal is anisotropic, which means the material has a different structure in different directions. The wire grid polarizer is anisotropic, and so are many crystal lattices.

We will not consider the exact structure of the calcite lattice. Instead, Figure 23.18 shows a simple

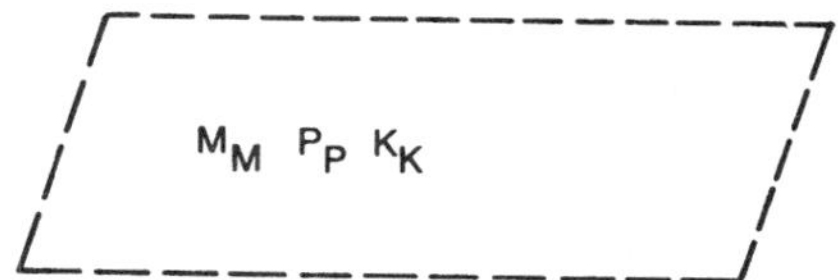

Figure 23.17 Double images of birefringence.

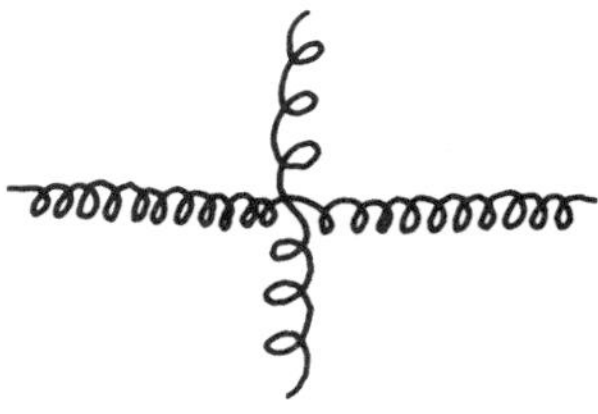
Figure 23.18 Representation of forces in an anisotropic material.

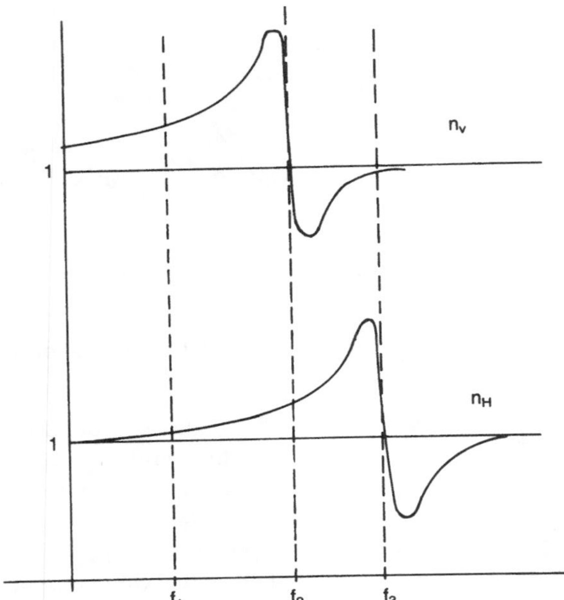

Figure 23.19 Dispersion curves for the vertical and horizontal components.

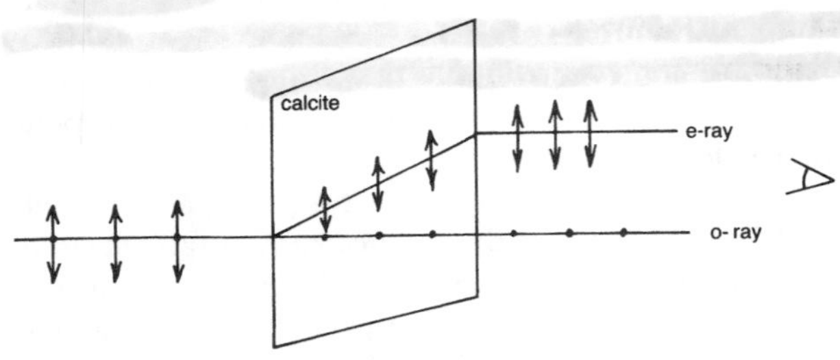

Figure 23.20 Extraordinary and ordinary rays for a calcite crystal.

spring model of an anisotropic lattice with a horizontal and a vertical axis. The horizontal set of springs represents a different molecular force than the vertical set of springs. Since the forces are different, the natural or resonant frequencies differ for vertically versus horizontally polarized light. The refractive index and the absorption strength for the vertically polarized light is determined by the vertical resonances, while the refractive index and the absorption strength for the horizontally polarized light is determined by horizontal resonances.

Figure 23.19 shows dispersion curves for both the vertical direction (i.e., the refractive index n_V versus frequency f) and the horizontal direction (n_H versus f). The vertical resonance occurs at frequency f_2, while the horizontal resonance occurs at frequency f_3. For incident frequency f_1, the anisotropic medium is transparent for both the horizontally and vertically polarized light. However, the refractive indices are different for the two polarizations. This difference in refractive index leads to the birefringence or double refraction phenomenon. When light propagates down the internal optical axis of a crystal, the different polarization components travel at different speeds due to the different indices of refraction.

Figure 23.20 shows unpolarized light incident normal to a calcite crystal where the light is traveling at an angle to the internal optical axis of the crystal (i.e., the crystal is cut so that the front surface is not perpendicular to the internal optical axis). The polarization component perpendicular to the plane of the paper (the dots) behaves as expected, and the associated ray is called the ordinary or o-ray. This component experiences an "ordinary" refractive index labeled n_o. The polarization component represented by the double-headed arrows does not behave as expected, instead it moves diagonally upward as it propagates through the crystal. The ray associated with this component is labeled the extraordinary or e-ray. This component experiences an "extraordinary" refractive index n_e. Figure 23.20 shows that the e-ray and the o-ray give the double images of Figure 23.17, and that these images are polarized perpendicular to each other.

While the o-ray (or o-wave) is easy to understand, the e-ray (or e-wave) is not. The following analogy supplies some intuition about the situation. Consider a truck that is parked along a North–South street. You are in the truck bed facing North and you are going to walk down a wide ramp to the ground. If the ramp happens to be a little icy, you may slip some as you go down the ramp, but you are still moving North as you go down it. This is analogous to the o-wave. Now suppose that some boxes are placed under the East side of the ramp (i.e., on your right) at the bottom and top. This makes the West side of the ramp lower than the East side (in addition to the ramp sloping down to the ground). When you attempt to walk straight down the somewhat icy ramp, your foot slips a little to the West (your left) with each step (as well as possibly slipping a little straight down the ramp). The net effect as you move down the ramp is that you now slip some

Table 23.1 Refractive Indices for some Birefringent Materials

	n_o	n_e
Calcite	1.658	1.486
Quartz	1.544	1.553
Sodium nitrate	1.585	1.337
Ice	1.309	1.313

to the West even though you are facing North, and your path proceeds diagonally down the ramp. This is analogous to the e-wave. Each polarization component of the light experiences a different set of molecular resonances and the different ramp orientations are analogous to the different resonances.

The refractive indices n_o and n_e can be specified independent of crystal orientation. Table 23.1 shows refractive indices for a few birefringent crystals.

For the frequency f_2 in Figure 23.19, the horizontal light is transmitted, while the vertical light experiences a resonance and is absorbed. A crystal that transmits one component and absorbs the other is called dichroic. J-sheet polaroid was made with dichroic herpathite crystals.

Before polaroid was invented, the most common polarizers were prisms made from birefringent materials. These included the Nicol, Glan-Thompson, and Wollaston prisms.

23.17 CIRCULAR POLARIZATION

Unpolarized light can be considered as composed of equal amounts of perpendicularly polarized light where the phase relations between the two components randomly fluctuate. Plane-polarized light can also be regarded as composed of two perpendicular components, but in this case the phases of the two components are correlated. Figure 23.21 shows the horizontal and vertical components for light that is plane-polarized at 45° to the vertical. As the time sequence advances from t_1 through t_5, the components oscillate in phase. When plane-polarized light is incident on an electrically charged particle, it drives the particle to oscillate in the plane of the polarization.

By using anisotropic materials, we can retard the phase of one component relative to the other. Figure 23.22 shows the effect of a 90° phase retardation. At t_1, the vertical component is maximally displaced, while the horizontal component has a zero displacement. At t_2, the vertical displacement is decreasing, while the horizontal displacement is increasing. At t_3, the horizontal component has reached maximum displacement while the vertical component is zero. As a function of time, the vector sum of the horizontal and vertical displacements gives a rotating arrow. In other words, the electric field vector of the electromagnetic wave is now circularly rotating as the light propagates through space. We call this light circularly polarized. When circularly polarized light is incident on an electrically charged particle, it drives the particle to rotate in a circle. For light coming out of the plane of the paper, Figure 23.23 shows the rotation directions for right versus left circularly polarized light.

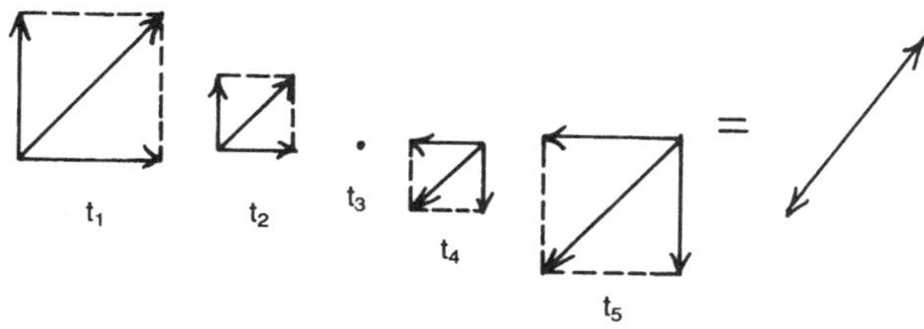

Figure 23.21 Motion picture sequence for the horizontal and vertical (correlated) components of linear polarized light.

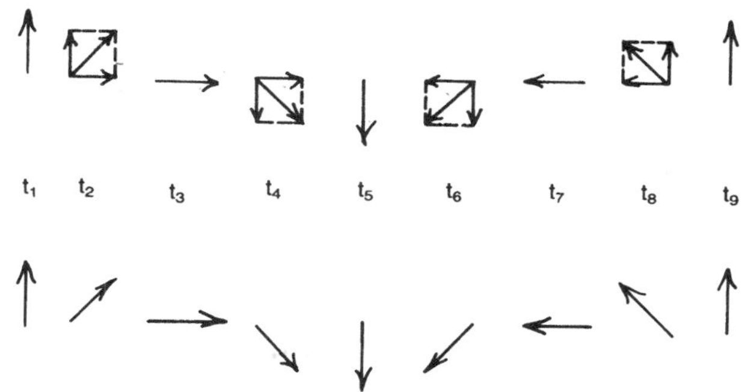

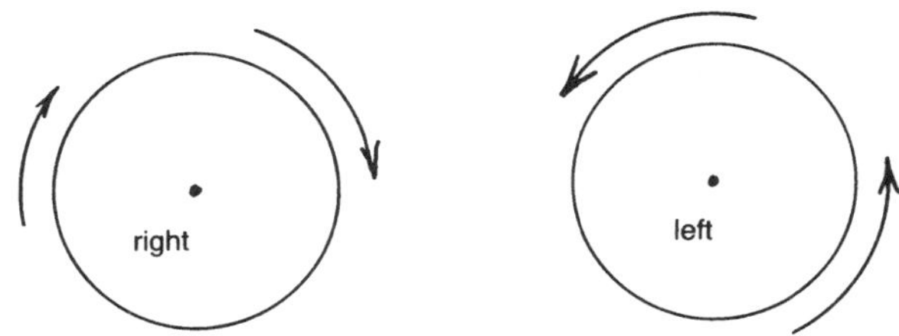

Figure 23.22 Motion picture sequence of a phase-retarded component resulting in circular polarization.

right
left

Figure 23.23 Right and left circular polarization directions for light coming out of the plane of the paper.

Circularly polarized light consists of equal amounts of plane-polarized components where the components are correlated and have a 90° phase difference. Other phase retardation values result in elliptical polarization. When elliptically polarized light is incident on an electrically charged particle, it drives the particle to rotate in an elliptical pattern. Actually, plane and circularly polarized light are special cases of elliptically polarized light.

Figure 23.24 shows the phase retardations needed to change the plane-polarized light on the left to each of the other polarization states. A phase retardation of either 90° or 270° gives circular polarization. A phase retardation of 180° gives plane polarization perpendicular to the original plane. A 360° phase retardation

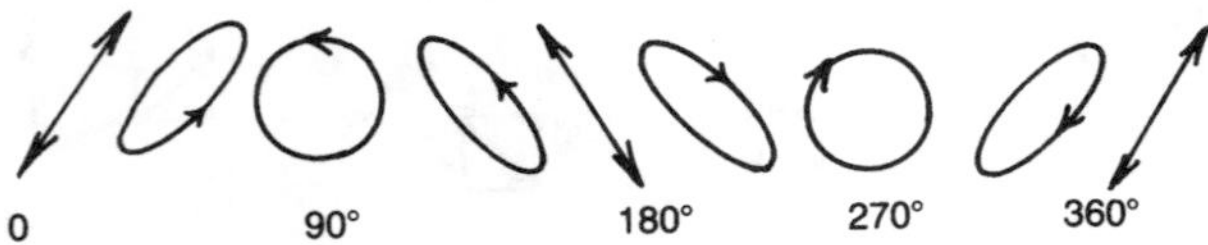

Figure 23.24 Phase retardations that give various polarization states.

gives the same polarization plane. Other phase retardation values give elliptically polarized light. The difference between the listed values gives the phase retardations needed to go from one state to another. For example, each circular polarization state differs from a plane-polarized state by a 90° phase retardation.

The above analysis shows how circularly polarized light can be made from two perpendicular plane-polarized components. A similar analysis shows that equal amounts of correlated right and left circularly polarized light can be combined to make plane polarized light.

23.18 PHASE RETARDERS

In an anisotropic material with a horizontal and vertical axis, a phase retardation between the horizontal and vertical polarization components is introduced because the wavelength of the light in the medium is different for each component (e.g., λ/n_H versus λ/n_v). The amount of phase retardation depends on these interior wavelengths plus the thickness of the material. Figure 23.25 shows horizontal and vertical components of wavelength λ incident on a halfwave plate. The plate thickness is equal to 1 interior wavelength for the horizontally polarized light and 1.5 times the interior wavelength for the vertically polarized light. The exiting components both have the same wavelength but now they are 180° out of phase. A quarterwave plate gives a 90° phase retardation, and a fullwave plate gives a 360° phase retardation.

If we neglect the violet leakage, then a polaroid with a 45° transmission axis followed by a polaroid with a 135° transmission axis does not transmit light. Suppose a fullwave plate for helium d light (587.56 nm or approximately 588 nm) has a horizontal and vertical axis and is placed between the two crossed polaroids. The 588 nm light leaving the first polaroid is plane-polarized, and the plate produces a 360° phase retardation, which gives the same polarization plane (Figure 23.24). The 588 nm light is not transmitted by the second polaroid (the analyzer).

However, the fullwave plate gives a 360° phase retardation only for 588 nm. For incident wavelengths different from 588 nm, the actual phase retardation produced by the fullwave plate differs from 360°. For the other phase retardation values, the light coming through the plate is elliptically polarized, and some of it is transmitted by the second polaroid. Since we are dealing with little or no transmission for some wavelengths, and some significant transmission for more distant wavelengths, the transmitted light is colored. A 588 nm fullwave plate between crossed polaroids gives a blue or a blue-green color. (In subtractive color terminology, this color is actually called cyan.) By adjusting the plate thickness, other colors may be obtained. These colors resemble those obtained from thin film interference, and hence are called interference colors.

For the appropriate incident wavelength, a halfwave plate placed between the two crossed polaroids flips the plane of polarization 90° resulting in 100% transmission at the second (ideal) polaroid. Wavelengths for which the plate is not quite a halfwave still have a high transmission at the second polaroid, so for incident white light the output remains white.

Mica and sheets of stretched polyvinyl alcohol are often used to make phase retarders. Common cellophane acts as a phase retarder (because of the stretching during its manufacture). Some isotropic transparent materials, such as plastic, can become anisotropic under stress. When these materials are placed

Figure 23.25 A halfwave plate.

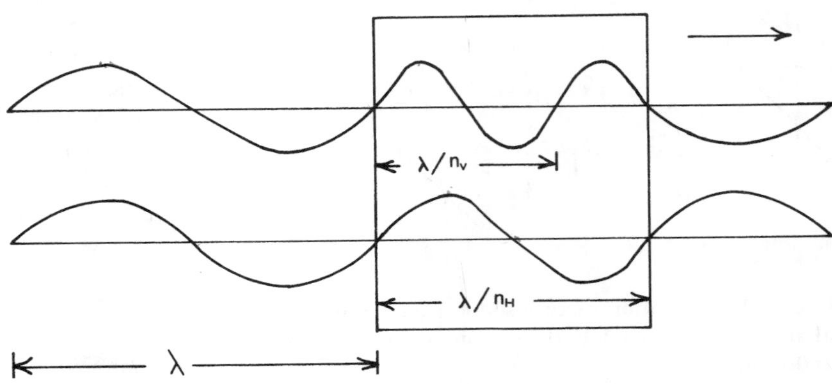

between two crossed polaroids, the differing areas of stress produce differing amounts of phase retardation, and the result is a colored map of the stress areas. This effect is called *photoelasticity* or *stress birefringence*. The stress patterns in heat-tempered glass can also be seen through crossed polaroids. (Sometimes a person wearing polaroid sunglasses can see the stress patterns in tempered automobile window glass. In this case, the scattering of the skylight serves as the polarizer, and the person's polaroids serve as the crossed polaroid analyzer.)

23.19 CIRCULAR POLARIZERS

We can make a right circular polarizer by placing a polaroid with a transmission axis at 135° in front of a quarterwave plate with a horizontal and vertical axis (Figure 23.26a). If the quarterwave plate is rotated 90° clockwise, the other polarization component is retarded and the combination is then a left circular polarizer (Figure 23.26b). The circular polarizer is definitely directionally dependent. Unpolarized light passing backwards through the circular polarizer remains unpolarized as it passes through the quarter-wave plate and then is plane-polarized by the polaroid.

Consider two identical right circular polarizers in which the quarterwave plates have a horizontal and vertical axis. Now rotate the second one 180° around a vertical axis so that it is backward relative to the first (Figure 23.27a). In this case, the two polaroids have perpendicularly crossed transmission axes, while the two quarterwave plates are still identically aligned. For light incident on the combination, the first polaroid plane polarizes the light. Then the two aligned quarter wave plates act like a single halfwave plate, and their effect is to flip the polarization plane by 90°, resulting in 100% transmission at the second polarizer. Note that the right circularly polarized light from the first polaroid and phase plate is highly transmitted when incident on the backwards right circular polarizer (i.e., the second combination).

If the first quarterwave plate is turned clockwise 90°, the first combination is a left circular polarizer (Figure 23.27b). Here the two quarterwave plates are perpendicularly crossed. One cancels the retardation of the other (zero net retardation), and they leave the polarization plane unchanged, resulting in no transmission at the second polaroid. In this case, the left circularly polarized light from the first combination is not transmitted through the backwards right circular polarizer.

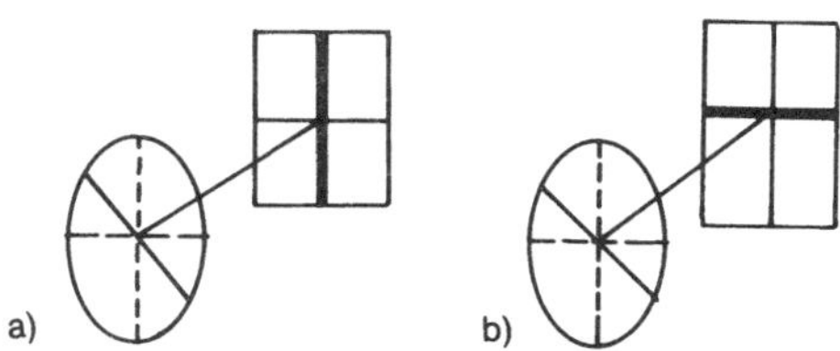

Figure 23.26 Polaroid and quarterwave plate that make a circular polarizer: a, right; b, left.

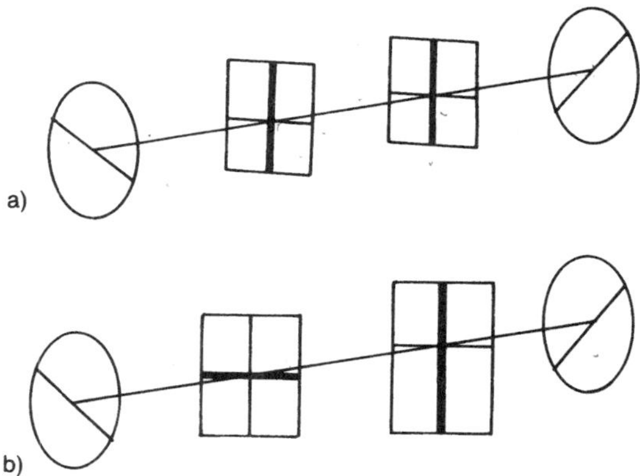

Figure 23.27 a, Right circular polarizers back to back (transmission); b, left and right circular polarizer back to back (no transmission).

Similarly, a backwards left circular polarizer transmits left circular polarized light, but does not transmit right circularly polarized light. Thus, backwards circular polarizers serve as analyzers for circular polarized light.

While linear polaroids eliminate glare due to specular reflection in the vicinity of Brewster's angle, they do not have the same property for light reflected at normal incidence. For normal incidence, we can use the polarizing–analyzing property of circular polarizers to reduce glare from reflection. Consider a video display terminal (VDT) with glare problems. When a right circular polarizer is placed over the VDT, the right circular polarized light incident on the VDT is specularly reflected as left circularly polarized light. This left circular polarized light cannot pass backwards through the right circular polarizer, so the glare is removed.

In a similar manner, circular polarizers have been used to control corneal reflex glare in direct ophthalmoscopy, and to improve the view of the corneal endothelium in slit-lamp biomicroscopy.

23.20 OPTICAL ACTIVITY AND INDUCED EFFECTS

Certain materials, particularly organic ones, rotate the plane of polarization of light that passes through them. This phenomenon is known as *optical activity*, and is important in organic chemistry and biochemistry. (You can investigate optical activity by placing common corn syrup between crossed polaroids.) When looking back toward the source, dextrorotatory (or *d*-rotatory) materials rotate the plane of polarization clockwise, and levorotatory (or *l*-rotatory) materials rotate the plane of polarization counter-clockwise.

Quartz crystal exists in two different mirror image forms. One of the mirror image forms is *l*-rotatory and the other is *d*-rotatory. There are also other crystals that have this same property.

Many organic compounds, such as sugar and turpentine, are optically active in solution or in the liquid state. When organic molecules are synthesized in the lab, equal numbers of *l*-rotatory and *d*-rotatory molecules (called stereoisomers) are produced. However, it is intriguing that many naturally occurring organic molecules consist of only one of the stereoisomers. For example, natural sugar is always *d*-rotatory. Similarly, the vast majority of amino acids, the building blocks of proteins, are *l*-rotatory.

In various circumstances, electric or magnetic fields applied to materials also rotate the plane of polarization. These are called *induced effects.* Induced effects are important in information storage, communication, and other electro-optical applications. Many calculators have liquid crystal displays that use the cross polaroid principal to make the numbers visible. I.e., when a small voltage is applied, the visible dark numbers are due to the crossed polaroid effect.

23.21 BINOCULAR VISION AND POLARIZED LIGHT

Polarized light is used clinically for studying binocular vision. Consider the letters END, where the E is covered with a vertically transmitting polaroid and the D is covered with a horizontally transmitting polaroid. Now consider a person wearing a horizontally transmitting polaroid over the left eye, and a vertically transmitting polaroid over the right eye. The person sees the N with both eyes (50% transmission). With the left eye, the person sees ND. With the right eye, the person sees EN. We can use this arrangement to tell if the person is suppressing, and if so which eye is being suppressed. For normals, we can also use this arrangement to compare clarity of the left and right images.

We can use a vectographic polaroid to actually superimpose letters that are perpendicularly polarized. A vectograph consists of two perpendicularly stretched sheets of polyvinyl alcohol. As such, there are no conduction electrons, and so, no polarizing properties. When iodine ink is used to print a letter, for example an O, on one side, the polaroid iodine chains are formed, and the O acts like a polarized O. The iodine ink can then be used to mark a different letter, say an X, on the other side, in which case the X is polarized perpendicular to the O. When a person looks through a polaroid at that spot on the vectograph, either the X or the O is seen depending on the polaroid's orientation. Vectographic slides are available for both far and near visual testing. When projecting the slide, one must make sure the screen does not depolarize the light.

Polarizers can also be used to present the slightly dissimilar views that serve as the stimulus for stereopsis. If the brain's stereopsis system is working, two flat slightly dissimilar targets result in a single three-dimensional perceived image. Systems that test this include the Worth four dot system and the stereofly.

23.22 OCULAR BIREFRINGENCE AND HAIDINGER'S BRUSH

Both the cornea and the crystalline lens are birefringent; however, there doesn't seem to be any clinical advantage to this birefringence. The macular area of the retina also has some birefringence. This results in the entoptic phenomenon called Haidinger's brush, which is clinically useful.

Suppose one stares through a polaroid at the blue sky. When the polaroid is suddenly rotated clockwise 90°, a yellowish brush appears momentarily and then fades. When the polaroid is continuously rotated at the right speed, a rotating yellowish brush is seen against the blue sky background. (The rotating brush resembles an airplane propeller.)

Haidinger's brush is due to the radially arranged nerve fiber layer of Henle, which lies over the rods and cones of the macular region. The nerve fibers are birefringent and act like a yellow radial polarizing filter. When the polarization plane is switched, the brush is visible, but then quickly fades as does any stabilized retinal image.

A Haidinger's brush apparatus consists of a blue filter and a rotating linear polaroid placed over a light bulb. It is used to detect, diagnose, and train amblyopia due to eccentric fixation. In eccentric fixation, acuity is reduced because the person fixates with a part of the peripheral retina instead of the macula. When a normal observer uses the Haidinger's brush apparatus, he or she sees the brush centered on the fixation target. When an eccentric fixator uses the apparatus, he or she sees the brush centered on a point different than the target point.

PROBLEMS

1. What is the relative Rayleigh scattering intensity for 500 nm light compared to 600 nm light?
2. Consider a multiple incoherent isotropic scattering medium in which the product of the scattering coefficient β and the thickness d is 6 (i.e., $\beta d = 6$). What is the transmission coefficient and albedo for this scattering medium?
3. Horizontally polarized light is incident on an ideal polaroid in which the transmission axis is rotated 30° from the horizontal. What percent of the incident light is transmitted?
4. Unpolarized light is incident on an ideal polaroid in which the transmission axis is rotated 60° from the horizontal. What percent of the incident light is transmitted?
5. Unpolarized light is incident on a two polaroid system. The transmission axis of the second polaroid is rotated 36° from that of the first. If the polaroids are ideal, what percent of the incident light is transmitted by the two polaroid system?
6. In a three polaroid system, the first and last polaroid have perpendicular transmission axes, while the middle polaroid has a transmission axis rotated 45° from the first. For ideal polaroids, what percent of the incident light is transmitted through the three polaroid system?
7. For light in air incident on high index plastic ($n = 1.66$), what incident angle results in 100% polarization in the reflected light?
8. For light in a medium index plastic ($n = 1.54$) incident on a glass–air interface, what incident angle results in 100% polarization in the reflected light?
9. What is Brewster's angle for polycarbonate ($n = 1.58$)?
10. What does the statement, "There is no blue in the sky nor white in the clouds" mean?
11. What is the physical explanation for Mikala Creampuff's green eyes (i.e., iris color)?
12. In terms of coherent scattering theory, why does an edematous cornea lose transparency?
13. Explain why light reflected from a dielectric surface at Brewster's angle is polarized.

CHAPTER 24

Emission, Absorption, Photons, and Lasers

24.1 THE DOPPLER SHIFT

Consider a stationary monochromatic point source in a uniform medium that emits spherical wavefronts of wavelength λ_s. In the cross sectional view of Figure 24.1a, the largest circle represents the first wavefront emitted, the next largest circle represents the second wavefront emitted, etc. The distance between successive wavefronts is λ_s.

Figure 24.1b shows the emitted wavefronts for a monochromatic point source that is moving quite fast to the right. The largest circle is centered on point 1 and represents the wavefront emitted when the point source was at position 1. The next largest circle is centered on position 2 and represents the wavefront emitted when the point source was at position 2. The next wavefront is the smallest shown and is centered on position 3. Figure 24.1b shows that the distance between the wavefronts (i.e., the wavelength) of the emitted light is shorter to the right or in front of the moving point source. Therefore for an observer looking at the source, the incident light shifted is shifted toward a shorter wavelength (a blue shift) when the source is traveling (quite fast) toward the observer. The distance between the wavefronts behind (to the left of) the moving point source is longer. Therefore to an observer looking at the source, the light is shifted toward a longer wavelength (a red shift) when the source is traveling (quite fast) away from the observer. This is called the *doppler shift*, after Johann Christian Doppler who proposed it for sound waves in 1842. When the velocity v of the source is much smaller than the speed of light c, it can be shown that the doppler shift $\Delta\lambda$ is given by

$$\Delta\lambda = \frac{v}{c}\lambda \tag{24.1}$$

where λ is the wavelength measured by an observer that is stationary with respect to the source.

EXAMPLE 24.1

One of the wavelengths strongly emitted by hot oxygen atoms is 513 nm. Consider a distant star that contains oxygen. From spectroscopy measurements on Earth, it is identified that the 513 nm wavelength is shifted to 525 nm. What is the speed of the distant star relative to Earth, and is the distant star moving toward earth or away from Earth?

The shift is toward a longer wavelength (a red shift), so the star is moving away from Earth at a speed v. From Eq. 24.1,

$$v = \frac{c\Delta\lambda}{\lambda} = \frac{(3 \times 10^8\ \text{m/s})(12\ \text{nm})}{513\ \text{nm}}$$

or

$$v = 7.02 \times 10^6\ \text{m/s} = 7020\ \text{km/s}$$

The fact that distant stars are all moving away from Earth (as measured by the doppler shift) is one component of the "Big Bang" theory of Astronomy.

The doppler shift in radar waves is used in speed detection of cars, trucks, and even clouds. The doppler shift of laser light has been used to measure the velocity of blood cells flowing through retinal blood vessels.

24.2 BLACKBODY RADIATION

A blackbody is a material that absorbs most of the incident light. By conservation of energy, the fraction A of the incident light intensity absorbed

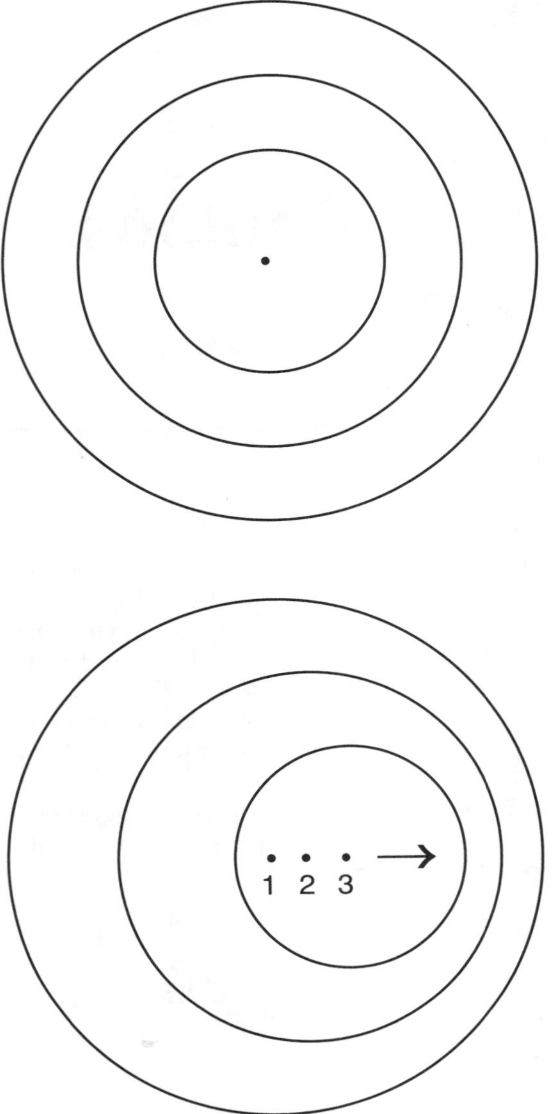

Figure 24.1 a, Stationary point source emitting spherical waves; b, Doppler shift by a point source moving to the right while emitting spherical waves. The wavelength in front of the point source is shifted to a shorter wavelength (a blue shift), while the wavelengths behind the point source are shifted to a longer wavelength (a red shift).

(the absorptance), the fraction R of the incident light intensity reflected (the reflectance), and the fraction T of the incident light intensity transmitted (the transmittance) must add to 1:

$$R + T + A = 1 \tag{24.2}$$

Scattered light is included in the reflectance or transmittance depending on its direction of travel. The absorptance A depends on the surface characteristics as well as the interior absorption strength k of the material. In particular, surfaces that diffusely reflect usually absorb more than smooth surfaces of the same material.

Metals have a high interior absorption strength k, but also a high reflectance R (see Eq. 23.12). Therefore, the absorptance A of a polished metal surface is small. On the other hand, solid carbon appears black because of its high absorptance A and low reflectance R.

You know from everyday experience that hot objects radiate light. The electromagnetic radiation from a hot object is called *thermal radiation*. The spectral distribution of thermal radiation is largely a function of the temperature of the source. We can investigate this temperature dependence by considering the thermal radiation from an ideal blackbody. To understand the emission properties of a blackbody, consider a ball suspended by an insulating string in a closed cavity (Figure 24.2). When the cavity is heated to a certain temperature, the walls emit electromagnetic radiation. This radiation is incident on the suspended ball, which in turn absorbs and re-radiates. Let I be the irradiance (intensity) of the radiation in the cavity. Let A_1 be the absorptance of the ball and E_1 the radiation emitted by the ball. When equilibrium is achieved, the suspended ball emits as much as it absorbs, or

$$E_1 = A_1 I$$

Now consider a second suspended ball in the cavity. The irradiance I is still the same, and for equilibrium

$$E_2 = A_2 I$$

It follows from the above two equations that

$$\frac{E_1}{A_1} = \frac{E_2}{A_2} \tag{24.3}$$

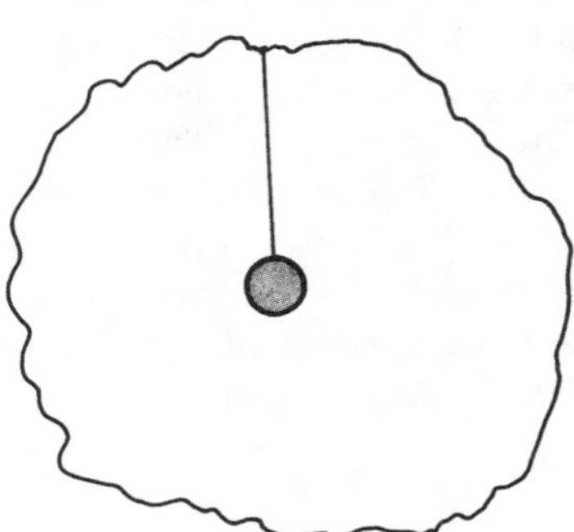

Figure 24.2 A ball suspended in a cavity.

The above relation, known as Kirchhoff's law, shows that the amount of emittance is directly proportional to the absorptance A. A ball that does not absorb much (small A) also does not emit much (small E). A ball that absorbs a lot (large A) also emits a lot (large E). A famous demonstration of Kirchhoff's law is to coat a Pyrex rod with lamp-black, and then heat the rod in a flame. When the rod is withdrawn the part coated with lamp-black glows a brighter red than the uncoated part.

It follows from Kirchhoff's law that an ideal blackbody ($A = 1$) is the strongest emitter. In an absorbing material, a cavity with a small opening approaches an ideal blackbody (Figure 24.3). When light is incident on the hole, it passes into the cavity and reflects back and forth from the interior cavity walls until it is absorbed. Very little light comes back out of the small opening. Hence, the opening appears to be an ideal black spot. (The pupil of your eye appears black for similar reasons.)

When the material is heated up, the surfaces radiate, and the cavity fills with electromagnetic radiation. Because there are many radiating points on the surface of the cavity, the radiation gets very concentrated in the cavity, and begins to leak out of the opening. The concentration of the radiation in the cavity makes the emittance at the cavity hole much higher than that of any other point on the outer surface.

For two temperatures, Figure 24.4 shows the irradiance I of the electromagnetic radiation emitted from the hole as a function of the frequency f. For an ideal blackbody cavity, this spectrum is independent of the specific absorbing material. For low temperatures, most of the radiation is in the infrared. You can feel this radiated "heat" with your hand, even though you cannot see it. As the temperature is increased, the emittance increases and moves toward the higher frequencies (shorter wavelengths). At about 800 K, some radiation becomes visible, and we say the object is red hot. (Recall that temperature on the Kelvin scale equals Celsius temperature plus 273.15, so 800 K is approximately 527 °C. The freezing point of water is 0 °C or 273.15 K, and the boiling point of water is 100 °C or 373.15 K.) As the temperature is increased still more, the trend continues—white hot at 6,000 K and blue hot at 10,000 K. (Thus a blue flame produced by a gas stove is burning at a higher temperature than a red flame.)

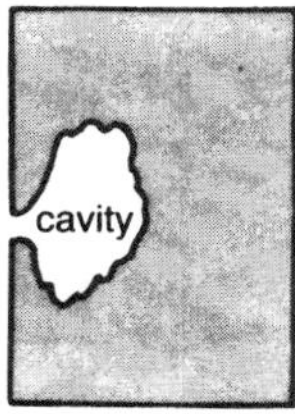

Figure 24.3 A cavity that serves as a blackbody radiator.

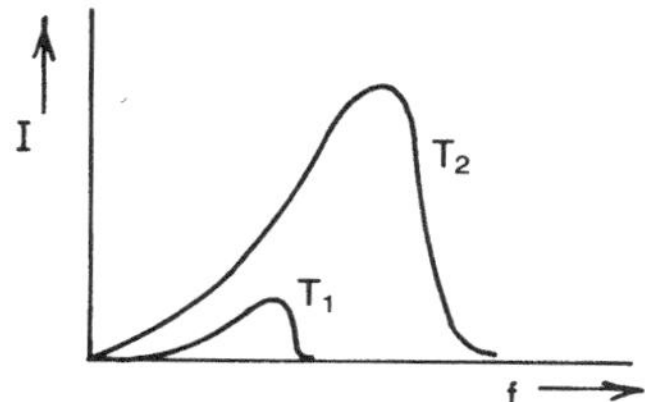

Figure 24.4 Blackbody irradiance distributions as a function of frequency for several different temperatures.

The sun's spectrum resembles that of a blackbody at 5,800 K. The spectrum of a candle flame resembles that of a blackbody at 1,800 K. A hot tungsten filament, called a greybody, produces a spectrum with the shape of a blackbody spectrum at 3,600 K, but the tungsten filament's irradiance has a magnitude of about one third of the blackbody irradiance.

One characteristic of blackbody radiation is that the peak wavelength λ_m is inversely proportional to the Kelvin temperature T_k of the blackbody. This is known as *Wien's displacement law*:

$$\lambda_m = \frac{2.90 \times 10^6 \text{ nm-K}}{T_k} \tag{24.4}$$

EXAMPLE 24.2a

What is the peak wavelength for a blackbody at 5,800 K (the sun)?

From Wien's displacement law,

$$\lambda_m = \frac{2.90 \times 10^6 \text{ nm-K}}{5800 \text{ K}} = 500 \text{ nm}$$

EXAMPLE 24.2b

The peak wavelength in a blackbody emission spectrum is 660 nm. Is the temperature of this blackbody hotter or cooler than that of the sun?

From Wien's displacement law,

$$T_k = \frac{2.90 \times 10^6 \text{ nm-K}}{660 \text{ nm}} = 4394 \text{ K}$$

which is cooler than the sun.

Another characteristic of blackbody radiation is that the total irradiance I_t is directly proportional to the fourth power of the temperature:

$$I_t = (\text{constant})(T_k)^4 \tag{24.5}$$

This is known as the *Stefan–Boltzman law*. The strong temperature dependence results in a dramatic increase in irradiance as T_k increases.

Because of the above two laws, care must be taken in judging apparent colors. A dim light may have a peak wavelength in the red. When a rheostat is turned to increase the current in a filament, the filament gets hotter and emits more light (Stefan–Boltzman). However, the peak wavelength emitted also shifts up (Wien displacement), so the incident light is bluer than before, and as a result an illuminated object may appear bluer.

24.3 PHOTONS

Classical electromagnetic wave theory correctly describes a wide range of everyday physical phenomena, but it breaks down at the atomic level. The blackbody radiation spectrum was one of the early breakdowns. In classical electromagnetic wave theory, the blackbody spectrum is analyzed by examining the standing wave modes set up in the cavity. The classical analysis correctly fits the low frequency part of the blackbody spectrum, but goes haywire at the higher frequencies (Figure 24.5). As a function of increasing frequency, the experimental curve peaks and turns down, while the classical prediction continues to grow. This is known as the *ultraviolet catastrophe* of classical electromagnetic wave theory. (In fact, according to the ever increasing function predicted by the classical theory, matter would radiate away all its energy and collapse. The estimated time for this to occur is about 17 s.)

Another breakdown in classical electromagnetic wave theory involved the *photoelectric effect*. In the photoelectric effect, electromagnetic radiation of high enough frequency incident on a metal results in the ejection of electrons. Classical theory predicts that electrons should be ejected, and that the mechanism is a "sunbathing" mechanism. In particular, classical

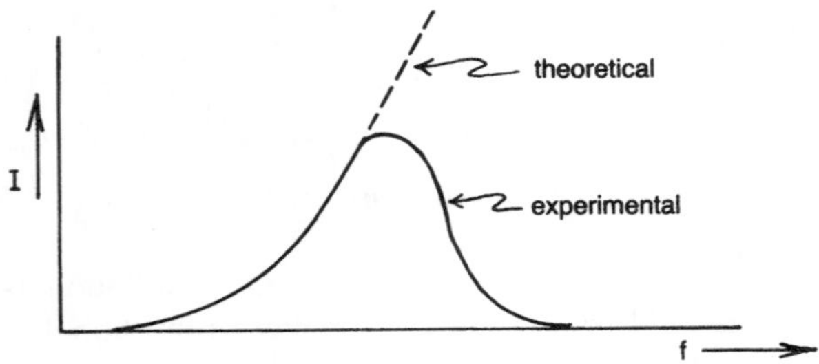

Figure 24.5 The ultraviolet catastrophe of classical electromagnetic wave theory.

electromagnetic theory says that the metal needs to sunbathe for awhile before the electrons come out (a time lag), that the effect should be frequency-independent, and that the maximum kinetic energy of the ejected electrons should be dependent on the irradiance of the light. The experimental results are: the effect is very frequency-dependent (it does not occur if the frequency is not high enough), the maximum kinetic energy of the ejected electrons is independent of the irradiance, and when the frequency is high enough the electrons are ejected immediately (no time lag).

Both of the above breakdowns are solved by the quantum theory of light. The quantum theory correctly describes electromagnetic radiation interactions at the atomic level, as well as encompassing and including the classical electromagnetic wave theory at the macroscopic level. A central feature of the quantum theory of light is that the energy carried by electromagnetic radiation is not continuous, but comes in packets called *photons*.

While photons appear to be particles, they also exhibit the interference and diffraction effects that we naively associate with waves. Other quantum particles, such as electrons, protons, neutrons, pions, etc., also exhibit interference and diffraction effects. (Some have felt that the term *wavicles* is a better name than quantum particles.)

For monochromatic electromagnetic radiation, the energy E carried by a single photon is directly proportional to the frequency f:

$$E = hf \tag{24.6}$$

where h is Planck's constant, which equals 6.63×10^{-34} J-s (Joule-seconds). Equation 24.6 was first introduced by Max Planck in 1901 to explain the blackbody radiation spectrum. However, Planck interpreted the equation as saying that while the radiation could have a continuous energy, the electrons in the blackbody walls could only emit the radiation in units of hf.

In 1905, Albert Einstein explained the photoelectric effect by saying that the radiation itself consisted of particles, each with energy hf. The radiation can consist of any integer number of particles, and hence the total radiated energy is an integer multiple of hf.

On an energy level diagram, a free electron with a kinetic energy of magnitude s is assigned a $+s$ value. A free electron with zero kinetic energy is assigned a zero value. An electron that is bound by an energy of magnitude w is assigned a value of $-w$ (Figure 24.6). According to Einstein, electrons bound in a metal can be freed by absorbing a single photon with enough

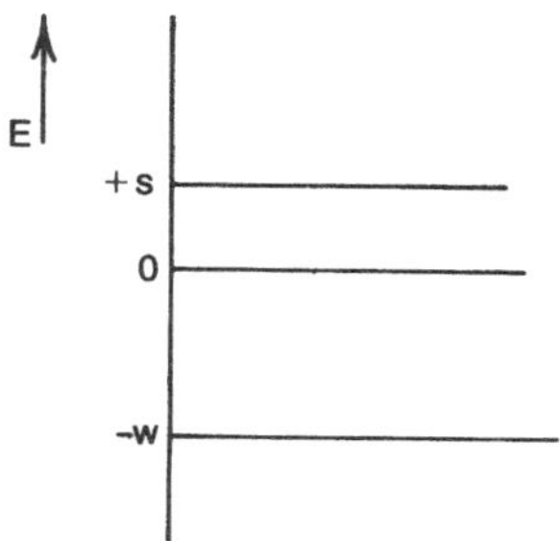

Figure 24.6 The energy level at +*s* is for a free electron with kinetic energy equal to *s*. The energy level at 0 is for a free electron with zero kinetic energy. The energy level at −*w* is for an electron in the metal that is bound by an energy that in magnitude equals *w*.

energy to overcome the binding energy ($hf \geq w$). When the photon does not have enough energy to free the electron ($hf < w$), the absorbed energy is dissipated as heat. Thus, the photoelectric effect is extremely frequency-dependent.

Since the electron is freed by absorbing one photon of high enough energy, the kinetic energy of that electron is the difference between the photon's energy (hf) and the binding energy w of the electron. This kinetic energy is independent of the irradiance. A higher irradiance means more electrons come out, but the maximum kinetic energy is still the same. Finally, when an incident photon has a high enough energy, an electron absorbs it and is immediately ejected (no time lag). Einstein's photon concept explained both the blackbody spectrum as well as the photoelectric effect. (It is interesting that Einstein received the Nobel Prize for his work on the photoelectric effect as opposed to the theory of relativity.)

Planck's constant is so small that the energy carried by a visible light photon is minute. Normal amounts of visible light consist of an incredible number of photons. A 60 W light bulb puts out about 10^{19} photons per second. Under these conditions, millions of photons can be added or subtracted without visual notice. However, when a person has been in a dark room long enough to fully dark-adapt, then a small flash consisting of only 5 to 10 incident photons is enough to trigger visual perception of that flash.

Since in a vacuum $\lambda f = c$, Eq. 24.6 can be rewritten as

$$E = \frac{hc}{\lambda} \tag{24.7}$$

The energy carried by a single photon is frequently expressed in terms of electron volts (eV). An *electron volt* is the amount of energy that an electron gains while moving through a potential difference of 1 V. Note that we are not saying that a photon is like an electron; we are only using the electron volt as a measure of energy. In other words, a 2 eV photon carries energy equal to that gained by an electron while moving through a potential difference of 2 V. In convenient units,

$$hc = 1239\ \text{nm-eV}$$

Therefore, Eq. 24.7 becomes

$$E = \frac{1239\ \text{nm-eV}}{\lambda} \tag{24.8}$$

EXAMPLE 24.3

What is the single photon energy for the C (red) line of the hydrogen spectrum ($\lambda = 656$ nm)?

From Eq. 24.8,

$$E = \frac{1239\ \text{nm-eV}}{656\ \text{nm}} = 1.89\ \text{eV}$$

What is the single photon energy for violet light of vacuum wavelength 413 nm?

From Eq. 24.8,

$$E = \frac{1239\ \text{nm-eV}}{413\ \text{nm}} = 3.00\ \text{eV}$$

Note that the shorter the wavelength, the higher the frequency, and the more energetic each photon is. Diagnostic *X*-rays have a wavelength of less than 0.1 nm. Consequently, their wave properties are not particularly noticeable, which is historically why they are referred to as rays rather than waves. The single photon energy for these *X*-rays is greater than 12,390 eV.

Photons are not electrically charged but are emitted and absorbed by electrically charged particles. Photons have a zero rest mass, but photons never occur at rest. Photons are always moving with the speed of light. Attempts to stop a photon (i.e., bring it to rest) simply result in its absorption.

A moving photon has a mass equivalent m that is found from Eq. 24.6 together with Einstein's relativity equation

$$E = mc^2$$

where E is the photon energy, m is the mass equivalent, and c is the speed of light. When we substitute Eq. 24.6 into the above equation and solve for m, the result is

$$m = (hf)/c^2$$

Since a photon has a mass equivalent, it carries momentum as well as energy. The momentum p of a particle is given by

$$p = mv$$

where m is the mass and v is the velocity. For a photon in a vacuum, $v = c$, and we can use the mass equivalent for m to obtain

$$p = (hf)/c$$

or

$$p = E/c \tag{24.9}$$

From $\lambda f = c$, it follows that

$$p = h/\lambda$$

Besides energy and momentum, a photon also carries angular momentum. A naive picture is that the photon is spinning as it moves through space. In the quantum theory, photons are spin 1 particles (as opposed to electrons, which are spin 1/2 particles, or pions, which are spin zero particles). It is the photon spin that is responsible for the polarization properties of light.

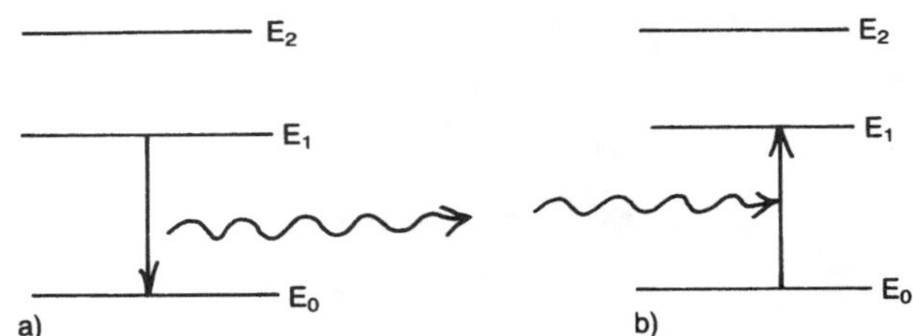

Figure 24.7 In both parts of the figure, there are three atomic electron energy levels. E_0 is the energy of the ground state, E_1 is the energy of the first excited state, and E_2 is the energy of the second excited state: a, in a radiative transition in which the electron jumps down from one energy level to another, it emits a single photon with an energy equal to the difference in energy levels; b, when an incident photon has an energy that matches an energy level difference, an electron can absorb the photon and jump to the higher energy level.

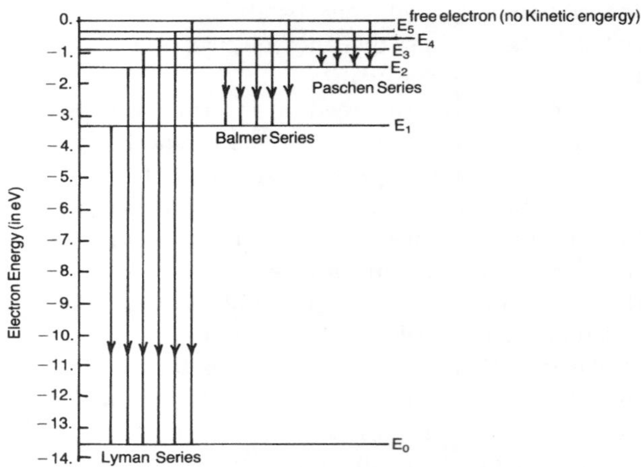

Figure 24.8 Transitions giving the hydrogen emission spectra.

24.4 BOHR MODEL OF THE ATOM

Besides thermal radiation, light is also emitted when a high voltage is placed across a tube of gas. Unlike the continuous blackbody spectrum, the spectrum from a low pressure gas discharge tube consists of a series of discrete wavelengths called a *line spectrum*. The line spectra are resolved by use of prisms or diffraction gratings (Figure 22.17). Line spectra were first explained by the Bohr model of the atom.

According to the Bohr model of the atom, the electrons that orbit the atomic nucleus exist only in discrete energy levels. An electron can jump to a lower energy level by emitting a photon (Figure 24.7a). Similarly, an electron can jump to a higher level by absorbing a photon (Figure 24.7b).

In the Bohr model, the allowed electron energy levels in the hydrogen atom are given by

$$E_m = \frac{-13.6\,\text{eV}}{(m+1)^2} \quad m = 0, 1, 2, \ldots \tag{24.10}$$

The lowest energy level, called the ground state, is given by $E_0 = -13.6\,\text{eV}$ (Figure 24.8). This means that an incident 13.6 eV photon has enough energy to free the ground state electron, thus ionizing the atom. In the absence of incident radiation, the ground state is the stable state of the atom. The higher states, called excited states, are not stable. The first excited state occurs at $E_1 = -13.6\,\text{eV}/2^2 = -3.4\,\text{eV}$. Similarly, the second excited state occurs at $E_2 = -13.6\,\text{eV}/3^2 = -1.51\,\text{eV}$

An electron typically stays in an excited state for less than 10^{-8} s and then jumps to a lower level emitting a photon in the process. This is called *spontaneous emission*. The energy of the emitted photon equals the difference in the energy levels. An electron can jump to a higher energy level by absorbing a photon that carries energy equal to that of the jump.

EXAMPLE 24.4a

What is the energy and wavelength of a photon emitted when an electron in hydrogen jumps from E_2 to E_1?

$$\Delta E = E_2 - E_1$$
$$= -1.51\,\text{eV} - (-3.4\,\text{eV}) = 1.89\,\text{eV}$$

The emitted photon has energy of 1.89 eV. From Eq. 24.8,

$$\lambda = 1239\,\text{eV-nm}/1.89\,\text{eV} = 656\,\text{nm}$$

These photons constitute the light in the C line of the hydrogen spectra.

EXAMPLE 24.4b

What is the energy and wavelength of a photon emitted when an electron in hydrogen jumps from E_3 to E_1?

The energy levels are farther apart than in Example 24.4a so the photon has more energy and the emitted light has a higher frequency (lower wavelength).

From the Bohr model,

$$E_3 = -13.6\,\text{eV}/(4)^2 = -0.85\,\text{eV}$$

Then the energy E of the emitted photon is

$$\Delta E = E_3 - E_1$$
$$= -0.85\,\text{eV} - (-3.4\,\text{eV}) = 2.55\,\text{eV}$$

From Eq. 24.8,

$$\lambda = 1239\,\text{eV-nm}/2.55\,\text{eV} = 486\,\text{nm}$$

These photons constitute the light in the F line of the hydrogen spectra.

Figure 24.8 shows the possible downward transitions for hydrogen. Those that end in the ground state (E_0) are referred to as the Lyman series. Those that end in the first excited state E_1 are referred to as the Balmer series, and those that end in the second excited state E_2 are referred to as the Paschen series. Table 24.1 gives the series, the initial and final states, and the vacuum wavelengths of the emitted photons. The jumps to the ground state are all large, and these transitions give ultraviolet photons. The visible wavelengths come from the Balmer series. The Paschen series has smaller energy jumps and gives infrared photons.

Because of the energy level structure, atoms absorb only those wavelengths that they can emit. Therefore, when visible light is incident on hydrogen with electrons in the first excited state E_1, the photons absorbed are those with the Balmer series wavelengths, and the electrons end up in the appropriate higher states. When the hydrogen gas is thick enough, the Balmer series wavelengths are deficient or missing from the transmitted radiation. Fraunhofer discovered the deficient or missing lines in the sun's spectrum and labeled them by letters. The deficient C and F lines are due to absorption by "cooler" hydrogen in the sun's outer atmosphere.

When an atomic electron is in a particular state, the electric charge density of the atom is constant with time. When the atom makes a transition between states of energy E_m and E_k, the electric charge density oscillates with a frequency f_{mk} where

$$f_{mk} = \left| \frac{E_m - E_k}{h} \right| \tag{24.11}$$

The frequencies f_{mk} are the resonance frequencies of the atom. (In the simple spring model of Chapter 23, the resonances appeared as the natural vibration frequencies of the spring.) Real atoms do have small damping factors. Thus, as discussed in Section 23.8, there may also be absorption or emission at some frequencies close to the resonance frequency. A simple model of this is to picture the damping factors causing a jiggle in the atom's energy levels, and this jiggle results in emission or absorption at a range of frequencies

Table 24.1 Hydrogen Energy Level Transitions and Emitted Wavelengths

Series	*Initial*	*Final*	*Wavelength (nm)*
Lyman	4	0	95
	3	0	97
	2	0	103
	1	0	122
Balmer	5	1	410
	4	1	434
	3	1	486
	2	1	656
Paschen	4	2	1,282
	3	2	1,875

around the f_{mk} resonance. This leads to a small natural linewidth (i.e. spread in the frequency or wavelength) for the light emitted when the electrons in atoms jump down from one energy level to another.

The *transition rate* between the different energy levels varies and is determined by the electromagnetic properties of the individual atom. Atoms that emit strongly at a certain wavelength have a high transition rate between the appropriate energy levels. Atoms that emit weakly at a certain wavelength have a low transition rate between the appropriate energy levels. In materials, transitions can also occur nonradiatively (e.g., by collisions between atoms), in which case the energy differences show up as heat loss or gain with no light emitted or absorbed.

When the pressure is increased in a gas discharge tube, the atoms bump into each other more, the transitions are disrupted, and the line spectra broaden into *band spectra*. If the pressure is increased still more, the band spectra broaden into a continuous spectra. Part of this broadening is related to the formation of molecules. Molecules provide many additional sets of energy levels for the electrons with the resulting increase in possible wavelengths that can be emitted and absorbed. In particular, organic dyes provide additional energy levels with very high transition rates. Liquids and solids have either a band spectrum or a continuous spectrum. The band absorption spectra are responsible for the color of many substances.

24.5 FLUORESCENCE AND PHOSPHORESCENCE

One sign of the contemporary world is the abundance of fluorescent colors. These colors stand out sharply because the luminous flux emitted at the fluorescent wavelengths by a fluorescent substance may be far greater than the luminous flux incident at those wavelengths. In most cases, the energy that drives the fluorescent radiation comes from an incident higher frequency radiation (such as ultraviolet).

Figure 24.9 shows the ray diagram for a fluorescent substance. Incident high frequency radiation causes the transition from E_0 to E_2. Assuming radiative jumps, the electron then spontaneously emits a lower frequency photon and jumps down to E_1. Finally, the electron spontaneously emits another lower frequency photon and jumps back to E_0. In terms of wavelengths, the incident radiation has a shorter wavelength than the emitted or fluorescent radiation.

In fluorescence, the higher frequency photon may be ultraviolet, while one or both of the lower frequency photons is visible. There are some cases where illumination by visible blue results in fluorescent radiation in the longer visible wavelengths (reds or oranges). The strength of the fluorescence depends on the transition rates between the different states.

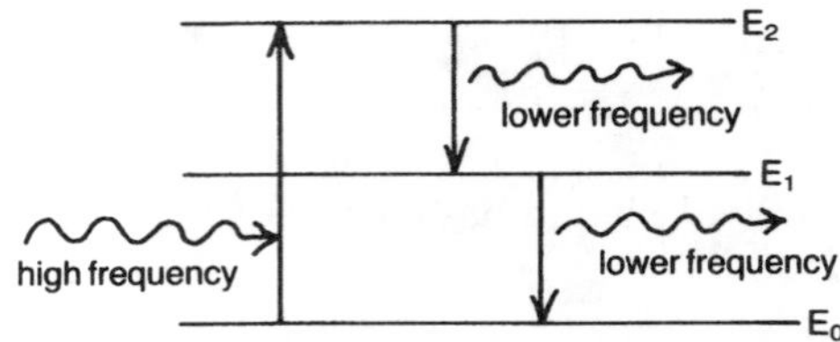

Figure 24.9 Energy levels for fluorescence. The emissions involved are all spontaneous.

EXAMPLE 24.5

A substance has energy levels of $E_0 = -10.0\,\text{eV}$, $E_1 = -8.0\,\text{eV}$, and $E_2 = -5.5\,\text{eV}$. Can this material fluoresce? If so, what incident wavelength is needed to excite the material? What wavelengths are emitted in the fluorescence?

For fluorescence, the incident radiation must have the energy needed for the electron to jump from the ground state to E_2. Therefore,

$$\begin{aligned}\Delta E &= E_2 - E_0\\ &= -5.5\,\text{eV} - (-10.0\,\text{eV}) = +4.5\,\text{eV}\end{aligned}$$

So,

$$\lambda = (1239\,\text{nm-eV})/4.5\,\text{eV} = 275\,\text{nm (ultraviolet)}$$

The electron in E_2 can spontaneously decay to E_1 by emitting a photon of wavelength

$$\lambda = \frac{1239\,\text{nm-eV}}{-5.5\,\text{eV} - (-8.0\,\text{eV})} = 496\,\text{nm (blue)}$$

Similarly, the electron in E_1 can spontaneously decay to E_0 by emitting a photon of wavelength

$$\lambda = \frac{1239\,\text{nm-eV}}{-8.0\,\text{eV} - (-10.0\,\text{eV})} = 620\,\text{nm (orangish-red)}$$

Here incident radiation of 275 nm can result in fluorescence at 496 nm and 620 nm.

Ultraviolet lamps (i.e., black lights) can be used to trigger fluorescence. Many minerals fluoresce naturally. Some white substances, such as paper or shirts, contain a fluorescent dye that emits in the blue end of the spectrum. This emission balances the natural longer wavelength emission of the material making it appear whiter under incandescent light. Many detergent whiteners contain a similar dye.

Sodium fluorescein is a fluorescent dye widely used in contact lens evaluations. Intact corneal epithelial cells do not absorb the dye because it is a water-soluble molecule that will not penetrate the lipid membranes of the cell. When these membranes are damaged (perhaps by the contact lens), the dye is absorbed, and these areas then fluoresce at a wavelength of about 522 nm when irradiated by near ultraviolet (365–470 nm). Fluorexon, a higher molecular weight dye, is used with those hydrophilic lenses that absorb sodium fluorescein.

The electron in an atomic excited state has a certain probability to decay or jump to a lower energy level. Usually these probabilities are such that the jump occurs within 10^{-8} s of excitation. However, there are some excited states, called *metastable states*, which have a very low probability of decay. Electrons may stay in the metastable excited states for milliseconds, seconds, minutes, or even hours. When a metastable state with a long lifetime is populated by incident radiation, the material may continue to glow or emit radiation long after the original source is removed. This is the phenomenon of *phosphorescence*. The distinction between fluorescence and phosphorescence is a matter of time. The material is classified as phosphorescent if it continues to fluoresce for more than 1 μs after the exciting radiation is shut off.

Clock hands that glow in the dark used to be a common example of phosphorescence. Television and video display terminals (VDTs) use short-acting phosphorescent materials. These phosphors are excited by an incident beam of electrons rather than by electromagnetic radiation, and they continue to emit visible light for a short period of time after the electron beam has passed on.

Since 1939, fluorescent lights have come into wide use. They consist of a gas discharge tube usually containing argon (with possibly some neon) and a small amount of mercury. The walls of the tube are coated with a phosphor. During the discharge, the ultraviolet emitted by the mercury (254 nm) excites the phosphor, which then emits visible light. Figure 24.10 compares the spectrum for a cool white fluorescent light (solid line) to the spectrum for a tungsten filament bulb (dashed line). The visible lines of the mercury spectrum are also passed by the tube and show up as spikes in the fluorescent spectrum. Fluorescent lights operate at the relatively low temperature of 40 °C and are more energy efficient than incandescent lights. The spectral distribution of a fluorescent light can be varied by using different phosphors on the tube.

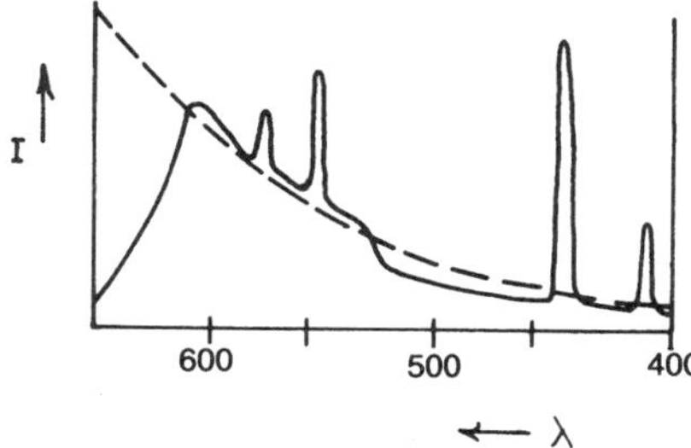

Figure 24.10 Emission by a fluorescence bulb (solid curve) versus a tungsten filament bulb (dashed curve).

24.6 STIMULATED EMISSION

According to the quantum theory, all states have some natural fluctuations. If an excited state happens to fluctuate too much, a downward jump results with the emission of a photon. This results in spontaneous emission and is responsible for the instability of the excited states.

Now consider absorption by an atom that has a resonance frequency f_{01} connecting the ground state E_0 and the first excited state E_1. When a photon of frequency f is incident on this atom, it perturbs the atom, causing the electrical charge density to oscillate with the frequency of the photon. When f equals f_{01}, the perturbation induces the electron to absorb the photon and jump to the first excited state E_1. In this sense, absorption might better be referred to as *stimulated absorption*.

Now suppose a photon of frequency f is incident on the excited atom in state E_1 where f equals the resonance frequency f_{01}. This photon again perturbs the atom causing the electric charge density to oscillate with the frequency f of the photon, but since this frequency is the resonance frequency f_{01} it induces the electron to emit a photon and jump down to E_0. The emitted photon is coherent with and travels in the same direction as the incident photon. (In other words, the emitted photon is indistinguishable from the stimulating photon). This is called *stimulated emission* (Figure 24.11).

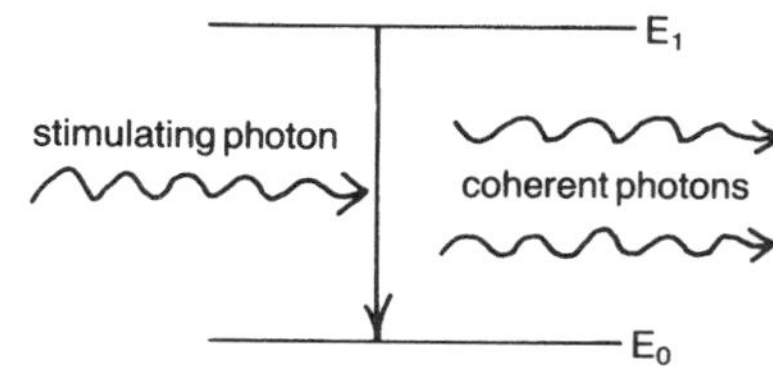

Figure 24.11 Stimulated emission. When the incident photon has an energy equal to the energy level difference ($E_1 - E_0$), it triggers the emission of a second photon that is coherent and traveling in the same direction as the stimulating photon.

Absorption (i.e., stimulated absorption) and stimulated emission are related processes, and the corresponding transition probabilities are identical in magnitude. Spontaneous emission is separate and has its own probability. Under normal light levels, the probability of spontaneous visible light emission is much higher than stimulated visible light emission. Therefore, stimulated emission was overlooked until Einstein pointed out its existence in 1916. Stimulated emission raised the possibility of a process whereby a large number of coherent photons could be produced. The modern result is the laser.

24.7 LASER THEORY

Lasers are sources of coherent electromagnetic radiation. Depending on the laser, the output beam might be in the visible light, infrared, or ultraviolet range. Some lasers produce low power beams, while others can generate enormous irradiances. The word LASER is actually an acronym for *Light Amplification by Stimulated Emission of Radiation*. Lasers were preceded by MASERs (Microwave Amplification by Stimulated Emission of Radiation). The maser was independently invented in the early 1950s by Charles Townes of the United States and Alexander Prokhorov and Nikolai Basov of Russia. These three men shared the 1964 Nobel Prize for their work on the maser. In 1958, Townes and Arthur Schawlow set forth the general conditions needed for a laser. Within two years (1960), Ted Maiman of the United States built the first successful laser. Arthur Schawlow received the 1981 Nobel Prize in Physics for his work on lasers and laser optics.

In a laser, a photon is used to trigger a stimulated emission resulting in two coherent photons that have the same wavelength and are traveling in the same direction. These two photons each trigger another stimulated emission resulting in four coherent photons all traveling the same direction. The four trigger more stimulated emissions resulting in eight coherent photons. If the process continues, an avalanche of coherent photons is produced (i.e., light amplification).

In a medium at a certain temperature, most atomic electrons are in the ground state E_0, the next most are in the first excited state E_1, and a decreasing number are in each successively higher excited state. Suppose we try to start an avalanche by stimulating a transition from E_1 to E_0. The initial coherent photon might be incident on an atom with an electron in state E_1, but it is more likely to be incident on an atom with an electron in the ground state. When the atom is in the ground state, the photon is absorbed and the avalanche is quenched. Therefore, in order to get an avalanche, we need more electrons in E_1 than in the ground state. This is a very unnatural situation called a *population inversion*.

Population inversions can be obtained by using metastable excited states, since on an atomic scale the metastable states live a very long time. The metastable states are populated by correctly "pumping" the medium. The pumping consists of supplying energy to the lasing medium. This can be accomplished by a variety of ways: ultraviolet radiation, white light illumination (i.e., flashlamps), radiation from another laser, electrical currents, atom–atom collisions, chemical reactions, etc.

Maiman's laser was a ruby laser, which is a three level laser pumped by a xenon flashlamp. Figure 24.12 shows the basics of an energy level diagram for a three level laser. The pump (incident light from the flashlamp) induces the transition from E_0 to E_2. The electron then makes a transition (possibly non-radiative) down to E_1. Since E_1 is metastable, the electrons tend to stay there, and hence with sufficiently vigorous pumping the number of electrons in E_1 can be built up until there are more in E_1 than in E_0 (the population inversion).

Eventually (on the atomic time scale), one of the metastable states spontaneously decays to the ground state and emits a photon. This photon is incident on another E_1 atom and stimulates the emission of a second photon that is coherent with the first. These two are then incident on two more E_1 atoms and stimulate the emission of two more coherent photons. The stimulated emission avalanche is now started. Since the pumping radiation operates at a different wavelength ($E_0 \rightarrow E_2$), it does not compete with the avalanche.

Usually, the lasing medium (or active medium) is placed between two reflectors so that the coherent photons travel back and forth across the medium, thus building the strength of the avalanche. Such a setup is

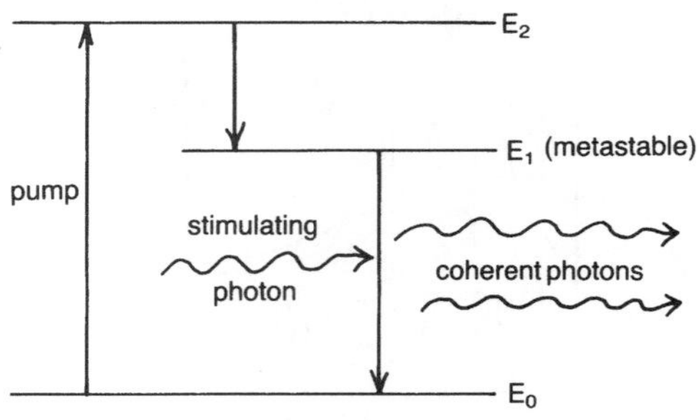

Figure 24.12 Energy level diagram for a three-level laser.

called a *cavity oscillator*. Figure 24.13 shows the active medium between two mirrors M and G. The pump feeds energy into the active medium to build and sustain the population inversion. The coherent light sweeping back and forth sets up a standing wave in the cavity between M and G. The increase in the number of the coherent photons as they sweep back and forth corresponds to increasing the amplitude of the standing wave. The mirror G may be partially transmitting, in which case a small percentage of the coherent light in the cavity is steadily drained off resulting in a *continuous beam laser*. In a *pulsed beam laser*, the mirror G contains an optical gate mechanism that when opened lets all the coherent light in the cavity out. Then the gate is closed and the laser needs to internally build up the coherent standing wave in the cavity before the gate is again opened. Many pulsed beam lasers operate at very fast repetition rates.

Two plane mirrors can define a laser cavity (e.g., M and G in Figure 24.13). This is the simplest cavity configuration. However, the plane mirrors have to be very precisely aligned in order to successfully build up a large amplitude standing wave. If the plane mirrors have some misalignment, the wave will "walk out" of the reflector (sometimes referred to as an unstable cavity). Figure 24.14a shows a confocal cavity in which two spherical converging mirrors are used with their focal points F coincident. The alignment of the mirrors in the confocal cavity is not as crucial as that of the plane mirrors. Figure 24.14b shows a hemispheric cavity where the center of curvature C of the left concave mirror occurs at the plane mirror on the right. The output beam characteristics of a laser depend on the cavity design, and there is a wide variety of other laser cavity designs.

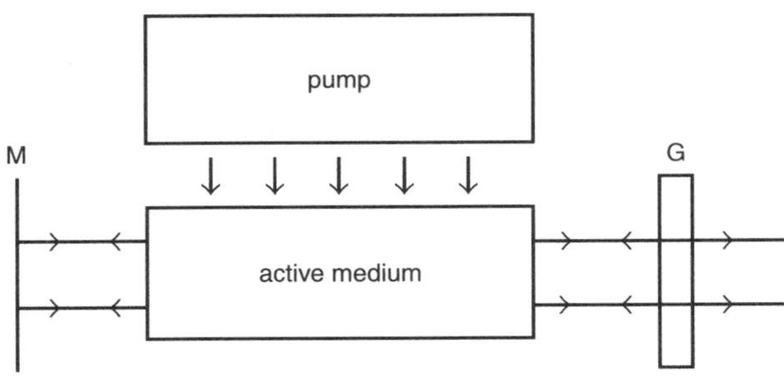

Figure 24.13 Schematic diagram of a laser cavity oscillator. *M* and *G* are mirrors. *G* is either a partially silvered mirror (or its equivalent) or an optical gate that can be opened or closed. The pump supplies the energy that creates a population inversion in the active medium. An amplification of the coherent light occurs as the stimulated photons sweep back and forth between *M* and *G*.

The *gain* of the active medium in the laser cavity is the net amount of coherent photons added to the beam in each sweep. The gain is a characteristic of the particular active medium and the cavity design. For a low gain active media, the laser cavity needs to be stable, so that the beam can sweep back and forth many times to build up the desired intensity. Unstable cavities can be used in the case of high gain active media in which only a few sweeps are needed. Then as the beam walks off, it encounters the outer areas of the cavity that were not initially involved and picks up more energy from them.

With the proper design and alignment, it is easy to set up a standing wave in a laser. Recall that the light emitted when an electron jumps to a lower energy level has a natural linewidth (i.e., a small spread in the wavelength or frequency). The laser cavity has a length L that is much longer than the wavelength λ_m of the light in the cavity medium. A standing wave can be set up when there is a wave node at each mirror, and this occurs whenever L is an integer multiple of half-wavelengths, i.e.,

$$L = j\left(\frac{\lambda_m}{2}\right) \tag{24.12}$$

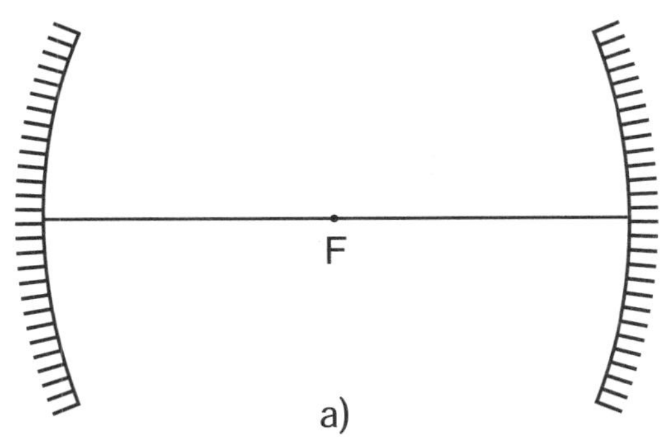

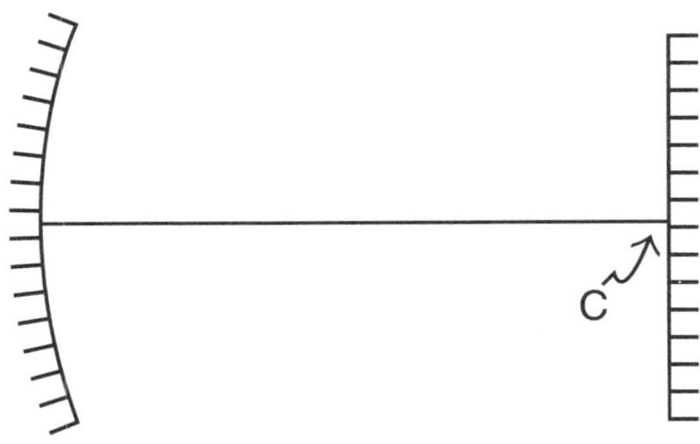

Figure 24.14 a, A confocal laser cavity; b, a hemispheric laser cavity.

where j is usually a large integer. (For simplicity, Figure 24.15 shows standing wave modes for the small integers of $j = 1$ to 3.) A 30 cm long helium–neon laser with an emission centered on 632.8 nm, j is of the order of 1,580,000. Values for j of 30,000–40,000 are common. Even for a semiconductor laser with a 0.25 mm length, j is still about 1,000. This means that there is a range of j values (i.e., j, $j \pm 1$, $j \pm 2$, etc) that will give standing waves that are within the natural linewidth of the stimulated emission. These different possible wavelengths are referred to as the *longitudinal modes* of the laser. In Figure 24.16a, the bell shaped curve gives the natural linewidth, and the vertical spikes are the longitudinal modes that fit in within the natural line width.

The longitudinal modes are often described in terms of the frequencies of the modes. Since $\lambda_m f = v_m$, where v_m is the velocity of light in the medium (i.e., $v_m = c/n$), Eq. 24.12 becomes

$$L = j\left(\frac{v_m}{2f}\right)$$

or

$$f = \frac{jc}{2Ln}$$

Then the frequency difference between two successive modes is

$$\Delta f = f_{j+1} - f_j = \frac{c}{2Ln}$$

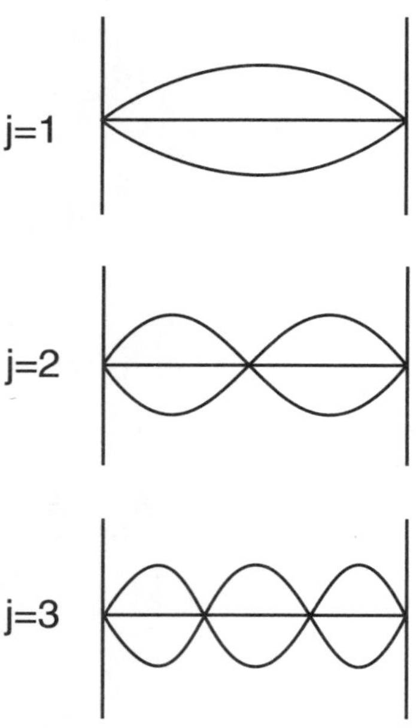

Figure 24.15 The first three possible standing waves (j=1, 2, 3) in a laser cavity oscillator.

An increase in the length L of the laser cavity (or an increase in the refractive index n) causes the modes to be closer together in frequency and consequently more modes can occur within the natural linewidth. A decrease in the length L of the laser cavity spreads the modes apart so that there are fewer allowed modes within the natural linewidth (Figure 24.16b). If needed, some cavities can be shortened until there is only one allowed mode. Alternatively, an interferometer-type device can be placed in a laser cavity that results in amplification of only one of the allowed modes.

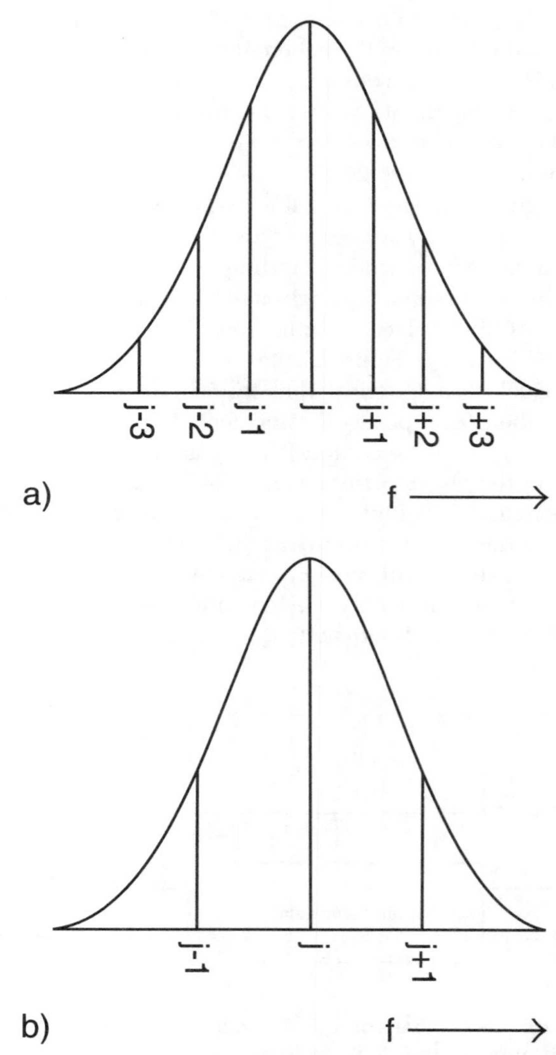

Figure 24.16 The bell shaped curve represents the natural linewidth of a stimulated emission: a, For a laser cavity oscillator, the vertical lines represent the possible standing waves (longitudinal modes) that can occur within the natural linewidth; b, a shorter cavity gives fewer possible modes within the natural linewidth.

Usually the width of the laser cavity is much smaller than its length, and then the standing waves in a laser cavity also have transverse electromagnetic (TEM) modes. The shape of the cavity determines the allowed TEM modes. Figure 24.17 shows an end view of some of the lower order transverse modes for a rectangular laser cavity. The TEM_{00} mode has lateral nodes only at the ends of the cavity (ie., no lateral nodes in the middle of the cavity). All parts of the standing wave in the cavity oscillate together. The TEM_{10} mode has one horizontal node and zero vertical nodes in the middle of the cavity. Here, there are separate standing wave oscillations on the left and right sides of the cavity, and these oscillations are 180° out of phase with each other. That is, when the standing wave on the left of the cavity is vibrating up, the standing wave on the right is vibrating down. The TEM_{01} mode has zero horizontal nodes and one vertical node in the middle of the cavity. Here, there are separate standing wave oscillations on the top and bottom of the cavity, and these oscillations are 180° out of phase with each other. The TEM_{11} mode has one horizontal node and one vertical node in the middle of the cavity. This results in 4 separate standing wave oscillations in the cavity. There are a whole series of other higher order modes (TEM_{21}, TEM_{22}, TEM_{23}, TEM_{33}, etc.) A cylindrical cavity has a corresponding set of modes.

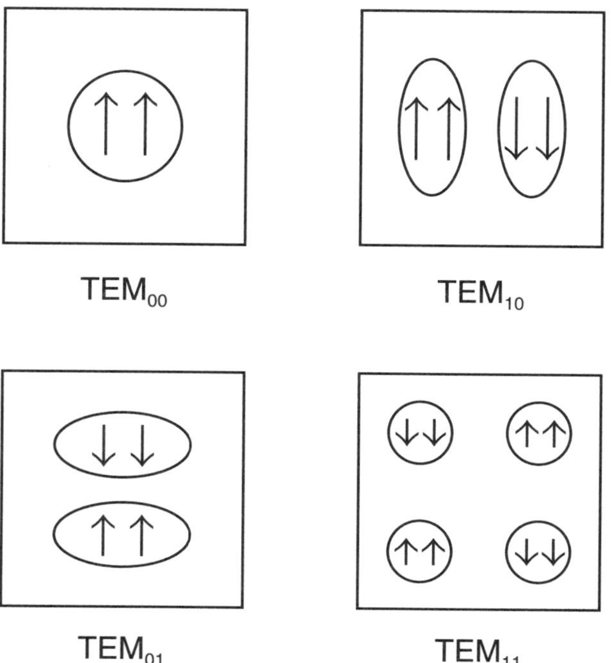

Figure 24.17 End view of a rectangular laser cavity showing the first four transverse electromagnetic modes (TEM).

In the TEM_{11} mode, there is no intensity in the middle of the beam (sometimes called the doughnut mode). Instead, the intensity is concentrated in the four areas symmetrically placed around the middle. As the mode number goes up (TEM_{22}, TEM_{33}, etc.), the intensity concentration moves farther away from the center of the beam. Many lasers are designed to operate in the TEM_{00} mode where the intensity is concentrated in the middle of the beam. The TEM_{00} mode can be focussed into a smaller spot size than the higher laser modes.

In a continuous beam laser, the output beam is only a small percentage of the light oscillating inside the tube. In a pulsed beam laser, there is a "gate" that lets most (or all) of the oscillating coherent light in the tube come out in a pulse. Then the gate closes, and the laser needs to recycle before it is ready to pulse again. Much higher intensities can be achieved with pulsed beam lasers. Lasers similar to the original ruby laser can have a pulse duration as fast as 1 ms (10^{-3} s). Nowadays, these are called *long-pulsed* lasers.

Much shorter pulses can be obtained by a method called *Q-switching*. In Q-switching the active medium is pumped while the Q-switch prohibits an oscillation. For example, when closed the Q-switch may be a photovoltaic absorber at one end of the cavity. Meanwhile in the cavity, some randomly directed stimulated emission occurs, but there is no sustained light amplification. In a suitable active media, this allows a huge population inversion to be built up. In other words, a large amount of energy is stored up in the active medium. Then when the Q-switch is triggered or opened (made transparent), the cavity oscillations can occur. This gives a rapid and large amplification, which results in a very short giant output pulse. In effect, the energy stored in the huge population inversion is rapidly "dumped" into the giant pulse. Q-switching results in pulses that are a few nanoseconds (10^{-9} s) in length. (The name Q-switch comes from the word "quality" as in quality of the laser cavity. When the quality is high, an excellent oscillation and amplification can occur. When the quality is low, the oscillation and amplification are inhibited or may not even occur.)

Even shorter pulses can be achieved in multi-mode lasers by a process called *mode locking*. In a mode locked laser, the various longitudinal modes are locked in a specific phase relationship. This is done by varying the quality of the laser cavity harmonically with time. Each of the longitudinal modes has a slightly different wavelength (Fig 24.18). When these waves are added together, the different wavelengths result in constructive interference in only a few places in the cavity. (In Figure 24.18, the superposition of the top three modes gives the bottom result, which begins to look like an ultra-short pulse. Adding more modes can make the "pulse" even shorter.) In a sense, the constructive interference has concentrated the laser light into the ultra-short pulses. Mode locking leads to a j-fold increase in the peak power of the pulses where j is the number of modes that are locked together. Mode locked lasers can produce pulses down to the femtosecond (10^{-15} s) range.

24.8 GAUSSIAN LASER BEAMS

A laser cavity operating in the TEM_{00} mode produces a cavity standing wave with a gaussian intensity distribution (or close to it). The output beam, usually well collimated, is a traveling wave that is a continuation of the gaussian wave. The specific type of laser cavity determines the characteristics of the gaussian wave. (Section 22.10 previously discussed waves with a gaussian intensity distribution.)

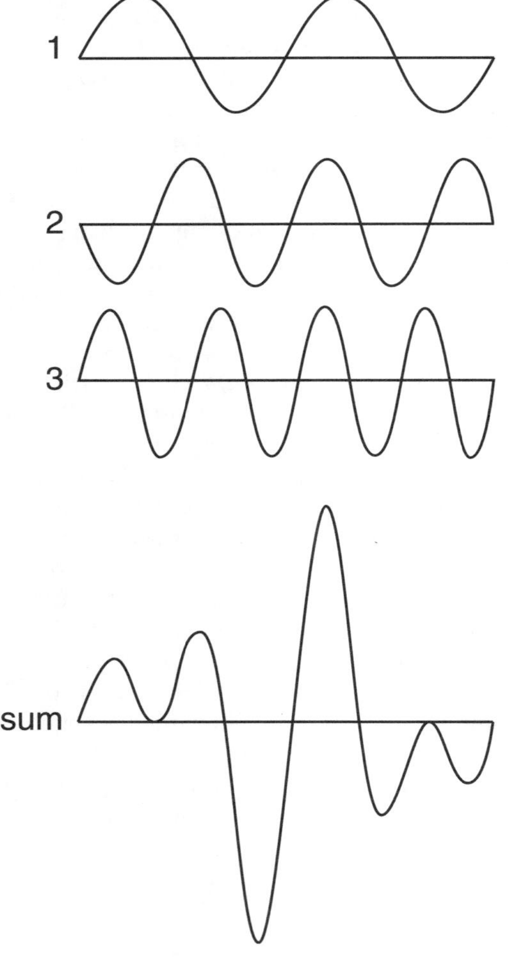

Figure 24.18 A number of locked longitudinal modes (standing waves). Their sum results in ultra-short pulses at the constructive interference zones, which occur only where the crests of the mode locked waves are all aligned.

Consider a concentric laser cavity that has two spherical mirrors with coincident centers of curvature. Figure 24.19a shows the first order geometric optics prediction for a photon starting in the middle of the cavity. The rays incident on the mirrors reflect straight back and predict a point concentration of the amplified light in the middle of the cavity. However because of diffraction, the coherent light does not concentrate into a point. Instead as the light sweeps back and forth in the cavity, it forms a standing wave that in the TEM_{00} mode has a lateral gaussian intensity distribution (Figure 24.19b).

The *beam waist* is the smallest lateral size of a gaussian standing wave. For the concentric cavity, the beam waist occurs at the middle of the cavity and has a non-zero semidiameter size parameter w_o. In the cavity, the wavefront curvature matches the curvature at each spherical mirror. The coherent wavefronts that reflect off the left mirror of the cavity are converging, but in the diffraction limited gaussian standing wave they flatten into a plane wave at the beam waist. Then to the right of the waist, they change to diverging and match the curvature of the right mirror when they reach it. When the right mirror is partially transmitting, the output beam is just a continuation of the gaussian beam in the cavity.

Assume that the laser output beam is traveling down the z axis, and let $z = 0$ at the beam waist. Then Eq. 22.9 specifies the semidiameter size parameter $w(z)$ of the gaussian laser beam at a distance z down the axis (including external to the laser). (Recall that at a position z along the axis, $w(z)$ is the radial distance to the position where the intensity drops to $1/e^2$ of the maximum.) Furthermore let

$$z_o = \frac{\pi w_o^2}{\lambda} \tag{24.13}$$

Then Eq. 22.9 can be rewritten as

$$w(z) = w_o\sqrt{1+\left(\frac{z}{z_o}\right)^2} \tag{24.14}$$

The gaussian beam equations also show that the radius of curvature $r(z)$ of the wavefronts as a function of the distance z along the axis is given by

$$r(z) = -z\left[1+\left(\frac{z_o}{z}\right)^2\right] \tag{24.15}$$

Equation 24.15 shows that at the waist ($z = 0$), the wavefront radius of curvature goes to infinity (i.e., the wavefront is a plane wavefront). Then from

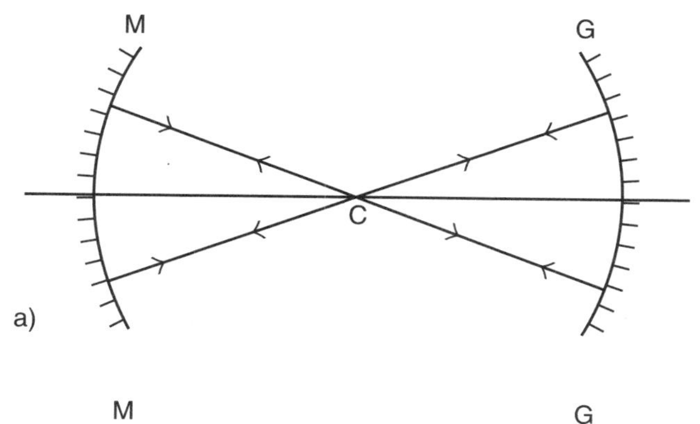

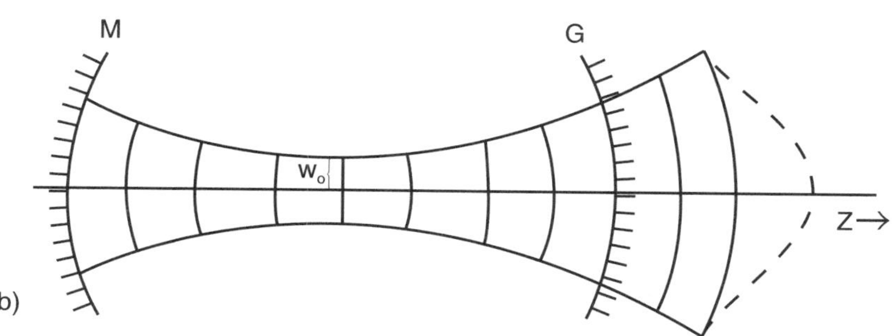

Figure 24.19 Concentric laser cavity: *M* and *G* are the respective left and right spherical mirrors, where *G* is partially transmitting. a, first order geometric optics prediction (diffraction neglected) for the oscillation in the concentric cavity; b, diffraction causes a Gaussian standing wave in the concentric cavity. The gaussian wave has a beam waist at the center with a finite size parameter w_o. The dashed curve on the right represents the Gaussian intensity distribution across the output beam.

the waist to $z = z_o$, the wavefronts gain curvature. At $z = z_o$, the wavefronts have their maximum curvature, and they flatten out again once past z_o. The area bounded by $\pm z_o$ is variously called the waist length, the near zone, or the Rayleigh range of the laser beam. The area well past z_o is called the far zone.

Equation 24.13 shows that large waist sizes (large w_o values) give large z_o values (large waist lengths). For a large z_o value, Eq. 24.15 shows that the wavefront radius of curvature is always large (in other words the wavefronts are always close to plane waves). For a very small z_o value (from a very small waist size w_o), Eq. 24.15 shows that the radius of curvature of the wavefronts is approximately equal to $-z$, which is the radius of curvature of a spherical diverging wavefront.

Similarly for a very small z_o value, Eq. 24.14 shows that $w(z)$ is initially increasing as a function of z, so the beam is spreading out or diverging. For a large z_o, Eq. 24.14 then shows that initially (i.e., small z values) $w(z)$ is equal to w_o, and the beam is well collimated.

The beam size represented by $w(z)$ is hyperbolic as a function of z. Far from the waist, the hyperbolas become asymptotic to straight lines, and the asymptotes diverge from the axis at the angle given by Eq. 22.10, or

$$\theta = \frac{\lambda}{\pi w_o} \tag{24.16}$$

The total laser beam diverges at an angle of 2θ, which is usually expressed in milliradians. (Note that 1 mrad = 3.44').

When the gaussian laser beam goes through an aberration free lens (or series of lenses), the beam emerging from the lens is also gaussian but with new parameters. In particular, the beam will have a new waist size and location, as well as a new beam divergence. Downstream from the laser, we may want to use a lens to focus the laser beam into a small spot (i.e., a small waist).

The waist is not actually an object, but nevertheless, the behavior of the gaussian laser beam can be described by equations that are similar to the thin lens imaging equations. In terms of lengths, the thin lens imaging equation is

$$\frac{1}{v} = \frac{1}{f_2} + \frac{1}{u}$$

A modification to find the new waist of a gaussian laser beam is

$$\frac{1}{v} = \frac{1}{f_2} + \frac{(u + f_2)}{u(u + f_2) + (z_o^2)} \tag{24.17}$$

where u is the (directed) distance from the lens to the old waist and v is the (directed) distance from the lens to the new waist. Equation 24.17 can be written as a $V = P + U$, where

$$U = \frac{(u + f_2)}{u(u + f_2) + (z_o^2)} \tag{24.18}$$

For a non-zero z_o, the gaussian beam equations can give results that are different from those of the thin lens imaging equations (where $U = 1/u$). For example, in geometric optics imaging, when an object point is at the primary focal point, the conjugate image point is at optical infinity. However for a gaussian beam waist in the primary focal plane of a lens, $u = f_1 = -f_2$. Then Eq. 24.17 gives $v = f_2$, and the new beam waist is in the secondary focal plane (Figure 24.20). One way to think of this is that the new waist is not the "image" of the old waist, but rather it is the diffraction pattern of the old waist.

Let w'_o be the semidiameter size parameter of the new waist, while w_o is the semidiameter size parameter of the old waist. Then we can define a gaussian beam lateral magnification as

$$|m| \equiv \frac{w'_o}{w_o} \tag{24.19}$$

From the diffraction equations for a gaussian beam,

$$|m| = \frac{f_2}{\sqrt{(u+f_2)^2 + z_o^2}} \tag{24.20}$$

For a fixed f_2 and u, Eqs. 24.19 and 24.20 show that a larger z_o value gives a smaller $|m|$ and thus a smaller new waist size. The equations also show that for a fixed z_o there are two ways to get a smaller waist (i.e., focus the laser beam into a smaller spot). One way is to minimize the numerator by using a shorter focal length lens (i.e., a higher dioptric power). The other way is to maximize the denominator, which can be done by increasing the distance u (i.e., move the lens farther away from the laser).

Let z'_o be the new waist length (Rayleigh range) after the beam goes through a lens. Then it follows from Eqs. 24.13 and 24.19 that

$$\frac{z'_o}{z_o} = \frac{(w'_o)^2}{(w_o)^2} = |m|^2 \tag{24.21}$$

Equation 24.21 is similar to the axial magnification equations (Section 9.10).

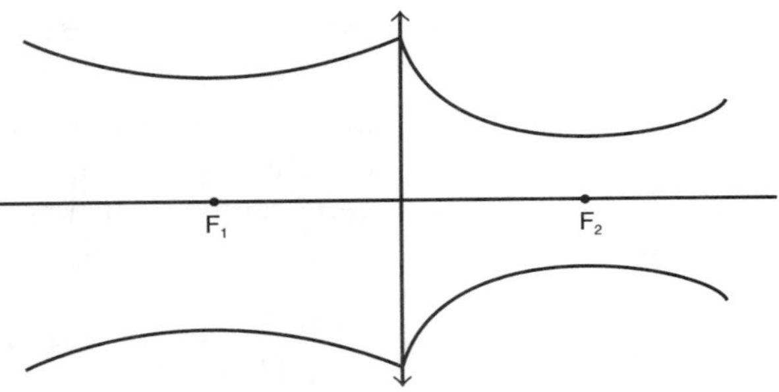

Figure 24.20 For a Gaussian beam waist at F_1, the thin lens forms a new gaussian beam waist at F_2.

For the special case of the old waist at f_1, which results in the new waist at f_2, Eq. 24.20 gives $|m| = f_2/z_o$. Then from Eqs. 24.13, 24.16, and 24.19, $w'_o = f_2\theta$, which shows that in this case the focussed spot size directly depends on the divergence of the laser beam. Spot sizes the order of a wavelength can be obtained with high power diffraction limited lenses.

If the coherent light could be concentrated into a single point (like a point source), then the waist size w_o equals 0, and Eq. 24.13 gives $z_o = 0$. Equation 24.17 then reduces to the thin lens imaging equation, and Eq. 24.20 for the gaussian beam magnification $|m|$ reduces to the lateral magnification equation $m = v/u = f_2/(u+f_2)$. Thus the difference between the gaussian beam equations and the thin lens equations is that the laser cavity acts like an *extended* coherent source where w_o is a representative measure of the extended source size, while the thin lens imaging equation is for a point source (zero size).

EXAMPLE 24.6a

A low power helium–neon laser ($\lambda = 632.8$ nm), operating in the TEM_{00} mode, has a beam divergence of 0.806 mrad (about 2.78′). What is the beam waist size and the waist length (Rayleigh range)?

The beam divergence equals 2θ, so $\theta = 0.403$ mrad. Equation 24.16 gives

$$w_o = \frac{632.8 \times 10^{-9}\,\text{m}}{\pi(0.403 \times 10^{-3})} = 5.0 \times 10^{-4}\,\text{m} = 0.50\,\text{mm}$$

Since w_o represents the semidiameter of the beam, the beam "diameter" is $2w_o$ or 1 mm. From Eq. 24.13,

$$z_o = \frac{\pi(0.50 \times 10^{-3}\,\text{m})^2}{632.8 \times 10^{-9}\,\text{m}} = 1.24\,\text{m}$$

EXAMPLE 24.6b

Suppose the He–Ne laser in the previous part has a waist produced inside the cavity at a distance of 20 cm from the partially transmitting output mirror, and a +10.00 D lens is then placed against the output mirror. Where is the new waist and what is its size? Also what is the new waist length (Rayleigh range)?

In this case, the beam waist is at $2F_1$ of the lens, so in a thin lens imaging situation, we would expect the image to be at $2F_2$ and the lateral magnification to be -1. Here $f_2 = 0.10$ m,

$u = -0.20\,\text{m}$, and $z_o = 1.26\,\text{m}$. From $V = P + U$, with U given by Eq. 24.18,

$$V = +10.00\,\text{D} + \frac{(-0.20\,\text{m} + 0.10\,\text{m})}{(-0.20\,\text{m})(-0.20\,\text{m} + 0.10\,\text{m}) + (1.24\,\text{m})^2}$$

Then,

$$V = +10.00\,\text{D} + \left(\frac{-0.10\,\text{m}}{1.56\,\text{m}^2}\right)$$
$$= +10.00\,\text{D} + (-0.064\,\text{D}) = +9.94\,\text{D}$$

and

$$v = 10.06\,\text{cm}$$

Unlike the imaging situation, the new beam waist is very near the secondary focal point of the $+10.00\,\text{D}$ lens, which is what we would expect for a well-collimated laser beam. From Eq. 24.19,

$$|m| = \frac{0.10\,\text{m}}{\sqrt{(-0.20\,\text{m} + 0.10\,\text{m})^2 + (1.24\,\text{m})^2}} = 0.0804$$

From Eq. 24.29, the size of the new waist semi-diameter is

$$w'_o = (0.0804)(0.50\,\text{mm}) = 40.2\,\mu\text{m}$$

so the waist diameter is $80.4\,\mu\text{m}$. From Eq. 24.13,

$$z_o = \frac{\pi(40.2 \times 10^{-6}\,\text{m})^2}{632.8 \times 10^{-9}}$$
$$= 8.02 \times 10^{-3}\,\text{m} = 8.02\,\text{mm}$$

The smaller waist size and waist length mean that once past the new waist, the beam has a larger spread (divergence) than it did before the focussing. In particular, with the new waist size, Eq. 24.16 gives

$$\theta = \frac{632.8 \times 10^{-9}\,\text{m}}{\pi(40.2 \times 10^{-6}\,\text{m})} = 5.01\,\text{mrad}$$

and the new beam divergence 2θ is 10.02 mrad.

EXAMPLE 24.7

In the previous example, a laser beam was focussed very near the secondary focal plane of the focussing lens. Now place a $+5.00\,\text{D}$ lens at a distance of 40 cm from the focussed waist. Where is the new waste and what is its size?

Here the initial focussed beam waist semidiameter is quite small ($40.2\,\mu\text{m}$), and the laser beam is diverging significantly once it passes the focussed waist. Therefore we might expect that the gaussian beam equations will act more like thin lens imaging equations in this case. For this case, $f_2 = 0.20\,\text{m}$, $u = -0.40\,\text{m}$, and $z_o = 8.02 \times 10^{-3}\,\text{m}$. From $V = P + U$, with U given by Eq. 24.18,

$$V = +5.00\,\text{D} + \frac{(-0.40\,\text{m} + 0.20\,\text{m})}{(-0.40\,\text{m})(-0.40\,\text{m} + 0.20\,\text{m}) + (8.02 \times 10^{-3}\,\text{m})^2}$$

Then,

$$V = +5.00\,\text{D} + \left(\frac{-0.20\,\text{m}}{0.080\,\text{m}^2}\right)$$
$$= +5.00\,\text{D} + (-2.50\,\text{D}) = +2.50\,\text{D}$$

and

$$v = 40.0\,\text{cm}$$

From Eq. 24.19,

$$|m| = \frac{0.20\,\text{m}}{\sqrt{(-0.40\,\text{m} + 0.20\,\text{m})^2 + (8.02 \times 10^{-3}\,\text{m})^2}} = 1.00$$

Indeed these results are identical to thin lens imaging results.

An afocal telescope is frequently used to expand the diameter of a well-collimated laser beam. Let M_{tel} be the magnification of the afocal telescope (so $M_{tel} = -P_{oc}/P_{obj} = -f_{obj}/f_{oc}$). Figure 19.11 shows the geometric optics ray behavior for plane waves incident on an afocal Keplerian telescope. The output beam also consists of plane waves but the beam diameter is M_{tel} times smaller than the incident beam diameter. Consequently when the beams are reversed in direction (arrows on the rays are reversed) and pass backward through the telescope, the telescope increases the beam diameter by a factor of M_{tel}.

Since the geometric optics rays do not take diffraction into account, let's consider an incident gaussian beam with its waist in the primary focal plane of the first lens of the backward telescope. Then the first lens forms a new beam waist of non-zero size in its secondary focal plane, which is also the primary focal plane of the second lens. The second lens then forms a beam waist at its secondary focal point, and this is the waist of the beam leaving the backward telescope. For lens 1 (the original ocular lens), Eq. 24.20 gives

$$|m|_1 = \frac{(f_2)_{oc}}{z_o}$$

where z_o is the waist length of the laser beam incident on the telescope. For lens 2 (the original objective lens),

$$|m|_2 = \frac{(f_2)_{obj}}{z'_o} = \frac{(f_2)_{obj}}{|m|_1^2 z_o}$$

where z'_o is the waist length of the beam between lenses 1 and 2. (The second equality comes from Eq. 24.21.) The total lateral magnification $|m|_t$ for the gaussian beam passing through the backward telescope is given by

$$|m|_t = |m|_1 |m|_2$$

Then from the above three equations,

$$|m|_t = |m|_1 \frac{(f_2)_{obj}}{|m|_1^2 z_o} = \frac{(f_2)_{obj}}{|m|_1 z_o}$$

and

$$|m|_t = \frac{(f_2)_{obj}}{(f_2)_{oc}} = |M_{tel}|$$

So the beam waist formed by the backward telescope is indeed M_{tel} times larger than the beam waist of the incident beam. From Eq. 24.16, this means that the output beam divergence is M_{tel} times smaller the input beam divergence. So a small diameter well-collimated input beam gives a larger diameter output beam that has even less divergence.

The above example was for the initial beam waist in the primary focal plane of the first lens of the backward telescope. For other initial waist locations, the details are a little different, but the overall results are similar for a well-collimated input beam.

For a high powered laser beam, there can be a high concentration of energy at the beam waist between the two lenses of a Keplerian telescope. This can lead to electrical breakdown of the air molecules at that position. This breakdown can be avoided by use of an afocal backward Galilean telescope to expand the laser beam.

24.9 COMMON LASERS

The standard lasers produce light that is coherent, highly monochromatic, and very well collimated. Furthermore, the laser irradiance output can be incredibly high. In addition, practically the entire power output can be concentrated into an extremely small area by focusing the laser beam.

Some of the laser applications are due to the coherence (e.g., precision measurement by interference, holography, and spatial filtering). Some are due to the monochromaticity (triggering of specific chemical reactions). Others are due to the ability to focus the laser radiation into such a small area (e.g., precision manufacturing, the optical "stylus" in a CD player). Still others are due to the brute force power applications that depend on large irradiances (e.g., welding, drilling, cutting hard materials such as diamond, vaporizing small amounts of material). Finally the fact that laser light can carry enormous amounts of information makes it the method of choice for transmitting information in computer networks, or even for just transmitting telephone signals.

There are a wide variety of lasers. Some are very small in size (pinhead or smaller), while others are very large (the size of a large building). Some are very low power (milliwatt output) while others are very high power (greater than 10^{13} W in a nanosecond pulse).

Continuous beam 632.8 nm helium–neon (He–Ne) gas lasers are a common low power (milliwatt) laser. The pump occurs in the helium, and the energy is then transferred to a metastable neon state by collisions between the helium and neon atoms. The neon lases at the 632.8 nm transition between two excited states, and then makes other transitions back down to the ground state. Recently, special cavity designs have resulted in green (543.5 nm), yellow (594.1 nm), and orange (612.0 nm) helium–neon lasers.

A more powerful (watt range) continuous beam gas laser is the argon ion laser, which generates its strongest outputs at either 488 nm (Argon blue) or 514.5 nm (Argon green). The krypton ion continuous beam gas laser has a strong output at 647.1 nm (krypton red). Both argon and krypton can be made to also lase at certain other wavelengths, but not as efficiently.

In terms of power output, the carbon dioxide (CO_2) gas laser is in a class by itself. The CO_2 laser emits in the infrared ($\lambda = 10{,}600$ nm). Even in continuous mode, it can emit in the kilowatt range, enough to cut through 2 cm of steel in a matter of seconds. The cavity of the CO_2 laser is actually a mixture of CO_2, nitrogen, and helium. The pump feeds energy to the nitrogen and helium, which in turn transfer the energy to the CO_2 for the stimulated emission.

Excimer lasers contain rare gas halides such as argon-fluoride (ArF). The word excimer is derived from excited state dimer. These substances are unusual in that they have no ground state, and are therefore automatically metastable. The excited state dimer can decay to the individual atoms giving off a photon in the process:

$$ArF^{\bullet} \rightarrow Ar + F + \text{photon}$$

An incident photon of the correct energy can stimulate this decay, in which case the emitted photon is coherent with the stimulating photon. Excimer lasers are exciting because they can lase in the ultraviolet region where each individual photon carries more energy. For example, the ArF excimer lases at 193 nm, while the KrF excimer lases at 248 nm, and the XeF lases at 350 nm. Typical power from the excimer lasers ranges from 50 W to 100 W, although they have reached powers as high as the megawatt range in very short pulses.

The ruby laser (the first laser) is a solid state laser, and is still used in pulsed mode at 694.3 nm. The ruby laser requires high pumping powers because the transitions terminate in the ground state, so the population inversion is hard to maintain (a 3 level laser). If the laser transition terminates in an excited state, the population inversion is easier to maintain and requires less pumping power. (Figure 24.21 shows a simplified energy level diagram for a 4 level laser.) A widely used 4 level laser is the solid state Nd:YAG laser, where a small percentage of neodymium (Nd) ions are dispersed as replacements for yttrium ions in yttrium aluminum garnet (YAG) crystals. (The terminology is that the crystal has been *doped* with neodymium.) The common Nd:YAG continuous beam laser can produce up to the kilowatt range at the infrared wavelength of 1,060 nm. Ultrashort pulsed Nd:YAG lasers can produce up to the terawatt range (10^{12} W).

The Nd:YAG laser has been a workhorse in several areas (manufacturing, military, surgical), and there are several other very similar lasers. These include the Nd:YLF (YLF = crystalline yttrium–lithium-fluoride) laser, the Nd:glass lasers, the holmium:YAG (Ho:YAG) laser, and the erbium YAG (Er:YAG) laser. Some laser surgery applications target the water in the body's cells. The Er:YAG laser emits at 2,940 nm, which is near the maximum absorption strength for water. The Ho:YAG emits at 2,100 nm, which is also well absorbed by water.

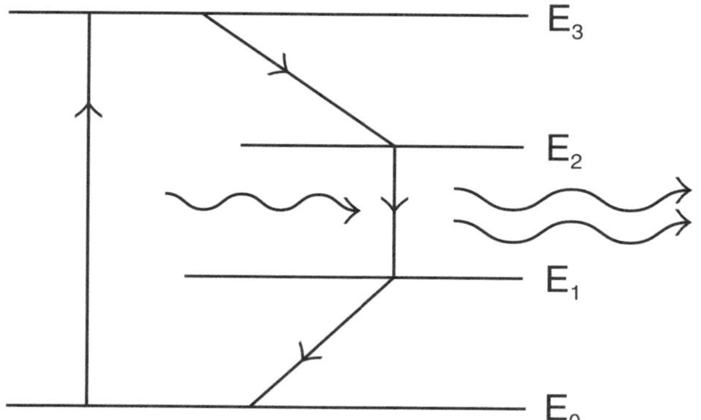

Figure 24.21 Energy level diagram for a four-level laser.

Semiconductor light emitting diodes (LEDs) can also be made to lase. Semiconductor lasers range in power from milliwatts to megawatts. Semiconductor lasers can be very small in size (millimeters down to a few microns). They are very common in such things as CD players and laser printers, and are the light sources for fiber optics Local Area (computer) Networks (LANs). The energy levels in a semiconductor diode are properties of the entire crystal as opposed to the individual atoms.

The active medium of a semiconductor diode laser is the boundary zone (a *pn* junction) between two parts of the semiconductor crystal with different replacement atoms (called impurities) through which an appropriate electrical current is flowing. Impurities with more electrons than the atoms they replace produce the *n* zone (negative charge carriers), while impurities with fewer electrons than the atoms they replace produce the *p* zone (positive charge carriers). In the *p* zone, the deficiency of electrons results in empty electron spaces or holes. When a neighboring electron moves into a hole, it leaves a new hole behind. As the process continues, the hole appears to propagate just as if it were a plus charge carrier.

When the negative voltage hookup is applied to the *n* side and the positive voltage hookup is applied to the *p* side, both the plus and minus charge carriers flow toward the junction (a process called injection). The electrons on the *n* side are in a higher energy level than the holes on the *p* side. In the junction area, electrons combine with the holes giving off energy (i.e. the electron jumps from a higher to a lower energy level). In silicon diodes, most of this energy is converted to heat and no light is produced. In a gallium arsenic (GaAs) diode, much of the energy is released as photons at 905 nm (infrared). GaAs has a 3.6 refractive index, so there are fairly strong reflections at the cleaved faces of the semiconductor diode. These reflections are usually used to form the laser cavity. The population inversion (more electrons than holes) is created by a combination of the proper doping (i.e., proper replacement of atoms) together with the appropriate current. The output beam can be switched to shorter wavelengths (including down into the visible red region) by adding aluminum to the GaAs diode (i.e., a GaAlAs semiconductor). Recently, the use of gallium nitride materials has resulted in semiconductor diode lasers that emit in the short wavelength (blue) end of the visible spectrum (around 400 nm). The nitride materials are so-called wide bandgap semiconductors.

The output beams from the small micro-sized semiconductor lasers are not well collimated (e.g., a total beam divergence angle of 158 mrad or 9°). For a horizontal *pn* junction, the original diode lasers emitted horizontally from the edge of the junction. Vertical-cavity surface emitting lasers (VCSELs) are newer micro-diode lasers in which the laser emission is vertical or perpendicular to the horizontal *pn* junction. The beam divergence can be made smaller with the VCSELs.

Liquid organic dye lasers, either flashlamp pumped or pumped by other lasers, can produce laser radiation that is tunable over a range of wavelengths. This occurs because the lower energy level in the stimulated emission transition is a group of a large number of very closely spaced molecular energy levels. Thus, the electron jump can be from the higher level to any of the lower levels. This gives a range of possible wavelengths. When the laser is tuned (by using a prism or diffraction grating in the cavity), the cavity amplification and output can be changed over this range of wavelengths. There are also some solid state tunable lasers.

When a high intensity (perhaps short or ultra short pulses) of laser light of frequency f is incident on certain nonlinear crystals, the output of the crystal may be coherent light at frequency $2f$, $3f$, $4f$, etc (see Section 25.14). When irradiated by a 1,064 nm beam from a Nd:YAG laser, a potassium titanyl phosphate (KTP) nonlinear crystal has a 532 nm coherent beam output. Thus if one has a sufficiently powerful Nd:YAG laser, one can put a KTP crystal in the beam to get a (lower energy) coherent beam at 532 nm. This is variously called a frequency doubled YAG laser, a KTP/YAG laser, a green YAG laser, or even KTP laser (even though the initial coherent light came from the Nd ions in the Nd:YAG laser).

24.10 OPHTHALMIC LASER SURGERY

The laser has become a valuable tool for a number of general surgical procedures, including some ophthalmic surgical procedures. The near infrared and visible laser wavelengths are transmitted by the cornea enabling large amounts of energy to be delivered to the interior of the eye without surgically cutting the eye open. Furthermore, this energy can be precisely focussed into a small area. To produce the surgical effect, the target tissue must absorb the laser light. (If there is no absorption, there is no energy gain in the target tissue, and therefore no effect.) The surgical effects of the laser beam depend on its wavelength (frequency) and on the amount of power delivered (which in turn depends on the laser pulse duration). The surgical effects produced by the laser are either photochemical, ionizing, or thermal. Most ophthalmic surgical lasers operate in the watt range.

For exposures longer than roughly 1 μs and low to moderate irradiances, laser radiation below 320 nm produces primarily photochemical reactions. For similar irradiances and exposure times, laser radiation at longer wavelengths usually produces thermal effects. At very high irradiances, generally produced by exposure times shorter than 20 ns, enough power is provided to tear electrons from atoms and molecules (ionization), and the resulting rapidly expanding electron plasma rips tissue apart (i.e., secondary mechanical damage or photodisruption).

Photochemical effects are divided into photoradiation and photoablation. Photoradiation is a process in which the absorption of light triggers a chemical reaction that produces the desired effect. For example, a chemical is injected into the blood stream. The particular chemical is taken up and retained by metabolically active tumor tissue. A specific laser with a wavelength that is absorbed by the chemical then subsequently irradiates the tissue. The absorbed energy triggers a chemical reaction that ultimately produces a cytotoxic derivative that kills the tumor tissue.

In photoablation, single photons of ultraviolet radiation have enough energy to break chemical bonds. When a surface is hit with a high irradiance of this ultraviolet radiation during a short exposure time, the bond breakage is very precise resulting in "clean" cuts with no collateral damage. These "cuts" cause ejection of molecular fragments (i.e., a "smoke" plume) at supersonic velocities (1,000–2,000 m/s). Since the etch depth per laser pulse is predictable, photoablation can remove material layer by layer in very thin layers. Photoablation is not a thermal effect and is considered a "cold" process.

Thermal effects can be divided into photocoagulation and photovaporization. The structure of biological tissue is stabilized by the relatively weak van der Waals force between molecules. Even at normal temperatures, some destabilization (or denaturation) may occur. Biological renewal processes "fix" this and maintain physiological equilibrium. A temperature increase of 10–20 °C overcomes the van der Waals force causing the coagulation (clotting) of the target tissue. (For example, think of the liquid material in an egg and how it changes when the egg is cooked.) The extent of the thermal injury is proportional to the product of the irradiance times the exposure time (i.e, the total energy delivered). A higher irradiance is required for an immediate effect. There may be damage to collateral tissue by either heat spreading or by scattered laser light.

When laser irradiances higher than those required for photocoagulation are applied to the target tissue, the tissue temperature may reach the boiling point of water, and rapidly expanding water vapor (an explosion) rips the tissue apart (tissue disruption) before coagulation can cauterize the tissue. This is called photovaporization. In many situations, cauterization will subsequently occur.

Usually incident electromagnetic waves have field strengths that are much lower than the electromagnetic field strengths of the atoms and molecules. However, this is not the case in the ultra high laser irradiances that result in ionization and subsequent secondary mechanical damage (photodisruption). The ultra high irradiances can be achieved with mode locked or Q-switched lasers focussed to small spot sizes. At the spot, the electromagnetic waves have electric field strengths that are large compared that of the atomic and molecular electrical fields. This energy frees the bound electrons (ionizes the material), and the resulting free electron plasma expands rapidly (an explosion) producing shock/acoustic pressure waves that rip the material apart. Latent stress can contribute further disruption of the material. Associated pressure spikes or liquid jets may damage adjacent tissue and membranes and/or subsequent thermal effects may also cause damage. A huge advantage of plasma formation (ionization) is that it does not depend on conventional absorption, so one can use it to operate on (i.e., disrupt) weakly absorbing or transparent materials.

A fairly common complication of a cataract removal and intraocular lens (IOL) implant is that the remaining lens capsule subsequently loses its transparency due to epithelial cell proliferation. In a capuslotomy, a Nd:YAG laser is used to "zap" (photodisrupt) the capsule causing it to split and pull back leaving a clear area of 3–4 mm in size. In cases of angle closure glaucoma due to a pupillary block, photodisruption by a Nd:YAG is also used for a peripheral iridectomy (opening a hole in the peripheral iris) on lightly colored (i.e., poorly absorbing) iris.

For darkly colored irises (better absorbers), a peripheral iridectomy can be achieved by photovaporization with an argon ion laser. The argon laser can also be used to photocoagulate blood vessels and thus control bleeding if needed. (This is an advantage of the argon ion laser over the Nd:YAG).

In cases of angle closure glaucoma, Argon ion lasers with a large spot size are used to create burns (photocoagulate) in the extreme periphery of the iris. The resulting burns cause tissue shrinkage, which then pulls the iris back and opens the angle. In glaucoma due to a lack of drainage through the trabecular meshwork, argon lasers are used to place burns at the juncture of the pigmented and non-pigmented trabeculum. The postulated theory is that the burns shrink the collagen, thereby tightening the ring of meshwork, and opening up the drainage spaces.

The argon ion laser is also commonly used for photocoagulation of the retina. This can seal/weld retinal holes and tears, and destroy new (leaky) blood vessel growth in diabetic retinopathy, age related maculopathy, or branch retinal vein occlusion. It may also be used in panretinal photcoagulation, which is a destruction of selected peripheral retinal tissue to decrease the demand for oxygen so that the new (leaky) blood vessel growth is inhibited.

In retinal photocoagulation near the macula, care must be taken not to damage the macula region, which is the region responsible for detail vision. Xanthophyll, the yellow pigment in the macular region, absorbs strongly for incident wavelengths below 500 nm, and only weakly for wavelengths above 500 nm. (Remember that something that looks yellow, orange, or red under white light illumination is generally absorbing blues better than reds, while something that looks blue is absorbing reds better than blues.) Therefore, an argon green laser (514.5 nm), or better a frequency doubled YAG (532 nm), or even better yet a krypton red (647 nm) laser would supply better protection against accidental damage to the macula than an Argon blue laser (488.0 nm).

Oxyhemoglobin strongly absorbs incident wavelengths below 630 nm, while hemoglobin absorbs strongly below 600 nm. Thus, in the presence of a hemorrhage, blood strongly absorbs Argon blue, Argon green, and frequency doubled YAG laser light. On the other hand, hemoglobin is a very weak absorber for krypton red (647 nm), while oxyhemoglobin is a moderately weak absorber (little less than 30%) of krypton red. Therefore, krypton red lasers are used for retinal photocoagulation through hemorrhages. Krypton red laser light also penetrates deeper into the choroid than either Argon blue or green laser light, and is thus used for photocoagulation of deeper choroidal structures.

The cornea is transparent to visible light, but absorbs (is opaque) out in the ultraviolet region. (Window glass is similar.) Therefore the ArFl excimer laser (193 nm) can be used to operate on the cornea by photoablation. In photorefractive keratectomy (PRK), the epithelial layer of the cornea is scraped away, and then the excimer is used to change the corneal curvature by removing material (laser sculpting) in a 5–9 mm diameter zone. In myopia, the cornea is flattened by removing more material in the center than at the edges of the zone. In moderate myopia up to 10% of the corneal thickness may be removed. In higher amounts of myopia, up to 30% of the corneal thickness may be removed. The material removed includes Bowman's membrane together with some stroma, and Bowman's membrane does not grow back. The wounded cornea must heal, and the steroid regimen that is used during the healing may also influence the final outcome. Regression occurs in some cases.

In laser in situ keratomileusis (LASIK), the cornea is flattened and a microkeratome is used to cut a thin slice in the anterior cornea, and the slice is then flapped back to expose the stroma. The ArFl excimer laser is then used to reshape the stroma, and the slice is then repositioned onto the reshaped stroma, where normal suction holds the flap in place. (Bowmen's membrane is in the flap, so it is not destroyed with LASIK.) LASIK is a riskier procedure than PRK, but appears to have a higher satisfaction rate.

Just as with any surgical procedures, there are sometimes complications with laser surgery. Besides major complications (loss of an eye, loss of detail vision, reduction in best corrected acuity, etc.), other laser refractive surgery complications might include glare, halos, starbursts, reduction in ability to see low contrast objects, and objects that are seen may not appear as crisp as before. Higher presurgery refractive errors, and wider ablation zones seem to result in more complications. Eyes that have undergone laser surgery currently have more optical third and higher order aberrations than presurgery eyes. At the start of the year 2000, a number of companies were conducting research and development on ways to incorporate aberration correction into laser corneal refractive surgery.

24.11 LASER SAFETY

High powered lasers are dangerous to any part of the human body. Low powered lasers, such as the milliwatt helium–neon lasers, are dangerous only to the eye. The laser beam is well collimated (very directional), and has a small enough beam diameter so that the entire undiverged beam can enter the eye. Furthermore, the eye focusses the collimated laser light into an even smaller area on the retina. A retinal burn may result even before the person can flinch. A foveal burn results in severe and irreversible loss in acuity. For this reason, care should be exercised in the vicinity of laser beams. Besides a direct exposure, the laser operator should avoid specular reflections of the laser beam that might cause an exposure from an unexpected direction. Interference filters are available that protect the eye by reflecting the laser wavelength while transmitting other wavelengths.

The American National Standards Institute (ANSI) divides lasers into 4 hazard classes. The classes include limits on infrared and ultraviolet exposures. Here only the visible light limits are quoted. Class I lasers are very lower power lasers ($\leq 0.5\,\mu$W) that present no eye or skin hazard from full day exposure, and are exempt from labeling requirements. Class II lasers produce low power (≤ 1 mW) visible radiation that cannot injure by a short accidental exposure, but retinal damage can occur if the beam is directly viewed for a long period of time. In more technical language, class II lasers present no eye hazard from intrabeam exposure within the aversion reflex time. Examples of class II lasers are sufficiently low power laser pointers and surveying lasers. Class IIIa lasers produce visible beams of power ≤ 5 mW capable of producing damage on accidental exposure through an optical aid. (More powerful laser pointers fall into this class.) Class IIIb lasers present an eye hazard from intrabeam exposure within the aversion reflex time (i.e., can cause a burn before the person can flinch). Diffuse reflections from a class IIIb laser may present eye and skin hazards. The beam should be viewed only via diffuse reflection, from a distance over 50 mm from the diffuse surface, for less than 10 s, and with the diffuse image diameter being greater than 5.5 mm. Class IV lasers present eye and skin hazard from intrabeam viewing and from diffuse reflection viewing, and are a fire hazard if combustible materials are exposed.

Required safety precautions include warning labels, signs, more careful operator behavior, and beam enclosure for the higher powers. The required precautions are obviously more stringent as the class number increases.

24.12 PHOTONS AND PROBABILITY

In classical harmonic wave theory, the energy carried by the wave is proportional to the square of the wave's amplitude. In the wave mechanics version of quantum theory, a single particle, including a photon, is represented by a wavepacket (Figure 24.22), and the square of the packet's wavefunction gives the probability of finding the photon at a particular position at a particular time. (In other words, the probability of finding the energy.)

In Figure 24.22a, the photon's wavefunction lies between *A* and *C*. We know the photon is somewhere between *A* and *C*, but we do not know exactly where.

The photon is most likely to be at the positions with a large wavefunction displacement and less likely to be at the small displacement positions.

Suppose the photon represented in Figure 24.22a is passing through an aperture that is rigged to close quickly at point B thereby dividing the photon's wavefunction into two parts. However, the photon itself is not divisible. So, does the photon get through the aperture or not?

Based on the wavefunction information, we do not know the answer. All we can determine is the probability of whether the photon gets through. Let us assume that 40% of the square of the wavefunction gets through. This means that the photon had a 40% chance of getting through and a 60% chance of not getting through. If we repeat this experiment many times, we cannot predict what happens to any one photon, but we do know that statistically the photon will get through in 40% of the cases and will not get through in 60%.

24.13 UNCERTAINTY

The beats shown in Figure 21.11b were the result of the superposition of two harmonic waves of slightly different frequencies. The photon wavepackets of Figure 24.22 can be made by the superposition of a number of harmonic waves each of slightly different frequency. Photons with a long emission time have wavepackets that resemble harmonic waves, and hence only a few harmonic waves need to be superposed to generate the photon wavepacket (Figure 24.22b). Thus, photons with long wavepackets have a relatively well-defined frequency and wavelength.

Many different harmonic waves are needed to make a short photon wavepacket (Figure 24.22a). So photons with short wavepackets have a large uncertainty in wavelength or frequency, i.e., the photon's frequency is $f \pm \Delta f$ where Δf is large. Since the photon's energy is related to its frequency, photons with a large uncertainty in frequency also have a large uncertainty in energy.

We can generalize these uncertainty relations by first noting that the uncertainty in frequency is inversely proportional to the emission time Δt. That is,

$$\Delta f \sim 1/\Delta t$$

or

$$\Delta f \Delta t \sim 1$$

Then,

$$h \Delta f \Delta t \sim h$$

where h is Planck's constant. Then from Eq. 24.6,

$$\Delta E \Delta t \sim h \qquad (24.22)$$

The length of a photon wavepacket, Δx in Figure 24.22, equals c times Δt, so Eq. 24.22 becomes

$$\Delta E[\Delta x/c] \sim h$$

Then from Eq. 24.9,

$$\Delta p \Delta x \sim h \qquad (24.23)$$

Equation 24.23 is the famous Heisenberg uncertainty principle, which couples the uncertainties in momentum and position together. A photon with a short wavepacket has a small Δx. Then since $\Delta p \sim h/\Delta x$, the uncertainty in momentum is large. Consider the photons that get through the aperture of Section 24.12. These photons have a shorter wavepacket than the incident photons. Thus, closing the aperture increased the uncertainty in the photon's momentum (and consequently in the energy).

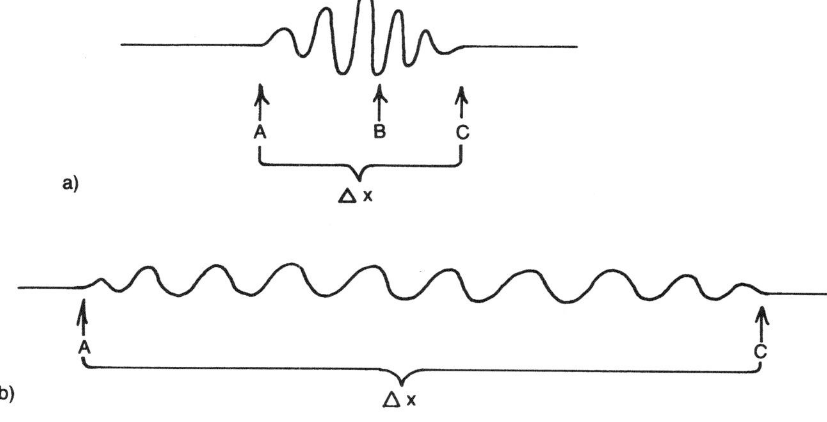

Figure 24.22 Single photon wave functions: a, short emission time; b, longer emission time.

Position measurements make Δx smaller, while momentum measurements make Δp smaller. Heisenberg's uncertainty principal says that when we make one uncertainty smaller, the other gets larger. In other words, the precise simultaneous knowledge of momentum and position is not possible. Basically, the measurement of position changes (increases the uncertainty in) the momentum and vice versa.

Heisenberg's uncertainty principle applies to all quantum particles. To understand the effect of a measurement, consider an electron moving with a well-defined momentum p. In general, one way to see objects is to shine light on them and then observe the diffusely reflected (scattered) light. So to see the electron, we will shine light on it and then observe the light that the electron scatters. However, an electron is so small that an incident photon hitting it is a significant collision. Therefore, while the scattered photon gives us information on the electron's position, we have now changed the electron's momentum increasing the uncertainty in Δp.

(The Vietnam War protests provide a real world analogy to the idea that measurements change the action. In theory, the television reporters with their cameras were present at the protests only to record (measure) the events. Presumably, the protest events would be exactly the same whether or not the television reporters were there. However, the protests seemed to gain momentum when the television crews showed up. So the measuring device, the television crews, influenced the event they were suppose to be measuring.)

24.14 DIFFRACTION AND SINGLE PHOTONS

When collimated light is incident on a narrow slit, we obtain a single-slit diffraction pattern on a distant screen. Now suppose the light level is decreased until only one photon at a time is incident on the slit. As time passes, the individual photons seem to land at random positions on the screen, but after awhile the cumulative effect of the energy delivered by the photons is equal to the irradiance of the classic single-slit diffraction pattern.

The irradiance on the screen is related to the square of the wavefunction. In the quantum theory, the square of the wavefunction tells the probability of where each individual photon will hit the screen. The most likely position for the photons to hit is at the central maximum. The least likely position for the photon to hit is at the minimum positions given by the photon's wavefunction.

We can relate the single-slit diffraction to the Heisenberg uncertainty principle. We know the position of the photons that pass through the slit within an uncertainty Δx equal to the slit width d. According to Heisenberg's uncertainty principle, the position measurement results in a momentum uncertainty perpendicular to the beam of

$$\Delta p \sim h/d$$

For a change in momentum Δp that is perpendicular to the beam direction, the angular deviation θ from the straight-ahead direction of the photons is given by

$$\tan\theta = \frac{\Delta p}{p}$$

or in the small angle approximation

$$\theta = \frac{\Delta p}{p}$$

Then the above three equations give

$$\theta = \frac{h/d}{p}$$

The photon's momentum p equals h/λ, and substitution and simplification results in

$$\theta = \frac{\lambda}{d}$$

This equation says that the increased uncertainty in momentum causes the photons to spread out in the angular zone bounded by λ/d, but this equation is just the small angle version of Eq. 22.1 for the first minimum in a single-slit diffraction pattern. So we see that the single slit makes a position measurement on the photons, and that position measurement changes the photon's momentum, which results in the angular spread that we classically call diffraction.

24.15 INTERFERENCE AND SINGLE PHOTONS

Consider a double-slit experiment in which only one photon at a time is incident on the double slits. The irradiance in the double-slit interference pattern is related to the square of the wavefunction and defines the probability of where the photon will hit the screen. The photon has a high probability of hitting the screen at or near the maximum positions and little or no probability of hitting the screen at or near the minimum positions.

We do not know exactly where any one photon will hit the screen, but we do know the probability. If we run enough identical photons through the double slits, we eventually end up with double-slit interference fringes. In Figure 24.23, each dot shown represents a photon hit on the screen. The first frame (a) shows the results after a few photons. The second frame (b) shows the results for more photons. Here the photon build up is already beginning to resemble the double-slit interference fringes.

From the single photon double-slit interference experiments, it is clear that interference is a single photon effect. As Paul Dirac said, "The photon interferes with itself." In fact, this is already evident in the single photon diffraction experiments. (Paul Dirac is also noted for his correct prediction of the existence of antimatter.)

For the double-slit interference experiment everything seems fine until someone asks, "Which slit does the photon go through?" The way to experimentally determine the answer is to rig the slits so that we can tell which slit the photon goes through. One possible way to do this is to put a red transmitting filter in front of one slit and a green transmitting filter in front of the other slit. Then we would look to see if the photon that hits the screen is green or red. When we do this, the interference fringes vanish. After all, even from classical wave theory, red and green light have different frequencies and are not mutually coherent.

Perhaps we can use monochromatic light and polarizing filters to tell which slit the photon goes through. Let us put a polaroid with a vertical transmission axis in front of one slit and a polaroid with a horizontal transmission axis in front of the other slit. Then we can measure the polarization of the photon incident on the screen to determine which slit the photon went through. When we do this, the interference fringes again vanish. After all, even from classical wave theory, plane-polarized light perpendicular to each other is not mutually coherent and so no interference occurs.

In fact, any experiment rigged to tell what slit the photon goes through destroys the coherence, and therefore, the interference does not occur. *Interference only occurs when we cannot tell which slit the photon goes through.* In general, interference is a single-particle phenomenon that occurs when there is more than one possible path for the particle, and it is not possible to tell which path the particle took. In order to make the correct predictions, we need to superpose the possible paths. Clearly, one approach is to use wave theory to give the superposition.

Figure 24.24a shows light from source *A* incident on a mirror. After reflecting, the light travels to the detector at *C*. Now by the law of reflection, the ray that leaves *A* and gets to *C* reflects at the position marked *B* on the mirror. Suppose the light level is cut until there is only one photon at a time incident on the mirror. Based on our discussions so far, we need to consider every

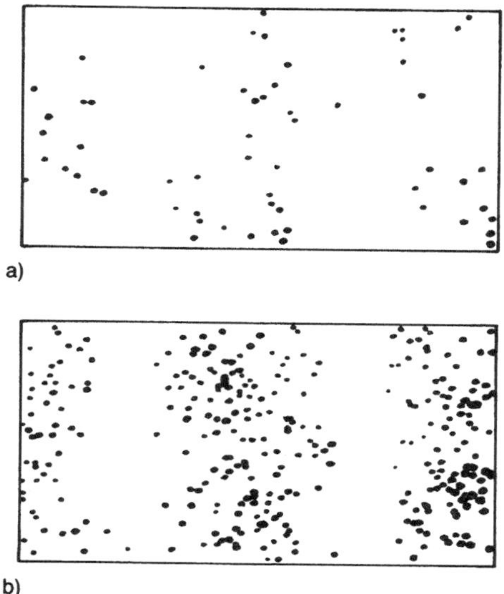

Figure 24.23 Single photon buildup of double-slit interference pattern; a, a few photons—interference fringes not obvious; b, more photons—interference fringes emerging.

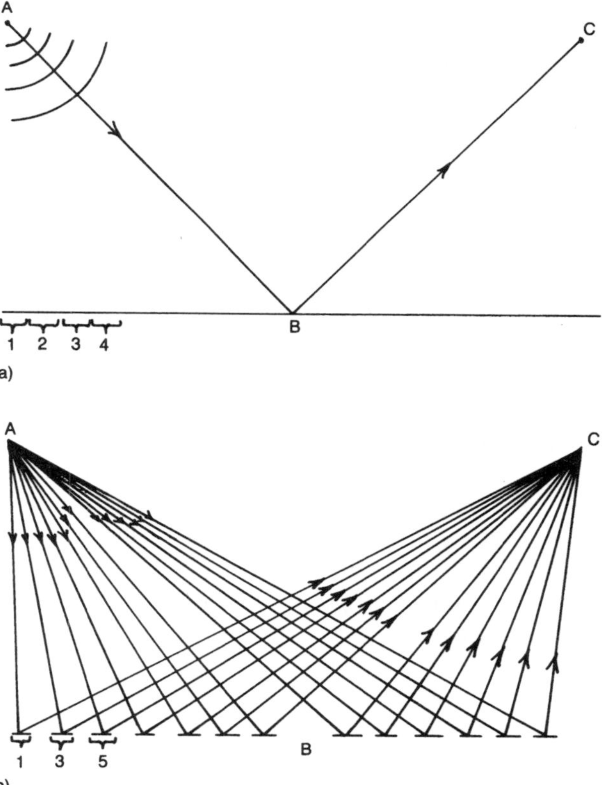

Figure 24.24 a, Contributions of various areas to single photon reflection; b, single photon paths for selected areas—a reflection grating.

possible path of the photon from A to the mirror to C. In wave theory, we superpose the waves reflecting from each small area of the mirror (1, 2, 3,...). The effect of the superposition is that the waves coming from area 1 destructively interfere with those from area 2, and those coming from area 3 destructively interfere with those coming from area 4. The only waves that do not destructively interfere are those that reflect from the area around B, the geometric optics reflection point. These paths give waves that constructively interfere at C, and so we say that the light is reflected from area B (the geometric optics law of reflection) but, in fact, this analysis shows that we do not really know exactly where the photon is reflected from. The result is a superposition of all the possible paths.

Suppose we section the mirror, and keep only those parts that would constructively interfere (i.e., areas 1, 3, 5, etc.). In particular, we will eliminate area B, the geometric optics reflection region (Figure 24.24b). Even though we have eliminated B, the photon still has a good probability of arriving at the detector C due to the constructive interference from the paths that we kept. That is, from wave theory, each small section acts like a point source that sends waves out in all allowed directions. At point C, the waves from the sections that we kept constructively interfere. So the sectored mirror is a reflection-type diffraction grating, and point C is a maximum of the diffraction grating. This process somehow occurs even for a single photon.

24.16 PHOTON FINALE

In these last photon sections, a discussion has been made of how photons and probability theory are intricately linked. Second, some single photon properties are shown, as well as how they merge with classical wave theory. There is much, much more to the quantum theory than indicated here, but the rest is beyond the scope of this book.

The conceptual interpretation of quantum theory is still a challenge. Nevertheless, the general quantum theory is a very successful physical theory, the products of which include antimatter, quarks, electron microscopes, lasers, nuclear power, radioactive isotopes for medical applications, and semiconductors (which have led to solid state electronics and many of the modern high tech devices that we enjoy, including personal computers, handheld calculators, and CD players).

PROBLEMS

1. What is the peak wavelength for a blackbody at 4,800 K? For a blackbody at 1,000 K?
2. What is the single photon energy for light of wavelength 500 nm? For light of wavelength 600 nm?
3. Describe the emission spectra for a low pressure gas with the following energy levels: −7.50 eV, −5.0 eV, and −3.0 eV.
4. The emission spectra of a low pressure source includes wavelengths at 510 nm and 610 nm. If the ground state energy level is at −15.00 eV, list two different possibilities for the other energy levels. How could one experimentally check which scheme is correct?
5. In terms of an energy level diagram, show why some rocks when irradiated by ultraviolet give off visible light. What is this called?
6. What does the word laser stand for?
7. What does the word excimer stand for?
8. For retinal photocoagulation, what factors influence the decision to use an argon green versus a krypton red laser?
9. A double-slit interference experiment is changed so that we can determine through which slit the light goes? How does the change affect the interference fringes?
10. Interference fringes are formed on a screen in a double-slit experiment. Then the light level is decreased to the smallest possible non-zero level. Describe the resulting illumination pattern on the screen, as a function of time.
11. A TEM_{00} beam from an argon green laser (wavelength 514.5 nm) has a waist with a 1.20 mm diameter and a 0.546 mrad beam divergence. When a +20.00 D lens is placed 5 cm from the beam waist, where is the new beam waist and what is its diameter? Also what is the resulting beam divergence?
12. Again consider the TEM_{00} beam from the argon green laser (wavelength 514.5 nm) that has a waist with a 1.20 mm diameter and a 0.546 mrad beam divergence. Assume that the incident beam waist is in the primary focal point of the first lens of a backward two-lens afocal telescope with an angular magnification that has a magnitude of 7×. For the laser beam leaving the backward telescope, where is the beam waist and what is its diameter? Also what is the resulting beam divergence?
13. Consider a TEM_{00} beam (wavelength 532 nm) from a frequency doubled Nd:YAG laser. This beam has a 0.80 mm beam waist and a 0.847 mrad divergence. A +5.00 D lens is placed 25 cm from the beam waist. Where is the new beam waist, what is its size, and what is the new beam divergence?
14. A TEM_{00} beam from an argon blue laser (wavelength 488 nm) has been focussed by a plus lens. The focussed beam waist is 30 μm in diameter, and the output beam has a 20.8 mrad divergence. A +5.00 D lens is placed 25 cm from the beam waist. Where is the new beam waist, what is its size, and what is the new beam divergence?

CHAPTER 25

Spatial Distribution of Optical Information

25.1 SPATIAL FREQUENCY

There is a variety of detail in the castle scene in Figure 25.1. The finest detail is in the grating on the entrance. The portals on the top of the castle walls constitute the next finest detail. Then in order of decreasing detail, we have the towers and the main blob of the castle itself, which is the grossest detail.

We can classify the detail in terms of the number of repetitions per unit distance. Across the width of the castle, the towers repeat three times, and the portals repeat 13 times. If the gate were the width of the entire castle, the grating would repeat about 75 times. The finest detail has the highest repetition rate, while the grossest detail has the lowest repetition rate. The repetition rate is more formally referred to as the *spatial frequency*. (Be careful not to confuse spatial frequency with the temporal frequency (cycles per second) of the light waves.)

It turns out that the quality of the information transferred from the object plane to the image plane by an optical system is a function of the spatial frequency. For example, consider an uncorrected low myope who looks at the distant castle but cannot resolve the detail on the entrance grating because of his blurred retinal image. This myope can still resolve the towers and possibly the portals. A person with added blur (perhaps an uncorrected medium myope) cannot resolve the portals, but can still count the three towers. With additional blur (perhaps an uncorrected high myope), the person loses the ability to resolve the three towers, but perhaps can still see the main gray blob of the castle itself. This example shows that information for the lower spatial frequencies can still be transferred by the optical system even though the higher spatial frequencies are wiped out.

To completely judge the quality of an optical system, we need to know how it images each of the spatial frequencies present in the object. The units for spatial frequency are repetitions per unit length, more commonly called cycles per unit length (e.g., cycles/mm = mm^{-1}). The spatial frequency information can also be converted to angular terms such as cycles per radian or cycles per degree.

25.2 SINE VERSUS SQUARE WAVE GRATINGS

A crude way to analyze the information transfer for a given spatial frequency is to use a chart consisting of

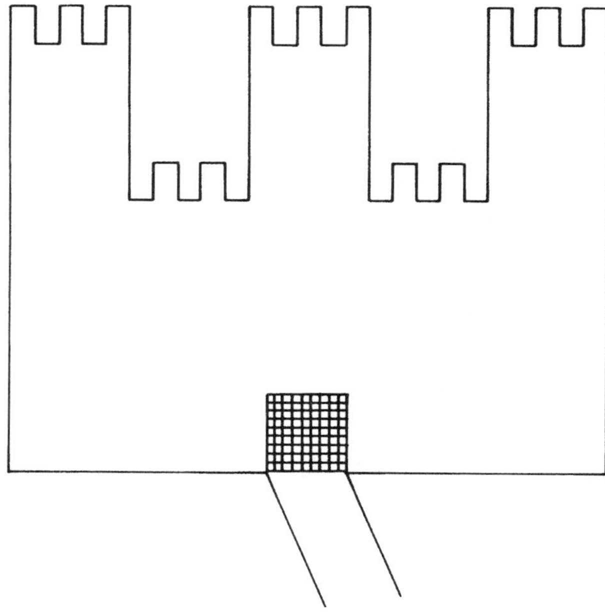

Figure 25.1 A castle scene with a variety of spatial frequency components.

Figure 25.2 a, A low frequency square wave grating; b, its luminance distribution; c, a higher frequency square wave grating; d, its luminance distribution.

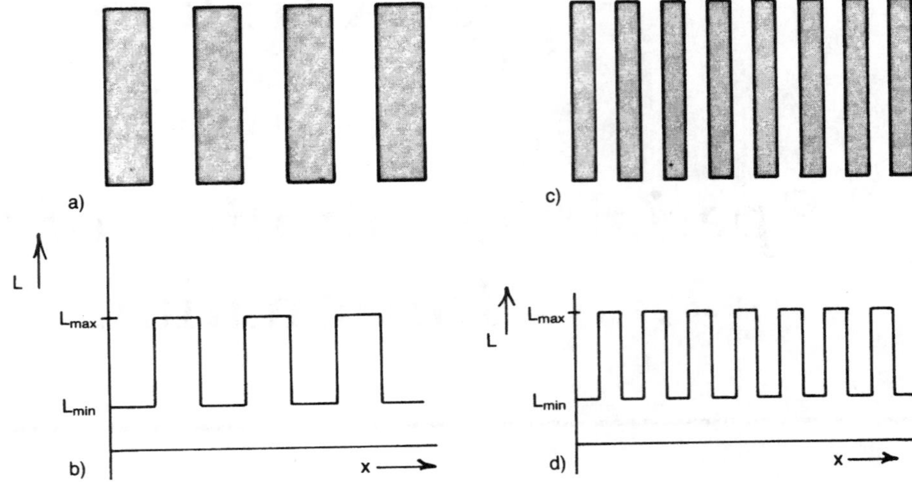

equally spaced black and white bars (Figure 25.2a). The repetition rate of each set of bars (one white and one black) determines the spatial frequency. Figure 25.2b shows a plot of the luminance for the bar chart as a function of distance across the chart. This luminance distribution is referred to as a square wave distribution, and the bar chart is called *a square wave grating*. Figures 25.2c and d show the bar chart and luminance distribution for a higher spatial frequency.

The method of analysis consists of comparing the modulation (also called visibility or contrast) in the object to the resulting modulation in the image. The *modulation M* is defined as

$$M = \frac{L_{max} - L_{min}}{L_{max} + L_{min}} \tag{25.1}$$

where L_{max} and L_{min} are the maximum and minimum luminances, respectively. *Contrast* is usually defined in terms of the luminance difference between the object L_o and the background L_b; i.e., contrast $= (L_o - L_b)/L_b$. When we specify that the mean luminance L_m serves as the background for the bar chart, then the modulation equals the contrast.

For a proper analysis of information transfer as a function of spatial frequency in an optical system using incoherent light, we need to use a grating chart with a sinusoidal luminance distribution. We refer to the sinusoidal chart as a *sine wave grating*. The solid curve in Figure 25.3a is the luminance distribution for a sine wave grating, while the dashed line is the luminance distribution for a square wave grating of the same frequency and amplitude.

As a function of the distance x across a sine wave grating, the luminance is described by

$$L_o(x) = L_m + a \sin(2\pi f x) \tag{25.2}$$

where the argument of the sine function is in radians. (There are 2π radians in a complete period, which is why the 2π appears in Eq. 25.2.) In Eq. 25.2, f is the spatial frequency of the sine wave grating, L_m is the mean luminance, and a is the amplitude of the deviation from the mean. The spatial period x_p of the sine wave grating is the reciprocal of f.

For a sine wave grating,

$$L_{max} = L_m + a \quad \text{and} \quad L_{min} = L_m - a$$

We can then substitute the above equations into Eq. 25.1 and with a little algebra obtain

$$M = \frac{a}{L_m} \tag{25.3}$$

For a sine wave grating, the absolute minimum luminance value is zero, in which case a equals L_m. For those sine wave gratings that have a minimum luminance greater than zero, a is less than L_m. Hence, the modulation M is always less than or equal to 1.

When we factor L_m out of Eq. 25.2 and use Eq. 25.3, we can write the luminance distribution for an object grating with modulation M_o as

$$L_o(x) = L_m[1 + M_o \sin(2\pi f x)] \tag{25.4}$$

Consider a misfocused optical system with a sine wave grating given by Eq. 25.4 as the object. One of the advantages of a sinusoidal object luminance distribution L_o is that for most optical systems the blurred image luminance distribution L_i is also sinusoidal.

The spatial period x'_p of the image grating is related to the spatial period x_p of the object grating by $x'_p = m x_p$, where m is the system's total lateral magnification. Since the spatial frequencies are reciprocals of the spatial periods, it follows that the spatial fre-

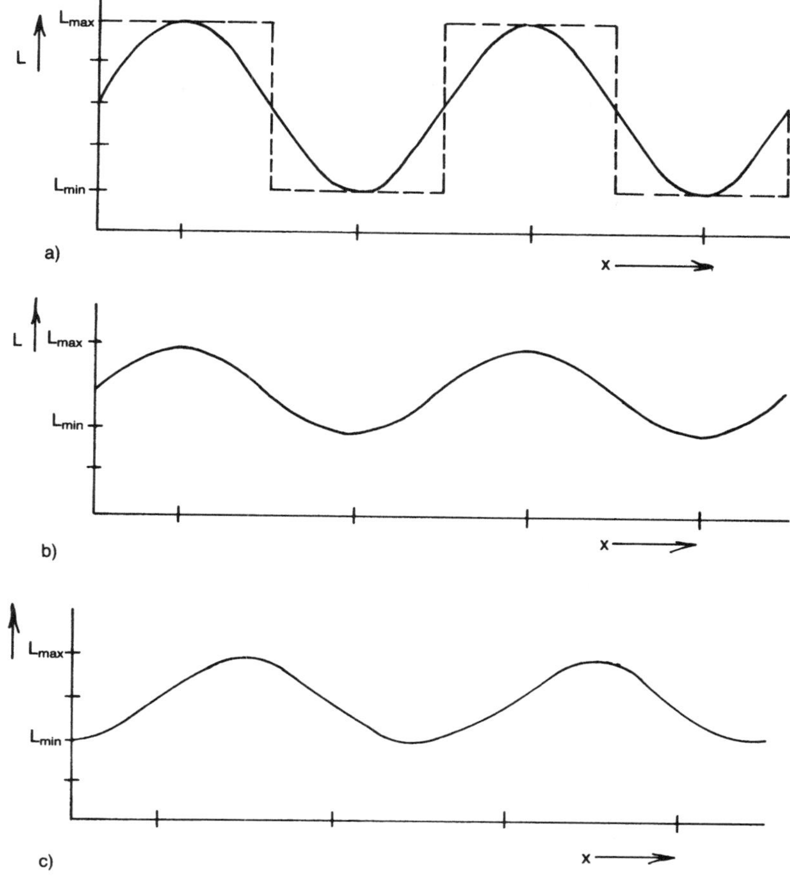

Figure 25.3 a, Object luminance distribution (solid) for as sine wave grating versus that of a square wave grating (dashed) of the same frequency; b, blurred image luminance distribution for sinusoidal object distribution of *a*; c, phase-shifted image.

quency f' of the image sine wave grating is related to the object spatial frequency f by $f' = f/m$. Due to the blur, the modulation M_i of the image grating is less than the modulation M_o of the object grating. Furthermore, if the blur happens to be asymmetric, such as would be given by the aberration coma, the image grating is phase shifted through an angle α relative to the object grating. So in general,

$$L_i(x) = L_m[1 + M_i \sin(2\pi f'x - \alpha)] \qquad (25.5)$$

When magnification occurs, f' is less than f. When minification occurs, f' is greater than f. For a lateral magnification of unit magnitude, $f' = f$.

Usually, the blur is symmetric, in which case there is no phase shift ($\alpha = 0$). Then,

$$L_i(x) = L_m[1 + M_i \sin(2\pi f'x)] \qquad (25.6)$$

For unit lateral magnification, Figure 25.3b shows the blurred image distribution for the sinusoidal object distribution given in Figure 25.3a. For completeness, Figure 25.3c shows the blurred image distribution for a 90° phase shift.

The fact that the blurred image of a sine wave grating of a single spatial frequency f is a sine wave grating of a single spatial frequency f', where $f' = f/m$, is a special property of sine wave gratings. In contrast to this, a blurred square wave grating is not imaged as a square wave grating. In fact for enough blur, a square wave grating is imaged as a sine wave grating. For example, the sine wave grating of Figure 25.3b could be the blurred image of the square wave grating represented by the dashed line in Figure 25.3a.

25.3 THE MODULATION TRANSFER FUNCTION

For incoherent light, the modulation transfer function (MTF) of the optical system as a function of the spatial frequency f is the ratio

$$\mathrm{MTF}(f) = \frac{M_i}{M_o} \qquad (25.7)$$

where M_i is the sinusoidal image modulation and M_o is the sinusoidal object modulation. A perfect optical system preserves the modulation, so the MTF is 1. For optical systems with blur, aberrations, scattering, etc., the image modulation is decreased, so the MTF is less than 1. When the image is completely blurred out, the information is lost and the MTF is zero. Hence, $0 \leq \text{MTF} \leq 1$.

EXAMPLE 25.1
Consider the following sinusoidal object luminance distribution with a spatial frequency of 3 cycles/mm (or $3\,\text{mm}^{-1}$).

$$L_o = 10.0 + 8.0\sin(2\pi 3x)$$

What is the image luminance distribution for an optical system with unit lateral magnification and a 0.40 MTF for 3 cycles/mm? (Assume a zero phase shift).

For unit magnification, the conjugate image distribution is a sinusoidal distribution of the same spatial frequency in which the modulation is decreased by a factor of 0.40. We can rewrite the object luminance distribution as

$$L_o = 10.0[1 + 0.80\sin(2\pi 3x)]$$

The object modulation M_o, is then 0.80, and the image modulation is

$$M_i = \text{MTF } 0.80 = (0.40)(0.80) = 0.32$$

Then the image luminance distribution is

$$L_i = 10.0[1 + 0.32\sin(2\pi 3x)]$$

or

$$L_i = 10.0 + 3.2\sin(2\pi 3x)$$

The transfer of information in a perfect optical system is limited by diffraction (i.e., a diffraction limited system). Diffraction has little effect on low spatial frequencies. As the spatial frequency is increased, diffraction causes an increasing loss of information, so that eventually very fine detail is completely lost. Figure 25.4 shows a plot of an MTF as a function of increasing spatial frequency *f*. Because of diffraction, the MTF eventually goes to zero at a frequency f_c called the cut-off frequency. All higher spatial frequencies are wiped out by the system. In a sense, the cut-off frequency f_c conveys information that is similar to Rayleigh's criterion of Chapter 22.

When other sources of blur are present, then the MTF is less than or equal to the diffraction-limited MTF at each spatial frequency. Depending on the amount and source of blur, the system may have an effective cut-off f_n sooner than the diffraction cut-off f_c.

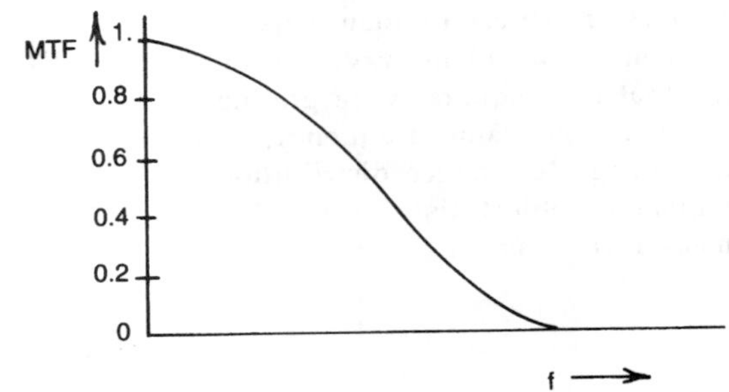

Figure 25.4 Modulation transfer function plotted versus spatial frequency *f*.

25.4 PERIODIC GRATINGS AND LINEAR SYSTEMS

Certainly one of the reasons that a sine wave grating is special is that most optical systems image it as a sine wave grating. There is a second reason why sine wave gratings are special. In technical terminology, the second reason relates to the fact that optical systems tend to function as linear systems.

Assume that the image luminance distribution for a sine wave grating L_1 of spatial frequency f_1 is the sine wave distribution A, and that the image luminance distribution for a sine wave grating L_2 of spatial frequency f_2 is the sine wave distribution B. Now let the object have a luminance distribution that consists of the sum $L_1 + L_2$. In a *linear system*, the resulting image luminance distribution is simply the sum $A + B$.

Note that for a linear system, a spatial frequency f' can appear in the image distribution only when the spatial frequency f (where $f = mf'$) appears in the object distribution. For a system with unit magnification, this means that the only spatial frequencies appearing in the image are those already present in the object.

Consider a series of sinusoidal distributions where the lowest spatial frequency is *f*, and the higher spatial frequencies are integer multiples of *f* (i.e., 2*f*, 3*f*, 4*f*, etc.) It is easy to show graphically that the resultant sum of such a series is always a periodic distribution (not sinusoidal) of spatial frequency *f*. In fact, any periodic distribution of spatial frequency *f* can be represented as the sum of a series of sinusoidals of integer multiples of *f*. The mathematical formulation of this statement is known as *Fourier's theorem*. In the Fourier sum, the sinusoidal with the lowest frequency (*f*) provides the gross shape of the periodic distribution and is called the fundamental harmonic. The sinusoidal of the next highest spatial frequency (2*f*) supplies finer detail, and each sinusoidal of higher spatial frequency supplies still finer detail.

As a result of Fourier's theorem, we can consider the luminance distribution $L_o(x)$ of any periodic grating of spatial frequency f as represented by the sum of sinusoidal distributions of frequencies which are integer multiples of f, or

$$L_o(x) = L_m[1 + M_1 \sin(2\pi fx - \phi_1) + M_2 \sin(2\pi 2fx - \phi_2) + M_3 \sin(2\pi 3fx - \phi_3) + \ldots] \quad (25.8)$$

The lowest frequency (f) component supplies the gross detail and is called the *fundamental harmonic*. Then finer and finer details are successively supplied by the higher frequency components. That is, the third harmonic ($3f$) supplies finer detail than the second harmonic ($2f$), and so on.

Figure 25.5a shows two cycles of a luminance distribution for a periodic grating described by the sum of two sine waves. The lower frequency sinusoidal distribution supplies the gross shape (the large slowly varying bumps), while the higher frequency sinusoidal supplies the fine detail (the little bumps).

The general equation for the luminance distribution of a periodic object grating with zero phase components is

$$L_o(x) = L_m[1 + M_1 \sin(2\pi fx) + M_2 \sin(2\pi 2fx) + M_3 \sin(2\pi 3fx) + \ldots] \quad (25.9)$$

Let us assume that the optical system is linear, has a lateral magnification of unit magnitude, and does not introduce any phase shifts. Then the image luminance distribution L_i is given by

$$L_i(x) = L_m[1 + N_1 \sin(2\pi fx) + N_2 \sin(2\pi 2fx) + N_3 \sin(2\pi 3fx) + \ldots] \quad (25.10)$$

where the MTF for each spatial frequency are

$$\text{MTF}(f) = N_1/M_1$$
$$\text{MTF}(2f) = N_2/M_2$$
$$\text{MTF}(3f) = N_3/M_3$$

etc.

EXAMPLE 25.2

Consider a system with unit lateral magnification and the following MTF values:

f	0	1	2	3
MTF	1.0	0.5	0.3	0.0

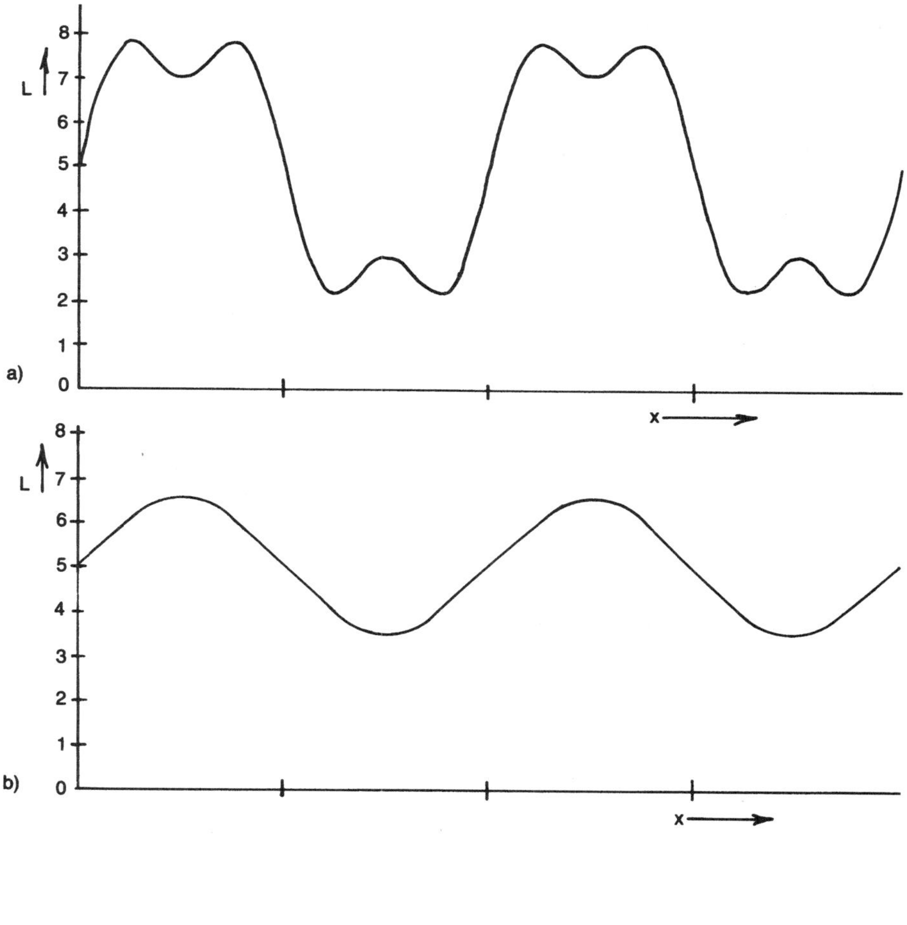

Figure 25.5 a, Object luminance distribution; b, conjugate image luminance distribution.

When the object has the luminance distribution of Figure 25.5a described by

$$L_o = 5 + 3\sin(2\pi x) + \sin(2\pi 3x)$$

what is the image luminance distribution? (Assume no phase shifts are introduced by the system.)

Here,

$$L_o = 5[1 + 0.60\sin(2\pi x) + 0.20\sin(2\pi 3x)]$$

and

$$N_1 = 0.5 \; M_1 = 0.5(0.60) = 0.30$$
$$N_2 = 0.3 \; M_2 = 0.3(0) = 0$$
$$N_3 = 0 \; M_3 = 0(0.20) = 0$$

Since the optical system is linear, the image distribution is

$$L_i = 5[1 + 0.30\sin(2\pi x)]$$

or

$$L_i = 5 + 1.5\sin(2\pi x)$$

The image luminance distribution is plotted in Figure 25.5b. The low frequency (large bumps) information is degraded but still present. The fine detail (small bumps) is blurred out.

EXAMPLE 25.3

The MTF for a linear optical system with a lateral magnification of unit magnitude is

f	0	1	2	3	4	5	6	7
MTF	1.0	1.0	0.9	0.8	0.6	0.3	0.1	0.0

When the object luminance distribution is given by

$$L_o = 6[1 + 0.50\sin(2\pi 2x) + 0.35\sin(2\pi 4x) + 0.25\sin(2\pi 6x)]$$

what is the image luminance distribution? (Assume no phase shifts are introduced by the system.)

Here the only spatial frequencies present in the object are 2, 4, and 6 cycles/mm. The transfers for these frequencies are:

$$N_2 = 0.9 \; M_2 = 0.9(0.50) = 0.45$$
$$N_4 = 0.6 \; M_4 = 0.6(0.35) = 0.21$$
$$N_6 = 0.1 \; M_6 = 0.1(0.25) = 0.025$$

Since the optical system is linear, the image distribution is then

$$L_i = 6[1 + 0.45\sin(2\pi 2x) + 0.21\sin(2\pi 4x) + 0.025\sin(2\pi 6x)]$$

The system transferred the fundamental harmonic well. There was some degradation of the middle spatial frequency, and the highest spatial frequency (the finest detail) was essentially lost. The solid curve in Figure 25.6 shows one cycle of the object luminance distribution, while the dashed curve shows one cycle of the image luminance distribution.

We previously said that the blurred image of a square wave grating is a sine wave grating. We can now show this mathematically. A square wave is periodic. The Fourier sine series for the square wave luminance distribution is

$$L_{square}(x) = L_m[1 + (C/1)\sin(2\pi fx) + (C/3)\sin(2\pi 3fx) + (C/5)\sin(2\pi 5fx) + \ldots]$$

where the constant C equals $4/\pi$. The $\sin(2\pi fx)$ term supplies the gross shape. Then each successive term ($3f$, $5f$, etc.) provides finer and finer detail. Figure 25.5a is the sum of the first two terms in the series, and we can see that the gross square wave shape is already emerging. The addition of the higher order terms sharpens the fine detail.

For an ideal system (diffraction neglected), the MTF is 1 and a square wave grating is imaged as a square wave grating. For a diffraction-limited system, the MTF falls to zero, and so some high frequency terms in the sum for L_{square} are missing. If the diffraction is small and the fundamental frequency f is low, then the lower order terms are not affected much and the image still looks like a square wave grating. However, if the diffraction is larger, the fundamental frequency f is higher, or another source of image degradation is present, then the lower order frequencies are affected and each is transferred by a different MTF factor. Here the luminance distribution of the image is no longer a square wave. Finally, when the diffraction (or other sources of blur) are large enough so that all the frequencies above the fundamental frequency are wiped out, then the image of the square wave grating becomes

$$L_i(x) = L_m + M_i \sin(2\pi fx) + 0$$

where M_i equals the MTF times the constant C. In this case the square wave grating has been imaged as a sine wave grating (Figure 25.5b).

In summary: this section pointed out that the luminance distribution for any periodic grating can be represented as the sum of a series of sinusoidal lumi-

Figure 25.6 Object (solid) and image (dashed) luminance distributions.

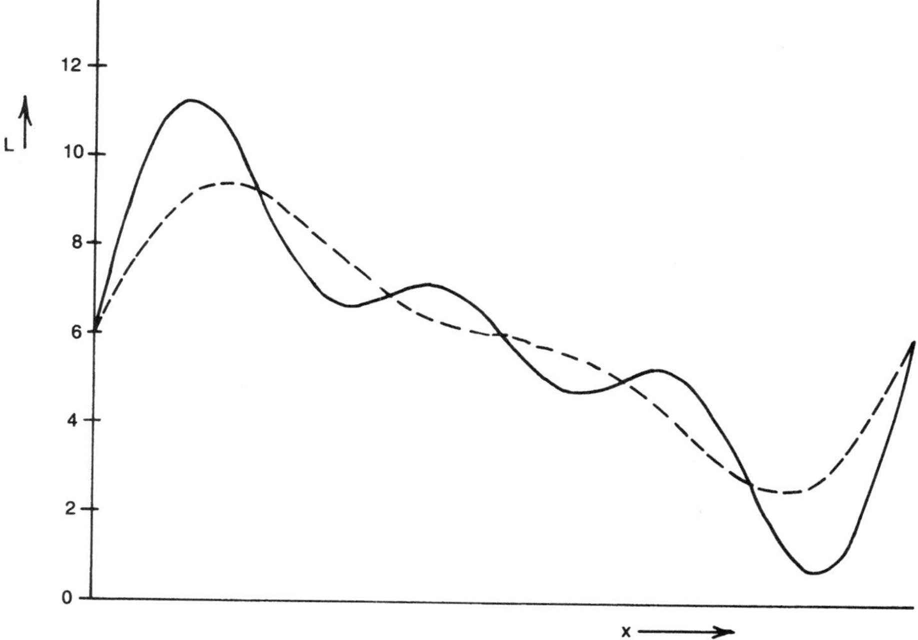

nance distributions. The lower frequency components are responsible for the gross detail, while the higher frequency components are responsible for the fine detail. In a linear optical system, each sinusoidal component is imaged by the system according to the MTF for that spatial frequency. The image then is the sum of the resulting sinusoidal image components.

Rayleigh's criterion supplies information roughly equivalent to the cut-off frequency f_c. The MTF analysis is much better than Rayleigh's criterion in the sense that it supplies information about the entire spatial frequency range from zero to f_c. Figure 25.7 shows MTFs for two optical systems (*A* and *B*). The MTF for system *B* has a lower cut-off frequency than the MTF for system *A*. However, over the middle spatial frequencies, the MTF for system *A* is less than that for system *B*. Suppose a human observer is to use these two systems, and the cut-off for the human observer is at f_d, which corresponds to the middle of the spatial frequencies transferred by the systems. For all spatial frequencies lower than f_d, system *B* has a better MTF. Therefore, optical system *B* is the better system for the observer to use even though a Rayleigh's criterion analysis would have said that system *A* is the better system. (This example is based on a dilemma that appeared in the development of television systems. The dilemma was that people preferred one system (*B*) over another (*A*) even though according to Rayleigh's criterion system *A* was better.)

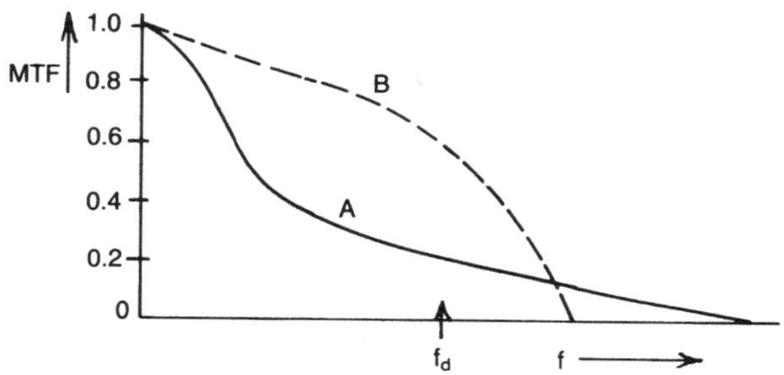

Figure 25.7 Modulation transfer functions for different systems.

25.5 SPREAD FUNCTIONS AND THE MTF

Ideally, the image of a point source is a point image. However, even in a properly focused system, diffraction and the aberrations cause the illuminance to spread out around the point image position. The *point spread function* is a relative measure of the luminous flux at the positions around the ideal point image. In a diffraction-limited system, the point spread function is determined by the Fraunhofer diffraction pattern (Airy's disk and its rings). In the presence of aberrations, defocus, or scatter, the light is spread even more.

The ideal image of a vertical line is a vertical line with zero horizontal width. However, due to the system's point spread function, the light in the image plane is spread horizontally (Figure 25.8). A horizontal plot of the spread $S(g)$ of the relative amounts of luminous flux is called the *line spread function* (Figure

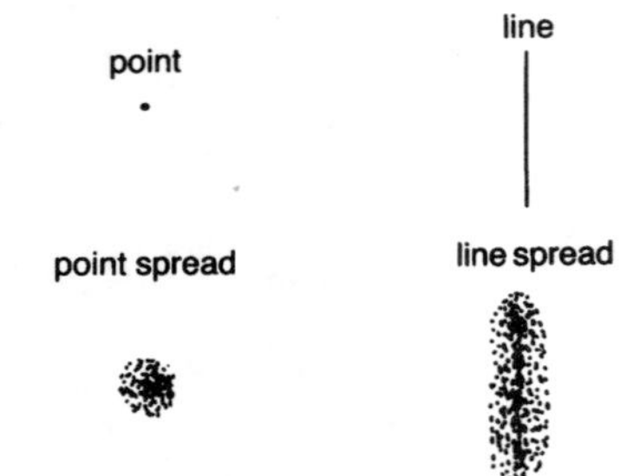

Figure 25.8 Point and line objects and resulting spreads in image plane.

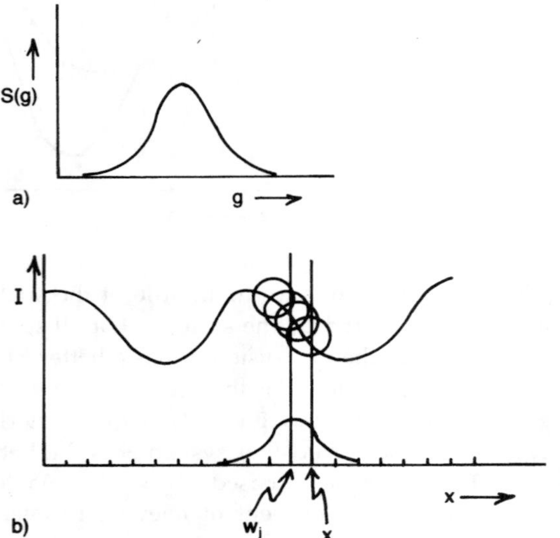

Figure 25.9 a, Line spread function; b, effect on sinusoidal luminance distribution.

25.9a). If the point spread function has been measured, then the line spread function can be calculated from the point spread function. Alternatively, the line spread function can be directly measured.

When the gratings of the previous section are imaged, the point spread function causes the degradation in the modulation. Because of the symmetry of the gratings, the blur is in the horizontal meridian, and we can work directly with the line spread function $S(g)$. Given a system with a line spread function, and a sine wave grating as an object, we want to show mathematically that, for incoherent light, the image is also a sine wave grating.

For simplicity, let us assume that the system has a lateral magnification of unit magnitude, and that the sinusoidal grating has a mean luminance of 1. With these assumptions, the object luminance distribution is

$$L_o(x) = 1 + M_o \sin(2\pi f x) \tag{25.11}$$

The perfect image distribution is identical to the object distribution. However, because of the line spread function $S(g)$, the illuminance from a number of the ideal horizontal image points overlaps, as represented by the overlapping circles in Figure 25.9b. Because the light is incoherent, the resultant illuminance is the sum of all the overlapping illuminances.

To analyze these contributions, first divide the image plane up into small vertical strips each of horizontal width Δg. Illuminance equals the luminous flux incident per unit area. So for the jth strip, the contribution to the illuminance from the line spread function equals $S(g)$ times Δg.

The contribution to the illuminance distribution at point x from the strip centered on point w_j equals the contribution from the line spread function times the ideal illuminance in the strip containing w_j, or

$$S(x - w_j)\{1 + M_o \sin[2\pi f w_j]\}\Delta g_j$$

Here,

$$g_j = x - w_j$$

and so can write the product as

$$S(g_j)\{1 + M_o \sin[2\pi f(x - g_j)]\}\Delta g_j$$

The line spread function can change as the object is moved further and further off axis. We will restrict ourselves to an area, called an isoplanatic patch, over which the line spread function does not change. Then the total distribution at point x is the sum of the distributions from each strip, or

$$L_i(x) = \sum_j S(g_j)\{1 + M_o \sin[2\pi f(x - g_j)]\}\Delta g_j$$

Once g_j is large enough, the line spread function $S(g_j)$ is zero, and the series can be terminated.

From the trigonometry relationship

$$\sin(a - b) = \sin a \cos b - \cos a \sin b$$

we have

$$L_i(x) = \sum_j S(g_j)\{1 + [M_o \sin(2\pi f x)\cos(2\pi f g_j) - \cos(2\pi f x)\sin(2\pi f g_j)]\}\Delta g_j$$

For simplicity, let us pick units so that the sum of the spread function is 1. In other words, the area under the line spread function is 1, or

$$\sum_j S(g_j)\Delta g_j = 1$$

Then we can bring the spread function inside the curly brackets and consider the sum term by term to obtain

$$L_i(x) = 1 + M_o F_c \sin(2\pi f x) - M_o F_s \cos(2\pi f x) \quad (25.12)$$

where,

$$F_s = \sum_j S(g_j) \sin(2\pi f g_j) \Delta g_j \quad (25.13)$$

$$F_c = \sum_j S(g_j) \cos(2\pi f g_j) \Delta g_j \quad (25.14)$$

The above two equations are similar to the sums of vector components, so the resultant sum also acts like a vector. Therefore,

$$F_c = |F| \cos\alpha \quad \text{and} \quad F_s = |F| \sin\alpha \quad (25.15)$$

where,

$$|F| = [F_c^2 + F_s^2]^{1/2} \quad (25.16)$$

and

$$\tan\alpha = F_s / F_c \quad (25.17)$$

We can use then Eqs. 25.15 through 25.17 together with Eq. 25.12 and

$$\sin(a - b) = \sin a \cos b - \cos a \sin b$$

to obtain

$$L_i = 1 + M_o |F| \sin(2\pi f x - \alpha) \quad (25.18)$$

Equation 25.18 shows that, in the presence of a line spread function $S(g)$, a sine wave grating is imaged as a sine wave grating with a possible phase shift α, and a modulation M_i where,

$$M_i = M_o |F| \quad (25.19)$$

From Eq. 25.7, we see that the MTF equals $|F|$.

So not only have we shown that sine wave gratings are imaged as sine wave gratings, we also see that the MTF is directly related to the line spread function $S(g)$ through the sums of Eqs. 25.13 and 25.14.

In the limit as the strip width, Δg_j, goes to zero, the sums given in Eqs. 25.13 and 25.14 become the integrals

$$F_s = \int_0^\infty S(g) \sin(2\pi f g)\, dg \quad (25.20)$$

$$F_c = \int_0^\infty S(g) \cos(2\pi f g)\, dg \quad (25.21)$$

The above integrals are called the Fourier sine and cosine transforms, and we say that *the MTF is the Fourier transform of the line spread function*. One of the results of Eqs. 25.16 through 25.21 is that whenever the spread function $S(G)$ increases (i.e., more blur, diffraction, aberrations, or scatter), the MTF decreases, and vice versa. (Numerical examples showing this are in the next section.)

The phase shift ϕ is also a function of the spatial frequency f. The MTF and the phase shift are considered two vector-like components of the *optical transform function* (OTF), i.e.,

$$\text{OTF} = (|F|, \alpha) \quad (25.22)$$

Since the MTF equals $|F|$, we see that the MTF is the modulus of the OTF. Equation 15.22 is the polar coordinate representation for the OTF. The rectangular component representation is

$$\text{OTF} = (F_c, F_s) \quad (25.23)$$

A simplification in the general theory results when the line spread function is symmetrical. Then the sum (or integral) F_s is zero, and Eq. 25.17 shows that the phase shift is either zero or 180° (depending on whether F_c is positive or negative). Hence, only nonsymmetrical line spread functions cause a phase shift other than 180° in the image grating.

A 180° phase shift is a phase reversal where the minimums replace the maximums and vice versa (like the negative of a photograph). So other than a possible phase reversal, the image grating is shifted relative to the object grating only for a nonsymmetrical line spread function. Off-axis blur patches, or asymmetric aberrations such as coma, cause a nonsymmetrical line spread function.

For a symmetric line spread function, we can simplify Eq. 25.18 to get

$$L_i(x) = 1 + M_i \sin(2\pi f x) \quad (25.24)$$

where,

$$M_i = M_o F_c \quad (25.25)$$

In this formulation F_c, is sometimes identified as the MTF,

$$\text{MTF} = F_c \quad (25.26)$$

even though the MTF is more properly defined as the absolute value of F_c.

What happens optically when F_c goes from positive to negative (Figure 25.10a)? For a positive F_c near zero, the grating is imaged with a decreased modulation

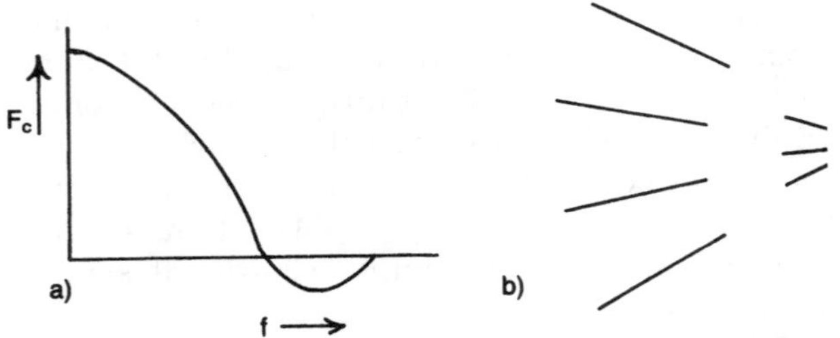

Figure 25.10 Spurious resolution for radial lines.

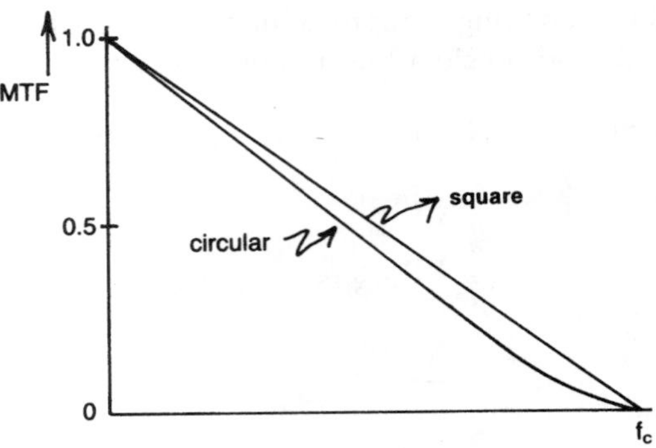

Figure 25.11 Diffraction-limited MTFs for a square and circular aperture.

and no phase shift. When F_c is zero, no modulation is transferred (the grating is blurred out). For the negative F_c, the grating reappears but is phase-reversed. This phenomenon is called *spurious resolution* and is shown in Figure 22.10b for the image of some radial lines. As the radial lines get closer, the spatial frequency increases. Frequently, the first zero is taken as the effective cut-off for the useful transferred spatial frequencies.

Let us summarize the crucial inputs into the derivation. We assumed a linear optical system, and that the light is incoherent. We also assumed that the point spread function does not change over the area that we are considering (called an isoplanatic patch). Finally, we assumed that the object was a sine wave grating. Given these assumptions, and the standard trigonometry behavior of cosines and sines, we showed that the image is a sine wave grating and that the MTF is related to the sum of cosines and sines times the line spread function. (In the calculus formulation, the sums are replaced by integrals, and we say that the MTF is the Fourier transform of the spread function.) It follows that anything (blur, aberrations, scatter, diffraction) that causes a larger spread function also decreases the MTF.

25.6 MTFS OF VARIOUS SYSTEMS

Consider a diffraction-limited system with a square aperture of width w. In this case, the Fourier transform equations can be used to derive an algebraic equation for the MTF. The result is the very simple equation:

$$\text{MTF}(f) = 1 - \frac{f}{f_c} \qquad (25.27)$$

where f_c is the incoherent cut-off frequency. According to Eq. 25.27, the (horizontal) MTF for an incoherent diffraction-limited system with a square aperture is a straight line that extends from 1 to 0 (Figure 25.11). A square aperture system with aberrations, defocus, scatter, etc., has an MTF that is less than the straight line given by Eq. 25.27.

In image space, the cut-off frequency is given by

$$f_c = \frac{w}{\lambda v} \qquad (25.28)$$

where v is the image distance. For a distant object, $v = f_2$, and v/w equals the system's f-number. Then,

$$f_c = 1/[\lambda(f\text{-number})] \qquad (25.29)$$

It is often convenient to express the image spatial frequency in cycles per mm. Let us take a wavelength of 555.55 nm as representative of the middle of the visual spectrum. Since 555.55 nm = 555.55×10^{-6} mm, the cut-off frequency becomes

$$f_c = \frac{1800\,\text{cycles/mm}}{f\text{-number}} \qquad (25.30)$$

For example, an $f/22$ system has an image space cut-off frequency of 81.8 cycles/mm, while an $f/1.8$ system has an image space cut-off frequency f_c of 1,000 cycles/mm. Because of diffraction, the spread function for the $f/22$ system is larger than that for the $f/1.8$ system. Clearly, f_c decreases when the spread function increases.

EXAMPLE 25.4

Consider an $f/4$ incoherent system with a square aperture. What is the MTF for an image space frequency of 200 cycles/mm?

The cut-off frequency is

$$f_c = (1800\,\text{cycles/mm})/4 = 450\,\text{cycles/mm}$$

Then from Eq. 25.28,

$$\text{MTF} = 1 - (200/450) = 0.56$$

We can also use the Fourier Transform equations to derive an algebraic equation for the incoherent MTF of a diffraction-limited system with a circular aperture. This equation is:

$$\mathrm{MTF} = \frac{2}{\pi}\{\cos^{-1}(f/f_c) - [f/f_c][1-(f/f_c)^2]^{1/2}\} \quad (25.31)$$

where the inverse cosine is in radians and the image space cut-off frequency is again given by Eq. 25.28. In the circular case the MTF initially decreases a little faster than the straight line MTF for the square aperture. Then the circular MTF gently curves and stretches out to the same cut-off (Figure 25.11). A degraded system with a circular aperture has an MTF that is less than that given by Eq. 25.31 at each spatial frequency.

EXAMPLE 25.5

Consider an incoherent $f/4$ system with a circular aperture. What is the MTF for an image space frequency of 200 cycles/mm? How does this compare to the previous example?

The cut-off frequency is the same as the previous example: $f_c = 450$ cycles/mm. So $f/f_c = 200/450 = 0.44$. Then,

$$\mathrm{MTF} = \frac{2}{\pi}\{\cos^{-1}(0.44) - [0.44][1-(0.44)^2]^{1/2}\}$$

Since the inverse cosine is in radians, this gives

$$\mathrm{MTF} = \frac{2}{\pi}\{1.11 - [0.44][0.90]\} = 0.45$$

The horizontal MTF for the square aperture was 0.56.

When blur by misfocus is introduced into a system, the MTF decreases from the diffraction-limited results. As the blur is increased, the middle of the MTF dips until an effective cut-off is reached earlier than f_c. This agrees with the castle scenario in Section 25.1.

Optically, a 60.00 D human eye with a 3 mm pupil acts like a $f/5.6$ optical system. If the eye were diffraction-limited, the cut-off frequency would be about 320 cycles/mm. The eye shows diffraction-limited behavior at a pupil sizes of the order of 1–2 mm, but at 3 mm, the effective cut-off f_n is typically about 200 cycles/mm (corresponding to a 20/10 visual acuity). The effective lower cut-off is due either to the aberrations and scatter present in the eye, or to the size and spacing of the retinal receptors (cones) in the foveal area.

When the blur circle is much larger than the diffraction pattern, a closed form equation for the MTF can be calculated. This equation is referred to as the geometric MTF and is not accurate for very small amounts of blur. For a square aperture, the horizontal geometric MTF is

$$\mathrm{MTF} = \frac{\sin(t)}{t} \quad (25.32)$$

where,

$$t = (8\pi B)(f/f_n)\ \mathrm{rad} \quad (25.33)$$

f_n equals the cut-off spatial frequency for no defocus, and B equals the diopters of defocus (i.e., the diopters of blur).

EXAMPLE 25.6a

Consider a system with a square aperture and a 200 cycle/mm cut-off for no defocus (except for the square pupil, this corresponds to the human eye). For 50 cycles/mm, what is the geometric MTF for a 1/4 D error, and a 1/2 D error?

For the 1/4 D error,

$$t = (8\pi)(1/4)(50/200) = \pi/2$$

where t is in radians. Then the geometric MTF is

$$\mathrm{MTF} = \sin(\pi/2)/(\pi/2) = 0.64$$

For the 1/2 D error,

$$t = (8\pi)(1/2)(50/200) = \pi$$

and the geometric MTF is

$$\mathrm{MTF} = \sin(\pi)/\pi = 0$$

EXAMPLE 25.6b

For the same system, what is the geometric MTF for a spatial frequency of 20 cycles/mm and a 1.00 D defocus?

For the 1.00 D error,

$$t = (8\pi)(1)(20/200) = 0.8\pi$$

where t is in radians. Then the geometric MTF is

$$\mathrm{MTF} = \sin(0.8\pi)/(0.8\pi) = 0.23$$

A geometric MTF can also be derived for a circular aperture, in which case it has the form $J_1(z)/z$ where J_1 is the first order Bessel function. Some calculated geometric MTFs for a schematic eye with a 3 mm pupil are given in Figure 25.12.

As mentioned, the geometric MTF equation is accurate only when the blur circle is much larger than Airy's disk. An approximation to the actual MTF for

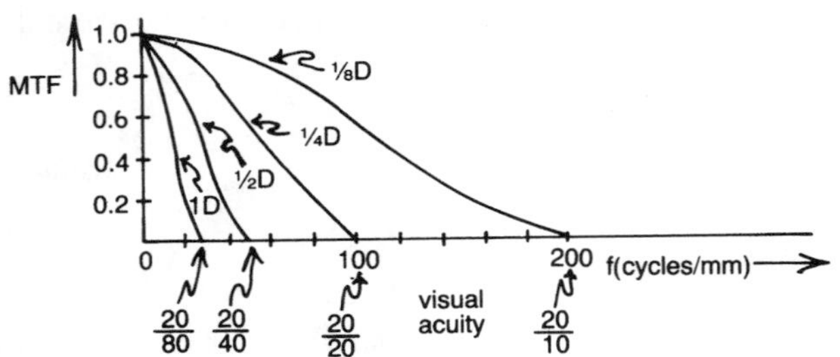

Figure 25.12 Geometric MTFs for a schematic eye with a 3-mm pupil.

smaller amounts of blur is the product of the geometric MTF and the diffraction limited MTF. That is, for a square aperture, this approximation for small amounts of blur would be the right side of Eq. 25.32 times the right side of Eq. 25.27. A similar approximation exists for circular apertures.

We can also determine MTFs for prisms. The aberrations of a thick prism introduce blur into the image so that the MTF for prisms decreases as the prism diopter value increases. Modulation transfer function also decrease due to scatter, as in the case of dirty windshields.

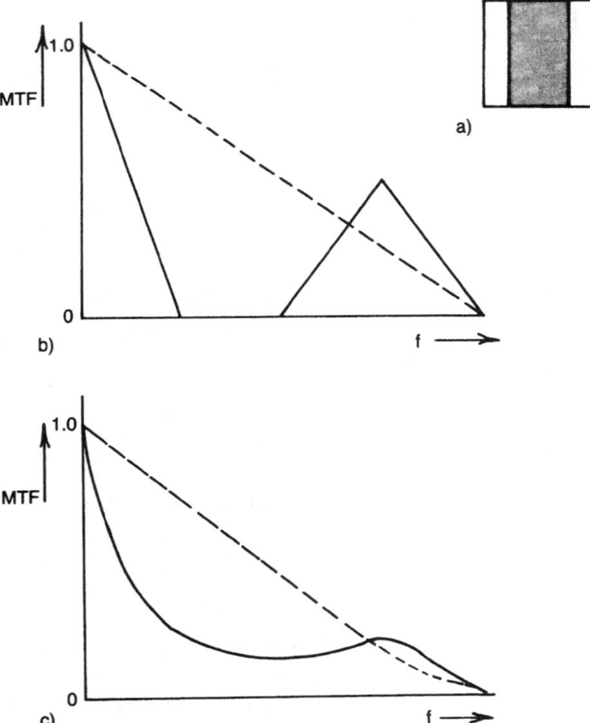

Figure 25.13 a, Square aperture with central obstruction; b, resulting MM; c, MTF for circular aperture with central obstruction.

An interesting situation occurs when there is a central obstruction in the system. A telescope with an objective mirror has such an obstruction. Consider the obstruction shown for the square aperture in Figure 25.13a. The corresponding diffraction limited MTF (solid lines in Figure 25.13b) drops to zero much quicker than that for a clear aperture (dashed lines) and then rises to a value greater than that for the clear aperture before it drops back to zero again. If the low frequency components are the most important in the object, then the obstruction degrades the image. If the higher frequency components are the most important, then the obstruction actually helps. The corresponding results for an annular aperture are shown in Figure 25.13c.

25.7 COUPLED SYSTEMS

Modulation transfer function theory can be applied to any linear system whether it is optical, electronic, or even film exposure and processing. Frequently, two linear systems are used in tandem. For example, for spatial frequency f, a camera lens has an MTF relating the object and image modulation:

$$M_i = (\mathrm{MTF})_1 M_o$$

Now if the film is operating in a linear range, the process of exposing and developing the film also has an MTF relating the image modulation to the modulation of the developed film.

$$M_{\mathrm{film}} = (\mathrm{MTF})_2 M_i$$

It is then easy to show that the MTF for the total process is the product of the individual MTFs, i.e., from the above two equations

$$M_{\mathrm{film}} = [(\mathrm{MTF})_2(\mathrm{MTF})_1]M_0$$

or

$$(\mathrm{MTF})_{\mathrm{tot}} = (\mathrm{MTF})_2(\mathrm{MTF})_1$$

Suppose, for a given spatial frequency, that a camera lens has an MTF of 0.85, and for that spatial frequency the film has an MTF of 0.71. Then the total MTF for the developed picture is the product $(0.85)(0.71) = 0.60$.

This analysis can also be applied to the human visual system provided the neural system is functioning linearly. Then the total MTF for the visual process is the product of the MTF for the optics of the eye and the MTF for the neural system. The MTF for the eye's optical system is a *low pass* system. In other words, lower spatial frequencies are transferred and higher spatial frequencies are not. On the other hand, the neural part of the visual system does not transfer very low spatial frequencies well, and transmits higher spatial frequencies better. Thus the MTF for the neural system is a *high pass* system. The product of the two MTFs is then peaked at a spatial frequency for which the human vision system is most sensitive.

Note that the MTF product does not apply to coherently coupled systems. For example, for two lenses, the total MTF is not the product of the MTFs for each individual lens. The reason is that the first lens may have a decreased MTF due to an aberration (e.g., positive spherical aberration), while the second lens has a decreased MTF due to the opposite aberration (e.g., negative spherical aberration). When used together the aberration of one lens may cancel the aberration of the other lens, so that the doublet has a better MTF than either lens by itself.

25.8 GENERAL OBJECTS

Consider a general object such as the castle in Figure 25.1. The castle is not periodic like a grating. Nevertheless, the luminance distribution of the castle scene can also be represented by a series of sine and cosine luminance distributions. In the periodic case, the spatial frequencies of the higher order sinusoidal components were integer multiples of the fundamental frequency. For a non-periodic object, such as the castle, there is a continuous range of frequencies in the higher order of components. These components can be computed with Fourier Transform methods.

Figure 25.14 shows a non-periodic object luminance distribution that has straight-line sides that extend out to a distance of $2x_o$ on either side of the central maximum. The maximum luminance value is A^2. The function $H(f)$ represents the continuous range of spatial frequency components in the object luminance distribution. The value of $H(f)$ represents the weighting of the component of spatial frequency f. In this case,

$$H(f) = [A \sin(2\pi x_0 f)/(\pi f)]^2$$

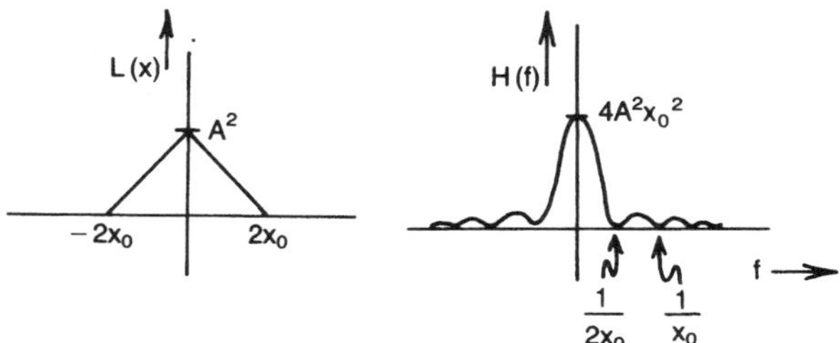

Figure 25.14 A nonperiodic object, $L(x)$, and its spatial frequency components $H(f)$.

Given an object, once we know the spatial frequency components we can apply the MTF theory to obtain the equation for the image luminance distribution. In that sense, the MTF analysis is theoretically independent of the exact object.

25.9 A NONLINEAR EXAMPLE

Consider a system with a lateral magnification of unit magnitude. One of the conditions for linearity of this system was that a spatial frequency f appears in the output if, and only if, the spatial frequency f appeared in the input. When a system is nonlinear the linear MTF theory does not apply.

Consider a tandem system consisting of the lenses and the photodetectors (electronic or neural). The photodetectors have a threshold. When the luminous flux falls below that threshold, the photodetector does not respond. Suppose the image is a single frequency sinusoidal grating (Figure 25.15a), and the mean luminance L_m of the image corresponds to the threshold. Then the detection system responds only to the luminance levels above L_m, and the detection system output (Figure 25.15b) consists of a periodic series of separated bumps. Now the output is no longer described by the sine wave of frequency f. According to Fourier's theorem, the periodic separated bumps can be represented by a sum of sine waves with spatial frequencies that are integer multiples of the fundamental frequency f. Thus, the photodetector threshold has resulted in the introduction of a number of spatial frequencies ($2f$, $3f$, $4f$, etc.) that were not present in the input. This is an example of a nonlinear response.

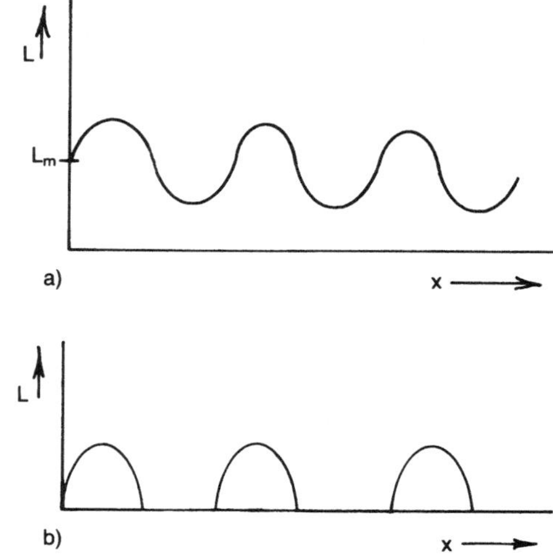

Figure 25.15 a, Sinusoidal object; b, above threshold part of the image.

25.10 MTFS IN TERMS OF CYCLES PER DEGREE

For applications to the eye, it is convenient to express spatial frequency in cycles per radian or cycles per degree. Consider a reduced (i.e., equivalent air) system. Let x_p be the length of one spatial period of a sine wave grating. In the paraxial approximation, x_p subtends an angle (expressed in radians) at the nodal point of the system given by

$$\phi = \tan\phi = \frac{x_p}{v}$$

where v is the (reduced) image distance. For the 60.00 D emmetropic eye, $v = 16.67$ mm. There are 57.30° rad, so ϕ in degrees for the 60.00 D emmetropic eye is

$$\phi = \frac{57.30x_p}{16.67\,\text{mm}} = 3.44\ x_p$$

where x_p is in mm. The spatial frequencies are the inverse of the spatial periods, so

$$f_\phi = \frac{f}{3.44} \tag{25.34}$$

where f_ϕ is in cycles per degree, while f is in cycles per mm.

In a 20/20 letter, the detail subtends an angle of 1′. So the dark horizontal bar of the letter E subtends an angle of 1′ and the white gap between the horizontal bars also subtends an angle of 1′. One spatial frequency in a corresponding sine wave grating then subtends a spatial frequency of 2′, or (2/60)°. The spatial frequency is then 30 cycles per degree. For a sine wave grating that corresponds to 20/10, the spatial frequency is 60 cycles per degree.

Even though images are usually different sizes than the conjugate object, the image subtends the same angle at the secondary nodal point N_2 as the object subtends at the primary nodal point N_1. It follows that an advantage of expressing spatial frequencies in cycles per degree (or in cycles per radian) is that the spatial frequencies are expressed by the same number in object space and in image space.

25.11 THE COHERENT TRANSFER FUNCTION

The previous MTF discussion was for incoherent light. We could repeat the discussion for coherent light, in which case we have to deal with sums of amplitudes (and constructive and destructive interference effects) rather than sums of intensities. In this case, we can define a transfer function, usually referred to as the coherent transfer function, for the amplitudes. One of the characteristics of the coherent transfer function is that its cut-off frequency (for the amplitude transfer) is one half that of the incoherent cut-off frequency f_c (which is for the intensity transfer). Therefore, when looking at the transfer function literature, pay attention to which cut-off frequency is being used. Sometimes the coherent cut-off is called f_c, in which case the incoherent cut-off is at $2f_c$.

The difference in cut-off frequencies (even though one is in amplitude and the other is in intensity) raises the question of which type of system transfers more information—coherent or incoherent. This is not a general answer to this question—since there are some objects for which a coherent system is better, and other objects for which an incoherent system is better.

25.12 ABBE THEORY OF IMAGE FORMATION

In the late 1800s Ernst Abbe was employed by the optical firm of Carl Zeiss to improve the optical properties of microscopes. In an effort to control the aberrations, Abbe worked on a number of designs with smaller and smaller apertures. Because of diffraction, Abbe expected the image to slowly get worse as the aperture size was decreased, but he found that for a certain aperture size the image abruptly vanished leaving only a uniformly illuminated background. This led Abbe to develop some rather different ideas about the image formation process.

For the compound microscope shown schematically in Figure 25.16a, a point source S provides the light, which is then collimated by a condensing lens. The collimated plane waves are incident on the microscope slide. In conventional theory, diverging light leaves the slide and is converged by the objective lens to form the magnified real image I inside the microscope.

Now let us consider Abbe's alternate formulation. Suppose the object on the microscope slide is a diffraction grating. When the collimated plane waves are incident, the diffraction grating generates a series of diffracted waves (the zero order along the axis, first order at an angle to the axis, second order at a larger angle, etc.). Each diffracted wave is considered a plane wave traveling at a different angle (Figure 25.16b). The objective lens of the microscope converges each diffracted wave to form a point image (actually an Airy's disk) in the secondary focal plane of the objective (marked by F_2). These point images are the diffraction grating maximums of Chapter 22. The zero order max-

Figure 25.16 a, Internal image formation by a microscope objective; b, optics of diffraction grating as a microscope slide.

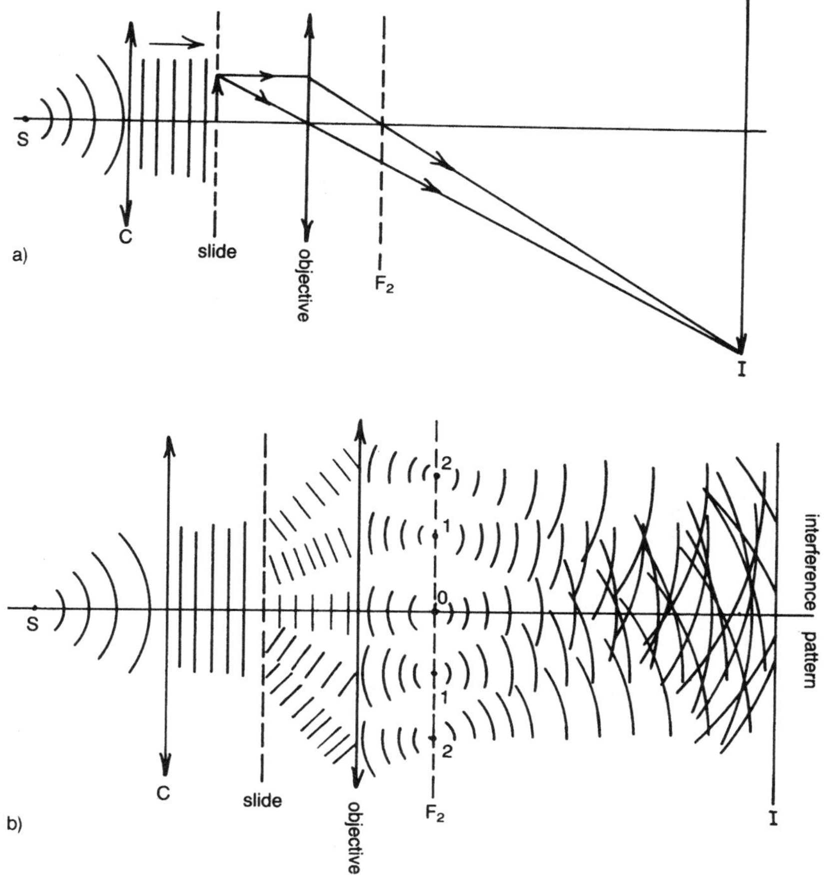

imum is labeled by 0, the first order maximums by 1, and the second order maximums by 2. The light then diverges away from the point images and the diverging waves overlap at the internal image plane. All the light originated from the point source *S*, and for small aperture sizes the coherence length of the overlapping light is such that interference effects occur. The result is a set of interference fringes in the internal image plane I. In fact, these interference fringes are the image of the diffraction grating.

Abbe realized that any small object diffracts light, so that the same theory can be applied, and the internal image is really an interference pattern. Abbe's theory explains why the image abruptly vanishes as the objective lens aperture is decreased in size. Once the aperture is small enough for the first and higher order diffracted waves to be blocked, there are not any waves for the zero order wave to interfere with. In this case there is no interference pattern and hence no image.

Figure 25.17 shows another ray diagram for the formation of the internal image. We can now interpret this ray diagram in two different ways. One way is the geometric optics method in which we follow the diverging rays from each object point until each bundle is converged to a point image. The second way is to follow each set of parallel rays leaving the grating at a particular angle to the axis, i.e., three parallel rays are traveling upward, three parallel to the axis, and three downward. These parallel rays correspond to the plane-diffracted waves, and they converge to form the series of point images (maximums) in the F_2 plane of the objective. The rays from each maximum then overlap at the internal image plane (where the interference forms the image).

Let us consider what additional image quality effects depend on the point images in the F_2 plane of the objective. When the aperture is large enough to pass the first order waves together with the zero order waves, interference occurs in the internal image plane. However, the interference fringes formed in this case have rounded edges. In effect, this "image" of the square wave diffraction grating is the sine wave grating of the same frequency (the fundamental harmonic). As the aperture size is increased so that the higher order diffracted waves are allowed through,

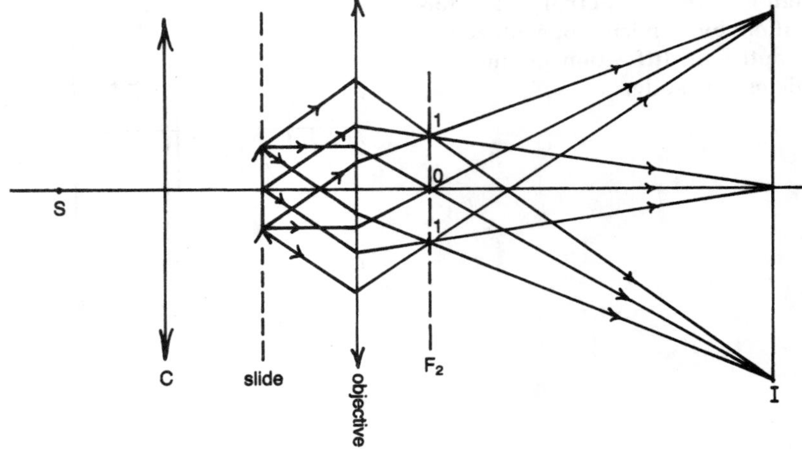

Figure 25.17 Rays for either the geometric or diffraction analysis.

the interference distribution builds into a square wave pattern just like a Fourier series, i.e., each higher order diffracted wave sharpens the fine detail.

We can further check the Fourier series analogy by isolating each of the orders of diffracted waves (e.g., the left and right first order diffracted waves, then the left and right second order diffracted waves, etc.). The interference fringes generated by each order are sine wave gratings, which are the Fourier components of the square wave grating. The position in the F_2 plane specifies the spatial frequency, and the intensity of the maximums specifies the magnitude of the sine wave component at that spatial frequency. This can be verified mathematically by showing that the light distribution in the F_2 plane is the Fourier transform of the square wave distribution of the original diffraction grating.

In the MTF sections, we noted that an optical system transferred information about each spatial frequency differently. Here we see that the information about each spatial frequency is in fact physically transferred through different positions in the F_2 or Fourier transform plane.

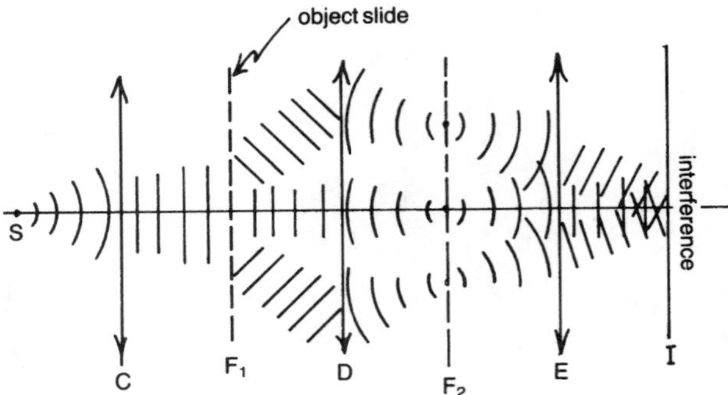

Figure 25.18 System with an accessible transform plane (F_2).

25.13 SPATIAL FILTERING

Given the Abbe theory of image formation, we can manipulate the resulting image by altering what happens in the transform plane. Figure 25.18 shows a system to perform this alteration. A point source S and condenser C collimate the incident light. (Laser light is easiest to use.) The object slide is placed at F_1 of lens D. Lenses D and E are separated by the sum of their focal lengths. From a geometric optics viewpoint, when an object is placed at F_1 of lens D, plane waves travel between the lenses, and lens E forms a conjugate image I in its secondary focal plane.

Now suppose the object slide is a diffraction grating. Diffracted plane waves leave the slide at various angles, and are converged by lens D to form a series of point images (maximums) at F_2. The composite of these point images is the diffraction pattern or Fourier transform of the object. The light diverges from these point images and is incident on lens E. Lens E converts the light into overlapping plane waves. The interference pattern formed at the secondary focal plane of lens E is the image I. Lens D took the diffraction grating object and formed the Fourier transform (the diffraction pattern) at F_2, while lens E takes the transform and forms the image.

When the diffraction grating consists of vertical lines, the Fourier transform (or diffraction pattern) at F_2 consists of a row of horizontal point images (Figure 25.19a). When the diffraction grating consists of horizontal lines, the Fourier transform consists of a row of vertical point images (Figure 25.19b). When the diffraction grating consists of crossed lines, then each horizontal point image is the center for a vertical row

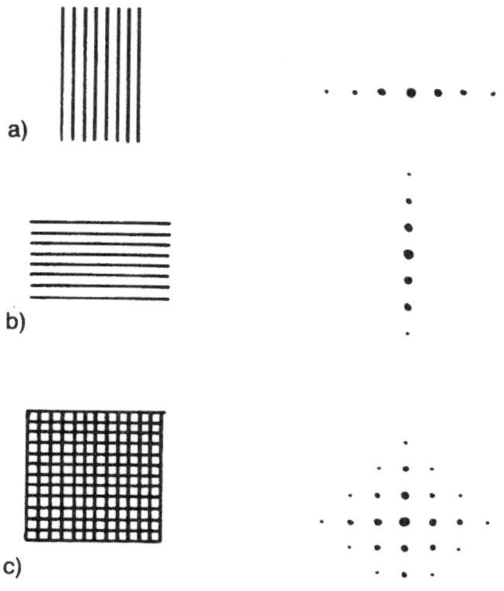

Figure 25.19 Objects and diffration patterns in the transform plane: a, vertical lines; b, horizontal lines; c, perpendicular lines.

of point images (or vice versa), and the result is a square array of point images (Figure 25.19c).

For the crossed grating, the interference pattern, which is the final image, also consists of crossed lines. When a horizontal slit is placed in the Fourier transform plane (at F_2 in Figure 25.18), the interference pattern in the image plane consists only of vertical lines, i.e., the object is the crossed grating in Figure 25.19c, but the horizontal slit passes only the maximums shown in Figure 25.19a, so the image is the vertical grating shown in Figure 25.19a. In this case, we say that the image was spatially filtered. When a vertical slit is placed in the transform plane, the interference pattern in the image plane consists only of horizontal lines.

Suppose a square aperture is placed in the transform plane and then decreased in size. Each of the point images in the image plane corresponds to one of the terms in the Fourier series (or transform) for the image. So if a square aperture is placed in the transform plane and decreased in size, the square wave luminance profiles in the image plane lose high frequency components and, hence, start to lose fine detail. When the square aperture is small enough to block all second and higher order diffracted waves, the interference pattern in the image plane is just the fundamental sine wave component of the object. In other words, the horizontal and vertical lines are now blurred to the point where they have a single sine wave distribution. When the square aperture is decreased further so that only the central maximum remains, the image abruptly vanishes and we have only uniform illumination in the image plane.

When no object is present in the object plane, lens D takes the incident collimated light and forms a point image in its F_2 plane. This point image is the zero order maximum. If a mask is made that just blocks this point image, the image plane is dark. Now when an object slide is placed in the object plane, higher order diffracted waves appear resulting in higher order maximums in the F_2 or transform plane. These higher order maximums are unaffected by the mask that blocks the zero order wave. The light from the higher order maximums passes through lens E to the image plane. The resulting interference in the image plane gives a phase reversed image in which high frequency information (edges), which were originally very faint, are now strongly evident. Figure 25.20 shows this for the case of a circular aperture; a is the object grating, while b is the filtered image grating. This principle is the basis for *dark field microscopy*. The phase reversal is understood by noting that dark areas in the unfiltered image are due to destructive interference between the zero order wave and the higher order waves. When the zero order wave is blocked, this destructive interference is removed.

A similar result is achieved in *phase contrast microscopy*. Suppose the object is essentially transparent but does have a variation in the refractive index. In the geometric optics image, these areas are still transparent and not visible. However, the phase variations do diffract a little light out of the zero order wave. Suppose a plate that introduces a phase shift is placed in the path of the zero order wave. Then the zero order wave is phase-shifted relative to the diffracted waves. Because of the shift, some destructive and constructive interference between the diffracted waves and the zero order waves occurs in the image plane. This interference makes the high spatial frequency phase information visible. The visibility is further enhanced when the phase plate is partially absorbing. (Sometimes

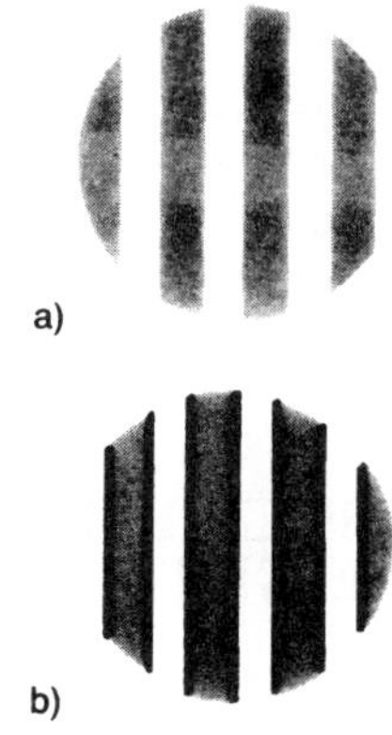

Figure 25.20 a, Object grating; b, spatially filtered image.

photochromic glass is used for the phase plate.) Some soft contact lens surface deposits that are hard to see with regular microscopy are readily visible with the phase contrast technique.

When laser light (highly coherent) is used as the illuminating light, spatial filtering can be performed with essentially any type of object slide. In this case, the light distribution in the F_2 plane of the objective is the Fourier transform of the object. By manipulating what happens in the transform plane, we can affect the image. For example, consider a magnified photograph of a television picture. The horizontal scan lines of the television are superimposed on the desired picture. These scan lines are periodic and so they give specifically placed vertical maximums in the Fourier transform plane. The rest of the light in the transform plane is the Fourier transform of the image. A mask can be made to block only the periodic maximums corresponding to the scan lines, while allowing all other light from the transform plane to pass on. The resulting interference pattern is the picture image without the scan lines.

When a laser beam is diverged, it typically gives a dirty illumination pattern because of diffraction from each dust particle or finger print. One way to clean the beam is to spatially filter it. First, the beam is converged to a focus. The light diffracted by the dust, fingerprints, etc. does not go to the point image but lies at some lateral position in the image plane. If a pinhole or small circular aperture is positioned to pass only the point image, then the diverging light leaving that image gives beautifully clean illumination.

Spatial filtering techniques can be used to enhance or depress certain spatial frequencies in an image. In fact, spatial filtering techniques have even been used to color code different spatial frequency information. In short, spatial filtering techniques give us tremendous power in recapturing hidden information.

It is possible to obtain artifacts in spatial filtering. Suppose for the crossed grating target of Figure 25.19c, a diagonal slit is placed in the transform plane (F_2 plane in Figure 25.18). Then a diagonal set of point images is transmitted through the slit. This results in a perpendicularly diagonal set of interference fringes in the image plane. In this case, we started with a target that has horizontal and vertical lines, and ended up with a filtered image that has diagonal lines.

25.14 FREQUENCY DOUBLING OF LASER LIGHT

In angular terms (e.g., cycles per degree), the image of a linear system contains only those spatial frequencies f_ϕ of the object for which there is a non-zero MTF. In particular, when a spatial frequency f_ϕ does not appear in the object, it cannot appear in the image. Section 25.9 gave an example of a system that was nonlinear because of threshold effects. In the nonlinear case, spatial frequencies (at $2f$, $3f$, $4f$, etc.) appeared in the image that were not present in the object.

The same type of phenomena also occurs in the temporal domain of light waves. In a linear system, when light waves of various temporal frequencies are incident on a system, the transmitted waves consist only of those incident frequencies that are transferred by the system. However in a nonlinear system, there may be temporal frequencies in the output that are not present in the input.

For incident electromagnetic radiation, certain crystals are nonlinear in character. Consider a coherent harmonic light wave of temporal frequency f_t incident on a particular nonlinear crystal. The electromagnetic light wave tries to impart a sinusoidal vibration to the electrons in the crystal. Suppose however the crystal forces on the electrons do not let them vibrate sinusoidally. For example, perhaps the crystal forces dampen out the top and bottom parts of the sinusoidal vibration. The result is a periodic vibration of the electrons that is not sinusoidal. By Fourier's Theorem, we can consider the periodic vibration as consisting of a sum of sinusoidal vibrations of temporal frequency f_t, $2f_t$, $3f_t$, $4f_t$, etc.

When the electrons in the nonlinear crystal re-radiate, they then emit light waves with frequencies f_t, $2f_t$, $3f_t$, $4f_t$, etc. The intensities of the higher order frequencies are usually very low. However there are crystals that result in sizable amounts of certain of the higher orders. The terms *second harmonic generation* refers to the case when the output light has a frequency of twice the input frequency (frequency doubling). Wavelength and temporal frequency are reciprocals—so when the frequency is doubled, the wavelength is halved. When irradiated by a 1064 nm coherent beam from a Nd:YAG laser, a potassium titanyl phosphate (KTP) nonlinear crystal produces a 532 nm coherent beam output (see Section 24.9)—in addition to a 1064 nm output. We can easily separate the two outputs with a diffraction grating or with a thick prism.

PROBLEMS

1. An optical system with unit lateral magnification has an object luminance distribution of

$$L_o = 13 + 8\sin(2\pi 4x)$$

When the MTF for 4 cycles/mm is 0.6, what is the image luminance distribution?

2. An optical system with unit lateral magnification has an object luminance distribution of

$$L_o = 15 + 4\sin(2\pi x) + 4\sin(2\pi 3x) + 4\sin(2\pi x)$$

The MTF for the system is given by $1 - 0.2f$. What is the image luminance distribution?
3. What is the image space cut-off frequency in cycles/mm for 633 nm light incident on an $f/5.6$ system? For 483 nm light incident?
4. A diffraction-limited system with a square aperture has a cut-off frequency of 600 cycles/mm. What is the MTF for a frequency of 400 cycles/mm?
5. A diffraction-limited system with a circular aperture has a cut-off frequency of 600 cycles/mm. What is the MTF for a frequency of 400 cycles/mm?
6. A system with a square aperture has an effective cut-off frequency of 240 cycles/mm. For 0.40 D of blur, what is the MTF for 60 cycles/mm?
7. A standard 60.00 D emmetropic eye has a sine wave grating on the retina with a 100 cycle/mm spatial frequency. What is the spatial frequency in cycles per degree?
8. For light of 633 nm incident on an eye with a 3 mm pupil, what is the diffraction limited cut-off frequency in cycles per degree?

Appendix A

Trigonometry Review

Figure A.1 shows an angle θ in a circle of radius r. The vertex of the angle is at point A, which is also the center of the circle. The bottom boundary of the angle is the horizontal line, which intersects the circle at point D. The top boundary of the angle is the diagonal line that intersects the circle at point B. The diagonal line segment AB has a length equal to the radius r. A vertical line drawn from point B down to the horizontal line intersects the horizontal line at point C, and the vertical line segment BC has length y. The horizontal line segment AC has length x.

In the international system of units (SI), the radian (abbreviated rad) is the unit for an angle in a plane. The angle in radians is the ratio of the subtended arc length on a circle to the radius of the circle. In Figure A.1, the subtended arc length is from B to D on the circle.

The circumference of a circle of radius r is $2\pi r$. So the subtended arc length for an angle that encompasses the whole circle is $2\pi r$, and the angle is 2π rad. The angle θ in Figure A.1 subtends only 1/8 of the circumference; so the subtended arc length is $2\pi r/8$, and resulting angle is $\pi/4$ rad. A right angle is an angle that subtends 1/4 of the circle; so the subtended arc length is $2\pi r/4$, and the resulting angle is $\pi/2$ rad. The radian is actually a unitless name that is convenient to use for angles.

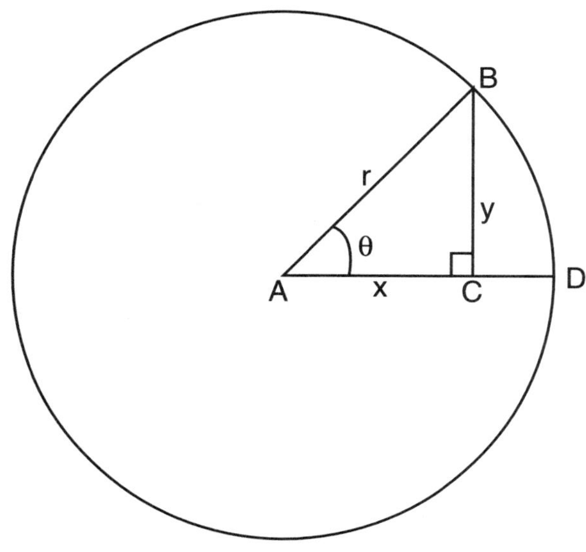

Figure A.1

Currently, people normally use a base 10 number system. At one time in history, a base 60 number system was in use. The fact that there are 60 min in an hour and 60 s in a minute is a leftover from the old base 60 number system. The degree-minute-second method of measuring angles is also a leftover from the base 60 number system. In the base 60 number system, each angle in an equilateral triangle was assigned the value of 60 degrees (written 60°). It follows that in the degree system, an angle that encompasses a full circle is 360°. Therefore a right angle, which subtends 1/4 of the circle, is 360°/4 or 90°. Each degree is further subdivided into 60 min (written 60′), and each minute is further subdivided into 60 s (written 60″).

It would make more sense to forget the degree-minute-second system, and just use the radian system. However in visual optics, there are aspects of the degree-minute-second that are deeply ingrained. Indeed the common spherocylindrical prescription has the cylinder axis expressed in degrees, and the 20/20 acuity system is related to minutes of subtended detail.

We can convert from radians to degrees by noting that

$$2\pi \text{ rad} = 360^\circ \tag{A.1}$$

or

$$\pi \text{ rad} = 180^\circ \tag{A.2}$$

It follows that

$$1 \text{ rad} = 57.29578^\circ \tag{A.3}$$

θ equal $\pi/4$ rad in Figure A.1. What is θ in degrees? From Eq. A.2,

$$\frac{\pi}{4}\text{ rad}\left(\frac{180^\circ}{\pi\text{ rad}}\right) = 45^\circ$$

Alternatively $\pi/4$ rad times $57.29578^\circ/\text{rad}$ also gives 45°.

The angle between a vertical line and a horizontal line is 90° and is called a right angle. What is the right angle in radians? From Eq. A.3,

$$\frac{90^\circ}{57.29578^\circ/\text{rad}} = 1.5708\text{ rad}$$

Alternatively, 90° times $(\pi\text{ rad}/180^\circ) = \pi/2$ rad, which equals 1.5708 rad.

The triangle *ABC* in Figure A.1, contains a right angle, and is said to be a right triangle. The side opposite the right angle (line segment *AB*) is called the hypotenuse. The Pythagorean Theorem relates the lengths of the sides of the right triangle by

$$x^2 + y^2 = r^2 \tag{A.4}$$

The basic trigonometry functions (sine, cosine, and tangent) of the angle θ in the right triangle *ABC* are defined as follows. The sine of θ is the length of the opposite side divided by the length of the hypotenuse, the cosine of θ is the length of the adjacent side divided by the length of the hypotenuse, and the tangent of θ is the length of the opposite side divided by the length of the adjacent side. In equation form:

$$\sin\theta = y/r \tag{A.5}$$

$$\cos\theta = x/r \tag{A.6}$$

$$\tan\theta = y/x \tag{A.7}$$

It follows that

$$\tan\theta = \sin\theta/\cos\theta \tag{A.8}$$

One can solve Eq. A.5 for y and Eq. A.6 for x, and then substitute the results into Eq. A.4 to get

$$\sin^2\theta + \cos^2\theta = 1 \tag{A.9}$$

The numerical values of the trig functions are readily available from hand held scientific calculators or from microcomputers. Calculators can be set to calculate the trig functions from the angle in radians or from the angle in degrees. Some computer programs also do that, but others need to have the angle in radians.

The cosine function varies from a maximum of +1 (at $\theta = 0$) to a minimum of -1 (at $\theta = 180^\circ$ or π rad). The sine functions varies from a maximum of +1 (at $\theta = 90^\circ$ or $\pi/2$ rad) to a minimum of -1 (at $\theta = 270^\circ$ or $3\pi/2$ rad). The sine of 0 is 0.

First quadrant angles are those between 0° and 90°, and in the first quadrant both the sine and the cosine are positive. Second quadrant angles are those between 90° and 180°, and in the second quadrant the cosine is negative while the sine is positive (e.g., $\cos 120^\circ = -0.50$). We can see this from Figure A.2, which shows a second quadrant angle θ. When the origin of the coordinate system is at the center of the circle (point *A*), the coordinate x is positive to the right of *A* and negative to the left of *A*. Then from Eq. A.6, the cosine is negative.

Third quadrant angles are those between 180° and 270°, and in the third quadrant both the sine and the cosine are negative. Fourth quadrant angles are those between 270° and 360°, and in the fourth quadrant the cosine is positive while the sine is negative (e.g., $\sin 300^\circ = -0.866$).

Consider an angle θ of 30°, and suppose that it is centered in a circle of radius 2 cm. (We'll use the same labeling as in Figure A.1). Since $\sin 30^\circ = 0.50$, Eq. A.5 shows that the length of the side opposite the 30° angle is 1/2 of the hypotenuse length, or for this case $y = 1$ cm. The Pythagorean Theorem (Eq. A.1) then gives the length x of the horizontal (adjacent) side as $\sqrt{3}$, which equals 1.7321. Here the polar coordinates (r and θ) of the point *B* are 2 and 30°, and the rectangular coordinates (x and y) of *B* are 1.7321 and 1. Scientific calculators include a button that converts from polar coordinates to rectangular coordinates, and vice versa.

Suppose the rectangular coordinates for point *B* (as in Figure A.1) are $x = +1.500$ and $y = +2.598$. What are the polar coordinates? From Eq. A.4,

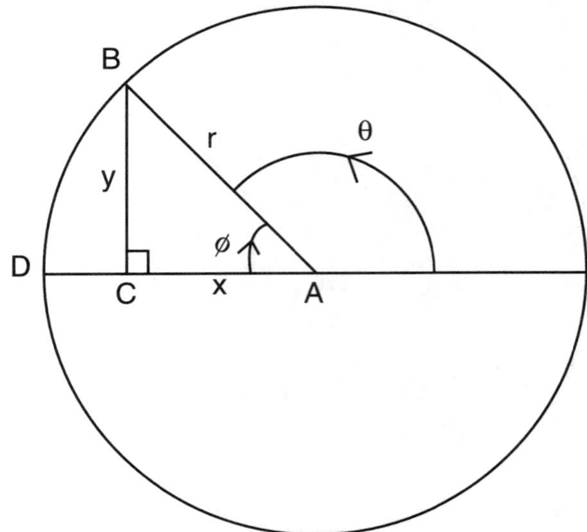

Figure A.2

$$r^2 = (+1.5000)^2 + (+2.598)^2$$
$$= 9.000 \quad \text{and} \quad r = 3.000$$

From Eq. A.7,

$$\tan\theta = \frac{+2.598}{+1.500} = 1.732$$

Then from a calculator, the inverse tangent gives $\theta = 60°$. So the polar coordinates of the point B are 3 and 60°.

Suppose the rectangular coordinates of a point are $x = -1.1472$ and $y = 1.6383$. This corresponds to the point B in Figure A.2. What are the polar coordinates? From Eq. A.4,

$$r^2 = (-1.1472)^2 + (1.6383)^2$$
$$= 4.000 \quad \text{and} \quad r = 2.0000$$

From the triangle ABC in Figure A.2, we can solve for the angle ϕ from

$$\tan\phi = \frac{y}{x}$$
$$= \frac{1.6383}{-1.1472} = -1.4281$$

On a calculator, the inverse tangent gives an angle ϕ of $-55°$. Here the angle ϕ is clockwise from the horizontal. To get the counter-clockwise angle θ, we need to add 180° to ϕ:

$$\theta = 180° + \phi$$

or

$$\theta = 180° + (-55°) = 125°$$

The polar coordinates of the point B are then 2 and 125°.

When the line segments AB represent vectors, the polar and rectangular coordinates of the vectors are found in the same way. Scientific calculators have a button that converts from rectangular to polar coordinates, and another button that converts from polar to rectangular coordinates.

When the angle θ *expressed in radians* is small, there is a series approximation for the sine, cosine, and tangent functions. For the sine, the approximation is

$$\sin\theta = \theta - \frac{\theta^3}{3!} + \frac{\theta^5}{5!} - \frac{\theta^7}{7!} + \cdots \qquad \text{(A.10)}$$

The exponent of θ is the order number of each term in the approximation. So the terms on the right are respectively the first order term, third order term, fifth order term, etc.

Consider $\theta = 30° = 0.5236$ rad. To 4 digits, a calculator gives

$$\sin 30° = \sin(0.5236\,\text{rad}) = 0.5000$$

The first, third, and fifth terms in the series approximation (Eq. A.10) give

$$\sin(0.5236) = 0.5236 - \frac{(0.5236)^3}{3!} + \frac{(0.5236)^5}{5!}$$
$$= 0.5236 - 0.0239 + 0.003 = 0.5000$$

Notice that each higher order term is much smaller than the pervious term, and to 4 digits the seventh and higher order terms are negligible.

For smaller angles, the fifth order term also becomes negligible. For example: $\theta = 15° = 0.2618$ rad. To 4 digits, a calculator gives

$$\sin 15° = \sin(0.2618\,\text{rad}) = 0.2588$$

The first and third order terms in the approximation give

$$\sin(0.2618) = 0.2618 - \frac{(0.2618)^3}{3!}$$
$$= 0.2618 - 0.0030 = 0.2588$$

For even smaller angles, even the third order term becomes negligible. Consider $\theta = 4° = 0.0698$ rad. To 4 digits, a calculator gives

$$\sin 4° = \sin(0.0698\,\text{rad}) = 0.0698$$

Here the first order term of the series approximation gives

$$\sin(0.0698) = 0.0698$$

In optics, we frequently deal with angles significantly smaller than 4°. For example, the height of a standard 20/20 letter subtends an angle of 5′ (or 0.0833°). For these small angles, the first order approximation to the sine is very accurate.

When θ *expressed in radians* is small, series approximations for the cosine and for the tangent are

$$\cos\theta = 1 - \frac{\theta^2}{2!} + \frac{\theta^4}{4!} - \frac{\theta^6}{6!} + \cdots \qquad \text{(A.11)}$$

and

$$\tan\theta = \theta + \frac{\theta^3}{3} + \frac{2\theta^5}{15} - \frac{17\theta^7}{315} + \cdots \qquad \text{(A.12)}$$

Note that for angles (expressed in radians) small enough that the first order approximation is accurate, the series approximations A.10 and A.12 give

$$\sin\theta = \tan\theta = \theta$$

Appendix B

Basic Matrix Algebra

When you go to a grocery store to buy a dozen oranges, you typically put the oranges in a bag to take home. The bag makes it easier to transport the oranges. In a sense, a matrix is a bag of numbers. We use the matrix (the bag) because it simplifies handling the numbers and enables us to do operations that are difficult to do without matrices.

A row number and a column number identify the individual numbers or elements of the matrix. Row numbers are written first. Consider a matrix with three row and two columns, a so-called 3×2 matrix.

$$\begin{matrix} & \text{column} & \text{column} & \\ & 1 & 2 & \\ \mathbf{A} = & \left(\begin{matrix} a_{11} \\ a_{21} \\ a_{31} \end{matrix}\right. & \left.\begin{matrix} a_{12} \\ a_{22} \\ a_{32} \end{matrix}\right) & \begin{matrix} \text{row 1} \\ \text{row 2} \\ \text{row 3} \end{matrix} \end{matrix}$$

For example, when

$$\mathbf{A} = \begin{pmatrix} 3 & 1 \\ -1 & 0 \\ 2 & 5 \end{pmatrix}$$

the individual elements are

$$\begin{matrix} a_{11} = 3 & a_{12} = 1 \\ a_{21} = -1 & a_{22} = 0 \\ a_{31} = 2 & a_{32} = 5 \end{matrix}$$

For a matrix **A**, we refer to the element in the ith row and jth column as a_{ij}.

MATRIX ADDITION

Matrices can be added together if, and only if, they have the same shape, that is, an $m \times n$ matrix can be added to another $m \times n$ matrix. For example, a 3×2 matrix can be added to another 3×2 matrix. A 3×2 matrix cannot be added to a 2×2 matrix.

In matrix addition, the individual elements are respectively added. The technical statement is:

Let **A**, **B**, and **C** be $m \times n$ matrices. Then $\mathbf{A} + \mathbf{B} = \mathbf{C}$ if and only if

$$a_{ij} + b_{ij} = c_{ij}$$

for all values of i and j.

EXAMPLE

Given the 3×2 matrices

$$\mathbf{A} = \begin{pmatrix} 3 & 1 \\ -1 & 0 \\ 2 & 5 \end{pmatrix} \quad \mathbf{B} = \begin{pmatrix} 4 & 3 \\ 1 & 9 \\ 6 & -6 \end{pmatrix}$$

Then,

$$\mathbf{C} = \mathbf{A} + \mathbf{B} = \begin{pmatrix} 7 & 4 \\ 0 & 9 \\ 8 & -1 \end{pmatrix}$$

In matrix addition, the mathematical properties of commutation and association hold.

$$\mathbf{A} + \mathbf{B} = \mathbf{B} + \mathbf{A} \quad \text{(commutation)}$$
$$(\mathbf{A} + \mathbf{B}) + \mathbf{C} = \mathbf{A} + (\mathbf{B} + \mathbf{C}) \quad \text{(association)}$$

SCALAR MULTIPLICATION

When a single number (a scalar) multiplies a matrix, then that number multiplies each element in the matrix. Let q be a number (scalar) and **A** be a matrix. Then,

$$\mathbf{C} = q\mathbf{A}$$

if and only if

$$c_{ij} = qa_{ij}$$

for all values of i and j. For example, let $q = 0.5$, and let **A** be the matrix used above. Then,

$$\mathbf{C} = q\mathbf{A} = 0.5\begin{pmatrix} 3 & 1 \\ -1 & 0 \\ 2 & 5 \end{pmatrix} = \begin{pmatrix} 1.5 & 0.5 \\ -0.5 & 0 \\ 1 & 2.5 \end{pmatrix}$$

MATRIX MULTIPLICATION

Matrix multiplication has some algebraic properties that differ from those of scalars (numbers). The learning of these special rules is the investment that enables one to harness the power of matrix algebra.

Two matrices can be multiplied together only when the number of columns of the left matrix equals the number of rows of the right matrix. The product matrix has the number of rows of the left matrix and the number of columns of the right matrix. That is, an $m \times n$ matrix can be multiplied from the right by an $n \times p$ matrix, and the product matrix is $m \times p$. As an example, a 3×2 matrix can be multiplied from the right by a 2×1 matrix, and the product matrix is a 3×1 matrix. A 3×2 matrix cannot be multiplied by another 3×2 matrix.

Consider an allowed matrix multiplication, $\mathbf{C} = \mathbf{AB}$. The element c_{ij} is obtained by taking the elements in the ith row of **A** and multiplying each by the corresponding element in the jth row of **B**, and then adding all the results together. This is algebraically stated as:

$$\mathbf{C} = \mathbf{AB}$$

if and only if

$$c_{ij} = \sum_k a_{ik} b_{kj}$$

EXAMPLE

$$\mathbf{A} = \begin{pmatrix} 3 & 1 \\ -1 & 0 \\ 2 & 5 \end{pmatrix} \quad \mathbf{B} = \begin{pmatrix} 7 \\ -4 \end{pmatrix}$$

Here **A** is a 3×2 matrix, and **B** is a 2×1 matrix. Then the product matrix **C**, where $\mathbf{C} = \mathbf{AB}$, is a 3×1 matrix. The corresponding algebraic equations are:

$$c_{11} = a_{11}b_{11} + a_{12}b_{21}$$

i.e., first row of **A** and first column of **B**,

$$c_{21} = a_{21}b_{11} + a_{22}b_{21}$$

i.e., second row of **A** and first column of **B**,

$$c_{31} = a_{31}b_{11} + a_{32}b_{21}$$

i.e., third row of **A** and first column of **B**.

The numerical results are:

$$\mathbf{C} = \begin{pmatrix} (3)(7) + (1)(-4) \\ (-1)(7) + (0)(-4) \\ (2)(7) + (5)(-4) \end{pmatrix} = \begin{pmatrix} 17 \\ -7 \\ -6 \end{pmatrix}$$

Note that for the matrices **A** and **B** above, **BA** is not defined. We cannot multiply a 2×1 matrix from the right by a 3×2 matrix.

2×2 *matrix examples*: Let

$$\mathbf{E} = \begin{pmatrix} 2 & 1 \\ 3 & 5 \end{pmatrix} \quad \text{and} \quad \mathbf{F} = \begin{pmatrix} -1 & -4 \\ 7 & 3 \end{pmatrix}$$

Then the product matrix **H**, where $\mathbf{H} = \mathbf{EF}$, is also a 2×2 matrix. The numerical results are:

$$\mathbf{H} = \mathbf{EF} = \begin{pmatrix} (2)(-1) + (1)(7) & (2)(-4) + (1)(3) \\ (3)(-1) + (5)(7) & (3)(-4) + (5)(3) \end{pmatrix}$$

or

$$\mathbf{H} = \begin{pmatrix} 5 & -5 \\ 32 & 3 \end{pmatrix}$$

For the matrices **E** and **F** above,

$$\mathbf{J} = \mathbf{FE} = \begin{pmatrix} -1 & -4 \\ 7 & 3 \end{pmatrix}\begin{pmatrix} 2 & 1 \\ 3 & 5 \end{pmatrix}$$
$$= \begin{pmatrix} (-1)(2) + (-4)(3) & (-1)(1) + (-4)(5) \\ (7)(2) + (3)(3) & (7)(1) + (3)(5) \end{pmatrix}$$
$$\mathbf{J} = \begin{pmatrix} -14 & -21 \\ 23 & 22 \end{pmatrix}$$

Note from the above two examples that $\mathbf{H} \neq \mathbf{J}$.

There are some exceptions, but in general matrix multiplication does *not* commute, i.e.,

$$\mathbf{AB} \neq \mathbf{BA}$$

Thus, the order of matrix multiplication is crucial.

There is an associative law for matrix multiplication:

$$(\mathbf{AB})\mathbf{C} = \mathbf{A}(\mathbf{BC})$$

There is also a distributive law:

$$\mathbf{A}(\mathbf{B} + \mathbf{C}) = \mathbf{AB} + \mathbf{AC}$$

THE UNIT MATRIX

Square matrices have the same number of rows and columns (e.g., 2×2, 3×3). The *diagonal elements* of a square matrix have the same row and column number (e.g., a_{11}, a_{22}, etc.). The *off-diagonal* elements have different row and column numbers (a_{ij} where $i \neq j$, as in a_{12} or a_{23}).

Consider square matrices. The unit matrix **1** has diagonal elements equal to 1 and off-diagonal elements equal to 0. The 3×3 unit matrix is

$$\mathbf{1} = \begin{pmatrix} 1 & 0 & 0 \\ 0 & 1 & 0 \\ 0 & 0 & 1 \end{pmatrix}$$

The 2×2 unit matrix is

$$\mathbf{1} = \begin{pmatrix} 1 & 0 \\ 0 & 1 \end{pmatrix}$$

For a square matrix **A**, the unit matrix has the property that

$$\mathbf{A1} = \mathbf{1A} = \mathbf{A}$$

Let us explicitly verify this for the matrix **F** above:

$$\mathbf{F1} = \begin{pmatrix} -1 & -4 \\ 7 & 3 \end{pmatrix}\begin{pmatrix} 1 & 0 \\ 0 & 1 \end{pmatrix}$$

The matrix multiplications give

$$\mathbf{F1} = \begin{pmatrix} (-1)(1) + (-4)(0) & (-1)(0) + (-4)(1) \\ (7)(1) + (3)(0) & (7)(0) + (3)(1) \end{pmatrix}$$

or

$$\mathbf{F1} = \begin{pmatrix} -1 & -4 \\ 7 & 3 \end{pmatrix} = \mathbf{F}$$

THE INVERSE MATRIX

Consider a square matrix **A**. If it exists, the inverse matrix $\mathbf{A}^{-1}$ is defined such that

$$\mathbf{AA}^{-1} = \mathbf{A}^{-1}\mathbf{A} = \mathbf{1}$$

For the special case of 2×2 matrices, i.e.,

$$\mathbf{A} = \begin{pmatrix} a_{11} & a_{12} \\ a_{21} & a_{22} \end{pmatrix}$$

the inverse matrix is given by

$$\mathbf{A}^{-1} = (1/\delta)\begin{pmatrix} a_{22} & -a_{12} \\ -a_{21} & a_{11} \end{pmatrix}$$

where δ stands for the determinant of **A**. For the 2×2 matrix, the determinant equals the product of the diagonal elements minus the product of the off-diagonal elements, or

$$\delta = a_{11}a_{22} - a_{12}a_{21}$$

Note that for the inverse matrix, the diagonal elements change place, the off-diagonal elements change sign, and all elements are divided by the determinant.

EXAMPLE

$$\mathbf{A} = \begin{pmatrix} 8 & 3 \\ 4 & 2 \end{pmatrix}$$

Then,

$$\delta = (8)(2) - (4)(3) = +4$$

and

$$\mathbf{A}^{-1} = (1/4)\begin{pmatrix} 2 & -3 \\ -4 & 8 \end{pmatrix} = \begin{pmatrix} 0.5 & -0.75 \\ -1 & 2 \end{pmatrix}$$

You should be able to verify this by explicitly checking that the product $\mathbf{AA}^{-1}$ equals the unit matrix **1**.

When a matrix has only diagonal elements, the inverse matrix also has only diagonal elements, where each element is the reciprocal of the corresponding element in the original matrix. For example, given

$$\mathbf{A} = \begin{pmatrix} 4 & 0 \\ 0 & 2 \end{pmatrix}$$
$$\mathbf{A}^{-1} = \begin{pmatrix} 0.25 & 0 \\ 0 & 0.50 \end{pmatrix}$$

If the determinant of a matrix is zero, then the matrix does not have an inverse and is called a singular matrix. A matrix that has an inverse is called a nonsingular matrix.

Suppose **A** and **C** are known matrices, and

$$\mathbf{AB} = \mathbf{C}$$

We can then find **B** by multiplying both sides from the left by $\mathbf{A}^{-1}$ (provided that the inverse exists):

$$\mathbf{A}^{-1}\mathbf{AB} = \mathbf{A}^{-1}\mathbf{C}$$
$$\mathbf{1B} = \mathbf{A}^{-1}\mathbf{C}$$

or

$$\mathbf{B} = \mathbf{A}^{-1}\mathbf{C}$$

Remember that the order of the matrices in the product is crucial.

VECTORS AND MATRICES

Vectors can be represented either as column matrices (i.e., $m \times 1$), or as row matrices (i.e. $1 \times m$). Consider the vector **G** with a horizontal component +2 and a vertical component −3. We could represent the vector as the 2×1 matrix

$$\mathbf{G} = \begin{pmatrix} +2 \\ -3 \end{pmatrix}$$

PROBLEMS

1. Find $\mathbf{C} = \mathbf{A} + \mathbf{B}$ where

$$\mathbf{A} = \begin{pmatrix} 3 & 4 \\ 5 & -2 \end{pmatrix} \quad \mathbf{B} = \begin{pmatrix} 7 & -6 \\ -5 & 3 \end{pmatrix}$$

2. Find $\mathbf{C} = q\mathbf{A}$, where $q = -0.4$ and

$$\mathbf{A} = \begin{pmatrix} 3 & 2 \\ 1 & -6 \\ 4 & 9 \end{pmatrix}$$

3. Find $\mathbf{C} = \mathbf{AB}$ where

$$\mathbf{A} = \begin{pmatrix} -2 & 5 \\ 3 & -1 \end{pmatrix} \quad \mathbf{B} = \begin{pmatrix} -3 \\ 7 \end{pmatrix}$$

4. Find $\mathbf{C} = \mathbf{AB}$ where

$$\mathbf{A} = \begin{pmatrix} 13 & 9 \\ 7 & -6 \end{pmatrix} \quad \mathbf{B} = \begin{pmatrix} 5 & -4 \\ 1 & 3 \end{pmatrix}$$

5. Use **A** and **B** from the previous problem to find $\mathbf{D} = \mathbf{BA}$. Check if **D** equals the product **C** of the previous problem, or not.
6. Find the product **E** where

$$\mathbf{E} = \begin{pmatrix} 5 & 3 \\ -4 & 2 \end{pmatrix} \begin{pmatrix} 1 & 0 \\ 0 & 1 \end{pmatrix}$$

7. Find the product **S** where

$$\mathbf{S} = \begin{pmatrix} 1 & 0 \\ 0.2 & 1 \end{pmatrix} \begin{pmatrix} 1 & -4 \\ 0 & 1 \end{pmatrix}$$

8. Label the following matrices as singular or nonsingular. Find the inverse matrix for those that are nonsingular.

$$\mathbf{A} = \begin{pmatrix} 3 & -4 \\ -3 & 5 \end{pmatrix}$$
$$\mathbf{B} = \begin{pmatrix} 1 & 1 \\ 1 & 1 \end{pmatrix}$$
$$\mathbf{C} = \begin{pmatrix} 2 & 0 \\ 0 & 2 \end{pmatrix}$$

9. Given the following equality, find the matrix **B**. (Hint: Use the inverse matrix.)

$$\begin{pmatrix} 2 & 3 \\ 5 & 4 \end{pmatrix} \mathbf{B} = \begin{pmatrix} 7 \\ -1 \end{pmatrix}$$

10. Given the following equality, find the matrix **A**. (Hint: Use the inverse matrix and watch the order.)

$$\mathbf{A} \begin{pmatrix} 9 & 7 \\ -3 & -2 \end{pmatrix} = \begin{pmatrix} 2 & 0 \\ 5 & 1 \end{pmatrix}$$

11. Find $\mathbf{C} = \mathbf{AB}$ where

$$\mathbf{A} = \begin{pmatrix} \cos\theta & \sin\theta \\ -\sin\theta & \cos\theta \end{pmatrix} \quad \mathbf{B} = \begin{pmatrix} \cos\theta & -\sin\theta \\ \sin\theta & \cos\theta \end{pmatrix}$$

(Hint: $\sin^2\theta + \cos^2\theta = 1$.) Does **B** have any special relationship to **A**?

12. The trace τ of a square matrix is defined as the sum of the diagonal elements. For a 2×2 matrix,

$$\mathbf{A} = \begin{pmatrix} a_{11} & a_{12} \\ a_{21} & a_{22} \end{pmatrix}$$
$$\tau = a_{11} + a_{22}$$

For 2×2 matrices: let $\mathbf{C} = \mathbf{A} + \mathbf{B}$. Then prove that the traces also add, i.e., trace **C** = (trace **A**) + (trace **B**).

Answers to Selected Problems

CHAPTER 1

(1) 1.67
(3) 31.2°, toward
(5) 5.32°, away
(7) yes
(11) abundance of short wavelengths (the blue end) incident on observer's eye. long wavelengths (red end) absorbed the most.

CHAPTER 2

(1) −12.50 D, −2.38 D, −0.81 D
(3) +12.16 D, −4.81 D
(5) +9.61 D
(7) −12.09 D, −6.33 D
(9) 12.5 cm, 16.67 cm
(11) 5.0 cm
(13) stays clear and gets larger

CHAPTER 3

(1) virtual, optically real, left
(3) *A*, virtual image, converging
(5) Lens 5, Lens 4
(7) Lens 3, Lens 2
(11) image formed by the spectacle lens, virtual, real

CHAPTER 5

(1) $v = +25.0$ cm, real, −0.5, $U_{5f} = -2.22$ D, $V_{5b} = +5.00$ D
(3) $v = -25.0$ cm, virtual, +2.5, $U_{5f} = -20.00$ D, $V_{5b} = -3.33$ D
(5) $v = +25.0$ cm, real, +0.36, $U_{5f} = +2.86$ D, $V_{5b} = +17.50$ D
(7) $v = -5.88$ cm, virtual, +0.59, $U_{5f} = -20.00$ D, $V_{5b} = -9.19$ D
(9) $v = 50.0$ cm, virtual, −2.5, $U_{5f} = +4.00$ D, $V_{5b} = -1.82$ D
(11) +7.15 cm, −12.5 cm
(13) −37.0 mm
(15) 0, 0
(17) virtual, +30.0 cm
(19) +60.98 cm, −15.24 cm
(21) +10.00 D, −1.25
(23) $u = -18.18$ cm
(25) +3.00 D
(27) 13.1 mm

CHAPTER 6

(1) far point real and 10.26 cm in front of cornea, near point real and 5.97 cm in front of cornea, myopia, −9.75 D, −11.42 D
(3) far point virtual and 40 cm behind cornea, near point real and 16.67 cm in front of cornea, hyperopia, +2.50 D, +2.41 D
(5) no, outside her far point
(7) yes, 1.00 D
(9) 5.26 D spectacle accommodative demand, 6.97 D exact ocular accommodative demand, 6.97 D approximate ocular accommodative demand
(11) real, 303–58.8 cm, +3.67 D, ∝ to 73 cm.
(13) 72.7 μm.

CHAPTER 7

(1a) +52 cm, −0.33, $U_{5f} = -1.05$ D, $V_{5b} = +3.32$ D
(1c) +136.5 cm, −2.50, $U_{5f} = -3.33$ D, $V_{5b} = +1.19$ D
(1e) +14 cm, +0.64, $U_{5f} = +5.26$ D, $V_{5b} = +17.33$ D
(1g) +33.78 cm, −0.35, $U_{5f} = -1.08$ D, $V_{5b} = +3.47$ D
(1i) −15.63 cm, +1.63, $U_{5f} = -15.60$ D, $V_{5b} = -4.85$ D
(2a) −25.33 cm, +0.33, $U_{5f} = -2.22$ D, $V_{5b} = -5.01$ D
(2c) +152 cm, +5.00, $U_{5f} = +4.00$ D, $V_{5b} = +1.03$ D
(2e) −9.92 cm, +0.60, $U_{5f} = -7.60$ D, $V_{5b} = -6.70$ D

(2g) −160.7 cm, −5.43, $U_{5f} = +3.04$ D, $V_{5b} = -0.60$ D
(3a) apparent depth is 5.58 cm
(3b) apparent depth is 22.78 cm
(5) −20.45 cm, 10.91 cm
(7) −1.99, +8.00 D
(9) +13.79 D
(11) 13.8 mm
(13) +5.00 D, +38.60 D
(15) +8.04 D

CHAPTER 8

(1) 24.6 cm, 188 cm
(3) −3.39 D, 10 cm
(5) in air 4.14 cm behind the plastic–air interface
(7) reduced system is a +10.00 D lens 4.49 cm in front of a −4.00 D lens, back vertex power is +14.12 D, neutralizing power is +6.61 D
(9) −50.00 D, +4.00 D
(11) −4.00 D
(13) +4.50 D

CHAPTER 9

(1) +3.22 D
(3) +5.36 D
(5) −5.74 D, −3.09 D
(7) +3.00 D, +33.33 cm from front vertex
(9) +52.20 D, 9.39 mm
(11) +5.16 D
(13) virtual, and 11.97 cm behind the cornea, +8.36 D
(15) +17.30 D
(17) −11.13 D, +13.13 D, +2.00 D

CHAPTER 10

(1) +50.0 cm, horizontal
(2) +40.0 cm (horizontal), +18.18 cm (vertical), +25.0 cm
(4a) vertical line, SMA, WTR, −2.00 × 180
(4c) horizontal blur ellipse, CHA, WTR, +4.00 ⊂ − 2.00 × 180
(4e) vertical blur ellipse, CMA, WTR, −2.00 ⊂ − 2.00 × 180
(7) −2.00 ⊂ − 2.50 × 20
(9) −3.00 ⊂ − 2.00 × 54
(11) −2.50 ⊂ − 2.00 × 60
(13) +2.75 D
(15) +13.68 ⊂ − 5.13 × 56
(16) 1.05 D (from approximations)

CHAPTER 11

52.9°, 32.4°, 28.1°, 28.1°, 27.2°, total internal reflection
(3) 23.2°, 19.2°
(5) 2.9°, 5.0^{Δ}
(7) 4.0^{Δ}
(9) 1.5^{Δ} BU
(11) 5.7^{Δ} BD & O @ 34.2
(13) 3.2^{Δ} BI, 5.1^{Δ} BU, left
(17) 9.4^{Δ}

CHAPTER 12

(1) 5.6^{Δ} BU
(3) 4.2^{Δ} BD & O @ 30
(5) 6.7 mm up
(7) 1.2^{Δ} BU
(9a) yes, 3.75 mm out
(9b) no
(9c) no
(11) 9.2^{Δ}
(14) 3.32^{Δ} BD, eye turns up, 1.9°

CHAPTER 13

(1) +5.00 D and +1.00 D, +3.68 D, 2.00 D and 0, 1.88 D
(3a) $\begin{pmatrix} -3.00\text{ D} & 0 \\ 0 & +1.00\text{ D} \end{pmatrix}$
(3c) $\begin{pmatrix} -2.00\text{ D} & +1.73\text{ D} \\ +1.73\text{ D} & 0 \end{pmatrix}$
(3e) $\begin{pmatrix} -1.00\text{ D} & +2.00\text{ D} \\ +2.00\text{ D} & -1.00\text{ D} \end{pmatrix}$
(5) −3.50 ⊂ − 2.00 × 180
(6a) +1.00 ⊂ − 4.00 × 160
(6c) +13.00 ⊂ − 4.00 × 135
(7) −1.08 ⊂ − 7.68 × 33.3
(9) +62.00 ⊂ − 5.00 × 108
(11) −10.00 D
(13) −4.00 ⊂ − 2.00 × 13, rotated by 13°, circle of least confusion
(15) +3.35 D
(16) 3.16 D, −1.00 D
(18) 5.05 D, −0.50 D

CHAPTER 14

(1a) +16.67 cm, real, −0.33
(1c) +40.91 cm, real, −2.27
(1e) +10.00 cm, real, +0.20
(2b) −6.00 cm, virtual, +0.40
(2d) −30.00 cm, virtual, −2.00
(2f) −12.50 cm, virtual, −0.25

(3) 50 cm behind mirror, +1, +1.00 D
(5) −6.25 D, −16.00 cm, −8.31 D, −16.00 cm
(7) 6.7%, 87.0%
(9) 2.1%, −3.68 mm, virtual, erect, +0.0184
(11) +1.65 D
(13) +64.64 D, 7.58 mm

CHAPTER 15

(1) +9.09 D, +12.50 D, +20.00 D, +15.08 cm, −0.92
(3) +82.71 cm, −2.22, +6.60 cm from the principal planes
(5) +10.06 D
(7) +8.85 D, +10.91 D, +6.90 D, the primary principal plane is 3.20 cm behind the front vertex, the secondary principal plane 7.10 cm in front of the back vertex, the nodal points are +4.79 cm from the principal planes
(9) +11.22 D, +11.05 D, +12.11 D, the primary principal plane is 1.40 mm in front of the front vertex, 6.55 mm in front of the back vertex

CHAPTER 16

(1) $\begin{pmatrix} 1.45 & -2.03\,\text{D} \\ 0.10\,\text{m} & 0.55 \end{pmatrix}$
+2.03 D, +3.68 D, +1.40 D

(3) $\begin{pmatrix} 0.82 & +3.56\,\text{D} \\ 0.06\,\text{m} & 1.48 \end{pmatrix}$
−3.56 D, −2.41 D, −4.13 D

(5) −6.69 D, +9.11 D

(7) $\begin{pmatrix} 0.72 & -4.40\,\text{D} \\ 0.26\,\text{m} & -0.20 \end{pmatrix}$
+4.40 D, −22.00 D, +6.11 D

(8) $\begin{pmatrix} -2.300 & -2.900\,\text{D} \\ 0.440\,\text{m} & 0.120 \end{pmatrix}$

(12) $\begin{pmatrix} -1.397 & +3.726\,\text{D} \\ 0.231\,\text{m} & -1.332 \end{pmatrix}$

CHAPTER 17

(1) 2.5×, relative distance magnification
(3) 7.0×
(5) No, Yes
(7) 6.4×
(9) −12.0×, 54.17 cm
(11) 107.14 cm
(13) 4.6×

CHAPTER 18

(1) virtual image of the aperture (located 13.33 cm behind the lens)
(3) entrance pupil 7.41 cm behind the +6.50 D lens, exit pupil 4.26 cm in front of the −3.50 D lens
(5) located 3.15 mm behind the cornea and 3.42 mm in size
(7) 9.8% loss
(9) 1.010 (or 1% gain), 0.939 (or 6.1% loss), 0.948 (or 5.2% loss)
(11) Many lenses will work. One is a CR-39 ($n = 1.495$) with a +9.87 D front surface and a 5.0-mm central thickness
(13) 1.049 (or 4.9% gain), 0.907 (or 9.3% loss)
(15) 5× in the horizontal meridian, 1× (or 0% gain) in the vertical meridian, as a rectangle that is 5× longer horizontally than vertically
(17) 17.6% gain in the vertical meridian, 9.9% gain in the horizontal meridian, a rectangle that is longer vertically
(19) 3.1% gain in the 135 meridian, 4.3% loss in the 45 meridian, parallelogram

CHAPTER 19

(1) 14.25°
(3a) 7.63°
(3b) 14.4°
(3d) 3.06°
(3f) 36.9°
(5) 0.72°
(7) 0.72°, 316.25 cm
(9) 18.1 mm
(11) f/2.1
(13) ±0.11 D
(15) 25 mm
(17) 16.1×
(19a) 5.6 cm
(19b) 41.9 cm
(19c) 6.4 cm
(19d) 13.5 mm, 9
(19e) −2.29
(19f) less magnification, larger field of view

CHAPTER 20

(1) +0.12 D, +0.23 D
(3) myopic for blue (F), hyperopic for red (C)
(5) 13.32$^{\Delta}$ BU ophthalmic crown, 8.32$^{\Delta}$ BD dense flint glass
(7) +9.86 ⊂⊃ − 0.67 × 180, gain, +8.81 ⊂⊃ − 0.60 × 90
(9) −5.31 ⊂⊃ − 1.16 × 154.6

CHAPTER 21

(1) 600 nm, orange, same frequency, 400 nm, no, same frequency
(3) 542.4 nm, green
(5) 17.7 mm, 3.54 mm
(7) decreases
(9) 108 nm
(11) 1.42 cm

CHAPTER 22

(1) 0.99°, 1.18°
(2) 0.39°, 55.1 mm, 0.33°, 45.4 mm
(3) 1.34 cm
(5) 20/17, 20/34
(7) semidiameter 7.2 mm, diameter 14.4 mm, smaller

CHAPTER 23

(1) 2.1
(2) 0.25, 0.75
(3) 75%
(4) 50%
(5) 33%
(7) 58.9°

CHAPTER 24

(1) 604 nm, 2,900 nm
(3) 275 nm, 500 nm, 620 nm
(11) 5 cm, 27.3 μm, 24 mrad
(13) 20.2 cm, 0.169 mm, 4 mrad
(14) 99.9 cm, 0.120 mm, 5.2 mrad

CHAPTER 25

(1) $13 + 4.8 \sin(2\pi 4x)$
(3) 282 cycles/mm, 370 cycles/mm
(5) 0.22
(6) 0.23
(7) 29

Index

Page numbers in *italics* indicate figures; page numbers followed by "t" indicate tabular material.